Copies of the laminated Equianalgesic Charts and Dosing Guides included with this manual can be printed from the Mosby PAIN Web site at **http://www.mosby.com/PAIN**

DATE DUE

OCT 0 2 2006	

PAIN
CLINICAL MANUAL
SECOND EDITION

Margo McCaffery, RN, MS, FAAN

Consultant in the Nursing Care of Patients With Pain

Chris Pasero, RN, MSNc

Pain Management Educator and Consultant

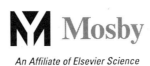 Mosby

An Affiliate of Elsevier Science

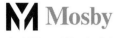

An Affiliate of Elsevier Science

Editor: Barry Bowlus
Developmental Editor: Barbara Watts
Project Manager: John Rogers
Production Editor: Mary Turner
Designer: Pati Pye, Amy Buxton
Manufacturing Manager: David Graybill
Cover Art: Pati Pye

Second edition

Mosby, Inc.
11830 Westline Industrial Drive
St. Louis, Missouri 63146

ISBN 0-8151-5609-X

02 03 / 9 8 7 6

In memory of
Alexandra Beebe
1951-1994

Co-author of the first edition of
Pain: Clinical Manual for Nursing Practice, 1989

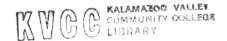

CONTRIBUTORS

Robin Burke Britt, RNC, WHCNP, CNS, Ed.D
Associate Professor
College of Nursing
Texas Woman's University
Houston, Texas

Peggy Compton, RN, PhD
Assistant Professor
UCLA School of Nursing
Los Angeles, California

Patrick J. Coyne, RN, MSN, CS, CRNH
Clinical Nurse Specialist, Oncology/Pain Management
Medical College of Virginia Hospitals
Virginia Commonwealth University
Richmond, Virginia

Pamela Stitzlein Davies, ARNP, MS
Adult/Geriatric Nurse Practitioner
Primary and Specialty Care
Puget Sound Health Care System
Veteran's Affairs Medical Center
Seattle, Washington

Linda Dunajcik, RN, MN, CS
Manager, St. John's Mercy Pain Therapy Center
Past President, American Society of Pain Management Nurses
St. Louis, Missouri

Anna DuPen, ARNP, MN
Pain Service
Swedish Medical Center
Bainbridge Island, Washington

Jane E. Faries, RN, MSN
Nurse Coordinator for the Acute Pain Service
Wellmon-Holston Valley Medical Center
Kingsport, Tennessee

Betty R. Ferrell, PhD, FAAN
Research Scientist
City of Hope National Medical Center
Duarte, California

Jan L. Frandsen, RN, BSN
Nurse Clinician II
Acute Pain Service
The Cleveland Clinic Foundation
Cleveland, Ohio

Russell L. George, RN, MSN, CCRN
Critical Care Educator—Burns
Parkland Health and Hospital System
Dallas, Texas

Mary Layman Goldstein, RN, MS, OCN
Clinical Nurse Specialist
Pain and Palliative Care Service
Memorial Sloan-Kettering Cancer Center
New York, New York

Debra B. Gordon, RN, MS
Senior Clinical Nurse Specialist
University of Wisconsin Hospital and Clinics
Madison, Wisconsin

Kathryn Hagen, RN, BA, BS
Rochester, Michigan

Anne Hughes, RN, MN, FNP, ACRN
Clinical Nurse Specialist, HIV Disease and Oncology
Community Health Network at San Francisco General Hospital
Assistant Clinical Professor of Nursing
University of California
San Francisco, California

Karen P. Kettelman, RN, BAHSA
Pain Management Coordinator
Doctors Medical Center
Modesto, California

Sharon Lauterback, RN, BS
Case Manager
Parkland Health and Hospital System
Dallas, Texas

Lora McGuire, RN, MS
Nursing Instructor and Pain Consultant
Joliet Junior College
Joliet, Illinois

Judith A. Paice, RN, PhD, FAAN
Clinical Nurse Specialist, Pain Management
Department of Neurosurgery
Rush Medical Center
Professor, College of Nursing
Rush University
Chicago, Illinois

Russell K. Portenoy, MD
Chairman, Department of Pain Medicine and Palliative Care
Beth Israel Medical Center
New York, New York

Linda Neuman-Potash, RN, MN
Executive Director
Ehlers-Danlos National Foundation
Registered Nurse
Children's Hospital—Los Angeles
Los Angeles, Calfornia

Barbara A. Reed, RN, MN, CGNP
Pain Management Specialist
Tucker, Georgia

Jaynie Bentz St. Pierre, RN, BSN
Pain Management Resource Leader/Coordinator
St. Frances Medical Center
Monroe, Louisiana

Marsha R. Stanton, RN, MS, CNS
Marketing Manager, Pain Management
Knoll Pharmaceutical Company
Mount Olive, New Jersey

Bonnie Stevens, RN, PhD
Associate Professor, Faculty of Nursing
University of Toronto
Toronto Prov., Ontario

April Hazard Vallerand, RN, PhD
Nurse Consultant
Novi, Michigan

Warren P. Vallerand, DDS, MD
Private Practice
Oral and Maxillofacial Surgery
Grosse Pointe, Michigan

Lia van Rijswijk, RN, ET
Nurse Consultant
Graduate Student School of Nursing, La Salle University
Philadelphia, Pennsylvania

REVIEWERS

Patrick J. Coyne, RN, MSN, CS, CRNH
Clinical Nurse Specialist, Oncology/Pain Management
Medical College of Virginia Hospitals
Virginia Commonwealth University
Richmond, Virginia

Terry DiMaggio, MSN, CRNP
Pain Management Advanced Practice Nurse
The Pain Management Program
Departments of Nursing and Anesthesia/Critical Care Medicine
The Children's Hospital of Philadelphia
Philadelphia, Pennsylvania

Jane E. Faries, RN, MSN
Nurse Coordinator for the Acute Pain Service
Wellmon-Holston Valley Medical Center
Kingsport, Tennessee

Betty R. Ferrell, PhD, FAAN
Research Scientist
City of Hope National Medical Center
Duarte, California

Debra B. Gordon, RN, MS
Senior Clinical Nurse Specialist
University of Wisconsin Hospital and Clinics
Madison, Wisconsin

Phala A. Helm, MD
Director (retired), Physical Medicine and Rehabilitation
Parkland Hospital
University of Texas Southwestern Medical School
Dallas, Texas

Lex Hubbard, MD
Department of Anesthesiology
Willis Knighton Medical Center
Shreveport, Louisiana

John L. Hunt, MD
Co-Director, Burn Unit
Parkland Hospital
University of Texas Southwestern Medical School
Dallas, Texas

Terry Karapas, RN, MS
Administrative Director
University of Chicago Center for Pain Treatment
Palo Heights, Illinois

Pamela Kedziera, RN, MSN, AOCN
Pain Management Center
Fox Chase Cancer Center
Philadelphia, Pennsylvania

Karen J. Kowalske, MD
Director, Physical Medicine and Rehabilitation
Parkland Hospital
University of Texas Southwestern Medical School
Dallas, Texas

Goldie Markowitz, RN, MSN, CNSC, CRNP
Pediatric Clinical Nurse Specialist
West Jersey Hospital
Voorhees, New Jersey

Lee Moore, RNC
Staff Nurse
Neonatal Intensive Care
West Jersey Hospital
Voorhees, New Jersey

Rhonda Nichols, RN, MS
Pain Management Nurse Clinician
San Francisco General Hospital
San Francisco, California

Gary F. Purdue, MD
Co-Director, Burn Unit
Parkland Hospital
University of Texas Southwestern Medical School
Dallas, Texas

Janice Rae, RN, BN
Coordinator, Acute Pain Service
Rockyview General Hospital
Calgary, Alberta, Canada

Susan L. Schroeder, RN, MS
Clinical Nurse Specialist, Acute Pain Service
Department of Anesthesiology
University of Wisconsin Hospital and Clinics
Madison, Wisconsin

John Smith
Birmingham, Alabama

Georgeanne V. Stilley, RN, MSN, AOCN
Our Lady of Lourdes Medical Center
Pain Management Service
Camden, New Jersey

Barbara Vanderveer, RN, MSN
Clinical Coordinator
Acute and Cancer Pain Management Services
University of Kentucky
Lexington, Kentucky

Korrine Van Keuren, RN-C, MS, PNP, ONC
Waltham, Massachusetts

Linda Vanni, RN, MSN
Coordinator, Pain Therapies
Detroit Medical Center—Harper Hospital
Detroit, Michigan

Kathleen G. Wallace, RN, PhD
Newport News, Virginia

Donna L. Wong, RN, PhD, PNP, CPN, FAAN
Nursing Consultant
Tulsa, Oklahoma

PREFACE

The science of pain is expanding rapidly and the care of patients with pain has become a specialty. At the same time, assessing and relieving pain is also the responsibility of *all* clinicians who care for patients with pain. The purpose of this manual is to provide current, scientifically based, practical information for nurses, physicians, pharmacists, and others who must manage pain in patients they encounter in their daily practice. Information is presented in a manner that can be readily applied to patients of all ages in all clinical settings. Through patient examples, practical guidelines, and reproducible forms, the manual teaches the reader how to use techniques and tools to provide the best possible pain management.

This revised edition of the manual includes both new and expanded content. Chapter 1 gives an update on current problems and progress in the field of pain management, emphasizing that much remains to be done to improve the care of patients with pain. Chapter 2 presents basic pain mechanisms that underlie the causes and effects of pain, pointing out the danger of assuming that pain has no harmful consequences. Chapter 3 covers a variety of practical assessment tools that are immediately useful in clinical practice, including some tools that are translated into foreign languages. Chapters 4 through 7 are devoted to pharmacology, covering the three analgesic groups (nonopioids, opioids, and adjuvants) and how to combine them. Chapter 9 covers practical nondrug approaches to pain management, including distraction techniques, relaxation strategies, and methods of cutaneous stimulation. Chapters 11 and 15, respectively, provide updates on the care of patients with chronic nonmalignant pain and management of pain in the elderly.

New additions to this manual include Chapter 8 on procedural pain, Chapter 10 on care of patients with both pain and substance abuse problems, Chapter 12 with brief descriptions of selected pain problems, Chapter 13 on the use of analgesics during pregnancy, childbirth, the postpartum period, and breast feeding, and Chapter 14 on special considerations in the management of pain in infants. The manual concludes with Chapter 16 that provides the information and tools needed to establish a multidisciplinary approach to building and maintaining institutional commitment to improving pain management.

Features of the text include:
- Terminology introducing each chapter to facilitate comprehension of content.
- Misconception tables that immediately identify and correct common misinformation.
- 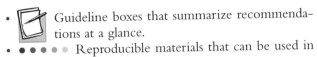 Pediatric icons that help the reader readily locate information pertinent to the care of children with pain.

- Guideline boxes that summarize recommendations at a glance.
- Reproducible materials that can be used in clinical practice.
- Patient examples that illustrate key points.
- Forms completed with patient information related to selected situations, illustrating how to use the forms.
- Numerous ready-to-use materials, such as patient medication information forms and instructions for nondrug pain management.
- Assessment forms and pain rating scales for all age groups that may be duplicated for use in clinical practice.
- Pain rating scales for children and adults in foreign languages that may be duplicated for use in clinical practice.
- Forms for numerous situations, such as monitoring IV, PCA, epidural analgesia, and pain care in the home.
- Forms and recommendations for pain care committees to use in improving pain management within the institution and to ensure ongoing continuous quality improvement, helping to meet JCAHO standards.
- Resources listed at the ends of most chapters so patients and clinicians can obtain additional information.
- Laminated equianalgesic chart to help with dose calculations when changing routes of administration or analgesics.

As with all publications, authors make certain assumptions that guide selection and presentation of content. One of our assumptions is that the care of patients with pain is best accomplished by a team approach. Therefore this manual presents information that is useful to most disciplines represented on the team. Content also aims to establish basic elements of collaborative practice. These include a common knowledge base shared by the patient, family members when appropriate, and all clinicians caring for the patient. Patient information forms and other patient teaching materials are included for this reason. A common language is necessary, and the use of pain rating scales by the patient and clinicians and adoption of standardized documentation forms are emphasized to facilitate communication. Common goals are essential to collaborative practice, and toward this end establishing comfort/function goals with patients is incorporated into assessment tools and patient teaching forms.

While the care of patients with pain ideally is a team approach, another one of our assumptions is that, in most cases, nursing care is the cornerstone. The nurse spends more time caring for people with pain than any other health team member. The nurse's role in this care most often includes implementing pain relief methods with and for the patient, identifying the need for change or the use of additional methods, obtaining them, and once again assessing the impact on the patient. The nurse is in a key position to tailor the application of pain relief approaches to meet the needs of the individual patient, regardless of where the approaches originate (e.g., with a physician's prescription for an analgesic or with the patient's desire for self-management techniques such as relaxation). We are convinced that it is through the efforts of the nurse that most patients with pain will receive assistance.

Both of us frequently speak on the topic of pain and have extended to our audiences an open invitation to write, fax, or telephone us regarding their views on patients with pain. We have learned much from this approach and invite our readers to contact us for assistance or to make comments and suggestions to us personally (no e-mail, please).

Margo McCaffery, RN, MS, FAAN
Consultant in the Nursing Care of Patients with Pain
8347 Kenyon Avenue
Los Angeles, California 90045
Phone: (310) 649-2219
Fax: (310) 649-0011

Chris Pasero, RN, MSNc
Pain Management Educator and Consultant
5045 Concord Road
Rocklin, California 95765
Phone: (916) 624-3928
Fax: (916) 624-4330

ACKNOWLEDGMENTS

Without our colleagues we would not have been able to write this book. Especially to those listed as contributors and reviewers, we wish to express deep appreciation for their insights and ideas. Many spent untold hours carefully preparing and critiquing the content of this book.

Our library researcher, Nancy K. Smith, provided invaluable help with literature searches. Thank you, Nancy, for your thoroughness and prompt response to our needs.

We are grateful to our family and friends who encouraged us. They also tolerated the social isolation that accompanied the writing of this book and were there for us when the writing was over.

Margo is especially grateful to her husband Rick, her friends Carol and Michael, and her computer consultant Craig.

Chris wishes to thank David, her husband, best friend, and partner in all aspirations. She is also forever grateful to her mentor and friend, Lex Hubbard, and to her colleagues, Linda, Lynda, Wanda, Ginger, Margaret, Terry, Susan, Bridget, Barbara, Maria, Kathy, and Tina, who helped establish the acute and chronic pain services at Schumpert Medical Center in Shreveport, Louisiana.

CONTENTS

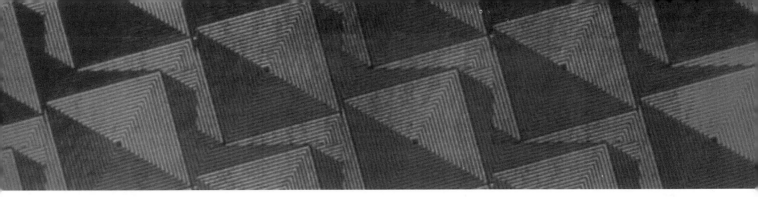

chapter one
PAIN MANAGEMENT
Problems and Progress

Margo McCaffery

CHAPTER OUTLINE

TERMINOLOGY: ACRONYMS

AACPI: American Alliance of Cancer Pain Initiatives

AAHPM: American Academy of Hospice and Palliative Medicine

AAPM: American Academy of Pain Medicine

ACEP: American College of Emergency Physicians

AHCPR: Agency for Health Care Policy and Research

AMA: American Medical Association

APS: American Pain Society

ASPMN: American Society of Pain Management Nurses

HPNA: Hospice and Palliative Nurses Association

IASP: International Association for the Study of Pain

JCAHO: Joint Commission on Accreditation of Healthcare Organizations

NHO: National Hospice Organization

WHO: World Health Organization

If you or a loved one has surgery or cancer that causes pain of moderate to severe intensity, a 50% chance exists that you or your loved one will unnecessarily suffer this pain about 50% of the time. Current survey data show that this is a conservative prediction.

Over the past decade enormous progress has been made in the field of pain. Unfortunately, this has had little effect on improving the care of patients with pain. As health care professionals, we must view this as an unforgivable failure. As human beings, we should take note of the personal impact this may have. In 1996 at the International Association for the Study of Pain's (IASP) Eighth World Congress on Pain, the president of IASP, John D. Loeser (1997), candidly described the current status of the clinical world of pain as "scary."

Following is an introduction to the undertreatment of pain, some of the barriers to using current knowledge and resources in the care of patients with pain, and potential remedies. Contrasting this is a discussion of some of the encouraging developments in pain management. (Some topics are discussed in greater detail later in the text.)

CONTINUING UNDERTREATMENT OF PAIN

The Agency for Health Care Policy and Research (AHCPR) states that institutions have a responsibility for pain management and this "begins with the affirmation that patients should have access to the best level of pain relief that may safely be provided" (Acute Pain Management Guideline Panel, 1992). Knowledge and resources exist to provide satisfactory and safe pain relief to approximately 90% of all people who suffer pain, but numerous studies document that this does not occur (Teoh, Stjernsward, 1992). A growing number of studies also document that progress in improving this situation is extremely slow, which suggests that forceful measures may be needed to correct the undertreatment of pain.

Studies of patients with cancer and other terminal illnesses reveal that needless suffering occurs in a variety of clinical settings. In 1990-1991 a study of 1308 outpatients with metastatic cancer from 54 cancer treatment centers found that 67% reported pain (Cleeland, Gonin, Hatfield et al., 1994). Of those who had pain, 62% had pain severe enough to impair their ability to function, and 42% were not prescribed analgesics capable of relieving their pain.

Beginning in 1989, a 4-year study was conducted in five teaching hospitals and included more than 9000 hospitalized terminally ill patients (The SUPPORT principal investigators, 1995). During the last 2 years of the study, efforts were made to correct pain management problems by improving communications among the patient, family, and physician. A nurse was provided to help facilitate discussions, provide information, and do whatever else seemed appropriate to achieve the pain management goals. However, physician behavior did not change, and these efforts were essentially unsuccessful. From the beginning to the end of the study, 50% of conscious patients who died in the hospital experienced moderate to severe pain at least half the time. This leads to the conclusion that changes in pain management will not occur with only marginal adjustments to the way patient care is provided (Issacs, Knickman, 1997). A sustained effort to change professional values and priorities is required.

Even in hospice settings, pain management is less than ideal. In a study of patients who were receiving hospice care in their homes, those who were reporting pain were asked 3 weeks after admission to rate their pain relief on a scale of 1 to 10 (1 = no relief, 10 = complete relief) (McMillan, 1996). Scores of 5 or less were reported by 42% of patients, meaning that only 50% or less of their pain was relieved.

Studies of patients with acute pain conditions also reveal undertreatment. Using a pain rating scale of 0 to 10 (0 = no pain, 10 = worst pain), 217 hospitalized adults with a variety of acute pain conditions in a university teaching hospital answered questions about their pain. More than half the patients, 61%, reported pain ratings of 7 to 10 during the last 24 hours, 49% had pain ratings of 4 to 10 "right now," and 20% had pain ratings of 4 to 10 even after receiving analgesics (Ward, Gordon, 1994). Following these findings, a variety of efforts were made throughout the institution to improve pain management, but a study 2 years later revealed little change in patients' pain ratings and physicians' analgesic orders (Ward, Gordon, 1996).

Adults from 500 households in the United States were interviewed about their experiences with postoperative pain (Warfield, Kahn, 1995). More than one quarter (27%) had had a surgical procedure during the past 5 years. Of those who experienced pain after surgery (77%), 80% experienced moderate to severe pain. Severe to extreme pain was reported by 31%. Even after receiving their first dose of medication, 71% continued to experience pain.

After more than 25 years, these findings are discouragingly similar to those of Marks and Sacher that were reported in 1973. In their study of medical inpatients, 73% had moderate to severe pain. They also found that physicians prescribed on the basis of incorrect information about analgesics. Clearly, progress in improving pain management is too little and too slow. Too many patients with pain are not yet benefiting from the tremendous advances in pain management.

CONTINUING BARRIERS TO PAIN MANAGEMENT

Barriers to pain management are numerous and complex, often poorly defined, and certainly resistant to current efforts to change them. They encompass problems related to three areas identified by AHCPR: the health care system, health care professionals, and patients (Jacox, Carr, Payne, et al., 1994).

The System: Lack of Accountability

Improving pain management requires that pain be recognized as a priority. Historically, this has not been the case. In the early 1970s, sociological analysis of acute pain management in various clinical settings revealed that health care team members did not seem to be held accountable for providing pain relief, but they felt responsible for controlling the patient's expression of pain (Fagerhaugh 1974; Strauss, Fagerhaugh, Glaser, 1974). For example, nurses attempted to control the expression of pain with statements such as, "Try to take control of yourself," "It's not as bad as you think," and "You're going to have to learn to handle this yourself." The patient was asked to suffer in silence and not bother the staff.

Evidence continues to demonstrate that health care systems do not hold clinicians accountable for assessing and relieving pain. In a study in which 353 hospitalized patients who experienced pain were interviewed, fewer than half of the patients with pain (45%) had a member of the health care team ask them about their pain or note it in their record (Donovan, Dillon, McGuire, 1987). In a more recent study of 242 hospitalized patients with pain, a review of their records revealed that no assessments of pain intensity were documented by any caregiver (Gu, Belgrade, 1993).

Making pain the fifth vital sign

In the studies just discussed, pain assessments were lacking in many of the patients, but it is probably safe to assume that all of them had their vital signs assessed, recorded, and attended to if they were abnormal. One simple strategy to increase accountability for pain is for an institution to make pain intensity ratings a routine part of assessment and documentation of vital signs. This suggestion comes from the American Pain Society (APS) and has been implemented in many hospitals, often simply by including pain on the vital sign record (American Pain Society Quality of Care Committee, 1995; McCaffery, Pasero, 1997). This makes pain visible and raises awareness of the problem. If pain ratings can be attached to an activity as routine as vital signs, clinicians will receive frequent reminders of existing pain problems.

Increasing focus on pain by the Joint Commission on Accreditation of Healthcare Organizations

Obviously, patients are likely to receive better pain relief if the health care system holds health care professionals responsible for assessing and relieving pain. "The traditional patterns of professional practice may be the most intractable barriers to effective pain management. A change in the standards to which healthcare organizations are held accountable should be a powerful force for change" (Berry, 1997, p. 2). A major determinant of what institutions emphasize in patient care is the Joint Commission on Accreditation of Healthcare Organizations (JCAHO).

In the 1992 standards manual issued by JCAHO, effective pain management was stated as one of the rights of a dying patient. In 1994, JCAHO broadened this statement to cover all patients, saying, "The management of pain is appropriate for all patients, not just dying patients" (JCAHO, 1994, p. 156). JCAHO accreditation visits began to include a focus on what institutions were doing about pain management.

In 1997, under a grant from the Robert Wood Johnson Foundation, JCAHO began working collaboratively with institutions to create standards for pain assessment and treatment, with plans to conduct national quality improvement programs to help health care facilities meet these standards (Berry, 1997; JCAHO grasps the initiative on pain: New standards within two years, 1997).

Harmful and expensive consequences of unrelieved pain

Other incentives for institutions to improve the standard of care for patients with pain are recognition that pain is harmful and that improved pain management is cost-effective. Evidence that pain has harmful consequences is certainly capable of elevating the importance of pain management. Contrary to our cultural attitude of "no pain, no gain," pain can kill. For example, pain may inhibit the immune system and even enhance tumor growth (Herzberg, Murtaugh, Beitz, 1994; Liebeskind, 1991). In patients having cardiovascular surgical procedures, those with greater pain intensity are more likely to have atelectasis (Puntillo, Weiss, 1994). In one study of patients with chronic nonmalignant pain, 50% had considered suicide (Hitchcock, Ferrell, McCaffery, 1994). (See Chapter 2 for a more thorough discussion of the harmful effects of pain.)

Not too surprisingly, unrelieved pain is expensive. Improving pain management costs less than continuing practices that result in inadequate treatment of pain. Several studies of acute pain problems demonstrated this. For example, the use of intravenous patient-controlled analgesia (IV PCA) and epidural anesthesia and analgesia (EAA) rather than intramuscular (IM) injections for postoperative pain relief results in a decrease in adverse effects and improved patient outcomes.

Studies have demonstrated shorter hospital stays when IV PCA rather than IM analgesia is used for pain management. For example, two studies showed that cholecystectomy patients were discharged 2 days sooner (Jackson 1989; Ross, Perumbeti, 1988). In another study patients having thoracotomy or lumbar laminectomy were discharged 4 days sooner (Ross, Perumbeti, 1988). In a study of trauma patients, discharge occurred up to 3 days sooner (Pierce, 1988).

Studies have also demonstrated the benefits of EAA compared with standard anesthesia and analgesia. Patients receiving EAA for high-risk intrathoracic, intraabdominal, or major vascular surgery had half the overall complication rate, were discharged more than 4 days sooner, and spent less time in the intensive care unit (ICU), resulting in a savings of $10,000 per patient (Yeager, Glass, Neff, et al., 1987). In another study patients who had cesarean sections and received EAA were discharged 0.74 days sooner (Grass, Zuckerman, Tsao, 1991).

Improving cancer pain management is also cost-effective. At City of Hope Medical Center in Duarte, California, the cost of hospital admissions for unrelieved cancer pain exceeded $5 million over 12 months in 1989-1990 (Ferrell, Griffith, 1994). However, nursing strategies to improve cancer pain management succeeded in reducing these admissions and resulted in an estimated savings of $2,719,245 during a 12-month period in 1992-1993 (Grant, Ferrell, Rivera et al., 1995).

Health Care Professionals

Barriers to improved pain management faced by clinicians include lack of education, poor pain assessment,

and concerns about opioids, especially addiction, respiratory depression, and regulatory scrutiny.

Lack of education

Because pain management is a newly developed science, it is imperative that clinicians critique their practice and ask, "Is there any scientific basis for the methods I use to assess and treat pain?" In the past, pain management was, of necessity, dictated by personal opinions, essentially anecdotal reports. Now these practices must be questioned. Current recommendations for pain management need to be incorporated into the basic education provided for all health care professionals, and continuing education must provide this information for clinicians currently in practice whose basic education did not include current pain management recommendations. However, educational preparation for pain management is still lacking.

Within the last decade, a survey of baccalaureate nursing programs accredited by the National League for Nursing revealed that 48% of the programs spent 4 hours or less on pain (Graffam, 1990). Even more alarming was a survey of graduating baccalaureate nursing students that revealed that only 13% thought cancer pain management should be taught as part of the nursing curriculum (Sheehan, Webb, Bower, et al., 1992). In other words, 87% of graduating nurses thought that information about cancer pain management was not relevant to their nursing practice, indicating that they did not consider pain management a nursing responsibility.

Educational resources for nurses require attention. A review of selected nursing textbooks revealed inaccurate, confusing, and often irrelevant information about pain, particularly addiction to opioid analgesics (Ferrell, McCaffery, Rhiner, 1992). A survey of nursing faculty knowledge about pain identified many weaknesses, especially knowledge about analgesics (Ferrell, McGuire, Donovan, 1993).

Several developments have occurred that may expedite education of health care professionals. These include innovative education courses, suggestions for curriculum content, and the publication of clinical practice guidelines.

Education Courses

In an attempt to improve the knowledge of faculty members in undergraduate nursing programs, a course to educate the educator was offered at City of Hope Medical Center, over a 3-day period (Grant, Rivera, Ferrell et al., 1994). Testing before and after the program revealed that faculty knowledge improved, suggesting that they would be able to offer more accurate and complete information about pain to their students.

In 1997 researchers at the City of Hope National Medical Center began a 3-year project, funded by the

Robert Wood Johnson Foundation, that was designed to strengthen nursing education in the areas of pain and end-of-life care. One intent of the project is to provide resources and support for state boards of nursing to enable them to better advise schools of nursing in curriculum content.

An example of an effective and efficient method of educating clinicians is the Cancer Pain Role Model Courses, which both instruct and involve participants. These are conducted for teams of nurses, physicians, and pharmacists. In one study, follow-up surveys at 4 and 12 months showed that participants in one role model course not only maintained knowledge and attitudes acquired in the program but also continued to improve on them. Furthermore, during the year after the program, the 50 program participants disseminated this knowledge to more than 4500 health care professionals (Janjan, Martin, Payne et al., 1996). To date, 23 courses have been conducted in 20 states (Dahl, 1997).

Another approach to educating health care professionals, developed at City of Hope Medical Center, consists of selecting a staff nurse from each clinical unit and designating that person as a pain resource nurse (PRN) (Ferrell, Grant, Ritchey et al., 1993). This is referred to as the PRN program. Other institutions have conducted educational courses patterned after this one (e.g., Ward, Gordon, 1996).

Curriculum Guidelines

Several groups have developed suggested curricula for professional education in pain. The International Association for the Study of Pain (IASP) has published a core curriculum for health care professionals (Fields, 1995). The Wisconsin Cancer Pain Initiative has published "Cancer Pain Management Competency Guidelines for Nursing Education and Practice" (1995). In 1994 the California Board of Registered Nursing adopted a Pain Management Policy and later developed curriculum guidelines for pain management content. Box 1.1 provides information on how to obtain these guidelines and other resources for developing a curriculum in pain management.

Clinical Practice Guidelines and Periodicals

The literature on pain is abundant. Before the introduction of the gate control theory in 1965 by Melzack and Wall, very little appeared in the health care literature about pain. By the mid 1970s this began to change, and today countless books are written on the subject, and professional journals in all the health care disciplines regularly feature articles on pain. Although the study of pain remains in its infancy, pain is now regarded as a science and as a field of specialization in health care. The knowledge and technology now available can provide safe and effective pain relief for most people who suffer pain.

To facilitate the dissemination of current information about pain management in various populations of people with pain, task forces, committees, and expert panels have developed guidelines for clinical practice. These documents may be used in the clinical area to establish a common base of knowledge and standards for patient care. Clinical practice guidelines have been developed by a number of organizations, notably AHCPR and APS (Box 1.2). The first widely used clinical practice guideline was *Cancer Pain Relief,* published in 1986 by the World Health Organization (WHO). More than 160,000 copies were printed in over 12 languages, and it has been revised (WHO, 1990).

To keep abreast of research and other developments in the field of pain, the number of periodicals focused on pain has increased. A partial list of these, along with addresses for subscribing, are in Box 1.3.

Pain assessment: Handling the subjectivity of pain

Clearly, for many years clinicians have been placed in a challenging situation: they have cared for patients who reported pain that could not be proved, and they had little education about what to do; certainly they had no standards for assessment and treatment. It is no wonder that most pain control has been inconsistent and often inadequate because it was, of necessity, dictated by personal opinion. Critical to correcting this is establishing a standard for assessing the existence and intensity of the patient's pain. Quite simply, if caregivers do not agree on a standard for assessing pain intensity (e.g., the patient's self-report), each is likely to assess pain differently. Consequently, the care of a single patient can vary from one caregiver to another, very likely resulting in unrelieved pain. Overall, research shows that nurses tend to underestimate severe pain (Zalon, 1993), and most physicians fail to appreciate the severity of pain as a problem for patients who rate it as moderate to severe (Grossman, Sheidler, Swedeen et al., 1991).

Probably the most humbling and challenging aspect of caring for the patient with pain is to accept that the sensation of pain is completely subjective. One definition of pain for use in clinical practice says that "Pain is whatever the experiencing person says it is, existing whenever he says it does" (McCaffery, 1968, p. 95). Statements from clinical practice guidelines have echoed the same approach to the patient's report of pain by statements such as, "The mainstay of pain assessment is the patient self-report" (Jacox, Carr, Payne et al., 1994, p. 3).

When a patient reports pain, the health care professional's responsibility is to accept and respect that report and to proceed with appropriate assessment and treatment. All reports of pain are taken seriously.

Text continued on p. 9.

● ● ● ● ●
BOX 1.1

Resources for Professional Education

Cancer Pain Assessment & Treatment Curriculum Guidelines: Teaching Syllabus & Slide Sets
American Society of Clinical Oncology
 435 N. Michigan Ave., Suite 1717
 Chicago, IL 60611
 (312) 644-0878
 Fax: (312) 644-8557
 See also:
 Ad Hoc Committee on Cancer Pain of the American Society of Clinical Oncology: Cancer pain assessment and treatment curriculum guidelines, *J Clin Oncol* 10:1976-1982, 1992.

Cancer Pain Management Competency Guidelines for Nursing Education and Practice
Wisconsin Cancer Pain Initiative
 1300 University Ave.
 Madison, WI 53706
 (608) 262-0978
 Fax: (608) 265-4014

Caring for the Dying: Identification and Promotion of Physician Competency: Educational Resource Document; Personal Narratives
American Board of Internal Medicine
 3624 Market St.
 Philadelphia, PA 19104
 (215) 243-1562
 Fax: (215) 382-4702

Curriculum Guidelines: Pain Management and Pain Management Policy
Board of Registered Nursing
 P.O. Box 94410
 Sacramento, CA 94244-2100
 (916) 322-3350

Fields HL, editor: Core Curriculum for Professional Education in Pain, ed 2, Seattle, 1995, IASP Press.
International Association for the Study of Pain
 909 N.E. 43rd St., Rm. 306
 Seattle, WA 98105-6021
 (206) 547-6409
 Fax: (206) 547-1703
 E-mail: *iasp@locke.hs.washington.edu*
 Web site: *//weber.u.washington.edu/~crc/IASP.html*

Mayday Pain Resource Center: A Clearinghouse for Materials Related to Pain
For index:
Mayday Pain Resource Center
 City of Hope Medical Center
 1500 E. Duarte Rd.
 Duarte, CA 91010
 (626) 359-8111, ext. 3829
 Fax: (626) 301-8941
 E-mail: *mayday_pain@smtplink.coh.org*

Network Project Teaching Modules
Topics include cancer pain assessment, cancer pain syndromes, opioid pharmacotherapy, use of nonopioids and adjuvant analgesics, pain in AIDS, and pediatric cancer pain. Each module includes a lecture with references and 25 to 40 color slides.
The Network Project
 Memorial Sloan-Kettering Cancer Center, Box 421
 1275 York Ave.
 New York, NY 10021
 (212) 639-3164
 Fax: (212) 752-7185

Oncology Nursing Society Position Paper on Cancer Pain
Oncology Nursing Society
 501 Holiday Dr.
 Pittsburgh, PA 15220-2749
 (412) 921-7373
 Fax: (412) 921-6565
 See also:
 Spross JA, McGuire D, Schmitt RM: Oncology Nursing Society position paper on cancer pain, part I, *Oncol Nurs Forum* 17(4):595-614, 1990.
 Spross JA, McGuire DB, Schmitt RM: Oncology Nursing Society position paper on cancer pain, part II, *Oncol Nurs Forum,* 17(5):751-760, 1990.
 Spross JA, McGuire DB, Schmitt RM: Oncology Nursing Society position paper on cancer pain, part III, *Oncol Nurs Forum,* 17(6):943-955, 1990.

Pain Resource Nurse (PRN) Curriculum
This is outlined in the following article:
Ferrell BR, Grant M, Ritchey KJ et al.: The pain resource nursing training program: A unique approach to pain management, *J Pain Symptom Manage* 8:549-556,1993.

UNIPACS
These are packets of information designed to help physicians provide effective end-of-life care for terminally ill patients and their families and include "UNIPAC Three: Assessment and Treatment of Pain in the Terminally Ill." Also available is Porter Storey's "Primer of Palliative Care," a guide to hospice/palliative medicine.
American Academy of Hospice and Palliative Medicine
 P.O. Box 14288
 Gainesville, FL 32604
 Fax: (352) 371-2349

The Williams & Wilkins Complete Library on Pain
These videotapes (approximately 30 minutes each) concentrate on various aspects of the nursing management of patients with pain, including pain assessment, preventing and managing opioid-induced respiratory depression, use of the three groups of analgesics, undertreatment of pain, pain in the elderly, pain in children, and physiology of pain.
Williams & Wilkins Electronic Media
 428 E. Preston St.
 Baltimore, MD 21202
 (800) 527-5597

● ● ● ● ●
BOX 1.2

Pain: Clinical Practice Guidelines

Agency for Health Care Policy and Research (AHCPR): Acute Pain, Cancer Pain, & Low Back Problems

I. Acute Pain Guidelines

Comment: These guidelines are widely accepted. They include specific information on assessment tools, opioids, nonopioids, and nondrug methods.

1. *Acute Pain Management in Adults: Operative Procedures,* Quick Reference Guide for Clinicians, 1992 (22 pages), DHHS Pub. No. AHCPR 92-0019.
2. *Acute Pain Management in Infants, Children, and Adolescents: Operative and Medical Procedures,* Quick Reference Guide for Clinicians, 1992 (22 pages), DHHS Pub. No. AHCPR 92-0020.
3. *Pain Control After Surgery,* Patient's Guide, 1992 (9 pages), DHHS Pub. No. AHCPR 92-0021.
4. *Acute Pain Management: Operative or Medical Procedures and Trauma,* Clinical Practice Guideline, 1992 (145 pages), DHHS Pub. No. AHCPR 92-0032.

II. Cancer Pain Guidelines

Comment: These guidelines are widely accepted. They include specific information on assessment tools, the three analgesic groups, and nondrug methods. In addition to ordering them free through AHCPR, they may also be obtained free by calling (800) 4-CANCER.

1. *Management of Cancer Pain: Adults,* 1994 (28 pages), AHCPR Pub. No. 94-0593.
2. *Managing Cancer Pain,* Patient Guide, 1994 (adults, 21 pages), AHCPR Pub. No. 94-0595.
3. *Management of Cancer Pain: Infants, Children, and Adolescents.* Not published. (For excerpts, see *Journal of Pharmaceutical Care in Pain & Symptom Control,* 2(1):75-103, 1994.
4. *Clinical Practice Guideline: Management of Cancer Pain,* 1994 (257 pages), AHCPR Pub. No. 94-0592.

III. Acute Low Back Problems

Comment: These guidelines are not widely accepted. For a discussion of areas of controversy, see de Jong, RH: Backlash: AHCPR practice guideline for acute low back pain, *Pain Digest* 6:1-2, 1996.

1. *Acute Low Back Problems in Adults: Assessment and Treatment,* Quick Reference Guide for Clinicians, 1994 (25 pages), AHCPR Pub. No. 95-0643.
2. *Understanding Low Back Problems,* Patient Guide, 1994 (13 pages), AHCPR Pub. No. 95-0644.

To order *all* of these AHCPR guidelines (free):

AHCPR, Publications Clearinghouse
P.O. Box 8547,
Silver Spring, MD 20907
(800) 358-9295
(From outside the United States, [410] 381-3150)
Hearing impaired TDD service (888) 586-6340.
To get copies off web site: *http://www.ahcpr.gov/guide/*

American College of Emergency Physicians: Acute Abdomen & Pediatric Analgesia

1. *Clinical Policy on Abdominal Pain,* Dallas, 1994, ACEP ($5.00)
2. *Pediatric Analgesia and Sedation,* Dallas, 1992, ACEP (reprint No. 47/1/53110, free)

To order:

ACEP
1125 Executive Cr.
Irving, TX 75038-2522
(800) 798-1822

Also see:

Proceedings from the First International Symposium on Pain Research in Emergency Medicine, Montreal, 1994, published in *Ann Emerg Med,* April 1996.

American Pain Society (APS): Acute and Cancer Pain

Principles of Analgesic Use in the Treatment of Acute Pain and Cancer Pain, ed 4, Skokie, Ill, 1999, APS (64 pages).

Comment: This guideline is widely accepted and is revised regularly. Content covers the three analgesic groups and provides well-documented and practical information.

To order ($3.00 members; $5.00 nonmembers; discount for larger orders):

APS
4700 W. Lake Ave.
Glenview, IL 60025-1485
Phone: (847) 375-4715
Fax: (847) 375-4777

International Association for the Study of Pain (IASP): Back Pain and Acute Pain

Fordyce WE, editor: *Back Pain in the Workplace,* Seattle, 1995, IASP Press.

Comment: This book has been the subject of considerable controversy; rejected by the Canadian Pain Society. For a discussion of the guidelines, see letters and editorials in *Pain* 65:5, 7-8, 111-114, 1996.

Ready LB, Edwards WT: *Management of Acute Pain: A Practical Guide,* Seattle, 1992, IASP Press.

To order:

IASP
909 N.E. 43rd St., Rm. 306
Seattle, WA 98105-6021
(206) 547-6409
Fax: (206) 547-1703

World Health Organization: Cancer Pain

Cancer Pain Relief and Palliative Care, 1990. Technical report series 804.

To order:

WHO Collaborating Center
UW-Comprehensive Cancer Center
1900 University Ave.
Madison, WI 53705
Fax: (608) 263-0259

● ● ● ● ●
BOX 1.3

Selected Periodicals on Pain

The American Journal of Hospice & Palliative Care
470 Boston Post Road
Weston, MA 02193

Analgesia (complimentary)
Abbott Laboratories, Hospital Products
Medical Dept., AP30; 1 Abbott Park Rd.
Abbott Park, IL 60064-3500

Cancer Pain Release (newsletter)
1900 University Ave.
Madison, WI 53705

The Clinical Journal of Pain
Lippincott-Raven Publishers
P.O. Box 1600
Hagerstown, MD 21741-9910

Current Review of Pain
Turpin Distribution Services Ltd.
Blackhorse Rd.
Letchworth, Hertfordshire SG6 1HN
UK

European Journal of Pain
Journals Subscription Dept.
Harcourt Brace & Company Ltd.
Foots Cray High St.
Sidcup, Kent DA14 5HP
UK

International Journal of Acute Pain Management
Saldatore Ltd.
Millars Three
Southmill Rd.
Bishop's Stortford, Herts CM23 3DH
UK

Journal of Pain & Symptom Management
Elsevier Science Publishing Co., Inc.
Journals Fulfillment Dept.
P.O. Box 882, Madison Square Station
New York, NY 10160-0200

Journal of Pharmaceutical Care in Pain & Symptom Control
The Haworth Press Inc.
10 Alice Street
Binghamton, NY 13904-1580

Network News (newsletter, cancer pain)
Network Project
MSKCC, Box 421
12175 York Ave.
New York, NY 10021

Pain (free to IASP members)
Elsevier Science Publishers
P.O. Box 211
1000 AE Amsterdam, The Netherlands

Pain Digest
Springer-Verlag New York, Inc.
Journal Fulfillment Services
P.O. Box 2485
Secaucus, NJ 07094

Pain Forum (journal of the American Pain Society; free to society members)
Churchill Livingstone, Inc.
P.O. Box 3217
Secaucus, NJ 07096-3217

The Pain Medicine Journal Club Journal
Lippincott-Raven Publishers
P.O. Box 1600
Hagerstown, MD 21741-9932

Pain Research & Management (journal of the Canadian Pain Society; free to society members)
Pulsus Group, Inc.
2902 South Sheridan Way
Oakville, Ontario, Canada L6J 7L6

Pain Reviews
Marketing Dept., Arnold
P.O. Box 386
Avenel, NJ 07001-0386

Palliative Care Letter (complimentary)
Roxane Laboratories, Inc.
P.O. Box 16532
Columbus, OH 43216

Palliative Medicine
Turpin Distribution Services Limited
Blackhorse Road
Letchworth, Hertfordshire SG6 1HN
UK

Topics in Pain Management (newsletter)
Williams & Wilkins
P.O. Box 23291
Baltimore, MD 21203-9990

On occasion, accepting and acting on the patient's report of pain is difficult. Pain cannot be proved or disproved, and health care professionals are vulnerable to being fooled by the patient who wishes to lie about pain. However, although accepting and responding to the report of pain will undoubtedly result in giving analgesics to some patients who do not have pain, it ensures that everyone who does have pain receives an attentive response. Many studies have shown that failure to assess pain or the existence of differences between the clinicians' pain ratings and those of patients is a major cause of unrelieved pain (e.g., Grossman, Sheidler, Swedeen et al., 1991; Von Roenn, Cleeland, Gonin et al., 1993). In a study of more than 1000 outpatients with metastatic cancer, the most powerful predictor of inadequate analgesia was the discrepancy between the physician's and the patient's estimate of pain severity (Cleeland, Gonin, Hatfield et al., 1994).

Opioid analgesics

Exaggerated Fears of Addiction and Respiratory Depression

In 1940 a consensus paper read at the annual meeting of the American Medical Association stated, "The use of narcotics in terminal cancer is to be condemned. . . . Morphine use is an unpleasant experience to the majority of human subjects because of undesirable side-effects. Dominant in the list of these unfortunate effects is addiction" (Reidenberg, 1996, p. 1278). Such authoritative statements are difficult to overcome.

For decades the dangers of opioid analgesics have received far more attention than their benefits. Opioids have a reputation for being very dangerous drugs that have the capacity to kill or change a person into an out-of-control addict. Although these are risks associated with the use of opioids, evidence is overwhelming that clinicians' fears of these events are greatly exaggerated.

The occurrence of addiction as a result of opioid use for pain relief is extremely rare (see Chapter 3, pp. 50-51). Several studies have concluded that the risk is far less than 1%. For example, in a prospective study of 11,882 hospitalized medical patients, only 4 patients could be documented as having become addicted as a result of receiving opioid analgesics (Porter, Jick, 1980). Even more convincing are studies of patients receiving heroin as an analgesic. In England two studies with more than 500 patients who received heroin for pain relief found that no patient could be documented as having become addicted (Twycross, 1974; Twycross, Wald, 1976).

Despite evidence to the contrary, addiction in particular remains an enormous concern of physicians, nurses, patients, and their families and tragically promotes the undertreatment of pain. A recent survey of nurses' knowledge of addiction revealed that 37.3% thought the overall likelihood of addiction occurring as a result of taking opioids for pain relief was 5% or greater (McCaffery, Ferrell, 1997). In patients who received opioid analgesics for 3 months or longer, concern about addiction increased dramatically, with 75.9% believing 5% or more of patients would become addicted.

In most instances respiratory depression can be prevented, and, if it is not, it can be treated (see Chapter 6, pp. 268-270). For example, in a study of 3785 patients who received IV opioid analgesics by PCA, the incidence of serious respiratory depression was 0.1% and no patient died (Ashburn, Love, Pace, 1994).

Regulatory Issues

Federal regulations for prescribing controlled substances such as opioids were established in the early 1970s and were not intended to interfere with the prescribing of opioids for intractable pain. Furthermore, no state has laws or regulations that consider use of opioids for intractable pain to be illegitimate (Joranson, 1995a).

Yet, a 1991 survey of members of state medical boards found that most members would discourage a physician from prescribing opioids for chronic noncancer pain, and approximately 30% would investigate this practice as a potential violation of law (Joranson, Cleeland, Weissman et al., 1992). With regard to chronic cancer pain, more board members responded that prescribing opioids was appropriate, but 24% regarded this practice as unacceptable or a probable violation of law. Not surprisingly, physicians have been inappropriately investigated and prosecuted for prescribing opioids for chronic pain, both noncancer and cancer. As a result of these survey findings, pain seminars were conducted for medical boards during 1994 and 1995, with participation of members of the APS (Joranson, 1995b).

In an effort to correct misunderstandings about the legitimate medical use of opioids for intractable pain and to protect physicians from inappropriate disciplinary action, several states have adopted intractable pain treatment acts (IPTA). However, IPTAs have not proved to be the ideal solution. In some cases they have placed additional restrictions on prescribing, and they have not successfully protected physicians from inappropriate investigation (Joranson, 1995a).

A more effective method of clarifying the role of opioids in chronic noncancer pain are guidelines and policies issued by state medical boards. Although such a guideline does not have the legal status of a law or regulation, it is an official statement by a medical board. Over the past 10 years a number of state medical boards have published guidelines pertaining to prescribing opioids for intractable pain. These guidelines may also be used to address physicians' fears of being investigated and disciplined by the board (Joranson, 1995b). Guidelines published by the Medical Board of California (1994) were endorsed by APS, with the exception of a provision that restricts prescribing opioids to substance abusers with pain (APS OK's California pain treatment guidelines, 1995).

In 1997 the American Academy of Pain Medicine and the American Pain Society published a consensus statement on the use of opioids for treatment of chronic nonmalignant pain, which stated that opioids are an essential part of management of chronic pain not caused by cancer.

APS has a committee on analgesic regulatory affairs. The Pain and Policy Studies Group, located at the University of Wisconsin-Madison, also addresses regulatory barriers to pain management.

The Patient and Family

Of all the barriers to providing adequate pain relief, the strangest may be that patients themselves are their own worst enemies. Following are results of surveys of the public, patients with cancer pain, and families of patients with cancer pain. All reveal strong negative attitudes about use of analgesics, especially "narcotics."

Attitudes of the layman

In August of 1993 a national telephone survey of 1000 Americans revealed that they have multiple fears related to pain medication (The Mayday Fund, 1993). Despite the widespread belief that Americans too readily take "pills" for pain relief, this survey revealed a negative attitude toward pain medicine. For example, 41% thought physicians tend to overprescribe, 66% said they simply endured severe pain the last time they experienced it, and 77% said they preferred to try "natural" techniques before turning to medication. Eighty-seven percent were fearful of becoming overreliant on pain medication, and 82% were concerned about becoming addicted. Many (72%) worried that pain medication would lose its effectiveness with continued use.

Interestingly, those who had experienced pain themselves or had close friends or family who had experienced severe pain were the most likely to believe that people should use pain-relieving drugs if they need them. However, some interesting inconsistencies were noted. Although 64% of those who had experienced severe pain (fracture, surgery) admitted they acted quickly to relieve the pain, most still insisted on their answer to another more general question, that they were more likely to bear pain than to seek relief.

Other findings in the study revealed that respondents were not optimistic about how much pain could be relieved. Less than half (41%) believed that all or almost all acute pain can be relieved, and only 21% believed that all or almost all chronic pain can be relieved.

The belief that very little can be done to relieve chronic pain may help explain the current public interest in euthanasia (intentionally administering a treatment to cause the patient's death with the patient's informed consent) and physician-assisted suicide (the provision of an agent [e.g., medication] with the intent that the patient will use it to commit suicide) (Humphry, 1996). The media coverage of this has been extensive. The public appears to be very fearful that suffering and death will be prolonged and that pain and other symptoms will not be addressed (Coyle, 1992). People seem to believe that death is painful and that people need to have control over their own deaths because health care professionals may keep them alive or let them die in pain.

Attitudes of patients with cancer pain and their families

Not surprisingly, attitudes expressed by the public are similar to those held by patients. A survey of 270 patients with cancer revealed a reluctance to report pain and to use analgesics, resulting in poor pain relief (Ward, Goldberg, Miller-McCauley et al., 1993). Inadequate pain relief was associated with concerns about addiction, side effects, injections, tolerance, believing that "good" patients do not complain, and believing that pain is inevitable. Respondents tended to agree with statements such as "Pain medicine cannot really control pain," "People get addicted to pain medicine easily," and "Good patients avoid talking about pain."

Family members of patients with pain have similar concerns about addiction. A study of 85 family caregivers of patients with cancer pain revealed that caregivers believed it was their responsibility to try to avoid addiction by limiting the amount of medication used (Ferrell, Cohen, Rhiner et al., 1991).

Need for education

Clearly, the public and patients and their families need education about what can be done to provide safe and effective pain relief. Fear and misinformation pose substantial barriers to patients with regard to reporting their pain and taking analgesics. Many patient education tools have been developed, but patients and families do not necessarily have easy access to them. Nurses are probably in the best position to obtain these materials and disseminate them (see Chapters 3 to 9 and 11 to 15 for patient/family education resources).

SIGNS OF PROGRESS

Another encouraging sign of progress is the growth of organizations and services that foster improvement of and access to pain management. Following are some examples of these developments.

Increase in Pain Facilities

Structured services for the delivery of care to patients with pain are now widespread. The first officially recognized hospices in the United States began operation in the mid-1970s. Now there are hundreds of hospice programs providing care to terminally ill patients throughout the United States. A directory of these is available from the National Hospice Organization (NHO).

Although nerve block clinics for pain relief have existed since the 1940s, it was not until the 1960s that multidisciplinary pain centers emerged. Two of the early ones were at University of Washington in Seattle (directed by John Bonica) and at City of Hope Medical Center (directed by Benjamin Crue, Jr.). Today numerous pain facilities exist for the treatment of chronic nonmalignant pain and cancer pain. The APS publishes a directory of pain facilities (*1996 Pain facilities directory*, 1996).

Creation of Acute Pain Services

Acute pain services for patients with acute pain related to surgery, trauma, or painful medical procedures who are receiving IVs, epidural, or intrathecal analgesics have become widespread over the last decade. One of the first acute pain services was started in 1986 at the University of Washington in Seattle by Brian Ready (Macintyre, Ready, 1996; Ready, Oden, Chadwick et al., 1988). Such services are now commonplace in most major hospitals, and research has shown that they provide a wide range of relatively invasive techniques for improving pain control without endangering patient safety (Schug, Torrie, 1993).

Growth of Professional Organizations That Focus on Pain

Founding of professional organizations concerned with pain management began in the 1970s (Box 1.4). IASP was founded on May 26, 1973. National chapters, including the Canadian Pain Society in 1976 and the APS in 1978, evolved shortly thereafter. Chapters now exist in 54 countries. The IASP and its chapters are multidisciplinary and have as their goals the promotion of education and research on pain. IASP meets every 3 years, and APS meets annually.

APS has committees on analgesic regulatory affairs, clinical practice guidelines, continuing education, and quality of care for acute pain and cancer pain. It has the following six regional chapters: Western, Eastern, Midwest, Southern, New England, and Greater Philadelphia.

NHO, formed in 1978, is dedicated to promoting quality care for terminally ill persons and their families. Pain control is one of several issues addressed. In 1986 the Hospice Nurses Association was formed, and it later became the Hospice and Palliative Nurses Association. The American Academy of Hospice and Palliative Medicine was organized in 1988.

The American Academy of Pain Medicine (AAPM) was founded in 1983. Membership includes physicians and surgeons from a variety of disciplines, including anesthesiologists, internists, and psychiatrists. The mission of AAPM is to provide quality care to patients with pain through research and through the education and training of all physicians. AAPM is the only pain organization with representation in the American Medical Association (AMA) House of Delegates. (Another organization—American Academy of Pain Management—has the same acronym. The two are sometimes confused with each other. The latter is multidisciplinary and is not affiliated with AMA, APS, or IASP. In this book, AAPM will refer only to the American Academy of Pain Medicine.)

The American Society of Pain Management Nurses (ASPMN) was founded in 1990. This is an organization of professional nurses dedicated to promoting and providing care to patients with pain through fostering education, standards, advocacy, and research. Regional chapters are beginning to form. ASPMN meets annually and publishes a newsletter.

Many specialty organizations in medicine and nursing have begun to focus on pain in their particular clinical areas. These include the Oncology Nursing Society, the American Society of Postanesthesia Nurses, the National Association of Orthopaedic Nurses, the American College of Emergency Physicians, and the American Academy of Pediatrics. Some have published position papers related to pain such as the placebo position statement and the cancer pain position paper issued by the Oncology Nursing Society. (Copies of these may be ordered from the organization; see Box 1.1, Resources for Professional Education.)

Growth of State Cancer Pain Initiatives

In 1986 the Wisconsin Cancer Pain Initiative, a group composed of health care professionals and volunteers, was organized for the purpose of improving cancer pain management. Shortly thereafter, other states began their own initiatives and now all 50 states have initiatives or are in the process of forming them. The American Alliance of Cancer Pain Initiatives (AACPI), a national organization for state cancer pain initiatives, was formed in 1996 to support and coordinate the activities of the states. In addition to promoting educational programs, the organization has also been active in addressing institutional and regulatory barriers to the treatment of cancer pain. The AACPI works collaboratively with many other organizations such as APS and the National Cancer Institute's Cancer Information Service. The ultimate goal is to make the cancer pain initiative movement a catalyst for change in the health care system (Dahl, 1996).

Certification for Pain Specialists

A task force of ASPMN is working toward certification of nurses who specialize in pain management.

● ● ● ● ●
BOX 1.4

Professional Organizations That Focus on Pain

American Academy of Hospice and Palliative Medicine
P.O. Box 14288
Gainesville, FL 32604-2288
(352) 377-8900
Fax: (352) 371-2349
E-mail: *aahpm@aahpm.org*
Web site: *www.aahpm.org*
Membership open to physicians only.
Membership includes newsletter, "Hospice Update."

American Academy of Pain Medicine
4700 W. Lake Ave.
Glenview, IL 60025
(847) 375-4731
Fax: (847) 375-4777
E-mail: *aapm@amctec.com*
Membership open to physicians only.
Membership includes newsletter.

American Board of Hospice and Palliative Medicine
1211 Avenue of the Americas, 15th Floor
New York, NY 10036
(212) 852-0400
Administers certification examination.

American Board of Pain Medicine
4700 W. Lake Ave.
Glenview, IL 60025
(847) 375-4731
Fax: (847) 375-4777
Offers pain medicine physicians certification as a Diplomat of the American Board of Pain Medicine.

American Pain Society
4700 W. Lake Ave.
Glenview, IL 60025-1485
(847) 375-4715
Fax: (847) 375-4777
Web site: *www.ampainsoc.org/*
E-mail: *info@ampainsoc.org*
Membership open to clinicians and researchers interested in pain.
Members receive a bimonthly bulletin, a copy of "Principles of Analgesic Use for Acute Pain and Cancer Pain," a copy of "Pain Facilities Directory," and a subscription to "Pain Forum."

American Society of Pain Management Nurses
7794 Grow Drive
Pensacola, FL 32514
(888) 34ASPMN ([888] 342-7766)
(850) 473-0233
Fax: (850) 484-8762
E-mail: *ASPMN@aol.com*
Membership open to registered nurses worldwide.
Membership includes newsletter.

Hospice and Palliative Nurses Association
(formerly Hospice Nurses Association)
National Office
Medical Center East, Suite 375
211 N. Whitfield St.
Pittsburgh, PA 15206-3031
(412) 361-2470
Fax: (412) 361-2425
E-mail: *HPNA@hpna.org*
Web site: *http://www.HPNA.org*
Membership open to registered nurses and volunteers. Membership includes quarterly newsletter "Fanfare" and provides a manual for preparation for the certification examination.

International Association for the Study of Pain (IASP)
909 N.E. 43rd St., Rm. 306
Seattle, WA 98105-6021
(206) 547-6409
Fax: (206) 547-1703
E-mail: *iasp@locke.hs.washington.edu*
Web site: *http://weber.u.washington.edu/~crc/IASP.html*
Membership includes newsletter, clinical updates, and a subscription to the journal *Pain*.

National Board for Certification of Hospice Nurses
Professional Testing Corporation
1211 Avenue of the Americas, 15th Floor
New York, NY 10036
(212) 852-0400
Provides information about certification.

National Hospice Organization
1901 N. Moore St., Suite 901
Arlington, VA 22209
(703) 243-5900
Has "Locator Directory of Hospices in America."

Pain & Policy Studies Group (Designated the World Health Organization Collaborating Center for Policy and Communications in Cancer Care)
UW Comprehensive Cancer Center
University of Wisconsin-Madison Medical School
1900 University Ave.
Madison, WI 53705
(608) 263-7662
Fax: (608) 263-0259

Resource Center for State Cancer Pain Initiatives and The American Alliance of Cancer Pain Initiatives
1300 University Ave., Room 4720
Madison, WI 53706
(608) 265-4013
Fax: (608) 265-4014
E-mail: *AACPI@AACPI.org*
Web site: *www.AACPI.org*

AAPM offers board certification for physicians who specialize in pain medicine. Physicians may elect fellowship status or become certified as a Diplomat of the American Board of Pain Medicine. Anesthesiologists may also obtain board certification in pain management through the American Board of Anesthesiology.

Certification for hospice registered nurses is available through the National Board for Certification of Hospice Nurses, sponsored by HPNA. Pain management comprises 15% of the examination.

The AAHPM sponsors a certification program for physicians. The examination is administered by the American Board of Hospice and Palliative Medicine. Pain in cancer and noncancer patients comprises 25% of the examination.

Recognition of the Rights of People With Pain

Because patients with pain are so often undertreated and sometimes stigmatized, several statements about the rights of patients with pain have emerged. In cooperation with the Iowa and Wisconsin Cancer Pain Initiatives, Cancer Care, Inc. developed a bill of rights for people with cancer pain (Box 1.5). This bill of rights was developed to encourage patients, their loved ones, and caregivers to learn the facts about pain and its treatment. The New York State Cancer and AIDS Pain Initiative has a similar 7–point statement of support for patients with pain, which is also available through Cancer Care, Inc. (Box 1.5). Patient education publications also often include a list of rights for patients with pain (e.g., Cowan, 1990; Cowles, 1993).

References

Acute Pain Management Guideline Panel: *Acute pain management in adults: operative procedures, quick reference guide for clinicians,* AHCPR Pub. No. 92-0019, Rockville, Md, 1992, Agency for Health Care Policy and Research, Public Health Service, U.S. Department of Health and Human Services.

American Academy of Pain Medicine, American Pain Society: The use of opioids for treatment of chronic pain, *Clin J Pain* 13:6-8, 1997.

American Pain Society: *1996 Pain facilities directory,* Glenview, Ill, 1996, American Pain Society.

APS OK's California pain treatment guidelines, *APS Bull* 5(2):20-21, 1995.

Ashburn MA, Love G, Pace NL.: Respiratory-related critical events with intravenous patient-controlled analgesia, *Clin J Pain* 10:52-56, 1994.

Berry P: JCAHO pain management standards, *Cancer Pain Update Issue* 45:2, 14, 1997.

Cleeland CS, Gonin R, Hatfield AK et al.: Pain and its treatment in outpatients with metastatic cancer, *N Engl J Med* 330:592-596, 1994.

Cowan P: *Workbook manual,* Rocklin, Calif, 1990, American Chronic Pain Association.

Cowles J: *Pain relief! How to say "no" to acute, chronic, and cancer pain,* New York, 1993, Mastermedia Limited.

Coyle N: The euthanasia and physician-assisted suicide debate: issues for nursing, *Oncol Nurs Forum* 19(Suppl) (7):41-46, 1992.

Dahl JL: State cancer pain initiatives form national organization: the American alliance of cancer pain initiatives, *APS Bull* 6(6):3, 1996.

Dahl JL: A decade of progress, *Cancer Pain Update Issue* 42:1-3, 6, 1997.

Donovan M, Dillon P, McGuire L: Incidence and characteristics of pain in a sample of medical-surgical inpatients, *Pain* 30:69-78, 1987.

Fagerhaugh SY: Pain expression and control on a burn unit, *Nurs Outlook* 22:645-650, 1974.

Ferrell B, McCaffery M, Rhiner M: Pain and addiction: an urgent need for change in nursing education, *J Pain Symptom Manage* 7:48-55, 1992.

Ferrell BR, Cohen MZ, Rhiner M et al.: Pain as a metaphor for illness part II: family caregivers' management of pain, *Oncol Nurs Forum* 18:1315-1321, 1991.

Ferrell BR, Grant M, Ritchey KJ et al.: The pain resource nursing training program: a unique approach to pain management, *J Pain Symptom Manage* 8:549-556, 1993.

Ferrell BR, Griffith H: Cost issues related to pain management: report from the cancer pain panel of the Agency for Health Care Policy and Research, *J Pain Symptom Manage* 9:221–234, 1994.

Ferrell BR, McGuire DB, Donovan MI: Knowledge and beliefs regarding pain in a sample of nursing faculty, *J Prof Nurs* 9:79-88, 1993.

Fields HL, editor: *Core curriculum for professional education in pain,* ed 2, Seattle, 1995, IASP Press.

Graffam, S: Pain content in the curriculum: a survey, *Nurse Educator* 15:20-23, 1990.

Grant M, Ferrell BR, Rivera LM et al.: Unscheduled readmissions for uncontrolled symptoms: a health care challenge for nurses, *Nurs Clin North Am* 30(4):673-682, 1995.

Grant M, Rivera LM, Ferrell BR et al.: Cancer pain management for nurse educators, *Canadian Oncol Nurs J* (Suppl):87, 1994.

Grass JA, Zuckerman RL, Tsao H et al.: Patient-controlled epidural analgesia results in shorter hospital stay after cesarean section, *Regional Anesthesia,* 15:S26, 1991.

Grossman SA, Sheidler VR, Swedeen K et al.: Correlation of patient and caregiver ratings of cancer pain, *J Pain Symptom Manage* 6:53-57, 1991.

Gu X, Belgrade M: Pain in hospitalized patients with medical illnesses, *J Pain Symptom Manage* 8:17-21, 1993.

Herzberg U, Murtaugh M, Beitz AF: Chronic pain and immunity: mononeuropathy alters immune responses in rats, *Pain* 59:219-225, 1994.

Hitchcock LS, Ferrell BF, McCaffery M: The experience of chronic nonmalignant pain, *J Pain Symptom Manage* 9(5):312-318, 1994.

Humphry D: *Final exit: the practicalities of self-deliverance and assisted suicide for the dying,* ed 2, New York, 1996, Dell.

Isaacs SL, Knickman JR: Editors' introduction. In Isaacs SL, Knickman JR, editors: *To improve health and health care 1997,* San Francisco, 1997, Jossey-Bass.

Jackson DA: A study of pain management: patient controlled analgesia versus intramuscular analgesia, *J Intravenous Nurs* 12(1):42-51, 1989.

Jacox A, Carr DB, Payne R et al.: *Management of cancer pain: adults quick reference guide,* No. 9. AHCPR Pub. No. 94-0593. Rockville, Md, 1994, Agency for Health Care Policy and Research, Public Health Service, U.S. Department of Health and Human Services.

Janjan NA, Martin CG, Payne R et al.: Teaching cancer pain management: durability of educational effects of a role model program, *Cancer* 77:996-1001, 1996.

JCAHO grasps the initiative on pain: new standards within two years, *Medical Ethics Advisor,* pp 113-116, 119, October 1997.

Joint Commission on Accreditation of Healthcare Organizations: *1992 Standards manual,* Oakbrook Terrace, IL, 1992, Joint Commission on Accreditation of Healthcare Organizations.

Joint Commission on Accreditation of Healthcare Organizations: *Accreditation manual for hospitals,* Oakbrook Terrace, IL, 1994, Joint Commission on Accreditation of Healthcare Organizations.

Joranson DE: Intractable pain treatment laws and regulations, *APS Bull* 5(2):1-3, 15-16, 1995a.

Joranson DE: State medical board guidelines for treatment of intractable pain, *APS Bull* 5(3):1-5, 1995b.

Joranson DE, Cleeland CS, Weissman DE et al.: Opioids for chronic cancer and noncancer pain: a survey of state medical board members, *Federation Bulletin: The Journal of Medical Licensure and Discipline* 79(4):15-49, 1992.

Liebeskind JC: Pain can kill, *Pain* 44:3-4, 1991.

Loeser JD: President's address to the 8th world congress on pain. In Jensen TS, Turner JA, Wiesenfeld-Hallin Z: Proceedings of the 8th world congress on pain. *Pain research and management,* vol 8, Seattle, 1997, IASP Press.

Marks RM, Sachar EJ: Undertreatment of medical inpatients with narcotic analgesics, *Ann Intern Med* 78:173–181, 1973.

The Mayday Fund: *1993 pain survey,* New York: 1993, Author.

Macintyre PE, Ready LB: *Acute pain management: a practical guide,* Philadelphia, 1996, WB Saunders.

McCaffery M: *Nursing practice theories related to cognition, bodily pain, and man-environment interactions,* Los Angeles, 1968, University of California at Los Angeles Students' Store.

McCaffery M, Ferrell BR: Nurses' knowledge of pain assessment and management: how much progress have we made? *J Pain Symptom Manage* 14:175-188, 1997.

McCaffery M, Pasero C: Pain ratings: the fifth vital sign, *Am J Nurs* 97(2):15-16, 1997.

McMillan SC: Pain and pain relief experienced by hospice patients with cancer, *Cancer Nurs* 19:298-307, 1996.

Medical Board of California: *New, easy guidelines on prescribing,* Medical Board of California Action Report 51:1, 8, Oct 1994.

Melzack R, Wall PD: Pain mechanisms: a new theory, *Science* 150:971-979, 1965.

Pierce JE: From all perspectives, patient-controlled analgesia seen as beneficial and profitable, *Pharmacy Practice News* 15(2):1988.

Porter J, Jick H: Addiction rare in patients treated with narcotics, *N Engl J Med* 302:123, 1980.

Puntillo K, Weiss SD J: Pain: its mediators and associated morbidity in critically ill cardiovascular surgical patients, *Nurs Res* 43:31-36, 1994.

Ready LB, Oden R, Chadwick IIS et al.: Development of an anaesthesiology-based postoperative pain management service, *Anesthesiology* 68:100-106, 1988.

Reidenberg MM: Barriers to controlling pain in patients with cancer, *Lancet* 347:1276, 1996.

Ross EL, Perumbeti P: Is it cost-effective when used for postoperative pain management? *Anesthesiology* 69:A710, 1988.

Schug SA, Torrie JJ: Safety assessment of postoperative pain management by an acute pain service, *Pain* 55:387-391, 1993.

Sheehan DK, Webb A, Bower D et al.: Level of cancer pain knowledge among baccalaureate student nurses, *J Pain Symptom Manage* 7:478-484, 1992.

Strauss A, Fagerhaugh SY, Glaser B: An organizational-work-interactional perspective, *Nurs Outlook* 22:560-566, 1974.

Teoh N, Stjernsward J: WHO cancer pain relief program: ten years on, *IASP Newsletter,* 1992.

The SUPPORT principal investigators: A controlled trial to improve care for seriously ill patients, *JAMA* 274:1591-1598, 1995.

Twycross RG: Clinical experience with diamorphine in advanced malignant disease, *Int J Clin Pharmacol* 9:184-198, 1974.

Twycross RG, Wald SJ: Long-term use of diamorphine in advanced cancer. In Bonica JJ, Albe-Fessard D, editors: *Adv Pain Res Ther* 1:653-661, 1976.

Von Roenn JH, Cleeland CS, Gonin R et al.: Physician's attitudes and practice in cancer pain management: a survey from the eastern cooperative oncology group, *Ann Intern Med* 119:121-126, 1993.

Ward SE, Goldberg N, Miller-McCauley V et al.: Patient-related barriers to management of cancer pain, *Pain* 52:319-324, 1993.

Ward SE, Gordon D: Application of the American Pain Society quality assurance standards, *Pain* 56:299-306, 1994.

Ward SE, Gordon D: Patient satisfaction and pain severity as outcomes in pain management: a longitudinal view of one setting's experience, *J Pain Symptom Manage* 11:242-251, 1996.

Warfield CA, Kahn CH: Acute pain management: programs in U.S. hospitals and experiences and attitudes among U.S. adults, *Anesthesiology* 83:1090-1094, 1995.

Wisconsin Cancer Pain Initiative: Cancer pain management competency guidelines for nursing education and practice, *Cancer Pain Update* (insert) Issue 35, 1995.

World Health Organization: *Cancer pain relief,* Geneva, 1986, World Health Organization.

World Health Organization: *Cancer pain relief and palliative care,* Geneva, 1990, World Health Organization.

Yeager MP, Glass DD, Neff KR et al.: Epidural anesthesia and analgesia in high-risk surgical patients, *Anesthesiology* 66:729-736, 1987.

Zalon ML: Nurses' assessment of postoperative patients' pain, *Pain* 54:329-334, 1993.

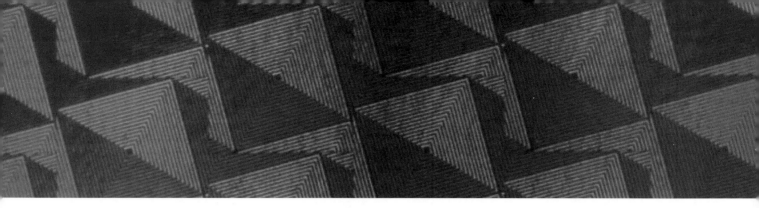

chapter two
BASIC MECHANISMS UNDERLYING THE CAUSES AND EFFECTS OF PAIN

Chris Pasero, Judith A. Paice, and Margo McCaffery

CHAPTER OUTLINE

TERMINOLOGY

Action potential: Cycle of electrical changes in cells by which an impulse is transmitted along a nerve fiber.

Allodynia: Pain caused by a stimulus that does not normally provoke pain.

Catabolism: The destructive phase of metabolism.

Central pain: Pain initiated or caused by a primary lesion or dysfunction in the central nervous system.

Depolarization: The inside of the cell becoming temporarily positive relative to the outside.

Endogenous opioids: Families of peptides (enkephalins, endorphins, and dynorphins) secreted naturally by the body ("morphine within"), capable of producing effects similar to exogenous opioids (e.g., inhibiting pain transmission).

Exogenous opioids: Drugs derived from opium administered to produce analgesia (e.g., morphine, codeine, methadone).

Modulation: The activation of descending pathways that exerts inhibitory effects on the cells responsible for pain transmission.

Morbidity: Pertaining to disease or complications.

Mortality: Death rate.

Neuralgia: Pain in the distribution of a nerve or nerves.

Neuropathic pain: Pain initiated or caused by a primary lesion or dysfunction in the nervous system.

Nociceptive pain: Pain resulting from the ongoing activation of primary afferent neurons by noxious stimuli. The nervous system is intact.

Nociceptor: A receptor preferentially sensitive to a noxious stimulus or to a stimulus that would be noxious if prolonged.

Noxious stimulus: A stimulus that is damaging or potentially damaging to normal tissue.

Pain perception: The process of recognizing, defining, and responding to pain.

Peripheral neuropathic pain: Pain initiated or caused by a primary lesion or dysfunction in the peripheral nervous system.

Primary afferent neuron: See definition of "nociceptor."

Repolarization: The inside of the cell becoming negative relative to the outside.

Resting potential: The normal physiochemical orientation of all body cells whereby the inside of the cell is negatively charged relative to the outside; a nonconducting state.

Somatic pain: Pain of the musculoskeletal system.

Synapse: Point of junction between two neurons.

Transduction: Conversion of one form of energy to another.

Transmission: The movement of pain impulses from the site of transduction to the brain.

Visceral pain: Pain of the body's internal organs.

Defining pain, distinguishing between the different types of pain, and understanding the way in which noxious stimuli are transmitted from the periphery to the part of the brain where pain is perceived are essential to assessing pain and providing adequate pain relief. The gate control theory (Melzack, Wall, 1965) stimulated intense interest in the anatomy and physiology of pain. This heightened interest led to a proliferation of research and discovery on the subject. Although great strides have been made in the past 30 years with regard to explaining the complexities of pain, much still remains unknown.

This chapter presents accepted definitions of pain and the distinctions between the various types of pain. It provides a basic foundation in the anatomy and physiology of pain and how this relates to several of the drugs commonly prescribed for pain control. Included is an overview of neuropathic pain. A discussion of the many harmful effects of unrelieved pain will underscore the necessity for adequate pain management. Misconcep-

tions related to the basic mechanisms underlying pain are presented and corrected in Table 2.1. Selected terms and definitions are listed at the beginning of this chapter to facilitate an understanding of the content. Box 2.1 provides resources for learning more about the physiology and effects of pain.

DEFINITIONS OF PAIN

The most widely accepted definition of pain, adopted by the International Association for the Study of Pain (IASP) and the American Pain Society (APS), is "Pain is an unpleasant sensory and emotional experience associated with actual or potential tissue damage, or described in terms of such damage" (APS, 1992; Mersky, Bogduk, 1994). This definition describes pain as a phenomenon with multiple components that makes an impact on a person's psychosocial and physical functioning. It acknowledges the complexity of the pain experience. Pain is not determined by tissue damage alone.

TABLE 2.1 ● ● ● ● ●

Misconceptions | **Pain Mechanisms**

MISCONCEPTION	CORRECTION
1. What we know about pain and its management is based on theory, not fact.	Considerable factual information is available regarding pain mechanisms and many other aspects of pain. Previously, the underlying causes of pain were often referred to as "theories" of pain mechanisms. Theories have been useful in stimulating research regarding pain and its management. The accepted guidelines (e.g., AHCPR and American Pain Society) have put forth recommendations for the management of pain that are based on facts, not theories.
2. Endorphins and enkephalins are effective analgesics.	Endorphins and enkephalins bind to opioid receptor sites and prevent the release of neurotransmitters inhibiting transmission of pain impulses. Unfortunately, endogenous opioids degrade too quickly to be considered useful analgesics. Although administering morphine and other opioids probably temporarily decreases production of endogenous opioids, belief that use of opioids, such as morphine, should be avoided for this reason is unfounded.
3. Pain never killed anyone.	Unrelieved pain may be dangerous and is, therefore, unacceptable. Research now shows that past attitudes of expecting surgery to hurt and believing that "pain never killed anyone" are no longer justified. Postoperative pain can kill by delaying healing and contributing to complications that can be life-threatening. Unrelieved postoperative pain must now be viewed and treated as a complication or risk, not as an acceptable consequence of surgery. Chronic pain also has many serious adverse effects such as suppressing immune function.

May be duplicated for use in clinical practice. From McCaffery M, Pasero C: *Pain: Clinical manual,* p. 17. Copyright © 1999, Mosby, Inc.

● ● ● ● ●

BOX 2.1

Resources for Learning More About the Physiology and Effects of Pain

Fine PG, Ashburn MA: Functional neuroanatomy and nociception. In Ashburn MA, Rice LJ, editors: *The management of pain,* pp 1-25, New York, 1998, Churchill Livingstone.

Kehlet H: Modification of responses to surgery by neural blockade. In Cousins MJ, Bridenbaugh PO, editors: *Neural blockade,* pp 129-175, Philadelphia, 1998, Lippincott-Raven.

Liu SS, Carpenter RL, Neal JM: Epidural anesthesia and analgesia: Their role in postoperative outcome, *Anesthesiology* 82(6):1474-1506, 1995.

Paice JA: Anatomy and physiology of pain: Practical aspects, *Hematol/Oncol Ann* 2(6):401-405, 1994.

Paice JA: *Physiology of pain: Unraveling the mystery,* Baltimore, 1994, Williams & Wilkins Electronic Media. For preview call (800) 527-5597.

Paice JA: Neuropathic pain, *Cope* 12(2):16-18, 1996.

Paice JA: *Pharmacologic management of pain: Tools for treatment,* Baltimore, 1994, Williams & Wilkins Electronic Media. For preview call (800) 527-5597.

Portenoy RK, Kanner RM, editors: *Pain management: Theory and practice,* Philadelphia, 1996, FA Davis.

May be duplicated for use in clinical practice. From McCaffery M, Pasero C: *Pain: Clinical manual,* p. 17. Copyright © 1999, Mosby, Inc.

In fact, no predictable relationship exists between identifiable tissue injury and the sensation of pain. For example, a patient's description of pain may be disproportionate to the evidence of tissue damage. In times of high stress and trauma, pain may be described as less severe than one might expect; whereas patients with chronic nonmalignant pain (CNP) may describe pain for which little or no tissue damage can be found. The latter may be due to abnormalities in the neural processing of stimuli. The inability to identify tissue damage sufficient to explain the pain is not proof that the pain is of psychologic origin (Portenoy, Kanner, 1996).

Because pain is a highly personal and subjective experience, Margo McCaffery's (1968) definition is apropos for use in clinical practice, "Pain is whatever the experiencing person says it is, existing whenever he says it does." In other words, the patient's self-report of pain is the single most reliable indicator of pain (AHCPR, 1992; Jacox, Carr, Payne et al., 1994).

TYPES OF PAIN

Clear distinctions between types of pain are not always possible. Simple classifications of pain invariably result in some omissions and overlap. General discussions of pain often refer simply to three types: (1) acute (relatively brief pain that subsides as healing takes place), (2) cancer, and (3) chronic nonmalignant pain. Another method of classifying pain is by inferred pathophysiology: (1) nociceptive pain (stimuli from somatic and visceral structures) and (2) neuropathic pain (stimuli abnormally processed by the nervous system) (Figure 2.1). The treatment of pain is affected by both of these methods of classifying pain.

Treatment Approaches

Acute pain usually is somatic and/or visceral, or nociceptive (e.g., surgical pain from traumatized skin, muscle, and visceral organs). However, chronic cancer pain and CNP may reflect both nociceptive and neuropathic pain. The treatment of pain requires assessment of these underlying mechanisms because pain caused by different mechanisms is likely to respond to different treatments.

Treatment of pain is also affected by how long it is expected to last. Both acute pain and cancer pain have somewhat predictable endings. The pain is expected to subside at some point. Healing or control of the disease may be expected to end the pain. For patients with cancer pain, death may mark the end of pain. When pain is of short duration or when prolonged pain is expected to have an endpoint, efforts to relieve pain tend to be more aggressive than when pain has no predictable ending, such as in CNP. For example, opioids are traditionally used more freely for acute or cancer pain than for CNP. Choice of route of administration is also affected by the duration of pain. Severe acute pain often is managed intravenously. Chronic pain, once it is under control, usually is managed by the oral route.

ANATOMY AND PHYSIOLOGY OF PAIN

Nociceptive Pain

Nociception is the term used to describe how pain becomes conscious. Four basic processes are involved in nociception: (1) transduction, (2) transmission, (3) perception, and (4) modulation (Figure 2.2). Transduction refers to changing noxious stimuli in sensory nerve endings to impulses; transmission refers to the movement of impulses from the site of transduction to the brain; perception refers to the processes involved in recognizing, defining, and responding to pain; and modulation involves the activation of descending pathways that exert inhibitory effects on pain transmission (Fields, 1987).

Transduction

Transduction is the first process involved in nociception. It begins at the periphery (skin, subcutaneous tissue, visceral, or somatic structures) where primary afferent neurons, called nociceptors, are distributed throughout. Nociceptors are free nerve endings with the capacity to distinguish between noxious and innocuous stimuli (Portenoy, 1996a). When exposed in sufficient quantity to mechanical (incision or tumor growth), thermal (burn), or chemical (toxic substance) noxious stimuli,

tissue damage or potential damage occurs. The trauma of this exposure causes the release of a number of substances that facilitate the movement of the pain impulse from the periphery to the spinal cord. These substances are principal sources of pain in the periphery and include prostaglandins, bradykinin, serotonin, substance P, and histamine (Fields, 1987).

Several pharmacologic approaches to pain relief involve minimizing the effects of substances released at the periphery. The most common approach for many types of pain is the use of nonsteroidal antiinflammatory drugs (NSAIDs) such as ibuprofen and naproxen (see Chapter 5). Another group of drugs are the corticosteroids, such as dexamethasone, which often are prescribed for cancer pain and CNP conditions (see Chapter 7). These drug groups work as analgesics primarily by interfering with the production of prostaglandins.

Prostaglandins are produced through a series of events beginning when cells are traumatized and release phospholipids. The enzyme phospholipase breaks down phospholipids into arachidonic acid. In turn, the enzyme cyclooxygenase breaks down arachidonic acid into prostaglandins. Corticosteroids block the action of phospholipase and NSAIDs block the action of cyclooxygenase, thereby interfering with the production of prostaglandins. Unfortunately, because prostaglandins maintain the protective layer of the gastric mucosa, one of the serious side effects of corticosteroids and NSAIDs is gastrointestinal erosion (Whittle, Bane, 1983).

For the pain stimulus to be changed to an impulse and move from the periphery to the spinal cord, an action potential must be created, so a general review of nerve conduction is in order. All cells in the body, including neurons, have a membrane potential. The inside of a neuron is negatively charged relative to the outside. This is called the resting membrane potential. In relation to pain transmission, sufficient amounts of noxious stimulation cause the membrane to become permeable to sodium ions, allowing the ions to rush into the cell and creating a temporary positive charge relative to the outside. This is called depolarization.

Other ion transfers also occur. For example, an efflux of potassium changes the charge inside the cell back to a negative one relative to the outside. This is called repolarization. If enough depolarization and repolarization occur, an action potential is created and the stimulus is converted to an impulse (see Figure 2.2). Transduction, which takes just milliseconds to occur, is then complete. The impulse is ready to be transmitted along the nociceptor fibers that extend from the nociceptor cell body.

Some analgesics relieve pain primarily by decreasing the influx of sodium and efflux of potassium at the neuron level, thereby slowing or stopping pain transmission. For example, anticonvulsants relieve some types of neuropathic pain, possibly by blocking or modulating

Text continued on p. 22.

CLASSIFICATION OF PAIN BY INFERRED PATHOLOGY

Two Major Types of Pain

I. Nociceptive Pain

A. Somatic Pain   B. Visceral Pain

II. Neuropathic Pain

A. Centrally Generated Pain   B. Peripherally Generated Pain

I. Nociceptive Pain: Normal processing of stimuli that damages normal tissues or has the potential to do so if prolonged; usually responsive to nonopioids and/or opioids.

A. Somatic Pain: Arises from bone, joint, muscle, skin, or connective tissue. It is usually aching or throbbing in quality and is well localized.

B. Visceral Pain: Arises from visceral organs, such as the GI tract and pancreas. This may be subdivided:

1. Tumor involvement of the organ capsule that causes aching and fairly well-localized pain.

2. Obstruction of hollow viscus, which causes intermittent cramping and poorly localized pain.

II. Neuropathic Pain: Abnormal processing of sensory input by the peripheral or central nervous system; treatment usually includes adjuvant analgesics.

A. Centrally Generated Pain

1. Deafferentation pain. Injury to either the peripheral or central nervous system. Examples: Phantom pain may reflect injury to the peripheral nervous system; burning pain below the level of a spinal cord lesion reflects injury to the central nervous system.

2. Sympathetically maintained pain. Associated with dysregulation of the autonomic nervous system. Examples: May include some of the pain associated with reflex sympathetic dystrophy/causalgia (complex regional pain syndrome, type I, type II).

B. Peripherally Generated Pain

1. Painful polyneuropathies. Pain is felt along the distribution of many peripheral nerves. Examples: diabetic neuropathy, alcohol-nutritional neuropathy, and those associated with Guillain-Barré syndrome.

2. Painful mononeuropathies. Usually associated with a known peripheral nerve injury, and pain is felt at least partly along the distribution of the damaged nerve. Examples: nerve root compression, nerve entrapment, trigeminal neuralgia.

May be duplicated for use in clinical practice. From McCaffery M, Pasero C: *Pain: Clinical manual*, p. 19. Copyright © 1999, Mosby, Inc.

● ● ● ● ●
FIGURE 2.1   A method of classifying pain is by inferred pathophysiology: *1*, nociceptive pain (stimuli from somatic and visceral structures); *2*, neuropathic pain (stimuli abnormally processed by the nervous system).

Information from Max MB, Portenoy RK: Methodological challenges for clinical trials of cancer pain treatments. In Chapman CR, Foley KM, editors: *Current and emerging issues in cancer pain: Research and practice*, pp 283-299, New York, 1993, Raven Press; Portenoy RK: Neuropathic pain. In Portenoy RK, Kanner RM, editors: *Pain management: Theory and practice*, pp 83-125, Philadelphia, 1996b, FA Davis.

A

NOCICEPTION: BASIC PROCESS OF NORMAL PAIN TRANSMISSION

1 **Transduction:** Conversion of one energy from another. This process occurs in the periphery when a noxious stimulus causes tissue damage. The damaged cells release substances that activate or sensitize nociceptors. This activation leads to the generation of an action potential.

   A. **Sensitizing substances** released by damaged cells:
   - Prostaglandins (PG)
   - Bradykinin (BK)
   - Serotonin (5HT)
   - Substance P (SP)
   - Histamine (H)

   B. An **action potential** results from:
   - Release of the above sensitizing substances (nociceptive pain)
       + a change in the charge along the neuronal membrane
                   or
   - Abnormal processing of stimuli by the nervous system (neuropathic pain)
       + a change in the charge along the neuronal membrane

   The change in charge occurs when Na^+ moves into the cell and other ion transfers occur.

2 **Transmission:** The action potential continues from the site of damage to the spinal cord and ascends to higher centers. Transmission may be considered in three phases:
   - Injury site to spinal cord. Nociceptors terminate in the spinal cord.
   - Spinal cord to brain stem and thalamus. Release of substance P and other neurotransmitters continues the impulse across the synaptic cleft between the nociceptors and the dorsal horn neurons. From the dorsal horn of the spinal cord, neurons such as the spinothalamic tract ascend to the thalamus. Other tracts carry the message to different centers in the brain.
   - Thalamus to cortex. Thalamus acts as a relay station sending the impulse to central structures for processing.

3 **Perception of pain:** Conscious experience of pain.

4 **Modulation:** Inhibition of nociceptive impulses. Neurons originating in the brain stem descend to the spinal cord and release substances such as endogenous opioids, serotonin (5HT), and norepinephrine (NE) that inhibit the transmission of nociceptive impulses.

● ● ● ● ●
F I G U R E 2.2   **A,** Outlines the four basic processes involved in nociception: *1,* transduction; *2,* transmission; *3,* perception; and *4,* modulation. **B,** Illustrates nociception.
Developed by McCaffery M, Pasero C, Paice JA. Reviewed by Kathleen G. Wallace.

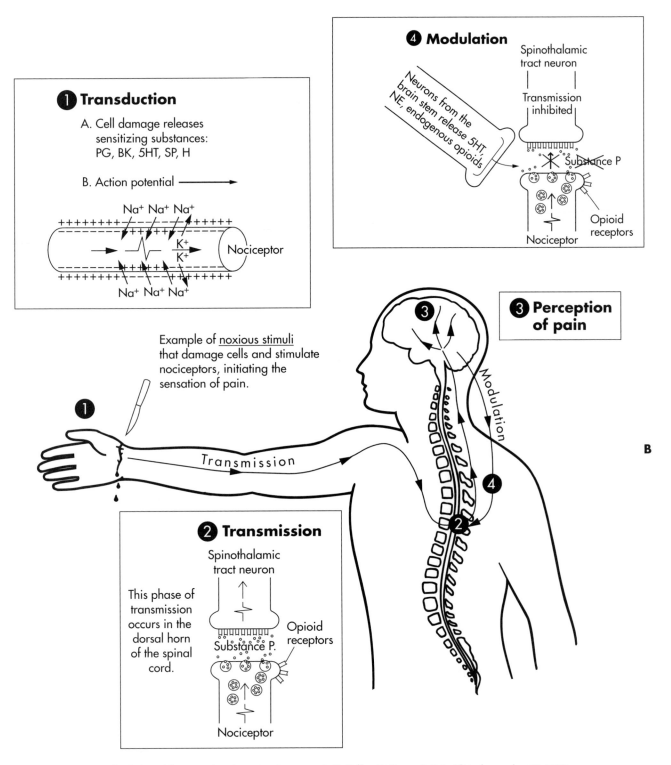

① **Transduction**

A. Cell damage releases sensitizing substances: PG, BK, 5HT, SP, H

B. Action potential ⟶

Na⁺ Na⁺ Na⁺
K⁺
K⁺
Nociceptor
Na⁺ Na⁺ Na⁺

Example of <u>noxious stimuli</u> that damage cells and stimulate nociceptors, initiating the sensation of pain.

Transmission

② **Transmission**

This phase of transmission occurs in the dorsal horn of the spinal cord.

Spinothalamic tract neuron

Opioid receptors

Substance P.

Nociceptor

④ **Modulation**

Spinothalamic tract neuron

Neurons from the brain stem release 5HT, NE, endogenous opioids

Transmission inhibited

Substance P

Opioid receptors

Nociceptor

③ **Perception of pain**

Modulation

B

May be duplicated for use in clinical practice. As appears in McCaffery M, Pasero C: *Pain: Clinical manual,* p. 21, 1999, Mosby, Inc.

● ● ● ● ●
FIGURE 2.2—cont'd **B,** Illustrates the four basic processes involved in nociception; *1,* transduction; *2,* transmission; *3,* perception; and *4,* modulation.
Developed by McCaffery M, Pasero C, Paice JA. Reviewed by Kathleen G. Wallace.

sodium channels and thus slowing the transmission of pain. Local anesthetics, which are also sodium channel blocking agents, are capable of completely stopping the transmission of pain, hence the lack of sensation patients report at the site of local anesthetic infiltration (Catterall, Mackie, 1996; Wallace, 1992) (see Chapters 6 and 7).

Transmission of pain

Transmission, the second process involved in nociception, is easier to understand when considered in three segments. The first segment, occurring after transduction is complete, is the transmission of the impulse along the nociceptor fibers to the level of the spinal cord. The second segment is transmission from the spinal cord to the brain stem and thalamus. The spinothalamic tracts are one example of neurons that ascend from the spinal cord to the thalamus. Other tracts terminate in different areas of the brain. The third segment involves transmission of the impulse through connections between the thalamus and the cortex (Fields, 1987) (see Figure 2.2).

Two types of nociceptor fibers are responsible for the transmission of pain from the site of transduction to the spinal cord, C fibers and A delta (δ) fibers. C fibers are unmyelinated, small-diameter, slow-conducting fibers, transmitting poorly localized, dull, and aching pain. The Aδ fibers are sparsely myelinated, large-diameter, fast-conducting fibers, transmitting well-localized, sharp pain. C fibers are sensitive to mechanical, thermal, and chemical stimuli, whereas Aδ fibers are sensitive primarily to mechanical and thermal stimuli (Fields, 1987; Portenoy, 1996a; Wallace, 1992).

The nociceptors carrying the impulse from the periphery terminate in the dorsal horn of the spinal cord. Because they stop there, neurotransmitters, such as adenosine triphosphate, glutamate, and substance P, are needed to continue the pain impulse across the synaptic cleft between the nociceptors and the dorsal horn neurons. It is at this site that exogenous and endogenous opioids play an important role in pain control by locking onto opioid receptors and blocking the release of neurotransmitters, principally substance P. Diffuse pain, carried by the C fibers, is particularly sensitive to opioids, whereas pain carried by the Aδ fibers is less sensitive (Portenoy, 1996a; Wallace, 1992).

A number of other drugs, which find their site of action at the synaptic cleft, are being investigated and developed for pain control. Included are the *N*-methyl-D-aspartate (NMDA) antagonists. These work by inhibiting the binding by excitatory amino acids, such as glutamate, that normally bind to the NMDA receptors in the dorsal horn facilitating the transmission of the pain impulse beyond the spinal cord level. An example of an NMDA antagonist currently used in pain control is ketamine. Unfortunately, the widespread use of NMDA antagonists has been limited by significant side effects, such

as dissociation and hallucinations (Max, Byas-Smith, Gracely et al., 1995) (see Chapter 7).

From the site of the dorsal horn, pain transmission is accomplished by a number of different ascending fiber tracts within the larger spinothalamic tract. These originate in the spinal cord and terminate in the brain stem and thalamic regions. For the final segment of transmission to take place, the thalamus acts as a relay station, sending the pain impulse to central structures where pain can be processed (Wallace, 1992).

Perception of pain

Perception, the third process in nociception, is the end result of the neural activity of pain transmission (see Figure 2.2). At this point pain is thought to become a conscious experience. The exact location in the brain where pain is perceived is unclear as are the reasons for the individual differences in the subjective experience of pain. A number of central structures are involved. For example, it is believed that the reticular system is responsible for the autonomic response to pain and for warning the individual to attend to it. The somatosensory cortex localizes and characterizes pain. The limbic system is thought to be responsible for the emotional and behavioral response to pain (Fields, 1987).

It is believed that pain perception occurs in the cortical structures. Therefore a number of cognitive-behavioral strategies can be applied to reduce the sensory and affective components of pain. For example, it is believed that the brain can accommodate a limited number of signals. When individuals use techniques such as distraction, relaxation, and imagery to control pain, they direct their attention away from the pain sensation. Theoretically, fewer signals associated with pain can be transmitted to the higher structures, and pain perception is modified (Wallace, 1992).

Modulation of pain

The fourth process involved in nociception is modulation, which refers to changing or inhibiting pain impulses. The pathways involved in modulation are referred to as the descending pain system because they involve neurons originating in the brain stem that descend to the dorsal horn of the spinal cord (Portenoy, 1996a) (see Figure 2.2). These descending fibers release substances, such as endogenous opioids, serotonin (5HT), norepinephrine (NE), γ-aminobutyric acid (GABA), and neurotensin, that have the capability of inhibiting the transmission of noxious stimuli and producing analgesia. Endogenous pain modulation helps to explain the wide variations in perception of pain seen from one person to the next (Basbaum, Fields, 1984; Fields, 1987; Hammond, 1986).

Endogenous opioids, also referred to as enkephalins and endorphins, are found throughout the central nervous system (CNS) and play an important role in basic survival mechanisms. Their discovery more than 20 years ago led to the explanation of pain-modulating systems (Portenoy, 1996a). Like exogenous opioids, endogenous opioids bind to opioid receptor sites and prevent the release of neurotransmitters, such as substance P, inhibiting the transmission of pain impulses. Unfortunately, endogenous opioids degrade too quickly to be considered useful analgesics (Wallace, 1992).

Clinicians apply an understanding of the modulatory systems when they prescribe tricyclic antidepressants, such as amitriptyline and desipramine, for chronic nonmalignant and cancer pain control. Serotonin and norepinephrine, substrates released by the descending fibers of the modulatory system, are normally taken up by the body, limiting their analgesic usefulness. Tricyclic antidepressants interfere with the reuptake of serotonin and norepinephrine, thereby increasing their availability to inhibit noxious stimuli and produce analgesia (Wallace, 1992; Walsh, 1983).

The rationale for administering baclofen for pain control comes from the ongoing research of an inhibitory neurotransmitter released by the body called GABA. GABA is localized in the dorsal horn of the spinal cord and interferes with the transmission of nociceptive impulses. Baclofen is a substrate of GABA receptors and can produce excellent analgesia for many chronic pain conditions, particularly those that are accompanied by spasms (Portenoy, 1996a).

A peptide released by the body called neurotensin is also concentrated in the dorsal horn. Its role in antinociception continues to be studied, but it is known that when administered intrathecally to mice, neurotensin produces an antinociceptive effect (Portenoy, 1996a).

Neuropathic Pain

Neuropathic pain is distinctly different from nociceptive pain (see Figure 2.1). It is pain sustained by abnormal processing of sensory input by the peripheral or central nervous system. A vast number of neuropathic pain syndromes exist, and they are often extremely difficult to treat. The pain reports of individuals who have neuropathic pain may be disproportionate to physical findings. In fact, a physical cause for reports of excruciating pain may not be evident on examination (Portenoy, Kanner, 1996).

Much research has been conducted on the pathophysiology of neuropathic pain, but the exact mechanisms involved remain unclear. It is thought that a chronic neuropathic pain state is initiated when pathophysiologic changes become independent of the inciting event (Portenoy, 1996a). One proposed explanation for some types of neuropathic pain is that the peripheral nervous system has become damaged in some way. An injury to the sensory neurons or axons can result in repetitive spontaneous depolarization and transmission of pain (Coderre, Melzack, 1995).

Another proposed pathologic theory includes a central mechanism. NMDA receptors are being investigated for their role in an important pain-related phenomenon called neuronal "wind-up." Wind-up is the progressive increase in the discharge of dorsal horn neurons (hyperexcitability) as a result of repeated, prolonged noxious stimuli. This spinal cord hyperexcitability and hypersensitivity can lead to chronic neuropathic pain states in which stimuli that are normally innocuous produce pain (allodynia). For example, light stroking of the hand may be felt as extremely painful. Most individuals with neuropathic pain describe a characteristic "burning, tingling, electric, shocklike, or shooting" quality to their pain (Eide, Stubhaug, Stenehjem, 1995; Portenoy, Kanner, 1996). Neuropathic pain usually requires adjuvant analgesics (see Chapter 7).

The types of neuropathic pain often are divided into categories on the basis of the mechanism thought to be primarily responsible for causing the pain (i.e., peripheral or central nervous system activity) (see Figure 2.1). Note that in some cases the original injury occurs in the peripheral nerves (e.g., amputation), but the mechanisms that underlie the pain (e.g., phantom pain) seem to be generated in the CNS.

HARMFUL EFFECTS OF UNRELIEVED PAIN: IMPACT OF AGGRESSIVE PAIN MANAGEMENT

Surgery, trauma, and tumor growth, and the pain associated with them, trigger a number of physiologic stress responses in the human body. These stress responses activate the sympathetic nervous system and alert the body to impending or existing harm. The purposes of the stress responses are protective in nature. These include preventing further damage, minimizing blood loss, maintaining perfusion to vital organs, promoting healing, and preventing and fighting infection. However, pain and stress responses, especially when prolonged, can also produce a number of harmful effects (Table 2.2).

It should be pointed out that providing adequate anesthesia and analgesia for surgical and trauma patients is just part of the picture of reducing the stress response and improving cardiac, pulmonary, gastrointestinal (GI), musculoskeletal, and cognitive function. Benefits gained from aggressive pain management are lost without a vigorous multimodal approach that focuses on enforced early mobilization and nutrition (Kehlet, 1998). Because the harmful effects of unrelieved pain are many and involve multiple systems, they are presented in a system-by-system format.

Endocrine and Metabolic System

The endocrine system works in conjunction with the nervous system to regulate metabolic activities that

● ● ● ● ○

TABLE 2.2   **Harmful Effects of Unrelieved Pain**

Domains affected	Specific responses to pain
Endocrine	↑ Adrenocorticotrophic hormone (ACTH), ↑ cortisol, ↑ antidiuretic hormone (ADH), ↑ epinephrine, ↑ norepinephrine, ↑ growth hormone (GH), ↑ catecholamines, ↑ renin, ↑ angiotensin II, ↑ aldosterone, ↑ glucagon, ↑ interleukin-1; ↓ insulin, ↓ testosterone
Metabolic	Gluconeogenesis, hepatic glycogenolysis, hyperglycemia, glucose intolerance, insulin resistance, muscle protein catabolism, ↑ lipolysis
Cardiovascular	↑ Heart rate, ↑ cardiac output, ↑ peripheral vascular resistance, ↑ systemic vascular resistance, hypertension, ↑ coronary vascular resistance, ↑ myocardial oxygen consumption, hypercoagulation, deep vein thrombosis
Respiratory	↓ Flows and volumes, atelectasis, shunting, hypoxemia, ↓ cough, sputum retention, infection
Genitourinary	↓ Urinary output, urinary retention, fluid overload, hypokalemia
Gastrointestinal	↓ Gastric and bowel motility
Musculoskeletal	Muscle spasm, impaired muscle function, fatigue, immobility
Cognitive	Reduction in cognitive function, mental confusion
Immune	Depression of immune response
Developmental	↑ Behavioral and physiologic responses to pain, altered temperaments, higher somatization, infant distress behavior; possible altered development of the pain system, ↑ vulnerability to stress disorders, addictive behavior, and anxiety states
Future pain	Debilitating chronic pain syndromes: postmastectomy pain, postthoracotomy pain, phantom pain, postherpetic neuralgia
Quality of life	Sleeplessness, anxiety, fear, hopelessness, ↑ thoughts of suicide

May be duplicated for use in clinical practice. From McCaffery M, Pasero C: *Pain: Clinical manual*, p. 24. Copyright © 1999, Mosby, Inc.
Information from Cousins M: Acute postoperative pain. In Wall PD, Melzack R, editors: *Textbook of pain*, ed 3, pp 357-385, New York, 1994, Churchill Livingstone; Kehlet H: Modification of responses to surgery by neural blockade. In Cousins MJ, Bridenbaugh PO, editors: *Neural blockade*, pp 129-175, Philadelphia, 1998, Lippincott-Raven; Mcintyre PE, Ready LB: *Acute pain management: A practical guide*, Philadelphia, 1996, WB Saunders.

maintain normal body growth and system function. For example, the endocrine system releases defined amounts of various hormones that are essential to the process of converting and using carbohydrates, proteins, and fats.

When a person is under stress, the endocrine system releases excessive amounts of hormones, including adrenocorticotrophic hormone (ACTH), cortisol, antidiuretic hormone (ADH), growth hormone (GH), catecholamines, and glucagon. Insulin and testosterone levels decrease. The resulting metabolic responses are numerous, including carbohydrate, protein, and fat catabolism (destruction), hyperglycemia, and poor glucose use (Anand, Hickey, 1987; Cousins, 1994; Page, 1996) (see Table 2.2). Inflammatory processes in combination with these endocrine and metabolic changes can produce weight loss, tachycardia, increased respiratory rate, fever, shock, and death (Anand, Hickey, 1992; Kehlet, 1998; Liu, Carpenter, Neal, 1995).

Unrelieved pain prolongs the stress response and can adversely affect a patient's recovery from trauma or surgery. Because the hormones that are released in response to stress can be detected in the blood and urine, researchers have been able to measure their amounts to determine the impact of the stress response on postoper-

ative morbidity and mortality. In addition, researchers are able to compare the effectiveness of various pain control methods in inhibiting the stress response.

Perioperative use of NSAIDs has been shown to slow the metabolic response to stress and improve protein catabolism (Kehlet, 1998). This provides support for the recommendation that unless contraindicated every postoperative patient should receive an around-the-clock (ATC) NSAID (AHCPR, 1992).

High doses of opioids also have been shown to attenuate the harmful hormonal and metabolic effects of stressors like surgery (Anand, Hickey, 1992). This was demonstrated dramatically in a study of neonates undergoing cardiac surgery. Researchers assigned 30 neonates to receive deep intraoperative anesthesia with high doses of the opioid sufentanil, followed postoperatively with an infusion of opioids for 24 hours. Another 15 neonates were assigned to receive lighter anesthesia with halothane and morphine followed postoperatively by intermittent morphine and diazepam. Hormonal and metabolic responses to surgery were evaluated before, during, and after surgery. The neonates who received light anesthesia plus intermittent postoperative opioids had more severe hyperglycemia and lactic acidemia during surgery and higher lactate and acetoacetate concentrations postoperatively compared with the neonates who received deep anesthesia and postoperative infusion of opioids. In addition, the neonates who received deep anesthesia had a decreased incidence of sepsis, metabolic acidosis, and disseminated intravascular coagulation. This group also experienced no postoperative deaths, whereas four deaths occurred in the 15 given light anesthesia. Although the effects of very high doses of opioids are impressive, only minor or no reduction in harmful neuroendocrine effects have been obtained with customary opioid doses (Kehlet, 1998).

Research has shown that intraspinal opioids alone are less effective than neural blockade with local anesthetics, and single intraspinal dose neural blockade has only a short-lasting inhibitory effect on the stress response. In addition, neural blockade appears to have a greater impact on reducing the stress response associated with lower body surgeries than upper body surgeries (Kehlet, 1998). Although data are limited, neural blockade reduces plasma aldosterone and renin responses during and after hip surgery. It also helps to reduce intraoperative lipolysis and the normal perioperative increase in blood lactate during lower abdominal surgery, such as hysterectomy. Neural blockade of T_{11}-L_1 inhibits the hyperglycemic response to both lower and upper abdominal surgery (Kehlet, 1998).

In a classic study epidural anesthesia and analgesia (EAA) reduced the stress response and resulted in decreased morbidity in high-risk surgical patients (Yeager, Glass, Neff et al., 1987). In this study patients received either epidural anesthesia plus postoperative epidural analgesia (EA) of local anesthetics and/or opioids or standard general anesthesia plus postoperative parenteral opioids on an "as-needed" basis after intraabdominal, intrathoracic, or major vascular surgery. Urinary cortisol excretion, which is elevated during times of stress, was significantly diminished during the first 24 postoperative hours in patients receiving EAA compared with the group receiving general anesthesia and parenteral opioids postoperatively. Those receiving EAA also experienced a reduction in the overall postoperative complication rate, incidence of cardiovascular failure, and major infectious complications.

Muscle protein synthesis decreases by approximately 40% after surgery or trauma. Under carefully controlled conditions of nociceptive block and nutritional intake, researchers studied the protein-sparing effect of epidural local anesthetics, specifically with regard to changes in muscle protein synthetic rate (Carli, Halliday 1997). Patients received either general anesthesia during colon surgery and subcutaneous morphine after (group 1) or epidural bupivacaine anesthesia started preoperatively and maintained during and after colon surgery (group 2). Although the sample size in this study was small ($n = 12$),

the researchers demonstrated that epidural infusion of local anesthetics as described significantly attenuates the decrease in muscle protein synthesis rate associated with surgery. Whereas muscle protein synthesis decreased significantly in group 1, it increased by 25% in group 2.

Cardiovascular System

The cardiovascular system responds to stress by activating the sympathetic nervous system. Activation of the sympathetic nervous system produces a number of effects, including hypercoagulation from decreased fibrinolysis, and increased heart rate, blood pressure, cardiac work load, and oxygen demand in the postoperative period (see Table 2.2). Hypercoagulation has a tremendous impact on patient morbidity and mortality because it is associated with unstable angina, intracoronary thrombosis, and myocardial ischemia and infarction. In fact, cardiac morbidity is the primary cause of death after anesthesia and surgery (Liu, Carpenter, Neal, 1995). Thus aggressive pain control interventions directed toward reducing cardiac workload and hypercoagulation and increasing myocardial oxygen supply and blood flow to the lungs and extremities could reduce thromboembolic complications and cardiac morbidity.

In a study of patients with cardiac disease, IV PCA hydromorphone (Dilaudid) was compared with on-demand IM meperidine (Demerol) for postoperative pain management after coronary artery bypass surgery (Searle, Roy, Bergeron et al., 1994). Although the duration and severity of ischemic attacks were similar in both groups, patients receiving IV PCA had a reduced incidence of myocardial ischemia, as well as lower pain ratings and a lower incidence of severe pain compared with those receiving conventional IM analgesia.

Parenteral analgesia and EAA were compared for their effects on postoperative cardiac morbidity in patients with ischemic cardiac disease undergoing elective surgery (Beattie, Buckley, Forrest, 1993). Compared with patients receiving parenteral analgesia, patients receiving EAA had a fourfold reduction in the relative risk for ischemic episodes and tachydysrythmias during the first 24 hours after surgery. The researchers concluded that epidural morphine reduces the risk of postoperative myocardial ischemia in patients with cardiac risk factors.

Coagulation and outcome after major vascular surgery in patients with atherosclerotic vascular disease were studied (Tuman, McCarthy, March et al., 1991). Patients received either general-epidural anesthesia with postoperative continuous epidural infusion of opioid and local anesthetic or general anesthesia with parenteral and/or oral on-demand opioid analgesia. The researchers found that hypercoagulability was attenuated in the general-EAA group and was associated with a lower incidence of thrombotic events, such as coronary artery and deep vein thrombosis. There was also a ninefold decrease in the incidence of vascular graft occlusion associated with EAA compared with conventional pain control. It has been suggested that these positive effects are not just a result of neural blockade afforded by EAA, but that the local anesthetics themselves may influence coagulation and fibrinolysis (Kehlet, 1998).

Although thoracic EA with opioids and local anesthetics is used most often as a postoperative pain management technique, it is helpful also in the management of some medical conditions. Several studies have demonstrated improved myocardial oxygen delivery with the use of thoracic EA in patients with myocardial ischemia refractory to conventional medical treatment (Liu, Carpenter, Neal, 1995).

Continuous EA has been used successfully to manage pain crises in patients with sickle cell disease, particularly those with pain localized to the trunk and lower extremities. It is thought that the effectiveness of regional technique is the result of improved blood flow to these areas from sympathetic blockade (Viscomi, Rathmell, 1998) (see quick reference guide, sickle cell disease, Chapter 12).

Respiratory System

Surgery and trauma, especially of the thoracic and abdominal regions of the body, can produce significant pain and result in respiratory dysfunction (see Table 2.2). Even when the source of pain is remote from the thoracic and abdominal region, respiratory dysfunction can occur (de Leon-Casasola, Lema, 1992). Involuntary responses to noxious stimuli cause reflex muscle spasm at the site of tissue damage and in muscle groups above and below the site. Patients with pain also voluntarily limit their thoracic and abdominal muscle movement ("splinting") and become immobile in an effort to reduce the pain they are experiencing (Cousins, 1994).

The measurable respiratory effects of severe pain are small tidal volumes and high inspiratory and expiratory pressures, as well as decreases in vital capacity, functional residual capacity, and alveolar ventilation. If adequate pain relief is not provided postoperatively, these effects can progress to significant pulmonary complications, such as atelectasis and pneumonia (Cousins, 1994). In addition, postoperative hypoxemia from decreased oxygen saturation can result in cardiac and wound complications and postoperative mental dysfunction (Rosenberg, Kehlet, 1993).

Numerous studies have been conducted comparing the effects of various pain management techniques on pulmonary function and the incidence of pulmonary complications. Consider the differences found between opioids administered by traditional "as-needed" IM injection and IV PCA. Better pulmonary function with higher forced vital capacity and peak expiratory flow was found in patients receiving morphine by IV PCA compared with morphine by IM injection after gastric bypass

(Bennett, Batenhorst, Foster et al., 1982). IM opioid administration was compared with IV PCA opioid administration in frail elderly men after major elective surgery (Egbert, Parks, Short et al., 1990). None of the patients receiving IV PCA opioids experienced any pulmonary complications, whereas 10% of the patients receiving IM opioids experienced severe pulmonary complications.

Nurses often report that their patients demonstrate improved mobility; are better able to perform pulmonary cleansing activities, such as coughing and deep breathing; and are more comfortable during painful procedures, such as physiotherapy, when IV PCA is used rather than IM opioids (Aitken, Kenny, 1990; Jackson, 1989). All these activities are extremely important in preventing pulmonary complications.

Patients themselves confirm these nursing observations. They cite numerous advantages of IV PCA over IM opioid administration, including less sedation, improved pain control and ability to ambulate and deep breathe, and overall greater satisfaction (Kenady, Wilson, Schwartz et al., 1992).

Glucocorticoids provide analgesia and also may alter some of the stress responses after surgery. At high doses they also appear to improve postoperative pulmonary function (Kehlet, 1998).

Support is strong for the use of aggressive pain control measures, such as EA, in patients with upper abdominal and thoracic incisions, thoracic trauma, preexisting pulmonary disease, advanced age, obesity, and those in severe pain. With the use of EA, these patients can experience improved diaphragmatic function, reduced frequency and severity of postoperative hypoxemia, and reduced pulmonary morbidity from better pain control than is possible with traditional pain management techniques (Liu, Carpenter, Neal, 1995). Neural blockade with local anesthetics or local anesthetics combined with opioids are more effective than opioids alone, and continuous infusion is more effective than single-dose blockade (Kehlet, 1998).

The effects of a variety of methods for delivering analgesics were studied in elderly patients after thoracic trauma (Wisner, 1990) Patients received either epidural, IV, IM, or oral opioids, or intercostal blocks with a long-lasting anesthetic agent. The use of EA was found to be an independent predictor of both decreased mortality and a decreased incidence of pulmonary complications in the patient sample. It was concluded that the increased costs associated with EA are minimal and justified by the improvements in outcome in this population of patients.

In another study of patients with multiple rib fractures, epidural fentanyl was shown to produce superior pain relief and improved ventilatory function compared with IV fentanyl (Mackersie, Karagianes, Hoyt et al., 1991). These findings led the researchers to recommend continuous epidural opioids as the preferred analgesic method for all patients at high risk of pulmonary complications developing after rib fractures.

Compared with other pain management methods, EA has been shown to decrease the time of intubation, time in the intensive care unit, and number of cardiac and pulmonary complications in patients after aortic aneurysmectomy (Major, Greer, Russell et al., 1995). This can lead to significant reductions in the cost of care associated with this expensive surgical procedure.

Obese surgical patients are at high risk for both pulmonary and cardiovascular complications postoperatively. In one study more obese patients receiving epidural morphine were able to sit, stand, or walk, and tolerate more vigorous physiotherapy postoperatively compared with obese patients receiving IM morphine (Rawal, Sjostrand, Christoffersson et al., 1984). This resulted in fewer pulmonary complications in this group of patients. Earlier postoperative recovery of peak expiratory flow and bowel function contributed to the significantly shorter hospital stay seen in the patients receiving EA.

The relationship between thermoregulation and oxygen consumption must be considered. Prevention of heat loss during anesthesia and postoperative recovery will help to maintain benefits gained in reducing the stress response with the use of aggressive pain control. In addition, clinicians should take advantage of excellent pain control and the opportunity to reduce pulmonary complications by enforcing vigorous use of incentive spirometers and early mobilization in their patients (Kehlet, 1998).

Genitourinary System

Hormones important in regulating urinary output, fluid and electrolyte balance, and in maintaining blood volume and pressure include catecholamines, aldosterone, ADH, cortisol, angiotensin II, and prostaglandins. As previously discussed, unrelieved pain can cause the excessive release of these hormones. This can result in retention of water and sodium ions, increased excretion of potassium ions, and decreased functional extracellular fluid with shifts of fluid to intracellular compartments (Mcintyre, Ready, 1996). Harmful effects include decreased urinary output, urinary retention, hypokalemia, fluid overload, increased cardiac work load, and hypertension (see Table 2.2). Further research is needed to better understand the impact of aggressive pain management on the genitourinary system (Kehlet, 1998).

Gastrointestinal System

The stress response causes an increase in sympathetic nervous system activity. When this occurs, intestinal secretions and smooth muscle sphincter tone increase and gastric emptying and intestinal motility decrease. This can result in temporary impairment of GI function (primarily the stomach and colon) and ileus (GI paralysis) (Cousins, 1994; Liu, Carpenter, Neal, 1995). Ileus usually

is discussed as a postoperative complication, but it can occur in any situation that causes an increase in sympathetic activity, such as when patients experience unrelieved pain (see Table 2.2).

Whereas opioids may cause delayed gastric emptying and contribute to the problem of impaired GI function and ileus (Cousins, 1994; Liu, Carpenter, Neal, 1995), NSAIDs and many adjuvant drugs can be administered for pain relief without fear of slowing the GI tract. When opioids are indicated, such as for moderate to severe pain, an NSAID or local anesthetic can be added to the pain management plan. NSAIDs and local anesthetics work synergistically with opioids, producing an opioid-sparing effect. It is then possible to decrease the opioid dose, and therefore the unwanted opioid effects, without jeopardizing patient comfort (see Chapters 5, 6, and 7 for more). Although research is needed, normalization of GI function after colon surgery has been observed with enforced oral nutrition during low-dose epidural opioid and local anesthetic infusion (Kehlet, 1998).

In addition to their opioid-sparing capabilities, local anesthetics, by a variety of routes, are associated with increased GI blood flow and motility. In fact, use of local anesthetics is suggested to shorten the duration of ileus (Morimoto, Cullen, Messick et al., 1995; Rimback, Cassuto, Faxen et al., 1986; Rimback, Cassuto, Tollesson et al., 1990).

Several explanations have been proposed for the positive effect local anesthetics have on GI function. Researchers suggest that, when instilled intraabdominally, bupivacaine inhibits the inflammatory response within the bowel wall, a response that can slow GI function (Rimback, Cassuto, Faxen et al., 1986). When given IV, the positive systemic effects include excitation of smooth muscle and suppression of the reflexes that inhibit GI function (Liu, Carpenter, Neal, 1995; Rimback, Cassuto, Tollesson, 1990). It is believed that, when given epidurally, local anesthetics exert a positive effect by inducing a sympathetic blockade, which is associated with increased GI blood flow (Kehlet, 1998; Liu, Carpenter, Neal, 1995). Continuous epidural local anesthetics appear to be more effective than single-dose epidural local anesthetics (Kehlet, 1998).

A number of researchers have studied the effect of EA, with and without local anesthetics, on GI function. A retrospective study was conducted to determine whether EA would speed recovery from postoperative ileus after proctocolectomy with ileal pouch-anal canal anastomosis (Morimoto, Cullen, Messick et al., 1995). Patients receiving epidural fentanyl supplemented with IV morphine were compared with those receiving only systemic morphine after this procedure. Researchers found that the use of EA resulted in less need for nasogastric suction and IV fluids, more rapid discharge of fecal content, more rapid return to oral intake, and shorter hospitalization. While studying postoperative pulmonary complications, Jayr and others (1993) demonstrated an earlier recovery of intestinal function in patients receiving epidural opioids and local anesthetic compared with those receiving parenteral opioids.

One group of researchers looked at the effects of perioperative analgesic technique and drugs on the rate of recovery in patients after colon surgery (Liu, Carpenter, Mackey et al., 1995). All patients were given general anesthesia and randomized into one of four different perioperative analgesic groups. They were given a preoperative epidural bolus of morphine and bupivacaine followed by an epidural infusion of morphine and bupivacaine (group 1), or a preoperative epidural bolus of morphine followed by an epidural infusion of morphine (group 2), or a preoperative epidural bolus of bupivacaine followed by an epidural infusion of bupivacaine (group 3), or a preoperative IV bolus of morphine followed by IV PCA morphine (group 4). Groups 1 and 3 (the bupivacaine groups) reported lower pain scores with cough and ambulation and recovered from postoperative ileus an average of 34 hours earlier than groups 2 and 4. As a result, the patients who received epidural bupivacaine were ready for discharge an average of 35 hours earlier than the patients who did not.

Time to ileus resolution may be influenced also by vertebral level of epidural catheter placement for EA. Patients in one study received either IV PCA opioid analgesia, lumbar EA, or thoracic EA after proctocolectomy (Scott, Starling, Ruscher et al., 1996). The epidural infusions were of opioids alone or in combination with local anesthetics. Pain rating scores were highest in the IV PCA group. Ileus resolution was comparable in patients receiving IV PCA analgesia or lumbar EA but was significantly faster in the thoracic EA group.

Liu, Carpenter, and Neal (1995) point out that factors other than pain and sympathetic activity contribute to ileus and that further research is needed to determine the best approach to ileus resolution. However, they recommend that when EA with local anesthetics is used, it should be continued for 48 to 72 hours after surgery when postoperative ileus is typically resolved.

Musculoskeletal System

Pain can cause muscle spasm, impaired muscle function, fatigue, and immobility (see Table 2.2). Poorly controlled pain can significantly influence a patient's short-and long-term recovery after orthopedic surgical procedures, primarily because it interferes with the patient's ability to perform physical therapy exercises. Good pain control with ATC scheduling of analgesic doses and supplemental doses for breakthrough pain and before and during times of expected discomfort can improve the patient's performance of the activities necessary for a smooth recovery.

Length of hospital stay usually is a reflection of patient outcome; patients with satisfactory outcomes usually will have a shorter length of hospital stay than those who do not. Regional anesthesia and analgesia techniques provide excellent postoperative analgesia and a window of opportunity to improve patient outcome. To appreciate the advantages of optimal pain control (e.g., better musculoskeletal function), clinicians must begin to enforce vigorous postoperative recovery programs that include early and increased mobilization. This is particularly important for patients at high risk for muscle loss and fatigue, such as the elderly. Such programs will require medical and nursing practice changes and the elimination of institutional barriers that foster a bedrest rather than an activity-oriented approach to delivering care (Kehlet, 1998) (see Chapter 16).

A significantly shorter hospitalization, as well as greater joint motion, was found in patients receiving EA compared with patients receiving parenteral analgesia after total knee arthroscopy (Mahoney, Noble, Davidson et al., 1990). In another study compared with IV PCA, EA significantly improved rehabilitation parameters, such as range of motion, ease of mobility, and independence in patients after total knee replacement (Pati, Perme, Trail et al., 1994).

A growing number of orthopedic procedures are being done on an outpatient basis today. Pain control is an important consideration in determining whether a patient is ready for discharge after outpatient surgery. In a double-blind study, the effect of intraarticular analgesia on pain relief after knee arthroscopy was evaluated (Joshi, McCarroll, O'Brien et al., 1993). Patients received intraarticular injections of morphine (group 1), or plain bupivacaine (group 2), or morphine plus bupivacaine (group 3), or a saline placebo (group 4). All patients could receive supplemental analgesia (opioid or NSAID) postoperatively on request. As one would expect, patients in group 4 had the highest pain scores and supplemental analgesic requirements. Patients in groups 1 and 3 had the lowest pain scores and supplemental analgesic requirements. The authors concluded that intraarticular morphine significantly reduces pain after knee arthroscopy, however, they found no advantage to adding bupivacaine by this route.

Cognitive Function

Transient reduction in cognitive function after surgery is common, especially in elderly patients. The reduction typically occurs on the second postoperative day usually with full recovery of cognitive function within 1 week (Liu, Carpenter, Neal, 1995). The administration of opioids often is implicated as the cause of cognitive impairment. When confusion is detected, especially in the elderly, opioids are likely to be abruptly discontinued. However, there is little to support the assertion that opioids directly cause cognitive impairment. In fact, pain (Duggleby, Lander, 1994; Lorenz, Beck, Bromm, 1997) and other factors (such as sleep disturbance, type of surgery, choice of opioid, and method of administering opioids) have been directly linked to cognitive impairment (see Table 2.2).

Duggleby and Lander (1994) studied the influences of postoperative pain and analgesics on mental status and the relationships among age, mental status, and pain in patients aged 50 to 80 years. Mental status declined after surgery for more than one third of the patients in this study. Pain was poorly managed in these patients. The researchers found that pain, not analgesic intake, predicted mental decline. Another interesting finding is that no correlation was found between age and pain, indicating that age is not a factor in pain perception. This study suggests that one reason for acute confusion in older patients after surgery is unrelieved pain and that improving pain management practices is one way to reduce confusion in these patients after surgery.

The effects of sustained-release morphine on pain, mood, and basic components of cognitive function at the beginning of long-term opioid treatment in patients with chronic nonmalignant pain were studied (Lorenz, Beck, Bromm, 1997). Findings included that even with sedation, the dosage of opioid required for subjective pain relief did not induce any signs of cognitive decline. Researchers suggested that pain relief may temper the sedative side effects of morphine and even lead to improved cognitive performance.

Sleeplessness after surgery may contribute to altered mental status (Duggleby, Lander, 1994; Rosenberg, Rosenberg-Adamsen, Kehlet, 1995). A number of factors contribute to sleeplessness, but patients cite incisional pain most often as the cause (Simpson, Lee, Cameron, 1996). Other causes include inability to get comfortable in the hospital bed, hypoxemia, and inability to perform usual routine activities before sleep. Several researchers have suggested changes be made in the patient's environment and nursing care routines that disturb sleep patterns (Rosenberg, Rosenberg-Adamsen, Kehlet, 1995; Simpson, Lee, Cameron, 1996). Changes may include providing better pain control with scheduled doses of analgesics, reducing environmental lighting and noise, encouraging patients to perform their usual routines before sleep, and coordinating nursing care activities to accommodate patients' sleep time as much as possible.

Theoretically, the use of epidural anesthesia, rather than general anesthesia, would benefit cognitive function because it would reduce the direct toxic effect of general anesthetics on the cerebral cortex (Kehlet, 1998). Unfortunately, it is quite common for practitioners to deny epidural anesthesia and/or analgesia to patients who might benefit the most. For example, for some types of surgery, the epidural route may actually be preferable to others for the elderly, cognitively impaired, or confused patients. Liu, Carpenter, and Neal (1995) point out that, ". . . previous studies have demonstrated less sedation in patients receiving epidural analgesia (local anesthetic or opioid) than those receiving parenteral opioid . . . these data suggest potential for reduction in postoperative cognitive dysfunction from use of epidural analgesia" (p. 1492).

Immune System

As part of the immune system, natural killer (NK) cells play a role in preventing tumor growth and controlling metastasis (Page, Ben-Eliyahu, 1997; Page, Ben-Eliyahu, Yirmiya et al., 1993). Stress and pain can suppress immune functions, including NK cell cytotoxicity (see Table 2.2). Immunosuppression also can predispose patients to postoperative infections, including pneumonia, wound infections, and sepsis (Liu, Carpenter, Neal, 1995; Page, Ben-Eliyahu, 1997). Local anesthetics and analgesic doses of opioids have been shown to block the immunosuppressive effects of pain and stress (Liebeskind 1991; Page, Ben-Eliyahu, Yirmiya et al., 1993).

Although the mechanism is not fully understood, neural blockade may reduce surgically induced impairment of various aspects of immunocompetence. For example, various types of neural blockade have been shown to improve monocyte function and leukocyte and neutrophil microbicidal activity in the perioperative period (Kehlet, 1998). Continuous EA has been shown to normalize lymphocytes and improve NK cell activity, as well as reduce cortisol and catecholamine responses after hysterectomy (Tonnesen, Wahlgreen, 1988). EAA provides better pain relief than parenteral and oral analgesics and is associated with a decreased incidence of postoperative infectious complications (Liu, Carpenter, Neal, 1995; Yeager, Glass, Neff et al., 1987).

A series of studies on rats were performed to explore the impact of morphine on surgery-induced tumor metastasis (Page, Ben-Eliyahu, Yirmiya et al., 1993). All the rats were subjected to abdominal surgery. Compared with rats that received no postoperative analgesia, rats that received morphine for 8 to 10 hours showed significantly fewer metastases 21 days after surgery. The researchers of this study concluded that if a similar relationship between pain and metastasis occurs in humans, pain control must be a vital component of postoperative care.

Because high doses of opioids can also be immunosuppressive, some researchers question the wisdom of using large doses of opioids to control some cancer pain (Shavit, Benzion, 1996). However, tolerance to immunosuppressive and tumor-enhancing effects of morphine develops rapidly, but no such tolerance develops to repeated exposure to unrelieved pain (Page, Ben-Eliyahu, Yirmiya et al., 1996). This led one expert to state,

". . . it is not only safe to use analgesic drugs for controlling cancer pain in man, it may be unsafe not to." (Liebeskind, 1991, p. 3).

Developmental Effects

Although pain itself cannot be remembered, the experiences associated with pain can be recalled (Anand, Hickey, 1987). Strong evidence suggests that neonates' memories of painful experiences persist long enough to influence later behavior (see Table 2.2 and Chapter 14). Preterm neonates exposed to repetitive pain show altered temperaments at 3 years of age and higher somatization scores at $4\frac{1}{2}$ years of age (Grunau, Whitfield, Petrie et al., 1994). Increased physiologic responses to neonatal heelsticks have been linked to infant distress behavior at 6 months of age (Gunnar, Porter, Wolf et al., 1995).

In a 1995 study of 42 healthy boys aged 4 to 6 months, the responses of circumcised and uncircumcised infants to routine diphtheria-pertussis-tetanus vaccination were compared (Taddio, Goldbach, Ipp et al., 1995). During and after vaccination, the boys who had been circumcised (none received anesthesia or analgesia) had higher pain scores and cried longer than those who had not. In a later study these findings were replicated and also showed that babies who had received topical anesthesia during circumcision subsequently had a milder pain response to vaccination than those who were circumcised without anesthesia (Taddio, Stevens, Craig et al., 1997).

In animal studies, repetitive neonatal pain showed a decreased pain threshold during development and a greater preference for alcohol in adulthood (Anand, 1996). Long-term effects lead to altered development of the pain system, increased vulnerability to stress disorders, addictive behavior, and anxiety states in rats. Similar abnormal behavior has been observed in studies of humans.

More than 500 children aged 4 months to 13 years were evaluated for incidence of behavioral changes during the 4 weeks after the day of surgery (Kotiniemi, Ryhanen, Moilanen, 1997). Severe pain on the day of surgery and mild pain at home were predictors of problematic behavioral changes in these children. Although problematic changes declined with time, pain on the day of operation predicted the occurrence of behavioral problems up to the fourth week after surgery, 2 to 4 weeks longer than the duration of the pain itself.

Future Pain

Poorly controlled acute pain can predispose patients to debilitating chronic pain syndromes (Bach, Noreng, Tjellden 1988; Tasmuth, Estlanderb, Kalso, 1996) (see Table 2.2). For example, some chronic pain syndromes have been linked directly to specific surgical procedures and often can be prevented with early physical rehabilitation and/or aggressive pain management. These include postmastectomy pain, postthoracotomy pain, and phantom pain. The predominant underlying mechanism of postsurgical chronic pain syndromes is neuropathic. Pain results from musculoskeletal changes and injury to peripheral nerves (Cherny, Portenoy, 1994; Foley, 1996).

The severity of postoperative pain may influence the development of postsurgical chronic pain syndromes. In 1996 researchers conducted a retrospective study of 93 women whose breast cancer was treated with modified radical mastectomy or breast resection (Tasmuth, Estlanderb, Kalso, 1996). One of the purposes of the study was to explore the relationship between a patient's memory of the intensity of acute postoperative pain and the development of chronic pain. Compared with women who did not develop chronic pain after surgery, those who developed chronic pain remembered their postoperative pain as more severe. This led the researchers to conclude that the amount of postoperative pain a person experiences may play a role in the development of chronic pain.

In a study of patients with long-term thoracotomy pain, early postoperative pain was the only factor that significantly predicted long-term pain (Katz, Jackson, Kavanaugh et al., 1996). Pain intensity 24 hours after thoracotomy, at rest, and after movement was significantly greater among patients who had long-term postthoracotomy pain compared with pain-free patients.

Failure to effectively control postsurgical chronic pain syndromes also can result in the development of other chronic pain syndromes. For example, poorly controlled postmastectomy and postthoracotomy pain can cause patients to flex the arm on the affected side and hold it close to the chest in an attempt to minimize the pain. This can lead to frozen shoulder and secondary reflex sympathetic dystrophy (RSD). (Refer to Chapter 12 for more on RSD.) Effective postoperative pain control and active mobilization of the joint soon after surgery can help prevent the development of frozen shoulder (Cherny, Portenoy, 1994; Foley 1996).

Phantom pain can occur after removal of a wide variety of body parts and is fairly common in patients after limb amputation, mastectomy, and abdominoperineal resection (phantom anal pain) (Bach, Noreng, Tjellden 1988; Cherny, Portenoy, 1994; Jensen, Rasmussen, 1994). Phantom pain can be severe and is described by some as continuous burning, cramping, throbbing, or crushing; others describe it as intermittent sharp or shooting pain (Portenoy, 1996b).

The incidence of phantom limb pain is significantly greater in patients who have had long-term pain before amputation and in patients who have pain on the day before the amputation (Cherny, Portenoy, 1994; Foley 1996; Jensen, Rasmussen, 1994; Nikolajsen, Ilkjaer, Kroner et al., 1997; Portenoy, 1996b). In a landmark study researchers showed that postoperative phantom limb pain can be reduced with preemptive analgesia (Bach, Noreng, Tjellden, 1988). (See Chapters 4 and 6 for more on preemptive analgesia.) The aim of their study was to reduce postoperative phantom limb pain by keeping their sample patients pain free for 72 hours before the amputation. They administered lumbar epidural blockade with morphine and bupivacaine to the study group of patients ($n = 11$), and the patients were pain free for 3 days before surgery. The control group ($n = 14$) was treated with various analgesics but none were pain free. The researchers found that 7 days after amputation, 27% of those who received blockade and 64% in the control group had phantom limb pain. After 6 months and 1 year, all patients in the blockade group were pain free, whereas in the control group, 36% and 21%, respectively, had phantom limb pain.

A relationship may also exist between the development of chronic pain and poorly controlled acute nonsurgical pain. One example is the development of postherpetic neuralgia (PHN) after acute herpes zoster (shingles). Herpes zoster represents reactivation of a latent virus originally acquired during acute varicella infection (chickenpox). It produces diffuse inflammation of peripheral nerves and is characterized by an erythematous rash, usually in the thoracic, lumbar, cervical, and ophthalmic regions (Portenoy, 1996b). Pain precedes the eruption of the rash and is the most common symptom of herpes zoster (Kost, Straus, 1996).

The pain of herpes zoster usually resolves spontaneously with time (Kost, Straus, 1996). However, approximately 10% of those who have acute herpes zoster develop PHN, which is characterized by persistent severe pain. The pain is described as burning dysesthesia (altered, painful sensitivity to touch), deep aching, itching, stabbing, and paroxysmal (Portenoy, 1996b).

A number of treatments have been proposed but not proven to prevent the development of PHN. Examples include a varicella vaccine and administration of antiviral drugs during the acute phase of herpes zoster (Kost, Straus 1996; Portenoy, 1996). Although research is lacking, some clinicians have strongly suggested that failure to relieve the pain associated with acute herpes zoster is likely to be a major element in the development of PHN (Elliott, 1996). Thus a critical factor in preventing PHN is aggressive treatment of herpes zoster with corticosteroids, NSAIDs, opioids, topical anesthetics, and nerve blocks (Portenoy, 1996b) (see quick guide on PHN, Chapter 12).

Survivors of serious and common illnesses, such as chronic obstructive pulmonary disorder (COPD), liver failure, and cancer, were studied to determine variables identified with later pain (Desbiens, Wu, Alzola et al., 1997). Level of pain during hospitalization was strongly associated with later pain. Researchers in this study concluded that better pain control during hospitalization and after discharge should be given a high priority and that pain during hospitalization should trigger future inquires about pain and its treatment.

Quality of Life

The impact of unrelieved cancer pain and CNP on quality of life (QOL) is significant. Effects range from decreased physical activity to thoughts of suicide (see Table 2.2).

In 1991 the National Chronic Pain Outreach Association (NCPOA) conducted a mailed survey to 500 of its members; 41% of whom responded (Hitchcock, Ferrell, McCaffery, 1994). The survey explored how subjects perceived the effect of their pain on various aspects of their QOL and their experiences with and perceptions of approaches to pain management, including the use of analgesics. Subjects' ages ranged from 19 to 90 years, and most were women. On average they had pain for 9.5 years. Most of the sample reported experiencing pain approximately 80% of the time, and 75% reported their usual pain intensity in the moderate to severe range.

Although 57% of the subjects with CNP rated their QOL as fair to good, they indicated by their responses to many other questions that this was a hard-won victory that was very likely in jeopardy. Several described their extreme distress when they encountered caregivers who did not believe their reports of pain, and many reported that their physicians had refused to prescribe more effective medication. At the same time 88% said it was important to them to keep others from noticing their pain. The fact that they tried hard not to "look like" they were in pain may have succeeded all too well (Hitchcock, Ferrell, McCaffery, 1994).

This group was somewhat unusual in that they had considerable financial and educational resources. For example, 91% had some college education, and the average annual household income was $43,000. Their responses indicated that they used active coping mechanisms, such as belonging to a self-help organization and using nondrug measures. Most alarming is the finding that in spite of their resources and active coping skills, 50% had felt hopeless enough about their pain to consider suicide. This certainly adds to the growing evidence that CNP is not only not "benign," but, on the contrary, can be life-threatening (Hitchcock, Ferrell, McCaffery, 1994).

Studies of patients with cancer pain have revealed that they have similar thoughts of suicide. In a survey study 69% of cancer patients reported that they would consider committing suicide if their pain was not treated adequately (Cleeland, 1989). Unfortunately, many patients with CNP or cancer pain do experience undertreated pain as a result of persistent misconceptions, such as exaggerated fears of addiction and respiratory depression.

Researchers found that for 50% of conscious patients who died in the hospital, family members reported moderate to severe pain at least half of the time (SUPPORT Principal Investigators, 1995). One reason for this may be failure to appreciate the development of tolerance to respiratory depression. Respiratory depression is rare in patients who have been receiving chronic opioid treatment (APS, 1992). Yet clinicians continue to worry about administering opioids to dying patients for fear that this will "hasten death." Consequently, these patients often receive less than therapeutic doses of opioid and, in many cases, no opioids at all (see Chapter 6).

Justification and reassurance are sufficient for the liberal use of opioids in dying patients (Brody, Campbell, Faber-Langendoen et al., 1997). Wilson and others (1992) studied terminally ill patients on ventilators who had not yet been declared brain dead. When life support was withdrawn, the median time until death for those receiving opioids and sedatives was 3.5 hours compared with 1.5 hours for those who received none. These findings suggest that the underlying disease process, not the opioid, usually determines the time of death (Brody, Campbell, Faber-Langendoen et al., 1997) (refer to Chapter 6).

Many patients who have cancer pain and are terminally ill live for months before death is imminent. During those months their QOL often is diminished by unrelieved pain. Many researchers have studied the impact of pain on the QOL of patients with cancer pain and caregivers of these patients. In one study of 41 patients with chronic cancer pain, pain was mentioned often in connection with a poor QOL (Padilla, Ferrell, Grant et al., 1990). Patients reveal that cancer pain means many losses, including the loss of control, autonomy, sexual activity, ability to work, and usefulness. One patient said it very simply, "The pain means I can't do the things I used to do." (Ferrell, Taylor, Satler et al., 1993).

A study of 80 women with pain related to breast cancer revealed similar findings (Arathuzik, 1991). Each of the following effects of pain on QOL were mentioned by more than half the women: fatigue; feelings of helplessness; disturbance of body functions; and interference with work, daily activities, and sleep.

The greatest area of burden for caregivers of patients with cancer was found to be concern about pain management. Caregivers expressed feelings of helplessness, frustration, and "heartbreak" (Ferrell, Grant, Chan, 1995). In another study that explored caregivers' perceptions of their roles in relation to pain medications, caregivers identified several areas of responsibility (Ferrell, Cohen, Rhiner et al., 1991). These included deciding what to give for pain relief, when to give it, and "night duty" that involved being awakened frequently. Many caregivers expressed fears of addiction and believed they were responsible for avoiding addic-

tion in their patients by limiting the amount of medication used.

Of all the adverse effects of unrelieved pain it may well be that decreased QOL in patients with chronic pain represents the greatest harm of all. It is also the most unforgivable. Chronic pain often is so easily treated, but, if not treated, it is completely dehumanizing to the patient and the family.

References

Acute Pain Management Guideline Panel: *Acute pain management: operative or medical procedures and trauma. Clinical practice guideline,* AHCPR Pub. No. 92-0032, Rockville, Md, Agency for Health Care Policy and Research, Public Health Service, U.S. Department of Health and Human Services, Feb 1992.

Aitken HA, Kenny GNC: Use of patient controlled analgesia in postoperative cardiac surgical patients: a survey of ward staff attitudes, *Intensive Care Nurs* 6:74-78, 1990.

American Pain Society (APS): *Principles of analgesic use in the treatment of acute and cancer pain,* ed 3, Glenview, Ill, 1992, APS.

Anand KJS: Long-term effects of pain in neonates and infants, Special Lecture Abstract 110, *Abstracts 8th World Congress on Pain,* Seattle, August 1996, International Association for the Study of Pain (IASP) Press.

Anand KJS, Hickey PR: Pain and its effects in the human neonate and fetus, *N Engl J Med* 317(21):1321-1329, 1987.

Anand KJS, Hickey PR: Halothane-morphine compared with high-dose sufentanil for anesthesia and postoperative analgesia in neonatal cardiac surgery, *N Engl J Med* 326(1):1-9, 1992.

Arathuzik D: Pain experience for metastatic breast cancer patients, *Cancer* 14(1):41-48, 1991.

Bach S, Noreng MF, Tjellden NU: Phantom limb pain in amputees during the first 12 months following limb amputation, after postoperative lumbar epidural blockade, *Pain* 33:297-301, 1988.

Basbaum AI, Fields HL: Endogenous pain control systems: brainstem spinal pathways and endorphin circuitry, *Ann Rev Neurosci* 7:309-338, 1984.

Beattie WS, Buckley DN, Forrest JB: Epidural morphine reduces the risk of postoperative myocardial ischaemia in patients with cardiac risk factors, *Can J Anaesth* 40(6):532-541, 1993.

Bennett R, Batenhorst RL, Foster TS et al.: Postoperative pulmonary function with patient-controlled analgesia, *Anesth Analg* 61(2):171, 1982 (abstract).

Brody H, Campbell ML, Faber-Langendoen K et al.: Withdrawing intensive life-sustaining treatment: recommendations for compassionate clinical management, *JAMA* 336(9):652-657, 1997 (sounding board).

Carli F, Halliday D: Continuous blockade arrests postoperative decrease in muscle protein fractional synthetic rate in surgical patients, *Anesthesiology* 86:1033-1040, 1997.

Catterall W, Mackie K: Local anesthetics. In Hardman JG, Limbird LE, editors: *Goodman and Gilman's the pharmacological basis of therapeutics,* ed 9, pp 331-347, New York, 1996, McGraw-Hill.

Cherny NI, Portenoy RK: Practical issues in the management of cancer pain. In Wall PD, Melzack R, editors: *Textbook of pain,* ed 3, pp 1437-1467, Edinburgh, 1994, Churchill Livingstone.

Cleeland CS: Pain control: public and physician attitudes. In Hill CS, Fields WS, editors: *Advances in pain research and therapy,* Vol 11, pp 81-89, New York, 1989, Raven Press.

Coderre TJ, Melzack R: The contribution of excitatory amino acids to central sensitization and persistent nociception after formalin-induced tissue injury, *J Neurosci* 12:3665, 1995.

Cousins M: Acute postoperative pain. In Wall PD, Melzack R, editors: *Textbook of pain,* ed 3, pp 357-385, New York, 1994, Churchill Livingstone.

de Leon-Casasola OA, Lema MJ: Spinal opioid analgesia: influence on clinical outcome. In Sinatra RS, Hord AH, Ginsberg B et al, editors: *Acute pain. Mechanisms and management,* pp 293-303, St. Louis, 1992, Mosby.

Desbiens NA, Wu AW, Alzola C et al.: Pain during hospitalization is associated with continued pain six months later in survivors of serious illness, *Am J Med* 103:269-276, 1997.

Duggleby W, Lander J: Cognitive status and postoperative pain: older adults, *J Pain Symptom Manage* 9(1):19-27, 1994.

Egbert AM, Parks LH, Short LM et al.: Randomized trial of postoperative patient-controlled analgesia vs intramuscular narcotics in frail elderly men, *Arch Intern Med* 150:1897-1903, September 1990.

Eide PK, Stubhaug A, Stenehjem AE: Central dyesthesia pain after traumatic spinal cord injury is dependent on n-methyl-d-aspartate receptor activation, *Neurosurgery* 37:1080, 1995.

Elliott KJ (presenter): *Herpes zoster and postherpetic neuralgia: new pharmacological approaches to treatment and prevention,* American Pain Society 15th Annual Scientific Meeting, Washington DC, November 14-17, 1996.

Ferrell BR, Cohen MA, Rhiner M et al.: Pain as a metaphor for illness Part II: family caregivers' management of pain, *Oncol Nurs Forum* 18(8):1315-1321, 1991.

Ferrell BR, Taylor EJ, Satler GR et al.: Searching for the meaning of pain, *Cancer Pract* 1(3):185-194, 1993.

Ferrell BR, Grant M, Chan J et al.: The impact of cancer pain education on family caregivers of elderly patients, *Oncol Nurs Forum* 22(8): 1211-1218, 1995.

Fields HL: *Pain,* pp 364, New York, 1987, McGraw-Hill.

Foley KM: Pain syndromes in patients with cancer. In Portenoy RK, Kanner RM, editors: *Pain management: theory and practice,* pp 191-215, Philadelphia, 1996, FA Davis.

Gunnar MR, Porter FL, Wolf CM et al.: Neonatal stress reactivity: predictions to later emotional temperament, *Child Dev* 66(1):1-13, 1995.

Grunau RVE, Whitfield MF, Petrie JH et al.: Early pain experience, child temperament and family characteristics as precursors of somatization: a prospective study of preterm and fullterm children, *Pain* 56:353-359, 1994.

Hammond DL: Control systems for nociceptive afferent processing: the descending inhibitory pathways. In Yaksh TL, editor: *Spinal afferent processing,* pp 363-390, New York, 1986, Plenum Press.

Hitchcock LS, Ferrell BR, McCaffery M: The experience of chronic nonmalignant pain, *J Pain Symptom Manage* 9(5):312-318, 1994.

Jackson D: A study of pain management patient controlled analgesia versus intramuscular analgesia, *J Intravenous Nurs* 12(1):42-51, 1989.

Jacox A, Carr D, Payne R et al.: *Management of cancer pain: clinical practice guideline* No. 9. AHCPR Publication No. 94-0592, Rockville, Md, Agency for Health Care Policy and Research, U.S. Department of Health and Human Services, Public Health Service, March 1994.

Jayr C, Thomas H, Rey A et al.: Postoperative pulmonary complications: epidural analgesia using bupivacaine and opioids versus parenteral opioids, *Anesthesiology* 78(4):666-676, 1993.

Jensen TS, Rasmussen P: Phantom pain and other phenomena after amputation. In Wall PD, Melzack R, editors: *Textbook of pain,* ed 3, pp 651-665, Edinburgh, 1994, Churchill Livingstone.

Joshi GP, McCarroll SM, O'Brien TM et al.: Intraarticular analgesia following knee arthroscopy, *Anesth Analg* 76:333-336, 1993.

Katz J, Jackson M, Kavanaugh B et al.: Acute pain after thoracic surgery predicts long-term post-thoracotomy pain, *Clin J Pain* 12:50-55, 1996.

Kehlet H: Modification of responses to surgery by neural blockade. In Cousins MJ, Bridenbaugh PO, editors: *Neural blockade,* pp 129-175, Philadelphia, 1998, Lippincott-Raven.

Kenady DE, Wilson JF, Schwartz RW: A randomized comparison of patient-controlled versus standard analgesic requirements in patients undergoing cholecystectomy, *Surgery* 174:216-220, 1992.

Kost RG, Straus SE: Postherpetic neuralgia: pathogenesis, treatment, and prevention, *N Engl J Med* 335(1):32-42, 1996.

Kotiniemi LH, Ryhanen PT, Moilanen IK: Behavioural changes in children following day-case surgery: a 4-week follow-up of 551 children, *Anaesthesia* 52:970-976, 1997.

Liebeskind JC: Pain *can* kill, *Pain* 44:3-4, 1991 (guest editorial).

Liu SS, Carpenter RL, Mackey DC et al.: Effects of perioperative analgesic technique on rate of recovery after colon surgery, *Anesthesiology* 83(4):757-765, 1995.

Liu SS, Carpenter RL, Neal JM: Epidural anesthesia and analgesia: their role in postoperative outcome, *Anesthesiology* 82(6):1474-1506, 1995.

Lorenz J, Beck H, Bromm B: Cognitive performance, mood and experimental pain before and during morphine-induced analgesia in patients with chronic non-malignant pain, *Pain* 73:369-375, 1997.

Mackersie RC, Karagianes TG, Hoyt DB et al.: Prospective evaluation of epidural and intravenous administration of fentanyl for pain control and restoration of ventilatory function following multiple rib fractures, *J Trauma* 31(4):443-451, 1991.

Mahoney OM, Noble PC, Davidson J et al.: The effect of continuous epidural analgesia on postoperative pain, rehabilitation, and duration of hospitalization in total knee arthroscopy, *Clin Orthop Related Res* 260:30-37, November 1990.

Major CP, Greer MS, Russell WL et al.: Postoperative pulmonary complications and morbidity after abdominal aneurysmectomy: a comparison of postoperative epidural versus parenteral opioid analgesia, *Am Surgeon* 62(1):45-51, 1995.

Max MB, Byas-Smith MG, Gracely RH et al.: Intravenous infusion of the NMDA antagonist, ketamine, in chronic posttraumatic pain with allodynia: a double-blind comparison to alfentanil and placebo, *Clin Neuropharmacol* 18(4):360-368, August 1995.

McCaffery M: *Nursing practice theories related to cognition, bodily pain, and man-environment interactions,* Los Angeles, 1968, UCLA Students Store.

Mcintyre PE, Ready LB: *Acute pain management: a practical guide,* pp 198, Philadelphia, 1996, WB Saunders.

Melzack R, Wall PD: Pain mechanisms: a new theory, *Science* 150:971-979, 1965.

Mersky H, Bogduk N, editors: *Classification of chronic pain,* ed 2, Seattle, 1994, IASP.

Morimoto H, Cullen JJ, Messick JM et al.: Epidural analgesia shortens postoperative ileus after ileal pouch-anal canal anastomosis, *Am J Surg* 169:79-83, January 1995.

Nikolajsen L, Ilkjaer S, Kroner K et al.: The influence of preamputation pain on postamputation stump and phantom pain, *Pain* 72:393-405, 1997.

Padilla GV, Ferrell B, Grant MM et al.: Defining the content domain of quality of life for cancer patients with pain, *Cancer Nurs* 13(2):108-115, 1990.

Page GG: The medical necessity of adequate pain management, *Pain Forum* 5(4):227-233, 1996.

Page GG, Ben-Eliyahu S: The immuno-suppressive nature of pain, *Semin Oncol Nurs* 13(1):10-15, 1997.

Page GG, Ben-Eliyahu S, Yirmiya R et al.: Morphine attenuates surgery-induced enhancement of metastatic colonization in rats, *Pain* 54: 21-28, 1993.

Pati AB, Perme DC, Trail M et al.: Rehabilitation parameters in total knee replacement patients undergoing epidural vs. conventional analgesia, *J Orthop Sports Phys Ther* 19(2):88-92, 1994.

Portenoy RK: Basic mechanisms. In Portenoy RK, Kanner RM, editors: *Pain management: theory and practice,* pp 19-39, Philadelphia, 1996a, FA Davis.

Portenoy RK: Neuropathic pain. In Portenoy RK, Kanner RM, editors: *Pain management: theory and practice,* pp 83-125, Philadelphia, 1996b, FA Davis.

Portenoy RK, Kanner RM: Definition and assessment of pain. In Portenoy RK, Kanner RM, editors: *Pain management: theory and practice,* pp 3-18, Philadelphia, 1996, FA Davis.

Rawal N, Sjostrand U, Christoffersson E et al.: Comparison of intramuscular and epidural morphine for postoperative analgesia in the grossly obese: influence on postoperative ambulation and pulmonary function, *Anesth Analg* 63:583-592, 1984.

Rimback G, Cassuto J, Faxen A et al.: Effect of intra-abdominal bupivacaine instillation on postoperative colonic motility, *Gut* 27:170-175, 1986.

Rimback G, Cassuto J, Tollesson P: Treatment of postoperative paralytic ileus by intravenous lidocaine infusion, *Anesth Analg* 70:414-419, 1990.

Rosenberg J, Kehlet H: Postoperative mental confusion: association with postoperative hypoxemia, *Surgery* 114(1):76-81, 1993.

Rosenberg J, Rosenberg-Adamsen S, Kehlet H: Post-operative sleep disturbance: causes, factors, and effects on outcome, *Eur J Anaesthesiol* 12(Suppl 10):28-30, 1995.

Scott AM, Starling JR, Ruscher AE et al.: Thoracic versus lumbar epidural anesthesia's effect on pain control and ileus resolution after restorative proctocolectomy, *Surgery* 120(4):688-697, 1996.

Searle NR, Roy M, Bergeron G et al.: Hydromorphone patient-controlled analgesia (PCA) after coronary artery bypass surgery, *Can J Anaesth* 41(3):198-205, 1994.

Shavit Y, Benzion B: Morphine: a double-edged sword, *Pain Forum* 5(4):237-239, 1996.

Simpson T, Lee ER, Cameron C: Patients' perceptions of environmental factors that disturb sleep after cardiac surgery, *Am J Crit Care* 5(3): 173-181, 1996.

SUPPORT Principal Investigators: A controlled trial to improve care for seriously ill hospitalized patients, *JAMA* 274(20):1591-1598, 1995.

Taddio A, Goldbach M, Ipp M et al.: Effect of neonatal circumcision on pain responses during vaccination in boys, *Lancet* 345:291-299, 1995.

Taddio A, Stevens B, Craig K et al.: Efficacy and safety of lidocaine-prilocaine cream for pain during circumcision, *N Engl J Med* 336(17):1197-1201, 1997.

Tasmuth T, Estlanderb A, Kalso E: Effect of present pain and mood on the memory of past postoperative pain in women treated surgically for breast cancer, *Pain* 68(2,3):343-347, 1996.

Tonnesen E, Wahlgreen C: Influence of extradural and general anaesthesia on natural killer cell activity and lymphocyte subpopulations in patients undergoing hysterectomy, *Br J Anaesth* 60:500, 1988.

Tuman KJ, McCarthy RJ, March RJ et al.: Effects of epidural anesthesia and analgesia on coagulation and outcome after major vascular surgery, *Anesth Analg* 73:696-704, 1991.

Viscomi CM, Rathmell JP: Pain management issues in the pregnant patient. In Ashburn MA, Rice LJ, editors: *The management of pain*, pp 263-381, New York, 1998, Churchill Livingstone.

Wallace K: The pathophysiology of pain, *Crit Care Nurs O* 15(2):1-13, 1992.

Walsh TD: Antidepressants in chronic pain, *Clin Neuropharmacol* 6(4):271-295, 1983.

Whittle BJR, Bane JR: Prostacyclin, thromboxanes, and prostaglandins: actions and roles in the gastrointestinal tract. In Glass GBJ, Sherlock P, editors: *Progress in gastroenterology*, New York, 1983, Grune & Stratton.

Wilson WC, Smedira NG, Fink C et al.: Ordering and administration of sedatives and analgesics during the withholding and withdrawal of life support from critically ill patients, *JAMA* 267(7):949-953, 1992.

Wisner DH: A stepwise logistic regression analysis of factors affecting morbidity and mortality after thoracic trauma: effect of epidural analgesia, *J Trauma* 30(7):779-805, 1990.

Yeager MP, Glass DD, Neff RK et al.: Epidural anesthesia and analgesia in high-risk surgical patients, *Anesthesiology* 66(6):729-736, 1987.

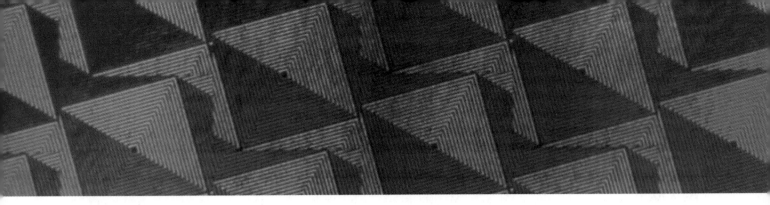

chapter three
ASSESSMENT
Underlying Complexities, Misconceptions, and Practical Tools

Margo McCaffery and Chris Pasero

CHAPTER OUTLINE

TERMINOLOGY

Addiction: Psychologic dependence. A pattern of compulsive drug use characterized by continued craving for an opioid and the need to use the opioid for effects other than pain relief. Physical dependence and tolerance are not the same as addiction.

DSM-IV: Diagnostic and Statistical Manual of Mental Disorders. A guide for clinical practice. Identifies mental disorders and lists diagnostic criteria.

Factitious disorder: Intentional production of physical symptoms (e.g., pain) but without clear motivation, except perhaps the need to assume the sick role.

Malingering: Intentionally produced symptom (e.g., pain) motivated by various factors (e.g., financial gain).

Numerical Rating Scale (NRS): The patient is asked to rate pain from 0 to 10, with zero equaling no pain and 10 equaling the worst possible pain. Scale may be presented visually with numbers placed along a vertical or horizontal line. Recommended for use in clinical practice.

Opioid: This term is preferred to "narcotic." Opioid refers to codeine, morphine, and other natural, semisynthetic, and synthetic drugs that relieve pain by binding to multiple types of opioid receptors in the nervous system.

Placebo: Any medication or procedure, including surgery, that produces an effect in a patient because of its implicit or explicit intent and not because of its specific physical or chemical properties.

Psychogenic pain: Term often used as a stigmatizing label. Presumed to exist when no nociceptive or neuropathic mechanism can be identified.

Somatoform disorders: Disorders in which physical symptoms, such as pain, suggest the existence of a disease, but demonstrable organic or objective findings are absent. Several are listed in the DSM-IV.

Supratentorial pain: Is not a recognized diagnosis and has no accepted definition. It is almost always used as a derogatory term to suggest that no physical cause exists for the pain or that the patient is lying about pain.

Titration: Adjusting the amount (e.g., adjusting the dose of opioid).

Visual Analog Scale (VAS): A horizontal (sometimes vertical) 10 cm line with word anchors at the extremes, such as "no pain" on one end and "pain as bad as it could be" or "worst possible pain" on the other end. Impractical for use in daily clinical practice.

UNDERLYING COMPLEXITIES OF PAIN ASSESSMENT

Failure of clinicians to ask patients about their pain and to accept and act on patients' reports of pain is probably the most common cause of unrelieved pain and unnecessary suffering. Basic pain assessment is a simple, but unfortunately, infrequently performed, task. Even when appropriate assessments are made, clinicians do not necessarily accept the findings and may not take appropriate action (Table 3.1).

Failure to Assess Pain

Some of the problems related to assessment of pain and decisions about treatment have been studied with vignettes such as the ones in Box 3.1. These vignettes are used in this chapter to illustrate several problems revealed by research and encountered in clinical practice. Take time now to review Box 3.1, p. 38, and answer the questions (without previewing the answers presented from the tabulated surveys, Table 3.2, p. 40).

As discussed in Chapter 1, many studies have shown that either lack of pain assessment or the existence of differences between the clinicians' pain ratings and those of patients is a major cause of inadequate pain management (Grossman, Sheidler, Swedeen et al., 1991; Von Roenn, Cleeland, Gonin et al., 1993). In one study of the skills of resident physicians in assessing chronic cancer pain, only 58% were deemed competent (Sloan, Donelly,

Schwartz et al., 1996). Assessment of simple characteristics of the pain were often omitted. For example, more than half the physicians failed to assess pain intensity.

In a study of 34 surgical oncology patients, 91% had been in pain during the prior 24 hours, but 28% said that a nurse had never asked them about their pain during their entire hospitalization (Paice, Mahon, Faut-Callahan, 1991). In this study patients, nurses, and physicians independently rated the patient's pain, but no correlation was found between nurse-patient, physician-patient, or nurse-physician pain assessments. As one would expect, clinicians could not accurately guess the patient's pain.

Overall, research shows that when clinicians do not obtain pain ratings from patients, they are likely to underestimate pain, especially moderate to severe pain (Graffam, 1981; Larue, Fontaine, Colleau, 1997; Zalon, 1993). In a study of 103 patients with cancer pain, the pain ratings of the patients were compared with those of nurses, house officers, and oncology fellows. All groups underestimated the patients' pain (Grossman, Sheidler, Swedeen et al., 1991). When pain was severe, only 7% of nurses, 20% of oncology fellows, and 27% of house officers correctly assessed the pain level. These caregivers were more accurate at rating moderate pain and even better at identifying mild pain. Interestingly, in another study nurses tended to overestimate mild pain (Zalon, 1993). In a study comparing pain ratings of children and nurses, nurses generally underestimated the children's

TABLE 3.1 ● ● ● ● ●

Misconceptions Barriers to the Assessment and Treatment of Pain

MISCONCEPTION	CORRECTION
1. The best judge of the existence and severity of a patient's pain is the physician or nurse caring for the patient.	The patient is the authority about his or her pain. The patient's self-report is the most reliable indicator of the existence and intensity of pain.
2. Clinicians should use their personal opinions and beliefs about the truthfulness of the patient to determine the patient's true pain status.	Allowing each clinician to act on personal beliefs presents the potential for different pain assessments by different clinicians, leading to different interventions from each clinician. This results in inconsistent and often inadequate pain management. It is essential to establish the patient's self-report of pain as the standard for pain assessment.
3. The clinician must believe what the patient says about pain.	The clinician must accept and respect the patient's report of pain and proceed with appropriate assessment and treatment. The clinician is always entitled to his or her personal opinion, but this cannot be allowed to guide professional practice.
4. Comparable noxious stimuli produce comparable pain in different people. The pain threshold is uniform.	Findings from numerous studies have failed to support the notion of a uniform pain threshold. Comparable stimuli do not result in the same pain in different people. After similar injuries, one person may suffer moderate pain and the other severe pain.
5. Patients with a low pain tolerance should make a greater effort to cope with pain and should not receive as much analgesia as they desire.	A stoic response to pain is valued in this society and many others. Research shows that clinicians often do not like patients with a low pain tolerance. However, imposing these values on the patient and withholding analgesics is inappropriate.
6. There is no reason for patients to hurt when no physical cause for pain can be found.	Pain is a new science, and it would be foolish of us to think that we will be able to determine the cause of all the pains that patients report.
7. Patients should not receive analgesics until the cause of pain is diagnosed.	Pain is no longer the clinician's primary diagnostic tool. Symptomatic relief of pain should be provided while the investigation of cause proceeds. Early use of analgesics is now advocated for patients with acute abdominal pain.
8. Visible signs, either physiologic or behavioral, accompany pain and can be used to verify its existence and severity.	Even with severe pain, periods of physiologic and behavioral adaptation occur, leading to periods of minimal or no signs of pain. Lack of pain expression does not necessarily mean lack of pain.
9. Anxiety makes pain worse.	Anxiety is often associated with pain, but the cause and effect relationship has not been established. Pain often causes anxiety, but it is not clear that anxiety necessarily makes pain more intense.
10. Patients who are knowledgeable about opioid analgesics and who make regular efforts to obtain them are "drug seeking" (addicted).	Patients with pain should be knowledgeable about their medications, and regular use of opioids for pain relief is not addiction. When a patient is accused of "drug seeking," it may be helpful to ask, "What else could this behavior mean? Might this patient be in pain?"
11. When the patient reports pain relief after a placebo, this means that the patient is a malingerer or that the pain is psychogenic.	About one third of patients who have obvious physical stimuli for pain (e.g., surgery) report pain relief after a placebo injection. Therefore placebos cannot be used to diagnose malingering, psychogenic pain, or any psychologic problem. Sometimes placebos relieve pain, but why this happens remains unknown.
12. The pain rating scale preferred for use in daily clinical practice is the VAS.	For patients who are verbal and can count from 0 to 10, the NRS pain rating scale is preferred. It is easy to explain, measure, and record, and it provides numbers for setting pain-management goals.
13. Cognitively impaired elderly patients are unable to use pain rating scales.	When an appropriate pain rating scale (e.g., 0-5) is used and the patient is given sufficient time to process information and respond, many cognitively impaired elderly can use a pain rating scale.

May be duplicated for use in clinical practice. From McCaffery M, Pasero C: *Pain: Clinical manual*, p. 37. Copyright © 1999, Mosby, Inc.
See text for references.

• • • • •

┌───┐
| BOX 3.1   **Survey—Assessment and Use of Analgesics: "Andrew—Robert"** |
└───┘

Directions: Please select one answer for each question.

PATIENT A

Andrew is 25 years old, and this is his first day after abdominal surgery. As you enter his room, he smiles at you and continues talking and joking with his visitor. Your assessment reveals the following information: BP, 120/80; HR, 80; R, 18; on a scale of 0 to 10 (0 = no pain/discomfort, 10 = worst pain/discomfort) he rates his pain as 8.

1. On the patient's record you must mark his pain on the scale below. Circle the number that represents your assessment of Andrew's pain:

   0   1   2   3   4   5   6   7   8   9   10

   No pain/   Worst pain/
   discomfort   discomfort

2. Your assessment, above, is made 2 hours after the patient received morphine, 2 mg IV. Half hourly pain ratings after the injection ranged from 6 to 8, and he had no clinically significant respiratory depression, sedation, or other untoward side effects. He has identified 2 as an acceptable level of pain relief. His physician's order for analgesia is "morphine IV 1 to 3 mg q1h PRN for pain relief." Check the action you will take at this time:
   _____ (a) Administer no morphine at this time.
   _____ (b) Administer morphine, 1 mg IV, now.
   _____ (c) Administer morphine, 2 mg IV, now.
   _____ (d) Administer morphine, 3 mg IV, now.

PATIENT B

Robert is 25 years old, and this is his first day after abdominal surgery. As you enter his room, he is lying quietly in bed and grimaces as he turns in bed. Your assessment reveals the following information: BP, 120/80; HR, 80; R, 18; on a scale of 0 to 10 (0 = no pain/discomfort, 10 = worst pain/discomfort) he rates his pain as 8.

1. On the patient's record you must mark his pain on the scale below. Circle the number that represents your assessment of Robert's pain:

   0   1   2   3   4   5   6   7   8   9   10

   No pain/   Worst pain/
   discomfort   discomfort

2. Your assessment, above, is made 2 hours after the patient received morphine, 2 mg IV. Half-hourly pain ratings after the injection ranged from 6 to 8, and he had no clinically significant respiratory depression, sedation, or other untoward side effects. He has identified 2 as an acceptable level of pain relief. His physician's order for analgesia is "morphine IV, 1 to 3 mg q1h PRN, for pain relief." Check the action you will take at this time:
   _____ (a) Administer no morphine at this time.
   _____ (b) Administer morphine, 1 mg IV, now.
   _____ (c) Administer morphine, 2 mg IV, now.
   _____ (d) Administer morphine, 3 mg IV, now.

May be duplicated for use in clinical practice. From McCaffery M, Pasero C: *Pain: Clinical manual,* p. 38. Copyright © 1999, Mosby, Inc.

pain, especially after the children had been given an analgesic (Romsing, Moller-Sonnergaard, Hertel et al., 1996).

Underestimation of pain by caregivers understandably contributes to undertreatment of pain. In a study of more than 1000 outpatients with metastatic cancer, the most powerful predictor of inadequate analgesia was the discrepancy between the physician's and the patient's estimate of pain severity (Cleeland, Gonin, Hatfield et al., 1994). For almost half the patients, physicians underestimated the extent to which pain interfered with the patients' activities.

Failure to Accept Patient's Report of Pain

When clinicians do obtain pain ratings from patients, they do not necessarily accept what the patients say. In a study of 24 surgical patients, the pain ratings of patients were compared with those documented on the PCA record by the nurses (Carey, Turpin, Smith et al., 1997). The nurses consistently documented lower pain ratings than those reported by patients. Once again, the greatest discrepancies occurred at the highest pain levels. Findings from other research using patient vignettes also reveal that even when patients report pain intensity as a specific

number on a pain rating scale, some nurses record a different number in the patient's record (McCaffery, Ferrell, 1991a,b; 1992a,b,c; 1997a).

The findings of several studies suggest that clinicians believe that patients exaggerate their pain. In one study, when medical and nursing staff were asked to rate what they believed were patients' pain intensities, they rated the pain lower than the patients did (Krivo, Reidenberg, 1995). However, when they were asked what pain rating they thought the patients would report, more than two thirds of the staff gave higher pain ratings that were much closer to those the patients gave, revealing that they thought the pain was really less than the patients said it was.

In a study of 22 adolescent patients with surgical pain and their nurses, pain ratings of the patients were compared with the pain ratings the nurses expected the patients to give (Favaloro, Touzel, 1990). The nurses believed that the male adolescents would rate their pain at a higher level than the nurses' ratings, whereas female adolescents were expected to give pain ratings similar to those of the nurses. Interestingly, in this particular situation, gender influenced the nurses' expectations of which patients would exaggerate pain, believing that male adolescents were more likely than females to overrate their pain. Contrary to these expectations, the pain ratings given by the males were significantly lower than those of the females.

In a comparison of oncology nurses and long-term care facility nurses, the latter were more likely to believe that patients with cancer pain over report their pain (Ryan, Vortherms, Ward, 1994). Nurses in long-term care facilities believed that about 25% of these patients were exaggerating the severity of their cancer pain. In another study of nurses across the United States, more than one third of the nurses believed that 20% or more of patients with cancer over report their pain (McCaffery, Ferrell, 1995b).

In a study of hospitalized oncology patients, physicians and nurses were asked to have patients rate their pain daily (Au, Loprinzi, Chodapkar et al., 1994). Compliance with this was poor, but when they did ask the patients for pain ratings, they tended to downgrade patient pain scores when they reported them verbally to the investigators.

Failure to Act on the Patient's Report of Pain

If clinicians believe patients overstate their pain, this would help explain why assessment of pain using patient self-report does not necessarily result in improved pain management. The clinicians may assess pain accurately but may be planning pain management on the basis of their own beliefs rather than what the patients say.

This possibility was illustrated in a study of pain ratings by nurses and surgical patients in the critical care setting (Puntillo, Miaskowski, Kehrie et al., 1997). These nurses consistently, although not significantly, underestimated mild to moderate pain. Most importantly, the amount of opioid administered was better correlated with the nurses' own pain ratings than those they obtained from the patients.

Failure to act on patients' reports of pain also is influenced by many other factors, in particular, institutional barriers, discussed in Chapter 16. For example, many hospitals do not have policies that allow nurses to titrate analgesic doses or to implement PRN analgesics ATC when pain is present most of the day. And, as mentioned throughout this book, many clinicians lack knowledge about appropriate pain management.

Focus of the Chapter

Clearly, many clinicians need instruction about how to conduct even the most basic pain assessments such as pain intensity. Clinicians also need education about the importance of regularly scheduled assessments, the responsibility of accepting what the patient says rather than downgrading reports of pain, and the necessity of planing action on the basis of patient reports of pain, not their own personal judgments.

The focus of this chapter is on assessment of the pain report itself, with some attention to how clinicians respond to these assessments. Misconceptions that hamper assessment and subsequent treatment of patients who report that they have pain will be discussed, followed by practical assessment tools for various clinical settings. These include pain rating scales and documentation forms, such as initial pain assessment tools and flow sheets. Communication strategies that use these tools are discussed. Finally, challenges in pain assessment are addressed and include patients who deny pain or refuse analgesics, patients of different cultural backgrounds, and cognitively impaired individuals.

The clinician is reminded that comprehensive, initial, and ongoing assessments of patients with pain also should include appropriate physical and neurologic examinations, as well as inquiries about psychosocial factors related to the pain such as the patient's and family's concerns about pain and the financial impact of pain. Every effort should be made to diagnosis the underlying mechanism or cause of pain not only initially, but also at regular intervals when the pain does not subside. Any significant increase in pain or change in the characteristics of pain should signal the need for another comprehensive physical assessment and possibly neurologic, psychosocial, and other examinations. Increases in pain should never be explained solely as drug-seeking behavior or as simply the result of tolerance to opioid analgesia or psychosocial problems.

MISCONCEPTIONS THAT HAMPER ASSESSMENT AND TREATMENT OF PATIENTS WHO REPORT PAIN

Regardless of what patients say about their pain, the subjectivity of pain seems to invite speculation from everyone—clinicians, families, and acquaintances—about the "true" nature of patients' pain. Numerous reasons are given by clinicians to explain why they find it difficult to accept some patients' reports of pain and why they fail to respond with appropriate treatment. These include lack of a known cause for the pain or lack of behavioral indicators, such as grimacing. Still other reasons remain less obvious, often below the level of awareness, but still cause clinicians to have doubts. For example, the patient's gender or ethnic origin may unknowingly influence clinicians' decisions about pain management.

Authority About Pain: Patient Versus Caregivers/Family

Who is the authority about the patient's pain? Whose pain is it? Clinicians sometimes believe they know more about the patient's pain than the patient does. No matter how appealing that belief may be, it is false. Nevertheless, privately or among themselves, clinicians may comment about a patient, "He doesn't have as much pain as he thinks he does," or "The pain is not that bad," implying that the clinician is the true authority about the patient's pain.

No objective measures of pain exist. The sensation of pain is completely subjective. Pain cannot be proved or disproved. One definition of pain for use in clinical practice says that, "Pain is whatever the experiencing person says it is, existing whenever he says it does" (McCaffery, 1968, p. 95). Statements from clinical practice guidelines have echoed the same approach to the patient's report of pain by statements such as:

- "The clinician must accept the patient's report of pain." (APS, 1992, p. 2)
- "The single most reliable indicator of the existence and intensity of pain—and any resultant distress—is the patient's self-report." (Acute Pain Management Guideline Panel, 1992a, p. 6)
- "The mainstay of pain assessment is the patient self-report." (Jacox, Carr, Payne et al., 1994b, p. 3)

The "gold standard" for assessing the existence and intensity of pain is the patient's self-report. No other source of information has ever been shown to be more accurate or reliable than what the patient says. The patient's behaviors, the opinions of nurses and physicians delivering care, the patient's vital signs—none of these is as reliable as the patient's report of pain and should never be used instead of what the patient says (Acute Pain Management Guideline Panel, 1992a).

The "Andrew-Robert" survey presented in Box 3.1 illustrates what happens when clinicians do not adopt the patient's self-report as the standard for assessment for pain intensity. This survey has been used by many nurse educators in hundreds of educational programs to illustrate the necessity of accepting the patient's report of pain as the standard for assessment. The survey has become so familiar to staff nurse educators that is it often referred to simply as the "Andrew-Robert" survey. Several publications have reported the results of studies using this survey and modifications of it (McCaffery, Ferrell, 1991a,b; 1992a,b; 1994a; 1997a; McCaffery, Ferrell, O'Neil-Page, 1992). A summary of survey findings over a 5-year period has been published by the originators of the survey, McCaffery and Ferrell (1997a).

The results of the Andrew-Robert survey as presented in Table 3.2 are based on the responses of 450 nurses throughout the United States. These were registered nurses with an average of 16.1 years of experience. In viewing the nurses responses to pain assessment (questions 1) it is apparent that not all nurses understood that the patient's self-report of pain is the single most reliable indicator of pain. Both of these patients reported their postoperative pain as 8, but only 73.8% of the nurses recorded 8 for the smiling patient. At least 26.2%, more

• • • • •

TABLE 3.2 **Nurses' Responses to the "Survey: Assessment and Use of Analgesics" (These data were collected in 1995; n = 450 nurses.)**

NURSES' RESPONSES TO		NURSES' RESPONSES TO
QUESTION 1. PAIN ASSESSMENT		
Smiling Andrew	Pain Rating	Grimacing Robert
2.0%	0	0%
2.4%	1	0.2%
4.0%	2	0.2%
5.6%	3	0.2%
3.8%	4	1.1%
5.3%	5	1.1%
2.9%	6	2.2%
0.2%	7	3.1%
73.8%	*8	87.1%
0%	9	2.9%
0%	10	1.8%
QUESTION 2. CHOICE OF OPIOID DOSE		
	Morphine IV	
10.0%	0	2.0%
16.7%	1 mg	7.6%
21.8%	2 mg	19.1%
51.5%	*3 mg	71.3%

May be duplicated for use in clinical practice. From McCaffery M, Pasero C: *Pain: Clinical manual,* p. 40. Copyright © 1999, Mosby, Inc.
* Correct answer.
Information from McCaffery M, Ferrell BF: *J Pain Symptom Manage* 14:175-188, 1997.

than one of four nurses, did not know the standard for assessment of pain intensity. When reviewing answers given for pain assessment, it is clear that when nurses do not agree with the patient, they do not agree with one another either. In fact, for the smiling patient, their answers included every pain rating from 0 to 7. Naturally this promotes confusion and inconsistency when a plan of action is considered. (The fact that these nurses responded differently to the two patients will be discussed in the following section on behavioral response to pain.)

This illustrates what is often seen in clinical practice—each person caring for the patient may have a different opinion about what the pain intensity is. Without a standard for assessing pain, chaos quickly ensues. For example, four different clinicians caring for the same patient may arrive at four different pain ratings, all of which are different from the patient's pain rating (usually underestimations of the patient's pain). How do you resolve five different pain ratings so that intervention can be planned?

The need to establish the patient's self-report as the standard becomes apparent. There appears to be no alternative. It is reassuring to realize that the validity and reliability of patients' self-reports of pain are testified to in the numerous double-blind studies of analgesics, in which the patients' pain ratings always determine the analgesic effect of the drugs being tested. Initial recommended doses of analgesics and equianalgesic charts have relied on such research for decades.

When a patient reports pain, the health care professional's responsibility is to accept and respect that report and to proceed with appropriate assessment and treatment. All reports of pain are taken seriously. When difficulties arise with accepting the patient's report of pain, some of the strategies listed in Box 3.2 may be helpful.

Considerations when doubts arise

On occasion, accepting and acting on the patient's report of pain are difficult. Because pain cannot be proved, health care professionals are vulnerable to being fooled by the patient who wishes to lie about pain. However, although accepting and responding to the report of pain will undoubtedly result in giving analgesics to some patients who do not have pain, it ensures that everyone who does have pain receives an attentive response. No health care professional has the right to deprive a patient of appropriate assessment and treatment simply because he or she believes the patient is lying.

An important distinction exists between believing the patient's report of pain and accepting that report. Following the recommendations of the clinical practice guidelines does not require that the clinician agree 100% with what the patient says. The clinician is merely required to accept what the patient says, convey acceptance to the patient, and take the appropriate action. The clinician is entitled to his or her personal doubts and

opinions. But these cannot be allowed to interfere with appropriate patient care.

Although accepting the patient's report of pain occasionally will result in being duped, no stigma or blame should attached to being duped. In any relationship, each party has certain responsibilities. Fault is assigned to that party who fails to meet his or her responsibility (Wesson, Smith, 1990). If the clinician fulfills his or her responsibility to respond to all reports of pain with appropriate assessment and treatment, the clinician will be able to say, "Although I was probably fooled by some patients, I never failed to help those who did have pain. No one can find fault with my behavior or professional conduct."

Furthermore, accepting the patient's report of pain avoids an adversarial relationship. When the clinician conveys to the patient that the report of pain is not accepted, this amounts to accusing the patient of lying. Understandably, this is upsetting and frightening to a patient who has asked the health care provider for help with pain. Much has been written in the literature about the distinction between suffering and pain. It is worth noting that in his analysis of suffering, Eric Cassell (1982) mentions that one source of suffering is physicians who do not validate the patient's pain, but rather ascribe it to psychologic causes or accuse the patient of faking. Clinicians ask patients to trust them. At some point clinicians must return the favor.

Invariably the term malingering is encountered when a patient's report of pain is doubted. Malingering may be defined as the conscious desire to deceive or misrepresent the facts, usually for monetary or other gains. Malingering seems to be suspected most often in patients with chronic nonmalignant pain, especially low back pain. In its core curriculum for professional education in pain, the International Association for the Study of Pain (IASP) cites several sources to support the conclusion that malingering occurs in 5% or fewer of patients with low back pain (Fields, 1995). In the IASP guideline for low back pain, clinicians are warned, "Interpreting inconsistencies or pain behaviors as malingering does not benefit the patient or the clinician. It is more useful to view such behavior and inconsistencies as . . . a plea for help" (Fordyce 1996, p. 46). The IASP further notes that the process of identifying malingering is, in the final analysis, a legal, not a medical, process (Mersky, Bogduk, 1994).

Secondary gain is another term that may be used to cast doubt on the patient's report of pain. This term is vague, ill defined, and often erroneously equated with malingering. Secondary gain usually suggests that the patient is somehow rewarded, perhaps economically or emotionally, by having pain. Sometimes the legitimacy of secondary gain is overlooked, such as the patient who is entitled to financial compensation after an injury caused by unsafe work conditions. Nevertheless, secondary gain tends to cause some clinicians to be suspicious of the

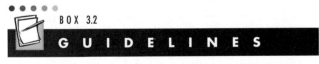

BOX 3.2

GUIDELINES

STRATEGIES WHEN THE PATIENT'S REPORT OF PAIN IS NOT ACCEPTED

Strategies: What do we do if the health care team does not respond positively to the patient's report of pain?
- Acknowledge that everyone is entitled to a personal opinion, but personal opinion does not form the basis for professional practice.
- Clarify that the sensation of pain is subjective and cannot be proved or disproved.
- Quote recommendations from clinical practice guidelines, especially APS and AHCPR.
- Ask: Why is it so difficult to believe that this person hurts?

May be duplicated for use in clinical practice. From McCaffery M, Pasero C: Pain: Clinical manual, p. 41. Copyright © 1999, Mosby, Inc.

patient's reports of pain and is often blamed for treatment failure. However, the clinician's suspicion of secondary gain may actually interfere with the treatment provided and cause treatment failures. The suggestion of secondary gain is also infuriating to patients who also frequently have secondary losses such as lower self-esteem and loss of job (Teasell, Merskey, 1997). In sum, the notion of secondary gain is of questionable value.

On reflection, one might ask whether it is justified to be suspicious of all patients in an attempt to avoid being fooled by the few who will lie. It is a burden to the clinician and an insult to the patient to wrestle with potential dishonesty at each encounter.

Pain Threshold: Uniform Versus Variable

Pain threshold may be defined as that point at which an increasing intensity of stimuli is felt as painful. Several decades ago, preliminary research erroneously suggested that everyone perceives the same intensity of pain from the same stimuli (Hardy, Wolff, Goodell, 1943). This has been called the uniform pain threshold. However, further research failed to support the uniform pain threshold theory (Beecher, 1956). For half a century it has been known that comparable stimuli in different people do *not* produce the same intensities of pain. A uniform relationship does not exist between tissue damage and pain. For example, a certain type of tissue damage may produce more or less pain than one might expect. Not only will pain intensity vary among patients, but duration and other characteristics will also vary.

One approach to explaining the lack of a uniform pain threshold is endorphins, which are naturally occurring substances in the body with morphine-like properties. Theoretically, when comparable stimuli are experienced, patients with low endorphin levels will feel more pain than those with high endorphin levels. Evidence suggests that constitutional differences may exist in the amount of endorphin present in different individuals (Tamsen, Sakurada, Wahlstrom et al., 1982). Other factors, such as physical exercise, sexual activity, or prolonged stress, may increase or decrease endorphin levels (Emrich, 1981; Janal, Colt, Clark et al., 1984; Terenius, 1981; Whipple, Komisaruk, 1985).

The misconception that, after repeated or prolonged experience with pain, the person feels less pain is also refuted by preliminary research with endorphins, which suggests that the opposite may be true (Kosten, Kleber, 1987). In one study the individual's endorphin response to each pain exposure was decreased with repeated episodes of pain, suggesting that repeated exposure to pain results in increasing pain. Also, endorphin levels tend to be low in patients with chronic pain (Puig, Laorden, Miralles et al., 1982).

The idea that a particular patient "does not hurt that much" probably is based on the misconception that comparable stimuli produce comparable pain in different people. A more appropriate appraisal might be that this painful event hurts this patient more than it seems to hurt others. Concluding that the patient is exaggerating the pain results in a number of potentially harmful effects such failing to detect a complication or providing inadequate analgesia.

When the patient reports pain that is considerably more than expected, it is always wise to reassess the patient. For example, a surgical patient may have a hematoma or infection. However, the patient should be given analgesia while being reassessed. As discussed later in this chapter, once pain has occurred and been assessed for intensity, location, and other characteristics, providing analgesia may facilitate a diagnosis because the patient is often better able to answer questions and cooperate with various tests. Masking the symptom of pain with analgesia rarely interferes with the continuation of an appropriate diagnostic workup.

Pain Tolerance: High Versus Low

Although pain threshold reflects the point at which the patient feels pain, pain tolerance may be defined as that duration or intensity of pain that a person is willing to endure. An example of high pain tolerance is the willingness to endure prolonged and severe pain without desiring relief, whereas low pain tolerance might be a desire for relief of brief, mild pain.

Pain tolerance varies from person to person and within the same person depending on numerous factors such as past experiences with pain, coping skills, motivation to endure pain, and energy level. For example, a patient may be willing to endure intense pain during childbirth to minimize the infant's exposure to medications, but may be unwilling to endure mild episiotomy pain later if she is not breast feeding.

Society places a high value on a high pain tolerance. The findings of one study suggest that nurses do not like patients who have severe pain or who are perceived as coping poorly with their pain (Salmon, Manyande, 1996). In this study nurses' estimates of their patients' pain intensity were fairly accurate, but when patients were perceived as being unable to cope with pain, they were evaluated by the nurses as demanding and were unpopular with the staff.

As distasteful as it may be to admit it, nurses and other clinicians probably tend to view patients who report pain as "bad" patients, hence the routine use of the phrase "complains of pain." Saying that the patient complains of pain suggests a much more negative evaluation of the patient than does saying that the patient reports pain. It might be worthwhile to make a conscious effort to avoid using the word complain. The reader may note that throughout this book, the authors never use the word "complain" in reference to patients' reports of pain.

One cannot escape the fact that this society and many others value a stoic response to pain, which is probably very closely aligned with valuing a high pain tolerance. No doubt this value is shared by most readers. However, health care providers must guard against requiring this of patients and certainly avoid criticizing patients who are unwilling or unable to meet this expectation. Pain tolerance may not be under the patient's direct control, and patients have a right to determine their own pain tolerance or willingness to endure pain. Nevertheless, misconceptions and judgmental statements about pain tolerance are heard in clinical practice.

Unfortunately, the use of the phrase "low pain tolerance" in clinical practice has not been well defined and researched, but almost every clinician is familiar with disdainful remarks made about patients with a low pain tolerance. For example, one or more clinicians may decide that an individual patient ought to be able to tolerate a particular painful experience. This may be a procedure, a chronic pain condition such as arthritis or low back pain, surgery, wound care, or a variety of other circumstances. The clinician may erroneously believe that the patient does not require analgesia, although the patient may report pain and request relief.

Clinicians may say that such a patient has a low pain tolerance and imply that the patient should not succumb to this. A low pain tolerance seems to be regarded as unnecessary, a weakness, a character flaw, a lack of will power, or perhaps even self-indulgent. The implication appears to be that the patient should be stronger and muster the energy to "cope better" with pain.

A common misconception is that increased experience with pain should teach a person to be more tolerant of it and better able to cope with it. However, repeated experience with pain usually teaches a person how severe pain may become and how difficult it is to get pain relief. Thus, a person who has repeated experiences with pain may have higher levels of anxiety and lower pain tolerance.

Furthermore, experience with pain does not necessarily result in less expressive behavioral responses. Observations of children 3 to 7 years of age revealed that those who experienced the most bumps, cuts, and scrapes common in childhood activities responded to them the most strongly (Fearon, McGrath, Achat, 1996). In other words, the more experience with pain, the more vigorous the behavioral response to pain. Similar findings have been reported in infants who undergo circumcision without anesthesia (Taddio, Katz, Ilersich et al., 1997). In adults, previous surgeries also appear to result in greater pain intensity and emotion during later surgical experiences (Wells, 1989).

Patients, as well as clinicians, value stoicism. When the patient is unable to meet his or her own expectation of tolerating pain or minimizing behavioral expressions of pain, the clinician can at least minimize the psychologic trauma to the patient by conveying that the patient's responses to pain are fully acceptable to us. Simply saying, "This is tough. You're doing well," may reduce the patient's distress considerably. If the patient wants help in coping with pain in another manner, or if it appears that teaching the patient certain coping strategies would result in less distress for the patient, this can certainly be offered. For example, some of the cognitive-behavioral techniques discussed in Chapters 8 and 9 can be considered.

Identifying the patient's pain tolerance is a critical part of providing pain relief. Setting pain rating and activity goals, discussed later in this chapter, is an effort to identify the level of pain the patient can endure without distress and still perform necessary activities.

Behavioral and Physiologic Responses to Pain: Acute Pain Model Versus Adaptation

The acute pain model says that if the patient has pain, visible signs of discomfort, behavioral and/or physiologic, will be present. Examples of behavior usually expected of patients with pain include grimacing, rigid body posture, limping, frowning, or crying. Physiologically, elevated vital signs are often expected. Clinicians and laymen alike usually fail to appreciate that both physiologic and behavioral adaptation occur, leading to periods of minimal or no signs of pain. Absence of behavioral or physiologic signs of pain does not necessarily mean absence of pain.

The acute pain model is of limited value. When pain is sudden or severe, behavioral and physiologic indicators may be present for a brief time. However, very quickly the patient may make an effort to cease behaviors such as crying or moaning. Behavioral adaptation or suppression of pain behaviors may occur because the patient values the stoic response or simply becomes exhausted. Physiologic indicators such as increased blood pressure or heart rate may also disappear. In a healthy individual the body will seek homeostasis or equilibrium, returning to the former physiologic state despite severe pain. Or, the patient may have a medical condition that causes low blood pressure, such as hypothyroidism or dehydration, that will have a much greater impact on vital signs than pain will have. In such patients sudden, severe pain may elevate the vital signs only briefly and minimally.

The AHCPR clinical practice guidelines for acute pain management and the guideline from the American Pain Society (APS) address the misconceptions about the acute pain model by stating the following:

- "Observations of behavior and vital signs should not be used instead of self-report." (Acute Pain Management Guideline Panel, 1992a, p. 7)

- "Physiological measures (e.g., heart rate and blood pressure). . . are neither sensitive nor specific as indicators of pain." (Acute Pain Management Guideline Panel, 1992b, p. 7)
- "The lack of objective signs may prompt the inexperienced clinician to say that the patient does not 'look' like he or she is in pain." (APS, 1992, p. 3)

Responses clinicians expect of patients with pain

Nurses' responses to the "Andrew-Robert" survey (see Table 3.2) reveal that patients' behavioral responses have a significant effect on nurses' pain assessments and treatment decisions (McCaffery, Ferrell 1997a). The only difference between Andrew and Robert is their behavior—Andrew smiles and laughs with visitors, whereas Robert lies in bed and grimaces. This simple difference has a startling effect on nurses' responses.

The vignettes state that both patients rated their pain as 8 out of 10. Thus a pain rating of 8 should have been recorded for both patients. For the smiling patient, only 73.8% recorded 8, but for the grimacing patient 87.1% recorded 8. Nurses were more likely to accept the report of pain from the grimacing patient than from the smiling patient.

Not too surprisingly, the nurses also were more likely to increase the morphine dose for the grimacing patient. Both patients had received morphine, 2 mg IV, 2 hours before, half hourly pain ratings had ranged from 6 to 8 out of 10, and no clinically significant side effects such as sedation had occurred. The pain rating goal was 2. Nurses were given a choice of administering no morphine or 1 mg, 2 mg, or 3 mg IV. Morphine, 3 mg IV, was the correct choice for both patients. However, only 51.5% of the nurses would increase the dose for the smiling patient, whereas 71.3% would increase the dose for the grimacing patient. At least 20% of the nurses knew that it was safe to increase the dose for the smiling patient, but they did not. Administering 2 mg of morphine IV is undertreatment, but more severe undertreatment was likely for the smiling patient, with 26.7% administering either no morphine or 1 mg, half the dose that was ineffective previously. For the grimacing patient, only 9.6% took this action. Other vignette surveys similar to "Andrew-Robert" have reported similar findings (McCaffery, Ferrell, 1994a).

These same biases about behavior also exist in the layman. A survey very similar to the "Andrew-Robert" survey was revised to be appropriate for a nonnurse audience and was administered to 85 college students who were not enrolled in a medical or nursing major (McCaffery, Ferrell, 1996a). College students' responses to assessment and relief of pain showed a trend similar to those of practicing nurses. The smiling patient's pain rating was accepted by 38% of the college students, whereas 55% accepted the grimacing patient's report of pain.

Vital signs also influence nurses' willingness to record the patient's report of pain. A survey using the same format as the "Andrew-Robert" survey was constructed in which the only difference between the patients was their vital signs (McCaffery, Ferrell, 1992a,b). One patient had low to normal vital signs, and the other patient had elevated vital signs. The responses of 166 nurses revealed that more nurses were willing to accept the report of severe pain from the patient with elevated vital signs than from the patient with low to normal vital signs.

Expectations that certain behaviors indicate pain also influences the prescribing of analgesics. To identify factors that affect physicians' decisions to prescribe opioids for chronic noncancer patients, a total of 191 patients referred to a pain center was examined by a variety of measures to determine pain severity, physical findings, pain duration, age, gender, observed pain behaviors, reported functional limitations, and affective distress (Turk, Okifuji, 1997). Of all these variables, only observed pain behaviors were significantly related to receiving opioid prescriptions. In other words, patients who exhibited pain behaviors were most likely to receive opioids for pain relief. The extent of physical findings and the severity of the pain did not appear to influence the decision to prescribe opioids. Because opioids are prescribed for the purpose of pain relief, it would seem more logical to find that severity of pain determined prescription of opioids, but this was not the case.

Similar findings also were reported regarding patients with low back pain. Decisions about lumbar surgery were not made on the basis of physical pathologic condition, but rather on behaviors demonstrated by patients during their evaluation (Waddell, Main, Morris et al., 1984). As summarized by Turk and Okifuji (1997), "physicians appear to believe that behavioral demonstrations of pain, such as limping and grimacing, indicate something important about the nature of the patient's pain and the need for prescribing specific treatments such as surgery and opioids" (p. 334).

Patients' Knowledge of Clinician's Expectations of Pain Behaviors

Interviews with patients who had used IV PCA for opioid administration after surgery revealed that a major reason for patient's valuing PCA was related to the fact that PCA decreased the need to interact with the nursing staff regarding pain (Hall, Salmon, 1997; Taylor, Hall, Salmon 1996a, 1996b). Not only did patients see PCA as better than waiting for the nurse to administer opioids IM, but they also believed it protected them from having to show distress to the nurses.

Apparently many patients with pain are aware of the behaviors expected of them, or they learn them quickly. Patients may learn from early childhood experiences with pain, television, the responses of their clinicians, and a variety of other sources how to behave to signal others that pain exists and that help is needed. It is a common observation that patients with pain change their behavior in the presence of clinicians and in other selected circumstances. Patients may appear calm and to read or have a lively telephone conversation, but as soon as the clinician enters, the patient may replace this activity with a solemn facial expression and may even grimace, moan, and restrict movement—just the behaviors the clinician wants to see when the patient reports pain, but not necessarily the behavior the patient prefers.

Consider what might happen if the patients in the "Andrew-Robert" survey were roommates. It would not take long for smiling Andrew to realize that grimacing Robert was receiving better pain relief, and the reason probably would be quite apparent to smiling Andrew. Andrew might take pride in looking energetic and happy in front of his visitors or may find that such distraction is very helpful as a coping mechanism. But, if he wants better pain relief, he may decide to change that behavior, at least during the time the clinicians are present. When clinicians see this change occur, they often regard the patient as manipulative, not realizing that it is the expectations clinicians convey to patients that causes this behavior change.

Taking this hypothetical situation further, by succumbing to expectations of pain behavior to obtain relief, Andrew may begin to jeopardize his recovery. For example, both patients might be told to ambulate. Smiling Andrew may walk the hall until he begins to hurt and then go to the nurses station and ask for something for relief. The staff may feel that if Andrew can be this active, he could not hurt enough to require an analgesic. Grimacing Robert, on the other hand, may remain in bed grimacing rather than ambulate and may also ask for an analgesic. Robert may very well be more likely to receive the analgesic than Andrew. Andrew may then learn to stay in bed, prolonging his recovery and increasing the risk of complications, but increasing his chances of receiving pain relief.

Comparable circumstances were observed in a study of cancer patients (Cleeland Gonin, Hatfield et al., 1994). The more active patients were most likely to receive inadequate pain management.

Because clinicians differ in how they expect patients to behave in response to pain, patients may have difficulty learning which behaviors will effectively convince which clinician. An analysis of staff and patient behavior on an orthopedic unit revealed that the staff assessed pain by observing patients' behaviors and that their expectations about how patients should express their pain varied within and between shifts (Wiener, 1975). Some, but not all, patients were adept at reading the explicit and implicit cues given by staff and changed their behavior accordingly. However, patients sometimes felt forced into using tactics that they believed were unacceptable but were expected by the staff and were necessary to obtain pain relief.

Expecting patients to behave in certain ways to verify their pain becomes more confusing when clinicians are especially particular about the intensity or type of behavior that the patient should display. Sometimes a clinician will say that a patient does not look like he or she is in pain, but, when the patient exhibits pain behavior, the clinician may say that the patient is making too much fuss over the pain.

Correction of the acute pain model misconception

One of the most interesting aspects of the misconception that the patient's behavioral response is more reliable than the patient's self-report of pain is that it is totally illogical. Virtually every human being has had the personal experience of trying to hide pain and function in spite of it, smiling when appropriate and even deliberately using humor as distraction. One of the oldest maxims in health care is that laughter is the best medicine. Why couldn't the nurses and college students responding to the "Andrew-Robert" survey use this folk wisdom and their own personal experiences with pain to realize that patients with severe pain most certainly may smile and laugh? Nurses are probably the largest group of clinician advocates for nondrug pain relief measures, of which distraction and laughter are highly ranked. And no research has ever even suggested that smiling and joking are incompatible with feeling pain. Why clinicians seem to have such difficulty accepting and acting on reports of pain from smiling and active patients remains a mystery, at least to these authors.

A substantial amount of research refutes the value of the acute pain model, showing that neither behavioral indicators nor physiologic responses are dependably related to the intensity of the patient's pain. Physiologic indicators appear to be even less valuable than the patient's behavioral responses to pain. Most nurses seem to have been taught to use elevated vital signs to assess or verify the presence of pain, especially severe pain. However, in a literature review, investigators found very little research that supported using physiologic manifestations as specific indicators of pain (Van Cleve, Johnson, Pothier 1996). They proceeded to study 90 infants and young children undergoing the painful procedures of venipuncture or intravenous cannulation. Heart rate, respiratory rate, and blood pressure were recorded before and immediately after the procedure. These physiologic indicators showed no significant change as a result of the painful procedure, except for the toddler group, which showed an increase in pulse rate after the procedure. They concluded that it was inappropriate to rely solely on physiologic data to measure pain.

Considerable research demonstrates that the behavioral expressions of pain that clinicians expect to see in patients are often absent. In the late 1970s investigators interviewed 102 adult patients with various types of pain, acute and chronic (Jacox, 1979). Many patients did not report pain and made strong efforts to conceal it. When the patients were asked whether they discussed pain with others, 70% said no, or they were ambivalent. When they were asked how they responded to pain, 66% said they tried to remain calm and not show pain. In another study of 45 patients with pain related to lung cancer, 42% of the patients revealed that they coped with pain by trying not to let others know about it (Wilkie, Keefe, 1991).

In a study of 3- to 7-year-old children after major surgery, findings revealed that behavior did not accurately reflect pain intensity (Beyer, McGrath, Berde, 1990). In 25 children, the behavioral responses to pain were compared with self-report of pain. Many children reported severe pain but manifested few of the expected behaviors.

Patients with pain may deliberately engage in certain behaviors that are incompatible with those of the acute pain model but are helpful in coping with pain. In a study of 13 patients with pain related to advanced cancer, the patients reported that behaviors they used to control their pain included watching television (nine patients) or chatting with family and friends (Wilkie, Lovejoy, Dodd et al., 1988). A questionnaire survey of 53 patients with chronic cancer pain asked them to identify and rate the effectiveness of the self-initiated, noninvasive pain control measures they used to cope with their pain (Fritz, 1988). Patients rated laughing as the most effective.

Sleep or sedation may be mistakenly equated with lack of pain, but even patients with severe pain may sleep. An appreciation of this is demonstrated in analgesic research. When the effectiveness of analgesics is studied, trained observers ask patients to rate their pain at specific intervals, such as every hour, after the administration of the analgesic. When the observer finds the patient asleep at the time a pain rating is required, the observer awakens the patient to obtain a pain rating (Forbes, 1991). Some patients use sleep to help control their pain (Wilkie, Lovejoy, Dodd et al., 1988). Sedation is not the same as analgesia. Many sedating drugs such as benzodiazepines and phenothiazines are given to patients with pain, but most of them provide no analgesia (see Chapter 7).

When a patient's report of pain is not accepted and acted on, an effective strategy is to ask, "Why is it so difficult to believe this patient has pain?" When the problem revolves around expecting the acute pain model to exist, the answer is likely to be, "He doesn't look like he's in pain." When you find yourself thinking this or hearing someone say it, try asking, "How would this person have to act for us to believe he has pain?" A clinician might answer that a patient in that much pain would grimace or be less active. Expecting the patient to "act like he is in pain" may lead to those behaviors and contribute to manipulative behavior and physical harm such as disability or complications from decreased function.

Cause of Pain: Known Versus Unknown Cause

When a patient reports pain and the cause clearly is established, clinicians are almost always more willing to treat the pain than when the cause of pain is in doubt. Surveys of nurses' responses to hypothetical patients who report pain show that nurses tend to attribute less intense pain when no physical pathologic condition is present (Halfens, Evers, Abu-Saad, 1990; Taylor, Skelton, Butcher, 1984) and when pain is chronic rather than acute (Burgess, 1980; Taylor, Skelton, Butcher, 1984). Also, nurses took fewer actions to relieve pain in those patients with chronic pain (Burgess, 1980).

Lack of physical evidence of pain

A previously suggested strategy for addressing clinicians' reluctance to accept a patient's report of pain is also useful here. Once again, try asking, "Why is it so difficult to believe this patient has pain?" If lack of a known physical cause is the reason, the answer is likely to be, "There's no reason for this patient to hurt." A more accurate and appropriately humble response would be, "We are unable to establish the cause of the pain. We simply don't know yet what causes it."

Statements that may help us reconsider our misconceptions include a reminder that pain is a new science and that it would be foolish of us to think that we will be able to determine the cause of all the pains that patients report. It also may be helpful to articulate the underlying thought process, which is, "We seem to be thinking that if there is pain, there is a cause. If there is a cause, we can find it. If we cannot find the cause, there is no pain." Once stated, we often began to recognize the absurdity of this idea.

Available assessment tools are not infallible and do not exhaust all possible means for determining the causes of pain. This is especially true of chronic nonmalignant pain. In a study of 60 patients with chronic pain referred to a diagnostic center, the overall rate of inaccurate or incomplete diagnosis at referral was 66.7% (Hendler, Kozikowski, 1993.) In particular, neuropathic pain, which is often severe burning or shooting pain, is not detectable with ordinary diagnostic tests because nerves, not muscles or other somatic structures, are involved.

Sometimes the physical cause of pain is known, but the pain is more intense or lasts longer than expected. In the 1980s a study examined the belief that postoperative pain subsides rapidly over the first 3 days and is negligible by the fourth day, but research did not support this. Of 88 patients on a general surgical unit, 31% had pain that persisted beyond day 4, often related to being older or to complications, such as infection. These patients typically received ineffective pain control because less potent analgesics were given (Melzack, Abbott, Zackon et al., 1987). Probably the staff believed there was no reason for the patient to hurt that much or that long.

Clearly, the cause of pain cannot always be determined. This does not mean that the pain is absent or that clinicians are entitled to ignore the patient's reports of pain. Pain is subjective, and it seems rather easy to engage in faulty reasoning about it. An analogy that may clarify our responsibility to such patients is our response to patients with objective symptoms with an unknown cause. For example, if a patient vomits, we may not know why this has occurred, but because it is objective (an undeniable symptom), we treat it anyway. The cause of the vomiting is sought, but meanwhile treatment, such as antiemetics, is provided. Pain deserves the same respect as objective symptoms.

Concern that analgesia will mask diagnostic information

For well over a century, clinicians have feared that treating pain of unknown origin will mask important diagnostic information. However, this concern is being reevaluated because research has demonstrated that much pain can be relieved during the diagnostic process without jeopardizing a diagnosis.

The American Pain Society (1992) notes that, "In cases in which the cause of acute pain is uncertain, establishing a diagnosis is a priority, but symptomatic treatment of pain should be given while the investigation is proceeding. With occasional exceptions (e.g., the initial examination of the patient with acute condition of the abdomen), it rarely is justified to defer analgesia until a diagnosis is made. In fact, a comfortable patient is better able to cooperate with diagnostic procedures" (p. 3). The American College of Emergency Physicians (1994) has published a clinical policy for the initial approach to patients presenting with a chief complaint of nontraumatic acute abdominal pain saying, "Early and appropriate use of analgesic medications is encouraged" (p. 907).

The results of two studies have shown that early administration of opioids to patients with acute abdominal pain did not alter the ability of physicians to accurately evaluate and treat patients (Attard, Corlett, Kidner et al., 1992; Burke, Mack, Coward, 1994). In fact, in one study the trend was toward more accurate diagnoses in the patients who received morphine compared with the control group who received normal saline (Burke, Mack, Coward, 1994).

Even analgesia for head injury is being reevaluated. Once ventilation has been controlled, the use of opioids and barbiturates may be beneficial in reducing cerebral oxygen requirements (Kistler, 1993). Incremental doses of opioids may be used to provide comfort and still monitor conscious level (Illingworth, Simpson, 1994). Intravenous fentanyl may be a particularly good choice because it has a minimal effect on hemodynamic parameters (Ducharme, 1994).

Questions that may help clinicians rethink the misconception that pain must be present to make a diagnosis include: "Now that we know the severity and location of the pain, how would pain relief interfere with the diagnostic process? If this patient were completely unconscious, would it be impossible to diagnose the cause of pain? Which of the diagnostic tests indicated will require that the patient be fully conscious and in pain?" Another point to remember is that analgesics do not render the patient anesthetic or comatose. Usually the pain is still present to some degree, or the dose can be adjusted so that the patient feels mild rather than severe pain. If a specific diagnosis is being investigated, such as a fracture or metastatic lesion, remind staff that the definitive diagnosis will depend on the radiographic or MRI findings, not on the continuing presence of pain.

Undertreatment in the emergency department is well documented. In a review of 198 patients admitted with a variety of acutely painful medical and surgical conditions, 56% received no analgesia (Wilson, Pendleton, 1989). Of those who did receive analgesia, more than 50% waited for more than 1 hour. In another study of patients with acute abdominal pain, more than half received no analgesia in the first 24 hours (Roughneen, Burns, Rowlands, 1986). The Canadian Association of Emergency Physicians now states that "it should be considered poor patient care not to treat pain while attempting to arrive at a diagnosis (Ducharme, 1994, p. 855).

For more than a century, medical textbooks have admonished physicians not to mask symptoms before a diagnosis is made. Medical science has progressed, however, and pain is no longer the clinician's primary diagnostic tool.

Belief that noncancer pain is not as painful as cancer pain

Even when the cause of pain is known, non-life-threatening pain is less likely to be treated than pain associated with a terminal illness. In one study of physicians treating patients with cancer, inadequate pain management was more likely when pain was not attributed to cancer (Cleeland, Gonin, Hatfield et al., 1994). Negative attitudes toward patients with low back pain have been recognized for many years (Burgess, 1980; Wiener, 1975). Disregard for noncancer pain is reflected in the statement, "It's not going to kill you. It couldn't hurt that much."

Public attitudes also reveal differing attitudes toward different types of pain. A telephone survey of 1000 Americans asked whether high doses of analgesics should be prescribed for any of these three conditions: severe chronic pain, cancer pain, and rheumatoid arthritis (The Mayday Fund, 1998). Approximately 80% supported high doses for cancer pain, approximately 70% for severe chronic pain, but only about 50% supported high doses for rheumatoid arthritis. Perhaps both the public and clinicians tend to believe that some types of pain should be tolerated or are not very painful. In any case the study reflects the tendency to provide less aggressive analgesia for noncancer pain.

However, non-life-threatening conditions can result in very intense and prolonged pain. In a survey of 204 people with chronic nonmalignant pain, respondents revealed that their average length of time in pain was 9.5 years, with a range of 6 months to 74 years (Hitchcock, Ferrell, McCaffery, 1994). They were in pain an average of 80% of the time. For 30% the usual intensity of pain was severe, with a rating of 4 to 5 out of 5.

A strategy for addressing these misconceptions about noncancer pain being less worthy of treatment is to ask, "Why are we more willing to treat pain in someone who is dying than in someone who will live, perhaps many years, with pain?" No doubt to some extent the answer involves an exaggerated fear of addiction, and this, of course, also will have to be addressed (see Chapter 10 for ideas).

Implication that anxiety or depression is the cause

When the physical cause of pain is unknown or seems insufficient to account for the severity of pain the patient reports, clinicians frequently attribute the pain to the patient's emotional state and cease treating the pain. Comments that suggest this are, "The patient is just upset" or "The pain is all in his head." Other labels, such as psychogenic pain, may be used. Interestingly, in a survey of the public's attitude toward stress and pain, 95% of respondents agreed with the statement that stress increases pain (The Mayday Fund, 1998).

Underlying such beliefs are several misconceptions. Actually, evidence that stress increases pain is limited. Also the belief that if pain is associated with an emotional or mental condition, the patient is at fault and is not deserving of treatment is mistaken.

An erroneous and simplistic view, promoted around the middle of the 20th century, was that physical and psychologic causes of pain were mutually exclusive, that is, that pain is caused by either organic or psychologic factors (IASP ad hoc Subcommittee for Psychology Curriculum, 1997). Trying to differentiate between psychogenic and physical pain is usually fruitless. Pain caused solely by psychogenic factors is rare, as is pain caused solely by physical causes. Most pain is a combination of physical and psychologic factors and is best treated a such.

Following is a discussion of the as yet unclear relationships between pain and anxiety or depression. Some of the problematic diagnoses and derogatory labels that may be assigned to patients with pain when physical findings are absent are also explored.

Relationships Between Pain and Anxiety or Depression

The International Association for the Study of Pain defines pain as "an unpleasant sensory and emotional experience which we primarily associate with tissue damage or describe in terms of such damage, or both" (Mersky, Bogduk, 1994, p. 210). By definition, pain is always unpleasant and always subjective, thus pain is always an emotional experience. But, what are the relationships between pain and various emotions? A common assumption is that anxiety or depression makes pain worse, but this is not always true.

For purposes of discussion, it is helpful to consider how anxiety and depression affect coping with pain as opposed to how they affect pain intensity. Although certain levels of anxiety are actually helpful in mobilizing appropriate coping mechanisms, high levels of anxiety and possibly any level of depression may adversely affect the patient's ability to cope with pain.

How anxiety and depression influence pain intensity, however, is an even more complicated issue. Anxiety certainly is associated with many types of pain, and depression is common in patients with chronic pain. However, the cause and effect relationship is unclear. Does anxiety cause pain or is it the result of pain? Is depression the cause or the result of pain? Some studies show a relationship between depression and pain and some do not. Likewise, anxiety has been correlated with increased pain in some studies but not in others. Anxiety unrelated to pain may actually decrease pain, possibly because the anxiety increases endorphins (Janssen, Arntz, 1996).

In a study of patients after coronary artery bypass graft surgery, the results showed that even in the range of low to moderate state anxiety, higher anxiety was associated with higher pain intensities (Nelson, Zimmerman, Barnason et al., 1998). Some studies have shown that postoperative anxiety is related to pain (Liu, Barry, Weinman, 1994). But the direction of causality has not been established.

One review of the literature found that research findings are conflicting and inconsistent regarding the relationship between depression and pain and between anxiety and pain (Zimmerman, Story, Gaston-Johansson et al., 1996). Another literature review pointed out that a high proportion of patients with chronic pain have some kind of depressive syndrome; however, the depression may precede, follow, or develop concomitantly with the chronic pain (Dellemijn, Fields, 1994). In a study of surgical patients, investigators found that preoperative anxiety was associated with greater pain postoperatively, and they pointed out that this result was consistent with some previous reports but not with others (Manyande, Salmon, 1992).

In another review of the literature investigators found little evidence that depression or anxiety is *strongly* related to pain and suggested that much more research is required to clarify these issues (McGuire, Sheidler, 1993). For example, in a study of 120 patients with cancer pain no difference was found in pain intensity measures or functional status between the depressed patients and those who were not depressed (Grossman, Sheidler, Sweeden et al., 1991). In other words, the depression associated with pain did not alter the patient's reports of the intensity of the pain. In another study of cancer patients, the presence of depression, hostility, and anxiety did not correlate with effectiveness of attempts at pain relief (Cleeland, 1984). Cleeland warns us that when patients do not respond to analgesics, clinicians should be wary of blaming this on the patient's depression rather than on inappropriate analgesic therapy.

The belief that anxiety causes pain is reflected in the common practice of combining anxiolytics and opioids. However, the findings in a study of postoperative patients who had access to IV PCA morphine and midazolam (Versed), separately, revealed that use of midazolam did not influence pain scores or amount of PCA morphine used (Egan, Ready, Nessly et al., 1992). In another study of postoperative pain, the administration of diazepam preoperatively was shown to have an ongoing antianalgesic effect on morphine analgesia (Gear, Miaskowski, Heller et al., 1997). In a double-blind study, combinations of various doses of midazolam and meperidine were administered to 150 patients with postoperative pain, and, once again, midazolam did not significantly enhance the analgesic effect of the opioid (Miller, Eisenkraft, Cohen et al., 1986).

Certainly no doubt exists that pain results in considerable distress for many patients, causing anxiety, depression, and hostility and interfering with all domains of quality of life (e.g., Ferrell, Grant, Funk et al., 1997; Zimmerman, Story, Gaston-Johansson et al., 1996). Until the relationship between pain and anxiety, depression, and other emotional states is clarified, the most practical initial approach to patients who are both in pain and anxious or depressed probably is to assume that pain causes these emotional responses rather than to assume that the emotional response causes or intensifies pain. Anxiety and depression appear to be normal responses to pain. When the patient is both in pain and anxious, initial intervention probably should be aimed at reducing the pain. This may well reduce the anxiety. Likewise, for patients who are in pain and depressed, the most logical initial approach probably is to relieve the pain, which may then reduce the depression. If anxiety or depression persists in the absence of pain, other interventions such as behavioral and pharmacologic approaches are indicated.

Psychogenic Pain and Other Labels

When no physical cause for pain can be identified, certain diagnoses or labels may be assigned to the patient. Psychogenic pain often is used as a stigmatizing label. As a diagnosis, it has become an obsolete term and is no longer listed in the DSM-IV manual (*Diagnostic and statistical manual of mental disorders,* 1994) nor in the International Association for the Study of Pain's Classification of Chronic Pain (Merskey, Bogduk, 1994). Rather, the DSM-IV describes criteria for several types of somatoform disorders such as hypochondriasis. These are disorders in which physical symptoms, such as pain, suggest the existence of a disease, but demonstrable organic or objective findings are absent. Patients do not consciously manufacture these disorders. The somatoform disorders are unintentional as opposed to malingering and factitious disorder, which are intentionally deceptive. To be diagnosed with any of these, the patient must be assessed carefully by a qualified clinician and must meet the criteria listed in the DSM-IV.

Unfortunately, the term psychogenic pain is still in common usage. Psychogenic pain "is presumed to exist when no nociceptive or neuropathic mechanism can be identified and there are sufficient psychologic symptoms to meet criteria for somatoform pain disorder, depression, or other DSM-IV diagnostic category commonly associated with complaints of pain" (Duarte, 1997, p. 6). However, it is most likely to be used as a derogatory label.

Clinicians must realize that the criteria for diagnosing somatoform disorders and those formerly used for psychogenic pain have several flaws. Diagnosing a mental disorder in a patient who reports pain for which no physical signs or neuropathic mechanisms are found is primarily a diagnosis of exclusion. In other words, the diagnosis is made simply because no other cause for the pain can be found. Pain with no underlying pathologic condition is unusual. Such diagnoses are not clinically useful because no specific therapy is suggested.

As discussed previously, the science of pain is new, and it is foolhardy to believe that all causes of pain can be identified. Pain in excess of organic pathologic processes probably is not a sound reason to diagnose a mental disorder because it is well known that pain is not proportional to tissue damage. Comparable stimuli in different people do not produce the same intensities of pain.

"Supratentorial pain" is a term that became popular on the 1990s. Supratentorial actually refers to a specific portion of the brain, and it appears to be a sophisticated term used to say that the pain is "all in the patient's head." However, it is not a recognized diagnosis and has no accepted definition. It is almost always used as a derogatory term to suggest that no physical cause for the pain exists or that the patient is lying about pain.

In a patient who reports pain, diagnosing or labeling the problem as a mental disorder also carries moral overtones, suggesting that the pain does not exist or that the patient is responsible for causing the pain. The diagnosis says that the patient is responsible for his or her suffering. This in turn relieves clinicians of the responsibility for further assessment and treatment of the problem. Saying that the patient has psychogenic pain or some other mental disorder invalidates the report of pain. This is communicated to the patient and family, as well as insurance companies, who are inclined to deny coverage for such problems.

When a the patient's pain is ascribed to a mental disorder, the questions should be asked, "Is this a label or a diagnosis?" If it is a diagnosis arrived at after careful assessment, clinicians should be mindful of the repercussions this may have for the patient, the family, the treatment plan, and insurance coverage. Diagnosis of a mental disorder in the patient with pain often has harmful consequences. Because this is a diagnosis of exclusion, meaning that it is made because no other cause could be found, clinicians must be vigilant about reassessment to determine whether any physical findings or neuropathic mechanisms can be identified.

Addiction: Seeking Drugs Versus Seeking Pain Relief

Perhaps the most common reason for not accepting and acting on a patient's report of pain is the belief that the patient is or will become addicted to an opioid/narcotic. A previously suggested strategy for addressing clinicians' reluctance to accept a patient's report of pain is to ask, "Why is it so difficult to believe this patient has pain?" Addiction is often the answer. Clinicians may say, "The patient is drug seeking," "He just wants drugs," or "He's getting addicted." At present, in many clinical settings, the term "drug seeking" is used synonymously with addiction. Although patients seek drugs for many legitimate purposes, such as treating an infection, diabetes, or heart disease, somehow the phrase drug seeking has become associated with seeking opioids for nonmedical purposes.

Questions that may be helpful in clarifying the confusion that surrounds beliefs about patients being addicted are:
- What is the definition of addiction?
- Does concern exist that use of opioids for pain relief causes addiction?

Various aspects of addiction are discussed throughout this book, particularly in Chapters 6 and 10. Some of the basic facts about addiction will be reiterated here so that the reader will not need to search for them before proceeding with the present discussion.

Definitions and likelihood of occurrence

Tolerance to opioids and physical dependence on opioids are not the same as addiction to opioids, but these three terms are often confused. Following are the definitions used by the APS (1992):
- Opioid addiction is psychologic dependence. It is "a pattern of compulsive drug use characterized by continued craving for an opioid and the need to use the opioid for effects other than pain relief" (p. 26) or for nonmedical reasons. In other words, taking opioids for pain relief is not addiction, regardless of the dose or length of time on opioids.
- Physical dependence is the occurrence of withdrawal symptoms when the opioid is suddenly stopped or an antagonist such as naloxone (Narcan) is given. Withdrawal symptoms usually are easily suppressed by gradual withdrawal of the opioid.
- Tolerance is a decrease in one or more effects of the opioid (e.g., decreased analgesia, sedation, or respiratory depression). Tolerance to analgesia may be treated with increases in dose. However, disease progression, not tolerance to analgesia, appears to be the reason for most dose escalations. Thus tolerance to analgesia poses very few clinical problems.

Each of the above is a separate entity requiring different treatment. Any one may occur alone, any two together, or all three together. Physical dependence and tolerance are a result of repeated administration of the opioid and should be expected if opioids are taken several times a day for a month or longer (APS, 1992). Addiction, however, is a rare consequence of using opioids for pain relief.

The findings of several studies have shown that addiction as a result of using opioids for pain relief occurs in less than 1% of patients. Possibly the most enlightening research in this area was conducted in the 1970s during a time when heroin was widely used as an analgesic in England. Heroin was used for a variety of types of pain, such as postoperative pain and pain associated with terminal illness. In fact, the popular "magic" mixture called Brompton Cocktail that originated in England contained heroin, cocaine, gin, and honey. It was modified and used in the United States for pain relief in terminal illness. Many clinicians are unaware that the Brompton Cocktail initially was used in England as an analgesic for postthoracotomy pain (Kerrane, 1975).

Thus the use of heroin as an analgesic was widespread in England in the 1970s. In two studies of more than

500 patients taking regular doses of heroin orally or parenterally for pain relief for weeks or months, no patients could be documented as having become addicted (Twycross, 1974; Twycross, Wald, 1976).

In a review of the literature on addiction as a consequence of taking opioid analgesics, findings revealed that more than 24,000 patients had been studied (Friedman, 1990). Yet only seven could be documented as having become addicted as a result of receiving opioids for pain relief.

The disease of addiction is complex and multicausal and occurs over time, certainly not as a result of one hospital experience. No single cause of addiction, such as taking an opioid for pain relief, has been found. However, several risk factors have been identified, such as genetic predisposition, abuse or neglect, and an environment of drug-using peers and celebrities (Cotton, 1994).

Addiction as a stigmatizing label

Unfortunately, drug abuse and addiction often are treated as crimes rather than public health problems (Cotton, 1994). Consequently, clinicians judgmentally regard addicts as bad people rather than focusing on addiction as a bad disease that requires treatment. Thus the label of addiction is stigmatizing and should be avoided. Addiction should be used only to refer to a brain disease that requires appropriate treatment.

When a patient is referred to as addicted or drug seeking, it is helpful to ask, "Has the patient been diagnosed as being an addict? If so, how does this affect our plan for pain relief?" If the patient is addicted, the patient still deserves the best possible pain relief that can safely be provided. The following position is *unethical:* I can provide safe and effective pain relief for this patient, but I will not because I do not believe the patient deserves it. (Chapter 10 and Appendix B address several approaches to pain relief in the addicted individual.)

Behaviors Mistaken as Indicators of Addiction

The focus here is on the patient who is labeled, not diagnosed, as being addicted. The patient has not been assessed appropriately for the presence of addiction, and a diagnosis of addiction probably is not written in the patient's chart. Yet clinicians may continue to refer to the patient as addicted or drug seeking. The stigmatizing label of addiction often influences the patient's pain treatment plan and other aspects of care. Clinicians may be reluctant to accept the patient's report of pain and opposed to providing pain relief.

To detect and correct this clinical situation, several questions may be explored:

- If this is a label, not a diagnosis, what has the patient done to cause us to believe he or she is drug seeking or addicted?

- Is there any other way to explain the behavior that seems to indicate drug seeking or addiction? In other words, might the patient behave in this way for some reason other than drug seeking?
- Could the patient be seeking pain relief rather than simply drugs for nonmedical use?

Some clinicians seem to believe that the addicted patient is easily identified by the presence of certain behaviors. Table 3.3 lists some of these behaviors and comments on what these behaviors may indicate other than addiction. Suggestions for remedying some problems are included. None of the behaviors listed in Table 3.3 are diagnostic of addiction. When addiction is suspected because of certain behaviors, an appropriate perspective may be to acknowledge that the behavior *may* mean addiction, but could it be something else?

Many of the suggestions and explanations included in Table 3.3 require knowledge about opioid analgesia, discussed in detail in Chapter 6. In that chapter the management of PCA, equianalgesic dosing, opioid naive versus opioid tolerant, and principles of titrating opioid analgesics are explained.

Other comments in Table 3.3 revolve around some complex issues that will be discussed here. These include clinicians accepting the responsibility for developing effective pain treatment plans and patients resisting changes in the analgesic treatment plan.

Blaming the Patient Instead of the Treatment Plan

Research has established that many clinicians lack knowledge about the principles of analgesic use (Chapter 1). No doubt this is a major reason that clinicians fail to assume responsibility for developing and tailoring pain treatment plans in some of the patient situations described in Table 3.3. Clinicians may believe that the pain relief provided for the patient should be effective. When it is not, clinicians tend to blame the patient rather than the treatment plan. For example, the patient who is a "clock watcher" probably should have a longer acting opioid or the interval between doses should be changed—the patient should not be blamed for trying to make the best of inadequate analgesia. Likewise, the patient should not be blamed for hitting the PCA button frequently. Rather, the bolus dose and/or lockout interval should be adjusted so that the patient need not push the button so often. Patients who receive inadequate analgesia in the emergency department (ED) or from a physician should not be blamed for seeking help elsewhere. For many patients, improving the pain treatment plan would negate the need to go to other physicians or EDs.

"Frequent flyers," or heavy users of the ED, are often regarded as problem patients. However, they tend to be a vulnerable population. In a study of 46 heavy ED users in two West Coast inner-city trauma center hospitals, findings revealed that many were homeless, poor, or

TABLE 3.3 ● ● ● ● ●

Misconceptions Behaviors Indicating Addiction	
BEHAVIORS THAT ARE OFTEN MISTAKEN AS INDICATORS OF ADDICTION	CORRECTION/COMMENTS—WHAT ELSE COULD IT BE?
1. The patient requests analgesics by name, dose, interval between doses, and/or route of administration e.g., "I'll need two Vicodin every 4 hours." "Morphine, 10 mg IV, works best for my headache."	This is likely to be a well-educated patient who probably has had pain previously or has chronic pain. Patients need to be educated about all their medications, including analgesics. If this patient were a diabetic talking about insulin requirements, it would be welcomed information. This patient is providing helpful information for the pain treatment plan.
2. The patient is "a frequent flyer," frequently visiting several emergency departments (EDs) to obtain opioid analgesics.	This is not desirable behavior, but it may be caused by inadequate pain treatment. If treatment at the ED results in poor pain relief or if staff convey that the patient comes too often, the patient may go to another ED for additional pain relief or to decrease the frequency of visits to a single ED. 　　The patient may have a chronic pain problem that is not well managed by the private physician, so the patient is forced to seek help in the ED. 　　If patients return often to the ED, a plan should be developed and on file to document previous assessments, the effectiveness of treatments, and recommendations for initiating pain relief on subsequent ED visits.
3. Patient obtains opioids from more than one physician.	This is not desirable behavior, but like the above, may reflect poor pain management. For example, a patient's physician may prescribe an opioid/nonopioid oral analgesic (e.g., Percocet or Tylenol No. 3). The patient may find that one dose in the morning effectively relieves his pain and helps him get moving so that he can work through the day. If the physician refuses to prescribe more than 30 tablets every 3 months and suggests no other methods of pain relief, the patient may seek drugs from another physician. 　　Improved assessment and pain treatment, including use of nonopioids and other modalities, may remedy this situation.
4. The patient requires higher doses of opioids than other patients. "He's hitting his PCA button too much."	There is no set dose of opioid that is safe and effective for all patients. Even a patient who has not received opioids regularly (opioid naive) may require 6 times more opioid than another patient. A patient who is tolerant to opioid analgesia may require 100 times more opioid than the opioid naive patient. 　　Some conditions, such as sickle cell crisis, are more painful than others. A patient may require much more opioid for a sickle cell crisis than for major abdominal surgery. 　　Frequent use of the PCA button indicates that the pump parameters need to be adjusted.
5. The patient has been taking opioids frequently.for a long time.	Length of time on opioids does not appear to increase the likelihood of developing addiction. Many patients with cancer or noncancer pain have taken opioids for months or longer and ceased taking them when the pain subsided. Physical dependence and tolerance may develop with prolonged use, but they are not the same as addiction.
6. The patient is a "clock watcher" and may ask for the analgesic in advance of a specified time. The patient may say, "I'll need my next dose in about 30 minutes."	Sometimes analgesics are prescribed at intervals longer than their duration. When the patient asks for a dose before the interval elapses, the clinician often tells the patient how much time he must wait. For example, "You can't have your next pill for 2 hours." Because the patient must wait in pain for 2 hours, he is likely to note the time and ask for the medication as soon as the 2 hours pass. The patient may then find that it takes the nurse another 30 minutes to deliver the dose. The patient may work with these realities by calculating when the next dose can be given and asking for it 30 minutes in advance. 　　This situation strongly suggests that the patient's opioid prescription should be changed to a longer acting opioid or the intervals between doses should be shortened.

TABLE 3.3—cont'd ● ● ● ● ●

Misconceptions	Behaviors Indicating Addiction

BEHAVIORS THAT ARE OFTEN MISTAKEN AS INDICATORS OF ADDICTION	CORRECTION/COMMENTS—WHAT ELSE COULD IT BE?
7. The patient "prefers the needle to the pill."	When the same dose given parenterally is given orally, the pain relief is likely to be much less. Using an equianalgesic chart often explains the problem. For example, if a patient has been receiving morphine, 10 mg IM or IV q4h, switching the patient to an opioid/nonopioid combination, such as one Tylenol No. 3, provides only ⅙ to ⅕ as much pain relief. The solution may be to use a single entity oral opioid such as morphine. A dose of 30 mg will provide approximately the same pain relief. If pain has decreased by 50%, morphine, 15 mg PO, is indicated.
8. The patient "enjoys his Demerol."	Once pain is relieved, it is natural for the patient to feel happier and engage in more activities such as talking and ambulating. By contrast, it may look like the patient is "high" or euphoric, but it is simply a return to normal mood, perhaps with some elation at being in less pain.
9. The patient says he is allergic to everything except one particular opioid.	Allergy to opioids is rare, but patients often mistake side effects such as nausea, vomiting, and itching for an allergy. These may have been poorly managed side effects, or the patient may have more severe side effects with some opioids than others. If the patient has more side effects with certain opioids, they should be avoided. If the patient is more convinced of the effectiveness of one opioid over others, it is possible that the patient will try to avoid the others by saying he is allergic to them. Even when an analgesic is not terribly effective, the patient may be afraid to try another analgesic for fear the results will be even worse. If it is not necessary for the patient to change to another opioid, the patient should receive what he prefers. If a change is necessary, perhaps because the opioid preferred by the patient has an active metabolite that is accumulating (a common problem with meperidine), then selection of another opioid will depend on careful assessment to determine whether the patient is allergic or whether he has experienced unmanaged or unmanageable side effects.

May be duplicated for use in clinical practice. From McCaffery M, Pasero C: *Pain: Clinical manual*, pp. 52-53. Copyright © 1999, Mosby, Inc. See text for references.

disabled (Malone, 1996). Many had no family and most had one or more chronic medical problems.

Some heavy users of the ED are seeking treatment for pain, and, if they visit the ED frequently, it is likely that they have a chronic pain condition. Migraine headache, sickle cell crisis, and flares of low back pain are common. Planning for the next visit is far more practical than feeling angry with the patient when he or she returns. Once again, a carefully developed treatment plan will greatly facilitate the patient's care and discourage the tendency to blame the patient for having a chronic problem.

An example of an innovative approach to the care of "frequent flyers" is the use of a "passport" document (small booklet or plasticized card) for patients with frequent sickle cell crises. The booklet summarizes the initial comprehensive clinical assessment and contains a written pain treatment plan that has been developed and agreed on by patient, family, and caregivers (Beyer, Platt, Kinney et al., 1994). The ED also may develop and have on file a protocol or individualized treatment plan for other patients who are seen regularly (Nichols, 1996).

Such treatment plans help clinicians realize the vast differences in opioid requirements. For identical painful problems, some patients will require six or more times what other patients require (American Pain Society, 1992). For certain types of pain, such as sickle cell crisis, a patient may require twice the dose for a crisis as that same patient requires for postoperative pain (Shapiro, Cohen, Howe, 1991).

Recognizing the limits of what can be done to help certain patients may enable clinicians to be less impatient and frustrated. It is not too surprising that vulnerable populations of patients, such as the homeless, disabled, or poor, might not follow up on prescribed treatment or suggestions to obtain additional help or to seek it from clinics or places other than the ED.

Patients Who Resist a New Treatment Plan

Oddly enough, developing and improving on a patient's analgesic treatment plan is sometimes met with resistance from the patient. This seems to be especially true of the patient who has had pain for a number of years. Unfortunately, this further reinforces the idea that the patient must be addicted.

For example, the patient may insist on receiving IM meperidine, a drug and route that are not recommended because of the active metabolite that may accumulate and the fibrosis caused by IM administration (APS 1992). The patient may even acknowledge that the IM meperidine did not provide adequate pain relief and muscles are now so hardened that it is difficult to find a place to inject the medication. To improve the safety and effectiveness of analgesia, the clinician may wish to substitute morphine or hydromorphone by the IV route. The new drug and route will provide more rapid onset of analgesia, the ability to titrate the dose upward more quickly, and less pain on administration. Yet, even after this is explained, the patient may adamantly refuse this option.

Why would a patient refuse a better method of pain relief? An obvious answer is that the patient may not believe that the new approach is in fact any better. The patient's reaction is a product of past experiences with clinicians. Patients with chronic pain often have been accused by clinicians of lying, drug seeking, and being at fault for having the pain. Trust has been eroded. New treatments are viewed with suspicion. Change is frightening, especially at a time of stress such as needing relief for sudden, severe pain. The patient may feel much safer with a previous, although not very effective, method of pain relief, rather than risking worse pain relief from an unfamiliar method.

Another interesting possibility is that patients become conditioned to experience pain relief from specific, complex set of stimuli. The way the drug is administered, such as rapid IV push versus continuous infusion, or the nonanalgesic effects of the drug, such as a certain type of mental clouding or heaviness in the chest, may be strongly associated in the patient's mind with experiencing pain relief. A new method of pain relief may be effective but may not feel like previously experienced pain relief. The patient may have difficulty trusting or adjusting to this new feeling. Switching drugs or changing some other aspect of analgesia may, in a sense, require the patient to learn to associate an entirely new set of circumstances with experiencing pain relief.

Patience and understanding are required to help patients make changes in well-established analgesic approaches. New pain relief methods are best introduced in the absence of stress and pain. Providing pain relief by the method preferred by the patient and then discussing changes in the treatment plan is apt to be met with more patient acceptance.

Pain Relief From Placebos

A placebo may be defined as any medication or procedure, including surgery, that produces an effect in a patient because of its implicit or explicit intent and not because of its specific physical or chemical properties. An example is a saline injection for analgesia. When the patient responds to a placebo in accordance with its intent, this is called a positive placebo response.

Placebos are often used as a control in preliminary research into the effects of a new medication. New drugs are compared with placebos and must demonstrate more favorable effects than placebos to warrant further investigation or marketing of the drug. In such studies patients or volunteers are informed of the nature of the project and told that a placebo may be given along with other medications. To be included in the study, the person must give informed consent. Unfortunately, placebos may be used clinically in a deceitful manner without informed consent.

Misconceptions about the meaning of a positive placebo response

Sometimes when the question is asked, "Why is it so difficult to believe this patient has pain?" the answer is that the patient reported satisfactory pain relief from a placebo. Pain relief from a placebo is mistakenly believed to invalidate the patient's report of pain.

Common misconceptions about pain relief from a placebo are that the patient is malingering (lying about pain) or the pain is "psychogenic" rather than physical in origin. The fallacy of this is apparent in the results of research using placebos as controls in the evaluation of potential analgesic drugs. Beginning in the 1950s, numerous placebo-controlled analgesic studies were conducted with postoperative patients. Thus we know the answer to this question: What percentage of patients will report adequate relief of pain from a placebo injection the day after abdominal surgery? The answer commonly quoted is 36% (Evans, 1974; Goodwin, Goodwin, Vogel, 1979), although no fixed percentage of the population responds to placebos (Wall, 1994).

If about one third of patients who have obvious physical stimuli for pain (abdominal surgery) report pain relief after a placebo injection, clearly placebos cannot be used to diagnose malingering, psychogenic pain, or any psychologic problem. Quite simply, all we can conclude is that sometimes placebos are effective in relieving moderate to severe pain of known physical origin.

Although it is well documented that positive placebo responses occur, *why* placebos relieve pain remains poorly understood. Many theories have been proposed, including operant conditioning, faith, anxiety reduction, and endorphin release (Grevert, Albert, Goldstein, 1983; Levine, Gordon, Fields, 1978; Richardson, 1994). Yet, none has been proved and the mystery remains.

Misconceptions about using placebos for pain relief

Because placebos do provide pain relief in a rather large portion of patients, why wouldn't they be a legitimate option for pain relief? One reason placebos are not appropriate as pain treatment is that a positive placebo response cannot be predicted in an individual, and a placebo may be effective at one time and not another. It is important, however, to distinguish between the placebo and the placebo effect. Although deceitful use of placebos is not recommended, efforts to enhance legitimate therapies with positive placebo effects is encouraged (Brody, 1997). This may be as simple as saying to the patient when an injection of morphine is administered, "This medication usually is a very effective way to relieve pain, and we can adjust it as necessary." Placebo effects occur with both inert substances such as saline injections and with proven analgesics such as opioids.

Another reason for not using placebos for pain relief is that they may produce harm as well as benefit. Research shows that placebos may mimic active drugs, produce side effects and toxic reactions, worsen symptoms (negative placebo effects), and directly affect many body organs (Lavin, 1991; Wolf, Pinsky, 1954). In pain management, placebos are most likely to be suggested as a substitute for an opioid analgesic opposed to a nonopioid or adjuvant analgesic. However, substituting a placebo for an opioid cannot be justified on the basis of avoiding side effects such as sedation or preventing addiction.

Unfortunately, placebos are most likely to be used in patients that the staff regards as difficult. The most extensive study of placebo use was undertaken in the 1970s (Goodwin, Goodwin, Vogel, 1979). Researchers surveyed placebo knowledge and use among 60 physicians and 39 nurses in a university teaching hospital. Most of the physicians (78%) had ordered a placebo, and most of the nurses (82%) had administered one. The reasons given for administering placebos revolved around proving the patient "wrong" and treating patients who were disliked, who did not obtain pain relief from standard treatment, or who had frustrated or angered the staff. Not only does this deceitful use of placebos in place of appropriate therapy violate patients' rights to the highest quality of care possible, it clearly poses a moral, ethical, and professional danger to the clinicians.

Perhaps the most important reason for not using placebos in the assessment and treatment of pain is that deception is involved. The clinician lies to the patient. Deceit is harmful to both patients and health care professionals. When discovered (and it usually is), it may permanently damage the patient's trust in health care professionals.

Legal and ethical considerations involved in the deceitful use of placebos in pain management include liability for fraud, malpractice, breach of contract, and medical negligence (Fox, 1994). Nurses should examine their nurse practice acts and the policies of their state boards of registered nursing for guidance. For example, in 1997, the Board of Registered Nursing in California specifically stated that the use "of placebos for management of pain would not fulfill informed consent parameters" (p. 12).

Placebo use violates the rights of all patients who receive them outside the context of an approved clinical trial in which the patient has given informed consent to participate. Even under these circumstances placebo use may not be justified when the study drug could be evaluated by comparing it with an effective medication instead of a placebo (Rothman, Michels, 1994).

There are no individuals and no conditions for which placebos are the recommended treatment. Literature review shows no basis for the assumption that placebo pain medication is useful to patients (Kleinman, Brown, Librach, 1994). Therefore the use of a placebo inevitably deprives the patient of more appropriate methods of assessment or treatment. In other words, a better way to assess and treat the patient with pain than to administer a placebo always exists.

Recommendations against the use of placebos

Avoidance of deceitful use of placebos is unanimously recommended in current clinical practice guidelines for pain management issued by the American Pain Society and the Agency for Health Care Policy and Research:

- "Do not use placebos to assess the nature of pain" and "The deceptive use of placebos and the misinterpretation of the placebo response to discredit the patient's pain report are unethical and should be avoided." (APS, 1992, p. 25)
- "Placebos should not be used in the management of cancer pain." (Jacox, Carr, Payne et al., 1994b, p. 17)

Nursing organizations have issued placebo policy statements that strongly recommend against the use of placebos in pain management. The first position statement was developed by the Oncology Nursing Society (ONS) (McCaffery, Ferrell, Turner, 1996). Soon after, 27 or more professional organizations, such as the National Association of Orthopaedic Nurses, endorsed the statement. The ONS position statement focuses on patients with diagnoses of cancer, but the article accompanying its publication verifies that the facts and ethical issues presented are equally applicable to other patients with pain regardless of their diagnoses.

The American Society of Pain Management Nurses (ASPMN) has adopted a position statement on placebo use that is similar to that of ONS, the primary difference being that the opposition to placebo use in pain management applies to all patients regardless of age or diagnosis. Box 3.3 summarizes the key elements of these position statements and provides information about how

● ● ● ● ●
BOX 3.3

Position Statements on the Use of Placebos for Pain Management

1. The Oncology Nursing Society's (ONS) position statement says:
   "Placebos should not be used
   1) To assess or manage cancer pain
   2) To determine if the pain is "real"
   3) To diagnose psychological symptoms, such as anxiety associated with pain
   Nurses should not administer placebos in these circumstances even if there is a medical order."

2. The American Society of Pain Management Nurses' (ASPMN) position statement says:
   The organization "adamantly opposes the use of placebos in the assessment and treatment of pain in all patients."

Copies of placebo position statements may be obtained by writing or calling:

ASPMN
7794 Grow Drive
Pensacola, FL 32514
(888) 34ASPMN ([888] 342-7766)
(850) 473-0233
Fax: (850) 484-8762

ONS
501 Holiday Drive
Pittsburgh, PA 15220-2749
(412) 921-7373
Fax: (412) 921-6565

Mayday Pain Resource Center (Example of placebo policy is also available)
City of Hope Medical Center
1500 E. Duarte Road
Duarte, CA 91010
(626) 359-8111, ext 3829
Fax: (626) 301-8941

May be duplicated for use in clinical practice. From McCaffery M, Pasero C: *Pain: Clinical manual,* p. 56. Copyright © 1999, Mosby, Inc.

to obtain copies along with other information pertaining to placebos.

Institutional policies about placebos

For the protection of patients and staff, written institutional policies about placebo use appear to be essential. The current frequency of deceitful placebo use in the assessment and treatment of pain is unknown, but it undoubtedly exists. Articles on this topic regularly appear in current professional literature, and misunderstandings persist (Fox, 1994; Fox, McCaffery, Ferrell et al., 1995; Haddad, 1993; Kleinman, Brown, Librach, 1994; McCaffery, Ferrell, 1994a; McCaffery, Ferrell, 1997b; McCaffery, Ferrell, Pasero, 1998; McCaffery, Pasero, 1995; Oh, 1994; Wall, 1993).

Surveys of nurses reveal that they are susceptible to becoming a part of deceitful placebo use. Surveys completed by nurses ($n = 601$) during 1995 revealed that a high percentage of these nurses exhibited a high level of readiness to participate in deceitful placebo use (McCaffery, Ferrell, 1996b). About one out of five nurses (19%) thought pain was a clinical problem for which placebos could be used. Even more respondents (27%) endorsed placebo use for anxiety. Twenty-five percent believed placebos were appropriate in patients whose symptoms (e.g. pain) were questionable. Clearly, if a placebo were suggested or prescribed, many nurses would participate in the action.

All hospitals and other health care agencies need a written policy that addresses unethical placebo use. When policies are in place, communication between health care providers is less difficult. If a physician prescribes a placebo, the nurse may use the existing placebo policy as a point of departure for communicating concerns about the patient's quality of care and for explaining why a nurse will not administer a placebo, even when a physician's order exits. A summary of key points about placebo use in pain management is found in Box 3.4.

Implications for Clinical Practice

The preceding discussion of misconceptions and misunderstandings that cause clinicians to doubt a patient's report of pain and refuse to take action to relieve pain covers only a few of many biases that may lead to inadequate pain management. Not only do many other misconceptions and biases exist, but some of them are well hidden from consciousness and very difficult to correct. Examples of hidden biases are provided below, followed by discussion of what may be done to protect patients from often unintentional, but nevertheless, inadequate pain management.

Hidden biases and other misconceptions

Biases and misconceptions that lead to inadequate pain management are not new. They are evident in recent history. In the late 1800s many physicians and scientists believed that cultural and intellectual development were accompanied by an increased sensitivity to pain (de Moulin, 1979). In 1892, Mitchell said, "The savage does not feel pain as we do." Mitchell suggested that increased capacity for feeling pain began at the end of the 18th century. Van den Berg (1963) was more exact, stating that pain sensitivity increased between 1780 and 1845. Racial and class prejudices were also apparent. In the Old South of the 1700s and 1800s, blacks were considered insensitive to pain and underwent limb amputation without anesthesia. However, upper-class white women were believed to have "delicate nerves," and the same surgeon would use ether or chloroform to deliver a baby (Pernick, 1985). No doubt many of these physicians believed that they were practicing medicine in professionally and ethically acceptable ways. Clinicians today

● ● ● ● ●

| BOX 3.4 | **Key Points About Placebo Use in Pain Management** |

1. Placebos can be effective in relieving pain, but this does not justify their use. On average, one third of patients who have obvious physical stimuli for pain (e.g., surgery) may report pain relief after administration of a placebo. However, a positive response varies between and within individuals and, therefore, cannot be predicted.
2. No medical conditions exist for which placebos are recommended as a method of assessment or treatment.
   a. Placebos cannot be used to diagnose malingering, psychogenic pain, or any psychologic problem.
   b. Use of placebos for pain relief does not prevent addiction to opioids.
   c. Placebo use deprives the patient of appropriate treatment or diagnostic measures.
3. Institutional policies that restrict the use of placebos to approved clinical trials in which informed consent is obtained are necessary not only to protect patients, but also to protect nurses and other staff from moral, ethical, and legal concerns.
   a. Placebos tend to be used in vulnerable patient populations (e.g., those with substance abuse or with pain that is difficult to diagnose or treat). This constitutes a dual standard of care.
   b. Deceitful placebo use endangers the patient's trust in caregivers and violates the patient's rights.
   c. Deceitful use of placebos violates informed consent and constitutes medical negligence, placing caregivers in a litigious position.
   d. Resorting to deceitful placebo use prevents caregivers from increasing their knowledge of more effective ways to assess and to treat pain.
   e. Deceit threatens the professional caregiver's own integrity.

May be duplicated for use in clinical practice. From McCaffery M, Pasero C: *Pain: Clinical manual*, p. 57. Copyright © 1999, Mosby, Inc.

believe the same thing, but what will be said of our pain management practices in the year 2099?

Do we know when our biases are showing? Following is a very brief overview of research findings related to some misconceptions that are likely to escape conscious awareness, but influence clinical practice:

- *Physical appearance.* Physicians infer more pain in unattractive patients and those who express pain (e.g., facial expression); they infer less pain in attractive patients and those who do not express pain (Hadjistavropoulos, Ross, von Baeyer, 1990).
- *Gender.* Workups by physicians in response to five common types of pain, including back pain, headache, and chest pain, were found to be significantly more extensive for men than they were for women (Armitage, Schneiderman, Bass, 1979). In a study of cancer patients, inadequate pain management was more likely in females than males (Cleeland, Gonin, Hatfield et al., 1994). Using vignettes of patients with surgical pain, nurses' medication choices

for men and women were compared, revealing that nurses were significantly more likely to undertreat pain in women than men (Cohen, 1980). However, gender biases are not always predictable. In one study of patients with chronic nonmalignant pain, men were no more likely than women to receive opioids (Turk, Okifuji, 1997).

The gender of the clinician may further complicate assessment. In one laboratory study, men reported significantly less pain to female experimenters than to male experimenters (Levine, De Simone, 1991).

- *Age.* In a study of 56 men age 65 and older undergoing major elective surgery, 16 received no parenteral postoperative analgesics (Short, Burnett, Egbert et al., 1990). The misconception that infants do not feel pain is longstanding. An analysis of 40 publications revealed that 77% of newborns undergoing surgical ligation of patent ductus arteriosus received no anesthesia, only muscle relaxants alone or with intermittent nitrous oxide (Anand, Sippell, Aynsley-Green, 1987). On the basis of vignette research, reports of severe pain are more likely to be accepted from elderly than young adult patients, but the elderly are less likely to receive an adequate dose of opioid analgesic (McCaffery, Ferrell, 1991b).
- *Race/culture.* In a survey of an ED in a large teaching hospital, Hispanic patients were twice as likely as non-Hispanic whites to receive *no* analgesia (Todd, Samaroo, Hoffman, 1993). In a study of outpatients with metastatic cancer treated at 54 treatment locations, patients seen at centers treating predominantly minorities were three times more likely than those treated elsewhere to have inadequate pain management (Cleeland, Gonin, Hatfield et al., 1994). In other words, at centers treating predominantly minorities, cancer patients were found to be three times more likely to have inadequate pain management (Cleeland, Gonin, Hatfield et al., 1994). In a study of outpatients with cancer pain, 65% of minority patients did not receive appropriate analgesic prescriptions for their pain compared with 50% of nonminority patients (Cleeland, Gonin, Baez et al., 1997). Hispanic patients in particular were less likely to experience adequate analgesia.

  In a study of 454 patients with postoperative pain receiving IV PCA opioids, the amount of opioid prescribed for Asians, blacks, Hispanics, and whites differed, with blacks and whites being prescribed more analgesic than Hispanics. No differences were found among these groups as to the amount of opioid self-administered (Ng, Dimsdale, Rollnik et al., 1996).
- *Personal experience with pain.* In a study of vignette descriptions of patients, nurses who had experienced

intense pain inferred higher levels of pain in patients than nurses who had not experienced intense pain (Holm, Cohen, Dudas et al., 1989).

- *"Irresponsible" lifestyle.* In a vignette survey nurses answers about assessments and analgesic choices for a patient described as a risk taker, consumer of alcohol, and unemployed were compared with their responses to a patient described as typically middle-class (McCaffery, Ferrell, O'Neil-Page, 1992). The nurses said they themselves would provide the same care for both patients, but they believed their colleagues would treat the patients differently, tending to disbelieve and undertreat the "irresponsible" patient. Nurses revealed they did not want personal values to interfere with their quality of care but they needed assistance (e.g., permission to say they do not like a certain patient and discussion about how to prevent this from interfering with care).

On a lighter note, to summarize these and other misconceptions, the following is what we could teach the patient to do, if possible, to increase the chances of clinicians accepting the patient's report of pain and providing pain relief: grimace, limp, report pain that is consistent with the diagnosis, report only minimal anxiety and depression, look elderly but hardy, do not admit to drug use of any kind, look unattractive, select clinicians who have had severe pain themselves, and beware of being female, an infant, or from an ethnic minority.

Protection for patients with pain

It is foolish to believe that we provide an equally high quality of care for all of our patients with pain regardless of our personal values, preferences, or painful experiences. All of us have many conscious and unconscious biases and misconceptions that may adversely affect the care we provide for patients with pain.

This sounds like a harsh judgment of mankind, but it may be true. A veritable mountain of literature over the past two decades attests to the undertreatment of pain. Much of this literature is consistent with the hypothesis that human beings, including the health care providers in all societies, have a strong tendency or motivation to deny or discount pain, especially severe pain, and to avoid relieving the pain. Certainly we should struggle to identify and correct personal tendencies that lead to inadequate pain management, but this may not be a battle that can be won. Perhaps it is best to assume that there are far too many biases to overcome and that the best strategy is to establish policies and procedures that protect patients and ourselves from being victims of these influences. Following are some simple tools that can be made mandatory in clinical practice as one way to hold clinicians accountable for assessing and treating pain.

ASSESSMENT TOOLS

Traditionally, asking patients about pain has been avoided. For example, as a profession, nursing has been charged for well over a century with bringing comfort to the patient. At the same time, nurses were cautioned not discuss the patient's condition with the patient and to divert the patient's attention away from illness (McIlveen, Morse, 1995).

Fear of causing pain by suggesting the possibility of pain or fear of increasing pain by focusing the patient's attention on it are but a few of the reasons given for not discussing pain. However, no studies have shown that asking the patient about pain increases the pain. A literature review resulted in the conclusion that when patients attend to and rate their pain levels, this usually lowers, not raises, the pain level (Cruise, Broderick, Porter et al., 1996). To explore this, these researchers asked patients with chronic rheumatoid arthritis to complete pain diaries for 1 week, rating their pain and mood seven times a day. The findings did not indicate that this intense self-assessment of pain increased pain, but pain was not lessened either.

No doubt questioning the patient about pain also has been avoided because it might identify a pain problem that the clinician did not know how to handle or was fearful of relieving. The clinician might fear that opioids would be necessary and that use of them would cause addiction or death by respiratory depression. "How are you feeling today?" is still about as close as many clinicians get to assessing pain. As one nurse explained, "I find it hard to talk about pain. I think it's the fear of stirring something up . . . If you're really going to talk about pain, you have to be able to handle things properly" (de Schepper, Francke, Abu-Saad, 1997, p. 425).

Thus routine assessment of pain is a relatively new idea and is recognized as essential in the prevention of inadequate pain relief. Following are practical tools for initial and ongoing assessments that may be used to facilitate regular pain assessment in a variety of clinical settings.

Tools for Initial Pain Assessment
Nursing admission assessment

When patients are admitted to a health care facility, such as a hospital or an outpatient clinic, nurses perform a general admission assessment. Along with other information such as the patient's self-care abilities and nutritional needs, a section should be included to identify pain problems. Patients may have chronic pain conditions for which they are already receiving treatment, or pain may be the primary reason for admission. Examples of questions that are appropriate for routine admission assessment tools are in Box 3.5.

BOX 3.5	**Questions About Pain to Be Included in the Routine Nursing Admission Assessment**

Do you have any ongoing pain problems? ____ Yes ____ No
Do you have pain now? ____ Yes ____ No
If yes to either of the above:
Location of pain: _____ (body figure drawing similar to the one in Form 3.1 may be included in the assessment form to mark location of pain)
Pain intensity on a scale of 0 to 10:
  Now: _____
  On average (usual): _____
  What, if any, medications do you take for pain relief?
  _____
  What, if any, other treatment do you receive for your pain? _____
  Is your pain satisfactorily controlled now? _____

NOTE: If a pain problem is identified and is not under satisfactory control, completion of a more comprehensive pain assessment tool, such as Forms 3.1 or 3.2, may be indicated.

May be duplicated for use in clinical practice. From McCaffery M, Pasero C: *Pain: Clinical manual*, p. 59. Copyright © 1999, Mosby, Inc.

The purpose of these questions is to identify new or ongoing pain problems. If a pain problem is ongoing and the patient already has an effective pain treatment plan, steps should be taken to ensure that this plan is continued. If a treatment plan needs to be developed, further assessment using the Initial Pain Assessment Tool (Form 3.1) or the Brief Pain Inventory (BPI) (Form 3.2) may be indicated.

Tools for initial overall pain assessment

Two tools widely used for overall initial pain assessments are referred to as Initial Pain Assessment Tool (see Form 3.1) and the BPI (see Form 3.2). Both of these are included in the cancer pain clinical guidelines published by the Agency for Health Policy and Research (Jacox, Carr, Payne et al., 1994a). These tools may be completed by the patient or the clinician. Another overall pain assessment tool often used in research and clinical practice is the short-form McGill Pain Questionnaire (Melzack, 1987).

These pain assessment tools need not be used for all patients with pain. The policies and procedures of a health care agency need to identify criteria for when these tools should be considered. Certainly if the patient has a chronic pain problem that is not satisfactorily controlled, an overall pain assessment tool should be completed. Hospices and pain treatment centers may need far more extensive initial overall assessment tools than those offered here. For patients with acute pain that is not easily controlled with the usual pain treatments (e.g., IV PCA following surgery), an overall assessment also is indicated.

Both the Initial Pain Assessment Tool and the BPI, described below, attempt to assess some aspects of suffering. Suffering, like pain, is subjective, but it goes beyond simply feeling pain. Pain may exist without suffering. Suffering eludes definition but has been characterized as an individual's experience of threat to self, a meaning given to events such as pain or loss (Kahn, Steeves, 1996). Suffering involves the person's evaluation of the significance or meaning of pain (Spross, 1993). To some extent suffering is similar to an impairment in quality of life. Items on the assessment tools directed at the effect of pain on various aspects of living are an attempt to assess the extent to which the patient suffers with pain.

Initial Pain Assessment Tool

The Initial Pain Assessment tool (Form 3.1) guides the clinician in collecting information about the patient's pain. A discussion of each assessment point follows:

1. *Location of pain.* This is most easily and quickly accomplished by asking the patient to mark the location on the figure drawings. Or, the clinician may ask the patient to point on his or her own body to the location of pain, and the clinician can mark the figure drawing. If there is more than one site of pain, letters (A, B, C, etc.) may be used to distinguish the different sites. These letters may be used in answering the remainder of the questions.

2. *Intensity.* The pain rating scale used by the patient is identified. The patient is asked to rate pain intensity for present pain, worst pain, best pain gets, and acceptable level of pain. If the patient has more than one site of pain, the letter designations mentioned above simplify recording. For example, for present pain intensity, the recording might be A = 4, B = 6. A time period may be specified for answering the next questions about pain intensity. For example, worst pain intensity may be asked in relation to the last 24 hours or the last week.

3. *Quality of pain.* This is helpful in diagnosing the underlying pain mechanism. Soreness is often more indicative of somatic pain, whereas burning or knifelike is more indicative of neuropathic pain. This information may have direct implications for the type of pain treatment chosen. For example, an anticonvulsant (an adjuvant analgesic, see Chapter 7) may be indicated for knifelike pain.

   If the patient has difficulty describing the pain, the clinician should ask the patient about the appropriateness of possible descriptors such as throbbing, shooting, sharp, cramping, aching, tender, pricking, burning, and pulling. For patients who continue to have difficulty, try asking the patient, "What could you do to me to make me feel the pain you have?"

4. *Onset, duration, variations, rhythms.* To detect variations and rhythms, ask the patient, "Is the pain better or

Text continued on p. 62.

Date _____

Patient's Name _____ Age _____ Room _____

Diagnosis _____ Physician _____

Nurse _____

1. LOCATION: Patient or nurse mark drawing.

2. INTENSITY: Patient rates the pain. Scale used _____

   Present: _____
   Worst pain gets: _____
   Best pain gets: _____
   Acceptable level of pain: _____

3. QUALITY: (Use patient's own words, e.g., prick, ache, burn, throb, pull, sharp) _____
   _____

4. ONSET, DURATION, VARIATIONS, RHYTHMS: _____
   _____

5. MANNER OF EXPRESSING PAIN: _____
   _____
   _____

6. WHAT RELIEVES THE PAIN? _____
   _____
   _____

7. WHAT CAUSES OR INCREASES THE PAIN? _____
   _____
   _____

8. EFFECTS OF PAIN: (Note decreased function, decreased quality of life.)
   Accompanying symptoms (e.g., nausea) _____
   Sleep _____
   Appetite _____
   Physical activity _____
   Relationship with others (e.g., irritability) _____
   Emotions (e.g., anger, suicidal, crying) _____
   Concentration _____
   Other _____

9. OTHER COMMENTS: _____
   _____

10. PLAN: _____
    _____

FORM 3.2 **Brief Pain Inventory**

Date _____ / _____ / _____   Time: _____

Name: _____ _____ _____
　　　　　　　 Last　　　　　　 First　　　　 Middle Initial

1) Throughout our lives, most of us have had pain from time to time (such as minor headaches, sprains, and toothaches). Have you had pain other than these everyday kinds of pain today?
   1. Yes　　2. No

2) On the diagram, shade in the areas where you feel pain. Put an X on the area that hurts the most.

3) Please rate your pain by circling the one number that best describes your pain at its **worst** in the past 24 hours.

0	1	2	3	4	5	6	7	8	9	10
No pain									Pain as bad as you can imagine	

4) Please rate your pain by circling the one number that best describes your pain at its **least** in the past 24 hours.

0	1	2	3	4	5	6	7	8	9	10
No pain									Pain as bad as you can imagine	

5) Please rate your pain by circling the one number that best describes your pain on the **average.**

0	1	2	3	4	5	6	7	8	9	10
No pain									Pain as bad as you can imagine	

6) Please rate your pain by circling the one number that tells how much pain you have **right now.**

0	1	2	3	4	5	6	7	8	9	10
No pain									Pain as bad as you can imagine	

7) What treatments or medications are you receiving for your pain?

_____

_____

8) In the past 24 hours, how much **relief** have pain treatments or medications provided? Please circle the one percentage that most shows how much relief you have received.

0%	10	20	30	40	50	60	70	80	90	100%
No relief										Complete relief

9) Circle the one number that describes how, during the past 24 hours, pain has **interfered** with your:

A. General activity

0	1	2	3	4	5	6	7	8	9	10
Does not interfere									Completely interferes	

B. Mood

0	1	2	3	4	5	6	7	8	9	10
Does not interfere									Completely interferes	

C. Walking ability

0	1	2	3	4	5	6	7	8	9	10
Does not interfere									Completely interferes	

D. Normal work (includes both work outside the home and housework)

0	1	2	3	4	5	6	7	8	9	10
Does not interfere									Completely interferes	

E. Relations with other people

0	1	2	3	4	5	6	7	8	9	10
Does not interfere									Completely interferes	

F. Sleep

0	1	2	3	4	5	6	7	8	9	10
Does not interfere									Completely interferes	

G. Enjoyment of life

0	1	2	3	4	5	6	7	8	9	10
Does not interfere									Completely interferes	

worse at certain times, certain hours during the day or night, or certain times of the month?"

5. *Manner of expressing pain.* Ask the patient if he or she prefers not to discuss the pain or tries to hide it from others. Ask the patient if using the pain rating scale is acceptable.

6. *What relieves the pain?* If the patient has had pain for a while, the patient may know which medications and doses are helpful and may have found some nondrug methods, such as cold packs, helpful. If appropriate, these should be continued.

7. *What causes the pain?* A variety of activities, body positions, and other events may increase the pain, and efforts can be made to avoid them or to provide additional analgesia at those times.

8. *Effects of pain.* These items help identify how pain affects the patient's quality of life or how pain interferes with recovery from illness. Information obtained in this section may be useful in developing pain management goals. If pain interferes with sleep, a major goal may be to identify a pain rating that will allow the patient to sleep through the night without being awakened by pain.

9. *Other comments.* No tool is comprehensive. This space simply allows for information the patient may wish to add.

10. *Plan.* Immediate and long-range plans can be mentioned here and developed in more detail as time passes.

Brief Pain Inventory (BPI)

The BPI assessment tool (Form 3.2) has been used extensively in research. It has reasonable validity and reliability (Daut, Cleeland, 1982; Daut, Cleeland, Flanery, 1983) and has proven useful in a variety of clinical settings (Cleeland, Gonin, Hatfield et al., 1994). It takes about 15 minutes to complete and has also been translated into other languages including Vietnamese (Cleeland, Ladinsky, Serlin et al., 1988), Chinese (Wang, Mendoza, Gao et al., 1996), the Philippine language, and French (Serlin, Mendoza, Nakamura et al., 1995).

Questions on the BPI focus on pain during the past 24 hours.

- Question 1 asks if the patient has experienced pain other than common everyday kinds of pain.
- Question 2 asks the patient to identify the location of that pain in the figure drawing.
- Questions 3 through 6 ask the patient to use a pain rating scale of 0 to 10 to rate pain at its worst and least in the past 24 hours and its intensity on average and right now.
- Question 7 asks about treatment or medication the patient is receiving for pain.
- Question 8 asks the percentage of pain relief provided by these treatments.
- Question 9 has seven parts that attempt to identify now much pain has interfered with the patient's life, including general activity, relations with other people, and sleep.

Pain Rating Scales

Pain rating scales used in daily clinical practice generally deal with pain intensity, that is, how much a person hurts. Numerous scales for measuring pain intensity exist, and they have been referred to by many different names. Each scale has no standardized title or definition. Following are definitions and descriptions used in this book to designate various scales:

- *Visual Analog Scale (VAS).* This is a horizontal (sometimes vertical) 10 cm line with word anchors at the extremes, such as "no pain" on one end and "pain as bad as it could be" on the other end (Figure 3.1). The patient is asked to make a mark along the line to represent pain intensity. Although this is easy to administer and has documented validity, scoring is time consuming. A number is obtained by measuring in millimeters up to the point the patient has indicated. In this book, the term VAS will refer only to a horizontal or vertical straight line with word anchors at the ends.
- *Graphic Rating Scale (GRS).* This scale builds on the VAS by adding to the measurement line either words or numbers between the extreme ends of the scale. If words are added, such as no pain, mild, moderate, and severe, it is called a verbal graphic rating scale. If numbers are added, such as 0 through

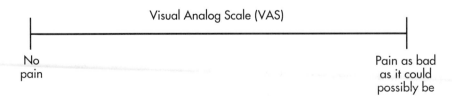

Visual Analog Scale (VAS)

No
pain

Pain as bad
as it could
possibly be

May be duplicated for use in clinical practice. From McCaffery M, Pasero C: *Pain: Clinical manual*, p. 62. Copyright © 1999, Mosby, Inc.

● ● ● ● ●
FIGURE 3.1 This horizontal visual analog scale (VAS) for rating pain intensity is a 10 cm line with word anchors. The patient is asked to mark on the line. Although the VAS is frequently used in research, it is not recommended for clinical practice because scoring is time-consuming.

10, it becomes a numerical graphic rating scale (Jensen, Karoly, 1992), which is the same as the visual representation of the numerical rating scale, (NRS) defined below.

- *Simple Descriptor Scale (SDS).* This is a list of adjectives describing different levels of pain intensity. A simple and clinically useful example is no pain, mild, moderate, and severe pain. These four words are easily understood and scored (assigning numbers 0 to 3) and have been used for many years in daily clinical assessments. SDSs with many words are not recommended because they are time consuming to administer and not all patients will be able to understand the words (Jensen, Karoly, 1992).

- *Numerical Rating Scale (NRS).* In clinical practice the term *numerical rating scale* is used loosely and may refer to a verbally administered 0 to 10 (or 0 to 5) scale or to a visually presented scale with both words and numbers along a vertical (Figure 3.2, *A*) or horizontal line (Figure 3.2, *B*). The patient is asked to rate pain from 0 to 10, with 0 equaling no pain and 10 equaling the worst possible pain. In this book, NRS will refer to all the possible combinations of pain rating scales that use numbers, whether they are verbally or graphically presented and whether they contain word descriptors or not. For additional discussion of NRS see below.

- *Faces rating scales.* Several faces rating scales exist and were developed primarily for use with young children. Among the more well known of these scales are the Oucher (six photographs of children with facial expressions suggesting various pain intensities [Beyer, Denyes, Villarruel, 1992]) and the Wong-Baker. Figure 3.3 illustrates the Wong-Baker faces rating scale with directions on how to present it to the patient. Figure 3.3 also provides translations in Chinese, French, Italian, Japanese, Portuguese, Romanian, Spanish, and Vietnamese. This scale may be used with children as young as the age of 3 years (Wong, Baker, 1988, 1995) and is also popular with many adults. Figure 3.4 demonstrates how the Wong-Baker faces rating scale may be displayed along with a numerical pain rating scale of 0 to 10.

Selection of a pain rating scale for daily clinical practice

All the scales described above have been documented as being valid measures of pain intensity, but some of the pain rating scales are more suitable for clinical practice

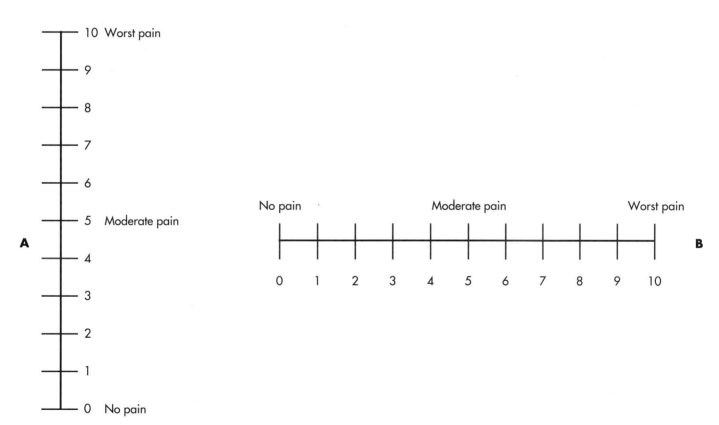

May be duplicated for use in clinical practice. From McCaffery M, Pasero C: *Pain: Clinical manual*, p. 63. Copyright © 1999, Mosby, Inc.

● ● ● ● ●
FIGURE 3.2   The vertical version **(A)** of the numerical rating scale may be more easily understood than the horizontal version **(B)**.

Which Face Shows How Much Hurt You Have Now?

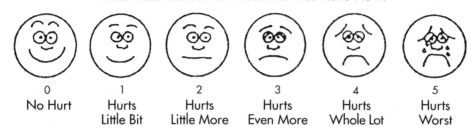

0	1	2	3	4	5
No Hurt	Hurts Little Bit	Hurts Little More	Hurts Even More	Hurts Whole Lot	Hurts Worst

F I G U R E 3.3 Explain to the person that each face is for a person who feels happy because he has no pain (hurt) or sad because he has some or a lot of pain. **Face 0** is very happy because he doesn't hurt at all. **Face 1** hurts just a little bit. **Face 2** hurts a little more. **Face 3** hurts even more. **Face 4** hurts a whole lot. **Face 5** hurts as much as you can imagine, although you don't have to be crying to feel this bad. Ask the person to choose the face that best describes how he is feeling.

Rating scale is recommended for persons age 3 years and older.

*The brief word instructions under each face can also be used. Point to each face using the words to describe the pain intensity. Ask the child to choose face that best describes own pain and record the appropriate number. *Note:* In a study of 148 children ages 4 to 5 years, there were no differences in pain scores when children used the original or brief word instructions.

Modified from Wong DL: *Whaley & Wong's essentials of pediatric nursing,* ed 5, pp. 1215-1216, St. Louis, 1997, Mosby.

Chinese

解釋給人聽用每張臉譜來代表著一個人的感覺是因為沒有疼痛〔傷痛〕而感快樂或是因為些許疼痛或者是許多疼痛而感傷心。第零張臉是很快樂的因為他一點也不覺得疼痛。第一張臉只痛一丁點兒。第二張臉又痛多了一些。第三張臉痛得更多了。第四張臉是非常痛了。第五張臉是為人們所能想像到的劇痛既使感到這樣難過，卻不一定哭出來。請這人選擇出最能代表他現在感覺的一張臉譜。此量表適用於三歲以上的人。

Italian

Spiegare a la persona che ogni facien è per una persona che si sente felice perchè non tiene dolore oppure triste perchè ha poco o molto dolore. **Faccia O** è molto felice perchè non tiene dolor. **Faccia 1** tiene poco dolore. **Faccia 2** tiene un po più di dolore. **Faccia 3** tiene più dolore. **Faccia 4** tiene molto dolore. **Faccia 5** tiene molto dolore che non puoi immaginare però non devi piangere per tenere dolore. Domandi ala persona di scegliere quale faccia meglio descrive come si sente.

Grado scale è raccomandata a la persona di tre anni in sù.

French

Expliquez à la personne que chaque visage représent un personne qui est heureux parce qu'elle n'a pas point du mal ou triste parce qu'il a un peu ou beaucoup du mal. **Visage 0** est trés heureux parce qu'elle n'a pas point du mal. **Visage 1** a un petit peu de mal. **Visage 2** a plus du mal. **Visage 3** a encore plus du mal. **Visage 4** a beaucoup du mal. **Visage 5** a autant mal que vous pouvez imaginer, bien que ces mauvais sentiments ne finissent pas nécessairement a vous faire pleurer. Demandez à la personne de choisir le visage qui convient le mieux avec ses sentiments.

Ces evaluations sont recommendés pour des personnes de trois ans et davantage.

Japanese

3歳以上の患者に望ましい。それぞれの顔は、患者の痛み(pain, hurt) がないのでご機嫌な感じ、または、ある程度の痛み・沢山の痛みがあるので悲しい感じを表現していることを説明して下さい。0＝痛みがまったくないから、とても幸せな顔をしている、1＝ほんの少し痛い、2＝もう少し痛い、3＝もっと痛い、4＝とっても痛い、5＝痛くて涙を流す必要はないけれども、これ以上の痛みは考えられないほど痛い。今、どのように感じているか最もよく表わしている顔を選ぶよう、患者に求めて下さい。

Continued.

Portuguese

Explique a pessoa que cada face representa uma pessoa que está feliz porque não têm dor, ou triste por ter um pouco ou muita dor. **Face 0** está muito feliz porque não têm nenhuma dor. **Face 1** tem apenas um pouco de dor. **Face 2** têm um pouco mais de dor. **Face 3** têm ainda mais dor. **Face 4** têm muita dor. **Face 5** têm uma dor máxima, apesar de que nem sempre provoca o choro. Peça a pessoa que escolhe a face que melhor descreve como ele se sente.

Esta escala é aplicável a pessoas de tres anos de idade ou mais.

Spanish

Expliquele a la persona que cada cara representa una persona que se siente feliz porque no tiene dolor o triste porque siente un poco o mucho dolor. **Cara 0** se siente muy feliz porque no tiene dolor. **Cara 1** tiene un poco de dolor. **Cara 2** tiene un poquito más de dolor. **Cara 3** tiene más dolor. **Cara 4** tiene mucho dolor. **Cara 5** tiene el dolor más fuerte que usted pueda imaginar, aunque usted no tiene que estar llorando para sentirse asi de mal. Pidale a la persona que escoja la cara que mejor describe su proprio dolor.

Esta escala se puede usar con personas de tres años de edad o más.

Romanian

Explică persoanei că fiecare faţă este specifică diferitelor stări fizice; o persoană este ferioita pentru că nu are nici o durere ori tristă pentru că suferă puţin sau mai mult. **Faţa 0** este foarte ferioită pentru că nu are absolut nici o durere. **Faţa 1** are un pic de durere. **Faţa 2** are ceva mai mult. **Faţa 3** suferă şi mai mult. **Faţa 4** suferă foarte mult. **Faţa 5** este greu de imaginat cât de mult suferă, căci nu trebuie neapărat să plângi, oricat de tare te-ar durea. Intreabă persoana să indice figura care-i desorie cel mai bine starea fizică.

Acest **grad de durere** este racomandat pentru persoanele de la 3 ani în sus.

Vietnamese

Xin cắt nghĩa cho mỗi người, từng khuôn mặt của một người cãm thấy vui vẽ tại vì không có sự đau đớn hoặc, buồn vì có chút ít hay rất nhiều sự đau đớn.

Cái **mặt** với **số 0** thì rất là vui tại vì mặt ấy không có sự đau đớn. **Mặt số 1** chỉ đau một chút thôi. **Mặt số 2** hơi đau hơn một chút nữa. **Mặt số 3** đau hơn chút nữa. **Mặt số 4** đau thật nhiều. **Mặt số 5** đau không thể tưởng tượng, mặc dù người ta không cần phải khóc mới cảm thấy được sự buồn khổ như thế.

Bạn hỏi từng người tự chọn khuôn mặt nào diễn tả được sự đau đớn của chính mình.

May be duplicated for use in clinical practice. As appears in McCaffery M, Pasero C: *Pain: Clinical manual,* pp. 64-65, 1999, Mosby, Inc.

● ● ● ● ●

F I G U R E 3.3 **Directions for use of faces pain rating scale: English and selected languages.** Spanish and Portuguese translations by Ellen Johnsen; French translation by Irene Sherman Liguori and Robert Marino; Italian translation by Madeline Mitchko and Ida DiPietropaolo; Romanian translation by Florin Nicolae; Vietnamese translation by Yen B. Isle; Chinese translation by Hung-Shen Lin; Japanese translation from *After the announcement of cancer,* Tokyo, 1993, Iwanami Shoten, Pub.

than others. The three pain rating scales most commonly used in the United States are numerical (NRS), word descriptors (SDS), and faces. Criteria to consider in selecting a pain rating scale for use in daily clinical practice are listed in Box 3.6. Following are research findings that assist in selecting a pain rating scale for an institution.

The pain rating scale selected must be reliable, meaning that the scale consistently measures pain intensity from one time to the next, and valid, meaning that the scale accurately measures pain intensity. The tool also should be sufficiently graded to capture changes in pain intensity, easily understood, easy to score, and liked by patients and staff.

Pain rating scales seem to invite creativity such as adding colors to a preexisting scale or developing a completely new scale. Many health care facilities do not have copiers that duplicate in color, and research on colors as indicators of pain intensity is limited. Such energy is better spent on promoting the routine use of a single, simple pain rating scale that has already been established as valid and reliable.

Patients tend to have more difficulty understanding and using a VAS than the other scales such as the NRS,

resulting in some clinicians recommending strongly against the use of the VAS (Jensen, Karoly, 1992). Also, without specific numbers arranged along the VAS line, it is difficult to use the scale to discuss pain rating goals with patients.

The NRS seems to be a suitable option. In a study of 60 patients in the immediate postoperative period, the verbally administered 0 to 10 scale was less difficult for patients to use than the VAS (DeLoach, Higgins, Caplan et al., 1998). Blurred vision, nausea, and residual anesthesia were some of the problems that interfered with use of the VAS.

The validity of the 0 to 10 NRS has been well established, and it is easy to score (Jensen, Karoly, 1992). In a study comparing the SDS, the VAS, and the NRS, the correlation between the VAS and the NRS was strong, supporting the validity of the verbally administered NRS (Paice, Cohen, 1997). The verbally administered 0 to 10 NRS is a particularly useful scale when visual contact between patient and clinicians cannot be made. An increasing amount of telephone contact is necessary because the care of patients with progressive disease and pain is moved into the home.

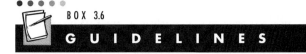

BOX 3.6

GUIDELINES

SELECTING A PAIN RATING SCALE FOR USE IN DAILY CLINICAL PRACTICE

- Research has established the tool is reasonably valid and reliable.
- Developmentally appropriate. Some scales commonly used with adults (e.g., 0 to 10 scale) are clearly inappropriate for children who cannot count. On the other hand, some scales, such as the Wong-Baker Faces Scale that are appropriate for young children may be appropriate for any age group, especially cognitively impaired patients.
- Easily and quickly understood by patients who have minimal formal education.
- Well-liked by patients.
- Well-liked by clinicians.
- Low burden on clinicians.
  —Quickly explained.
  —Easily scored and recorded.
- Easily used with the patient to set pain management goals (i.e., comfort/function goals).
- Inexpensive.
- Multiple copies easily created for distribution to clinicians, patients, and their families.
- Easily disinfected (or inexpensive enough to discard, e.g., scales that are photocopied).
- Readily available. Multiple copies are easily and inexpensively made for distribution to clinicians, patients, and their families.
- Appropriate for patients from different cultures.
- Tool is available in various languages spoken in that clinical setting (or may be translated easily).

May be duplicated for use in clinical practice. As appears in McCaffery M, Pasero C: *Pain: Clinical manual*, p. 66, 1999, Mosby, Inc.

Modified from Hester NO: Integrating pain assessment and management into the care of children with cancer. In McGuire DB, Yarbro CH, Ferrell BR: *Cancer pain management*, pp. 231-271, Boston, 1995, Jones and Bartlett Publishers, pp. 247-248.

The NRS is easily administered either orally or in writing and is easy to score and record. The NRS is also more reliable than other scales, such as the SDS, with less educated patients (Ferraz, Quaresma, Aquino et al., 1990). Some clinicians are now recommending universal adoption of the 0 to 10 scale with adults who do not have cognitive disorders (Dalton, McNaull, 1998).

Both the 0 to 5 and 0 to 10 scales are widely used in clinical practice. Of concern is how many points are necessary to measure pain intensity. The VAS, when measured in millimeters, is a 0 to 100 scale (101 points). The 0 to 10 scale is 11 points; the 0 to 5 scale, 6 points. Investigators have found that patients usually treat a 0 to 100 point scale as they would a 0 to 10 scale (Jensen,

Turner, Romano, 1994). Thus a scale with 101 points seems unnecessary. However, one study found that patients' pain ratings on the VAS and a 0 to 5 NRS were not mathematically equivalent. VAS ratings were lower than NRS ratings (Carpenter, Brockopp, 1995). Thus correlation between a 0 to 5 point scale and the 1 to 100 VAS is lower than with the 0 to 10 scale. Further, 0 to 10 is potentially more sensitive to changes in pain intensity than is 0 to 5. Consequently, a NRS of 0 to 10 seems indicated.

It is customary to present the NRS visually as a horizontal line. However, research findings indicate that the vertical VAS (see Figure 3.1) is more sensitive and easier for patients to use, especially patients who are under stress with a narrowed visual field (Gift, 1989; Gift, Plaut, Jacox, 1986). In a small study of children ranging in age from 4.5 to 17 years, correlations between scores on vertical and horizontal VAS were strong enough to suggest that either would be acceptable in the clinical setting (Walco, Ilowite, 1991). Therefore the vertical (see Figure 3.2, *A*) visual NRS may be advisable for some patient populations or may be presented as an alternative to patients who have difficulty with the horizontal scale (see Figure 3.2, *B*).

The Wong-Baker faces scale is widely used because it is easily photocopied and is popular among children and adults. In a study of 267 hospitalized patients ranging in age from 16 to 91 years, almost half preferred the Wong-Baker faces pain rating scale to the 0 to 10 numeric scale or the VAS (Carey, Turpin, Smith et al., 1997).

In this book the NRS and the Wong-Baker faces scale have been selected for patient examples. We also recommend these choices for most clinical settings. Figure 3.4 shows how these may be combined and standardized as a 0 to 10 pain rating scale to be used throughout an institution.

Another advantage to using the 0 to 10 NRS and the Wong-Baker faces scale is that they have been translated into several languages. For translations of the Wong-Baker faces scale, see Figure 3.3. Figure 3.5 presents translations for the 0 to 10 NRS.

Whichever pain rating scale is chosen, it should be used consistently with the patient. Obviously, using the same scale is easier for the patient than switching from one scale to another. Certainly, standardization is helpful within a given health care system, so that the same scale is used in the ED, the hospital, and the outpatient care services. A standard pain rating scale minimizes confusion for both patients and staff.

The frequency with which pain ratings are obtained obviously depends on the situation. When pain is out of control, such as a 10 on a scale of 0 to 10, and a rapidly acting analgesic is used, pain ratings every 15 minutes may be appropriate. However, initially, at the beginning of treatment, asking the patient for a pain rating may

Pain Rating Scales

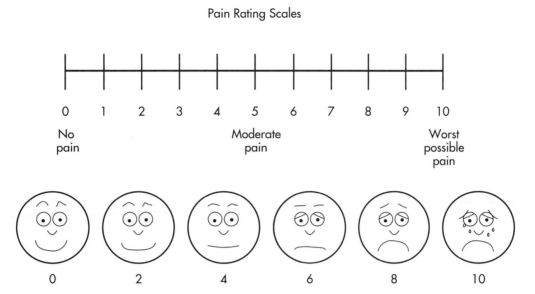

May be duplicated for use in clinical practice. As appears in McCaffery M, Pasero C: *Pain: Clinical manual*, p. 67, 1999, Mosby, Inc.

● ● ● ● ○

F I G U R E 3.4   Example of how some clinical settings combine the horizontal numerical rating scale (NRS) with word anchors and the Wong-Baker faces scale. These are placed on one card or piece of paper so that the patient has a choice of pain rating scales. If the numerical scale with word descriptors is not easily understood, the faces scale is likely to be. The numbers beneath the faces have been changed from 0 to 5 to a 0 to 10 scale so that the recording of pain intensity is consistently on a 0 to 10 scale.

Faces pain rating scale modified from Wong DL: W*haley & Wong's essentials of pediatric nursing*, ed 5, pp. 1215-1216, St. Louis, 1997, Mosby.

be entirely inappropriate. When patients are obviously in pain or not focused enough to learn to use a pain rating scale, pain treatment should proceed without a pain rating. Once pain is well controlled, however, in a hospitalized patient, pain ratings every 8 to 12 hours may be sufficient. In home care, once pain is controlled, patients are not ordinarily asked to keep a record of pain ratings.

Teaching the patient/family how to use the pain rating scale

It is not unusual for clinicians to claim that patients cannot use pain rating scales. However, even in cognitively impaired elderly patients in nursing homes, 83% who report pain are able to use at least one type of pain rating scale (Ferrell, Ferrell, Rivera, 1995). Therefore most adolescents and adults, and probably schoolage children, who are not cognitively impaired, should be able to learn to use a pain rating scale. It is simply a matter of having a plan that assures that when patients are admitted to a clinical setting, someone is responsible for teaching each patient the pain rating scale, having the patient demonstrate an understanding of this, and documenting this in the record.

Steps for teaching the 0 to 10 NRS are in Box 3.7. Steps 1, 2, and 3 provide information, steps 4 and 5 ask the patient to demonstrate an understanding of the information, and Step 6 focuses on the goal for com-

fort and function/recovery. Along with each step are specific examples of what may be said to the patient/family.

Patients tend to have a narrow concept of the word pain, often restricting its use to excruciating and intolerable sensations. The patient's concept of pain may be expanded by explaining that pain includes several different uncomfortable sensations, such as tightness and pressure, and by using the words aching and hurting (Step 3). In a study of four different ethnic groups, Hispanics, American Indians, blacks, and whites, participants were asked to describe and rate painful experiences. Findings revealed that in all groups the word ache was used for mild pain, hurt for moderate pain, and pain for the most intense discomfort (Gaston-Johansson, Albert, Fagan et al., 1990).

The primary reason for using pain rating scales is to evaluate the effectiveness of the pain treatment plan. To do this, it is essential to set goals. The expected outcomes of pain management should be as clearly identified as possible. As described in Box 3.7, Step 6, the goal includes both comfort and function. For most patients only one pain rating goal needs to be set. In other words, one pain rating goal usually is applicable to most functions or activities the patient needs to perform. The goal is based on the pain rating required for the patient to perform activities related to satisfactory recovery or improved quality of life. This process helps set realistic goals because zero pain is not always possible. Once the

Text continued on p. 74.

English

Please point to the number that best describes your pain.

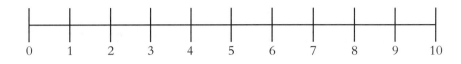

0   1   2   3   4   5   6   7   8   9   10

No pain   Terrible pain

Chinese ★

請指出那個數字反映你痛的程度

Please point to the number that best describes your pain.

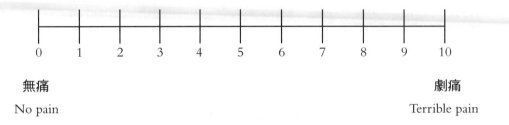

0   1   2   3   4   5   6   7   8   9   10

無痛   劇痛
No pain   Terrible pain

French ★★

S'il vous plaît, indiquez le chiffre qui décrit le mieux votre douleur.

Please point to the number that best describes your pain.

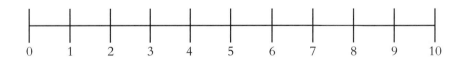

0   1   2   3   4   5   6   7   8   9   10

Pas de douleur   **Douleur intense**
No pain   Terrible pain

May be duplicated for use in clinical practice. As appears in McCaffery M, Pasero C: *Pain: Clinical manual*, pp. 68-73, 1999, Mosby, Inc.

Continued.

● ● ● ● ●
FIGURE 3.5 **Translations of 0-10 pain rating scales.** Most of the translations of the pain rating scales were done by volunteers. No back and forth translation has been done, so the reader is advised that errors may occur. However, these scales have been used extensively by the facilities that submitted them.

Courtesy:

★ Pain Management Committee, St. Francis Medical Center, Honolulu, HI.

★★ Compiled by Josephine Musto, RN, MS, ONC, Nursing Care Manager, Pain Management Service and members of Nursing Department, Saint Vincent's Hospital and Medical Center, New York, NY.

German ★★

Bitte markieren Sie die Nummer, die Ihren Schmerz am besten beschreiben.

Please point to the number that best describes your pain.

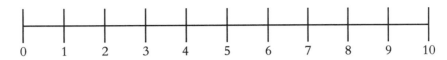

Kein Schmerz		**Unerträglicher Schmerz**
No pain		Terrible pain

Greek ★★

Παρακαλώ, δείξετε με το δάκτυλό σας τον
αριθμό που δείχνει πόσο πόνο έχετε.

Please point to the number that best describes your pain.

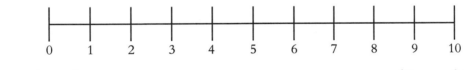

Δεν έχω πόνο		΄Εχω πολύ πόνο
No pain		Terrible pain

Hawaiian ★

E koho a kuhi ʻoe i ka helu pololei ma ke ʻano o ka ʻeha i pili ia ʻoe, ina ʻole (0) ka ʻeha ʻole a ʻumi (10) ka ʻeha palena ʻole.

Please point to the number that best describes your pain.

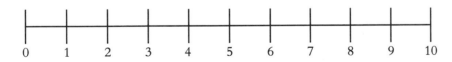

Ka ʻeha ʻole		**Ka ʻeha palena ʻole**
No pain		Terrible pain

May be duplicated for use in clinical practice. As appears in McCaffery M, Pasero C: *Pain: Clinical manual*, pp. 68-73, 1999, Mosby, Inc.

● ● ● ● ●

FIGURE 3.5—cont'd **Translations of 0-10 pain rating scales.** Most of the translations of the pain rating scales were done by volunteers. No back and forth translation has been done, so the reader is advised that errors may occur. However, these scales have been used extensively by the facilities that submitted them.

Courtesy:

★ Pain Management Committee, St. Francis Medical Center, Honolulu, HI.

★★ Compiled by Josephine Musto, RN, MS, ONC, Nursing Care Manager, Pain Management Service and members of Nursing Department, Saint Vincent's Hospital and Medical Center, New York, NY.

Continued.

Hebrew ★★

בבקשה תשימו אצבע על המספר מאפס עד עשר:
שמראה לנו כמה חזק הכאב

Please point to the number that best describes your pain.

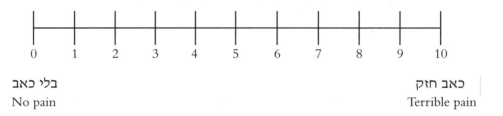

בלי כאב
No pain

כאב חזק
Terrible pain

Ilocano ★ (spoken in the Philippines)

Paki tudo ti numero nga mangipakita ti kinasakitna.

Please point to the number that best describes your pain.

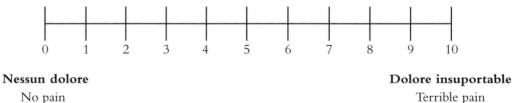

Awan sakit na
No pain

Nakasaksakit unay
Terrible pain

Italian ★★

Segna il numero che indica il level del dolore.

Please point to the number that best describes your pain.

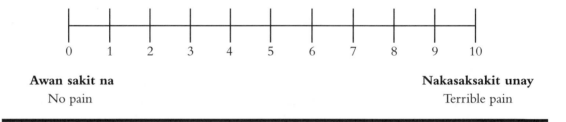

Nessun dolore
No pain

Dolore insuportable
Terrible pain

May be duplicated for use in clinical practice. As appears in McCaffery M, Pasero C: *Pain: Clinical manual,* pp. 68-73, 1999, Mosby, Inc.

● ● ● ● ●

FIGURE 3.5—cont'd   **Translations of 0-10 pain rating scales.** Most of the translations of the pain rating scales were done by volunteers. No back and forth translation has been done, so the reader is advised that errors may occur. However, these scales have been used extensively by the facilities that submitted them.

Courtesy:

* Pain Management Committee, St. Francis Medical Center, Honolulu, HI.

** Compiled by Josephine Musto, RN, MS, ONC, Nursing Care Manager, Pain Management Service and members of Nursing Department, Saint Vincent's Hospital and Medical Center, New York, NY.

Continued.

Japanese ★★

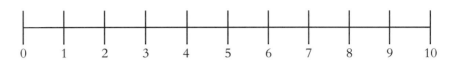

痛みの強さの度合を0～10までの階段で示して下さい。

Please point to the number that best describes your pain.

```
0   1   2   3   4   5   6   7   8   9   10
```

ゼロ　全く痛みがない   激痛 敦痛

　　　No pain   Terrible pain

Korean

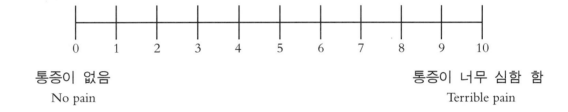

현재 통증의 강도를 가장 잘 나타내는 번호에 표시하십시오.

Please point to the number that best describes your pain.

```
0   1   2   3   4   5   6   7   8   9   10
```

통증이 없음   통증이 너무 심함 함

　No pain   Terrible pain

Pakistan ★★

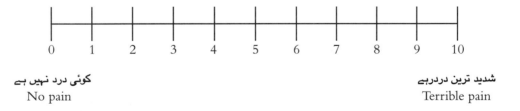

برائے مہربانی اپنے درد کی شدت بتانے کے لیے نیچے لکھے ہوئے
نمبروں میں سے کسی ایک کی طرف اپنی انگلی سے اشارہ کریں ۔

Please point to the number that best describes your pain.

```
0   1   2   3   4   5   6   7   8   9   10
```

کوئی درد نہیں ہے   شدید ترین دردہے

　No pain   Terrible pain

May be duplicated for use in clinical practice. As appears in McCaffery M, Pasero C: *Pain: Clinical manual*, pp. 68-73, 1999, Mosby, Inc.

Continued.

● ● ● ● ●

F I G U R E 3.5—cont'd **Translations of 0-10 pain rating scales.** Most of the translations of the pain rating scales were done by volunteers. No back and forth translation has been done, so the reader is advised that errors may occur. However, these scales have been used extensively by the facilities that submitted them.

Courtesy:

* Pain Management Committee, St. Francis Medical Center, Honolulu, HI.

** Compiled by Josephine Musto, RN, MS, ONC, Nursing Care Manager, Pain Management Service and members of Nursing Department, Saint Vincent's Hospital and Medical Center, New York, NY.

Polish ★★

Proszę wskazać numer, który najlepiej określa jak silny jest ten ból.

Please point to the number that best describes your pain.

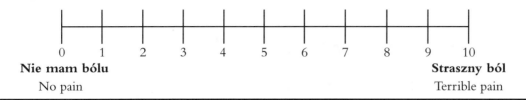

Nie mam bólu
No pain

Straszny ból
Terrible pain

Russian ★★

Выбирите число, которое указывает вашу боль по десятибальной системе.

Please point to the number that best describes your pain.

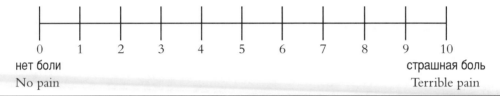

нет боли
No pain

страшная боль
Terrible pain

Samoan ★

Fa'amolemole ta'u mai le numera e fa'amatala ai le itu-aiga tiga o loo e lagonaina.

Please point to the number that best describes your pain.

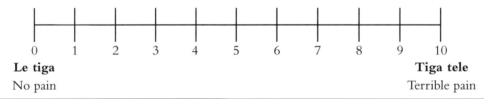

Le tiga
No pain

Tiga tele
Terrible pain

Spanish ★★

Por favor senale al numero que mejor describe su dolor. (Mas grande el numero mayor su dolor).

Please point to the number that best describes your pain.

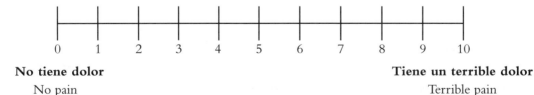

No tiene dolor
No pain

Tiene un terrible dolor
Terrible pain

Continued.

● ● ● ● ●

F I G U R E 3.5—cont'd **Translations of 0-10 pain rating scales.** Most of the translations of the pain rating scales were done by volunteers. No back and forth translation has been done, so the reader is advised that errors may occur. However, these scales have been used extensively by the facilities that submitted them.

Courtesy:

* Pain Management Committee, St. Francis Medical Center, Honolulu, HI.

** Compiled by Josephine Musto, RN, MS, ONC, Nursing Care Manager, Pain Management Service and members of Nursing Department, Saint Vincent's Hospital and Medical Center, New York, NY.

Tagalog ★★ (spoken in the Philippines)

Ituro po ninyo ang numerong nagpapaliwanag kung gaano kasakit.

Please point to the number that best describes your pain.

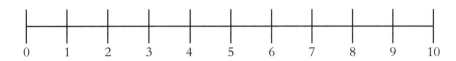

| 0 | 1 | 2 | 3 | 4 | 5 | 6 | 7 | 8 | 9 | 10 |

Walang masakit
No pain

Napakasakit
Terrible pain

Tongan ★★ (spoken in Tonga, an island in the south Pacific)

I he ngaahi fika koena, fakailongai mai ai e tuunga ho falangaaki.

Please point to the number that best describes your pain.

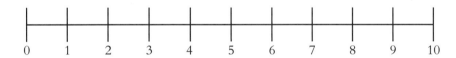

| 0 | 1 | 2 | 3 | 4 | 5 | 6 | 7 | 8 | 9 | 10 |

Ikai ha felangaaki
No pain

Ikai matuuaki'e langa
Terrible pain

Vietnamese

Xin chỉ số mô tả đúng nhất sự đau nhức của quý vị

Please point to the number that best describes your pain.

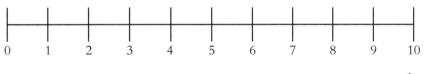

| 0 | 1 | 2 | 3 | 4 | 5 | 6 | 7 | 8 | 9 | 10 |

Không đau
No pain

Đau rất nhiều
Terrible pain

May be duplicated for use in clinical practice. As appears in McCaffery M, Pasero C: *Pain: Clinical manual,* pp. 68-73, 1999, Mosby, Inc.

● ● ● ● ●

FIGURE 3.5—cont'd **Translations of 0-10 pain rating scales.** Most of the translations of the pain rating scales were done by volunteers. No back and forth translation has been done, so the reader is advised that errors may occur. However, these scales have been used extensively by the facilities that submitted them.

Courtesy:

* Pain Management Committee, St. Francis Medical Center, Honolulu, HI.

** Compiled by Josephine Musto, RN, MS, ONC, Nursing Care Manager, Pain Management Service and members of Nursing Department, Saint Vincent's Hospital and Medical Center, New York, NY.

B O X   3.7

G U I D E L I N E S

TEACHING THE PATIENT/FAMILY HOW TO USE A PAIN RATING SCALE

- *Step 1. Show the pain rating scale to the patient/family and explain its primary purpose.*

    Example: "This is a pain rating scale that many of our patients use to help us understand their pain and to set goals for pain relief. We will ask you regularly about pain, but anytime you have pain you must also let us know. We don't always know when you hurt."

- *Step 2. Explain the parts of the pain rating scale.* If the patient does not like it or understand it, switch to another scale (e.g., vertical scale or faces).

    Example: "On this pain rating scale, 0 means no pain and 10 means the worst possible pain. The middle of the scale around 5 is moderate pain. A 2 or 3 would be mild pain, but 7 and higher is severe pain."

- *Step 3. Discuss pain as a broad concept that is not restricted to a severe and intolerable sensation.*

    Example: "Pain refers to any kind of discomfort anywhere in your body. Pain also means aching and hurting. Pain can include pulling, tightness, burning, knifelike, and other unpleasant sensations."

- *Step 4. Verify that the patient understands the broad concept of pain.*

    Ask the patient to give two examples of pain he or she has experienced.

    If the patient is already in pain that requires treatment, use the present situation as the example.

    Example of what to say if patient is not now in significant pain: "I want to be sure that I've explained this clearly, so would you give me two examples of pain you've had recently?"

    If the patient's examples include different parts of the body and different pain characteristics, that indicates that the patient understands pain as a fairly broad concept. The patient might say, "I have a mild, sort of throbbing headache now, and yesterday my back was aching."

- *Step 5. Ask the patient to practice using the pain rating scale with his or her present pain or select one of his examples.*

    Example: "Using the scale, what is your pain right now?" "What is it at its worst?" Or "Using the pain rating scale and one of your examples of pain, what is that pain usually?" "What is it at its worst?"

- *Step 6. Set goals for comfort and function/recovery.* Ask the patient what pain rating would be acceptable or satisfactory to him or her, considering the activities required for recovery or for maintaining a satisfactory quality of life. (Research strongly suggests that pain rating goals of 4 or more on a 0 to 10 scale are not appropriate.)

    Example for a surgical patient: "I have explained the importance of coughing and deep breathing to prevent pneumonia and other complications. Now we need to determine the pain rating that will not interfere with this so you may recover quickly. If you're not sure, you can guess, and we can change it later."

    Example for the terminally ill patient: "What do you want to do that pain keeps you from doing? What pain rating would allow you to do this?"

goal is achieved, such as a pain rating of 2, the possibility of even better pain relief can always be considered. Over time or with experience, goals may change. For example, if the patient finds that the pain rating is too high to allow uninterrupted sleep, it should be changed to a lower number.

The patient should be assured that a reported pain rating above the goal will result in consideration of additional intervention:

The clinical practice guidelines are explicit about the need for goals:

- "Determine the level of pain above which adjustment of analgesia or other interventions will be considered." (Acute Pain Management Guideline Panel, 1992a, p. 7)
- "Document . . . the goals for pain control (as scores on a pain scale) in the patient's pain history." (Jacox, Carr, Payne et al., 1994b, p. 3)

How much pain is too much pain? When the clinician works with the patient to set comfort/function

goals, the patient must understand that the intent is not to identify the highest pain level the patient can tolerate, but rather to identify how much pain can exist without interfering with function. Research helps guide this process by suggesting that certain pain levels are more than the patient should attempt to tolerate.

The findings of several studies of different cultures have found that on a 0 to 10 pain rating scale, pain ratings of 5 or more interfere significantly with daily function (Cleeland, 1984; Cleeland, Gonin, Hatfield, 1994; Serlin, Mendoza, Nakamura et al., 1995). Further research suggests that 4, rather than 5, is the point at which pain significantly interferes with function. The results using the Brief Pain Inventory to assess 111 patients with pain and advanced cancer showed that on a 0 to 10 scale, pain ratings of 4 or greater interfered markedly with activity, and interference with enjoyment increased markedly between scores of 6 and 7 (Twycross, Harcourt, Bergl, 1996). This study and others, combined with clinical experience, has led many clinicians to the conclusion that a pain rating greater than 3 signals the need to revise the pain treatment plan with higher doses of analgesics or different medications and other interventions (Cleeland, Syrjala, 1992; Syrjala, 1993). In addition, even temporary pain at a level of 6 or more should mandate immediate intervention.

One practical implication of these studies is that when patients and staff are determining the comfort/function goal, pain ratings goals greater than a 3 should be avoided. Thus pain ratings of 4 or more are not appropriate unless they are temporary or intermediary goals. In other words, for a patient with a pain rating of 10, achieving a pain rating of 5 within 8 hours might be a way to mark progress toward a lower pain rating such as a 3 within the next 24 hours. Or, a pain rating of 5 may be appropriate for a brief procedure. However, patients who set ongoing goals greater than 3 need to be reminded that recovery or quality of life requires that they easily perform certain activities. Emphasize to the patient that satisfactory pain relief is a level of pain that is noticeable but not bothersome. Also, explain that a pain rating equal to or less than the goal should be maintained as much of the time as possible. Once again, be specific about the activities that accompany the pain rating goal. Ask the patient what pain rating would make it easy to sleep, eat, or perform other physical activities.

Not only does setting a comfort/function goal help the entire team, including the patient and family, know what the pain treatment plan should achieve, but it also helps the patient see how pain relief contributes to recovery or improves quality of life. As discussed in Chapter 1, many patients do not expect to have their pain relieved, are frightened of taking opioid analgesics, and value a stoic response to pain. By setting pain rating goals that correspond to function, patients learn that pain relief helps them recover faster from illness such as surgery. In the case of chronic pain, patients learn that pain control puts them back in control of their daily lives rather than allowing pain to control their lives.

The patient's comfort/function goal should be visible on all records where pain ratings are recorded, such as a bedside flow sheet. Whether the goal has been achieved or not should also be routinely included at change-of-shift report, perhaps as the fifth vital sign along with other vital signs.

Neuropathic Pain Scale

Until recently, no tool existed to assess the unique qualities of neuropathic pain. The Short Form McGill Pain Questionnaire (Melzack, 1987) contains items that capture the multiple descriptions of neuropathic pain, but it does not provide information about the degree to which the sensation is felt. A new assessment tool for neuropathic pain has been developed that is brief yet comprehensive (Form 3.3) (Galer, Jensen, 1997). Studying

288 patients with neuropathic pain, the researchers identified eight common qualities of neuropathic pain: sharp, hot, dull, cold, sensitive (like raw skin or a sunburn), itchy, and deep versus surface pain. Each item is rated on a 0 to 10 scale (0 = none; 10 = most imaginable). The tool is easy for most patients to learn, takes about 5 minutes to complete, and is sensitive to the effects of treatment.

Although this neuropathic pain scale is in the developmental stages, it appears to have implications for diagnosis and treatment. The words used by the patient to describe pain may indicate the underlying pain mechanism. For example, postherpetic neuralgia is more likely to be described as sharp, less cold, and more sensitive and itchy than other types of neuropathic pain (Galer, Jensen, 1997). Patients with diabetic neuropathy who described sharp and shooting pain were found in one study to be more likely to respond to clonidine than those who did not (Byas-Smith, Max, Muir et al., 1995).

Clinically, it appears that the neuropathic pain scale will be useful in the initial assessment of patients with chronic pain. Early identification of the existence of these sensations may facilitate the diagnosis and treatment of neuropathic pain. The scale could be used on follow-up to evaluate the effectiveness of treatment.

For patients who do not initially have neuropathic pain, routine pain assessment tools completed at each visit to the clinician might include a list of the eight descriptors on the neuropathic pain scale. The patient could be asked to indicate whether any of these sensations has been noted since the last visit. In that way, patients who did not originally have neuropathic pain might be identified, and changes in the progression and underlying pathologic condition of the patient may be more quickly assessed and treated.

Assessment of Breakthrough Pain

Chronic pain that is more or less stable and continuous may be accompanied by intermittent episodes of increased pain. In patients with chronic cancer pain who are already receiving opioids, these flares of pain are referred to as breakthrough pain. In these patients, severe breakthrough pain is very common, occurring in approximately two thirds of patients (Portenoy, Hagen, 1990). Although the term breakthrough pain is most often used in relation to patients with chronic cancer pain who are receiving ATC opioids, the occurrence of intermittent increases in pain is important to assess in all patients.

Two types of breakthrough pain are incident pain and end of dose failure. Pain that occurs spontaneously without warning or as a result of an identifiable event, such as coughing, is known as incident pain. These pain exacerbations may vary in duration from seconds to hours, may occur once a day or many times, and may be slow or sudden in onset. Incident pain may be handled with a quick-acting analgesic of short duration. When the

Text continued on p. 78.

● ● ● ● ●

FORM 3.3 **Neuropathy Pain Scale**

Date _____   Name _____

There are several different aspects of pain which we are interested in measuring: pain **sharpness, heat/cold, dullness, intensity,** overall **unpleasantness** and **surface vs. deep** pain.

The distinction between these aspects of pain might be clearer if you think of taste. For example, people might agree on how *sweet* a piece of pie might be (the *intensity* of sweetness), but some might enjoy it more if it were sweeter while others might prefer it to be less sweet. Similarly, people can judge the loudness of music and agree on what is more quiet and what is louder, but disagree on how it makes them feel. Some prefer quiet music and some prefer it louder. In short, the *intensity* of a sensation is not the same as how it makes you feel. A sound might be unpleasant and still be quiet (think of someone grating their fingernails along a chalkboard). A sound can be quiet and "dull" or loud and "dull."

Pain is the same. Many people are able to tell the difference between many aspects of their pain: for example, *how much* it hurts and *how unpleasant* or annoying it is. Although often the intensity of pain has a strong influence on how unpleasant the experience of pain is, some people are able to experience more pain than others before they feel very bad about it.

There are scales for measuring different aspects of pain. For one patient, a pain might feel extremely hot, but not at all dull, while another patient may not experience any heat, but feel like their pain is very dull. We expect you to rate very high on some of the scales below and very low on others. We want you to use the measures that follow to tell us exactly what your experience of pain has been, on average, *during the past week.*

● ●

Instructions: Please think about each sensation listed below and rate that sensation as the *average* you have experienced *during the past week.* Place an "X" through the number that best describes this.

1. Please use the scale below to tell us how **intense** your pain has been on average during the past week.

| No pain | 0 | 1 | 2 | 3 | 4 | 5 | 6 | 7 | 8 | 9 | 10 | The most **intense** pain sensation imaginable |

2. Please use the scale below to tell us how **sharp** your pain has felt on average during the past week. Words used to describe "sharp" feelings include: "like a knife," "like a spike," "jabbing" or "like jolts."

| No pain | 0 | 1 | 2 | 3 | 4 | 5 | 6 | 7 | 8 | 9 | 10 | The most **sharp** sensation imaginable ("like a knife") |

3. Please use the scale below to tell us how **hot** your pain has felt on average during the past week. Words used to describe very hot pain include: "burning" and "on fire."

| Not hot | 0 | 1 | 2 | 3 | 4 | 5 | 6 | 7 | 8 | 9 | 10 | The most **hot** sensation imaginable ("on fire") |

4. Please use the scale below to tell us how **dull** your pain has felt on average during the past week. Words used to describe very dull pain include: "like a dull toothache," "dull pain," "aching" and "like a bruise."

| Not dull | 0 | 1 | 2 | 3 | 4 | 5 | 6 | 7 | 8 | 9 | 10 | The most **dull** sensation imaginable |

May be duplicated for use in clinical practice. As appears in McCaffery M, Pasero C: *Pain: Clinical manual,* pp. 76-77, 1999, Mosby, Inc.   *Continued.*
From Galer BS, Jensen MP: Development and preliminary validation of a pain measure specific to neuropathic pain: The neuropathic pain scale, *Neurology* 48:337-338, 1997.

FORM 3.3 **Neuropathy Pain Scale—cont'd**

5. Please use the scale below to tell us how **cold** your pain has felt on average during the past week. Words used to describe very cold pain include: "like ice" and "freezing."

| Not cold | 0 | 1 | 2 | 3 | 4 | 5 | 6 | 7 | 8 | 9 | 10 | The most **cold** sensation imaginable ("freezing") |

6. Please use the scale below to tell us how **sensitive** your skin has been to light touch or clothing on average during the past week. Words used to describe sensitive skin include "like sunburned skin" and "raw skin."

| Not sensitive | 0 | 1 | 2 | 3 | 4 | 5 | 6 | 7 | 8 | 9 | 10 | The most **sensitive** sensation imaginable ("raw skin") |

7. Please use the scale below to tell us how **itchy** your pain has felt on average during the past week. Words used to describe itchy pain include: "like poison oak" and "like a mosquito bite."

| Not itchy | 0 | 1 | 2 | 3 | 4 | 5 | 6 | 7 | 8 | 9 | 10 | The most **itchy** sensation imaginable ("like poison oak") |

8. Which of the following best describes the **time** quality of your pain on average during the past week? **Please check only one: a, b, or c.**
   a. ❑ I felt background pain <u>all of the time</u> **and** occasional flare-ups (break-through pain) <u>some of the time</u>.

   Describe the background pain: _____
   Describe the flare-up (break-through pain): _____

   b. ❑ I felt a single type of pain <u>all of the time</u>. Describe this pain: _____

   c. ❑ I felt a single type of pain <u>only sometimes</u>. Describe this pain: _____

9. Now that you have told us the different physical aspects of your pain, the different types of sensations, we want you to tell us overall how **unpleasant** your pain has been. Words used to describe very unpleasant pain include: "miserable" and "intolerable." Remember, pain can have a low intensity, but still feel extremely unpleasant, and some kinds of pain can have a high intensity but be very tolerable. Please use the scale below to tell us how **unpleasant** your pain has felt on average during the past week.

| Not unpleasant | 0 | 1 | 2 | 3 | 4 | 5 | 6 | 7 | 8 | 9 | 10 | The most **unpleasant** sensation imaginable ("intolerable") |

10. Lastly, we want you to give us an estimate of the severity of your deep versus surface pain. We want you to rate each location of pain separately. We realize that it can be difficult to make these estimates, and most likely it will be a "best guess," but please give us your best estimate.

HOW INTENSE HAS YOUR **DEEP** PAIN BEEN ON AVERAGE DURING THE PAST WEEK?

| No **deep** pain | 0 | 1 | 2 | 3 | 4 | 5 | 6 | 7 | 8 | 9 | 10 | The most **intense** **deep** pain sensation imaginable |

HOW INTENSE HAS YOUR **SURFACE** PAIN BEEN ON AVERAGE DURING THE PAST WEEK?

| No **surface** pain | 0 | 1 | 2 | 3 | 4 | 5 | 6 | 7 | 8 | 9 | 10 | The most **intense** **surface** pain sensation imaginable |

patient is receiving ATC analgesics, especially controlled-release opioid formulations, pain that returns toward the end of the dosing interval is termed end of dose failure. This pain may be eliminated by increasing the dose of analgesic or shortening the intervals between doses.

No tool has been developed specifically for the assessment of breakthrough pain. However, use of a 24-hour record, such as a flow sheet that includes pain ratings, patient activities, and analgesic administration, is useful in capturing the characteristics of breakthrough pain. In brief, the breakthrough pain assessment includes identification of the following:

- Duration
- Intensity
- Quality, characteristics (e.g., aching, shooting)
- Precipitating factors (if any), such as bowel movement, change in the weather
- Factors that relieve the pain
- Sudden or slow onset
- Occurrence in relation to time of analgesic doses
- Frequency (numbers of occurrences in 24 hours)

Flow Sheets

Flow sheets for pain management are work sheets that document progress toward achieving and maintaining pain management goals. They are used for ongoing assessment and evaluation. Typically, flow sheets include, at a minimum, columns for time, pain ratings, facts about the analgesic administered (e.g., dose route), and side effects pertinent to the situation. Side effects pertinent to the use of opioids for severe pain in an opioid naive patient include sedation level and respiratory status. Side effects important with chronic opioid administration include constipation and nausea.

Flow sheets must be tailored to the patient population, clinical setting, and type of pain being managed. Some are designed for staff to complete on hospitalized patients using IV PCA for severe pain. Others are designed for the patient and/or family to use at home.

One important reason for using flow sheets for pain ratings is that recall of pain is poor. For example, in a study of 60 patients being discharged from the postanesthesia care unit, many were unable to recall the pain ratings they gave when they were admitted to the unit (DeLoach, Higgins, Caplan et al., 1998). In a study of 125 patients with a long history of facial pain, self-reported dates of onset of pain were compared with onset dates patients reported 7 years earlier (Raphael, Marbach, 1997). The dates reported differed by more than a year in 74% of the patients. As time went by, patients underestimated how chronic their pain was. They recalled pain as having begun more recently than was actually recorded in their records. Thus information about pain should be obtained and recorded near the time of event, whenever possible.

Research has verified that the use of pain flow sheets, compared with the routine narrative charting in nursing notes, is effective in improving pain management (e.g., decreasing pain intensity and sedation) (Brown, 1992; Faries, Mills, Goldsmith et al., 1991; McMillan, Williams, Chatfield et al., 1988).

Obtaining pain ratings before and after administration of analgesics is especially important because a tendency exists for clinicians to assume that analgesics are effective. For example, a study of 100 children and their nurses revealed that nurses overestimated the effectiveness of analgesics (Romsing, Moller-Sonnergaard, Hertel et al., 1996). However, when the patient is obviously in severe pain (e.g., following trauma or surgery), a pain rating need not be obtained initially. An analgesic should be given and pain ratings collected when the patient is better able to participate.

Following are explanations of two types of flow sheets, one for an acute care setting where patients with severe pain are being treated with opioids and another for home care situations. Patient examples accompany each.

Characteristics of the flow sheet for analgesic infusions

The flow sheet for analgesic infusions provides a quick and easy assessment and evaluation tool. It is used primarily in the hospital setting where nurses are responsible for recording the information. The information required on the analgesic infusion flow sheet varies widely from one institution to another.

Most flow sheets are designed to prevent duplicate documentation. Space can be provided on the back of the flow sheet for documenting detailed information (e.g., description of how severe pain or a side effect was brought under control) (see Form 3.4, *B*, on pp. 83-84). A mechanism can be incorporated in the flow sheet for referring other members of the health care team to this detailed information. For ease in using the flow sheet, the order of the information recorded in the columns of the flow sheet should correspond with the order in which the information is displayed on the screens of the institution's infusion pump.

An example of a flow sheet for analgesic infusions is Form 3.4, *A*, on pp. 79-80. Each space and column of the flow sheet is numbered to match the numbered explanations that follow.

1. *Route of administration.* Analgesic infusion therapies are given by either the IV, subcutaneous (SC), or epidural route of administration.
2. *Comfort goal.* The comfort goal is a pain level that will enable the patient to participate in recovery activities (e.g., 2/10 to 3/10). The patient is encouraged to set a comfort goal, and it is recorded in the space provided at the top right-hand corner

Text continued on p. 81.

FORM 3.4A 24-Hour Pain Management Flow Sheet for Analgesic Infusions

① IV ———— SC ———— Epidural ————

② Comfort Goal ————

③ Date	④ Time	⑤ Drug	⑥ Drug Concentration	⑦ Rem Vol	⑧ # INJ	⑨ # ATT	⑩ Given Vol	⑪ PCA Dose	⑫ Delay	⑬ Basal Rate	⑭ 1 Hr Limit	⑮ Clinician Bolus	Patient Assessment				⑳ Signature
													⑯ Pain Rate	⑰ Resp Rate	⑱ LOS S/1-4	⑲ S/E	

EPIDURAL CATHETER REMOVAL ㉑

"Epidural catheter site clean, dry, no redness, no edema, no back soreness or tenderness. Black mark visible on catheter tip."

(✓ = agree; ✱ = See comments)

Time ———— Signature ————

INFUSION SYSTEM ASSESSMENT (✓ = agree; ✱ = See comments) ㉒

"Infusion system securely taped, tubings patent, reservoir has volume, and parameters are set as prescribed." PCA/PCEA: "Patient button within reach, connected to pump, and functioning properly." Initials ———— Initials ————

NEW TUBING ———— Time ———— Initials ————

CODES FOR PATIENT ASSESSMENT

ASK PATIENTS TO RATE THEIR PAIN: ㉓

No pain .... Worst possible pain

LOS = LEVEL OF SEDATION ㉔

S = Sleep
1 = Alert, easy to arouse
2 = Occasionally drowsy; easy to arouse
3 = Frequently drowsy
4 = Somnolent, difficult to arouse

S/E = SIDE EFFECTS ㉕

M = Medicated
N = Nausea
V = Vomiting
P = Pruritis
UR = Urinary retention
SL = Sensory loss
MW = Muscle weakness

RECORD OF WASTE ㉖

DATE	TIME	DRUG	AMT	SIGNATURE	WITNESS

May be duplicated for use in clinical practice. As appears in McCaffery M, Pasero C: *Pain: Clinical manual*, pp. 79-80, 1999, Mosby, Inc. Copyright Chris Pasero, 1994; faces pain rating scale modified from Wong DL: *Whaley & Wong's essentials of pediatric nursing*, ed 5, pp. 1215-1216, St. Louis, 1997, Mosby.

Continued.

● ● ● ● ●

FORM 3.4A	**24-Hour Pain Management Flow Sheet for Analgesic Infusions—cont'd**	
DATE	TIME	COMMENTS

May be duplicated for use in clinical practice. As appears in McCaffery M, Pasero C: *Pain: Clinical manual*, pp. 79-80, 1999, Mosby, Inc.

Backside of 24-Hour Pain Management Flow Sheet provides space for comments when patient or infusion system assessment is outside of the norm. Comments can be made at any time by any member of the health care team and do not necessarily coincide with the flow sheet.

of the flow sheet. Pain ratings greater than the patient's comfort goal should trigger further assessment and possible intervention (see Chapter 6). This information can be used for quality assurance and improvement purposes (see Chapter 16).

3. *Date.* A new flow sheet can be started at 12 midnight (2400) every 24 hours or when space runs out for documentation.

4. *Time.* Pain ratings, respiratory status, level of sedation (LOS), and side effects usually are monitored every 1 to 2 hours for the first 12 to 24 hours of analgesic infusion therapies in opioid naive patients. After that time, these parameters usually can be monitored every 4 hours. The analgesic prescription (also called pump parameters) (numbers 5 to 15) is recorded typically only every 4 to 8 hours. An asterisk just to the left of the time column means that other members of the health care team should read comments on the back of the flow sheet.

5. *Drug.* After checking the drug reservoir label, the name of the drug or drugs in the drug reservoir are recorded in this column every 4 to 8 hours.

6. *Drug concentration.* The concentration of drug to solution (e.g., $\mu g/ml$, mg/ml) in the drug reservoir is recorded every 4 to 8 hours. The drug concentration programmed in the pump is checked for accuracy against the drug concentration recorded on the drug reservoir label.

7. *Remaining volume.* The amount of solution remaining in the drug reservoir is recorded every 4 to 8 hours. (This feature is not available on all pumps.)

8-9. *Injections and attempts.* Injections are the number of times the patient self-administers a PCA dose. Attempts are the number of times the patient presses the PCA button, whether a dose is delivered or not. These amounts are recorded for patients receiving PCA/PCEA. Most PCA pumps store in memory the number of injections and attempts every hour. This hourly information is added up and documented every 4 to 8 hours (i.e., the number recorded should reflect the number of injections and attempts since the last recording). This information is used to help determine the type of intervention that would benefit the patient the most (e.g., patient teaching, increase dose) (see Chapter 6).

10. *Given volume.* The amount of solution delivered since the start of therapy or since the last time the amount was cleared is recorded every 4 to 8 hours. (This feature is not available on all pumps.)

11. *PCA dose.* The amount the patient will receive each time a PCA bolus dose is self-administered is recorded every 4 to 8 hours.

12. *Delay interval.* The number of minutes that must elapse between PCA doses administered is recorded every 4 to 8 hours. This is the same as the "lockout interval."

13. *Basal rate.* The amount of the continuous analgesic infusion is recorded every 4 to 8 hours. Many pumps bypass this display screen if a basal rate has not been programmed.

14. *Hour limit.* The total amount the patient can receive in 1 hour by PCA dose and basal rate is recorded every 4 to 8 hours.

15. *Clinician bolus.* Clinician-administered bolus doses (supplemental doses) are recorded when administered.

16. *Pain rating.* The patient's pain rating is usually recorded every 1 to 2 hours during the first 12 to 24 hours, then every 4 hours if pain is controlled. The pain rating scale used in this institution is provided in the bottom left corner of the flow sheet. A pain rating higher than the patient's comfort goal (upper right-hand corner of flow sheet) should trigger further assessment and action.

17. *Respiratory rate.* One of the most important physical parameters for the opioid naive patient, respiratory rate (nurse monitored), is recorded every 1 to 2 hours during the first 12 to 24 hours, then every 4 hours if the respiratory status is stable. After this time, significant increases in opioid dose warrant a return to respiratory monitoring every 1 to 2 hours until a stable respiratory pattern is observed. The rate and depth of respirations should be compared with the baseline. Depending on the respiratory rate and depth, further action may be warranted (see Chapter 6).

18. *Level of sedation (LOS).* In opioid naive patients, LOS is as important to monitor as respiratory rate. LOS is usually recorded every 1 to 2 hours during the first 12 to 24 hours, then every 4 hours if the LOS is stable. After this time, significant increases in opioid dose warrant a return to LOS monitoring every 1 to 2 hours until a stable LOS is observed. The sedation scale used in this institution is at the bottom of the flow sheet. On this scale, a sedation level of 3 should trigger further assessment and a decrease in the opioid dose (see Chapter 6).

19. *Side effects (S/E).* Using the code for side effects (bottom of flow sheet), the presence of side effects is recorded every 1 to 2 hours during the first 12 to 24 hours, then every 4 hours if the patient has no side effects. The letter "M" recorded above or next to a side effect signifies that the patient was given medication to treat the side effect. Depending on the side effect, further action may be warranted and noted in the comment section

on the back of the flow sheet (see Form 3.4, *B*, on pp. 83-84) (see also Chapter 6).

20. *Signature.* The signature of the clinician who performs the assessment is recorded with each entry.

21. *Epidural catheter removal.* This section is used to document the removal of the epidural catheter. A check mark in the space provided signifies normal assessment findings and epidural catheter removal (agreement with the quoted statement). An asterisk in the space means that detailed information is provided in the comment section on the back of the flow sheet. Space is provided for the signature of the clinician removing the epidural catheter.

22. *Infusion system assessment.* This section is used to document that the infusion system, from patient access to the infusion pump, has been assessed and is functioning properly. This is documented usually as often as IV site assessment is documented in the institution (e.g., every 8 hours or every shift). A check mark in the space provided signifies normal assessment findings (agreement with the quoted statement). An asterisk in this space means that detailed information is provided in the comment section on the back of the flow sheet. Space is provided to record analgesic infusion pump tubing changes.

23. *Pain rating scale.* An example of the 0 to 10 NRS and the Wong-Baker Faces Pain Rating Scale is shown for clinicians' reference.

24. *Sedation scale.* The sleep/0 to 4 sedation scale is shown for clinicians' reference.

25. *Side effects.* The codes for recording the side effects are shown for clinicians' reference.

26. *Record of waste.* The amount of solution left in the drug reservoir that is discarded when a reservoir is changed or when therapy is discontinued is recorded in this section. Space is provided for the signature of the clinician who discards the solution and the person who witnesses the discard.

When patients are switched from analgesic infusions to oral pain medication, the medication record is used to document analgesic use. Wherever vital signs are recorded is the most logical place to document pain ratings. Space should be provided for recording the institution's minimum standard for pain assessment (e.g., pain rating every 8 hours), and pain ratings at the time an analgesic is administered and 1 hour later. When pain is difficult to control, the Pain Control Record (Form 3.5, *B*, p. 88) can be kept at the bedside for closer monitoring.

Examples of using the analgesic infusion flow sheet for a patient receiving IV PCA (see Form 3.4, *B*) and a patient receiving epidural analgesia (see Form 3.4, *C*) are shown on pp. 83 to 86.

Pain control records for outpatient care

Increasing numbers of patients with pain are being cared for on an outpatient basis. Patients with severe and sometimes escalating pain related to cancer are often cared for at home by family caregivers. Patients with moderate to severe pain related to surgical procedures are discharged from the hospital quickly, sometimes on the same day of their surgery. Because flow sheets for these patients are kept by the patient and/or family, they must be especially easy to use. Form 3.5, *A,* (p. 87), presents a flow sheet designed for these circumstances.

To avoid burdening the patient and family, certain criteria should be established regarding when to keep the record and for how long. The instructions for the pain control record in Form 3.5, *A,* stipulate that the record is to be kept only until an effective pain management plan is developed. This pain control record is designed for the home care of patients with pain related to progressive disease, typically patients who are terminally ill (see Patient example, Form 3.5, *B*).

By altering the instructions, the same form may be used for patients being discharged from the hospital with potentially significant pain. For example, in ambulatory surgery, patients are usually discharged before there is time to establish the effectiveness of the oral analgesics they will be taking at home. Such patients may be asked to complete this form about every 2 hours for the remainder of the day until the clinician calls that evening. With the pain control record, patients can report their status. If a patient encounters unrelieved pain or troublesome side effects such as nausea, this will be detected before the patient spends an uncomfortable night and develops complications from poorly managed pain or other problems. Information from the pain control record will be helpful in correcting the problem. For example, unrelieved pain may be due to failure to take the analgesic or the analgesic prescription may be inadequate.

For a hospitalized patient for whom the switch from parenteral or spinal analgesia to oral analgesia is not going smoothly, this pain control record may be modified and kept by the patient at the bedside. The information may be summarized in the nursing notes. Pain ratings every 2 hours may expedite identification of an effective oral analgesic plan.

For certain periods of time a daily pain control record may be indicated for patients with chronic nonmalignant pain, such as headaches. This type of record is especially important when medications or other treatments are being evaluated for continued use or are being adjusted to improve effectiveness.

Poor recall of pain underscores the importance of asking some patients under certain circumstances to keep a record of pain management in the outpatient setting. The patient's recall of pain often influences both the diagnosis and treatment of pain. In one study of patients with

FORM 3.4B 24-Hour Pain Management Flow Sheet for Analgesic Infusions

Patient A

IV ✓ SC ____ Epidural ____ Comfort Goal 3

Date	Time	Drug	Drug Concentration	Rem Vol	# INJ	# ATT	Given Vol	PCA Dose	Delay	Basal Rate	1 Hr Limit	Clinician Bolus	Pain Rate	Resp Rate	LOS S/1-4	S/E	Signature
4/10	2400	Morphine	1 mg/1 ml	175	9	10	20	1 mg	8 min	0	7 mg	—	3	18	1	0	N. Nurse
	0200													16	S	0	N. Nurse
	0400													16	S	0	N. Nurse
* 0500	0500	Morphine	1 mg/1 ml		1	1		1 mg	8 min	add 1 mg	8 mg	2 mg	8	18	1	0	N. Nurse
* 0515	0515	Morphine	1 mg/1 ml		1	1						2 mg	6	18	1	0	N. Nurse
* 0530	0530				1	1						—	4	18	1	0	N. Nurse
* 0600	0600				2	2							2	16	1	0	N. Nurse
	0800	Morphine	1 mg/1 ml	160	3	3	35	1 mg	8 min	1 mg	8 mg	—	2	18	1	0	U. Nurse
	1000													18	S	0	U. Nurse
	1200												2	16	1	0	U. Nurse
* 1600	1600	Morphine	1 mg/1 ml	142	10	12	53	1 mg	8 min	1 mg	8 mg	—	2	18	1	0	C. Nurse

EPIDURAL CATHETER REMOVAL

"Epidural catheter site clean, dry, no redness, no edema, no back soreness or tenderness. Black mark visible on catheter tip." (✓ = agree; * = See comments)

Time ____ Signature ____

INFUSION SYSTEM ASSESSMENT (✓ = agree; * = See comments)

"Infusion system securely taped, tubings patent, reservoir has volume, and parameters are set as prescribed." (PCA)/PCEA: "Patient button within reach, connected to pump, and functioning properly." Initials N.N. ✓ Initials U.N. ✓ Initials C.N. ✓

NEW TUBING ____ Time ____ Initials ____

CODES FOR PATIENT ASSESSMENT

LOS = LEVEL OF SEDATION

S = Sleep
1 = Alert, easy to arouse
2 = Occasionally drowsy, easy to arouse
3 = Frequently drowsy
4 = Somnolent, difficult to arouse

S/E = SIDE EFFECTS

M = Medicated
N = Nausea
V = Vomiting
P = Pruritis
UR = Urinary retention
SL = Sensory loss
MW = Muscle weakness

RECORD OF WASTE

DATE	TIME	DRUG	AMT	SIGNATURE	WITNESS

ASK PATIENTS TO RATE THEIR PAIN:

No pain										Worst possible pain
0	1	2	3	4	5	6	7	8	9	10
0		2		4		6		8		10

Continued.

• • • • •

FORM 3.4B **24-Hour Pain Management Flow Sheet for Analgesic Infusions—cont'd**		
DATE	TIME	COMMENTS
4/10	0500	Called to room by patient who reported he was awakened by severe pain. No PCA doses last 5 hours while asleep. Given bolus dose & basal rate added. N. Nurse
	0515	Improved but still uncomfortable. Bolus repeated. N. Nurse
	0530	Patient reports "I feel much better." States he will use PCA to reduce pain further. Told to call me whenever needed. N. Nurse
	0600	Patient reports good pain control & is pleased with addition of basal rate. N. Nurse
	1600	Stable at 24 h post op. Switched to q 4 h resp. rate, LOS, pain rating & side effects. C. Nurse

May be duplicated for use in clinical practice. As appears in McCaffery M, Pasero C: *Pain: Clinical manual*, pp. 83-84, 1999, Mosby, Inc.

Backside of 24-Hour Pain Management Flow Sheet provides space for comments when patient or infusion system assessment is outside of the norm. Comments can be made at any time by any member of the health care team and do not necessarily coincide with the flow sheet.

FORM 3.4B   Patient assessment columns show that the patient had satisfactory pain control while awake, but after 5 hours of sleep and no self-administering PCA, the patient was awakened by pain. Pain was brought under control with two clinician-administered bolus doses and the addition of a basal rate. Note that the number of injections and attempts (e.g., 9 and 10 at 2400 and 10 and 12 at 1600) reflect the total number of injections and attempts since the last recording. The patient's pain, respiratory rate, LOS, and side effects are recorded every 2 hours during the first 24 hours after surgery, and pump parameters are recorded only every 8 hours.

---

chronic headache, pain ratings from daily pain diaries kept over approximately 1 week were compared with patients' memories of pain felt during that time (Eich, Reeves, Jaeger et al., 1985). Recall of pain intensity for maximum, usual, and minimum levels was influenced by the pain intensity felt at the time of the interview. The patients recalled their previous levels of pain as being more severe than they actually had been when the intensity of their present pain was high, but as less severe when their present pain intensity was low. In another study of patients with chronic pain, results with regard to recall of pain were similar (Smith, Safer, 1993). In addition, findings revealed that patients with lower present pain ratings also recalled their medication use as less than it actually was.

In a study of patients receiving nerve blocks for pain, pain ratings were obtained before and after the block as well as 2 days and 2 weeks after the procedure (Porzelius, 1995). Findings revealed that memory distortions were common. At 2 days and 2 weeks after the block, many patients recalled pain immediately after the block as higher than they had reported. No correlations were found between memory distortions and gender, litigation, psychologic factors, and other variables.

In outpatient care it is common to ask patients about their average or usual pain over the last week. Clinicians must realize that when precise information about pain ratings is needed to determine further treatment, daily records will be more accurate than recall. Under these circumstances, a daily pain control record is indicated. In Form 3.5, *B*, the patient was awakened by moderate to severe pain. It would be difficult to expect accurate recall of the variations in pain ratings and the times when supplemental doses were taken.

Communication Strategies

Pain is best managed by a team approach. Seldom does any one clinician possess the time, knowledge, and skill to provide all the care required by a patient with pain. Usually the care of a single patient requires at least the involvement of a physician, nurse, and pharmacist, and sometimes many other health care professionals representing various disciplines. Working as a team becomes increasingly important as pain management becomes incorporated in the current health care system of managed care.

Nurses have emerged as pivotal members of the team with respect to pain management. As has been known in the palliative care setting for decades, the nurse is the cornerstone of the team approach to caring for patients with pain. The nurse uses, as necessary, the expertise of all team members, applies their recommendations to the care of the individual patient, and reports to team

FORM 3.4C 24-Hour Pain Management Flow Sheet for Analgesic Infusions

Patient **B**   IV _____   SC _____   Epidural **✓**   Comfort Goal **2**

Date	Time	Drug	Drug Concentration	Rem Vol	# INJ	# ATT	Given Vol	PCA Dose	Delay	Basal Rate	1 Hr Limit	Clinician Bolus	Pain Rate	Resp Rate	LOS S/1-4	S/E	Signature
4/10	2400	Fentanyl & Bupivacaine	10 µg/ml & 0.0625%	162	1	1	33	10µg	15 min	40 µg	80 µg	—		18	S		N. Nurse
	0200													16	S		N. Nurse
*	0400	Fentanyl & Bupivacaine	10 µg/ml & 0.0625%		0	0		10µg	15 min	30 µg→	70 µg	—	0	18	2	M P	N. Nurse
	0600												0	18	2	0	N. Nurse
*	0800	Fentanyl & Bupivacaine	10 µg/ml & 0.0625%	133	1	1	62	10µg	15 min	20 µg→	60 µg	—	0	16	2	M P	U. Nurse
	1000												0	16	1	0	U. Nurse
	1200													18	S		U. Nurse
	1400												1	18	2	0	U. Nurse
	1600	Fentanyl & Bupivacaine	10 µg/ml & 0.0625%	113	4	4	82	10µg	15 min	20 µg	60 µg	—	1	16	1	0	C. Nurse
*	2000													18	S		C. Nurse

EPIDURAL CATHETER REMOVAL

"Epidural catheter site clean, dry, no redness, no edema, no back soreness or tenderness. Black mark visible on catheter tip."   (✓ = agree; * = See comments)

Time _____   _____ Signature

INFUSION SYSTEM ASSESSMENT (✓ = agree; * = See comments)

"Infusion system securely taped, tubings patent, reservoir has volume, and parameters are set as prescribed." PCA (PCEA) "Patient button within reach, connected to pump, and functioning properly."   Initials _N.N._ ✓   Initials _U.N._ ✓   Initials _C.N._ ✓

NEW TUBING   Initials _____   Time _____

CODES FOR PATIENT ASSESSMENT

LOS = LEVEL OF SEDATION

S = Sleep
1 = Alert, easy to arouse
2 = Occasionally drowsy, easy to arouse
3 = Frequently drowsy
4 = Somnolent, difficult to arouse

S/E = SIDE EFFECTS

M = Medicated
N = Nausea
V = Vomiting
P = Pruritus
UR = Urinary retention
SL = Sensory loss
MW = Muscle weakness

ASK PATIENTS TO RATE THEIR PAIN:

No pain   0 1 2 3 4 5 6 7 8 9 10   Worst possible pain

0   2   4   6   8   10

RECORD OF WASTE

DATE	TIME	DRUG	AMT	SIGNATURE	WITNESS

May be duplicated for use in clinical practice. As appears in McCaffery M, Pasero C: Pain: Clinical manual, pp. 85-86, 1999, Mosby, Inc.
Copyright Chris Pasero, 1994; faces pain rating scale modified from Wong DL: Whaley & Wong's essentials of pediatric nursing, ed 5, pp. 1215-1216, St. Louis, 1997, Mosby.

Continued.

● ● ● ● ●

FORM 3.4C **24-Hour Pain Management Flow Sheet for Analgesic Infusions—cont'd**		
DATE	TIME	COMMENTS
4/10	0400	Patient reports discomfort from facial & neck itching. No rash or redness. Given Benadryl & basal rate decreased. N. Nurse
	0800	Patient reports return of facial "itchiness" No rash or redness. Given Benadryl & basal rate decreased. U. Nurse
	2000	24 h post op. To q 4 h pain rating, resp. rate, LOS, & side effects. Stable. C. Nurse

May be duplicated for use in clinical practice. As appears in McCaffery M, Pasero C: *Pain: Clinical manual*, pp. 85-86, 1999, Mosby, Inc.

Backside of 24 Hour Pain Management Flow Sheet provides space for comments when patient or infusion system assessment is outside of the norm. Comments can be made at any time by any member of the health care team and do not necessarily coincide with the flow sheet.

FORM 3.4C   Patient assessment columns show that the patient had very adequate pain control with pain ratings of 0 to 1, which are less than the patient's comfort goal of 2, and that the analgesic dose was safe with a LOS of S or 1 to 2. Itching is the only side effect and was handled by decreasing the basal rate. Note that the patient's pain, respiratory rate, LOS, and side effects are recorded every 2 hours during the first 24 hours after surgery, and pump parameters are recorded only every 8 hours.

---

members regarding the success of the plan or problems that emerge requiring revision of the plan.

The assessment tools previously discussed are important methods of fostering a team approach. They provide a method of communication between team members. Standardization of these tools plus other communication formats facilitates communication and avoids delays in making appropriate changes in the pain treatment plan.

Such a team approach requires collaboration among the clinicians and the patients and their families. In simple terms, collaborative practice means working together, not against. Following are some basic requirements for a team/collaborative approach to pain management (Summary in Box 3.8 on p. 89), many of which have already been incorporated in the assessment tools presented in this chapter:

1. *Common goals.* Two aspects of establishing a common goal concern setting goals for individual patients and acknowledging the rights of all patients with pain.

    In each specific situation the physician, nurse, patient, and others involved in the care must agree on a common goal, referred to in Box 3.8 as the comfort/function goal. This is often a simple matter of identifying activities the patient values or needs to perform and the pain rating that would be necessary for engaging in these activities. An example is the surgical patient who requires a pain rating of 3 on a scale of 0 to 10 to ambulate for 10 minutes.

    Underlying agreement on specific, common goals is an agreement on the rights of all patients

with pain. Some agencies formulate a list of patients' rights that addresses pain management. In the absence of such a list the statement of patients' rights published by the Joint Commission on Accreditation of Healthcare Organizations (JCAHO) is useful (Accreditation manual for hospitals, 1994). JCAHO states that all patients have a right to effectively managed pain. The Agency for Health Care Policy and Research (AHCPR) states in its guideline for pain management that "patients should have access to the best level of pain relief that may safely be provided" (Acute Pain Management Guideline Panel 1992b, p. 13).

2. *Common language.* Obviously, communication is facilitated when all people involved are using the same words to refer to important elements of the situation. Pain rating scales are an example of using a common language. One of the most essential components of pain management is assessment of pain intensity. Pain rating scales that are valid, reliable, and easy to understand and use have been discussed in this chapter. For each individual patient a single pain rating scale appropriate for the patient should be used by all team members when they discuss pain management among themselves and with the patient and family.

    Among clinicians, another component of a common language is using standardized assessment tools and formats for written communication and documentation. Examples of these, already discussed in this chapter, are the flow sheets.

FORM 3.5A **Pain Control Record**

This is a record of how your pain medicines are working. Please keep this record until you and your nurse/ doctor find the dose and frequency of medicine that provides satisfactory pain relief for you most of the time. After that, you only need to keep this record when you have problems related to your pain medicines.

Name: _____ Date: _____

GOALS Satisfactory pain rating: _____ Activities: _____

My pain rating scale:

|---|---|---|---|---|---|---|---|---|---|---|
| 0 | 1 | 2 | 3 | 4 | 5 | 6 | 7 | 8 | 9 | 10 |

No
pain

Moderate
pain

Worst
possible
pain

Directions: Rate your pain before you take pain medicine and 1 to 2 hours later.

Time:	Pain rating:	Medicine I took:	Side effects (drowsy? upset stomach?)	Other:

If pain is greater than _____ , or if you have other problems with your pain medicine, call:

Nurse: Name/phone _____

Doctor: Name/phone _____

Continued.

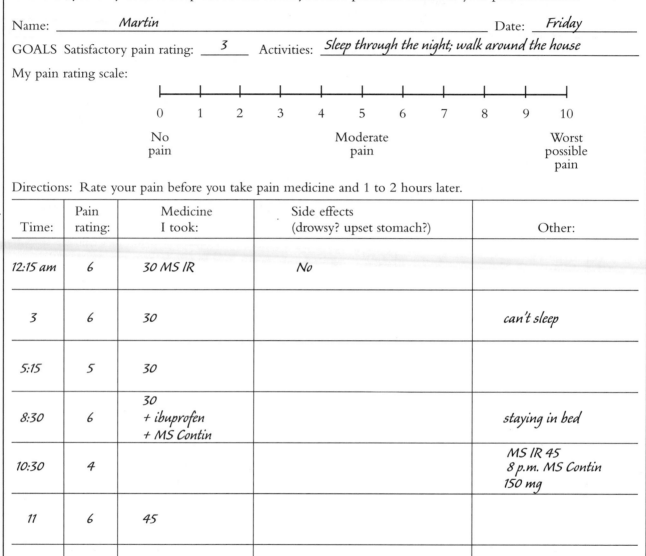

FORM 3.5B **Pain Control Record: Patient Example**

This is a record of how your pain medicines are working. Please keep this record until you and your nurse/doctor find the dose and frequency of medicine that provides satisfactory pain relief for you most of the time. After that, you only need to keep this record when you have problems related to your pain medicines.

Name: _____Martin_____   Date: _Friday_

GOALS Satisfactory pain rating: ___3___   Activities: _Sleep through the night; walk around the house_

My pain rating scale:

| 0 | 1 | 2 | 3 | 4 | 5 | 6 | 7 | 8 | 9 | 10 |

No pain   Moderate pain   Worst possible pain

Directions: Rate your pain before you take pain medicine and 1 to 2 hours later.

Time:	Pain rating:	Medicine I took:	Side effects (drowsy? upset stomach?)	Other:
12:15 am	6	30 MS IR	No	
3	6	30		can't sleep
5:15	5	30		
8:30	6	30 + ibuprofen + MS Contin		staying in bed
10:30	4			MS IR 45 8 p.m. MS Contin 150 mg
11	6	45		
12	3			

If pain is greater than ___5___ , or if you have other problems with your pain medicine, call:

Nurse: Name/phone   _C. Adams   555-1234_

Doctor: Name/phone   _Jones   555-4321_

FORM 3.5 B   Patient example. This patient has been receiving the following analgesics ATC every day: ibuprofen, 400 mg qid; amitriptyline, 100 mg HS; MS Contin, 100 mg q12h (8 AM and 8 PM). His supplemental (breakthrough, rescue) dose is morphine immediate release (MS IR), 30 mg PO q2h. He usually takes two supplemental doses a day. This has relieved his pain to a 3 or less, and he has been able to sleep through the night uninterrupted by pain and walk around his home. The record reveals that his pain ratings now are greater than 3 and that he is taking supplemental doses every 3 to 4 hours. Pain keeps him awake and he stays in bed. The patient talks with the nurse at 10:30 AM. The nurse contacts the physician and the decision is to increase his morphine doses by 50% to 45 mg MS IR q2h and to MS Contin 150 mg q12h. (This dose of MS Contin requires five 30-mg tablets. However, depending on the tablet strength the patient has on hand, the MS Contin dose may be slightly more or less than 150 mg.) When an opioid dose is safe but ineffective, a 50% increase will usually produce a moderate increase in pain relief. When the patient takes more than two supplemental doses during a 12-hour period, the controlled-release should be increased.

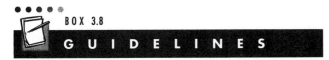

ESTABLISHING A TEAM/COLLABORATIVE APPROACH TO PAIN MANAGEMENT

1. Common goals:
   Agreement on comfort/function goals for pain relief (e.g. pain rating, activities)
   Agreement on patient's rights
2. Common language:
   Pain rating scale
   Standardized assessment tools
3. Common knowledge base:
   Clinical practice guidelines (e.g., AHCPR)
   Patient education
4. Regular communication:
   Regular contact (e.g., daily progress report, weekly fax, notes)
   Standardized report format

May be duplicated for use in clinical practice. From McCaffery M, Pasero C: *Pain: Clinical manual,* p. 89. Copyright © 1999, Mosby, Inc.

3. *Common knowledge.* Because pain is a new scientific discipline, lack of education about pain management is expected. For this reason, clinical practice guidelines (see Chapter 1, p. 7 for a list) have been developed. Those from the American Pain Society and AHCPR may be used to provide clinicians with a quick summary of current recommendations for pain management. One or more of these can be distributed to clinicians and referred to for guidance each time a question arises about the assessment and treatment of pain. Although a considerable amount of essential information is contained in the clinical practice guidelines, the single most important directive is that clinicians must accept the patient's report of pain. Repeated reference to this recommendation is often necessary.

The clinical practice guidelines from AHCPR have companion patient guides that summarize current pain management recommendations in language the patients and families can understand. When the clinician guidelines are used in conjunction with the patient guides, all members of the team share common knowledge.

4. *Regular communication.* All the above needs to be shared by team members on a regular, predictable basis. In some instances, such as the care of patients with chronic pain, this is a weekly team meeting. In other situations, such as the care of surgical patients, it may be the recording of pain ratings every 8 hours on the vital sign sheet and including this information at the change of shift report. Home health care agencies may use a standardized format to fax updates to referring physicians and follow up with telephone calls when there are problems. Care should be taken, however, to report the positive, not just the problems.

Virtually all communications about pain should include reference to the goal (e.g., pain rating and activities). A format for communicating pain management problems and a patient example are presented in Form 3.6, *A,* and Form 3.6, *B* (patient example). This form may be used in either inpatient or outpatient settings and for patients with either acute or chronic pain. A format for communicating verbally and a patient example are presented in Box 3.9. All of these patient examples are from the pain control record on Form 3.5, *B,* on p. 88.

CHALLENGES IN PAIN ASSESSMENT

Some patients with pain are unable or unwilling to report or discuss their pain. Patients with pain who are able to communicate verbally may deny having pain or refuse analgesia. Other patients are simply incapable of providing a self-report of pain. They may be cognitively impaired or unconscious. Such circumstances necessitate using other less reliable indicators of pain, always being mindful of the fact that in the absence of self-report all else is an educated guess.

Patients Who Deny Pain or Refuse Pain Relief

When a patient denies pain, clinicians must accept this because the patient's self-report is the single most reliable indicator of pain. However, when the patient's behaviors, known pathologic condition, or other findings suggest the existence of pain, clinicians are responsible for exploring this seeming contradiction with the patient and family. Sometimes the patient will acknowledge the pain but refuse analgesics. Clinicians must respect this decision but, again, the reasons should be discussed with the patient and family. Providing information or considering other approaches to pain management may result in the admission of pain or the acceptance of measures to relieve it.

Reluctance to report pain or to use analgesics obviously results in poor pain relief. The reasons patients may do this have been shown to be associated with a variety of specific concerns (Ward, Goldberg, Miller-McCauley et al., 1993), many further supported by a survey of laymen's attitudes (Mayday Fund, 1993). The relationships between patient's attitudes about pain and its treatment and their willingness to report pain and take analgesics were investigated using the Barriers Questionnaire (BQ) (Ward, Goldberg, Miller-McCauley et al., 1993) (Form 3.7 on p. 93.) The patients in the study had chronic cancer pain. The patients' responses to the BQ revealed that poor pain control was related to concerns about addiction, side effects, and tolerance (the need to "save" the pain medicine); the belief that increased pain

Text continues on p. 92.

● ● ● ● ●

FORM 3.6A **Pain Report**

To: _____   From: _____   Date: _____

Patient: _____   HOSPICE PATIENT?   YES ____   NO ____

Current analgesic dose:	Supplemental dose:

Pain rating <u>goal</u>: (Circle)

   0   1   2   3   4   5   6   7   8   9   10

Frequency of supplemental use:

Current pain rating:

   0   1   2   3   4   5   6   7   8   9   10

Comments:

Requested analgesic dose:	Requested supplemental dose:

(PHYSICIAN: SIGN BELOW IF AGREE WITH Rx AS REQUESTED AND/OR SUPPLY OTHER Rx:)

Rx AS REQUESTED _____

OTHER _____   Rx:

May be duplicated for use in clinical practice. As appears in McCaffery M, Pasero C: *Pain: Clinical manual*, p. 90, 1999, Mosby, Inc.

FORM 3.6A   Example of a form for standardizing nurse-physician reporting of pain management problems. The form may be faxed from one clinician to another, sent by electronic mail, and/or become part of the patient's record.

Modified from Hospice of Lubbock, Lubbock, TX.

● ● ● ● ●

FORM 3.6B **Pain Report**

To: _R. Jones, M D_   From: _C. Adams_   Date: _Friday_

Patient: _Martin_   HOSPICE PATIENT?   YES ✔   NO ___

Current analgesic dose:	Supplemental dose:
ibuprofen 400 mg qid amitriptyline 100 mg HS MS Contin 100 mg q 12 h	MS IR (morphine immediate release) 30 mg q 2 h

Pain rating <u>goal</u>: (Circle)

0   1   2   ③   4   5   6   7   8   9   10

Frequency of supplemental use:

q 3-4 h

Current pain rating:

0   1   2   3   ④   5   6   7   8   9   10

Comments: Goal of 3 enables pt. to sleep through night & walk around his home. In spite of supplemental doses, pain ↑ 4-6. He remains alert. Pain kept pt. awake last night & he's unable to get out of bed. Cancer guideline recommends 25-50% ↑ in opioid doses that are safe but ineffective. See request below.

Requested analgesic dose:	Requested supplemental dose:
MS Contin 150 mg q 12 h	MS IR 45 mg q 2 h

(PHYSICIAN: SIGN BELOW IF AGREE WITH Rx AS REQUESTED AND/OR SUPPLY OTHER Rx:)

Rx AS REQUESTED _____

OTHER _____   Rx: _____

May be duplicated for use in clinical practice. As appears in McCaffery M, Pasero C: *Pain: Clinical manual,* p. 91, 1999, Mosby, Inc.

F O R M   3.6 B   Pain report: patient example. This example of the nurse's written communication to the physician concerning a pain management problem is based on the patient's Pain Control Record on Form 3.6A.

Modified from Hospice of Lubbock, Lubbock, TX.

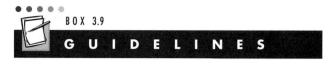

BOX 3.9

G U I D E L I N E S

NURSE-PHYSICIAN COMMUNICATION AND PATIENT EXAMPLE

Communication steps
1. Identify physician by name.
2. Give your name.
3. State the general nature of the call.
4. Identify the patient by name and diagnosis.
5. State the pain management goal: pain rating and activities.
6. Summarize the current pain ratings and effect of pain on activities.
7. List the current analgesic doses and relevant side effects.
8. Suggest a solution (on the basis of a clinical practice guideline, if possible).

Patient example (on the basis of Pain Control Record in Form 3.5B):
The numbers correspond to the above.
1. Hello, Dr. Jones.
2. This is Cindy Adams.
3. I am calling regarding a pain management problem
4. with your patient, Martin, who has prostate cancer with metastasis.
5. The pain management goal for Martin is to keep his pain ratings at 3 or less on a scale of 0 to 10 so he can sleep through the night and get out of bed to walk around his home.
6. His pain ratings over the past several hours have been 4 to 6, and he has been unable to sleep or get out of bed.
7. His current dose of MS Contin is 100 mg q12h with a supplemental dose of MS IR 30 mg q2h. He has had to take four supplemental doses since midnight. He remains very alert but in pain. He also takes ibuprofen, 400 qid, and amitriptyline, 100 mg hs.
8. The cancer pain guideline says that opioid doses that are safe but ineffective may be titrated up by 25% to 50%. What do you think about increasing Martin's morphine doses by 50%? That would mean 150 mg MS Contin q12h and 45 mg MSIR q2h PRN.

May be duplicated for use in clinical practice. From McCaffery M, Pasero C: *Pain: Clinical manual,* p. 92. Copyright © 1999, Mosby, Inc.

meant increased disease; concern that complaining about pain would distract the physician from curing the illness; and the belief that "good" patients do not complain about pain. Many of these attitudes and fears are discussed in greater detail in Chapters 1 and 6.

The BQ is recommended for use with patients and their families to help identify what may be causing the patient to deny pain or refuse analgesics. For patients newly diagnosed with a disease that may become painful eventually, the BQ may be administered before pain occurs to identify barriers to pain control before problems arise. Depending on the patient population, clinicians may wish to adapt the BQ by omitting some items and

adding others, such as concerns about finances, hiding pain from the family and others, distrust of caregivers, not being a "sissy," or wanting to avoid highly technologic methods of pain control.

Immediately after the BQ is administered, clinicians should discuss the results with the patient. The patient and family should be assured that many others have similar concerns, but that these need not be problems. Appropriate patient teaching should follow. Most patient teaching literature about pain control covers the concerns listed in the BQ. However, one session of patient teaching will not be sufficient to reassure the patient and family, especially about concerns related to addiction. (See Chapter 6 for ways of addressing fears of addiction.)

One of the most frustrating occurrences in pain management is knowing that a patient with pain does not have to suffer, yet the patient refuses help. The BQ may help clinicians begin the process of exploring why a particular patient has decided to endure pain.

Interestingly, denial of pain is not always deliberate or conscious. Sometimes patients have a narrow concept of pain and will deny it when asked. Following up with other terms such as aching or hurting may uncover the existence of pain.

Other situations where pain is denied are related to the energizing effect of visits from physicians or health team members. Before and after the visit, the patient may report pain. But, the encounter during hospital rounds or a clinic visit sometimes has a powerful positive placebo effect, and the patient honestly reports feeling fine at the time. Clinicians must remember to question the patient further and to check the patient's record to determine what occurred before the visit.

Some patients who have experienced pain for a long time seem to lose their frame of reference. Oddly, they may forget what it is like not to have pain. As one patient reported after reluctantly taking an analgesic, "I didn't know I had pain. I guess I had been in pain too long to know the difference."

Sometimes pain will not be reported, not because of any wish to deny pain, but because the patient believes that the health care providers know about the pain. The patient may reason that the clinicians know about his or her disease or surgery and know that pain is present. Therefore it is unnecessary to tell them. For example, a study comparing adolescents' pain ratings with their perceptions of nurses' evaluations of their pain revealed that adolescents perceived that nurses know how much pain they are experiencing (Favaloro, Touzel, 1990).

Patients With Impaired Communication

This group of patients covers a wide range of communication difficulties, from those who are conscious but unable to speak or are nonverbal to those who are both unconscious and unable to speak. Examples are

● ● ● ● ●

FORM 3.7 **Barriers Questionnaire**

We are interested in learning more about your attitudes toward treatment of pain. There are no right or wrong answers, we just want to know what *you* think. Please answer all the questions. For each of the items below, please *circle the number* (0, 1, 2, 3, 4, or 5) that comes closest to *how much you agree* with that item.

1) Pain medicine cannot really control pain.

        0   1   2   3   4   5

    Do not agree   Agree very

        at all   much

2) People get addicted to pain medicine easily.

        0   1   2   3   4   5

    Do not agree   Agree very

        at all   much

3) Good patients avoid talking about pain.

        0   1   2   3   4   5

    Do not agree   Agree very

        at all   much

4) The experience of pain is a sign that the illness has gotten worse.

        0   1   2   3   4   5

    Do not agree   Agree very

        at all   much

5) It is easier to put up with pain than with the side effects that come from pain medicine.

        0   1   2   3   4   5

    Do not agree   Agree very

        at all   much

6) Pain medicine should be "saved" in case the pain gets worse.

        0   1   2   3   4   5

    Do not agree   Agree very

        at all   much

7) Pain builds character—it's good for you.

        0   1   2   3   4   5

    Do not agree   Agree very

        at all   much

8) Complaining about pain could distract a doctor from curing my problem.

        0   1   2   3   4   5

    Do not agree   Agree very

        at all   much

FORM 3.7 Barriers Questionnaire (BQ). If the patient agrees with any of these items, it could result in the patient failing to report pain or not taking analgesics. As soon as the patient (and family, if possible) has completed this, the clinician must begin appropriate patient teaching, accompanied by written materials.

Information from Gordon DB, Ward SE: Correcting patient misconceptions about pain, *Am J Nurs* 95(7):43-45, 1995; Ward SE, Goldberg N, Miller-McCauley V et al: Patient-related barriers to management of cancer pain, *Pain* 52:319-324, 1993.

infants and those children and adults who have cognitive impairment, severe emotional disturbance, dementia, delirium, psychosis; who are frail or among the oldest-old (>85 years); who are intubated; who speak a different language; or whose educational or cultural background is significantly different from that of the health care team (Acute Pain Management Guideline Panel, 1992a; American Pain Society, 1992).

Cognitively impaired elders

Because self-report is the most reliable indicator of pain, every effort should be made to obtain pain ratings. Sometimes clinicians prematurely conclude that the patient cannot report pain or use a pain rating scale. In a study of 758 cognitively impaired nursing home residents investigators concluded that although these patients "may slightly underreport experienced pain, their self-reports are generally no less valid than those of cognitively intact individuals" (Parmelee, Smith, Katz, 1993, p. 517).

Furthermore, even patients with substantial cognitive impairment may be able to use a pain rating scale. A study of 217 patients in skilled nursing homes who were dependent in most activities of daily living, had a mean age of 84.9 years, and had substantial cognitive impairment (Mean Folstein Mini-Mental State examination score = 12.1) revealed that many reported pain and were able to use a pain rating scale (Ferrell, Ferrell, Rivera, 1995). Of these patients, 62% reported pain, mostly musculoskeletal and neuropathic, and 83% who reported pain could complete at least one of five pain rating scales that were explained to them. The pain rating scale completed by the most patients (65%) was the McGill's Present Pain Intensity scale, a 0 to 5 scale with word anchors. Before patients were considered unable to respond to a specific scale, they were given at least 30 seconds to reply, and the scale was repeated at least three times.

These findings suggest that teaching cognitively impaired patients to use a pain rating scale is best accomplished by allowing sufficient time for the patient to process the information and then respond. It also appears that a 0 to 5 scale may be preferable to a 0 to 10 scale for these patients.

Unconscious patients

Some patients are mistakenly believed to be unconscious or pain-free. For example, patients with endotracheal tubes or those who have received a neuromuscular blocking agent, such as pancuronium (which does not alter sensitivity to pain), may be fairly alert and fully capable of feeling pain. Health care professionals must suspect pain in these individuals. In a sample of 24 patients in the intensive care unit, 63% recalled moderate to severe pain; those who could not talk (80% had endotracheal tubes) described numerous behaviors they used in

an attempt to tell staff they were in pain, such as signaling with their eyes and moving their legs up and down (Puntillo, 1990). These patients should be offered writing materials and taught to use a pain rating scale. The call button should be placed within easy reach. For those who receive a neuromuscular blocking agent, analgesics should be provided routinely for any procedure, injury, or disease that ordinarily causes pain.

If unconsciousness is defined as no awareness of self or environment, how is it possible that an unconscious patient could feel pain and suffer from it? The problem is that unconsciousness is not easily determined, and there appear to be varying levels of unconsciousness. Anecdotal evidence and some research strongly suggest that quite a few patients who appear to be unconscious and unresponsive to painful stimuli actually feel and recall pain. Thus clinicians should assume that the unconscious patient may feel pain, and, once again, provide analgesia if anything known to be painful is present.

In a study of 100 critically ill patients whose records indicated they were unconscious, interviews with the patients revealed that only about one quarter were actually unaware of themselves and their surroundings (Lawrence, 1995). The remaining three quarters had some awareness of themselves and their environment, and about 25% were able to hear and to feel pain (Lawrence, 1995).

An anecdotal report illustrates the tragedy of assuming an unconscious patient does not feel pain. A terminally ill patient was receiving morphine IV for cancer-related pain; as her disease progressed, she gradually became unresponsive to voices and no longer grimaced during position changes, which were previously painful to her. Because she appeared to be unconscious and unresponsive to painful stimuli, morphine was no longer administered. After 3 days the patient regained consciousness and immediately asked for morphine. The patient reported that during the apparent "coma," she had heard voices and felt intense pain (Stephens, 1994).

Regarding pain in terminally ill patients who appear to be unconscious, a recommendation made in the 1980s is worth repeating: "When patients are no longer able to verbally communicate whether they are in pain or not, the best approach is to assume that their cancer is still painful and to continue them on their regular medications. . . . a therapeutic narcotic level should be maintained. . . . continued narcotics simply ensure that the death will be as peaceful and painless as possible" (Levy, 1985, pp. 397-398).

Whether patients in a persistent vegetative state feel pain remains controversial. This state is defined as complete unawareness of self and environment, including lack of the cortical capacity to feel pain. However, some have voiced reservations about assuming that patients in a vegetative state do not feel pain and have suggested that, until it can be proved otherwise, clinicians should assume that such patients feel pain and should treat that pain (Bushnell, 1997; Klein, 1997).

Assessment strategies

A suggested hierarchy of importance of basic measures of pain intensity is presented in Box 3.10. Note that when a patient is unable to report pain, the existence of a pathologic condition or procedures known to be painful is a strong indicator that pain may be present. In the nonverbal patient, that information alone may be sufficient to justify administering analgesics. For this reason, regular and thorough physical assessments, perhaps every 3 months, are indicated in nonverbal patients.

Clinical practice guidelines offer the following recommendations:

- "If there is reason to suspect pain, an analgesic trial can be diagnostic as well as therapeutic." (Acute Pain Management Guidelines Panel, 1992b, p. 41)
- "Patients who are unable to communicate and who undergo a procedure that would be painful for others should be treated for pain preemptively." (APS, 1992, p. 3)

When patients are unable to provide self-reports of pain, family members, close friends, or clinicians familiar with the patient may be asked to rate the pain, called a proxy pain rating. Families and close friends of patients may be better able than clinicians to identify behaviors in a loved one that suggest the possibility of pain. They may also be more sensitive to changes in behavior. Just as pa-

tients must be taught to use the pain rating scale so must those who will be providing proxy pain ratings (see Box 3.7 for steps in teaching). Whenever possible, especially initially, the proxy pain rating is accompanied by the clues used by the rater to arrive at the pain rating number. The behaviors in Box 3.11 may be helpful. For example, a family member may guess that the patient's pain is a 6 because the patient is frowning and no longer moving about in bed.

Proxy pain ratings are understood to be merely a guess, and they are never used for determining pain management when the patient can provide pain ratings. Ordinarily, proxy pain ratings are not used along with the patient's pain ratings because this violates the foundation of pain assessment—only the patient can feel the pain. However, in a confused or demented patient who occasionally or irregularly reports pain or gives inconsistent information, the patient's pain ratings may be used along with proxy pain ratings.

Behavioral and physiologic responses are, of course, potential indicators of pain. In a study of 31 surgical patients in the critical care setting, patients' pain ratings were compared with those arrived at by nurses who used a structured scale of behavioral and physiologic indicators of pain (Puntillo, Miaskowski, Kehrie et al., 1997). The systematic use of the scale resulted in nurses ascribing pain ratings that were similar to those of the patients, although the nurses consistently underestimated the pain. Behavioral and physiologic indicators that appeared to be useful in assessing pain included absence of movement, facial expressions of grimacing or frowning, restlessness, and increased heart rate or blood pressure. (A copy of their pain assessment tool is included in the published article.)

The practicality of using behavioral indicators in patients who are unable to provide a self-report is illustrated in a pilot study using a list of 25 observable pain behaviors to assess pain in nonverbal elderly patients

Text continued on p. 98.

• • • • •

BOX 3.10 **Hierarchy of Importance of Basic Measures of Pain Intensity**

1. Patient's self-report using a pain rating scale (e.g., 0-10).
2. Pathologic conditions or procedures that usually cause pain.
3. Behaviors (e.g., facial expressions, body movements, crying).
4. Report of pain from parent, family, or others close to patient. These individuals may be asked to give proxy pain ratings—guesses about the intensity of the patient's pain.
5. Physiologic measures. These are the least sensitive indicators of pain.

Information from Acute Pain Management Guideline Panel: *Acute pain management in adults: Operative procedures. Quick reference guide for clinicians*, AHCPR Pub. No. 92-0019, Rockville, Md, Agency for Health Care Policy and Research, Public Health Service, US Department of Health and Human Services, 1992; Acute Pain Management Guideline Panel: *Acute pain management in infants, children and adolescents: Operative and medical procedures. Quick reference guide for clinicians*, AHCPR Pub. No. 92-0019, Rockville, Md, Agency for Health Care Policy and Research, Public Health Service, US Department of Health and Human Services, 1992; McGrath PJ, Beyer J, Cleeland C et al.: Report of the subcommittee on assessment and methodological issues in the management of pain in childhood cancer, *Pediatrics* 86(Suppl)(5):814-817, 1990.

May be duplicated for use in clinical practice. From McCaffery M, Pasero C, *Pain: Clinical manual*, p. 95. Copyright © 1999, Mosby, Inc.

• • • • •

BOX 3.11 **Behaviors Potentially Indicative of Pain**

This list is a simple guide to behavioral assessment of pain in patients who are unable to provide a self-report of pain. It is not an exhaustive list.
Facial expressions: frown (wrinkled forehead), grimace, fearful, sad, muscle contraction around mouth and eyes
Physical movements: restlessness, fidgeting, absence of movement, slow movements, cautious movements, guarding, rigidity, generalized tension (not relaxed), trying to get attention (beckoning someone)
Vocalizations: groaning, moaning, crying, noisy breathing

May be duplicated for use in clinical practice. From McCaffery M, Pasero C, *Pain: Clinical manual*, p. 95. Copyright © 1999, Mosby, Inc.

• • • • •

FORM 3.8A **Pain Screen**

1. Patient self-report: Unable: _____   Occasionally: _____   Inconsistent: _____

   Other: _____

2. Physical findings indicative of pain:

   a. Disease processes _____

   _____

   _____

   _____

   b. Painful procedures _____

   _____

3. Family (caregiver) assessment: 0 to 10 and why: _____

   _____

4. Behaviors indicative of pain: _____

   _____

   _____

   _____

May be duplicated for use in clinical practice. From McCaffery M, Pasero C: *Pain: Clinical manual,* p. 96. Copyright © 1999, Mosby, Inc.

FORM 3.8 A   Pain Screen. This form coordinates information that may be used in the initial assessment of pain in a patient who is unable to provide a self-report.

• • • • •

FORM 3.8B **Pain Screen: Patient Example**

1. Patient self-report: Unable: ✔   Occasionally: _____   Inconsistent: _____

   Other: _____

2. Physical findings indicative of pain:

   a. Disease processes _____*Venous stasis ulcer left leg; Hx of arthritis treated with ibuprofen*_____

   _____

   _____

   b. Painful procedures _____*Dressing change daily*_____

3. Family (caregiver) assessment: 0 to 10 and why: _____*Wife guesses ongoing pain = 5; RN guesses*

   *dressing change = 7*_____

4. Behaviors indicative of pain: _____*Ongoing pain suggested by lack of movement, resists getting out of*

   *bed. With dressing change, pt. groans, frowns, and attempts to move leg away.*_____

   _____

   _____

May be duplicated for use in clinical practice. From McCaffery M, Pasero C: *Pain: Clinical manual,* p. 96. Copyright © 1999, Mosby, Inc.

FORM 3.8 B   Pain Screen: Patient example. The patient described above is in a long-term care facility. He is 78 years old and has been nonverbal since a cerebrovascular accident 6 months ago. He does not appear to be oriented to his environment, but he seems to recognize his wife, who visits several times a week.

FORM 3.9A **Flow Sheet: Ongoing Pain Assessment in the Absence of Self-Report**

Patient: _____ Date _____

Analgesics: _____

Time:	Proxy pain rating:	Analgesics:	Possible pain behaviors:	Possible comfort behaviors:	Plan:

May be duplicated for use in clinical practice. From McCaffery M, Pasero C: *Pain: Clinical manual*, p. 97. Copyright © 1999, Mosby, Inc.

FORM 3.9A Flow sheet: ongoing pain assessment in the absence of a self-report. The above is used after completion of the Pain Screen, Form 3.8A.

FORM 3.9B **Flow Sheet: Ongoing Pain Assessment in the Absence of Self-Report**

Patient: _____ Date _____

Analgesics: _____ *ibuprofen 400 mg tid; Percocet τ-π PRN for dressing change* _____

Time:	Proxy pain rating:	Analgesics:	Possible pain behaviors:	Possible comfort behaviors:	Plan:
0800	*Wife 5*	*ibuprofen 400 mg*	*resists getting out of bed*		
1000	*Wife 2*			*willing to get out of bed*	*continue ibuprofen 400 mg tid*
1200	*Wife 3*	*Percocet τ*		*Still out of bed; walking occ.*	
1300	*RN = 4 during dressing change*		*one groan; does not pull away; occ. frown*		*↑ Percocet π for tomorrow's dressing change*

May be duplicated for use in clinical practice. From McCaffery M, Pasero C: *Pain: Clinical manual*, p. 97. Copyright © 1999, Mosby, Inc.

FORM 3.9B Flow sheet: ongoing pain assessment in the absence of self-report: patient example. The above patient is the one described in the example of the Pain Screen in Form 3.8B. The proxy pain ratings suggest that ibuprofen relieves his arthritis pain and that one tablet of Percocet given 1 hour before his dressing change decreases some but not all of the pain associated with the dressing change. Therefore the plan is to continue the ibuprofen and increase the Percocet to two tablets for the next dressing change. Behavioral observations indicating the presence or absence of his ongoing pain should be recorded at least every 8 hours, as well as before and during the dressing change.

(Simons, Malabar, 1995). In all instances the nurses were able to identify one of the behaviors to support their belief that the patient was in pain (The behavioral list is included in the published article.) Furthermore, when analgesics were administered, the behaviors either changed or the analgesic was modified, resulting in behavior change. In most instances, attempts at pain relief changed the pain behaviors to nonpain behaviors.

A scale to assess pain in patients with advanced Alzheimer's disease has been developed and consists of nine items: noisy breathing, absence of a look of contentment, looking sad, looking frightened, frowning, absence of relaxed body posture, looking tense, and fidgeting (Hurley, Volicer, Hanrahan et al., 1992). A brief list of these and other behaviors that may indicate pain is presented in Box 3.11.

In patients with dementia (impairment of intellectual function), however, caution is necessary when using behavioral and physiologic indicators of pain. Increased dementia is associated with blunting of physiologic responses to pain, and facial expressions may be difficult to interpret (Porter, Malhotra, Wolf et al., 1996).

To coordinate the information that may be used to assess pain in a patient who is unable to provide a self-report, a pain screen may be useful (Form 3.8, A). A patient example is provided in Form 3.8, B. Accompanying this is a flow sheet and a patient example of ongoing assessment and the use of a trial analgesic (Forms 3.9, A, and 3.9, B). Note that in the flow sheet, a column for possible comfort behaviors is included. In particular, it is helpful to note behavior that is the opposite of the behavior indicative of pain.

In summary, assessment of patients who are unable to provide a self-report of pain requires that clinicians rely on indicators that are less reliable. These include the presence of pathologic processes or procedures that are ordinarily painful, behavioral and physiologic indicators of pain, and the best guesses of family and caregivers. Suspicion of pain should be maintained in the care of these patients. It is well to remember that clinicians undertreat pain even in those who can and do report it. It is likely that those who cannot report pain will be even more undertreated.

Cultural Considerations

As racial and cultural diversity increases in the United States, clinicians are increasingly likely to care for patients from backgrounds quite different from their own. There is little doubt that different ethnic groups express pain and suffering differently. The same can be said of people in general. Fortunately, many of the pain assessment tools used in the United States can be used successfully in other countries if they are translated into the appropriate languages. Culture affects behavioral responses to pain and treatment preferences. However, patients from many different cultures may be assessed using similar pain assessment tools and the findings will have similar meanings across cultures.

Three terms—pain, hurt, and ache—seem to be used similarly across cultures to describe pain intensity. The term pain is usually used for the most intense pain, followed by hurt, with ache meaning the least pain. This was shown to be true in a study of Hispanics, American Indians, blacks, and whites (Gaston-Johansson, Albert, Fagan et al., 1990). These terms are also basic words used in the Swedish language to describe pain intensity (Gaston-Johansson, 1984), as well as the Dutch language (Francke, Theeuwen, 1994). Thus persons with diverse ethnic-cultural and educational backgrounds use similar words to describe pain intensity.

This chapter provides translations of the horizontal 0 to 10 NRS and the Wong-Baker faces scale into a number of different languages. However, some minor changes may be made when necessary. For example, a study of Chinese patients' responses to a VAS revealed that it was a suitable method for assessing pain intensity but that the vertical presentation was more quickly understood than the horizontal line, probably because traditionally the Chinese read vertically downwards and from right to left, not left to right (Aun, Lam Collett, 1986). If difficulties are encountered with the horizontal Chinese translation in Figure 3.5, readers are encouraged to make a vertical presentation with 10 at the top.

The Brief Pain Inventory has also consistently demonstrated a high degree of reliability and validity when administered to cancer patients from other countries besides the United States, namely, Singapore (Cleeland, Ryan, 1994), France, the Philippines, and China (Cleeland, Nakamura, Mendoza et al., 1996). The findings of several studies of different cultures have found that on a 0 to 10 pain rating scale, pain ratings of 5 or more interfere significantly with daily function (Cleeland, 1984; Cleeland, Gonin, Hatfield, 1994; Serlin, Mendoza, Nakamura et al., 1995). Although behavioral expression of pain may differ considerably among cultures, pain ratings and the impact of pain on quality of life appears to be very similar.

However, the usefulness of basic pain assessment tools across cultures is not sufficient to ensure a high quality of care for patients of different cultural backgrounds. To enhance cultural sensitivity, clinicians must work closely with patients and their families to identify mutual goals of care that take into account different preferences, such as relative values placed on being free of pain versus being fully alert. Whenever possible, health care practices desired by the patient that are specific to the patient's cultural group should be included in the patient's care. Teaching materials in the patient's own language may be secured or developed, and cultural resources such as interpreters may be useful (McGuire, Sheidler, 1993).

Clinicians must be particularly mindful of the fact that the more difference there is between the patient and the clinician, the more difficult it is for the clinician to assess and treat the patient. As an example, in a study of 50 hospitalized patients who spoke Arabic, a comparison of the patients' pain ratings with those of nurses who shared the mother tongue and those who did not revealed that nurses sharing a mother tongue with the patient were much more likely to provide pain ratings similar to those of their patients than were the other nurses (Harrison, Busabir, Al-Kaabi et al., 1996).

Far too many cultures are represented in the patient population to allow a consideration of each in this section. Clinicians are encouraged to seek information about the specific cultural backgrounds of their patients through exploration with the patients and through publications such as the following. A helpful guide to cultural assessment is provided by Fong (1985). Information about health and illness beliefs of 27 different cultures, including many Asian groups, is available in a pocket guide (Lipson, Dibble, Minarik, 1996). Care of oncology patients of Hispanic and Japanese American background is discussed by Kagawa-Singer (1987). Other articles address pain in the Arab American (Reizien, Meleis, 1986), the Chinese (Louie, 1985), and Afro-Americans (Capers, 1985).

CONCLUSION

Chapter 3 is the most important chapter in this book. The essential message about pain assessment is easy to summarize: Ask patients about their pain, accept and respect what they say, intervene to relieve their pain, and ask them again about their pain. It is a circle of assessment, intervention, and reassessment. Without assessment of the patient with pain, none of the pain relief measures presented in the following chapters will be useful. Approximately half the people who suffer moderate to severe pain will continue to suffer primarily because clinicians fail to assess pain.

References

Acute Pain Management Guideline Panel: *Acute pain management in adults: operative procedures. Quick reference guide for clinicians,* AHCPR Pub. No. 92-0019, Rockville, Md, Agency for health Care Policy and Research, Public Health Service, U.S. Department of Health and Human Services, 1992a.

Acute Pain Management Guideline Panel: *Acute pain management in infants, children and adolescents: operative and medical procedures. Quick reference guide for clinicians,* AHCPR Pub. No. 92-0019, Rockville, Md, Agency for health Care Policy and Research, Public Health Service, U.S. Department of Health and Human Services, 1992b.

American College of Emergency Physicians: Clinical policy for the initial approach to patients presenting with a chief complaint of nontraumatic acute abdominal pain, *Ann Emerg Med* 23:906-922, 1994.

American Pain Society (APS): *Principles of analgesic use in the treatment of acute pain and cancer pain,* ed 3, Skokie, Ill, 1992, The Society.

Anand KJS, Sippell WG, Aynsley-Green A: Randomized trial of fentanyl anaesthesia in preterm babies undergoing surgery: effects on the stress response, *Lancet* 1:62-66, Jan. 10, 1987.

Armitage KJ, Schneiderman LJ, Bass RA: Response of physicians to medical complaints in men and women, *JAMA* 241(20):2186-2187, May 1979.

Attard AR, Corlett MJ, Kidner NJ et al.: Safety of early pain relief for acute abdominal pain, *BMJ* 305:554-556, Sept. 1992.

Au E, Loprinzi C, Chodapkar M et al.: Regular use of a verbal pain scale improves the understanding of oncology inpatient pain intensity, *J Clin Oncol* 12:2751-2755, 1994.

Aun C, Lam YM, Collett B: Evaluation of the use of visual analogue scale in Chinese patients, *Pain* 25:215-221, 1986.

Beecher HK: Limiting factors in experimental pain, *J Chron Dis* 4:11-21, 1956.

Beyer JE, Denyes MJ, Villarruel AM: The creation, validation, and continuing development of the oucher: a measure of pain intensity in children, *J Pediatr Nurs* 7:335-346, 1992.

Beyer JE, McGrath PJ, Berde CB: Discordance between self-report and behavioral pain measures in children age 3-7 years after surgery, *J Pain Symptom Manage* 5:350-356, Dec. 1990.

Beyer JE, Platt A, Kinney T et al.: Assessment of pain in adults and children with sickle cell disease. In Shapiro BS, Schechter NL, Ohene-Frempong K, editors: *Sickle cell disease related pain assessment and management: conference proceedings,* pp. 10-17, Mt. Desert, Maine, 1994, New England Regional Genetics Group.

Brody H: The doctor as therapeutic agent: a placebo effect research agenda. In Harrington A, editor: *The placebo effect: an interdisciplinary exploration,* pp. 77-92, Cambridge, 1997, Harvard University Press.

Brown J: Nurses' analgesic choices and postoperative patients' perceived pain: the effect of a pain flow sheet, *Am J Pain Manage* 2:192-197, 1992.

Burgess MM: Nurses' pain ratings of patients with acute and chronic low back pain, Unpublished master's thesis, Univ. of Virginia School of Nursing, May 1980.

Burke T, Mack S, Coward B: The use of intravenous morphine for early pain relief in patients with acute abdominal pain, Abstract presented at the 1994 Society of Academic Emergency Medicine Annual Meeting, 1994.

Bushnell MC: Commentaries, *Eur J Pain* 1:167, 1997.

Byas-Smith MG, Max MB, Muir J et al.: Transdermal clonidine compared to placebo in painful diabetic neuropathy using a two-stage "enriched enrollment design", *Pain* 60:267-274, 1995.

California Board of Registered Nursing (BRN): BRN focuses on pain management, *BRN Report* 10(1):12, 1997.

Capers CF: Nursing and the Afro-American client, *Top Clin Nurs* 7:11-17, 1985.

Carey SJ, Turpin C, Smith J et al.: Improving pain management in an acute care setting, *Orthop Nurs* 16(4)29-36, 1997.

Carpenter JS, Brockopp D: Comparison of patients' ratings and examination of nurses' responses to pain intensity rating scales, *Cancer Nurs* 18:292-298, 1995.

Cassell EJ: The nature of suffering and the goals of medicine, *N Engl J Med* 306:639-645, 1982.

Cleeland CS: The impact of pain on the patient with cancer, *Cancer* 54:2635-2641, 1984.

Cleeland CS, Gonin R, Baez L et al.: Pain and treatment of pain in minority patients with cancer: The Eastern Cooperative Oncology Group Minority Outpatient Pain Study, *Ann Intern Med* 127:813-816, 1997.

Cleeland CS, Gonin R, Hatfield AK et al.: Pain and its treatment in outpatients with metastatic cancer, *N Engl J Med* 330:592-596, 1994.

Cleeland CS, Ladinsky JL, Serlin JRD et al.: Multidimensional measurement of cancer pain: comparisons of US and Vietnamese patients, *J Pain Symptom Manage* 3:23-27, 1988.

Cleeland CS, Nakamura Y, Mendoza TR et al.: Dimensions of the impact of cancer in a four country sample: new information from multidimensional scaling, *Pain* 67:267-273, 1996.

Cleeland CS, Ryan KM: Pain assessment: global use of the brief pain inventory, *Ann Acad Med* 23:129-138, 1994.

Cleeland CS, Syrjala KL: How to assess cancer pain. In Turk DC, Melzack R, editors: *Handbook of pain assessment,* pp. 362-387, New York, 1992, The Guilford Press.

Cohen FL: Postsurgical pain relief: patients' status and nurses' medication choices, *Pain* 9:265-274, 1980.

Cotton P: "Harm reduction" approach may be middle ground, *JAMA* 271(21):1641-1645, 1994.

Cruise CE, Broderick J, Porter L et al.: Reactive effects of diary self-assessment in chronic pain patients, *Pain* 67:253-258, 1996.

Dalton JA, McNaull F: A call for standardizing the clinical rating of pain intensity using a 0 to 10 rating scale, *Cancer Nurs* 21:46-69, 1998.

Daut RL, Cleeland CS: The prevalence and severity of pain in cancer, *Cancer* 50:1913-1918, 1982.

Daut RL, Cleeland CS, Flanery RC: Development of the Wisconsin Brief Pain Questionnaire to assess pain in cancer and other diseases, *Pain* 17:197-210, 1983.

Dellemijn PLI, Fields HL: Do benzodiazepines have a role in chronic pain management? *Pain* 57:137-152, 1994.

DeLoach LJ, Higgins MS, Caplan AB et al.: The visual analog scale in the immediate postoperative period: intrasubject variability and correlation with a numeric scale, *Anesth Analg* 56:102-106, 1998.

de Moulin D: A historical-phenomenological study of bodily pain in western man, *Bull Hist Med* 48(4)540-570, Winter 1979.

de Schepper AME, Francke AL, Abu-Saad HH: Feelings of powerlessness in relation to pain: ascribed causes and reported strategies, *Cancer Nurs* 20: 422-429, 1997.

Diagnostic and statistical manual of mental disorders, 4th ed, Washington, DC, 1994, American Psychiatric Association.

Duarte RA: Classification of pain. In Kanner R: *Pain management secrets*, pp. 5-7, Philadelphia, 1997, Hanely & Belfus.

Ducharme J: Emergency pain management: a Canadian Association of Emergency Physicians (CAEP) consensus document, *J Emerg Med* 12:855-866, 1994.

Egan KJ, Ready, LB, Nessly M et al.: Self-administration of midazolam for postoperative anxiety: a double blinded study, *Pain* 49:3-8, 1992.

Eich E, Reeves JL, Jaeger B et al.: Memory for pain: relation between past and present pain intensity, *Pain* 23:375-379, 1985.

Emrich HM, editor: The role of endorphins in neuropsychiatry, vol 17. In Ban TA et al., editors: *Modern problems of pharmacopsychiatry*, New York, 1981, Basal.

Evans FJ: The placebo response in pain reduction. In *Advances in Neurology*, vol. 4, pp. 289-296, New York, 1974, Raven Press.

Faries JE, Mills DS, Goldsmith KW et al.: Systematic pain records and their impact on pain control: a pilot study, *Cancer Nurs* 14:306-313, 1991.

Favaloro R, Touzel B: A comparison of adolescents' and nurses' postoperative pain ratings and perceptions, *Pediatr Nurs* 16:414-417, 1990.

Fearon I, McGrath PJ, Achat H: `Booboos': the study of everyday pain among young children, *Pain* 68:55-62, 1996.

Ferraz MB, Quaresma MR, Aquino LR et al.: Reliability of pain scales in the assessment of literate and illiterate patients with rheumatoid arthritis, *J Rheumatol* 17:1022-1024, 1990.

Ferrell BA, Ferrell BR, Rivera L: Pain in cognitively impaired nursing home patients, *J Pain Symptom Manage* 10:591-598, 1995.

Ferrell BR, Grant M, Funk B et al.: Quality of life in breast cancer. Part I: physical and social well-being, *Cancer Nurs* 20:398-408, 1997.

Fields HL, editor: *Core curriculum for professional education in pain*, ed 2, Seattle, 1995, IASP Press.

Fong CM: Ethnicity and nursing practice, *Top Clin Nurs* 7:1-10, 1985.

Forbes JA: The nurse-observer: observation methods and training. In Max MB, Portenoy RK, Laska EM, editors: *Adv Pain Res Therapy* 18:607-620, 1991.

Fordyce WE, editor: *Back pain in the workplace*, Seattle, 1995, IASP Press.

Fox AE (pseudonym): Confronting the use of placebos for pain, *Am J Nurs* 94(9):42-46, 1994.

Fox AE (pseudonym), McCaffery M, Ferrell B et al.: A place for placebos? Reply, *Am J Nurs* 95(2):18, 1995.

Francke AL, Theeuwen I: Inhibition in expressing pain: a qualitative study among Dutch surgical breast cancer patients, *Cancer Nurs* 17:193-199, 1994.

Friedman DP: Perspectives on the medical use of drugs of abuse, *J Pain Symptom Manage* 5:S2-S5, Feb. 1990.

Fritz DJ: Noninvasive pain control methods used by cancer outpatients, *Oncol Nurs Forum* (Suppl.) p. 108, 1988 (abstract).

Galer BS, Jensen MP: Development and preliminary validation of a pain measure specific to neuropathic pain: the neuropathic pain scale, *Neurology* 48:332-338, 1997.

Gaston-Johansson F: Pain assessment: differences in quality and intensity of the words pain, ache, and hurt, *Pain* 20:69-76, 1984.

Gaston-Johansson F, Albert M, Fagan E et al.: Similarities in pain descriptions of four different ethnic-culture groups, *J Pain Symptom Manage* 5:94-100, 1990.

Gear RW, Miaskowski C, Heller PH et al.: Benzodiazepine mediated antagonism of opioid analgesia, *Pain* 71:25-29, 1997.

Gift A: Visual analogue scales: measurement of subjective phenomena, *Nurs Res* 38:286-288, 1989.

Gift AG, Plaut DM, Jacox AK: Psychologic and physiologic factors related to dyspnea in subjects with chronic obstructive pulmonary disease, *Heart Lung* 15:595-601, 1986.

Goodwin JS, Goodwin JM, Vogel AA: Knowledge and use of placebos by house officers and nurses, *Ann Intern Med* 91:106-110, 1979.

Gordon DB, Ward SE: Correcting patient misconceptions about pain, *Am J Nurs* 95(7):43-45, 1995.

Graffam S: Congruence of nurse-patient expectations regarding nursing intervention in pain, *Nurs Leadership* 4(2):12-15, 1981.

Grevert P, Albert LH, Goldstein A: Partial antagonism of placebo analgesia by naloxone, *Pain* 16:129-143, 1983.

Grossman SA, Sheidler VR, Sweeden K et al.: Correlation of patient and caregiver ratings of cancer pain, *J Pain Symptom Manage* 6:53-57, 1991.

Haddad A: Ethics in action: What would you do? *RN* 56(3) 21-24, 1993.

Hadjistavropoulos HD, Ross MA, von Baeyer CL: Are physicians' ratings of pain affected by patients' physical attractiveness? *Soc Sci Med* 31(1):69-72, 1990.

Halfens R, Evers G, Abu-Saad H: Determinants of pain assessment by nurses, *Int J Nurs Stud* 27(1):43-49, 1990.

Hall GM, Salmon P: Patient-controlled analgesia: who benefits? *Anaesthesia* 52:401-402, 1997.

Hardy JD, Wolff HG, Goodell H: Pain threshold in man, *Proc Assoc Res Nerv Men Dis* 23:1, 1943.

Harrison A, Busabir AA, Al-Kaabi AO et al.: Dose sharing a mother-tongue affect how closely patients and nurses agree when rating the patient's pain, worry and knowledge? *J Adv Nurs* 24:229-235, 1996.

Hendler NH, Kozikowski JG: Overlooked diagnoses in chronic pain patients involved in litigation, *Psychosomatics* 34(6):494-504, 1993.

Hester NO: Integrating pain assessment and management into the care of children with cancer. In McGuire DB, Yarbro CH, Ferrell BR: *Cancer pain management*, pp. 231-271, Boston, 1995, Jones and Bartlett Publishers.

Hitchcock LS, Ferrell BR, McCaffery M: The experience of "chronic nonmalignant pain" *J Pain Symptom Manage* 9(5):312-318, July 1994.

Holm K, Cohen F, Dudas S et al.: Effect of personal pain experience on pain assessment, *Image J Nurs Scholar* 21:72-75, 1989.

Hurley AC, Volicer BJ, Harahan PA et al.: Assessment of discomfort in advanced Alzheimer patients, *Res Nurs Health* 15:369-377, 1992.

IASP ad hoc Subcommittee for Psychology Curriculum: *Curriculum on pain for students in psychology*, Seattle, 1997, International Association for the Study of Pain.

Illingworth KA, Simpson KH: *Anaesthesia and analgesia in emergency medicine*, New York, 1994, Oxford University Press.

Jacox A: Assessing pain, *Am J Nurs* 79:895-900, 1979.

Jacox A, Carr DB, Payne R et al.: *Management of cancer pain: clinical practice guideline No. 9*, AHCPR Pub. No. 94-0592, Rockville, Md, Agency for healthcare policy and research, U.S. Department of Health and Human Services, Public Health Service, 1994a.

Jacox A, Carr DB, Payne R et al.: *Management of cancer pain: adults. Quick reference for clinicians. Clinical practice guideline No. 9*, AHCPR Pub. No. 94-0593, Rockville, Md, Agency for healthcare policy and research, U.S. Department of Health and Human Services, Public Health Service, 1994b.

Janal MN, Colt EWD, Clark WC et al.: Pain sensitivity, mood and plasma endocrine levels in man following long-distance running: effects of naloxone, *Pain* 19:13-25, 1984.

Janssen SA, Arntz A: Anxiety and pain: attentional and endorphinergic influences, *Pain* 56:145-150, 1996.

Jensen MP, Karoly P: Self-report scales and procedures for assessing pain in adults. In Turk DC, Melzack R, editors: *Handbook of pain assessment*, pp. 135-151, New York, 1992, The Guilford Press.

Jensen MP, Turner JA, Romano JM: What is the maximum number of levels needed in pain intensity measurement? *Pain* 58:387-392, 1994.

Joint Commission on Accreditation of Healthcare Organizations: *Accreditation manual for hospitals,* Oakbrook Terrace, IL, 1994, The Commission.

Kagawa-Singer M: Ethnic perspectives of cancer nursing: Hispanics and Japanese- Americans, *Oncol Nurs Forum* 14:59-65, 1987.

Kahn DL, Steeves RH: The experience of suffering. In Ferrell BR: *Suffering,* pp. 3-27, Boston, 1996, Jones and Bartlett Publishers.

Katz ER, Sharp B, Kellerman J et al.: Beta-endorphin immunoreactivity and acute behavioral distress in children with leukemia, *J Nerv Ment Dis* 170:72-77, 1982.

Kerrane TA: The Brompton Cocktail, *Nurs Mirror* 140:59, May 1, 1975.

Kistler P: Analgesia for the victim of trauma. In Ferrante FM, VadeBoncouer TR, editors: *Postoperative pain management,* pp. 589-598, New York, 1993, Churchill Livingstone.

Klein M: Perception of pain in the persistent vegetative state? *Eur J Pain* 1:165-167, 1997.

Kleinman I, Brown P, Librach L: Placebo pain medication, *Arch Fam Med* 3: 453-457, 1994.

Kosten TF, Kleber HD: Control of nociception by endogenous opioids. In Aronoff GM, editor: *Mediguide to pain* 8:1-5, New York, 1987, DellaCorte Publications.

Krivo S, Reidenberg MM: Assessment of patient's pain, *N Engl J Med* 334: 59, 1995.

Larue F, Fontaine A, Colleau SM: Underestimation and undertreatment of pain in HIV disease: multicentre study, *BMJ* 3144:23-28, 1997.

Lavin MR: Placebo effects on mind and body, *JAMA* 265:1753-1754, 1991.

Lawrence M: The unconscious experience, *Am J Crit Care* 4:227, 1995.

Leavitt F, Sweet JJ: Characteristics and frequency of malingering among patients with low back pain, *Pain* 25:357-364, 1986.

Levine FM, De Simone LL: The effects of experimenter gender on pain report in male and female subjects, *Pain* 44:69-72, 1991.

Levine JD, Gordon NC, Fields H: The mechanism of placebo analgesia, *Lancet* 2:654-657, 1978.

Levy M: Pain management in advanced cancer, *Semin Oncol* 12:394-410, 1985.

Lipson JG, Dibble SL, Minarik PA, editors: *Culture and nursing care: a pocket guide,* San Francisco, 1996, UCSF Nursing Press.

Liu R, Barry JES, Weinman J. Effects of background stress and anxiety on postoperative recovery, *Anaesthesia* 49:382-6, 1994.

Louie KB: Providing health care to Chinese clients, *Top Clin Nurs* 7:18-25, 1985.

Malone RE: Almost `like family': emergency nurses and `frequent flyers,' *J Emerg Nurs* 22:3:176-183, 1996.

Manyande A, Salmon P: Recovery from minor abdominal surgery: a preliminary attempt to separate anxiety and coping, *Br J Clin Psychol* 31:227-237, 1992.

The Mayday Fund: *1993 Pain Survey,* New York, NY, 1993, The Mayday Fund.

The Mayday Fund: *Pain in America: a survey of American attitudes toward pain,* New York, NY, 1998, The Mayday Fund.

McCaffery M: *Nursing practice theories related to cognition, bodily pain, and man-environment interactions,* Los Angeles, 1968, University of California at Los Angeles Students' Store.

McCaffery M, Ferrell, B: How would you respond to these patients in pain? *Nurs* (6):21:34-37, 1991a.

McCaffery M, Ferrell BR: Patient age: does it affect your pain-control decisions? *Nurs* 21(9):44-48, 1991b.

McCaffery M, Ferrell BR. Does the gender gap affect your pain-control decisions? *Nurs* 22(8):48-51, 1992a.

McCaffery M, Ferrell BR. How vital are vital signs? *Nurs* 22(1):42-46, 1992b.

McCaffery M, Ferrell B: Opioid analgesics: addiction, *Age Concern* 1(5):1 & 4, 1992c.

McCaffery M, Ferrell BR: Opioid analgesics: nurses' knowledge of doses and psychological dependence, *J Nurs Staff Development* 8(2):77-84, 1992d.

McCaffery M, Ferrell B: Nurses' assessment of pain intensity and choice of analgesic dose. *Contemporary Nurse* 3(2):June, 1994a.

McCaffery M, Ferrell BR: Say no to placebos, *Am J Nurs* 94 (11):20, 1994b.

McCaffery M, Ferrell B: Are nurses' analgesic choices influenced by the pain rating scale used? 0-5 versus 0-10. *ASPMN Pathways* 4:1:3, 6, 1995a.

McCaffery M, Ferrell BR: Nurses' knowledge about cancer pain: a survey of five countries, *J Pain Symptom Manage* 10(5):356-369, 1995b.

McCaffery M, Ferrell BR: Correcting misconceptions about pain assessment and use of opioid analgesics: educational strategies aimed at public concerns. *Nurs Outlook* 44(4):184-190, 1996a.

McCaffery M, Ferrell, BR: Current placebo practice and policy, *ASPMN Pathways* 5(4):1:12-14, Winter 1996b.

McCaffery M, Ferrell BR: Nurses' knowledge of pain assessment and management: how much progress have we made? *J Pain Symptom Manage* 14(3):175-188, 1997a.

McCaffery M, Ferrell, BR: Pain and placebos: ethical and professional issues, *Orthop Nurs* 16(5):8-11, 1997b.

McCaffery M, Ferrell BR, O'Neil-Page E: Does life-style affect your pain-control decisions? *Nurs* 22(4):58-61, 1992.

McCaffery M, Ferrell BR, Pasero CL: When the physician prescribes a placebo, *Am J Nurs* 98(1):52-53, 1998.

McCaffery M, Ferrell BR, Turner M: Ethical issues in the use of placebos in cancer pain management, *Oncol Nurs Forum* 23:1587-1593, 1996.

McCaffery M, Pasero C: Are there circumstances that justify deceitful placebo use? *Pediatr Nurs* 21:6:588, Nov-Dec 1995 (To The Editor).

McCaffery M, Vourakis C: Assessment and relief of pain in chemically dependent patients, *Orthop Nurs* 11(2):13-27, 1992.

McGrath PJ, Beyer J, Cleeland C et al.: Report of the subcommittee on assessment and methodological issues in the management of pain in childhood cancer, *Pediatrics* 86(Suppl)(5):814-817, 1990.

McGuire DB, Sheidler VR: Pain. In Groenwald SL, Frogge MH, Goodman M et al., editors: *Cancer nursing: principles and practice,* ed 8, pp. 499-556, Chicago, 1993, Jones and Bartlett.

McIlveen KH, Morse JM: The role of comfort in nursing care: 1900-1980, *Clin Nurs Res* 4:127-148, 1995.

McMillan SC, Williams FA, Chatfield R et al.: A validity and reliability study of two tools for assessing and managing pain, *Oncol Nurs Forum* 15:735-741, 1988.

Melzack R, Abbott FV, Zackon W et al.: Pain on a surgical ward: a survey of the duration and intensity of pain and the effectiveness of medication, *Pain* 29:67-72, 1987.

Melzack R: The short-form McGill Pain Questionnaire, *Pain* 30:191-197, 1987.

Merskey H, Bogduk N, editors: *Classification of chronic pain,* ed 2, Seattle, 1994, IASP Press.

Miller R, Eisenkraft JB, Cohen M et al.: Midazolam as an adjunct to meperidine analgesia for postoperative pain, *Clin J Pain* 2:37-43, 1986.

Mitchel SW: Civilization and pain, *JAMA* 18:108, 1892.

Nelson FV, Zimmerman L, Barnason S et al.: The relationship and influence of anxiety on postoperative pain in the coronary artery bypass graft patent, *J Pain Symptom Manage* 15:102-109, 1998.

Ng B, Dimsdale JE, Rollnik JD et al.: The effect of ethnicity on prescriptions for patient-controlled analgesia for post-operative pain, *Pain* 66:9-12, 1996.

Nichols R: Pain during sickle-cell crises, *Am J Nurs* 96:59-60, 1996.

Oh VMS: The placebo effect: can we use it better? *BMJ* 309:69-70, 1994.

Paice JA, Cohen FL: Validity of a verbally administered numeric rating scale to measure cancer pain intensity, *Cancer Nurs* 20:88-93, 1997.

Paice JA, Mahon SM, Faut-Callahan M: Factors associated with adequate pain control in hospitalized postsurgical patients diagnosed with cancer, *Cancer Nurs* 14:298-305, 1991.

Parmelee PA, Smith BD, Katz IR: Pain complaints and cognitive status among elderly institution residents, *J Am Geriatr Soc* 41:517-522, 1993.

Pernick MS: A calculus of suffering, New York, 1985, Columbia Univ. Press.

Portenoy RK, Hagen NA: Breakthrough pain: definition, prevalence and characteristics, *Pain* 41:273-281, 1990.

Porter FL, Malhotra KM, Wolf CM et al.: Dementia and response to pain in the elderly, *Pain* 68:413-421, 1996.

Porzelius J: Memory for pain after nerve-block injections, *Clin J Pain* 11:112-120, 1995.

Puig, MM, Laorden ML, Miralles FS et al.: Endorphin levels in cerebralspinal fluid of patients with postoperative and chronic pain, *Anesthesiology* 57:1-4, 1982.

Puntillo KA: Pain experiences of intensive care unit patients, *Heart Lung* 19(5):526-533, Sept. 1990.

Puntillo KA, Miaskowski C, Kehrie K et al.: Relationship between behavioral and physiological indicators of pain, critical care patients' self-reports of pain, and opioid administration, *Crit Care Med* 25:1159-1166, 1997.

Raphael KG, Marbach JJ: When did your pain start? Reliability of self-reported age of onset of facial pain, *Pain* 13:352-359, 1997.

Reizien A, Meleis AI: Arab-Americans' perceptions of and responses to pain, *Crit Care Nurs* 6:30-37, 1986.

Richardson PH: Placebo effects in pain management, *Pain Reviews* 1:15-32, 1994.

Romsing J, Moller-Sonnergaard J, Hertel S et al.: Postoperative pain in children: comparison between ratings of children and nurses, *J Pain Symptom Manage* 11:42-46, 1996.

Ross RS, Bush JP, Crummette BD: Factors affecting nurses' decisions to administer PRN analgesic medication to children after surgery: an analog investigation, *J Pediatric Psychol* 16:151-167, 1991.

Rothman KJ, Michels KB: The continuing unethical use of placebo controls, *N Engl J Med* 331:394-397, 1994.

Roughneen PT, Burns HJ, Rowlands BJ: Adequate analgesia for acute pain, *BMJ* 292:663, 1986.

Ryan P, Vortherms R, Ward S: Cancer pain: knowledge, attitudes of pharmacologic management, *J Gerontol Nurs* 20(1):7-16, 1994, January.

Salmon P, Manyande A: Good patients cope with their pain: postoperative analgesia and nurses' perceptions of their patients' pain, *Pain* 68:63-68, 1996.

Serlin RC, Mendoza TR, Nakamura Y et al.: When is cancer pain mild, moderate or severe? Grading pain severity by its interference with function, *Pain* 61:277-284, 1995.

Short LM, Burnett ML, Egbert AM et al.: Medicating the postoperative elderly: how do nurses make their decisions? *J Gerontol Nurs* 16(7):12-17, 1990.

Simons W, Malabar R: Assessing pain in elderly patients who cannot respond verbally, *J Adv Nurs* 22:663-669, 1995.

Sloan PA, Donelly MB, Schwartz RW et al.: Cancer pain assessment and management by housestaff, *Pain* 67:475-481, 1996.

Smith WB, Safer MA: Effects of present pain level on recall of chronic pain and medication use, *Pain* 55:355-361, 1993.

Spross JA: Pain, suffering, spiritual well-being: assessment and interventions, *Qual Life* 2:71-79, 1993.

Stephens, ST: A promise to Billie, *Nurs* 24(4):96, 1994.

Syrjala KL: The measurement of pain. In Yarbo CH, McGuire DB, editors: *Cancer pain: nursing management*, pp. 133-150, Orlando, 1987, Grune & Stratton.

Syrjala KL: Integrating medical and psychological treatments for cancer pain. In Chapman CR, Foley KM, editors: *Current and emerging issues in cancer pain: research and practice*, pp. 393-409, New York, 1993, Raven Press.

Taddio A, Katz J, Ilersich AL et al.: Effect of neonatal circumcision on pain response during subsequent routine vaccination, *Lancet* 349:599-603, 1997.

Tamsen A, Sakurada T, Wahlstrom A et al.: Postoperative demand for analgesics in relation to individual levels of endorphins and substance P in cerebrospinal fluid, *Pain* 13:171-183, June 1982.

Taylor NM, Hall GM, Salmon P: Is patient-controlled analgesia controlled by the patient? *Soc Sci Med* 43:1137-1143, 1996a.

Taylor NM, Hall GM, Salmon P: Patients' experiences of patient controlled analgesia, *Anaesthesia* 51:525-528, 1996b.

Taylor AG, Skelton JA, Butcher J: Duration of pain condition and physical pathology as determinants of nurses' assessments of patients in pain, *Nurs Res* 33:4-8, 1984.

Teasell RW, Merskey H: Chronic pain disability in the workplace, *Pain Res Manage* 4:197-205, 1997.

Terenius L: Endorphins and pain. In Rees LH, van Wimersma Greidanus TB, editors: *Frontiers of hormone research*, vol 8, pp. 162-177, Karger, 1981, Basel.

Todd KH, Samaroo N, Hoffman JR: Ethnicity as a risk factor for inadequate emergency department analgesia, *JAMA* 269(12):1537-1539, 1993.

Turk DC, Okifuji A: What factors affect physicians' decisions to prescribe opioids for chronic noncancer pain patients? *Clin J Pain* 13:330-336, 1997.

Twycross RG: Clinical experience with diamorphine in advanced malignant disease, *Int J Clin Pharmacol* 9:184-198, 1974.

Twycross R, Harcourt J, Bergl S: A survey of pain in patients with advanced cancer, *J Pain Symptom Manage* 12:273-282, 1996.

Twycross RG, Wald SJ: Long-term use of diamorphine in advanced cancer. In Bonica JJ, Albe-Fessard D, editors: *Advances in pain research and therapy*, Vol 1, pp. 653-661, New York, 1976, Raven Press.

Van Cleve L, Johnson L, Pothier P: Pain responses of hospitalized infants and children to venipuncture and intravenous cannulation, *J Pediatr Nurs* 11:161-168, 1996.

Van den Berg JH: *Leven in meervoud*, pp. 248-253, Nijkerk, 1963, G. F. Callenback.

Von Roenn JH, Cleeland CS, Gonin R et al.: Physician attitudes and practice in cancer pain management: a survey from the Eastern Cooperative Oncology Group, *Ann Intern Med* 119:121-126, 1993.

Waddell G, Main CJ, Morris EW et al.: Chronic low-back pain, psychological distress, and illness behavior, *Spine* 9:209-213, 1984.

Walco GA, Ilowite NT: Vertical versus horizontal visual analogue scales of pain intensity in children, *J Pain Symptom Manage* 6:200, 1991.

Wall PD: Reply to E. Leskowitz, *Pain* 53(1):115, 1993.

Wang XS, Mendoza TR, Gao S-Z et al.: The Chinese version of the Brief Pain Inventory (BPI-C): its development and use in a study of cancer pain, *Pain* 67:407-416, 1996.

Ward SE, Goldberg N, Miller-McCauley V et al.: Patient-related barriers to management of cancer pain, *Pain* 52:319-324, 1993.

Wells N: Management of pain during abortion, *J Adv Nurs* 14:56-62, 1989.

Wesson DR, Smith DE: Prescription drug abuse: patients, physician, and cultural responsibilities, *West J Med* 152(5):613-616, 1990.

Wiener CL: Pain assessment on an orthopedic ward, *Nurs Outlook* 23:508-516, 1975.

Wilkie DF, Keefe FJ: Coping strategies of patients with lung cancer-related pain, *Clin J Pain* 7:292-299, 1991.

Wilkie D, Lovejoy N, Dodd M et al.: Cancer pain control behaviors: description and correlation with pain intensity, *Onc Nurs Forum* 15(6):723-731, 1988.

Wilson JE, Pendleton JM: Oligoanalgesia in the emergency department, *Am J Emerg Med* 7:620-623, 1989.

Whipple B, Komisaruk BR: Elevation of pain threshold by vaginal stimulation in women, *Pain* 21:357-367, 1985.

Wolf S, Pinsky RH: Effects of placebo administration and occurrence of toxic reactions, *JAMA* 155:339-341, May 22, 1954.

Wong D, Baker C: Pain in children: comparison of assessment scales, *Pediatr Nurs* 14:9-17, 1988.

Wong D, Baker C: *Reference manual for the Wong-Baker FACES pain rating scale*, Tulsa, 1995, Wong & Baker.

Zalon ML: Nurses' assessment of postoperative patients' pain, *Pain* 54:329-334, 1993.

Zimmerman L, Story KT, Gaston-Johansson F et al.: Psychological variables and cancer pain, *Cancer Nurs* 19:44-53, 1996.

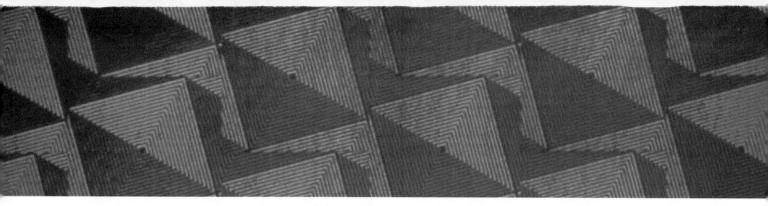

chapter four

OVERVIEW OF THREE GROUPS OF ANALGESICS

Margo McCaffery and Russell K. Portenoy

CHAPTER OUTLINE

TERMINOLOGY

Adjuvant analgesic: A drug that has a primary indication other than pain (e.g., antidepressant or anticonvulsant) but is also analgesic for some painful conditions.

Analgesic ceiling: A dose beyond which additional analgesia is not obtained.

Balanced analgesia: Also referred to as continuous, multimodal analgesia. Balanced analgesia often includes drugs from each of the three analgesic groups, such as nonsteroidal antiinflammatory drugs (NSAIDs), opioids, and local anesthetics, that may be given by several different routes of administration.

Mu agonist: A type of opioid, includes morphine and other opioids that relieve pain by binding to the mu receptor sites in the central nervous system. Used interchangeably with the terms full agonist, pure agonist, and morphine-like drug.

Narcotic: Obsolete term used to refer to what is now called opioid. Current usage is primarily in a legal context to refer to a wide variety of substances of potential abuse.

Nonopioid: Preferred to "nonnarcotic." Refers to acetaminophen and NSAIDs.

NSAID: An acronym for nonsteroidal antiinflammatory drug. (Pronounced "in said.")

Opioid: Preferred to "narcotic." Refers to codeine, morphine, and other natural, semisynthetic, and synthetic drugs that relieve pain by binding to multiple types of opioid receptors in the nervous system.

In clinical practice analgesics are divided into three groups: nonopioids, opioids, and adjuvants. For an overview of each group and its subgroups, see Figure 4.1.

The purpose of this chapter is to provide a framework for understanding the expanding world of analgesics and to identify some practical guidelines for selecting and combining analgesics from the different groups. A brief discussion of each analgesic group is provided and is derived from information presented in considerably more detail in Chapter 5 on nonopioids, Chapter 6 on opioids, and Chapter 7 on adjuvants. Therefore documentation is kept to a minimum in this chapter, and the reader is referred to the other chapters for a more comprehensive review with accompanying references.

Over the past 10 years numerous analgesics have been added to the list of commonly used analgesics and some of the related terminology has also changed. The most obvious changes are the substitution of the term opioid for narcotic and the addition of the adjuvant analgesic group. Terminology and misconceptions about combining analgesics (Table 4.1) are provided at the beginning of this chapter.

The term "opioid" is now preferred to the word "narcotic," and the term "nonopioid" is substituted for "nonnarcotic." Narcotic is an obsolete term, in part because the media and government use the term loosely to refer to a variety of substances of potential abuse, some of which do not fit the pharmacologic definition of a narcotic analgesic. For example, cocaine is a local anesthetic with a central nervous system (CNS) stimulant effect, not a narcotic analgesic. Yet, the media and federal regulations refer to cocaine as a narcotic.

The term "opiate" is sometimes used by pharmacologists to describe any naturally occurring substances (that is, alkaloid compounds originating from the poppy) that bind to opioid receptors. The term opiate is legally distinguished from narcotic and refers specifically to drugs similar to morphine (it does not include cocaine).

More recently, the term opioid supplanted opiate and is now the preferred term. Opioid clearly distinguishes these drugs from others, includes synthetic drugs and compounds that already exist in the body (also known as endorphins), and appropriately suggests that the effects of these compounds are mediated through opioid receptor sites.

Opioid analgesics are divided into two major subgroups. The largest subgroup and the one most often used as an analgesic is referred to as the morphine-like agonist. The terms morphine-like drug, mu agonist, pure agonist, and full agonist refer to the same group of analgesics, and the terms may be used interchangeably. The other subgroup of opioids is referred to as agonist-antagonist and is further subdivided into the mixed agonist-antagonists (pentazocine, nalbuphine, butorphanol, dezocine) and the partial agonists (buprenorphine).

The nonopioid analgesic group includes acetaminophen and nonsteroidal antiinflammatory drugs (NSAIDs). Sometimes all nonopioids are loosely referred to as NSAIDs. However, acetaminophen should be distinguished from NSAIDs because it seems to relieve pain by mechanisms quite different from NSAIDs. Although NSAIDs appear to have a prominent action on inflammatory processes in the peripheral tissues, acetaminophen seems to have a central effect and has very little antiinflammatory effect.

Adjuvant analgesics refer to a diverse group of drugs that have a primary indication other than pain but are also analgesic in some painful conditions. An example is amitriptyline, which has a primary indication for depression but also has proven analgesic effects for many types of pain, such as the continuous neuropathic pain with burning and aching qualities that patients with diabetic

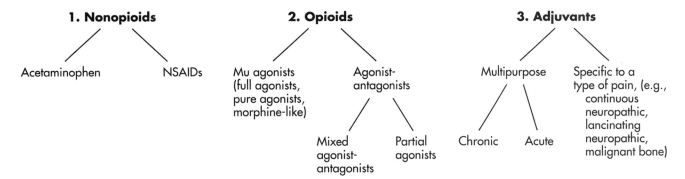

May be duplicated for use in clinical practice. From McCaffery M, Pasero C: *Pain: Clinical manual,* p. 105. Copyright © 1999, Mosby, Inc.

● ● ● ● ●
F I G U R E 4.1   Three analgesic groups with subgroups.

T A B L E 4.1 ● ● ● ● ●

Misconceptions	**Combining Analgesics**
MISCONCEPTION	CORRECTION
1. Use only one analgesic for pain control.	Use of one analgesic from each of the three groups is often more effective and safer in the treatment of acute or chronic pain than using only one analgesic. However, only one NSAID should be used, and, when possible, only one morphine-like drug.
2. If a nonopioid does not provide satisfactory pain relief, discontinue the nonopioid and switch to an opioid.	Whenever pain is severe enough to require an opioid, always consider adding a nonopioid, especially if the patient previously obtained some relief from the nonopioid. Among other benefits, this reduces the amount of opioid required, thereby reducing opioid-induced side effects.
3. It is dangerous to administer an opioid and a NSAID at the same time.	Administering the opioid and the NSAID at different times during the day is unnecessary. They have different side effects. If each one is safe for the patient, it is safe and more convenient to administer them at the same time.
4. It is unacceptable polypharmacy to administer a NSAID, opioid, and one or more adjuvant analgesics (e.g., anticonvulsant, antidepressant) for pain control.	Each group of analgesics relieves pain by a different mechanism. It is acceptable polypharmacy to administer several drugs if each one is for a specific purpose.

May be duplicated for use in clinical practice. From McCaffery M, Pasero C: *Pain: Clinical manual,* p. 105. Copyright © 1999, Mosby, Inc.

neuropathy experience. Adjuvant analgesics are sometimes referred to as "coanalgesics," particularly in the palliative care literature.

Although the three analgesic groups are referred to as nonopioids, opioids, and adjuvants, this terminology is not exact and does not adequately distinguish between the groups. For example, an argument could be made that NSAIDs are adjuvants because their primary indication is antiinflammatory, not analgesic. Or perhaps NSAIDs and acetaminophen should not comprise one group but two groups because they relieve pain by different mechanisms. Nonopioid is also a problematic category because theoretically it should include all analgesics, including adjuvants, that are not opioids.

Furthermore, the adjuvant group encompasses such a wide variety of drugs, ranging from antidepressants to topical anesthetics, that it is impossible to identify characteristics common to all. The adjuvant group is almost equivalent to a miscellaneous category (that is, a dumping ground for whatever does not fit in the opioid or nonopioid group). Another confusing feature of this terminology is that an adjuvant drug usually refers to a drug given in addition to another drug, not a drug given alone. Yet many adjuvant analgesics are used alone, not as adjuvants to any other treatment.

① **Transduction:** Conversion of one energy form to another. This process occurs in the periphery when a noxious stimulus causes tissue damage. The damaged cells release substances that activate or sensitize nociceptors. This activation leads to the generation of an action potential.

> A. **Sensitizing substances** released by damaged cells:
> - Prostaglandins (PG)
> - Bradykinin (BK)
> - Serotonin (5HT)
> - Substance P (SP)
> - Histamine (H)
>
> *Nonopioids: At the site of injury NSAIDs inhibit PG production, causing a decrease in pain.*
>
> B. An **action potential** results from
> - Release of the above sensitizing substances (nociceptive pain)
>   + a change in the charge along the neuronal membrane
>   or
> - Abnormal processing of stimuli by the nervous system (neuropathic pain)
>   + a change in the charge along the neuronal membrane.
>
> The change in charge occurs when Na^+ moves into the cell and other ion transfers occur.
>
> *Adjuvants: Local anesthetics and many anticonvulsants reduce pain by blocking Na^+, thereby decreasing the action potential.*

A

② **Transmission:** The action potential continues from the site of damage to the spinal cord and ascends to higher centers. Transmission may be considered in three phases:

- Injury site to spinal cord. Nociceptors terminate in the spinal cord.
- Spinal cord to brain stem and thalamus. Release of SP and other neurotransmitters continues the impulse across the synaptic cleft between the nociceptors and the dorsal horn neurons. From the dorsal horn of the spinal cord, neurons such as the spinothalamic tract ascend to the thalamus. Other tracts carry the message to different centers in the brain.

> *Opioids: Morphine-like drugs bind to mu opioid receptors and block the release of SP, preventing the impulse from crossing the synapse.*

- Thalamus to cortex. Thalamus acts as a relay station sending the impulse to central structures for processing.

③ **Perception of pain:** Conscious experience of pain is decreased by actions of the nonopioids, adjuvants, and opioids.

④ **Modulation:** Inhibition of nociceptive impulses. Neurons originating in the brain stem descend to the spinal cord and release substances such as endogenous opioids, serotonin (5HT), and norepinephrine (NE) that inhibit the transmission of nociceptive impulses.

Adjuvants: Tricyclic antidepressants enhance normal modulation by interfering with the reuptake of 5HT and NE.

May be duplicated for use in clinical practice. As appears in McCaffery M, Pasero C: *Pain: Clinical manual,* p. 106, 1999, Mosby, Inc.

● ● ● ● ●
F I G U R E 4.2   **A,** Outlines analgesic action sites. **B,** Illustrates this.
Developed by McCaffery M, Pasero C, Paice JA.

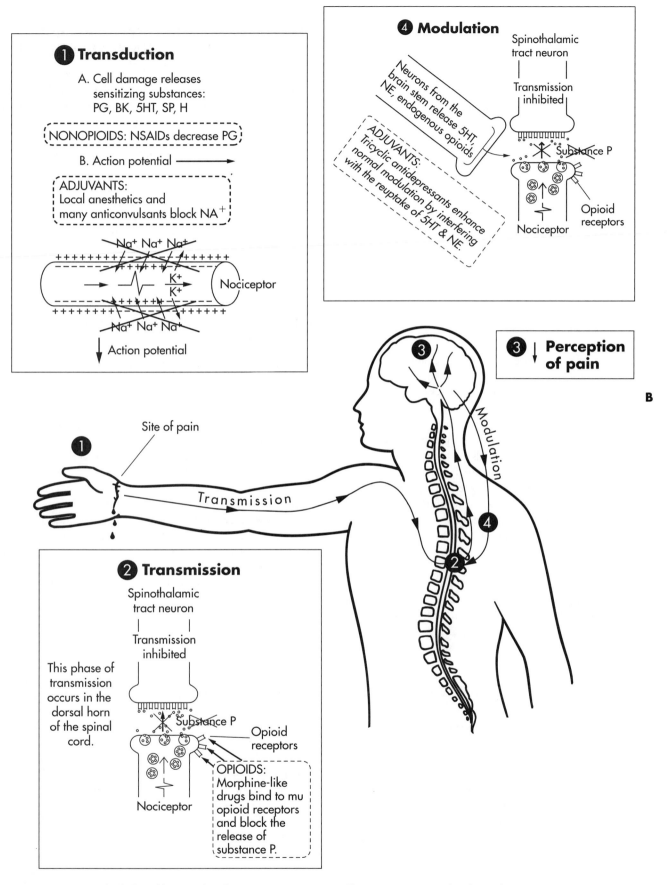

① Transduction

A. Cell damage releases sensitizing substances: PG, BK, 5HT, SP, H

NONOPIOIDS: NSAIDs decrease PG

B. Action potential ⟶

ADJUVANTS:
Local anesthetics and many anticonvulsants block NA$^+$

Na$^+$ Na$^+$ Na$^+$

K$^+$
K$^+$

Nociceptor

Na$^+$ Na$^+$ Na$^+$

↓ Action potential

④ Modulation

Neurons from the brain stem release 5HT, NE, endogenous opioids

ADJUVANTS:
Tricyclic antidepressants enhance normal modulation by interfering with the reuptake of 5HT & NE.

Spinothalamic tract neuron

Transmission inhibited

Substance P

Opioid receptors

Nociceptor

③ ↓ Perception of pain

Site of pain

Transmission

Modulation

B

② Transmission

Spinothalamic tract neuron

Transmission inhibited

This phase of transmission occurs in the dorsal horn of the spinal cord.

Substance P

Opioid receptors

OPIOIDS:
Morphine-like drugs bind to mu opioid receptors and block the release of substance P.

Nociceptor

May be duplicated for use in clinical practice. As appears in McCaffery M, Pasero C: *Pain: Clinical manual*, p. 107, 1999, Mosby, Inc.

● ● ● ● ●
F I G U R E 4.2 **B,** Illustrates analgesic action sites.

Developed by McCaffery M, Pasero C, Paice JA.

Thus the explanations and definitions suggested here are best regarded as a reflection of current customary usage of the terms in the clinical practice of pain management. In the near future analgesic groupings and terminology will no doubt undergo much refinement.

PAIN MECHANISMS AFFECTED BY EACH ANALGESIC GROUP

It is useful to distinguish among analgesics that relieve pain by different mechanisms. This has clinical significance. Because different analgesics relieve pain in different ways, it is sometimes logical to combine analgesics from different groups to relieve one specific type of pain or to relieve different types of pain occurring in the same patient. Following is a brief description of selected mechanisms of action thought to be unique to each analgesic group (see Figure 4.2).

1. *Nonopioids: acetaminophen and NSAIDs.* The analgesia produced by acetaminophen appears to be related to events in the CNS that are not well understood. NSAIDs also work in the CNS but their better characterized actions are peripheral (at the site of injury), where they may exert analgesic effects through the inhibition of prostaglandin (PG) production. Prostaglandin is an inflammatory mediator released when cells are damaged that sensitizes nerves that carry information about pain.

2. *Opioids.* Opioids probably relieve pain mainly by action in the CNS, binding to opioid receptor sites in the brain and spinal cord. Multiple opioid receptor sites are present, but the ones most frequently mentioned in relation to pain relief are mu, kappa, and delta. When a drug binds to any of these sites as an agonist, pain relief occurs. When a drug attaches to these opioid receptor sites as an antagonist, pain relief and other effects are blocked. A well-known opioid antagonist is naloxone (Narcan), which antagonizes (blocks or reverses) the action of all opioids, both full agonists and agonist-antagonists.

3. *Adjuvant analgesics.* No one mechanism of action for pain relief can be identified for this analgesic group. This group is composed of diverse classes of drugs that relieve pain by a variety of mechanisms, many of them as yet not understood. For example, certain antidepressants appear to relieve pain by blocking the reuptake of serotonin, making more serotonin present and thereby inhibiting the transmission of nociceptive impulses. Oral local anesthetics such as mexiletine and certain anticonvulsants such as carbamazepine are sodium channel blocking agents, and this may be part of the mechanism underlying their ability to relieve certain types of pain.

CLINICAL CONSIDERATIONS FOR USE OF EACH OF THE THREE ANALGESIC GROUPS

Certain characteristics of the analgesic groups have a major impact on how the drugs may be used effectively in clinical situations. These include the presence or absence of an analgesic ceiling (a dose beyond which no further analgesia will occur), expected onset of analgesia, acceptability of side effects, degree of difficulty in managing or preventing adverse side effects, availability of various routes of administration, and whether or not repeated administration will cause tolerance or physical dependence. The cost of analgesics within each group varies considerably, but each analgesic group contains some inexpensive formulations.

Following is an overview of selected characteristics of each analgesic group (see Chapters 5, 6, and 7 for more details). Refer to Table 4.2 for examples of analgesics within each group.

Nonopioids: Acetaminophen and NSAIDs

Acetaminophen (e.g., Tylenol)

Acetaminophen is a nonopioid, but it is not a NSAID. It differs from the NSAIDs in that it has considerably fewer adverse effects. It does not affect platelet function, rarely causes gastrointestinal problems, and can be given to patients who are allergic to aspirin or other NSAIDs. However, it has very little antiinflammatory effect. It may cause liver toxicity and should be used with caution in patients who regularly consume large amounts of alcohol or have liver disease. The analgesia of acetaminophen has a ceiling, and the total daily dose is restricted. For adults, the usual recommendation is that the dose should not exceed 4000 mg/24 hr (APS, 1992). Some clinicians extend that limit to 6000 mg/24 hr in appropriately monitored patients (Portenoy, Kanner, 1996). It is available without a prescription.

NSAIDs

These were, of course, originally marketed for inflammatory conditions such as rheumatoid arthritis. Over the years it has become increasingly apparent that they are also multipurpose analgesics. For example, they are effective with postoperative pain, cancer pain, headache, menstrual cramps, and a variety of other painful conditions. Aspirin is available without a prescription as are an increasing number of other NSAIDs such as ibuprofen (Advil, Nuprin), ketoprofen, and naproxen sodium (Aleve).

Indications

- Nonopioids have a role in a wide spectrum of acute and chronic painful situations.
- Nonopioids may be used with both nociceptive (somatic and visceral) pain and neuropathic pain (see Chapter 2). They seem to be more effective

THREE ANALGESIC GROUPS: EXAMPLES WITHIN EACH GROUP

Nonopioids Two Groups Are:	Opioids Two Groups Are:	Adjuvants Several Groups; Examples Are:

a. *Acetaminophen* (Tylenol)
b. *NSAIDs*
  Examples:
  Aspirin
  Carprofen (Rimadyl)
  Choline magnesium trisalicylate
    (Trilisate)
  Choline salicylate (Arthropan)
  Diflunisal (Dolobid)
  Etodolac (Lodine)
  Fenoprofen calcium (Nalfon)
  Ibuprofen (Motrin, Advil)
  Ketorolac (Toradol)
  Ketoprofen (Orudis)
  Meclofenamate sodium (Meclomen)
  Mefenamic acid (Ponstel)
  Nabumetone (Relafen)
  Naproxen (Naprosyn)
  Naproxen sodium (Anaprox, Aleve)
  Piroxicam (Feldene)
  Salsalate (Disalcid)
	a. *Mu agonists* (full agonists, pure
	    agonists, morphine-like)
	  Examples:
	  Codeine (as in Tylenol No. 3)
	  Fentanyl (Duragesic patch)
	  Hydrocodone (as in Lortab,
	    Vicodin)
	  Hydromorphone (Dilaudid)
	  Levorphanol (Levo-Dromoran)
	  Meperidine (Demerol)
	  Methadone
	  Morphine
	  Oxycodone (OxyContin; as in
	    Percocet)
	  Propoxyphene (Darvon)
	b. *Agonist-antagonists*
	  Examples:
	  Buprenorphine (Buprenex)
	  Butorphanol (Stadol)
	  Dezocine (Dalgan)
	  Nalbuphine (Nubain)
	  Pentazocine (Talwin)
		a. *Multipurpose for chronic pain:*
		  Examples:
		  Antidepressants, e.g.,
		    Amitriptyline (Elavil)
		    Desipramine (Norpramin)
		    Nortriptyline (Aventyl, Pamelor)
		  Corticosteroids, e.g.
		    Dexamethasone (Decadron)
		  Psychostimulants, e.g.
		    Dextroamphetamine (Dexedrine)
		    Methylphenidate (Ritalin)
		b. *Multipurpose for moderate to severe*
		  acute pain
		  Examples:
		  Lidocaine
		  Ketamine
		c. *Continuous neuropathic pain:*
		  Examples:
		  Antidepressants, e.g.,
		    Amitriptyline (Elavil)
		  Oral local anesthetics, e.g.,
		    mexiletine
		d. *Lancinating neuropathic pain:*
		  Examples:
		  Anticonvulsants, e.g.,
		    Gabapentin (Neurontin)
		    Carbamazepine (Tegretol)
		    Phenytoin (Dilantin)
		    Clonazepam (Klonopin)
		    Valproic acid (Depakene)
		  Baclofen (Lioresal)
		e. *Malignant bone pain:*
		  Examples:
		  Corticosteroids, e.g.,
		    Dexamethasone (Decadron)
		  Calcitonin

with nociceptive pain, particularly somatic pain such as muscle and joint pain.

• Used alone, acetaminophen or a NSAID often provides adequate relief for mild pain.

• Although acetaminophen has very little antiinflammatory effect, it is often an effective analgesic for inflammatory conditions.

• Used alone, a NSAID may provide adequate relief for moderate pain.

• Used alone, some NSAIDs at high doses may provide adequate relief for severe pain. However, NSAIDs alone often are not sufficient for severe pain.

• Nonopioids are often combined with opioids for their additive analgesic effects, or conversely, their opioid dose-sparing effect. In other words, adding a nonopioid to an opioid may allow the opioid dose to be lowered without compromising pain relief. When pain is severe enough to require an opioid, the addition of a nonopioid can be helpful if opioid-related side effects are troublesome. The nonopioid may handle residual pain and obviate the need for more opioid or even allow reduction of the opioid dose with lessening of the side effects.

Choice of drug

- Whichever NSAID has worked well for the patient in the past and has caused minimal or no side effects is often the best place to begin with drug selection.
- Patients vary in response to NSAIDs. If one NSAID is ineffective after a few days of appropriate dosage adjustment, it is worthwhile to try another NSAID. This is referred to as sequential trials.
- If the patient is hypersensitive ("allergic") to aspirin or any other NSAID, all NSAIDs are contraindicated, but acetaminophen may be given.
- Acetaminophen is probably the safest nonopioid for most patients unless the patient has liver disease or a history of regular moderate to heavy alcohol intake.
- When NSAIDs are used as a single dose at low doses or for only a short period of time (e.g., postoperatively), side effects are less problematic than with long-term use.
- The risk of gastric ulcers from NSAIDs can be reduced by coadministration of misoprostol, a prostaglandin analog. Unproven alternatives include some combination of a H2 blocker (e.g., cimetidine [Tagamet] or ranitidine [Zantac]), sucralfate (Carafate), and antacids.
- Most NSAIDs interfere with platelet aggregation. In patients with bleeding diatheses such as hemophilia and in some patients undergoing surgery or cancer treatment, it may be important to minimize increased bleeding. Acetaminophen has no effect on platelet aggregation. On theoretical grounds, NSAIDs that have minimal or no effect on platelet aggregation such as choline magnesium trisalicylate (Trilisate), salsalate (Disalcid), and nabumetone (Relafen), may be preferable when bleeding is a concern. None of these drugs have been proven safe in the setting of a bleeding diathesis, however.
- Nonprescription formulations are usually less expensive than prescription formulations. Acetaminophen, aspirin, and an increasing number of NSAIDs, such as ibuprofen (Advil, Nuprin), ketoprofen (Orudis), and naproxen sodium (Aleve), are available over the counter.

Routes and dosing

- Acetaminophen and all NSAIDs are available orally. Only a few are commercially available for rectal administration, but most oral dose forms can be given rectally.
- Currently only ketorolac (Toradol) is available in the United States in adult doses for parenteral administration, IM or IV. It is indicated for short-term use only.

- Acetaminophen and NSAIDs may be given as needed (PRN) for occasional pain or around-the-clock (ATC) for ongoing pain.
- Acetaminophen has a short half-life and usually must be given every 4 hours for ongoing pain.
- The half-lives of NSAIDs differ, and dosing intervals range from every 4 hours to once a day. For chronic pain, infrequent dosing (e.g., once or twice a day) is usually more convenient for patients and more likely to result in the patient taking all prescribed doses. When patients are taking other analgesics or medications, consider selecting NSAIDs that allow for scheduling as many doses as possible at the same time.
- A ceiling or limit exists on the analgesia provided by acetaminophen and NSAIDs.
- For NSAIDs the ceiling dose for analgesia varies from one individual to another. If careful dose selection is desired, half the recommended dose may be given and then increased every few days until a further increase provides no additional pain relief or results in undesirable side effects. Then one may drop back to the previous dose. However, the dose should not exceed 200% of the recommended daily starting dose.
- For acetaminophen, potential hepatotoxicity limits the maximum dose to 4000 to 6000 mg/day.
- Dosing of acetaminophen and NSAIDs is not affected by physical dependence and tolerance because these do not develop with repeated administration.

Opioids

Opioids available in the United States may be divided into two groups, full mu agonists and mixed agonist-antagonists. These two subgroups of opioids are used very differently in the clinical setting. Whereas the mu agonists are beneficial in the management of a wide spectrum of acute and chronic painful conditions, the agonist-antagonists have a very limited role. Thus the two groups are discussed together and separately.

Mu agonists and agonist-antagonists

- Physical dependence should be expected in patients who receive opioids regularly for several days or longer.
- Physical dependence is manifested by withdrawal syndrome when the opioid is abruptly discontinued or when an antagonist (e.g., naloxone) is administered. Withdrawal can be suppressed with a gradual reduction in dose over 7 to 10 days. The withdrawal syndrome also can be suppressed by administering as little as 25% of the previous dose. Physical dependence requires no treatment unless withdrawal symptoms occur or are anticipated.
- Tolerance to some side effects, such as sleepiness and nausea, usually occurs after a few days. Tolerance to

analgesia occurs but is rarely a problem. The opioid dose usually stabilizes if the pain is stable. Tolerance to analgesia, if it does occur, such as pain escalation from progressive disease, is managed by increasing the opioid dose and sometimes by shortening of the interval between doses. Tolerance to respiratory depression occurs routinely if doses are increased slowly. Thus if the patient requires a higher opioid dose because of increased pain, it is usually safe.

Mu agonist opioids (full agonist, pure agonists, morphine-like drugs)

Mu agonist opioids are the largest group of opioids and the most commonly used. They include codeine, morphine, hydromorphone (Dilaudid), fentanyl, methadone, oxycodone, levorphanol, meperidine (Demerol), and propoxyphene (Darvon). See Table 4.2 for other examples.

Indications

- Mu agonists are the mainstay of analgesia for acute pain and cancer pain. They are also appropriate for some patients with chronic nonmalignant pain.
- All types of pain are responsive to opioids. However, some types of pain are more responsive than others. Nociceptive pain (i.e., somatic or visceral pain) is more responsive to opioids than neuropathic pain.
- Breakthrough pain is almost always best treated with a mu agonist. This is pain that "breaks through" the pain relief provided by ongoing, ATC analgesics. Breakthrough analgesics are often referred to as the rescue or supple tary dose when the route is oral and as a bolus dose when the route is IV or intraspinal.

Choice of Drug

- One mu agonist by one route of administration should be used whenever possible. Unfortunately, it is still common practice for patients to receive more than one opioid by more than one route. Usually this is unnecessary, and often it is confusing and expensive.
- Because all mu agonists relieve pain by attaching to mu opioid receptor sites, very little difference exists in their overall ability to relieve pain. However, patients vary in their responsiveness (that is, their ability to achieve a favorable balance between pain relief and side effects) to the different drugs. This is the reason that it may be rational to switch from one mu agonist to another. This should only be done, however, if the dose of the first drug has been gradually increased to determine whether it actually can provide adequate relief without intolerable

side effects. Without dose titration to treatment-limiting side effects, the responsiveness of the patient to the drug is not known. It is usually not appropriate to switch to a new opioid until the responsiveness has been determined. Unrelieved pain per se is not usually a sound reason to switch to another mu agonist.
- The terms "weak" opioid and "strong" opioid are incorrect. A more appropriate designation is opioids usually used for mild pain and opioids usually used for moderate to severe pain.
- All mu agonists have the same side effects. Although, theoretically, the side effects should be the same at equianalgesic doses (doses that provide the same pain relief), variability is the rule. Some individuals will have different side effects or more severe side effects from one mu agonist than another. This cannot be predicted except on the basis of the patient's previous experience with the drug.
- The appearance of unmanageable and unacceptable side effects from a mu agonist is one of the major reasons for switching to another mu agonist. Before switching, determine whether the side effects are unmanageable (e.g., nausea cannot be managed with antiemetics) or simply unmanaged (e.g., no attempt was made to treat the nausea).
- If the dose of a mu agonist relieves pain but causes unmanageable and unacceptable side effects, another mu agonist should be used. Sequential trials may be necessary because considerable interindividual variability exists in the occurrence, severity, and manageability of side effects.
- Another major reason for switching from one mu agonist to another is the occurrence of or likelihood of accumulation of an active metabolite, such as norpropoxyphene (from propoxyphene [Darvon]) or normeperidine (from meperidine [Demerol]), that causes unmanageable or unacceptable effects.
- In summary, as a general rule, the two main reasons for selecting one morphine-like drug over another are as follows:
  1. Unmanageable side effects
  2. Potential toxicity from accumulation of an active metabolite
- A true allergy to mu agonist opioids is rare. Side effects are often erroneously referred to by the patient as an allergy. If the patient has a true allergy to an opioid, such as morphine, another opioid, such as methadone or fentanyl, may be tolerated.
- For breakthrough pain, the mu agonist opioid selected should have a rapid onset and short duration of action, such as immediate-release morphine. Whenever possible, the opioid for breakthrough pain should be the same as the opioid used for ongoing pain. For example, if controlled-release morphine

is given for ongoing pain, use immediate-release morphine for breakthrough pain. Or if the patient is receiving epidural analgesia, provide additional analgesia by the same route rather than administering opioids IV.

Routes and Dosing

- Routes of administration for mu agonist opioids are multiple. Most are available orally and parenterally. Some (not all) are used intrathecally, epidurally, or for subcutaneous continuous infusion. New delivery systems include controlled-release morphine (MS Contin, Oramorph SR) and oxycodone (OxyContin) and transdermal fentanyl (Duragesic).
- Mu agonists may be given PRN for occasional pain or ATC for ongoing or chronic pain.
- If a dose of mu agonist is safe but ineffective, it is usually safe and appropriate to increase the dose by 25% to 50% until pain relief occurs or until unmanageable and unacceptable side effects occur.
- No ceiling exists on the analgesia of mu agonists. However, some opioids such as propoxyphene and meperidine have active metabolites that increase the risks of higher doses and therefore limit their doses; all opioids have side effects that ultimately limit dose escalation.
- If the dose relieves pain but causes unmanageable and unacceptable side effects, one strategy is to decrease the dose by 25% and consider adding another type of analgesic such as acetaminophen or a NSAID. Another strategy is to switch to another mu agonist.

Agonist-antagonists

The agonist-antagonists are further subdivided into mixed agonist-antagonists (pentazocine [Talwin]), nalbuphine [Nubain], butorphanol [Stadol], dezocine [Dalgan]) and partial agonists (buprenorphine [Buprenex]).

Indications

- Agonist-antagonists may be appropriate for acute nociceptive pain (visceral or somatic) of moderate to severe intensity.
- Agonist-antagonists are inappropriate for severe, escalating pain.
- Avoid buprenorphine in labor. Respiratory depression is not readily reversed by naloxone (APS, 1992).
- Butorphanol nasal spray may be appropriate for outpatient treatment of moderate to severe acute migraine headache pain or some types of postoperative pain.
- Use agonist-antagonists with caution in patients who are receiving mu-agonists. Because of their antagonist properties at the mu opioid receptor site

("Narcan-like" effect), agonist-antagonists may cause the following problems if given to a patient already taking a mu agonist:

1. Analgesia from the mu agonist may be reduced.
2. Withdrawal-like symptoms may be precipitated in patients who are physically dependent on mu agonists. Physical dependence should be expected after the patient has been on regular doses of mu agonist opioids for several days or longer.

Choice of Drug

- Some of the mixed agonist-antagonists are especially likely to cause psychotomimetic effects such as agitation, dysphoria, and confusion.
- Nalbuphine has a lower incidence of psychotomimetic effects than pentazocine (APS, 1992).
- Nalbuphine is the most likely agonist-antagonist to be used to reverse side effects of opioids administered epidurally.

Routes and Dosing

- Routes of administration are limited to parenteral except for oral pentazocine and butorphanol nasal spray.
- Agonist-antagonists may be given PRN for occasional pain or ATC for ongoing pain.
- A ceiling exists on the analgesia and respiratory depressant effects of the mixed agonist-antagonists and partial agonists.
- If a dose of agonist-antagonist is safe but ineffective, increase the dose by 25% to 50% until the analgesic ceiling is reached, pain relief occurs, or unmanageable and unacceptable side effects occur.

Adjuvant Analgesics

Adjuvant analgesics are drugs with other specific indications that have been found to be effective analgesics for selected types of pain. They have been used to treat other conditions before the discovery of their analgesic properties. Originally, the adjuvant analgesic group was composed mainly of drugs used for chronic pain, particularly neuropathic pain. Now the group has expanded to include drugs for a wider variety of painful conditions.

Indications

Multipurpose for Chronic Pain

Some of the more useful multipurpose drugs include the following drug groups:

- Antidepressants. Tricyclic antidepressants, particularly amitriptyline (Elavil), are more effective analgesics than the selective serotonin reuptake inhibitors (SSRIs). At present antidepressants have no role in acute pain management, primarily because of delayed analgesia (owing to the need to start with low doses, escalate slowly, and allow several days for accumulation), but are used for a variety of chronic pain conditions, especially continuous neuropathic pain.

- Corticosteroids. These may be used for a variety of types of cancer-related pain, such as metastatic bone pain or neuropathic pain associated with tumor compression. For example, dexamethasone (Decadron), 16 mg/day, or its equivalent may be useful when opioids are ineffective.
- Psychostimulants. These also relieve a variety of types of pain, ranging from cancer-related pain to headache. Dextroamphetamine (Dexedrine) and methylphenidate (Ritalin) have been used in cancer patients both to reduce sedation and to increase pain relief.

Multipurpose for Moderate to Severe Acute Pain

Opioids are usually the mainstay of treatment for moderate to severe acute pain. However, recent indications of the value of establishing multimodal, continuous analgesia preoperatively (preemptive analgesia) in the surgical patient have resulted in an increased use of local anesthetics in addition to opioids, such as infiltration of the surgical site with lidocaine before incision and bupivacaine added to epidural opioids for postoperative pain management. Other adjuvants used for acute pain, sometimes alone or in addition to opioids, include IV lidocaine (e.g., for burn pain), ketamine by various routes, and EMLA, a topical anesthetic for procedural pain.

Chronic Continuous Neuropathic Pain

First-line treatment is usually antidepressants and/or oral local anesthetics such as mexiletine (Mexitil).

Chronic Lancinating Neuropathic Pain

First-line treatment includes anticonvulsants and baclofen (Lioresal).

Chronic Malignant Bone Pain

Treatment includes corticosteroids, biphosphonates (osteoclast inhibitor to reduce bone resorption [e.g. pamidronate]), calcitonin, and radiopharmaceuticals (strontium-89 and samarium-153).

Choice of drug

- The type of pain being treated determines the choice of drug group (see above). Within each drug group, selection is made on the basis of multiple patient characteristics, such as age and other medical conditions.
- If one adjuvant is ineffective or causes unacceptable and unmanageable side effects, another adjuvant analgesic in that drug group or in another group

should be used. Individuals vary in their responses to these drugs. In other words, sequential trials are often necessary because considerable interindividual variability exists.

Routes and dosing

- Almost all adjuvant analgesics are available orally and some may be given parenterally, epidurally, intrathecally, or transdermally.
- Generally a ceiling effect exists on the analgesia of adjuvants, but it is individual. Most must be titrated upward slowly. Thus for many of the adjuvants, analgesia is delayed until the appropriate dose is reached and the drug accumulates. The maximum analgesic effect may not occur for several days or longer.

What Is Not Analgesic?

Note what is *not* included in the discussion of any of the analgesic groups: phenothiazines and benzodiazepines. These are avoided because, with few exceptions, they increase sedation without enhancing analgesia.

- Phenothiazines do not relieve pain, except for methotrimeprazine (Levoprome), and they do not potentiate opioid analgesia (APS, 1992). The combination of meperidine and promethazine (Phenergan) or DPT (Demerol, Phenergan, and Thorazine) are no longer recommended for pain relief.
- Benzodiazepines, such as diazepam (Valium) and lorazepam (Ativan), may be useful for muscle spasm and terminal dyspnea. Clonazepam (Klonopin), an anticonvulsant, may relieve sharp neuropathic pain. Otherwise, benzodiazepines are not effective analgesics. Titration of the opioid should be done before use of benzodiazepines (APS, 1992).

COMPARISON OF CHARACTERISTICS OF THE THREE ANALGESIC GROUPS

The analgesic groups have some characteristics in common, whereas other characteristics differ significantly, affecting the feasibility of using them in the clinical situation. Table 4.3 summarizes some of the clinically relevant similarities and differences between the three analgesic groups.

The most flexible of all the analgesics are the mu agonist opioids (morphine-like, full agonists, pure agonists). Virtually all types of pain can be relieved to some degree by these drugs, and they have no ceiling on their analgesia. Mu agonists are available by numerous routes of administration, and onset of analgesia is immediate, within minutes by some routes. Although a dozen or more mu agonists are commercially available in the United States, for the individual patient it is usually only necessary to use one mu agonist by one route of administration.

● ● ● ● ●
TABLE 4.3

COMPARISON OF CHARACTERISTICS OF THE THREE ANALGESIC GROUPS

	Nonopioids	Opioids		Adjuvants
		mu Agonists	Agonist-Antagonists	
Characteristics				
1. Indications	Multipurpose, especially mild musculoskeletal pain	Multipurpose; mainstay of acute and cancer pain	Theoretically multipurpose but rarely first line choice	Variable; specific types, e.g., neuropathic; usually chronic pain; some for acute
2. Onset of analgesia	Immediate	Immediate	Immediate	Delayed (some exceptions)
3. Analgesic ceiling	Yes	No	Yes	Yes
4. Routes of administration	Oral, some rectal or parenteral	Numerous	Parenteral (some exceptions)	Oral for most; routes vary with drug
5. Dose titration if safe but ineffective at recommended dose	If acetaminophen, discontinue; if NSAID, typically acceptable to increase dose up to twice recommended starting dose or switch to another NSAID	Increase by 25%-50% until unmanageable and unacceptable side effects; analgesia dose related	Discontinue	Increase dose; switch to another adjuvant; add another adjuvant
6. Use of more than one drug from the same analgesic group	No, except acetaminophen may be combined with any NSAID	No need — Avoid combining mu agonist with agonist-antagonist (some exceptions)	No need	May be beneficial
7. Combining a drug from this analgesic group with a drug from another analgesic group	Yes, combine with any analgesic group*	Yes, combine with any analgesic group		Yes, combine with any analgesic group*
8. Development of tolerance and physical dependence	No	Yes (seldom problematic)	Yes (seldom problematic)	No (some exceptions)

May be duplicated for use in clinical practice. From McCaffery M, Pasero C: *Pain: Clinical manual*, p. 114. Copyright © 1999, Mosby, Inc.

*NSAID coadministered with a corticosteroid increases risk of gastric ulceration fourfold. NSAID coadministered with phenytoin or other anticonvulsants requires careful monitoring (Portenoy RK, Kanner RM: Nonopioid and adjuvant analgesics. In Portenoy RH, Kanner RM, editors: *Pain management: Theory and practice*, pp. 219-249, Philadelphia, 1996, F.A. Davis).

Although mu agonists cause tolerance and physical dependence after repeated administration, these are seldom difficult clinical problems. The mu agonists can also be combined with practically any of the other analgesics in the nonopioid and adjuvant groups.

The least flexible of all the analgesics are the agonist-antagonist opioids. Although their analgesic effect is immediate, there is a ceiling on their analgesia, and their routes of administration are limited to parenteral except for oral pentazocine and butorphanol nasal spray. They may be combined with nonopioids or adjuvants, but combining them with mu agonists may precipitate withdrawal or reduce analgesia.

Nonopioids are fairly flexible analgesics in that they may be used for a variety of acute and chronic painful conditions of mild to moderate intensity. Onset of analgesia is immediate (often within an hour), and tolerance and physical dependence do not occur with repeated administration. Any one nonopioid is compatible with most other analgesics from the other two analgesic groups. Most may be administered orally or rectally, but only a few are available parenterally, limiting their usefulness with many types of severe pain in which the patient cannot take medication orally. Further limiting their usefulness is the fact that a ceiling on their analgesia exists.

As a group, adjuvants are less reliable analgesics than opioids or nonopioids. Although this group contains multipurpose analgesics for acute and chronic pain, no single adjuvant is appropriate for all types of pain or even a wide variety of pains. Overall, a small percentage of patients report effective analgesia from adjuvants, but a higher percentage of patients have troublesome side effects. Most adjuvants have a slow onset of analgesia, often because of the need to start with low doses to avoid side effects. Thus many adjuvants are not appropriate for acute or severe pain. If adjuvants with delayed analgesia are used for severe pain, other analgesics such as opioids should be relied on for pain relief until the adjuvant analgesic becomes effective. For example, for cancer patients, opioid therapy should be maximized before adding an adjuvant. It is not possible to predict which patient will respond to adjuvant analgesics or which will develop side effects. Considerable intraindividual variability exists in response to different drugs, including those within the same class (Portenoy, 1998). The usefulness of adjuvant analgesics is further limited by lack of research.

COMBINING ANALGESICS
Rationale

Appropriate reasons for considering the use of more than one analgesic for the management of an individual patient's pain include the following:
- The combination of two or more drugs attacks more of the underlying pain mechanisms than can be achieved by using only one analgesic.
- The combination allows for smaller doses of each analgesic than would be required if only one analgesic is used, thereby reducing the side effects from any one analgesic. For example, using a nonopioid along with an opioid has an opioid dose-sparing effect, and the lower opioid dose may significantly decrease opioid side effects such as sedation.
- The patient has several different types of pain such as sharp neuropathic pain and also musculoskeletal pain, and they are not both responsive to a single analgesic.

Warnings about polypharmacy cause many clinicians to be suspicious of the wisdom of combining two or more analgesics (see Table 4.1). Box 4.1 offers a quick guide to combining analgesics from different analgesic groups and within drug groups.

If drugs are physically combined, their stability and compatibility must be determined. For long-term epidural or intrathecal administration, morphine hydrochloride, bupivacaine hydrochloride, and clonidine hydrochloride were found to be physically and chemically stable for up to 90 days (Wulf, Gleim, Mignat, 1994). In another study combinations of bupivacaine and morphine and bupivacaine and buprenorphine were found to be stable for at least 30 days (Nitescu, Hultman, Applegren et al., 1992). Fentanyl citrate combined with bupivacaine hydrochloride is also stable and compatible for up to 30 days (Tu, Stiles, Allen, 1990).

Analgesics, including opioids, also may be combined for parenteral administration. For example, a patient with cancer pain being cared for at home may be receiving a subcutaneous continuous infusion of an opioid along with another drug. A study of the injectable mu agonist opioids fentanyl, hydromorphone, methadone, and morphine showed that over a 48-hour period they are physically compatible with dexamethasone, ketorolac, and diazepam, but not phenytoin (Chandler, Trissel, 1996).

WHO Analgesic Ladder for Cancer Pain Relief

Because drugs are often coadministered separately, physical compatibility is not usually an issue. The issue with this approach is safety and efficacy. Probably the most well-known example of combining analgesics from the three analgesic groups is the WHO analgesic ladder (Figure 4.3) proposed in the early 1980s as a guide to the management of chronic cancer pain. It has been endorsed by the United States Agency for Health Care Policy and Research (1994) and the American Pain Society (1992). The analgesic ladder focuses on selecting analgesics on the basis of the intensity of the pain using analgesics from each of the analgesic groups and, to some extent, building on previously effective analgesics.

Steps 1, 2, and 3

The three steps of the WHO analgesic ladder address different intensities of pain. However, patients do not always have mild pain at the bottom of the ladder and do not necessarily progress through each of the three levels of pain intensity. Some patients with cancer pain will have moderate to severe pain initially, whereas others may progress directly from mild pain to severe pain. Therefore treatment of cancer pain does not necessarily begin with step 1, progress to step 2, and follow with step 3. If the patient initially has severe pain, step 3 treatment considerations are appropriate.

Step 1 of the analgesic ladder addresses mild pain by suggesting a nonopioid analgesic and the possibility of an

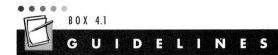

BOX 4.1

GUIDELINES

COMBINING ANALGESICS

Acetaminophen + Any Other Analgesic = Acceptable, Common Practice

Acetaminophen may be given along with any of the NSAIDs, opioids, or adjuvants.

Acetaminophen + NSAID = Acceptable, Common Practice

Acetaminophen may be given with any of the NSAIDs. Including acetaminophen usually adds analgesia without increasing side effects.

NSAID + NSAID = Not Recommended

This is not recommended. The additional pain relief is minimal and the risk of side effects is considerable.

Corticosteroid + NSAID = Caution

Prolonged administration of this combination increases the risk of side effects such as peptic ulcer.

Opioid + Nonopioid (Acetaminophen and/or NSAID) = Highly Recommended

Giving a nonopioid along with an opioid (either mu agonist or agonist-antagonist) is highly recommended. For all analgesic regimens, consider including a nonopioid, even if pain is severe enough to require an opioid. Many opioids given orally for mild to moderate pain, such as codeine and oxycodone, are compounded with a nonopioid, either aspirin or acetaminophen.

mu Agonist + Agonist-Antagonist = Rarely Appropriate

Very few situations exist when use of a mu agonist should be followed by an agonist-antagonist. This sequence may reverse analgesia of the mu agonist or precipitate withdrawal in a physically dependent patient. However, in an opioid-naive patient experiencing side effects such as itching or sedation from spinal opioids, nalbuphine is sometimes used to reverse these supraspinal side effects.

mu Agonist + mu Agonist = Usually Not Necessary

Few situations exist when more than one mu agonist should be administered to a patient. However, any or all of the mu agonists may be combined or given to the same patient. Side effects and analgesia simply will be additive.

Adjuvant + Opioid + Acetaminophen/NSAID = Often Appropriate for Chronic Pain, Sometimes Appropriate for Acute Pain

This combination may be very appropriate for a patient with chronic pain. (If the adjuvant analgesics provide a reasonably rapid onset of analgesia, this combination may be appropriate for acute pain.)

Adjuvant + Adjuvant = Sometimes Appropriate for Chronic Pain

An adjuvant from one group of drugs may be combined with an adjuvant from another group of drugs and is sometimes helpful in relieving chronic cancer pain or chronic noncancer pain. For example, there might be a patient who would benefit from a combination of all of the following: dexamethasone (Decadron), a corticosteroid; dextroamphetamine (Dexedrine), a psychostimulant; amitriptyline (Elavil), a tricyclic antidepressant; and clonazepam (Klonopin), an anticonvulsant.

adjuvant analgesic. It should be noted, however, that the term adjuvant, when used in this ladder refers to both the adjuvant analgesics and the adjuvant drugs that are added to analgesics to reduce side effects (e.g., laxatives for opioid-induced constipation).

If pain is mild to moderate and not relieved by a nonopioid (with or without an adjuvant), step 2 recommends adding an opioid. In other words, the next level of analgesia builds on the previous analgesics. If a nonopioid relieves some but not enough pain, it is continued and an opioid is added. A common mistake at this juncture is to stop the nonopioid and start an opioid rather than add an opioid to the nonopioid. Note that by step 2 of the ladder, when pain may still be only mild to moderate, consideration of an analgesic from each of the three groups is recommended.

Pharmacologically, no difference exists between step 2 and step 3. Because the same three groups of anal-

gesics are considered at both steps, the ladder could be reduced to only 2 steps. In clinical practice, the difference between steps 2 and 3 is choice of opioid analgesic. The reason for having step 2 is that many of the opioids that are customarily prescribed for mild to moderate pain are not appropriate for severe, escalating pain. For example, mild to moderate pain is often treated with oral analgesics in a fixed combination of opioid and nonopioid, usually acetaminophen or sometimes aspirin. The problem with fixed combinations is that the dose of acetaminophen (or other nonopioid) limits the escalation of the opioid dose. Common examples of opioid/nonopioid fixed combinations are:

Lortab 5/500 (hydrocodone, 5 mg, and acetaminophen, 500 mg)

Percocet (oxycodone, 5 mg, and acetaminophen, 325 mg)

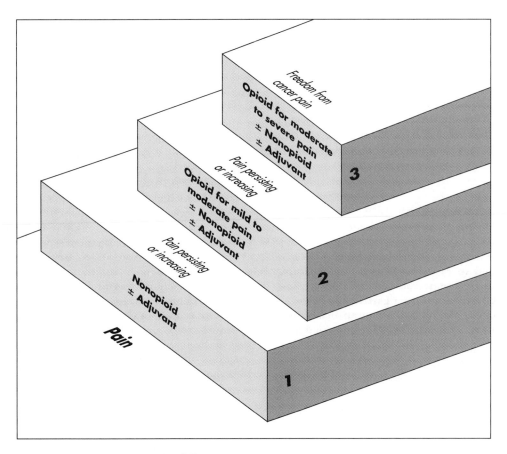

FIGURE 4.3 The WHO three-step analgesic ladder.

Reproduced by permission of WHO, from: *Cancer pain relief*, 2nd ed. Geneva, World Health Organization, 1996.

Tylenol No. 3 (codeine, 30 mg, and acetaminophen, 300 mg)

Tylox (oxycodone, 5 mg, and acetaminophen, 500 mg)

Vicodin (hydrocodone, 5 mg, and acetaminophen, 500 mg)

To avoid exceeding the recommended maximum daily dose of 4 to 6 g of acetaminophen, the patient cannot take more than 8 to 12 tablets per day of those containing 500 mg of acetaminophen or 12 to 18 tablets per day of those containing 325 mg of acetaminophen.

Oxycodone is commonly used in these fixed combinations and is also considered a step 3 drug, a useful opioid for escalating pain. Therefore if a fixed combination of acetaminophen and oxycodone is used at step 2, plain oxycodone may be continued at step 3. Plain acetaminophen can also be continued at appropriate doses.

To avoid step 2 and the need to change opioids or formulations as pain increases, mild to moderate pain may be treated with low doses of plain oxycodone, morphine, or hydromorphone. These mu agonists may be continued through the course of therapy because doses of these may be escalated for the relief of increasingly severe pain.

Opioid analgesics recommended at step 3 should be available orally and by a variety of other routes of administration so that the opioid need not be changed if the route of administration must change. For example, if a patient taking oral morphine has a temporary episode of nausea and vomiting, morphine may be continued by administering it by other routes, such as rectally or subcutaneously. Hydromorphone is also available by a variety of routes of administration.

Opioids used at step 3 also should have a short half-life so they can be titrated upward rapidly for severe, escalating pain. At the same time, for chronic pain it is advantageous if the short half-life opioid is available in a controlled-release formulation so that dosing intervals can be lengthened after the appropriate dose is determined with immediate-release formulations. For example, morphine and oxycodone have fairly short half-lives, 2 to 3 hours (Deglin, Vallerand, 1997), and are available in controlled-release formulations that allow dosing every 12 hours.

The opioid should have no problematic active metabolites. Opioids meeting these criteria include morphine, oxycodone, hydromorphone, fentanyl, and others. Morphine does have an active metabolite (morphine-6-glucuronide, M6G) that accumulates in patients with renal dysfunction and can cause opioid toxicity (Osborne, Joel, Slevin, 1986). Hydromorphone (Dilaudid) is a common alternative to morphine and soon should be available in a controlled-release formulation.

Other important recommendations that accompany the WHO analgesic ladder are to administer analgesics orally whenever possible and to administer them "by the clock," or ATC, to prevent the return of pain.

The patient example that follows illustrates the application of principles related to the WHO analgesic ladder to manage pain associated with progressive metastatic cancer.

Patient Example

A 59-year-old man has arm, shoulder, and chest pain as a result of invasion of the chest wall and brachial plexus by an apical lung cancer. He has not responded to radiation therapy and chemotherapy. History is remarkable for a major gastrointestinal hemorrhage from a gastric ulcer 2 years earlier. Analgesic use is limited to an occasional acetaminophen for headaches. He is married and has two adult children.

Patient Encounter 1

Pain severity and descriptors: Mild, aching (1 to 2/10) in arm, shoulder, and chest.

Inferred pain pathophysiology: Somatic and neuropathic.

Analgesic selection: Acetaminophen, 650 mg orally (PO), every 4 hours.

Step on analgesic ladder: 1.

Rationale: Step 1 of the "analgesic ladder" indicated because patient had mild pain. Analgesic history indicated that he had done well with acetaminophen in the past. NSAIDs relatively contraindicated because of history of ulcer. (NOTE: if patient's pain was moderate to severe on the first encounter, it would have been appropriate to start the patient on Step 2 or Step 3 of the "analgesic ladder.")

Potential side effects: None.

Outcome: Good pain relief for 3 to 4 weeks.

Patient Encounter 2

Pain severity and descriptors: The patient returns to the clinic with reports of escalating chest wall pain. The pain was described as aching and constant, moderate in severity (5 to 6/10).

Inferred pain pathophysiology: Somatic.

Analgesic selection: Oxycodone begun in addition to acetaminophen and given in combination form (oxycodone, 5 mg, + acetaminophen, 325 mg {Percocet}). To take 1 to 2 tablets PO, every 4 hours.

Step on analgesic ladder: 2.

Rationale: Step 2 chosen because pain was moderate to severe.

Potential side effects: Constipation, sedation, nausea.

Outcome: Pain progressed over the next 2 to 3 days and its quality changed. Percocet intake was 12 tablets per day. No side effects were reported.

Patient Encounter 3

Pain severity and descriptors: Aching, burning, constant, radiating from chest and shoulder into arm, moderate to severe (7 to 8/10). Disturbed sleep and ability to concentrate.

Inferred pain pathophysiology: Neuropathic and somatic.

Analgesic selection; Percocet was changed to morphine sulfate, 15 mg, + acetaminophen, 650 mg PO, every 4 hours, around the clock, with morphine sulfate, 15 mg, "rescues" every 1 to 2 hours as needed (PRN). An adjuvant, amitriptyline, 25 mg, was added at night.

Step on analgesic ladder: 3.

Rationale: Step 3 of the analgesic ladder was selected because the patient's pain was severe. An adjuvant drug was added because of the neuropathic component of the pain. The opioid dose was determined as follows: 10 mg of morphine PO is considered to be equianalgesic to 7 to 10 mg of oxycodone PO (= 2 Percocet). Because the pain was not controlled, the equianalgesic dose was increased by 50%. The "rescue" dose of morphine sulfate of 15 mg PO every 1 to 2 hours PRN was selected on the basis of a 5% to 15% ratio of his 24-hour baseline morphine dose. The dose, 15 mg, is in fact 17% of the 24-hour dose but was chosen because of the available tablet size.

Possible side effects: Constipation, sedation, nausea, dry mouth.

Outcome: Thirty-six hours later the patient called to say that his pain control had markedly improved but only in the setting of frequent "rescue" doses. Overall, with "rescues," pain was 75% better. He had required nine "rescue" doses in the previous 24 hours (15 mg × 9 = an additional 135 mg of morphine). Consequently, his baseline morphine dose was increased by approximately the equivalent amount, to 30 mg PO every 4 hours. The dose chosen was a slightly lower dose than the total of the baseline plus "rescues" but reflected the available tablet size and was considered likely to provide adequate analgesia. Rescue medication continued to be available. His "rescue" dose was adjusted to reflect 5% to 15% of the new 24-hour baseline dose of 180 mg, at 30 mg every 2 hours PRN. Again, this dose, 30 mg, is in fact 17% of the 24-hour dose but was chosen because of the available tablet size. Adjustment was undertaken because the 15 mg dose was not providing effective analgesia.

Good pain control was reached with "rescue" doses used only once or twice a day in relation to a specific activity. Once stable pain relief was established, he was switched to a controlled-release oral morphine preparation, allowing for 12-hour dosing. The equivalent dose he received was 90 mg q12h; the "rescue" dose was left unchanged. The amitriptyline was increased every 3 to 4 days until the analgesia it provided seemed maximal and he was sleeping well; the dose reached was 100 mg qhs. Mild nausea and mental clouding resolved after a few days. Constipation was treated with a bowel regimen (refer to Chapter 6 for management).

He did relatively well for several months; however, his disease was progressing, and intermittent upward titration of his baseline dose was undertaken on the basis of his "rescue" requirement. Four months later he was taking controlled-release morphine, 180 mg every 12 hours, and the "rescue" dose remained at 30 mg immediate-release morphine every 1 to 2 hours PRN (within 5% to 15% of baseline and providing effective analgesia).

Patient Encounter 4

A fall at home resulted in a fractured femur. The patient elected to have surgery as a means of allowing prompt mobilization that could facilitate an improved quality of life. Preoperatively his leg pain was severe, and analgesic therapy needed to be adjusted.

Pain severity and descriptors: Sharp, 9 to 10/10 on movement.

Inferred pain pathophysiology: Somatic. Acute pain superimposed on chronic chest wall and arm pain.

Analgesic selection: Morphine was continued, but the route of administration was changed from an oral to an IV infusion. His infusion rate was started at 7.5 mg/h with 4 mg "rescues" available every 30 minutes PRN.

Step on analgesic ladder: 3.

Rationale: Because of the severity of the pain, the equianalgesic dose was increased by 50% when switching from the oral to the route. Using a 3:1 oral/IV ratio, his infusion rate was started at 7.5 mg/h (360 mg + 180 mg = 540 mg oral morphine/24 h = 180 mg IV morphine/24 h = 7.5 mg/h), with 4 mg "rescues" available every 30 minutes PRN. (The total hourly rescue was approximately 5% of the total daily dose, and the first dose given provided effective analgesia. If it had not, the rescue dose would have been escalated by 30% to 50%.) Although several "rescues" were required in the first few hours, the need for these subsided. Surgical recovery was uneventful. Five days after surgery, he was able to take PO medications and was using very occasional "rescue" doses. He was, however, anxious about the planned switch to oral pain medication and requested that it be done gradually. The IV infusion was initially decreased to approximately half (3.5 mg/hr) and he was given the equivalent oral dose, 130 mg every 12 hours, in a controlled-release oral morphine preparation. He continued to have IV "rescues" available to him as before. Forty-eight hours later his IV infusion had been discontinued, and he was taking the equivalent controlled-release morphine dosage of 260 mg every 12 hours by mouth. "Rescue" doses of oral morphine sulfate immediate-release, 60 mg (5% to 15% of 24-hour opioid dose) were available to him every 1 to 2 hours PRN. Amitriptyline was restarted at 25 mg qhs and gradually titrated up

to its previous level of 100 mg.

Outcome: The patient's pain remained well controlled at home on oral analgesics until his death 4 weeks after discharge. Ongoing assessment and reassessment by the nurse in liaison with the patient's primary physician were critical components in managing the analgesic approach to this man's pain. The assessment included the effectiveness of relief, the duration of relief, the effectiveness of "rescue" doses, and the presence and management of side effects.

From Coyle N, Portenoy RK: Pharmacologic management of cancer pain. In McCorkle R, Grant M, Frank-Stromborg M, Baird, editors: *Cancer nursing: A comprehensive textbook,* pp. 1035-1055, Philadelphia, 1996, WB Saunders Co., pp. 1050-1051.

Effectiveness of the WHO analgesic ladder

Studies of the effectiveness of the WHO analgesic ladder have revealed that this approach has improved management of chronic cancer pain. In a 10-year study of 2118 patients with cancer-related pain, use of the WHO guidelines for relieving pain resulted in clinically significant pain reduction, usually within the first week (Zech, Grond, Lynch et al., 1995). Good to satisfactory pain relief was maintained in 88% of the patients over the entire treatment period. Only 12% required invasive procedures for pain relief, such as nerve blocks. Of note is the fact that both opioids and nonopioids were prescribed in 73% of the patients. Also, oral opioid doses reported in this study suggest that the clinicians understood that no ceiling exists on the analgesia of mu agonists because some patients received up to 2400 mg/day of oral morphine. A willingness to titrate upward beyond the usual recommended doses of oral morphine is essential if unnecessary invasive procedures are to be avoided.

Other studies of the effectiveness of the WHO analgesic ladder have reported adequate analgesia in 69% to 100% of patients. Although it is true that controlled studies are needed to estimate more accurately the effectiveness of the WHO guidelines (Jadad, Browman, 1995), it is also true that they have achieved widespread acceptance and are believed to be a positive force in improving cancer pain management (Ventafridda, Caraceni, Sbanotto, 1996).

Multimodal, Continuous Analgesia: Balanced Analgesia

Over the past decade, research on the management of postoperative pain, especially in high-risk patients such as the frail elderly, has led to the recommendation of a multimodality approach, commonly called "balanced analgesia." Balanced analgesia often includes drugs from each of the three analgesic groups, such as NSAIDs, opioids, and local anesthetics. Lower doses of several analgesics reduces the likelihood of significant side effects from a single agent or method. This maximizes postoperative pain control and minimizes side effects. Drug choices and routes of administration are carefully determined along with establishing the lowest possible effective doses. For example, severe postoperative pain is often treated with opioid and local anesthetic combinations administered by the epidural route (Dahl, Rosenberg, Dirkes et al., 1990; Dahl, Kehlet, 1991, Kehlet, Dahl, 1993; Pasero, McCaffery, 1996).

The true benefits of continuous multimodality analgesia are realized only when patient teaching emphasizes the patient's role in recovery activities, continuous balanced analgesia starts preoperatively, and early enteral nutrition and mobilization occur (Kehlet, 1994). The ultimate goal of the pain management plan is to take advantage of the benefits of optimal pain control to improve the patient's outcome. This decreases the cost of care and reduces the length of hospital stay (Box 4.2).

Preemptive analgesia is the preoperative phase of continuous multimodality analgesia with the three drug groups, NSAIDs, opioids, and local anesthetics, by a variety of routes to treat pain before it occurs. In a review of the clinical trials of preemptive analgesia, Woolf and Chong (1993) state that ideal preoperative, intraoperative, and postoperative treatment would include "NSAIDs to reduce the activation/centralization of nociceptors, local anesthetics to block sensory inflow, and centrally acting drugs such as opiates." (p. 367) Such a multimodality approach to preemptive analgesia, as opposed to a single entity approach, may be preferred in some patient populations.

Well-controlled research on the long-lasting benefits of specific types of preemptive analgesia is still lacking. To date, research does not suggest that this treatment alone has a major impact on postoperative pain control. Improved outcomes are much more likely to be demonstrated when preemptive analgesia is one of several components in the plan for postoperative pain control (Kehlet, 1994).

Preemptive analgesia should be considered whenever postoperative pain management is expected to be difficult (Portenoy, 1992), such as for frail, debilitated, elderly patients who are at particularly high risk for opioid-induced side effects. Health care providers are often reluctant to administer adequate doses of analgesics to the frail elderly for fear of causing side effects, especially respiratory depression. Consequently, elders suffer unrelieved pain. Preemptive analgesia may provide some solutions to this dilemma (Pasero, McCaffery, 1996).

Several studies have shown that postoperative pain and analgesic requirements can be reduced by implementing various preemptive approaches. For example, preoperative regional anesthesia by nerve block has been shown to reduce analgesic requirements after various orthopedic surgeries, such as knee joint surgery (Ringrose, Cross, 1984; McQuay, Carroll, Moore, 1988; Woolf, Chong, 1993). Opioid premedication may not only reduce pain and analgesic requirements but also increase the time to first request for postoperative analgesia (McQuay, Carroll, Moore, 1988; Woolf, Chong, 1993). Even single doses of NSAIDs administered preoperatively can reduce postoperative pain (Campbell, Kendrick, Patterson, 1990; Dueholm, Forrest, Hjortoso et al., 1989; Woolf, Chong, 1993).

In a 1991 study the effects of epidural fentanyl administered before surgical incision were compared with its effects when administered after surgical incision. Thirty patients scheduled for elective thoracotomy were randomized and studied prospectively in a double-blind fashion. The study group received an epidural fentanyl infusion (4 μg/kg in 20 ml normal saline) before surgical incision followed by a normal saline infusion (20 ml) 15 minutes after incision. The control group received these in the reverse order (i.e., epidural normal saline infusion before the surgical incision followed by an epidural fentanyl infusion 15 minutes after incision). No other drugs were given before or during surgery, and

---

● ● ● ● ●

BOX 4.2 *Clinical Application of Balanced Analgesia*

DEFINITION OF BALANCED ANALGESIA

Balanced analgesia is a concept involving the continuous use of more than one method of controlling a patient's pain; continuous delivery of combined analgesic regimens. This may include more than one drug and more than one route of administration. Also referred to as multimodal (as opposed to unimodal) continuous analgesia. Usually refers to analgesia for acute pain, but the concept applies equally well to all other types of pain.

CLINICAL EXAMPLES OF BALANCED ANALGESIA
- Systemic NSAID + systemic opioid (e.g., ibuprofen PO + morphine PO)
- Systemic NSAID + epidural opioid and local anesthetic (e.g., ketorolac IV + fentanyl/bupivacaine epidurally)
- Local infiltration of anesthetic + systemic NSAID + systemic opioid (e.g., lidocaine infiltration of surgical site + ketorolac IV + IV PCA morphine)
- Regional block + systemic NSAID + epidural opioid and local anesthetic (e.g., epidural anesthetic during surgery; postoperatively epidural fentanyl/bupivacaine + ketorolac IV)

EXAMPLES OF IMPROVED OUTCOMES FOR THE PATIENT WITH ACUTE PAIN (E.G., POSTOPERATIVE PAIN OR TRAUMA)
- Early ambulation
- Early enteral feeding
- Increased participation in recovery activities (e.g., coughing, physical therapy)
- Early discharge

anesthesia was the same for both groups. IV PCA morphine was used to manage postoperative pain. At 6 hours after surgery when plasma fentanyl concentrations were at subtherapeutic levels, the study group, which received epidural fentanyl before surgical incision, had significantly less pain as measured by visual analog scale. Between 12 and 24 hours after surgery, PCA morphine use was significantly higher in the control group than in the study group, although pain scores during that time were not significantly different. These findings suggest that administration of a preoperative opioid may prevent central sensitization that can result from surgical incision and other noxious perioperative events (Katz, Kavanaugh, Sandler et al., 1992).

Woolf and Chong (1993) conclude that further research on preemptive analgesia is warranted, but "Treating pain in advance of its manifestation should become a goal for all personnel involved in postoperative pain care" (p. 374).

Principles of balanced analgesia should also extend into the plan for postoperative care after discharge from the hospital. For example, if pain is only mild to moderate, a fixed combination of opioid and nonopioid, such as oxycodone and acetaminophen, might be sufficient. For moderate to severe pain, the patient might take plain oxycodone or morphine along with an ATC nonopioid, such as ibuprofen or naproxen.

KEY PRINCIPLES OF ANALGESIC THERAPY

Effective pharmacologic management of pain requires application of two principles: individualize the regimen and optimize administration. These principles are followed in the treatment of many conditions such as diabetes, hypertension, and asthma. However, what is common sense in the management of these conditions is sometimes regarded as revolutionary in pain management. All too often when analgesics are used to relieve pain, patients receive inadequate doses at intervals that allow for the return of the problem. A comparable situation would not be tolerated in a diabetic patient requiring insulin. Insulin doses would be titrated to achieve the desired effect, and the insulin would be administered on a regular basis to keep the condition under control.

Following are reminders of aspects of these principles that apply to all three analgesic groups.

Individualizing the Regimen

Drug choice

First, determine the analgesic group most likely to satisfy the immediate goals of pain management and select an analgesic from that group. Within each analgesic group there are a variety of drugs from which to select. The specific analgesic chosen obviously depends on numerous considerations, particularly the type of pain being treated and the patient's medical condition. Second, determine the long-range goals of pain management and, when indicated, add appropriate analgesics one at a time so that each can be evaluated carefully.

For example, a patient with severe somatic, visceral, and neuropathic pain related to metastatic cancer requires an opioid such as morphine to provide some immediate pain relief. The long-range plan may include the addition of a nonopioid to relieve musculoskeletal pain and later an adjuvant analgesic to relieve neuropathic pain. The nonopioid alone probably would not relieve the severe pain and the adjuvant probably will take some time to become effective as the dose is adjusted and the drug accumulates.

The drug selected as a rescue, breakthrough, or supplementary medication for chronic pain (the drug prescribed as the PRN analgesic to be given as needed in addition to the ATC analgesics) is almost always a mu agonist. Because the purpose of a rescue dose is to relieve pain that increases above pain addressed by the ongoing analgesics, the drug should have a fairly rapid onset of action and short duration. Thus a controlled-release formulation of a mu agonist is inappropriate for rescue dosing. For example, if a patient is receiving a controlled-release formulation of morphine orally ATC, the rescue dose should be immediate-release oral morphine, not controlled-release morphine.

The practice of using nonopioids as rescue doses for patients receiving opioids ATC usually is not logical. The reason commonly given for using nonopioids as rescue doses is to avoid side effects such as sedation that occur when an additional dose of opioid is given. However, if a nonopioid is indicated, it should be given ATC along with the opioid.

Route of administration

The oral route is often the optimal route, especially for chronic pain treatment, because of its convenience, flexibility, and the relatively steady blood levels produced. However, the IV route is usually necessary when a quick onset of analgesia is desired or when the patient is unable to take oral medication. When the pain is under control, the patient might then be switched to equianalgesic doses by the oral route.

The IM route should be avoided, especially repeated IM administration, because this is painful and may cause fibrosis of muscle and soft tissue and sterile abscesses. IM administration of opioids is associated with wide fluctuations in absorption, including delayed absorption in postoperative patients, making it an ineffective and potentially dangerous method of managing pain (AHCPR, 1992, 1994; APS, 1992; Austin, Stapleton, Mather, 1980).

Dose

Titrate to effect. Opioid doses must be titrated to optimize the balance between analgesia and side effects. The dose of virtually all other analgesics also must be titrated.

Dose increases typically are made at the onset or peak effect of the analgesic. For IV opioids, titration may occur as often as every 5 minutes, whereas titration of a tricyclic antidepressant may occur only every 4 to 5 days. Generally, the goal is to use the smallest dose that relieves the maximum amount of pain with the fewest side effects. Thus dose titration may maximize the amount of pain relief obtained from a given drug while ensuring that the dose is no higher than necessary.

The nonopioids and adjuvants have a ceiling on their analgesia, but the mu agonist opioids do not. Therefore with opioids it is especially important to focus on the effect, not the milligrams. No set amount of mu agonist opioid is optimum or maximum. For example, some cancer patients have required 30,000 to 40,000 milligrams of IV morphine equivalents per 24 hours (Weinstein, 1994). Even in opioid-naive postoperative patients, research continues to reveal large differences (up to 10-fold) in the amount of opioid required (Macintyre, Jarvis, 1995).

Mu agonist opioids should be titrated up to pain relief or the appearance of limiting side effects (APS, 1992). Titration of mu agonist opioids is usually done in 25% to 100% increments. If the previous opioid dose is safe but pain remains severe, the mu agonist may be increased by 50% to 100%. If pain is moderate, the dose may be increased by 25% to 50% (AHCPR 1994; Levy, 1996).

For ongoing pain, the repeated occurrence of breakthrough pain and the frequent need for rescue doses indicate the need to increase the ATC analgesia. Often it is the opioid dose that is increased, but sometimes the NSAID dose may be increased or an adjuvant may be added.

A guide for calculating rescue or supplemental doses of mu agonists is to allow a large enough dose at frequent enough intervals to double the opioid dose for the dosing period or the 24-hour period. For example, if a patient with chronic cancer pain has a continuous infusion of morphine at 12 mg/hr, PCA bolus doses could be 3 mg q15 minutes, allowing the patient to bolus enough in 1 hour (12 mg) to double the hourly infusion dose (12 mg/hr + 12 mg possible by PCA doses). For oral opioids, the recommendation for calculating the rescue or supplemental dose is $\frac{1}{10}$ to $\frac{1}{6}$ (10% to 15%) the total daily dose given every hour if needed (APS, 1992; Levy, 1996). This may more than double the 24-hour dose.

Optimize Administration

Stay on top of the pain. A preventive approach means that the analgesic(s) should be given before pain occurs or increases (that is, before a painful event such a wound debridement) or ATC (regularly scheduled doses) if pain is present most of the day.

Ongoing pain

Giving the next dose before the last dose wears off has long been recommended for the control of prolonged pain in terminally ill patients in hospice settings, and it is also recommended for acute pain, such as the control of postoperative pain. If pain awakens the patient at night or if the patient wakes in the morning with pain out of control, administer a dose during the night before pain awakens the patient. Failing to awaken the patient may cause a resurgence of pain as blood levels of the analgesic decline (AHCPR, 1992, 1994; APS, 1992).

Because the goal of pain management is to maintain an optimum level of pain relief, analgesics should be scheduled to prevent the recurrence of pain. A rule of thumb is if the pain is expected to be present 12 or more hours out of the next 24 hours, consider ATC dosing. Along with ATC dosing, supplementary analgesia (that is, a rescue dose) should also be available (APS, 1992).

Depending on the analgesic and whether it is a controlled release formulation, an ATC schedule may mean once daily dosing or dosing every 4 hours or more often. Some NSAIDs and adjuvants require only one daily dose and some opioids with a short half-life are formulated in controlled-release tablets for once or twice a day dosing.

Duration of action of all opioids, especially when given parenterally or in immediate-release oral formulations, will vary from one patient to another for many reasons that are not always predictable. Age appears to greatly influence duration of action. The younger the patient, the shorter the duration of action tends to be (Kaiko, 1980). Opioids tend to have a longer duration of action in elderly patients. Therefore, intervals between doses must be individualized after observing the patient's response.

Because both pain and analgesic duration of action may be unpredictable, nurses play a pivotal role in the appropriate use of PRN analgesics. Two ways nurses may use PRN analgesics are: (1) implement PRN analgesics ATC to control ongoing pain, and (2) administer PRN analgesics in addition to those given ATC to relieve pain that breaks through ATC dosing. The latter, often referred to as rescue doses, has been discussed earlier.

Can nurses implement PRN analgesics ATC? Yes, if assessment of the patient reveals that they are needed ATC to keep pain under control. This simply requires a broad understanding of what is currently meant by "as needed." Unfortunately, some nurses have been taught that PRN analgesics should be given only if patients request them or only if the pain is severe. Current clinical practice guidelines make it clear that this is not a sound method for managing pain. State boards of nursing have reassured nurses that PRN analgesics may be implemented ATC. For example, the California Board of Registered Nursing's "Pain Management Policy," 1994, states that nurses should recognize "that prn medications may be given around-the-clock" and "treat pain before the pain becomes severe."

PRN means as needed, requiring assessment to determine when it is needed. Once the safe and effective dose and interval have been determined for the individual patient, PRN analgesics should be implemented ATC for ongoing pain. If pain cannot be predicted, a PRN medication should be used as soon as pain begins and before it becomes severe. Patients must be taught to request pain medication before pain occurs (if it can be predicted) or as soon as pain occurs and before it increases.

Painful procedures

Before a painful event, the patient should receive analgesia and/or local anesthesia. See Chapter 8 on procedural pain. Sedatives may be added but should not be the only agent if the procedure is painful. Opioids and sometimes nonopioids may be given before the procedure at a time that permits the drugs to reach their peak effect just before the painful procedure is performed.

GUIDELINES FOR IMPLEMENTING PHARMACOLOGIC PAIN MANAGEMENT

Assessment of Analgesic History

Form 4.1 offers an example of an analgesic history. This information may be obtained by interviewing the patient, by asking the patient to write down the answers, or by a combination of these. Some initial pain assessment tools simply include a question asking, "What pain relievers have you taken for this pain (or, for pain in the past)? For each one, list the name, dose, how effective it was, and any troublesome side effects." In some clinical situations, this type of questioning is sufficient. Sometimes the patient is told which analgesics are planned, such as morphine for postoperative pain, and asked, "Have you ever had this before? If so, did you have any problems with it?"

Before launching into a multifaceted pharmacologic plan for chronic pain management, many problems can be avoided by conducting a thorough analgesic history. Patients with chronic pain may say, "I've taken everything," but they are unlikely to be aware of all the possibilities. Therefore it is important to assess this more carefully by providing a list of a variety of analgesics, especially the adjuvants, including both generic and common brand names (Form 4.2). This list may be presented as a reference for the patient rather than being contained within the actual written assessment tool. Another approach to assessment of analgesic history and present use is to ask the patient to bring in all medications in their original bottles.

When patients say, "I've taken that and it didn't work," it is essential to find out the details, such as what doses were taken and for how long, before determining that the drug is useless for this patient. Many unfavorable experiences with analgesics are a result of inappropriate dose adjustment.

Patient/Family Teaching

Analgesic regimens for ongoing pain, especially those that include a number of different analgesics, require patient and family teaching to ensure that the patient actu-

ally adheres to the plan. Evaluation of the analgesic regimen and favorable outcomes depend on the patient's willingness to follow through with instructions.

It is not safe to assume that patients with pain will take their medications as prescribed. Unfortunately, little research concerning patient compliance with analgesic regimens exists (Chapman, 1996; Turk, Rudy, 1991). However, literature from other fields has revealed that noncompliance for all types of drugs ranges from 13% to 93% among adults (Sclar, Tartaglione, Fine, 1994). Nurse counseling and printed materials have been shown to increase the likelihood that patients will take their pain medicine on the correct schedule and at the correct dosage (Rimer, Levy, Keintz et al., 1987). Form 4.3, *A,* provides a tool that may assist with patient teaching in the home care setting. Form 4.3, *B,* is an example of the completed tool, using the patient described on p. 118 at the point his pain was well controlled.

Following are selected components of patient teaching that apply to a variety of analgesic regimens for various types of pain.

- Discuss the harmful effects of unrelieved pain. Give examples specific to the patient's situation, such as pain makes it difficult to get a restful night of sleep or pain interferes with using the incentive spirometer to prevent pneumonia. Identify specific goals of pharmacologic pain management: pain rating desired and any related increase in function. An example of such a goal is "pain rating of 2/10 or better to participate in physical therapy."
- If the analgesics are used for different types of pain, specify this. For example, a NSAID may be used mainly for aching musculoskeletal pain in the lower back and an adjuvant may be primarily used for sharp shooting pain radiating down the leg.
- Provide the patient and family with written instructions listing all analgesics by name, dosage, and dose times.
- Explain and emphasize the importance of maintaining control of the pain with ATC dosing. Work with the patient and family to identify specific times for doses. For example, rather than tell the patient to take the medication twice a day, find out what the patient's schedule is for sleeping and meals and correlate doses with those events.
- Because taking more than one analgesic increases the risk of the patient not taking all doses, coordinate dose times when possible (e.g., give analgesics that have the same dosing intervals at the same time). Emphasize to the patient and family that taking several doses at one time is not dangerous and is simply more convenient.
- When new analgesics are added to the regimen, provide written information about possible side effects, which side effects should be reported, which side effects can be managed and how, when pain

● ● ● ● ●

FORM 4.1 Assessment of Analgesic History

Experience With Pain Medications

Name: _____ Date: _____

Purpose: To find out what you are taking now for pain relief, what you have taken for pain in the past, and how these medicines worked for you.

Directions: Please answer the following questions as completely as possible. Include pain medications that require a prescription, as well as those that do not.

1. What medications are you taking *now* for pain relief?

Drug, dose (or color)	Number of pills taken at one time	How often do you take this?	Any relief?	Any problems?
_____	_____	_____	_____	_____
_____	_____	_____	_____	_____
_____	_____	_____	_____	_____
_____	_____	_____	_____	_____
_____	_____	_____	_____	_____

2. What medications have you taken in the *past* for pain relief?

Drug, dose (or color)	Number of pills taken at one time	How often do you take this?	Any relief?	Any problems?
_____	_____	_____	_____	_____
_____	_____	_____	_____	_____
_____	_____	_____	_____	_____
_____	_____	_____	_____	_____
_____	_____	_____	_____	_____

3. What has provided you with the *best* pain relief so far?

4. Are you allergic to any pain medications?   _____ yes   _____ no
   If yes, please list.

5. Comments.

_____
_____
_____
_____
_____
_____

●●●●●

FORM 4.2 **List of Analgesics to Assist With Assessment of Analgesic History**

List of Pain Relievers

Please review this list and identify which pain relievers you have taken.

1. Examples of pain relievers that *do not require a doctor's prescription*

   Acetaminophen (Tylenol)
   Anacin
   Aspirin
   BC Powder
   Bufferin
   Doan's Pills
   Excedrin
   Ibuprofen (Advil, Motrin)
   Naproxen (Aleve)

2. Examples of common pain relievers that *require a doctor's prescription* and are often taken at home

   Codeine
   Darvon, Darvocet, Darvon-N (propoxyphene)
   Fiorinal
   Levo-Dromoran (levorphanol)
   Lortab
   MS Contin
   Methadone (Dolophine)
   Oramorph SR
   OxyContin
   Percocet
   Percodan
   Roxanol (liquid)
   Talwin
   Tylenol No. 3 or No. 4
   Tylox
   Vicodin
   Wygesic
   Anaprox (naproxen)
   Ansaid (flurbiprofen)
   Daypro (oxaprozin)
   Dolobid (diflunisal)
   Feldene (piroxicam)
   Indocin (indomethacin)
   Lodine (etodolac)
   Nalfon (fenoprofen)

   Orudis (ketoprofen)
   Relafen (nabumetone)
   Trilisate
   Voltaren (diclofenac)
   Duragesic Patch (fentanyl patch)
   Stadol Nasal Spray

3. Examples of pain relievers often given by injection for relief of moderate to severe pain, especially *in the hospital*

   Fentanyl
   Hydromorphone (Dilaudid)
   Ketorolac (Toradol)
   Meperidine (Demerol)
   Methadone
   Morphine

4. Examples of pain relievers the doctor may prescribe for *specific types of pain*

   Amitriptyline (Elavil)
   Desipramine (Norpramin)
   Doxepin (Sinequan)
   Imipramine (Tofranil)
   Nortriptyline (Aventyl, Pamelor)
   Fluoxetine (Prozac)
   Paroxetine (Paxil)
   Sertraline (Zoloft)
   Trazodone (Desyrel)
   Carisoprodol (Soma)
   Cyclobenzaprine (Flexeril)
   Carbamazepine (Tegretol)
   Clonazepam (Klonopin)
   Phenytoin (Dilantin)
   Valproic acid (Depakene)
   Dexamethasone (Decadron)
   Dextroamphetamine (Dexedrine)
   Methylphenidate (Ritalin)
   Sumatriptan (Imitrex)
   Hydroxyzine (Atarax, Vistaril)
   Clonidine
   Diazepam (Valium)
   Alprazolam
   Mexiletine (Mexitil)

May be duplicated for use in clinical practice. From McCaffery M, Pasero C: *Pain: Clinical manual*, p. 125. Copyright © 1999, Mosby, Inc.

---

relief is expected (e.g., an hour after dose, after several days of accumulation or dose escalation), and when dose titration is appropriate.

- The patient and family should be told whom and when to call regarding any questions or problems with analgesics.

Nurse's Role

Nurses have an active and pivotal role in analgesic use. Teaching the patient and family about the analgesic

plan is critical to success. The nurse is in an ideal position to initiate patient teaching and to reinforce this over time.

Considering the great variability in patients' responses to all analgesics, titration of doses and intervals between doses is necessary to achieve maximum pain relief with minimal side effects. Again, the nurse is in an ideal position to assume responsibility for titrating doses and adjusting intervals between doses. This occurs within the context of an interdisciplinary approach to pain management,

Text continued on p. 128.

● ● ● ● ●

FORM 4.3A **Patient/Family Information**

Daily Schedule for Taking Pain Medicines at Home

To: _____ (Patient's name)   Date: _____

Purpose: This form is to help you follow the plan for using pain medicines to control your pain at home. You want to be sure to take all your pain medicines and to take them at the right times so that you can achieve your goals.

Your pain rating and activity goal(s): _____

1. *Daily Pain Medicine Schedule:*

    Time/Activity: Medication(s):

    _____   _____

    _____   _____

    _____   _____

    _____   _____

    _____   _____

    _____   _____

    _____   _____

    _____   _____

    _____   _____

    _____   _____

    _____   _____

    _____   _____

    _____   _____

2. *"Rescue" doses* (additional pain medicine to be taken if the above is not enough pain relief):

    Medication: _____   Dose: _____   How often? _____

Important Points:
- More than one pain medicine may be used because different medicines attack pain in different ways.
- Two or more of your pain medicines may be scheduled at the same time because it is safe and more convenient. If you are concerned about taking several pills at once, talk with your nurse or doctor.
- For pain that is present most of the day, pain medicine is scheduled at regular times to stay on top of the pain. This is called "around the clock" dosing.
- "Rescue" doses are taken when around the clock doses do not relieve enough pain. When you take a rescue dose, continue to take all of your around the clock doses at the scheduled times.
- Take your "rescue" dose before pain becomes bad. Trying to "wait a little longer" only allows the pain to get worse and means that it will take longer to control it.

Contact the following person if your pain rating is above a _____ for more than a few hours or if you must take more than _____ rescue doses a day:

_____ (RN, MD)   Phone: _____

● ● ● ● ●

FORM 4.3B **Patient/Family Information**

Daily Schedule for Taking Pain Medicines at Home

To: _____ *Mr. X* _____ (Patient's name) Date: ___*9-20*___

Purpose: This form is to help you follow the plan for using pain medicines to control your pain at home. You want to be sure to take all your pain medicines and to take them at the right times so that you can achieve your goals.

Your pain rating and activity goal(s): ___*3/10: Sleep through night and walk a few blocks*___

1. *Daily Pain Medicine Schedule:*

Time/Activity:	Medication(s):
9 a.m. - after breakfast	*MS Contin 90 mg - 3 purple tablets*
9 p.m. - after dinner	*MS Contin 90 mg - 3 purple tablets*
	& Amitriptyline 100 mg - 1 pink tablet

2. *"Rescue" doses* (additional pain medicine to be taken if the above is not enough pain relief):

Medication: ___*MS IR*___ Dose: ___*30 mg - 1 white tablet*___ How often? ___*every 2 hours when needed*___

Important Points:

- More than one pain medicine may be used because different medicines attack pain in different ways.
- Two or more of your pain medicines may be scheduled at the same time because it is safe and more convenient. If you are concerned about taking several pills at once, talk with your nurse or doctor.
- For pain that is present most of the day, pain medicine is scheduled at regular times to stay on top of the pain. This is called "around the clock" dosing.
- "Rescue" doses are taken when around the clock doses do not relieve enough pain. When you take a rescue dose, continue to take all of your around the clock doses at the scheduled times.
- Take your "rescue" dose before pain becomes bad. Trying to "wait a little longer" only allows the pain to get worse and means that it will take longer to control it.

Contact the following person if your pain rating is above a ___*5*___ for more than a few hours or if you must take more than ___*4*___ rescue doses a day:

_____*A. B.*_____ (RN, MD) Phone: ___*555-1234*___

---

and the nurse's role requires effective communication with other team members, especially the patient and family, the physician, and the pharmacist. Effective communication regarding analgesics includes the following:

- Flow sheet or daily pain log that organizes pertinent data, such as pain ratings, sedation level, dosages, intervals between doses, and the pain rating and activity goals (see examples in Chapter 3, pp. 83-86, 88).
- Ability to provide appropriate documentation for recommendations. Clinical practice guidelines are ideal for this purpose, especially those published by APS (1992) and AHCPR (1992, 1994).
- Persistence.

For nurses to perform these activities and be effective team members, it is essential that agency policies, education, and resource materials enable them to work with flexible analgesic doses and intervals, to teach the patient and family, and to communicate efficiently with other team members.

References

AHCPR: *Acute pain management in adults: operative procedures, quick reference guide for clinicians,* DHHS Pub. No. AHCPR 92-0019, 1992.

AHCPR: *Management of cancer pain: adults, quick reference guide for clinicians,* AHCPR Pub. No. 94-0593, 1994.

American Pain Society (APS): *Principles of analgesic use in the treatment of acute pain and cancer pain,* ed 3, Skokie, Ill, 1992, The Society.

Austin KL, Stapleton JV, Mather LE: Multiple intramuscular injections: a major source of variability in analgesic response to meperidine, *Pain* 8:47-62, 1980.

Board of Registered Nursing: *Pain management policy,* Sacramento, April 1994, State of California Department of Consumer Affairs.

Campbell WI, Kendrick R, Patterson C: Intravenous diclofenac sodium, *Anaesthesia* 45:763-766, 1990.

Chandler SW, Trissel LA: Combined administration of opioids with selected drugs to manage pain and other cancer symptoms: initial safety screening for compatibility, *J Pain Symptom Manage* 12:68-171, 1996.

Chapman CR: Compliance with pain medication: a hidden problem? *APS Bull* 6(6):11, 1996.

Dahl JB, Kehlet H: Non-steroidal anti-inflammatory drugs: rationale for use in severe postoperative pain, *Br J Anaesth* 66:703-712, 1991.

Dahl JB, Rosenberg J, Dirkes WE et al.: Prevention of postoperative pain by balanced analgesia, *Br J Anaesth* 64:518-520, 1990.

Deglin JH, Vallerand AH: *Davis's drug guide for nurses,* ed 5, Philadelphia, 1997, FA Davis.

Dueholm S, Forrest M, Hjortoso N-C et al.: Pain relief following herniotomy: a double-blind randomized comparison between naproxen and placebo, *Acta Anaesthesiol Scand* 33:391-394, 1989.

Jadad AR, Browman GP: The WHO analgesic ladder for cancer pain management, *JAMA* 274:1870-1873, 1995.

Kaiko RF: Age and morphine analgesia in cancer patients with postoperative pain, *Clin Pharmacol Ther* 28:823-826, 1980.

Katz J, Kavanaugh BP, Sandler AN et al.: Preemptive analgesia: clinical evidence of neuroplasticity contributing to postoperative pain, *Anesthesiology* 77:439-446, 1992.

Kehlet H: Postoperative pain relief: what is the issue? *Br J Anaes* 72:374-378, 1994 (editorial).

Kehlet H, Dahl, JB: Are perioperative nonsteroidal anti-inflammatory drugs ulcerogenic in the short term? *Drugs* 44 (suppl 5):38-41, 1992.

Kehlet H, Dahl JB: The value of "multimodal" or "balanced analgesia" in postoperative pain treatment," *Anesth Analg* 77:1048-1056, 1993.

Levy MH: Pharmacologic treatment of cancer pain, *N Engl J Med* 335:1124-1132, 1996.

Macintyre PE, Jarvis DA: Age is the best predictor of postoperative morphine requirements, *Pain* 64:357-364, 1995.

McQuay HJ, Carroll D, Moore RA: Postoperative orthopaedic pain: the effect of opiate premedication and local anaesthetic block, *Pain* 33:291-295, 1988.

Nitescu P, Hultman E, Appelgren L et al.: Bacteriology, drug stability and exchange of percutaneous delivery systems and antibacterial filters in long-term intrathecal infusion of opioid drugs and bupivacaine in "refractory" pain, *Clin J Pain* 8:324-337, 1992.

Osborne RJ, Joel SP, Slevin ML: Morphine intoxication in renal failure: the role of morphine-6-glucuronide, *Br J Med* 292:1548-1549, 1986.

Pasero C, McCaffery M: Postoperative pain management in the elderly. In Ferrell BR, Ferrell BA, editors: *Pain in the elderly,* pp. 45-68, Seattle, 1996, IASP Press.

Portenoy RK: Clinical application of opioid analgesics. In Sinatra RS, Hord AH, Ginsberg B, Preble LM, editors: *Acute pain mechanisms and management,* pp. 93-101, St. Louis, 1992, Mosby Inc.

Portenoy RK: Adjuvant analgesics in pain management. In Doyle D, Hanks GWC, MacDonald N, eds: *Oxford textbook of palliative medicine,* ed 2, pp. 361-390, New York, 1998, Oxford University Press.

Portenoy RK, Kanner RM: Nonopioid and adjuvant analgesics. In Portenoy RK, Kanner RM, editors: *Pain management: theory and practice,* pp. 219-247, Philadelphia, 1996, FA Davis.

Rimer B, Levy MH, Keintz MK et al.: Enhancing cancer pain control regimens through patient education, *Patient Educ Counseling* 10:267-277, 1987.

Ringrose NH, Cross, MJ: Femoral nerve block in knee joint surgery, *Am J Sports Med* 12:398-402, 1984.

Sclar DA, Tartaglione TA, Fine MJ: Overview of issues related to medical compliance with implications for the outpatient management of infectious diseases, *Infect Agents Dis* 3:266-273, 1994.

Tu Y-H, Stiles ML, Allen LV: Stability of fentanyl citrate and bupivacaine hydrochloride in portable pump reservoirs, *Am J Hosp Pharm* 47:2037-2040, 1990.

Turk DC, Rudy TE: Neglected topics in the treatment of chronic pain patients: relapse, noncompliance, and adherence enhancement, *Pain* 44:5-28, 1991.

Ventafridda V, Caraceni A, Sbanotto A: Cancer pain management, *Pain Rev* 3:153-179, 1996.

Weinstein SM: In patients with chronic pain, what is the suggested maximum dose of sustained-release morphine? *Primary Care Cancer* 14:1:15, 1994.

Woolf CJ, Chong M-S: Preemptive analgesia: treating postoperative pain by preventing the establishment of central sensitization, *Anesth Analg* 77:362-379, 1993.

Wulf H, Gleim M, Mignat C: The stability of mixtures of morphine hydrochloride, bupivacaine hydrochloride, and clonidine hydrochloride in portable pump reservoirs for the management of chronic pain syndromes, *J Pain Symptom Manage* 9:308-311, 1994.

Zech DFJ, Grond S, Lynch J et al.: Validation of World Health Organization guidelines for cancer pain relief: a 10-year prospective study, *Pain* 63:65-76, 1995.

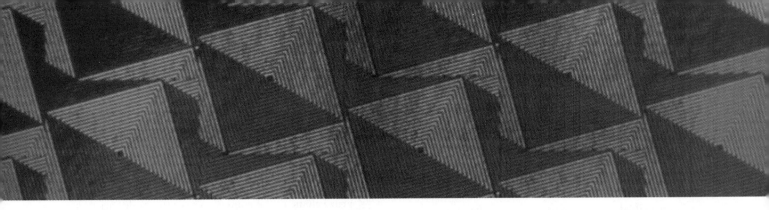

chapter five
NONOPIOIDS
Acetaminophen and Nonsteroidal Antiinflammatory Drugs (NSAIDs)

Margo McCaffery and Russell K. Portenoy

CHAPTER OUTLINE

TERMINOLOGY

Acetaminophen: Other generic names include paracetamol and acetylparaaminophenol (APAP). Also referred to as "aspirin-free."

Analgesic ceiling: A dose beyond which further increases in dose do not provide additional analgesia.

Nonopioid: Used instead of nonnarcotic. Refers to acetaminophen and nonsteroidal antiinflammatory drugs (NSAIDs).

NSAID: An acronym for nonsteroidal antiinflammatory drug. (Pronounced "in said.") Also referred to as "aspirin-like" drugs.

Opioid: This term is now used instead of narcotic. Narcotic has become an obsolete term. Narcotic is used primarily in a legal context to refer to a wide variety of substances of potential abuse.

Opioid dose-sparing effect: The dose of opioid may be lowered when a nonopioid is added.

The nonopioid analgesic group includes acetaminophen and nonsteroidal antiinflammatory drugs (NSAIDs). All nonopioids are analgesic and antipyretic; NSAIDs are also antiinflammatory. Although they share many of the same effects, they are a mixed group of drugs that differ in chemical structure.

Sometimes all nonopioids are loosely referred to as NSAIDS, but acetaminophen is not a NSAID. Acetaminophen should be distinguished from NSAIDs because it seems to relieve pain by different mechanisms and has minimal antiinflammatory effect. Acetaminophen may be referred to as an aspirin-free drug and NSAIDs as aspirin-like drugs. Other generic names for acetaminophen are APAP (acetylparaaminophenol) and paracetamol. Review Table 5.1: Misconceptions about nonopioids.

MECHANISMS UNDERLYING ANALGESIA OF ACETAMINOPHEN AND NSAIDS

Acetaminophen

The mechanism of action for acetaminophen is different from that of aspirin and the other NSAIDs. Analgesia appears to result primarily from a central mechanism rather than a peripheral one (Coyle, Cherny, Portenoy, 1995; Piletta, Porchet, Dayer, 1991). Very little else is known about how acetaminophen relieves pain.

NSAIDs

Although NSAIDs relieve pain through multiple mechanisms, including a central nervous system (CNS) mechanism, their best characterized action is in the periphery at the site of injury. Tissue damage initiates a complex set of events leading to activation of primary afferent nociceptors and eventually to pain.

Transduction is the first process involved in nociception, or the sensation of pain (refer to pp. 18-22, Chapter 2, for more detail). It begins at the periphery (skin, subcutaneous tissue, visceral or somatic structures), where primary afferent neurons, called nociceptors, are distributed throughout. When tissue damage or potential damage results from mechanical (e.g., incision or tumor growth), thermal (e.g., burn), or chemical stimuli, noci-

ceptors are activated. These stimuli may also cause the release of a number of substances that facilitate the activation of nociceptors. Most of these substances at the site of injury are inflammatory mediators; they play a major role in pain transmission. They include prostaglandins (PG), bradykinin (BK), serotonin (5HT), substance P (SP), and histamine (H) (Paice, 1991; Paice, 1994).

NSAIDs relieve pain by interfering with the production of PGs. PGs are produced through a series of events beginning when cells are traumatized and release phospholipids. The enzyme, phospholipase, breaks down phospholipids into arachidonic acid. In turn, the enzyme, cyclooxygenase, breaks down arachidonic acid into PGs. NSAIDs block the action of cyclooxygenase, thereby interfering with the production of PGs, ultimately decreasing pain (Figure 5.1). Thus NSAIDs are cyclooxygenase inhibitors.

Unfortunately, NSAIDs reduce PGs throughout the body, and this may cause certain side effects. For example, because PGs maintain the protective layer of the gastric mucosa, one possible side effect of NSAIDs is gastrointestinal erosion (Paice, 1991; Paice, 1994). Methods of minimizing the occurrence of this side effect and others are discussed later in this chapter.

In an effort to reduce side effects from NSAIDs, a new type of NSAID is being developed. Most currently available NSAIDs inhibit both cyclooxygenase 1 and 2 (COX-1 and COX-2). Inhibition of COX-2 seems to be related to the analgesic and antiinflammatory effects of NSAIDs. The inhibition of COX-1 is thought to be responsible for many of the side effects such as gastric ulcers. Thus efforts are underway to develop NSAIDs that inhibit COX-2 but not COX-1. At present only one drug, nabumetone (Relafen), that preferentially inhibits COX-2 is available (Insel, 1996).

PRINCIPLES OF ADMINISTRATION OF NONOPIOID ANALGESICS

Clinical decisions about the use of nonopioids are made by considering indications, side effects, the individual being treated, and dosing and titration. Miscon-

TABLE 5.1 ● ● ● ● ●

| *Misconceptions* | Nonopioids |

MISCONCEPTION	CORRECTION
1. Regular daily use of NSAIDs is much safer than taking opioids.	Side effects from long-term use of NSAIDs are considerably more severe and life-threatening than the side effects from daily doses of oral morphine or other opioids. The most common side effect from long-term use of opioids is constipation, whereas NSAIDs can cause gastric ulcers, increased bleeding time, and renal insufficiency. Acetaminophen can cause hepatotoxicity.
2. Nonopioids are not useful analgesics for severe pain.	Nonopioids alone are rarely sufficient to relieve severe pain, but they are an important part in the total analgesic plan. One of the basic principles of analgesic therapy is: Whenever pain is severe enough to require an opioid, adding a nonopioid should be considered.
3. A nonopioid should not be given at the same time as an opioid.	It is safe to administer a nonopioid and opioid at the same time. Giving a dose of nonopioid at the same time as a dose of opioid poses no more danger than giving the doses at different times. In fact, many opioids are compounded with a nonopioid (e.g., Percocet [oxycodone and acetaminophen]).
4. Administering NSAIDs rectally or parenterally prevents gastric ulcers.	Regardless of the route of administration, NSAIDs inhibit PGs that are necessary to maintain the protective barrier in the GI tract. Rectal or parenteral administration will only avoid the local irritation that occurs with oral administration.
5. Administering antacids with NSAIDs is an effective method of reducing gastric distress.	Administering antacids with NSAIDs can lessen distress but may be counter productive. Antacids reduce the absorption and therefore the effectiveness of the NSAID by releasing the drug in the stomach rather than in the small intestine where absorption occurs.
6. For patients receiving long-term treatment with NSAIDs, H_2 blockers such as cimetidine (Tagamet) provide effective protection against gastric and duodenal ulcers.	H_2 blockers at higher than standard doses may be helpful, but misoprostol (Cytotec) is the only proven method to reduce the occurrence of gastric and duodenal ulcers.
7. Gastric distress (e.g., abdominal pain) is indicative of NSAID-induced gastric ulceration.	Most patients with gastric lesions have no symptoms until bleeding or perforation occurs.

May be duplicated for use in clinical practice. From McCaffery M, Pasero C: *Pain: Clinical manual*, p. 131. Copyright © 1999, Mosby, Inc. See text for references.

ceptions that hamper the appropriate use of nonopioids as analgesics are listed in Table 5.1 and corrected in this chapter.

Indications for Administration of Acetaminophen or NSAIDs

Nonopioids are fairly flexible analgesics. They may be used for a wide spectrum of acute and chronic painful conditions of mild to moderate intensity. Nonopioids may relieve both nociceptive (somatic and visceral) pain and neuropathic pain, but they seem to be more effective with nociceptive pain, particularly somatic pain such as muscle and joint pain. Onset of analgesia is rapid (within an hour for many). Box 5.1 provides a summary of indications for nonopioids based on the discussion that follows.

Acetaminophen and aspirin have long been recognized as multipurpose analgesics, but their analgesic ability is frequently underestimated. As shown in Table 5.2, 650 mg of aspirin or acetaminophen may relieve as much pain as 50 mg of meperidine by mouth or 3 to 5 mg of oxycodone by mouth. Although NSAIDs other than aspirin were originally marketed for inflammatory conditions such as rheumatoid arthritis, it has become increasingly apparent that they, too, are multipurpose analgesics.

One principle of analgesic use is to start with a nonopioid if pain is mild. Acetaminophen or a NSAID alone often provides adequate relief. Note that despite having very little antiinflammatory effect, acetaminophen still may be an effective analgesic for inflammatory conditions.

When pain is moderate to severe, nonopioids are frequently ignored, but pain of any severity may be at least

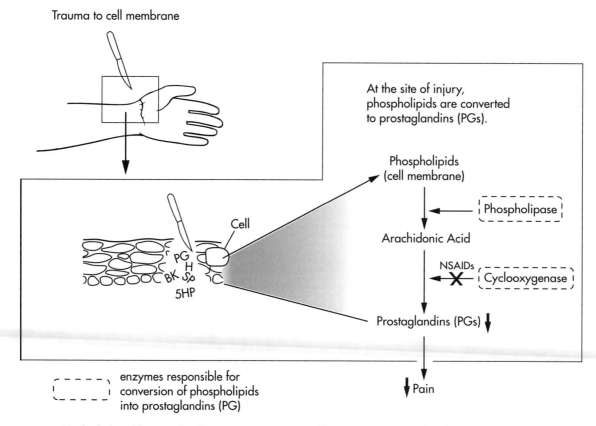

Trauma to cell membrane

At the site of injury, phospholipids are converted to prostaglandins (PGs).

Phospholipids (cell membrane)

Phospholipase

Arachidonic Acid

NSAIDs — Cyclooxygenase

Prostaglandins (PGs) ↓

↓ Pain

PG H BK S₀ 5HP

Cell

┌ ─ ─ ─ ─ ┐
¦ ¦ enzymes responsible for
└ ─ ─ ─ ─ ┘ conversion of phospholipids into prostaglandins (PG)

May be duplicated for use in clinical practice. As appears in McCaffery M, Pasero C: *Pain: Clinical manual,* p. 132, 1999, Mosby, Inc.

● ● ● ● ●
F I G U R E   5.1   An analgesic action of NSAIDs is cyclooxygenase inhibition. (See Figure 2A & B, pp. 20-21, for an overview of analgesic action sites for nonopioids, opioids, and adjuvants.) When cells are traumatized, they release phospholipids. Phospholipase breaks down phospholipids into arachidonic acid. Cyclooxygenase breaks down arachidonic acid into PGs, substances that facilitate pain transmission. NSAIDs block the action of cyclooxygenase, thereby inhibiting the production of PGs and ultimately decreasing pain.

Developed by McCaffery M, Pasero C, and Paice JA, 1998.

partially relieved by a nonopioid. For some types of moderate pain, especially muscle and joint pain, NSAIDs alone may provide adequate relief. However, a NSAID alone should not be expected to relieve severe pain in all patients. Severe pain may require two or more analgesics. Any of the nonopioids is compatible with most other opioid and adjuvant analgesics.

Although the mechanisms of pain relief no doubt differ between many of the NSAIDs, no well-controlled clinical trials demonstrate that combining one NSAID with another provides an analgesic effect superior to either one alone. Combining two NSAIDs increases risk of side effects and drug interactions. Adding aspirin to a NSAID may result in decreased or increased effect, but the result is not predictable. For these and other reasons, combinations of NSAIDs are not recommended (Merry, Power, 1995; Mohamed, Mohamed, Borsook, 1996). However, the small daily aspirin dose for prevention of myocardial infarction appears to pose no problem for patients taking another NSAID.

Giving acetaminophen as an analgesic supplement to ongoing NSAID therapy is fairly common. Research neither supports this practice nor warns against it. Some clinicians find it to be a questionable practice (Sunshine, Olson, 1994).

Acute pain

Headache, including muscle contraction (tension) headache, vascular or migraine headache, mixed headache, sinus headache, hangover headache, and various muscle or joint pains are among the acute pain problems that may respond to a nonopioid alone (Lipman, 1996).

Ketorolac (Toradol) is the first NSAID available in the United States for parenteral administration. In many acute pain situations such as trauma or surgery, the patient is unable to take a nonopioid orally. Thus ketorolac is an appropriate consideration but does not relieve moderate to severe pain in all patients. Many will require an opioid as well.

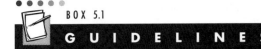

BOX 5.1

GUIDELINES

INDICATIONS FOR NONOPIOID ANALGESICS

1. Mild pain. Start with a nonopioid. Acetaminophen or a NSAID alone often provides adequate relief.
2. Moderate to severe pain. Pain of any severity may be at least partially relieved by a nonopioid. For some types of moderate pain, especially muscle and joint pain, NSAIDs alone may provide adequate relief. However, a NSAID alone usually does not relieve severe pain.
3. Postoperative pain. Perioperative use of a NSAID, especially parenteral ketorolac, may be part of preemptive analgesia or ongoing balanced analgesia.
4. Chronic pain. All types of chronic pain, including neuropathic pain, deserve a trial with a NSAID. All types of cancer pain, especially cancer-related bone pain, are usually partly responsive to a NSAID.
5. Pain that requires an opioid. Whenever pain is severe enough to require an opioid, always consider adding a nonopioid for the following reasons:
   - Opioid dose-sparing effect (i.e., opioid dose may be lowered without decreasing pain relief. Reduces opioid-induced side effects). A common example is IV ketorolac (Toradol) plus opioid postoperatively.
   - Opioids and nonopioids relieve pain by different mechanisms.

May be duplicated for use in clinical practice. From McCaffery M, Pasero C: *Pain: Clinical manual*, p. 133. Copyright © 1999, Mosby, Inc.

Recent research on preemptive analgesia with surgical procedures has produced evidence of the possible benefit of NSAID administration preoperatively and continuing intraoperatively and postoperatively as a part of ongoing multimodal, balanced analgesia. Balanced analgesia usually includes not only nonopioids, but also opioids and local anesthetics. Several studies have shown that preemptive analgesia reduces postoperative pain and improves outcomes. This combination allows doses of each to be lower, thereby producing fewer side effects and achieving comparable or greater analgesia than may be achieved with any single analgesic (Kehlet, 1994; Kehlet, Dahl, 1993; McQuay, Carroll, Moore, 1988; Woolf, Chong, 1993). Although the manufacturer does not recommend the use of ketorolac preoperatively, it is becoming common practice and has been used safely and effectively (Varrassi, Panella, Piroli et al., 1994). (See Chapter 6, pp. 174-175, and the end of this chapter, pp. 146-148, for further information on preemptive analgesia.)

In addition to use as a perioperative analgesic, parenteral ketorolac is also likely to be used in emergency departments (EDs). Many indications for parenteral ke-

TABLE 5.2

EQUIANALGESIC CHART: APPROXIMATE EQUIVALENT DOSES OF NONOPIOIDS AND OPIOIDS FOR MILD TO MODERATE PAIN	
ANALGESIC	PO DOSAGE (MG)
Nonopioids	
Acetaminophen	650
Aspirin (ASA)	650
Choline salicylate	870
Magnesium salicylate	1000
Sodium salicylate	1000
Opioids	
Codeine	32-60
Hydrocodone	5
Meperidine (Demerol)	50
Oxycodone	3-5
Pentazocine (Talwin)	30-50
Propoxyphene hydrochloride (Darvon)	65
Propoxyphene napsylate (Darvon-N)	100

From McCaffery M, Pasero C: *Pain: Clinical manual*, p. 133. Copyright © 1999, Mosby, Inc.

Information from American Pain Society (APS): *Principles of analgesic use in the treatment of acute pain and cancer pain*, ed 3, Skokie, Ill., 1992, The Society; Beaver WT, Wallenstein SL, Rogers A et al.: Analgesic studies of codeine and oxycodone in patients with cancer. I. Comparisons of oral with intramuscular codeine and of oral with intramuscular oxycodone, *J Pharmacol Exp Ther* 207: 92-100, 1978; Houde RW: Systemic analgesics and related drugs: Narcotic analgesics. In Bonica JJ and Ventafridda V, editors: *Advances in pain research and therapy*, vol 2, pp 263-273, New York, 1979, Raven Press; Kaiko R, Lacouture P, Hopf K et al.: Analgesic efficacy of controlled-release (CR) oxycodone and CR morphine, *Clin Pharmacol Ther* 59:130, 1996; Lipman AG: Internal analgesic and antipyretic products. In *Handbook of nonprescription drugs*, pp. 45-74, Washington DC, 1996, American Pharmaceutical Association; Moertel CG: Relief of pain with oral medications, *Aust NZ J Med* 6(suppl 1): 1-8, 1976.

torolac exist in this clinical setting (e.g., renal colic), but sometimes it is used primarily because of the staff's fear of being duped by an addict. Appropriate prescribing, of course, is made on the basis of the patient's condition, not on the staff's suspicions.

Chronic pain

Those NSAIDs that are restricted to short-term use and are not appropriate therapy for chronic pain include ketorolac (Toradol, limited to 5 days) and mefenamic acid (Ponstel, limited to 7 days). Longer use is associated with increased adverse effects. Other NSAIDs may be considered for long-term therapy. Any patient with chronic pain, including those with neuropathic pain, is a candidate for a trial of NSAIDs. All types of cancer pain, especially cancer-related bone pain, may respond to a NSAID (Portenoy, Kanner, 1996).

Although ketorolac is recommended only for short-term use, case reports of terminally ill patients with intractable pain showed that some have benefited from continuous subcutaneous or intravenous infusion of ketorolac (Middleton, Lyle, Berger, 1996). In one case report of a patient unresponsive to opioids and adjuvants, a subcutaneous continuous infusion of ketorolac, 120 mg/24 h, was administered for 75 days without any significant renal or gastric side effects. Misoprostol was also given. Pain relief was achieved with ketorolac alone (Ripamonti, Ticozzi, Zecca et al., 1996).

The practice of using nonopioids as rescue doses for patients receiving opioids around the clock (ATC) usually is not logical. The reason commonly given for this practice is to avoid side effects such as sedation that occur when the rescue dose is an opioid. However, the most logical plan is to give both the opioid and nonopioid ATC to reduce the daily dose of opioid and thereby reduce the opioid-related side effects on an ongoing basis. An opioid is used for the rescue dose. (For patients receiving ATC NSAIDs but no opioids, acetaminophen may be an appropriate drug for rescue doses.)

Nonopioid plus opioid

A basic principle of analgesic use is that whenever pain is severe enough to require an opioid, always consider adding a nonopioid (APS, 1992). Nonopioids are often combined with opioids for their opioid dose-sparing effect. As described earlier, adding a nonopioid to an opioid allows the opioid dose to be lowered without compromising pain relief. A lower opioid dose in turn decreases the occurrence or severity of opioid-induced side effects such as sedation. Furthermore, a combination of opioid and nonopioid may provide more effective pain relief than either one alone because the combination attacks pain at both the peripheral and CNS levels.

Mild to moderate pain is often treated with oral analgesics in a fixed combination of opioid and nonopioid, usually acetaminophen and sometimes aspirin. The problem with fixed combinations is that the dose of acetaminophen (or other nonopioid) limits the escalation of the opioid dose. Common examples of opioid/nonopioid fixed combinations are (see inside cover for more examples):

  Lortab 5/500 (hydrocodone, 5 mg, and acetaminophen, 500 mg)
  Loracet 10/650 (hydrocodone, 10 mg, and acetaminophen, 650 mg)
  Percocet (oxycodone, 5 mg, and acetaminophen, 325 mg)
  Tylenol No. 3 (codeine, 30 mg, and acetaminophen, 300 mg)
  Tylox (oxycodone, 5 mg, and acetaminophen, 500 mg)
  Vicodin (hydrocodone, 5 mg, and acetaminophen, 500 mg)
  Vicoprofen (hydrocodone, 7.5 mg, and ibuprofen, 200 mg)

The advantage of these combinations is that each analgesic component can be used at a reduced dose, resulting in reduced adverse reactions. However, this advantage is lost when higher doses are required to relieve pain. To avoid exceeding the recommended maximum daily dose of 4 to 6 g of acetaminophen, the patient cannot take more than 8 to 12 tablets per day of those containing 500 mg of acetaminophen or 12 to 18 tablets per day of those containing 325 mg of acetaminophen.

Unfortunately, a tendency to prescribe opioid/nonopioid combinations for patients who experience only marginal relief and have reached the maximum recommended daily dose of nonopioid exists. This inappropriate prescribing is especially likely with fixed combinations that include codeine or hydrocodone. Because they are not Schedule II drugs, physicians may be more comfortable prescribing them. However, when the ceiling dose of nonopioid is reached and the patient's pain is not adequately controlled, the recommended strategy is to discontinue the combination drug, give the nonopioid separately at fixed doses ATC (if indicated), and prescribe an opioid as a single drug. The opioid dose may then be increased without concern about exceeding the recommended dose of nonopioid.

Side Effects of Acetaminophen and NSAIDs

In contrast to opioids repeated use of acetaminophen or a NSAID does not result in tolerance or physical dependence. Furthermore, they cause no respiratory depression and no cardiovascular depression.

Occasional use of nonopioids at the recommended doses for analgesia, especially in a healthy individual, generally does not result in significant side effects. However, a variety of known and unknown risk factors may cause the side effects discussed in the following. A summary of side effects and their treatment or prevention is provided in Box 5.2.

Side effects of acetaminophen

Acetaminophen differs from the NSAIDs in that it has considerably fewer adverse effects. It does not affect platelet function, rarely causes gastrointestinal (GI) problems, and can be given to patients who are hypersensitive ("allergic") to aspirin or other NSAIDs. Chronic use may cause stomach upset (Portenoy, Kanner, 1996).

Although acetaminophen is probably the safest nonopioid for most patients, it poses a danger in certain instances. Even at the recommended therapeutic doses, acetaminophen can cause severe hepatotoxicity (liver toxicity) in patients with chronic alcoholism, recent fasting, or liver disease (Coyle, Cherny, Portenoy, 1995;

BOX 5.2

G U I D E L I N E S

SIDE EFFECTS OF NONOPIOIDS AND THEIR TREATMENT/PREVENTION

Acetaminophen

1. Hepatotoxicity; occurs with an overdose. At recommended doses, certain individuals are also at risk. Preventive strategy is to avoid or use with caution in the following patients:
   - Malnourishment, recent fasting
   - Alcoholism, regular and heavy use of alcohol
   - Preexisting liver disease
   - Concomitant use of other potentially hepatotoxic drugs
2. Renal disease. Questions remain about the association of acetaminophen with renal disease.

NSAIDs

1. Gastric side effects associated with acute local irritation from orally administered NSAIDs. Uncomfortable (e.g., heartburn) but rarely indicative of serious injury. May resolve with continued use. Treatment options:
   - Lower the dose.
   - Switch to another NSAID.
   - Use enteric-coated NSAIDs.
   - Use an H_2 blocker (e.g., ranitidine [Zantac]).
   - Take the NSAID with food or a large glass of water.
   - Antacids may reduce symptoms, but they also reduce absorption of the NSAID.
2. Gastrointestinal side effects associated with the systemic effect of NSAIDs, regardless of route of administration. NSAIDs interfere with PG synthesis throughout the body. PG reduction impairs the protective barrier in the GI tract and allows injury to occur. Often asymptomatic until bleeding or perforation occurs.
   Preventive strategies for all patients:
   - Select NSAIDs with low risk (e.g., ibuprofen, diclofenac, choline magnesium trisalicylate [Trilisate], salsalate [Disalcid], nabumetone [Relafen]).
   - Use the lowest effective dose.
   Risk factors warranting use of gastroprotective therapies:
   - History of NSAID-induced ulcer
   - Prior ulcer disease

   - Advanced age (>60 years)
   - Concomitant corticosteroid therapy
   - Concomitant anticoagulant therapy
   - High doses of NSAID
   - Patient unlikely to survive a GI complication
   Gastroprotective therapies:
   - Misoprostol (Cytotec). This is the only method shown to reduce the occurrence of gastric and duodenal ulcers.
   - For patients who cannot afford or tolerate misoprostol, use some combination of H_2 blocker (e.g., ranitidine [Zantac], sucralfate [Carafate]), and antacids.
   - A single strategy such as antacids, buffered tablets, or enteric-coated tablets does not provide sufficient protection.
3. Hematologic side effects (e.g., bleeding). Preventive strategies when bleeding is a concern:
   - Use NSAIDs that have minimal or no effect on bleeding time, such as choline magnesium trisalicylate (Trilisate), salsalate (Disalcid), and nabumetone (Relafen).
   - Use acetaminophen instead of a NSAID.
   - To decrease bleeding associated with operative procedures, stop aspirin therapy 1 week before surgery, and stop most other NSAIDs 2 to 3 days before surgery. Aspirin has an irreversible effect on platelets but other NSAIDs do not.
4. Renal effects. Renal insufficiency is uncommon, and acute renal failure is rare, but chronic NSAID use at high doses may cause end-stage renal disease. Preventive strategies in patients with impaired renal function:
   - Avoid indomethacin (Indocin).
   - Consider aspirin.
   - Use low doses.
   - Monitor kidney function.
5. Cognitive dysfunction (CNS effect). Treatment options:
   - Lower the dose.
   - Discontinue the NSAID.
   - Switch to another NSAID.

May be duplicated for use in clinical practice. From McCaffery M, Pasero C: *Pain: Clinical manual*, p. 135. Copyright © 1999, Mosby, Inc.

Seeff, Cuccherini, Zimmerman et al., 1986; Whitcomb, Block, 1994).

In one study of patients with hepatotoxicity, all took more than 4000 mg/day of acetaminophen, and recent fasting was more common than recent alcohol use (Whitcomb, Block, 1994). Very ill patients may be malnourished or may go through periods of inability or lack of desire to eat, yet may continue to take acetaminophen rectally or orally (e.g., liquid). The total daily dose of acetaminophen should be carefully monitored in these patients.

Acetaminophen is a metabolite of phenacetin, an analgesic known to be associated with renal failure. Until the 1970s, phenacetin was a common ingredient in nonprescription analgesics (e.g., APC, a combination of aspirin, phenacetin, and caffeine). When its association with renal failure became apparent, it was removed from the market. Questions remain as to whether acetaminophen is also associated with renal disease.

In a study of 716 patients with end-stage renal disease, acetaminophen appeared to contribute to approximately

10% of the cases. Taking more than one pill a day or a cumulative lifetime dose of 1000 pills doubled the risk of end-stage renal disease. Patients who took a cumulative lifetime dose of 5000 or more acetaminophen pills were considerably more likely to have end-stage renal disease. Aspirin use did not increase the risk of end-stage renal disease, and use of NSAIDs had only a relatively weak association with end-stage renal disease (Perneger, Whelton, Klag, 1994).

These data suggest a significant correlation between acetaminophen consumption and end-stage renal disease. However, it is not clear from these data, or other data in the literature, whether the increased risk applies to individuals with preexisting underlying renal dysfunction, to individuals with normal renal function, or both.

From the standpoint of renal dysfunction, aspirin appears to be a much safer alternative for patients requiring prolonged nonopioid therapy who are also at high risk for renal failure.

Multiple trade names of acetaminophen-containing medications, both prescription and nonprescription, contribute to the likelihood that patients will unknowingly take high doses of acetaminophen. Patients must be cautioned about hidden acetaminophen in analgesics and other types of medications such as cold remedies.

A study of 100 patients with chronic pain presenting to a pain center revealed that more than half were taking one or more acetaminophen-containing analgesics. On the basis of patient self-report, some were taking more than the maximum recommended daily dose. Interestingly, only 7% had plasma concentrations of acetaminophen reported to be within the therapeutic range and none reached a toxic blood concentration or showed signs of acetaminophen toxicity (Heavner, Shi, Diede et al., 1996). Although this sounds reassuring, the study had numerous limitations and the problem requires further study.

Side effects of NSAIDs

The side effects of NSAIDs remain the same regardless of the condition being treated. However, when NSAIDs are used as a single dose, at low doses, or for only a short period of time (e.g., postoperatively) side effects are less problematic. When NSAIDs are used at high doses or for a prolonged time, the following side effects are more likely to occur.

GI Effects

The most common side effects for most NSAIDs are GI. Gastric damage by NSAIDs occurs by at least two distinct mechanisms.

Local Effect

One mechanism is acute local irritation from the orally administered NSAIDs. Symptoms include heartburn and upper abdominal pain. Mild gastritis or local irritation often resolves with continued NSAID use. Minor GI symptoms may also be resolved by lowering the dose, changing to another NSAID, or using a gastroprotective drug such as misoprostol, an antacid, sucralfate (Carafate), an H_2 blocker (cimetidine [Tagamet]; or ranitidine [Zantac]), or omeprazole (Prilosec).

Local injury resulting from contact with the mucosa may be avoided by use of enteric-coated NSAIDs. All patients taking NSAIDs should also be taught to take each dose with food or, at the very least, a large glass of water.

Systemic Effect

The other mechanism by which NSAIDs cause gastric damage is a systemic effect that occurs without the NSAID actually being in contact with the mucosa. Regardless of the route of administration, NSAIDs interfere with PG synthesis throughout the body. The protective barrier in the GI tract depends on PG synthesis. Reduction in PG impairs the protective barrier in the GI tract and allows injury to occur (Bjorkman, 1996). This may lead to life-threatening adverse effects, such as ulceration, bleeding, and perforation.

Unfortunately, GI symptoms such as heartburn or burning upper abdominal discomfort have little relationship to more serious adverse effects such as ulcerations. For example, dyspepsia occurs rather often in chronic aspirin therapy, but it does not necessarily indicate intestinal blood loss or injury to the gastric mucosa (Sunshine, Olson, 1994). However, persistent burning should not be ignored because it may be associated with a serious pathologic condition. Conversely and equally important, absence of GI symptoms should not reassure the clinician that no ulceration is occurring. Most patients with gastric lesions have no symptoms until bleeding or perforation occurs. Even positive fecal occult blood testing is not helpful in diagnosing ulcers caused by NSAIDs (Bjorkman, 1996).

Clinically important adverse GI effects, such as ulceration and bleeding, occur in about 10% of patients treated with NSAIDs (Portenoy, Kanner, 1996). The risk of serious GI complications is influenced by several interrelated factors: specific NSAID, dose of NSAID, length of time on NSAID, and patient characteristics.

Different NSAIDs carry different risks for serious GI complications, but the dose also influences the risk of the specific NSAID. In a review of 11 studies concerning relative risk of GI complications with different NSAIDs, ibuprofen and diclofenac ranked low in adverse effects, whereas ketoprofen and piroxicam ranked high. However, the risk of bleeding ulcer was dose related. Thus even low-risk NSAIDs may become high risk when the dose is increased. For example, in these studies the usual dose of ibuprofen was 1600 mg daily. At higher doses, ibuprofen may be high risk. In contrast, NSAIDs that appear to be high risk may become low risk when the doses are lowered (Henry, Lim, Rodriguez et al., 1996).

Although gastric injury is not common with short-term use of most NSAIDs, GI complications again vary with different NSAIDs (Henry, Lim, Rodriguez et al.,

1996). Short-term use of ibuprofen (Lanza, 1984) or ketoprofen (Rahbek, 1976), (e.g., 3 days or less) was found to produce little or no injury to the gastric mucosa. Endoscopic studies of gastric injury indicate that 1600 to 2400 mg of ibuprofen daily, given for 3 days or less, produces little or no injury to the gastric mucosa. In contrast, 3 days or less of aspirin 600 mg every 4 hours (3600/day) produces gastric injury (Lanza, 1984).

A study of GI bleeding related to aspirin revealed no substantial differences in the risk of major GI bleeding according to type of aspirin preparation used. In other words, the risk of gastric or duodenal bleeding is approximately the same for buffered, plain, or enteric-coated aspirin. Apparently, the benefit of one type of aspirin tablet versus another is overwhelmed by systemic effects of aspirin on the GI tract (Kelly, Kaufman, Jurgelon et al., 1996).

The findings of the study just cited are consistent with endoscopic studies showing no difference between buffered and plain aspirin in relation to gastric injury. However, they are not consistent with those of endoscopic studies of young, healthy volunteers in which enteric-coated aspirin caused less gastric injury than plain aspirin. This raises the question of whether gastric injury seen in endoscopic studies of healthy individuals is relevant to clinical outcomes. Patients taking aspirin for therapeutic purposes may be elderly with concurrent illnesses and taking multiple medications (Kelly, Kaufman, Jurgelon et al., 1996).

More research is needed to identify which specific NSAIDs at what doses for what duration pose the most and the least risk. On the basis of the studies just quoted along with literature reviews (Bjorkman, 1996; Sunshine, Olson, 1994), the consensus is that overall the NSAIDs least likely to cause GI injury are diclofenac, ibuprofen, nonacetylated salicylates (e.g., Trilisate), and nabumetone. Those NSAIDs most likely to produce adverse GI effects are aspirin, meclofenamate, piroxicam, indomethacin, and tolmetin.

Different patients have different degrees of risk. The best defined risk factors for ulcerations and erosions are history of a NSAID-induced ulcer complication, prior ulcer disease, advanced age ($>$75 years, some say $>$60 years), concomitant corticosteroid therapy, or concomitant anticoagulant therapy. Prophylactic therapy is strongly recommended for these patients and should also be considered in patients on high doses of NSAID or those who would be unlikely to survive a GI complication (Bjorkman, 1996; Borda, 1992). Young healthy patients without prior GI problems have a low risk of serious GI problems.

As mentioned previously, regardless of the route of administration, NSAIDs inhibit PGs that protect the GI mucosa. Obviously, the treatment of choice for NSAID-induced ulcers is discontinuation of the NSAID (Bjorkman, 1996). However, gastroprotective therapy may prevent the occurrence of GI complications.

Gastroprotective Therapies During NSAID Therapy

Patients who should receive prophylactic therapy to prevent serious GI complications are those who are at increased risk (as mentioned previously) and those who might not survive a GI complication should it occur (Coyle, Cherny, Portenoy, 1995; Coyle, Portenoy, 1996).

For both short- and long-term NSAID therapy, coadministration of misoprostol (Cytotec) is the only method thus far that has been shown repeatedly to reduce the occurrence of gastric and duodenal ulcers (Bjorkman, 1996; Koch, Dez, Ferrario et al., 1996). For example, in one study, cancer patients received diclofenac (200 to 300 mg/day) and either 200 μg misoprostol twice daily or 150 mg ranitidine (Zantac) twice daily. After 4 weeks endoscopy revealed a significantly lower incidence of GI lesions in the group taking misoprostol (Valentini, Cannizzaro, Polette et al., 1995).

The manufacturer's recommended dose of misoprostol for an adult is 200 μg four times daily with food. If this is not tolerated, a dose of 100 μg may be used. This drug is expensive and some patients experience side effects (e.g. diarrhea). Side effects may subside after 1 week or may necessitate discontinuation of the drug. The likelihood of diarrhea may be decreased by starting with small doses and increasing the dose gradually (Bjorkman, 1996). Misoprostol is taken for the duration of NSAID therapy and does not relieve dyspepsia (e.g., heartburn).

If the NSAID is given twice or three times a day, the patient must be reminded that dose times for misoprostol taken four times a day will not coincide with NSAID dosing. Patients are likely to think that misoprostol should be taken at the same time as the NSAID. Some NSAIDs are combined with misoprostol (e.g., diclofenac and misoprostol [Arotec]).

For patients who cannot afford or tolerate misoprostol, an alternative to misoprostol is some combination of an H_2 blocker (e.g., cimetidine [Tagamet] or ranitidine [Zantac]), sucralfate (Carafate), and antacids. Data are insufficient to recommend sucralfate for prophylactic therapy, but it is commonly recommended together with H_2 blockers (Portenoy, Kanner, 1996). H_2 blockers at standard doses prevent duodenal ulcers but not gastric ulcers (Koch, Dez, Ferrario et al., 1996). Higher doses of H_2 blockers are required to decrease gastric ulcers (Bjorkman, 1996). In a study of 285 patients on long-term NSAID therapy, famotidine (Pepcid), 40 mg twice daily, significantly reduced the incidence of both gastric and duodenal ulcers (Taha, Hudson, Hawkey et al., 1996).

No data support the use of antacids alone to prevent NSAID-induced ulcers. In fact, administering antacids with NSAIDs is somewhat counterproductive. Antacids reduce the absorption and therefore the effectiveness of the NSAID by releasing the drug in the stomach rather than in the small intestine where absorption occurs (Sunshine, Olson, 1994).

Hematologic Effects

Most NSAIDs interfere with platelet aggregation. Aspirin has an irreversible effect on platelets and will increase bleeding time for up to 7 days after the last dose (i.e., until the platelets are replaced). For that reason, aspirin therapy should be stopped 1 week before surgery. Other NSAIDs have reversible effects on platelets so that inhibition of platelet aggregation only lasts as long as it takes to eliminate a sufficient quantity of the drug from the system (Sunshine, Olson, 1994).

In patients with bleeding diatheses such as hemophilia and in some patients undergoing surgery or cancer treatment, it may be important to minimize increased bleeding time. Those NSAIDs that have minimal or no effect on platelet aggregation are choline magnesium trisalicylate (Trilisate), salsalate (Disalcid), and nabumetone (Relafen) (Blower, 1992; Insel, 1996).

Renal Effects

Although uncommon, NSAIDs can cause renal insufficiency and significant nephrotoxicity. Acute renal failure is rare. End-stage renal disease may occur with chronic NSAID use at high doses (Portenoy, Kanner, 1996). Indomethacin is associated with a high incidence of adverse renal effects. Aspirin does not appear to adversely affect renal function in normal individuals, but it nonetheless should be used with caution in patients with impaired renal function (Sunshine, Olson, 1994).

Impaired renal function is only a relative contraindication to the use of NSAIDs. Such patients should be given lower doses, and kidney function should be monitored closely. Some drugs, such as sulindac and etodolac, are referred to as "renal sparing," but the clinical relevance of this term is unclear because studies of full dose ranges in patient populations are lacking (Portenoy, Kanner, 1996).

CNS Effects

Mild dizziness and drowsiness are relatively common side effects (Eisenberg, Berkey, Carr et al., 1994). Cognitive dysfunction may also be a side effect of any of the NSAIDs. Symptoms include decreased attention span and loss of short-term memory. Cognitive dysfunction has been noted in the elderly in response to naproxen and ibuprofen, even when doses are within the accepted range (Sunshine, Olson, 1994). Symptoms are usually mild and rapidly reversible (Coyle, Cherny, Portenoy, 1995).

The elderly are especially reluctant to report these symptoms, probably because they are not aware that these are reversible side effects of a drug and not an irreversible effect of aging. Often these symptoms will be detected only on direct questioning of the patient or by observing the patient's responses to routine questions.

Individualizing the Selection of Nonopioid Analgesics

The goal of nonopioid selection is to find a single nonopioid at a dose that offers satisfactory pain relief with a low risk of side effects. Once the patient's risk factors for side effects are assessed, drug selection and dosing requires consideration of certain characteristics of the drug. Quite a few NSAIDs are now commercially available. Table 5.3 is a guide to generic and brand names of nonopioids and may be used in conjunction with Table 5.4, which details dosing information for acetaminophen and NSAIDs.

Acute versus chronic pain

When NSAIDs are used as a single dose, at low doses, or for only a short period of time (e.g., postoperatively),

● ● ● ● ●
TABLE 5.3

NONOPIOIDS LISTED ALPHABETICALLY BY GENERIC NAME FOLLOWED BY BRAND NAME

GENERIC NAME(S)	BRAND NAME(S)
Acetaminophen (APAP, paracetamol)	Tylenol, many other brands
Aspirin	Bayer, many other brands
Choline magnesium trisalicylate	Trilisate
Choline salicylate	Arthropan
Diclofenac	Cataflam (immediate release for acute pain)
	Voltaren Delayed Release, Voltaren-XR, (extended release for chronic therapy)
Diflunisal	Dolobid
Etodolac	Lodine
Fenoprofen calcium	Nalfon
Flurbiprofen	Ansaid
Ibuprofen	Motrin, Advil, many other brands
Indomethacin	Indocin
Ketoprofen	Orudis, Oruvail Extended-Release
Ketorolac	Toradol
Meclofenamate sodium	Meclomen
Mefenamic acid	Ponstel
Nabumetone	Relafen
Naproxen	Naprosyn
Naproxen sodium	Aleve
Oxaprozin	Daypro
Piroxicam	Feldene
Salsalate	Disalcid
Sulindac	Clinoril
Tolmetin	Tolectin

May be duplicated for use in clinical practice. From McCaffery M, Pasero C: *Pain: Clinical manual*, p. 138. Copyright © 1999, Mosby, Inc.

TABLE 5.4

ACETAMINOPHEN AND NSAIDS: DOSING INFORMATION*

Chemical Class	Generic Name	Half-Life (hours)	Dosing Schedule	Recommended Starting Dose Oral (mg)	Maximum Oral Dose Recommended (mg/day)	Comments
P-Aminophenol derivatives	Acetaminophen	2	q4-6h	650	6000	Overdosage produces hepatic toxicity. No GI or platelet toxicity. Available as liquid and for rectal administration.
Salicylates	Aspirin	3-12	q4-6h	650	6000	Standard for comparison. May not be as well tolerated as some of the newer NSAIDs. Available for rectal administration.
	Diflunisal	8-12	q12h	500	1500	Less GI toxicity than aspirin.
	Choline magnesium trisalicylate	9-17	q12h	500-1000	4000	Minimal GI toxicity. No effect on platelet aggregation. Available as liquid.
	Choline salicylate	2-3	q3-6h	870	5352	Liquid. Minimal effect on platelet function.
	Magnesium salicylate		q4-6h	1000	4000	
	Salsalate	16	q12h	500-1000	4000	
Proprionic acids	Ibuprofen	2	q6h	400	3200	Available as a suspension.
	Naproxen	13	q12h	250	1025-1375	
	Fenoprofen	2-3	q6-8h	200	3200	
	Ketoprofen	2-3	q6-8h	25	300	Available for rectal administration and as a topical gel.
	Flurbiprofen	5-6	q12h	100	300	
	Oxaprozin	40	q24h	600	1800	
Acetic acids	Indomethacin	4-5	q8h	25	150	Higher incidence of GI and CNS side effects than proprionic acids. Available in slow-release preparations, and for rectal administration.
	Tolmetin	2-5	q8h	200	2000	
	Sulindac	14	q12h	150	400	Not recommended for prolonged use because increased risk for GI toxicity.
	Diclofenac	2	q8h	25	150	
	Ketorolac	4-7	q6h	10	40	Use limited to 5 days. Recommended parenteral dose ≤30 mg; total daily dose ≤120 mg.
Oxicams	Piroxicam	50	q24h	20	40	
Fenamates	Mefenamic acid	2	q6h	250	1000	Use limited to 7 days.
	Meclofenamate	2	—	—	400	Not recommended for analgesia.

May be duplicated for use in clinical practice. As appears in McCaffery M, Pasero C: *Pain: Clinical manual*, pp. 139-140, 1999, Mosby, Inc.   *Continued.*

● ● ● ● ●
TABLE 5.4—cont'd

ACETAMINOPHEN AND NSAIDS: DOSING INFORMATION*

Chemical Class	Generic Name	Half-Life (hours)	Dosing Schedule	Recommended Starting Dose Oral (mg)	Maximum Oral Dose Recommended (mg/day)	Comments
Pyranocarboxylic acids	Etodolac	7	q8h	200	1200	
Other	Nabumetone	24	q24h	1000	2000	Minimal effect on platelet aggregation.

May be duplicated for use in clinical practice. As appears in McCaffery M, Pasero C: *Pain: Clinical manual*, pp. 139-140, 1999, Mosby, Inc.

q, every; *h*, hour.

*Table based on clinical experience of the authors and a variety of published sources, including:

AHCPR: *Management of cancer pain: adults. Quick reference guide for clinicians*, 1994. AHCPR Pub. No. 94-0593; American Pain Society (APS): *Principles of analgesic use in the treatment of acute pain and cancer pain*, ed 3, Skokie, Ill., 1992, The Society; Insel PA: Analgesic-antipyretic and antiinflammatory agents and drugs employed in the treatment of gout. In Hardman JL, Limbird LE: *Goodman and Gilman's the pharmacological basis of therapeutics*, ed 9, pp 617-657, New York, 1996, McGraw-Hill; Portenoy RK, Kanner RM: Nonopioid and adjuvant analgesics. In Portenoy RK, Kanner RM, editors: *Pain management: Theory and practice*, p 221, Philadelphia, 1996, FA Davis; Sunshine A, Olson NZ: Nonnarcotic analgesics. In Wall PD, Melzack R, editors: *Textbook of pain*, ed 3, pp 923-942, New York, 1994, Churchill Livingstone.

Modified from Coyle N, Cherny NL, Portenoy RK: Pharmacologic management of cancer pain. In McGuire DB, Yarbro CH, Ferrell BR, editors: *Cancer pain management*, ed 2, pp 91-92, Boston, 1995, Jones & Bartlett Publishers.

Clinical Relevance of Information Presented in Table 5.4:

- Half-life. Half-life is the time required for 50% of the dose to be eliminated from the body. A short half-life (approximately 2 to 7 hours) is recommended for some patients, such as the elderly. Drugs with a short half-life are usually preferred for occasional or unexpected pain because they tend to have a quicker onset of analgesia than drugs with a long half-life.
- Dosing schedule. Dosing intervals may range from every 4 hours to once a day. Drugs with short half-lives have shorter dosing intervals than those with long half-lives. If patients can tolerate a drug with a long half-life, dosing once or twice a day is usually preferred. The fewer the doses, the more likely the patient will remember to take the drug.
- Recommended starting dose. This dose should be reduced by one half to two thirds in the elderly, those taking multiple drugs, or those with renal insufficiency.
- Maximum dose recommended. Data are lacking, but the dose listed is thought to be the maximum needed by most patients for analgesia and the dose beyond which side effects are more likely. However, in some patients careful dose titration may identify patients who need and tolerate 50% to 100% more than the maximum dose recommended. Others may require or tolerate less. For some patients at risk for side effects, the maximum daily dose may be one half or less that recommended.

side effects are less problematic than with long-term use. Compared with single doses of NSAIDs, side effects increase dramatically with multiple dosing over 7 to 10 days (Eisenberg, Berkey, Carr et al., 1994). Therefore the importance of careful nonopioid selection increases over time.

Analgesic history

Whichever NSAID has worked well for the patient in the past and has caused minimal or no side effects is often the best place to begin with drug selection.

Current analgesic response

Patients vary in response to NSAIDs. If one NSAID is ineffective after appropriate dose adjustment, it is worthwhile to try another NSAID. This is referred to as sequential trials. An NSAID should not be considered a failure until it has been administered at the maximum tolerated dose. Many clinicians believe that it takes up to 1 week to evaluate the analgesia of a NSAID (Duarte,

1997). Others recommend waiting only 24 to 48 hours (Mayer, Struthers, Fisher, 1997).

Frequency of dosing

Acetaminophen and NSAIDs may be given PRN for occasional pain or ATC for ongoing pain. The half-life of the drug is associated with frequency of dosing. The longer the half-life, the less frequent the dosing. Acetaminophen has a short half-life and usually must be given every 4 hours for ongoing pain.

The half lives of NSAIDs differ, and dosing intervals range from every 4 hours to once a day. For chronic pain the use of once or twice a day dosing is clearly advantageous. Infrequent dosing is usually more convenient and more likely to result in the patient taking all prescribed doses. This requires a NSAID with a long half-life or one that is formulated for extended release. When patients are taking other analgesics or medications, consider selecting NSAIDs that allow for scheduling as many doses as possible at the same time.

Routes

All NSAIDs are available orally, and a few are available rectally, parenterally, or topically. Rectal formulations of NSAIDs are used far more in other countries. In the United States very few are available commercially for rectal administration, but most pharmacies can compound them as rectal suppositories. Oral formulations can also be administered rectally, either by using the intact tablet or by crushing the tablet and placing it in a gelatin capsule (McCaffery, Martin, Ferrell, 1992).

Currently in the United States the only NSAIDs available for parenteral administration are ketorolac (Toradol) and indomethacin (Indocin). Ketorolac is widely used parenterally as an analgesic, but parenteral indomethacin is used primarily in infants for closure of patent ductus ateriosus. Other countries have many nonopioids available parenterally, including acetaminophen, ibuprofen, aspirin, ketoprofen, and diclofenac.

Cost

Nonprescription generic brands of aspirin and acetaminophen are almost always less expensive than brand names and prescription nonopioids. See the following for a discussion of over-the-counter analgesics.

Cost of prescription NSAIDs varies from one pharmacy to another, but the newer NSAIDs without generic equivalents tend to be more expensive. On the basis of information published by Portenoy and Kanner in 1996, the least expensive NSAIDs are often salsalate (Disalcid), diflunisal (Dolobid), diclofenac (Cataflam, Voltaren), indomethacin (Indocin), and choline magnesium trisalicylate (Trilisate). However, the prices of some of these may range into the more expensive realm, depending on the pharmacy. Those that tend to be more expensive include ketoprofen (Orudis), fenoprofen (Nalfon), flurbiprofen (Ansaid), etodolac (Lodine), piroxicam (Feldene), and nabumetone (Relafen). The cost to the patient of any of these drugs also depends on the required dose. If drug costs are a significant issue, prices should be checked with the pharmacy.

Choice of Starting Dose and Dose Titration

Acetaminophen

For adults, the total daily dose of acetaminophen should not exceed 4000 mg/24 h because of potential hepatotoxicity (APS, 1992). Some clinicians extend that limit to 6000 mg/24 h in selected patients (Coyle, Cherny, Portenoy, 1995). In patients at high risk for he-patotoxicity (e.g., liver disease), low doses of acetaminophen are indicated.

There is a ceiling on the analgesia of acetaminophen. Increasing each dose greater than 1000 mg will result in very little added analgesia (Sunshine, Olson, 1994).

NSAIDs

For most patients, the dose of NSAID recommended by the manufacturer is chosen. However, the analgesic dose is usually less than the antiinflammatory dose. For example, 400 mg of ibuprofen is usually recommended for analgesia, but doses as high as 800 mg four times a day may be necessary for an antiinflammatory effect.

There is a ceiling to the analgesia of each NSAID, but it varies from one person to another. There is no certainty about the minimal effective analgesic dose, the ceiling dose, or the toxic dose for the individual patient. Analgesic doses may be higher or lower than those recommended. Higher doses are associated with a higher incidence of side effects (Eisenberg, Berkey, Carr et al., 1994). To avoid giving a patient a higher dose than is needed, dose titration is sometimes warranted.

Dose titration is recommended for those with increased risk of NSAID toxicity, such as the elderly. Chronic NSAID therapy may also be an indication for dose titration so that the patient does not receive unnecessarily high doses over a long period of time. In most other patients the usual starting doses can be used. In patients with severe pain who are not at high risk for side effects, the dose can be increased to 50% to 100% higher than the conventional starting dose (Coyle, Cherny, Portenoy, 1995; Portenoy, Kanner, 1996).

To titrate NSAID doses, begin with half the recommended dose and increase by approximately 50% increments. With each dose escalation, a period of 5 to 7 days is needed to evaluate the response. The occurrence of increased analgesia after a dose increase implies that the ceiling dose has not been reached. Continue titration until a further dose increase provides no additional pain relief or results in undesirable side effects. Then drop back to the previous dose. However, the dose should not exceed 200% of the recommended daily starting dose (Portenoy, Kanner, 1996). The lowest dose that provides satisfactory pain relief should be maintained.

Acute pain

NSAIDs vary in time to onset and duration of analgesia. Generally, the longer the half-life of a NSAID, the slower the onset of analgesia. Usually the higher the dose the faster the onset, the higher the peak effect, and the longer the duration. Therefore in patients with acute pain there appears to be an advantage in starting with the highest approved dose of a short half-life drug and then adjusting the dose downward (Sunshine, Olson, 1994). This strategy is not recommended for patients at high risk for side effects.

Chronic pain

Although some clinicians recommend a priming dose of a long half-life drug to increase blood levels and shorten onset of analgesia (Sunshine, Olson, 1994), others start with low doses to minimize side effects, especially in those patients at risk for side effects such as the elderly.

Several weeks are necessary to evaluate the effectiveness of a NSAID when it is used to treat grossly inflammatory conditions such as rheumatoid arthritis, but a week or less is usually sufficient to evaluate the analgesic effect. If any analgesia occurs, it will be evident to most patients within 1 to 3 hours of the first dose.

The foregoing discussion of selection and dosing of nonopioids is summarized in Box 5.3.

Special Circumstances

Pregnancy and breast feeding

NSAIDs are not recommended for use during pregnancy. Short-term use is probably safe. However, a literature review revealed a few reports about maternal use of indomethacin being associated with renal failure in the newborn (Merry, Power, 1995). If a NSAID is necessary, low doses of aspirin are probably the safest. Although no evidence exists that moderate doses of aspirin damage the fetus, long-term use is associated with reduced birth weight (Insel, 1996). During the third trimester of pregnancy, salicylates and other NSAIDs should be avoided because they delay onset of labor and increase the possibility of prepartum and postpartum hemorrhage. Misoprostol, a gastroprotective therapy coadministered with NSAIDs to prevent ulcers, should not be used during pregnancy because it may induce a spontaneous abortion (Bjorkman, 1996).

Acetaminophen is considered safe for use during pregnancy and while breast feeding (Lipman, 1996).

Generally NSAIDs are not recommended for use in nursing mothers because of the possible adverse effects on the infant. The American Academy of Pediatrics Committee on Drugs (1994) published a statement on drugs in human milk. Nonprescription analgesics that the committee identified as usually compatible with breast feeding include acetaminophen, ibuprofen, naproxen, and ketoprofen.

If a NSAID is required, drug exposure for the child can be minimized by taking the drug just before breast feeding. Plasma drug levels will be lowest at that time. Under these conditions, an appropriate choice of NSAID is one with a short half-life and inert metabolites that are rapidly excreted, such as ibuprofen (Brooks, Needs, 1992).

Pain in children

 When nonopioid analgesics are used for children, the same principles that are suggested for adults are followed.

Table 5.5 gives nonopioid dosing recommendations for children. Nonprescription pediatric formulations of oral aspirin and acetaminophen are included in Table 5.7 and rectal formulations are included in Table 5.8. Nonprescription NSAIDs for children are included in Table 5.9. Those available in a liquid form include acetaminophen, choline

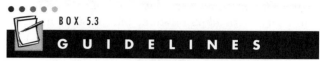

BOX 5.3

GUIDELINES

SELECTION AND DOSING OF NONOPIOIDS FOR ANALGESIA

After identifying the patient's risk factors for side effects, the following are relevant to drug selection and dosing.

Drug selection
1. Acute versus chronic pain. Importance of careful drug selection increases over time.
2. Analgesic history. Whenever possible, select a NSAID that has worked well for the patient.
3. Current analgesic response. If one NSAID is ineffective, try another.
4. Frequency of dosing. For PRN use, 4 hourly dosing is acceptable. For ATC use, dosing once or twice a day is preferred.
5. Routes. All are available orally, most can be formulated for rectal administration, and ketorolac (Toradol) is available parenterally.
6. Cost. Certain NSAIDs are considerably more expensive than others. Those that tend to be the least expensive are salsalate (Disalcid), diflunisal (Dolobid), diclofenac (Cataflam, Voltaren), indomethacin (Indocin), and choline magnesium trisalicylate (Trilisate).

Starting dose and dose titration: (NOTE: Nonopioids have an analgesic ceiling that varies from one individual to another.)
1. Acetaminophen. Usual recommended dose is 650 mg q4h, not to exceed 4000 mg/24 h.
2. NSAID for acute pain. Use the recommended starting dose for analgesia. For rapid onset of oral analgesia, use a short half-life drug and/or a loading dose (50% to 100% higher than recommended dose).
3. NSAID for frail elderly patients, others at risk for side effects, and chronic therapy. Start with 50% or less of the usual recommended dose.
4. NSAID dose titration. For patients who are started on a low dose, increase the dose in 50% increments at least weekly until analgesia is satisfactory or a ceiling dose is identified. Do not exceed 200% of the recommended daily dose.

Evaluation of analgesia
1. Acetaminophen. Pain relief may be evaluated within 2 hours.
2. NSAIDs. Initial pain relief may be evaluated within 3 hours. Maximum pain relief with repeated dosing may be evaluated in 2 to 7 days, depending on the half-life of the drug.

magnesium trisalicylate (Trilisate), ibuprofen, naproxen, and indomethacin. Those available as a rectal suppository include aspirin, acetaminophen, and indomethacin.

Acetaminophen is the most commonly used analgesic in children. Although acetaminophen elimination in neonates is significantly slower than in adults, it need not be withheld from newborns because of concern about hepatic toxicity. The immaturity of hepatic metabolism reduces the production of toxic metabolites and may diminish the risk of toxicity (Berde, Kain, 1996). Reportedly, acetaminophen has a high therapeutic ratio in children and adolescents, meaning that it is very safe (Rumack, 1978). The likelihood of renal and hepatic damage is minimal (except in the case of overdose). In children, 75 to 90 mg/kg per 24 hours is generally accepted as the safe upper limit of acetaminophen (Penna, Dawson, Penna, 1993; Yaster, Krane, Kaplan et al., 1997).

Rectal absorption of acetaminophen is poor compared with oral, and doses of 35 mg/kg every 4 hours are recommended by some (Rusy, Houck, Sullivan et al., 1995). Others suggest a loading dose of 25 to 40 mg/kg followed by 10 to 15 mg/kg every 4 hours (Yaster, Krane, Kaplan et al., 1997).

Aspirin and other salicylates are avoided in young children, especially those with varicella infections or influenza-like illness because aspirin is associated with an increased risk of Reye's syndrome developing (Yaster, Krane, Kaplan et al., 1997). However, another fairly common concern, aspirin-induced asthma, is rare in children (Merry, Power, 1995).

Findings from several studies have demonstrated the effectiveness of nonopioids for different types of pain in children. The usefulness of acetaminophen, alone or in combination with an opioid, is illustrated in a study of 395 acutely burned children (from infancy through adolescence) (Meyer, Nichols, Cortiella et al., 1997). Doses of 10 to 15 mg/kg per 4 hours were used for control of postburn background pain. Although assessment of children younger than 3 years is difficult, acetaminophen alone appeared to be sufficient for relief of background pain in 74% of this age group. For children older than 3 years, acetaminophen alone was sufficient in only about one third of the children. Scheduled doses of morphine were added when acetaminophen alone was insufficient.

In a study of children aged 4 to 15 years, with migraine, a single dose of either acetaminophen (15 mg/kg orally) or ibuprofen (10 mg/kg orally) was often effective in reducing pain within 2 hours of administration. However, pain reduction was twice as likely with ibuprofen as acetaminophen (H"am"al"ainen, Hoppu, Valkeila et al., 1997).

Ibuprofen at doses of 4 to 8 mg/kg per dose every 6 hours has been used by some clinicians to relieve chronic pain in children, such as arthritis, and was found to be safe (Berde, Kain, 1996). Hepatic and renal dysfunction are rare with chronic use, but children should be appropriately monitored with complete blood counts, hepatic and renal function tests, and urinalysis twice yearly.

As with adults, the use of nonopioids for postoperative pain appears to decrease the opioid dose required. However, nonopioids do not eliminate the need for opioids. A study of the effectiveness of rectal ibuprofen as preemptive analgesia in children aged 1 to 4 years undergoing elective surgery showed that ibuprofen compared with placebo provided superior pain relief during the first hour after surgery and significantly reduced the need for morphine during the first 24 hours (Kokki, Hendolin, Maunuksela et al., 1994). Blood loss was negligible and side

● ● ● ● ○
TABLE 5.5

NONOPIOID DOSING RECOMMENDATIONS FOR CHILDREN

Drug Generic (Brand)	Single Dose (mg/kg)	Dosing Interval	Maximum Dose (mg/kg/day)
Acetaminophen (e.g., Tylenol)	10-15 PO	q4h	60-90
	35-40 rectal 1st dose, then 20	q4h	Unknown
Aspirin	10-15 PO	q4h	60
Choline magnesium trisalicylate (Trilisate)	25 PO	q12h	50
Ibuprofen (e.g., Motrin)	5-10 PO	q6-8h	40
Indomethacin (Indocin)	0.5-1 IV, PO, rectal	q8h	3
Ketorolac (Toradol)	0.5 IV, IM	q6h	2
	Adolescents: 10 mg/PO dose	q6-8h	40 mg/day short term use only
Naproxen (Naprosyn)	5-8 PO	q12h	15

May be duplicated for use in clinical practice. From McCaffery M, Pasero C: *Pain: Clinical manual*, p. 143. Copyright © 1999, Mosby, Inc.

Information from Berde CB, Kain ZN: Pain management in infants and children. In Motoyama EK, Davis PJ, editors: *Smith's anesthesia for infants and children*, ed 6, pp 385-402, St. Louis, 1996, Mosby; Houck CS: The management of acute pain in the child. In Ashburn MA, Rice LJ, editors: *The management of pain*, pp 651-666, New York, 1998, Churchill Livingstone; Penna AC, Dawson KP, Penna CV: Is prescribing paracetamol `pro re nata' acceptable? *J Pediatr Child Hlth* 29:104-106, 1993; Yaster M, Krane EJ, Kaplan RF et al., editors: *Pediatric pain management and sedation handbook*, St. Louis, 1997, Mosby.

effects were mild. Doses of ibuprofen were 10 to 13 mg/kg rectally every 6 hours, beginning intraoperatively.

Parenteral ketorolac has been used postoperatively in children. In one children's hospital widespread use (3000 instances) resulted in only rare episodes of gastritis and nephropathy (Houck, 1998). The clinicians suggest that these risks may be reduced by limiting the dose to less than 0.5 mg/kg IV every 6 hours for no longer than 48 hours and avoiding children with hypovolemia or risk factors for gastritis.

Parents, of course, are the ones responsible for providing analgesics for children on an outpatient basis. Little is known about parents' attitudes toward using medication to treat children's pain. However, it appears that parents often have unwarranted fears about nonopioids. A survey of the attitudes of 298 mothers regarding use of acetaminophen in children ages 5 to 7 years of age revealed a surprising level of concern about tolerance and side effects from acetaminophen (Forward, Brown, McGrath, 1996). Undertreatment would be likely because more than one third of the mothers agreed that acetaminophen worked best if used as little as possible and that it should be saved for severe pain. Mothers with more positive attitudes were more likely to medicate than those with less positive attitudes. These findings suggest that education about tolerance and side effects might improve mothers' attitudes about acetaminophen and result in more willingness to medicate children for pain.

Unfortunately, preliminary research on the effect of giving parents a booklet about pain assessment and treatment improved attitudes but not drug administration. This may be partly related to the finding that less than 50% of the parents were told to give acetaminophen regularly after surgery (Chambers, Reid, McGrath et al., in press).

Need for minimal antipyretic effect

Occasionally, the antipyretic effect of NSAIDs is an undesirable side effect because it could mask an infection. In that case diflunisal (Dolobid) may be an alternative because it has minimal antipyretic effects (Insel, 1996). The beneficial effect of NSAID analgesia must be carefully weighed against the risk of masking an infection. Most infections can be detected by means other than a fever (e.g., visual inspection, increased pain, and elevated white blood cell count). Furthermore, short half-life NSAIDs or acetaminophen can be used, and a temperature reading may be obtained at the end of the drug's duration of action.

Hemophiliacs and others at high risk for bleeding

Choice of NSAIDs for patients with bleeding disorders, such as hemophilia, is limited because most interfere with platelet function and increase bleeding time. However, the exceptions are nabumetone (Relafen) and nonacetylated salicylates such as choline magnesium trisali-

cylate (Trilisate), magnesium salicylate (Arthriten, Backache), and salsalate (Disalcid). Compared with other NSAIDs, these are largely devoid of significant adverse effects associated with PG inhibition, such as gastric ulceration, inhibition of platelet function, and broncho-spasm (Abramson, 1991). They are preferred in patients who have a predilection for bleeding because they have less effect on platelet aggregation and no effect on bleeding time at the usual clinical doses (Blower, 1992; Danesh, Saniabadi, Russell et al., 1987; Estes, Kaplan, 1980; Insel, 1996).

Aspirin allergy/intolerance/hypersensivity

Aspirin intolerance and aspirin hypersensitivity are more acceptable terms than allergy because the exact mechanism underlying the phenomena is not known (Sunshine, Olson, 1994). Patients may erroneously report an allergy simply because they have experienced side effects such as heartburn or nausea after aspirin use. However, true aspirin intolerance or hypersensitivity involves far more serious symptoms.

Two subgroups of aspirin-sensitive patients have been reported. One subgroup develops a respiratory reaction with rhinitis, asthma, or nasal polyps. The other subgroup develops urticaria, wheals, angioedema, and hypotension. These effects occur within minutes to an hour after ingestion (Coyle, Cherny, Portenoy, 1995).

Patients who are sensitive to aspirin may also develop sensitivity to other NSAIDs (Coyle, Cherny, Portenoy, 1995). Such patients should be advised to use acetaminophen. Some patients who are allergic to aspirin may be able to tolerate nonacetylated salicylates such as choline magnesium trisalicylate (Trilisate) (Lipman, 1996). Trials of nonopioids other than aspirin should be carefully monitored. Obviously, patients with aspirin hypersensitivity should be warned about possible sensitivity to other NSAIDs and to read the labels of nonprescription products to detect "hidden" aspirin.

Perioperative NSAID Use
Effectiveness

Recent research has produced evidence of the possible benefit of NSAID administration perioperatively as part of ongoing multimodality, balanced analgesia. Ketorolac (Toradol) is often the NSAID used because it is the only one available parenterally in the United States. Overall, many (but not all) studies of thoracic, abdominal, and major orthopedic surgery have supported the use of NSAIDs as part of the analgesic regimen. Benefits have included improved analgesia, earlier recovery of GI function, reduced need for antiemetic therapy, and better preservation of respiratory function. Side effects have not been a major problem. Studies of NSAID use in minor or same-day surgery, such as oral surgery or minor gynecologic surgery, have been especially encouraging (Merry, Power, 1995).

Balanced analgesia may begin preoperatively and continue through the postoperative period. It usually includes three groups of analgesics: nonopioids, opioids, and local anesthetics. This combination allows doses of each to be lower, thereby producing fewer side effects and achieving comparable or greater analgesia than may be achieved with any single analgesic. Moreover, some studies show that when it is begun preoperatively, it reduces postoperative pain and improves surgical outcomes (Dahl, Rosenberg, Dirkes et al., 1990; Kehlet, 1994; Kehlet, Dahl, 1993; Woolf, Chong, 1993). Although the manufacturer does not recommend the use of ketorolac preoperatively, it has been used safely and effectively (Varrassi, Panella, Piroli et al., 1994). (See Chapter 6, pp. 174-175, for further information on preemptive analgesia.)

Opioid-naive patients being treated for severe pain with an opioid (the typical scenario for surgical patients) are at risk for life-threatening opioid-induced respiratory depression. The risk may be reduced by using a NSAID along with the opioid because the nonopioid has an opioid dose-sparing effect, allowing lower opioid doses without decreasing pain relief. Typically, studies of NSAID use along with IV patient-controlled analgesia (PCA) opioid have demonstrated about a 30% reduction in opioid use (Merry, Power, 1995).

Many NSAIDs have been examined for their effectiveness in relieving postoperative pain. Because the studies involve different drugs used under different conditions and at different doses, a comparison of effectiveness is not possible. Those that have been shown in some (but not necessarily all) studies to be effective for postoperative pain include indomethacin, ketorolac, diclofenac, ketoprofen, and naproxen (Alon, Niv, Varrassi et al., 1996; Dueholm, Forrest, Hjortso et al., 1989; McGlew, Angliss, Gee et al., 1991; Plummer, Owen, Ilsley et al., 1996). Ketorolac may be administered parenterally, but other NSAIDs may be administered rectally in patients who are unable to take oral medication.

Parenteral ketorolac usually is not sufficient as the sole agent for postoperative analgesia after certain procedures such as intraabdominal surgery (Cepeda, Vargas, Ortegon et al., 1995). When pain relief is not adequate with ketorolac alone, appropriate doses of opioids are indicated.

One approach to NSAID use in ambulatory surgery is to administer 15 mg of parenteral ketorolac intraoperatively, once again postoperatively, and discharge the patient with oral ibuprofen. Opioids are used as necessary in addition to the NSAIDs.

Oral doses of ketorolac are not nearly as effective as parenteral doses. Ketorolac, 10 mg orally, is approximately equianalgesic to ibuprofen, 400 mg (Forbes, Kehm, Godein et al., 1990). It is recommended only as a continuation of parenteral ketorolac. The maximum length of time on parenteral or oral ketorolac is 5 days.

Wound infiltration with ketorolac has shown promising results (Ben-David, Katz, Gaitini et al., 1995).

Adverse effects

Short-term use of NSAIDs is rarely associated with serious effects on the GI system, platelets, renal function, or bleeding processes (Alon, Niv, Varrassi et al., 1996; Dahl, Kehlet, 1991). However, perioperative NSAID use is contraindicated in patients with active or recent GI ulcers (Kehlet, Dahl, 1992). Acetaminophen may be an effective alternative (Alon, Niv, Varrassi et al., 1996).

Hematologic Effects

Obviously, the possibility of increased bleeding time is of special concern when NSAIDs are used for surgical pain. Aspirin has an irreversible effect on platelets and will increase bleeding time for up to 7 days after the last dose (i.e., until the damaged platelets are replaced by new ones). For that reason, aspirin therapy should be stopped 1 week or longer before surgery (Insel, 1996), and aspirin is not recommended for perioperative use. Those NSAIDs that have minimal or no effect on platelet aggregation and therefore may be preferable for preoperative use are choline magnesium trisalicylate (Trilisate), salsalate (Disalcid), and nabumetone (Relafen). With other NSAIDs, platelet function is restored as the drug is eliminated from the body. Several studies of NSAIDs, including diclofenac, indomethacin, and ketorolac, show increases in bleeding times that nevertheless remain within the normal range (Alon, Niv, Varrassi et al., 1996).

GI Bleeding and Bleeding at the Operative Site

Thus far, studies that use a variety of NSAIDs perioperatively suggest that blood loss is not significant in the postoperative period (Kenny, 1992; Lindgren, Djupso, 1985; Serpell, Thomson, 1989; Strom, Berlin, Kinman et al., 1996a; Taivainen, Hiller, Rosenberg et al., 1989). In a review article about NSAID use for postoperative pain, the authors conclude that "short-term treatment with nonsteroidal anti-inflammatory drugs, such as that utilized for postoperative pain management, is not associated with any clinically significant adverse events, but that their use should be carefully monitored in patients with preexisting risk factors" (Alon, Niv, Varrassi et al., 1996, p. 147).

Cumulative data from 15 studies with a total of 927 patients have also been reassuring about the adverse effects of the perioperative use of NSAIDs. Patients in these studies underwent a variety of surgical procedures, varying from herniotomy to abdominal surgery, and received NSAIDs perioperatively for 2 to 7 days. The NSAIDs were ketorolac, indomethacin, diclofenac, and piroxicam. Only one case of significant GI toxicity was identified. The authors conclude that less than 1 week of NSAID treatment causes superficial injury to the GI mucosa, but so far no evidence exists of an increased risk of serious GI complications. Also, the various NSAIDs studied showed no clinically important differences in the risk of serious GI side effects (Kehlet, Dahl, 1992).

Attention tends to center on the perioperative use of ketorolac because it is the only NSAID currently available parenterally in the United States. In a larger study involving 35 hospitals between 1991 and 1993, a total of 10,272 courses of parenteral ketorolac (9900 patients) were compared with 10,247 courses of a parenteral opioid (10,247 patients). Both ketorolac and opioids were used primarily for postoperative pain. Analysis of data showed relatively little difference in the risk of GI bleeding, operative site bleeding, and other adverse effects in patients receiving ketorolac versus those treated with opioids. As Table 5.6 shows, both groups had a very similar incidence of adverse events (Strom, Berlin, Kinman et al., 1996a).

Use of ketorolac in patients younger than 65 years at an average dose of 105 mg/day or lower for 5 or fewer days was not associated with a detectable increase in risks. Factors that increased the risk of bleeding in the ketorolac group were advanced age (65 years with significant increase at 75 years), higher doses (120 mg/day or more), and therapy lasting longer than 5 days. Because ketorolac has been shown to provide effective analgesia with doses as low as 10 mg, the authors recommend using the lowest dose needed to obtain the desired analgesic effect rather than following a specific regimen. The current commercially available dosage of 15 mg parenteral ketorolac given q6h would fulfill the criteria of keeping the dose at less than 105 mg/24 hr while providing potentially effective analgesia. Like opioids, ketorolac can be titrated to effect. An initial loading dose is not necessary and should be avoided. Elderly patients should be started and maintained on lower dosages than those recommended for younger patients (Strom, Berlin, Kinman et

al., 1996a). Overall, the recommendation for minimizing NSAID-induced side effects is to administer the lowest possible dose for the shortest period of time.

Nevertheless, the effect of NSAIDs on the degree of blood loss during surgery remains controversial (Alon, Niv, Varrassi et al., 1996). Some clinicians have raised concerns about ketorolac causing increased bleeding in tonsillectomies and other surgical procedures of the ear, nose, and throat. However, data analysis does not confirm that an increased risk from ketorolac in those undergoing surgery on mucosal surfaces (Strom Berlin, Kinman et al., 1996b).

When operative site bleeding occurs in a patient receiving ketorolac, it is tempting to blame the NSAID. Anecdotal reports of such events may lead the clinician to suspect that ketorolac is more dangerous than the studies indicate. Thus research helps contrast ones own clinical impressions with what actually happens when the problem is studied in much larger groups of patients.

In theory, increased bleeding at the surgical site is a possibility when ketorolac is used as a postoperative analgesic, but in clinical practice it does not appear to materialize. However, bleeding at the operative site is a serious potential side effect of ketorolac, and further research is needed to resolve this issue (Merry, Power, 1995; Thwaites, Nigus, Bouska et al., 1996).

Renal Effects

The effect of perioperative NSAID use on renal function is minimal and reversible on discontinuation of the NSAID (Nuutinen, Laitenen, Salomaki, 1993). In fact, the actual surgical procedure appears to be more closely linked to adverse renal effects than is the administration of NSAIDs (Kenny, 1992). However, volume depletion should be corrected before treatment with ketorolac. In patients with moderately elevated serum creatinine, the daily dose of ketorolac should be reduced by half and should not exceed 60 mg/day. Ketorolac is contraindi-

●●●●○

TABLE 5.6 **Occurrence of Adverse Effects in Surgical Patients Treated With Parenteral Ketorolac Versus Those Treated With Opioids and No Ketorolac**

	PATIENTS WHO HAD ADVERSE EFFECTS (%)	
ADVERSE EFFECTS	KETOROLAC-TREATED PATIENTS (N = 9900)	OPIOID-TREATED PATIENTS; NO KETOROLAC: (N = 10,247)
GI bleeding		
Overall incidence (%)	4.0	3.6
Clinically serious (%)	1.3	1.0
Operative site bleeding		
Overall incidence (%)	39.6	38.6
Clinically significant (%)	1.5	1.8
Acute renal failure (%)	0.6	0.8
Allergic reactions (%)	4.6	5.5

May be duplicated for use in clinical practice. From McCaffery M, Pasero C: *Pain: Clinical manual*, p. 146. Copyright © 1999, Mosby, Inc.
Modified from Strom BL, Berlin JA, Kinman JL et al.: Parenteral ketorolac and risk of gastrointestinal and operative site bleeding, *JAMA* 275:376-382, 1996.

cated in patients with advanced renal impairment and in those at risk for renal failure owing to volume depletion (Physicians' Desk Reference, 1997).

Bone Formation

Another concern is related to the orthopedic patient and bone formation. NSAIDs, particularly indomethacin, have been used to inhibit heterotopic bone formation. In one study of patients with total hip arthroplasty, an increase in problems such as loosening of cementless hip prostheses did not appear to be increased by NSAID therapy (Kjaersgaard-Andersen, Schmidt, 1991). The nonunion rate after spinal fusion may increase with increasing doses of ketorolac (Glassman, Rose, Dimar et al., 1998).

Reducing adverse effects

One means of reducing adverse effects of NSAIDs is to reduce the dose. Initially the recommended parenteral dosing for ketorolac postoperatively was up to 60 mg as a loading dose followed by up to 30 mg q6h. A loading dose is no longer recommended. For patients younger than 65 years, 30 mg ketorolac every 6 hours is recommended, and the total daily dose should not exceed 120 mg. Dose recommendations for older patients and those weighing less than 50 kg (110 lb) is 15 mg every 6 hours with a daily maximum dose of 60 mg. IV PCA administration of ketorolac appears to be safe, but data do not show that it is any more effective than intermittent dosing (Cepeda, Vargas, Ortegon et al., 1995). The recommended total daily dose of oral ketorolac is 40 mg, significantly lower than the parenteral dose.

For many patients, parenteral doses of 10 to 15 mg of ketorolac may provide significant pain relief. In a study of postoperative pain relief ketorolac, 15 mg q6h, was almost as effective as 30 mg q6h, indicating that a relatively low dose of ketorolac may be effective, reducing the risk of dose-related side effects (Sevarino, Sinatra, Paige et al., 1992). Another study confirmed that, for some patients, lower doses of parenteral ketorolac (e.g., an average of 12 mg q6h) are effective and cause no adverse GI effects (Cepeda, Vargas, Ortegon et al., 1995).

To reduce the risk of renal failure, volume depletion must be corrected before treatment with ketorolac. In patients with moderately elevated serum creatinine, the daily dose of ketorolac should be reduced by half and should not exceed 60 mg/day. Ketorolac is contraindicated in patients with advanced renal impairment and those at risk for renal failure caused by volume depletion *(Physicians' Desk Reference,* 1997).

Although potential benefits to the use of NSAIDs for analgesia in surgical patients exist, serious concerns also exist. The use of a NSAID may allow a lower opioid dose and thereby reduce opioid-related side effects, but this must be balanced against potential adverse effects such as GI bleeding and operative site bleeding. Cost per dose of the NSAID, particularly parenteral ketorolac,

versus an opioid is also a consideration, although less of one as generic equivalents of ketorolac become available. Higher cost of the NSAID must be balanced against potential savings, such as decreased length of stay (Gillis, Brogden, 1997). Further research is necessary to resolve issues of safety and effectiveness. Box 5.4 summarizes

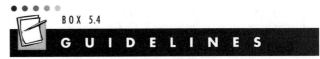

BOX 5.4

GUIDELINES

USE OF KETOROLAC FOR ANALGESIA IN THE SURGICAL PATIENT

Potential Benefits
- Opioid dose sparing. Lower doses of opioids may be used without compromising analgesia. This reduces opioid-induced side effects:
  - ↓ Sedation
  - ↓ Constipation
  - ↓ Respiratory depression
  - ↓ Nausea and vomiting
  - ↓ Duration of postoperative ileus
- Earlier mobilization
- Decreased length of stay

Potential Adverse Events
- GI bleeding
- Operative site bleeding
  NOTE: The incidence of GI bleeding and operative site bleeding in patients receiving ketorolac is only slightly higher than the incidence in patients receiving opioids and no ketorolac.
- Acute renal failure
- Allergic reactions

Prevention of Adverse Effects
- Use low doses of 105 mg/day or less (customary dosing of 30 mg q6h is slightly higher; alternatives are 30 mg q8h or 15 mg q6h).
- Do not use a loading dose.
- Use for 5 days or less.
- Correct volume depletion before use.
- Use less than 105 mg/day and shorter duration of treatment in patients 65 years or older (e.g., ketorolac, 10 mg IV q6h or q8h for one day only).
- Use no more than 60 mg/day in patients with moderately elevated serum creatinine.
- Do not use in patients with advanced renal impairment.
- Do not use in patients with active or recent GI ulcers.

May be duplicated for use in clinical practice. From McCaffery M, Pasero C: *Pain: Clinical manual,* p. 147. Copyright © 1999, Mosby, Inc.

Information from Cepeda MS, Vargas L, Ortegon G et al.: Comparative analgesic efficacy of patient-controlled analgesia with ketorolac versus morphine after elective intraabdominal operations, *Anesth Analg* 80:1150-1153, 1995; Sevarino FB, Sinatra RS, Paige D et al.: The efficacy of intramuscular ketorolac in combination with intravenous PCA morphine for postoperative pain relief, *J Clin Anesth* 4:285-288, 1992; Strom BL, Berlin JA, Kinman JL et al.: Parenteral ketorolac and risk of gastro-intestinal and operative site bleeding, *JAMA* 275:376-382, 1996.

various clinical considerations when ketorolac is used for analgesia in the surgical patient.

NONPRESCRIPTION NONOPIOIDS

Judging from the rows of nonprescription analgesics found in a well-stocked pharmacy, millions of Americans are self-medicating with nonopioids to treat their aches and pains. As a group, these analgesics are marketed to the public as "pain relievers." Those available without a prescription (over-the-counter, OTC) include many formulations and brands of aspirin and acetaminophen as well as ibuprofen, naproxen, and ketoprofen (Tables 5.7,

5.8, 5.9). More NSAIDs are likely to become available as OTC analgesics. Clinicians need to be familiar with doses and ingredients of those used by the individual patient. Clinicians should also know that sometimes a nonprescription NSAID (e.g., ibuprofen) will be less expensive than the same dose by prescription.

As the tables reveal, many nonprescription pain relievers are merely different doses of either acetaminophen or aspirin. Quite a few contain both aspirin and acetaminophen. The combination of acetaminophen and aspirin has raised concern about enhanced renal toxicity, and some find this combination questionable (Sunshine,

TABLE 5.7

NONPRESCRIPTION ANALGESICS: ORAL ACETAMINOPHEN, ASPIRIN, AND COMBINATION ANALGESICS (SELECTED BRANDS FOR ADULTS AND CHILDREN)

ACETAMINOPHEN ONLY, ORAL

Brand Name	Dose of Acetaminophen	Dosage Form
Acetaminophen Oral Solution	160 mg/5 ml	Solution (flavors: cherry AL*; lime, some alcohol)
Alka-Seltzer	500 mg	Caplet
Anacin Aspirin Free Maximum Strength	500 mg	Tablet
APAP Extra Strength	500 mg	Tablet, caplet
APAP, Children's	80 mg/2.5 ml	Elixir AL, suspension AL
APAP, Children's	80 mg	Chewable tablet
APAP Infant's	80 mg/0.8 ml	Drops AL
Arthritis Foundation Aspirin Free	500 mg	Caplet
Aspirin Free Pain Relief	325 mg, 500 mg	Tablet caplet
Bromo-Seltzer	325 mg/capful	Granular effervescent
Excedrin Aspirin Free	500 mg	Caplet, geltab
Panadol Junior Strength	80 mg	Caplet
Panadol Maximum Strength	500 mg	Caplet, tablet
Panadol, Children's	32 mg/ml	Liquid, fruit flavor AL
Panadol, Children's	80 mg	Chewable tablet, fruit flavor
Panadol, Infants's	80 mg/0.8 ml	Drops, fruit flavor AL
Percogesic Coated	325 mg	Tablet
Stanback AF Extra-Strength	950 mg	Powder
Tempra 1	80 mg/0.8 ml	Drops, grape flavor AL
Tempra 2	160 mg/5 ml	Syrup, grape flavor AL
Tempra 3	80 mg, 160 mg	Chewable tablet, grape flavor
Tylenol Extended Relief	650 mg	Timed-release caplet
Tylenol Extra Strength	500 mg	Caplet, gelcap, geltab, tablet
Tylenol Extra Strength Adult	166.7 mg/5 ml	Liquid (alcohol 7%)
Tylenol Extra Strength Headache Plus	500 mg	Caplet
Tylenol Regular Strength	325 mg	Caplet, tablet

(Tylenol brand is also available in a variety of doses for children and infants as chewable tablets [grape or fruit flavor], suspension, elixir, and drops.)

ASPIRIN ONLY, ORAL

Brand Name	Dose of Aspirin	Dosage Form
Alka-Seltzer Extra Strength	500 mg	Effervescent tablet (588 mg sodium)
Alka-Seltzer Original	325 mg	Effervescent tablet (567 mg sodium)
Arthritis Foundation Safety Coated Aspirin	500 mg	Tablet

May be duplicated for use in clinical practice. As appears in McCaffery M, Pasero C: *Pain: Clinical manual*, pp. 148-149, 1999, Mosby, Inc.

Olson, 1994). Other common ingredients in nonprescription pain relievers are buffering agents, caffeine, and antihistamines.

Buffered Aspirin

Buffered aspirin has been compared with nonbuffered aspirin, and endoscopic evaluation shows no difference in the amount of gastric damage produced by either. Enteric-coated aspirin may be more effective in reducing the amount of local gastric irritation produced by aspirin (Lipman, 1996). However, a multicenter case-control study suggests that when clinicians recommend enteric-

coated or buffered aspirin, they should not assume that these are any safer than plain aspirin with respect to protecting the patient from a major upper GI bleeding episode (Kelly, Kaufman, Jurgelon et al., 1996).

Caffeine

Caffeine appears to augment the analgesia of most nonopioids. In studies involving more than 10,000 patients with pain, results unequivocally attest to the analgesic efficacy of combining caffeine with either acetaminophen or aspirin. When these analgesics were given without caffeine, the doses had to be about 40% larger to

● ● ● ● ●
TABLE 5.7—cont'd

NONPRESCRIPTION ANALGESICS: ORAL ACETAMINOPHEN, ASPIRIN, AND COMBINATION ANALGESICS (SELECTED BRANDS FOR ADULTS AND CHILDREN)

ASPIRIN ONLY, ORAL—cont'd

Brand Name	Dose of Aspirin	Dosage Form
Arthritis Pain Formula	500 mg	Caplet
Ascriptin Arthritis Pain	325 mg	Caplet
Ascriptin Maximum Strength	500 mg	Caplet
Ascriptin Regular Strength	325 mg	Tablet
Aspergum, Cherry or Orange	227 mg	Gum
Aspirin, Enteric Coated	650 mg	Tablet

COMBINATION ANALGESIC BRANDS

Brand Name	Dose of Acetaminophen	Dose of Aspirin	Other Analgesic Ingredients/Dose	Dosage Form
Arthriten	250 mg		Magnesium salicylate, 250 mg, caffeine, 32.5 mg	Tablet
Bayer Select Aspirin-Free Headache	500 mg		Caffeine, 65 mg	Caplet
Excedrin Extra Strength	250 mg	250 mg	Caffeine, 65 mg	Caplet, tablet, geltab
Anacin		400 mg	Caffeine, 32 mg	Tablet, caplet
Anacin Maximum Strength		500 mg	Caffeine, 32 mg	Tablet
BC		650 mg	Caffeine, 32 mg	Powder
BC		325 mg	Caffeine, 16 mg	Tablet
BC Arthritis Strength		742 mg	Caffeine, 36 mg	Powder
Cope		421 mg	Caffeine, 32 mg	Tablet
Goody's Extra Strength	130 mg	260 mg	Caffeine, 16.25 mg	Tablet
Goody's Extra Strength Headache	260 mg	520 mg	Caffeine, 32.5 mg	Powder
Rid-a-Pain with Codeine	97.2 mg	226.8 mg	Caffeine, 32.4 mg, codeine, 1 mg	Tablet
Stanback, Original Formula		650 mg	Caffeine, 32 mg, salicylamide, 200 mg	Powder
Vanquish	194 mg	227 mg	Caffeine, 35 mg	Caplet

May be duplicated for use in clinical practice. As appears in McCaffery M, Pasero C: *Pain: Clinical manual*, pp. 148-149, 1999, Mosby, Inc.

*AL, alcohol-free liquids.

From *Nonprescription products: Formulations & features '96-97*, ed 11, Washington, DC, 1996, American Pharmaceutical Association.

NONPRESCRIPTION ANALGESICS: RECTAL SUPPOSITORIES FOR ADULTS AND CHILDREN

Acetaminophen Rectal Suppositories

BRAND NAME	DOSE OF ACETAMINOPHEN
Acephen	120 mg, 325 mg, 650 mg
Acetaminophen Uniserts	120 mg, 325 mg, 650 mg
APAP	650 mg
APAP, Pediatric	120 mg
Feverall Adult Strength	650 mg
Feverall Junior Strength	325 mg
Feverall, Children's	120 mg
Feverall, Infant's	80 mg
Neopap	125 mg

Aspirin Rectal Suppositories

BRAND NAME	DOSE OF ASPIRIN
Aspirin	120 mg
Aspirin	125 mg, 300 mg, 600 mg

May be duplicated for use in clinical practice. As appears in McCaffery M, Pasero C: *Pain: Clinical manual,* p. 150, 1999, Mosby, Inc.

From *Nonprescription products: Formulations & features '96-97,* ed 11, Washington DC, 1996, American Pharmaceutical Association.

obtain the same degree of pain relief as was obtained when the analgesics were given in combination with caffeine. For each 650 to 1000 mg dose of aspirin or acetaminophen, the recommended additional dose of caffeine is 100 to 200 mg. On a long-term basis, adding caffeine to each 650 mg daily dose of aspirin or acetaminophen is believed by some to be safer than repeatedly giving larger doses without caffeine (Beaver, 1984; Laska, Sunshine, Mueller et al., 1984.) See Table 5.10 for the caffeine content of common beverages.

Other research confirms these findings. In six studies totaling 2400 patients with moderate to severe headache pain, caffeine-containing analgesics were significantly superior to placebo and to 1000 mg acetaminophen. The caffeine-containing analgesics were of two types: (1) 500 mg acetaminophen, 500 mg aspirin, and 130 mg caffeine; and (2) 1000 mg acetaminophen and 130 mg caffeine (Migliardi, Armenia, Freedman et al., 1994).

A double-blind study compared a combination of caffeine and ibuprofen with plain ibuprofen for relief of postoperative dental pain. A single dose of ibuprofen, 100 mg or 200 mg, with 100 mg caffeine was more than twice as effective as ibuprofen alone (Forbes, Beaver, Jones et al., 1991).

Research has not confirmed the optimal dose of caffeine for increasing the analgesia of nonopioids, but the minimal effective dose appears to be 65 mg. The addition of 100 to 200 mg of caffeine per dose of nonopioid seems well tolerated by most adults (Beaver, 1984). However, some adults are very sensitive to caffeine and respond to even small doses with tremors, increased heart rate, and insomnia.

An inexpensive way to reap the benefits of a caffeine/nonopioid combination is to avoid commercially compounded preparations and simply buy generic forms of the ingredients separately (e.g., aspirin and acetaminophen) and ordinary caffeine-containing beverages as a source of the dose of caffeine required for enhanced analgesia. Table 5.10 lists common dietary sources of caffeine. Stimulant products also often contain a sufficient amount of caffeine (e.g., No-Doz has 100 mg caffeine).

Despite negative publicity about caffeine as a food additive, it is generally a safe drug (Laska, Sunshine, Mueller et al., 1984). Because caffeine is a CNS stimulant, the effect of caffeine on the cardiovascular system has been a concern. Most research confirms that small doses of caffeine (e.g., 200 mg or less [the amount required to augment nonopioid analgesia]) in normal subjects and in subjects with heart disease did not significantly affect heart rate; blood pressure; and/or cardiac rhythm (Schneider, 1987). Allowance should be made for the possibility that caffeine users and nonusers react differently.

Chocolate lovers may be dismayed to learn that most chocolate contains very little caffeine (e.g., 4 to 5 mg). However, 1 ounce of dark, semisweet chocolate contains 20 mg, requiring about 5 ounces to obtain the desired analgesic effect (Hallal, 1986).

Antihistamines

Research has also demonstrated enhanced analgesia when various antihistamines are combined with nonopioids. The combination of phenyltoloxamine citrate, 60 mg, and acetaminophen, 650 mg, has been found to be more effective than acetaminophen alone (Lipman, 1996, Sunshine, Zighelbolm, Sorrentino et al., 1989). We were unable to locate a nonprescription analgesic with this combination. However, many diet pills and cold remedies contain phenyltoloxamine. Thus it is possible to formulate one's own nonprescription combination.

Another antihistamine that enhances analgesia of nonopioids is orphenadrine (Lipman, 1996). It is available by prescription only (e.g., Norgesic [orphenadrine, 25 mg; aspirin, 385 mg; caffeine, 30 mg]).

OVERDOSE

Aspirin and acetaminophen are widely used as self-medication for pain relief, and many products marketed for other conditions such as cold and flu (e.g., Actifed Cold & Sinus tablets) contain one or more of these nonopioids. Patient/family teaching about these products should warn the patient about the maximum rec-

TABLE 5.9

NONPRESCRIPTION NSAIDS OTHER THAN ASPIRIN (SELECTED BRANDS)			
Brand Name	Ingredient	Dose	Dosage Form
Actron	Ketoprofen	12.5 mg	Caplet, tablet
Advil	Ibuprofen	200 mg	Caplet, tablet, gelcap
Aleve	Naproxen sodium	220 mg	Caplet, tablet
Arthropan	Choline salicylate	174 mg	Liquid
Backache from the makers of Nuprin	Magnesium salicylate tetrahydrate	580 mg	Caplet
Doan's Regular Strength	Magnesium salicylate tetrahydrate	377 mg	Tablet
Midol IB Cramp Relief	Ibuprofen	200 mg	Tablet
Motrin IB	Ibuprofen	200 mg	Caplet, tablet, gelcap
Motrin, Children's	Ibuprofen	100 mg/5 ml	Suspension
Nuprin	Ibuprofen	200 mg	Caplet, tablet
Orudis KT	Ketoprofen	12.5 mg	Caplet, tablet

May be duplicated for use in clinical practice. As appears in McCaffery M, Pasero C: *Pain: Clinical manual,* p. 151, 1999, Mosby, Inc.
From *Nonprescription products: Formulations & features '96-97,* ed 11, Washington, DC, 1996, American Pharmaceutical Association.

TABLE 5.10

BEVERAGES CONTAINING CAFFEINE		
	Approximate Amounts of Caffeine	
Beverages	Range (mg)	Average (mg)
Coffee (brewed) 1 cup*	40–180	100
Coffee (instant) 1 cup	30–120	65
Coffee (decaffeinated) 1 cup	2–5	3
Tea 1 cup	20–110	50
Soft drinks 12 oz.	38–54	45

May be duplicated for use in clinical practice. As appears in McCaffery M, Pasero C: *Pain: Clinical manual,* p. 151, 1999, Mosby, Inc.
*1 cup = 5 oz
From Hallal JC: Caffeine, *Am J Nurs* 86:422-425, 1986.

Clinical Relevance of Information Presented in Table 5.10:
The analgesia of a dose of nonopioid may be augmented by 65 to 200 mg of caffeine. The ideal caffeine dose has not been established.

ommended doses and the signs of overdose and alert them to sources of "hidden" aspirin and acetaminophen.

Acetaminophen

Acetaminophen toxicity is also generally a result of taking more than the recommended dose. Acute overdose is most likely to occur in children and, unless observed by an adult, may go undetected because only mild symptoms occur for the first day or two. Early symptoms include nausea, vomiting, drowsiness, confusion, and abdominal pain. First aid for acute overdose is to induce vomiting (Lipman, 1996). The antidote for acute over-

dose is acetylcysteine (Mucomyst, Mucosol) given orally within the first 36 hours after ingestion. The earlier it is given the more effective it is (Insel, 1996).

Clinical manifestations of hepatotoxicity begin 2 to 4 days after ingestion. At this time, jaundice occurs and laboratory findings reveal increased plasma bilirubin and plasma transaminases and prolonged prothrombin time. If the dose is not fatal, liver damage is reversible over a period of weeks or months. If the dose is fatal, death usually occurs from hepatic necrosis. In adults a single dose of 10 to 15 g of acetaminophen may result in toxicity. Acetaminophen in a single dose of 25 g or more can be fatal (Flower, Moncada, Vane, 1985). A 25 g dose translates into approximately 77 regular strength tablets (325 mg each) or 50 extra strength tablets (500 mg each).

Chronic overdose of acetaminophen results in hepatotoxicity and may occur with doses as low as 4 to 10 g/day. Patients at increased risk are those who do not eat regularly (fasting), who regularly consume alcohol, and those with preexisting liver disease who are taking other potentially hepatotoxic drugs (Lipman, 1996).

Aspirin and Other Salicylates

Toxicity related to aspirin and other salicylates is also generally a result of taking higher than recommended doses (i.e., overdosing). Symptoms of toxicity from chronic use include headache, dizziness, ringing in the ears, difficulty hearing, dim vision, confusion, drowsiness, and sweating. Toxicity may go undetected because some of these symptoms mimic the disease being treated. All are reversible by lowering the dose (Lipman, 1996).

If salicylate toxicity is acute, symptoms may include lethargy, ringing in the ears, nausea and vomiting, and convulsions. Children are prone to high fever developing. Initial emergency treatment usually consists of inducing vomiting with ipecac syrup (Lipman, 1996).

Other NSAIDs

An overdose of a proprionic acid derivative, such as ibuprofen, ketoprofen, or naproxen, usually produces minimal symptoms of toxicity and is rarely fatal. Common symptoms of overdose include nausea, vomiting, and abdominal pain, but many patients are asymptomatic. Massive doses appear to be required to produce serious toxicity. First aid treatment is to induce vomiting. Overdose of other NSAIDs appears to be similar to that seen with the proprionic acid derivatives (Insel, 1996).

PATIENT/FAMILY TEACHING TOOLS

Use of acetaminophen and NSAIDs for pain relief is usually on an outpatient basis. Patients are often discharged from the hospital with nonopioids, and they are frequently prescribed or recommended to patients during an office or clinic visit. Because many are available without a prescription, the patient may decide independently to use them.

NSAIDs are more likely than acetaminophen to cause side effects, some of them quite serious. NSAIDs are also likely to be dosed on a regularly daily schedule. Patients and families need information to help them adhere to the plan of treatment and to do so safely. The usual patient teaching about drug name, dose, timing, and side effects is important. Written information may be particularly helpful because it reminds the patient of what was said. It can be shared with interested family members and any health care providers the patient may see.

Boxes 5.5 and 5.6 are patient teaching tools specific to a particular drug. One is for the NSAID ibuprofen and the other for the NSAID choline magnesium trisalicylate. This same format may be used to develop information on other frequently used NSAIDs. Form 5.1, *A*, may be used for all patients taking NSAIDs and may be individualized for the specific drug and patient. Form 5.1, *B*, provides a completed example.

● ● ● ● ●
BOX 5.5

PATIENT MEDICATION INFORMATION

Ibuprofen (generic name)

BRAND NAMES: Advil, Motrin, Nuprin, Rufen, Ibu-Tab, Ibupren

TYPE OF PAIN MEDICINE: Nonsteroidal antiinflammatory drug (NSAID), nonopiod (not a narcotic)

DESCRIPTION:
Ibuprofen comes in regular tablets, film-coated tablets, and liquids.
Nonprescription strength—200 mg.
Prescription strength tablets—300 mg, 400 mg, 600 mg, 800 mg.
Nonprescription strength liquid—100 mg/teaspoon (5 ml).

USES:
Relieves mild to moderate pain.
Decreases inflammation.
Reduces fevers.
Treats bone pain and symptoms of arthritis.

DOSAGE AND ADMINISTRATION:
- Take only as directed.
- Take this medicine with food, milk, or an antacid.
- May be taken with other pain medicines as directed by your doctor.
- Be sure to tell your doctor if you are taking aspirin, steroids, or other antiinflammatory medicines.
- If you miss a dose of your medicine, take it as soon as possible. If it is almost time for the next dose, skip the missed dose. Do not take two doses at one time to make up for your missed dose.

POSSIBLE SIDE EFFECTS: Call your doctor or nurse if these happen to you.
- Stomach irritation (indigestion): This can usually be prevented by taking ibuprofen with food, milk, or an antacid.
- Nausea and vomiting: This can be controlled with other medicines.
- Change in color of bowel movement.
- Ringing sound in your ears.

PRECAUTIONS:
- Discuss the use of this medicine with your doctor or nurse. This medicine can possibly interact with other medicines you are taking.
- Do not take aspirin, steroids, or other antiinflammatory medicines unless you discuss it with your doctor. Always tell your doctor what other medicines you are taking.
- If you are going to have surgery, ask your doctor if you need to stop this medicine before surgery.
- Avoid alcohol while taking ibuprofen. Alcohol combined with ibuprofen can increase your risk of stomach irritation.
- Notify your doctor or nurse if pain increases or if you do not get pain relief.

May be duplicated for use in clinical practice. As appears in McCaffery M, Pasero C: *Pain: Clinical manual*, pp. 153-154, 1999, Mosby, Inc. *Continued.*

● ● ● ● ●
BOX 5.5—cont'd

PATIENT MEDICATION INFORMATION—cont'd

Ibuprofen (generic name)

BRAND NAMES: Advil, Motrin, Nuprin, Rufen, Ibu-Tab, Ibupren

STOPPING MEDICATIONS: Do not suddenly stop taking your medicine. Call your doctor or nurse before you stop taking your medicine.

REMEMBER!
- Don't run out of medicine.
- Keep count of your pills.
- Buy more medicine a few days before you run out.
- If your ibuprofen is by prescription, get it refilled or phoned into your pharmacy or drug store a few days before you run out of medicine.

COMMENTS:

WARNING: Keep this and all medicines out of the reach of children!

May be duplicated for use in clinical practice. As appears in McCaffery M, Pasero C: *Pain: Clinical manual,* pp. 153-154, 1999, Mosby, Inc. Modified from Fox Chase Cancer Center/Pain Management, Philadelphia, 1997.

PATIENT MEDICATION INFORMATION

Choline Magnesium Trisalicylate (generic name)

BRAND NAME: Trilisate

TYPE OF PAIN MEDICINE: Nonsteroidal antiinflammatory drug (NSAID), nonopiod (not a narcotic)

DESCRIPTION:
Trilisate comes as a tablet and a liquid.
Tablets are scored (a line down the center) and come in three strengths:
   500 mg—pale pink
   750 mg—white
   1000 mg—red
Liquid (cherry flavored)—500 mg/teaspoon (5 ml).
Generics (nonbrand names)—may look different.

USES:
Relieves mild to moderate pain.
Decreases inflammation.
Reduces fevers.
Treats bone pain and symptoms of arthritis.

DOSAGE AND ADMINISTRATION:
- Take only as directed.
- Usually taken twice a day, sometimes taken three times a day.
- Take this medicine with food, milk, or an antacid.
- May be taken with other pain medicines as directed by your doctor.
- Be sure to tell your doctor if you are taking aspirin, steroids, or other antiinflammatory medicines.
- If you miss a dose of your medicine, take it as soon as possible. If it is almost time for the next dose, skip the missed dose. Do not take two doses at one time to make up for your missed dose.
- Trilisate is best used on a regular basis for chronic pain.

POSSIBLE SIDE EFFECTS: Call your doctor or nurse if these happen to you.
- Stomach irritation (indigestion): This can usually be prevented by taking Trilisate with food, milk, or an antacid.
- Nausea and vomiting: This can be controlled with other medicines.
- Ringing sound in your ears.

PRECAUTIONS:
- Do not take aspirin, steroids, or other antiinflammatory medicines unless you discuss it with your doctor. Always tell your doctor what other medicines you are taking.
- Avoid alcohol while taking Trilisate. Alcohol combined with Trilisate can increase your risk of stomach irritation.
- Notify your doctor or nurse if pain increases or if you do not get pain relief.

May be duplicated for use in clinical practice. As appears in McCaffery M, Pasero C: *Pain: Clinical manual,* pp. 155-156, 1999, Mosby, Inc.   *Continued.*

PATIENT MEDICATION INFORMATION—cont'd

Choline Magnesium Trisalicylate (generic name)

BRAND NAME: Trilisate

STOPPING MEDICATIONS: Do not suddenly stop taking your medicine. Call your doctor or nurse before you stop taking your medicine.

REMEMBER!
- Don't run out of medicine.
- Keep count of your pills.
- Get your prescription refilled by or phoned into your pharmacy or drug store a few days before you run out of medicine

COMMENTS:

WARNING: Keep this and all medicines out of the reach of children!

May be duplicated for use in clinical practice. As appears in McCaffery M, Pasero C: *Pain: Clinical manual,* pp. 155-156, 1999, Mosby, Inc.
Modified from Fox Chase Cancer Center/Pain Management, Philadelphia, 1997.

FORM 5.1A **Patient/Family Information: Using Your Nonsteroidal Antiinflammatory Drug (NSAID)**

To _____   Date _____
                        (patient's name)

Name of pain medicine: _____

Description: _____

Other names: _____

Why you are receiving this medicine: _____

Dose: _____   (number of pills per dose _____)

How often: _____

    _____ Every day without skipping a dose.

    _____ When you need it.

Get more medicine before you run out. To obtain more medicine:

    _____ Pharmacy can refill this prescription _____ time(s).

    _____ Call your doctor.

    _____ Make an appointment with your doctor.

    _____ You may obtain this medicine without a prescription.

Heartburn and stomach discomfort are common side effects. To avoid stomach upset or stomach injury (ulcer):

- Never take a medication dose on an empty stomach or with an alcoholic beverage.
- Take each dose of medicine with food or at least a full glass of water.
- An antacid may be helpful if you have indigestion.
- Do not take any other NSAID or aspirin-like drug. However, it is safe to take a daily dose of aspirin to prevent a heart attack, occasional doses of acetaminophen, and opioid (narcotic) pain medicine.
- Watch for nonprescription medicines with "hidden aspirin," such as some cold remedies or sinus medications. Read the labels on all nonprescription medications.

Other side effects that may occur are:

- Nausea and vomiting (If it looks like coffee grounds or is bloody, stop the medicine and report this side effect to your doctor or nurse at once.)
- Breathing problems (Stop the medicine and report this side effect to your doctor or nurse at once.)
- Dark stool (Stop the medicine and report this side effect to your doctor or nurse at once.)
- Headache
- Drowsiness
- Dizziness
- Ringing in the ears
- Blurred vision
- Swelling of the ankles
- Diarrhea or constipation
- Rash

Report all side effects to your doctor or nurse. You may need other medicines to control the side effects, or you may need a different pain medicine.

Your pain rating scale is: _____

If your pain is _____ after _____ days, notify your doctor or nurse.

If you have any questions or problems, contact:

Nurse: _____   Phone: _____

Doctor: _____   Phone: _____

Office hours: _____

Please report to your nurse or doctor by telephone: _____

Your next appointment is: _____

FORM 5.1B Patient/Family Information: Using Your Nonsteroidal Antiinflammatory Drug (NSAID)

To _____ *Ann M.* _____ Date _*May 10*_
(patient's name)

Name of pain medicine: _*ibuprofen*_

Description: _*tablet - usually white or brown*_

Other names: _*Advil, Nuprin, Motrin*_

Why you are receiving this medicine: _*neck & back pain*_

Dose: _*400 mg*_ (number of pills per dose _*2*_)

How often: _*4 times a day - with breakfast, lunch, dinner, bedtime snack*_

_✓_ Every day without skipping a dose.

_____ ~~When you need it.~~

Get more medicine before you run out. To obtain more medicine:

_____ Pharmacy can refill this prescription _____ time(s).

_____ Call your doctor.

_____ Make an appointment with your doctor.

_✓_ You may obtain this medicine without a prescription.

Heartburn and stomach discomfort are common side effects. To avoid stomach upset or stomach injury (ulcer):

• Never take a medication dose on an empty stomach or with an alcoholic beverage.
• Take each dose of medicine with food or at least a full glass of water.
• An antacid may be helpful if you have indigestion.
• Do not take any other NSAID or aspirin-like drug. However, it is safe to take a daily dose of aspirin to prevent a heart attack, occasional doses of acetaminophen, and opioid (narcotic) pain medicine.
• Watch for nonprescription medicines with "hidden aspirin," such as some cold remedies or sinus medications. Read the labels on all nonprescription medications.

Other side effects that may occur are:

• Nausea and vomiting (If it looks like coffee grounds or is bloody, stop the medicine and report this side effect to your doctor or nurse at once.)
• Breathing problems (Stop the medicine and report this side effect to your doctor or nurse at once.)
• Dark stool (Stop the medicine and report this side effect to your doctor or nurse at once.)
• Headache
• Drowsiness
• Dizziness
• Ringing in the ears
• Blurred vision
• Swelling of the ankles
• Diarrhea or constipation
• Rash

Report all side effects to your doctor or nurse. You may need other medicines to control the side effects, or you may need a different pain medicine.

Your pain rating scale is: _*0 - 10*_

If your pain is _*5+*_ after _*2*_ days, notify your doctor or nurse.

If you have any questions or problems, contact:

Nurse: _*Mary*_ Phone: _*555-1234*_

Doctor: _*Jones*_ Phone: _*555-4321*_

Office hours: _*9 - 12 & 2 - 5*_

Please report to your nurse or doctor by telephone: _*Friday, May 14*_

Your next appointment is: _*May 24*_

References

Abramson S: Therapy with and mechanisms of nonsteroidal anti-inflammatory drugs, *Curr Opin Rheumatol* 3:336-340, 1991.

AHCPR: *Acute pain management in adults: operative procedures, Quick reference guide for clinicians,* 1992, DHHS Pub. No. AHCPR 92-0019.

AHCPR: *Management of cancer pain: adults. Quick reference guide for clinicians,* 1994, AHCPR Pub. No. 94-0593.

Alon E, Niv D, Varrassi G et al.: Nonsteroidal anti-inflammatory drugs in the control of postoperative pain, *Pain Digest* 6:145-152, 1996.

American Academy of Pediatrics Committee on Drugs: Transfer of drugs and other chemicals into human milk, *Pediatrics* 93:137-150, 1994.

American Pain Society (APS): *Principles of analgesic use in the treatment of acute pain and cancer pain,* ed 3, Skokie, Ill., 1992, The Society.

Beaver WT: Aspirin and acetaminophen as constituents of analgesic combinations, *Arch Intern Med* 141:293-300, 1981.

Beaver W: Caffeine revisited, *JAMA* 251:1732-1733, 1984.

Beaver WT, Wallenstein SL, Rogers A et al.: Analgesic studies of codeine and oxycodone in patients with cancer. I. Comparisons of oral with intramuscular codeine and of oral with intramuscular oxycodone, *J Pharmacol Exp Ther* 207:92-100, 1978a.

Beaver WT, Wallenstein SL, Rogers A et al.: Analgesic studies of codeine and oxycodone in patients with cancer. II. Comparisons of intramuscular oxycodone with intramuscular morphine and codeine, *J Pharmacol Exp Ther* 207:101-108, 1978b.

Ben-David B, Katz E, Gaitini et al.: Comparison of i.m. and local infiltration of ketorolac with and without local anaesthetic, *Br J Anaesth* 75:409-412, 1995.

Berde CB, Kain ZN: Pain management in infants and children. In Motoyama EK, Davis PJ, editors: *Smith's anesthesia for infants and children,* ed 6, pp 385-402, St. Louis, 1996, Mosby.

Bjorkman DJ: Nonsteroidal anti-inflammatory drug-induced gastrointestinal injury, *Am J Med* 101 (suppl 1A): 25S-32S, 1996.

Blower PR: The unique pharmacologic profile of nabumetone, *J Rheumatol* 9(suppl 36):13-19, 1992.

Borda IT: The spectrum of adverse gastrointestinal effects associated with nonsteroidal anti-inflammatory drugs. In Borda IT, Koff RS, editors; *NSAIDs: a profile of adverse effects,* pp 25-80, St. Louis, 1992, Mosby.

Brooks PM, Needs CJ: NSAIDs in lactating women. In Famaey JP, Paulus HE, editors: *Therapeutic applications of NSAIDs subpopulations and new formulations,* pp 157-162, New York, 1992, Marcel Dekker.

Cepeda MS, Vargas L, Ortegon G et al.: Comparative analgesic efficacy of patient-controlled analgesia with ketorolac versus morphine after elective intraabdominal operations, *Anaesth Analg* 80:1150-1153, 1995.

Chambers CT, Reid GJ, McGrath PJ et al.: Parents' attitudes and management of postoperative pain in children following a pain education booklet, *Children's Health Care.* In press.

Coyle N, Cherny NI, Portenoy RK: Pharmacologic management of cancer pain. In McGuire DB, Yarbro CH, Ferrell BR, editors: *Cancer pain management,* ed 2, pp 89-130, Boston, 1995, Jones & Bartlett Publishers.

Coyle N, Portenoy RK: Pharmacologic management of cancer pain. In McCorkle R, Grant M, Frank-Stromborg M, Baird SB, editors: *Cancer nursing: a comprehensive textbook,* ed 2, pp 1035-1055, Philadelphia, 1996, WB Saunders.

Dahl JB, Kehlet H: Non-steroidal anti-inflammatory drugs: rational for use in severe postoperative pain, *Br J Anaesth* 66:703-712, 1991.

Dahl JB, Rosenberg J, Dirkes WE et al.: Prevention of postoperative pain by balanced analgesia, *Br J Anaesth* 64:518-520, 1990.

Danesh BJZ, Saniabadi AR, Russell RI et al.: Therapeutic potential of choline magnesium trisalicylate as an alternative to aspirin for patients with bleeding tendencies, *Scot Med J* 32:167-168, 1987.

Duarte RA: Nonsteroidal anti-inflammatory drugs. In Kanner R: *Pain management secrets,* pp 167-171, Philadelphia, 1997, Hanley & Belfus.

Dueholm S, Forrest M, Hjortoso N-C et al.: Pain relief following herniotomy: a double-blind randomized comparison between naproxen and placebo, *Acta Anaesthesiol Scand* 33:391-394, 1989.

Eisenberg E, Berkey C, Carr D et al.: Efficacy and safety of nonsteroidal anti-inflammatory drugs for cancer pain: a meta-analysis, *J Clin Oncol* 12:2756-2765, 1994.

Estes D, Kaplan K: Lack of platelet effect with the aspirin analog, salsalate, *Arthritis Rheum* 23:1303-1307, 1980.

Flower RJ, Moncada S, Vane JR: Drug therapy of inflammation. In Gilman AG, Goodman LS, Rale TW et al., editors: *Goodman and Gilman's the pharmacological basis of therapeutics,* ed 7, pp. 674-715, New York, 1985, Macmillan Publishing Co., Inc.

Forbes JA, Beaver WT, Jones KF et al.: Evaluation of caffeine on ibuprofen analgesia in postoperative oral surgery pain, *Clin Pharmacol Ther* 49:674-684, 1991.

Forbes JA, Kehm CJ, Godein CD et al.: Evaluation of ketorolac, ibuprofen, acetaminophen, and an acetaminophen-codeine combination in postoperative oral surgery pain, *Pharmacotherapy* 10(6[pt 2]):94s-105s, 1990.

Forward SP, Brown TL, McGrath PJ: Mothers' attitudes and behavior toward medicating children's pain, *Pain* 67:469-474, 1996.

Gillis JC, Brogden RN: Ketorolac: a reappraisal of its pharmacodynamic and pharmacokinetic properties and therapeutic use in pain management, *Drugs* 53:139-188, 1997.

Glassman SD, Rose M, Dimar JR et al: The effect of postoperative nonsteroidal antiinflammatory drug administration on spinal fusion, *Spine,* 23:834-838, 1998.

H"am"al"ainen ML, Hoppu K, Valkeila E et al.: Ibuprofen or acetaminophen for the acute treatment of migraine in children: a double-blind, randomized, placebo-controlled, crossover study, *Neurology* 48:103-107, 1997.

Hallal JC: Caffeine, *Am J Nurs* 86:422-425, 1986.

Heavner JE, Shi B, Diede J et al.: Acetaminophen (paracetamol) use and blood concentration in pain patients, *Pain Digest* 6:215-218, 1996.

Henry D, Lim LL-Y, Rodriguez LAG et al.: Variability in risk of gastrointestinal complications with individual non-steroidal anti-inflammatory drugs: results of a collaborative meta-analysis, *BMJ* 312:1563-1566, 1996.

Houck CS: The management of acute pain in the child. In Ashburn MA, Rice LJ, editors: *The management of pain,* pp 651-666, New York, 1998, Churchill Livingstone.

Insel PA: Analgesic-antipyretic and antiinflammatory agents and drugs employed in the treatment of gout. In Hardman JL, Limbird LE: *Goodman & Gilman's the pharmacological basis of therapeutics,* ed 9, pp 617-657, New York, 1996, McGraw-Hill.

Kaiko R, Lacouture P, Hopf K et al.: Analgesic efficacy of controlled-release (CR) oxycodone and CR morphine, *Clin Pharmacol Ther* 59:130, 1996.

Kehlet H: Postoperative pain relief-what is the issue? *Br J Anaes* 72:374-378, 1994 (editorial).

Kehlet H, Dahl JB: Are perioperative nonsteroidal anti-inflammatory drugs ulcerogenic in the short term? *Drugs* 44(Suppl 5):38-41, 1992.

Kehlet H, Dahl JB: The value of "multimodal" or "balanced analgesia" in postoperative pain treatment, *Anesth Analg* 77:1048-1056, 1993.

Kelly JP, Kaufman DW, Jurgelon JM et al.: Risk of aspirin-associated major upper-gastrointestinal bleeding with enteric-coated or buffered product, *Lancet* 348:1413-1416, 1996.

Kenny GNC: Potential renal, haematological and allergic adverse effects associated with nonsteroidal anti-inflammatory drugs, *Drugs* 44(suppl 5):31-37, 1992.

Kjaersgaard-Andersen P, Schmidt SA: Total hip arthroplasty: the role of antiinflammatory medications in the prevention of heterotopic ossification, *Clin Orthop* 263:78-86, 1991.

Koch M, Dez I, Ferrario F et al.: Prevention of nonsteroidal anti-inflammatory drug-induced gastrointestinal mucosal injury: a meta-analysis of randomized controlled clinical trials, *Arch Intern Med* 11:2321-2332, 1996.

Kokki H, Hendolin H, Maunuksela E-L et al.: Ibuprofen in the treatment of postoperative pain in small children: a randomized double-blind-placebo controlled parallel group study, *Acta Anaesth Scand* 38:467-472, 1994.

Lanza FL: Endoscopic studies of gastric and duodenal injury after the use of ibuprofen, aspirin, and other nonsteroidal anti-inflammatory agents. Proceedings of a symposium-motrin ibuprofen, past, present, and future, *Am J Med* 77:19-24, 1984.

Laska EM, Sunshine A, Mueller F et al.: Caffeine as an analgesic adjuvant, *JAMA* 251:1711-1718, 1984.

Lindgren J, Djupso H: Diclofenac for pain after hip surgery, *Acta Anaesthesiol Scand* 56:28-31, 1985.

Lipman AG: Internal analgesic and antipyretic products. In *Handbook of nonprescription drugs,* pp 45-74, Washington DC, 1996, American Pharmaceutical Association.

Mayer DK, Struthers C, Fisher G: Bone metastases: part II: nursing management, *Clin J Oncol Nurs* 1:37-44, 1997.

McCaffery M, Martin L, Ferrell BR: Analgesic administration via rectum or stoma, *J ET Nurs* 19(4):114-121, 1992.

McGlew IC, Angliss DB, Gee GJ et al.: A comparison of rectal indomethacin with placebo for pain relief following spinal surgery, *Anaesth Intensive Care* 19:40-45, 1991.

McQuay HJ, Carroll D, Moore RA: Postoperative orthopaedic pain: the effect of opiate premedication and local anaesthetic block, *Pain* 33:291-295, 1988.

Merry A, Power I: Perioperative NSAIDs: towards greater safety, *Pain Rev* 2:268-291, 1995.

Meyer SJ, Nichols RJ, Cortiella J et al.: Acetaminophen in the management of background pain in children post-burn, *J Pain Symptom Manage* 13:50-55, 1997.

Middleton RK, Lyle JA, Berger DL: Ketorolac continuous infusion: a case report and review of the literature, *J Pain Symptom Manage* 12:190-194, 1996.

Migliardi JR., Armenia DU, Freedman M et al.: Caffeine as an analgesic adjuvant in tension headache, *Clin Pharmacol Ther* 56(5):576-586, 1994.

Mohamed SA, Mohamed K, Borsook D: Choosing a pharmacotherapeutic approach: nonopioid and adjuvant analgesics. In Borsook D, LeBel AA, McPeek B: *The Massachusetts general hospital handbook of pain management*, pp 76-104, Boston, 1996, Little, Brown & Co.

Nuutinen LS, Laitenen JO, Salomaki TE: A risk-benefit appraisal of injectable NSAIDs in the management of postoperative pain, *Drug Safety* 9:380-393, 1993.

Paice JA: Anatomy and physiology of pain: practical aspects, *Hemtol/Oncol Ann* 2:401-406, 1994.

Paice JA: Unraveling the mystery of pain, *Oncol Nurs Forum* 18:843-849, 1991.

Penna AC, Dawson KP, Penna CV: Is prescribing paracetamol 'pro re nata' acceptable? *J Pediatr Child Hlth* 29:104-106, 1993.

Perneger TV, Whelton PK, Klag MJ: Risk of kidney failure associated with the use of acetaminophen, aspirin, and nonsteroidal antiinflammatory drugs, *N Engl J Med* 331:1675-1679, 1994.

Physicians' desk reference: ed. 51, Montvale, NJ, 1997, Medical Economics Company.

Piletta P, Porchet HC, Dayer P: Central analgesic effect of acetaminophen but not of aspirin, *Clin Pharmacol Ther* 49:350-354, 1991.

Plummer JL, Owen H, Ilsley AH et al: Sustained-release ibuprofen as an adjunct to morphine patient-controlled analgesia, *Anesth Analg* 83:92-96, 1996.

Portenoy RK, Kanner RM: Nonopioid and adjuvant analgesics. In Portenoy RK, Kanner RM, editors: *Pain management: theory and practice*, pp 219-247, Philadelphia, 1996, FA Davis.

Rahbek I: Gastroscopic evaluation of the effect of a new antirheumatic compound, ketoprofen (19,583 RP) on the human gastric mucosa, *Scand J Rheumatol* 5(suppl 141):63, 1976.

Ripamonti C, Ticozzi C, Zecca E et al.: Continuous subcutaneous infusion of ketorolac in cancer neuropathic pain unresponsive to opioid and adjuvant drugs: a case report, *Tumori* 82:413-415, 1996.

Rumack B: Aspirin versus acetaminophen: a comparative view, *Pediatrics* 62:943, 1978.

Rusy LM, Houck CS, Sullivan IJ et al.: A double blind evaluation of ketorolac tromethamine versus acetaminophen in pediatric tonsillectomy: analgesia and bleeding, *Anesth Analg* 80:226, 1995.

Schneider JR: Effects of caffeine ingestion on heart rate, blood pressure, myocardial oxygen consumption, and cardiac rhythm in acute myocardial infarction patients, *Heart Lung* 16(2):167-174, 1987.

Seeff LB, Cuccherini BA, Zimmerman HI et al.: Acetaminophen hepatotoxicity in alcoholics, *Ann Intern Med* 104:399-404, 1986.

Serpell MG, Thomson MF: Comparison of piroxicam with placebo in the management of pain after total hip replacement, *Br J Anaesth* 63:354-356, 1989.

Sevarino FB, Sinatra RS, Paige D et al.: The efficacy of intramuscular ketorolac in combination with intravenous PCA morphine for postoperative pain relief, *J Clin Anesth* 4:285-288, 1992.

Strom BL, Berlin JA, Kinman JL et al.: Parenteral ketorolac and risk of gastrointestinal and operative site bleeding, *JAMA* 275:376-382, 1996a.

Strom BL, Berlin JA, Kinman JL et al.: Risk of operative site bleeding with parenteral ketorolac, *JAMA* 276:372, 1996b.

Sunshine A, Zighelboim I, Sorrentino JV et al.: Augmentation of acetaminophen analgesia by the antihistamine phenyltoloxamine, *J Clin Pharmacol* 29:660-664, 1989.

Sunshine A, Olson NZ: Nonnarcotic analgesics. In Wall PD, Melzack R, editors: *Textbook of pain*, ed 3, pp 923-942, New York, 1994, Churchill Livingstone.

Taha AS, Hudson N, Hawkey CJ et al.: Famotidine for the prevention of gastric and duodenal ulcers caused by nonsteroidal antiinflammatory drugs, *N Engl J Med* 334:1435-1439, 1996.

Taivainen T, Hiller A, Rosenberg PH et al.: The effect of continuous intravenous infusion on bleeding time and postoperative pain in patients undergoing emergency surgery of the lower extremities, *Acta Anaesthesiol Scand* 33:58-60, 1989.

Thwaites BK, Nigus DB, Bouska GW et al.: Intravenous ketorolac tromethamine worsens platelet function during knee arthroscopy under spinal anesthesia, *Anesth Analg* 82:1176-1181, 1996.

Valentini M, Cannizzaro R, Polette M et al.: Nonsteroidal antiinflammatory drugs for cancer pain: comparison between misoprostol and ranitidine in prevention of upper gastrointestinal damage, *J Clin Oncol* 13:2637-2642, 1995.

Varrassi G, Panella L, Piroli A et al.: The effects of perioperative ketorolac infusion on postoperative pain and endocrine-metabolic response, *Anesth Analg* 78:514-519, 1994.

Whitcomb DC, Block GD: Association of acetaminophen hepatoxicity with fasting and ethanol use, *JAMA* 272:1845-1850, 1994.

Woolf CJ, Chong M-S: Preemptive analgesia: treating postoperative pain by preventing the establishment of central sensitization, *Anesth Analg* 77:362-379, 1993.

Yaster M, Krane EJ, Kaplan RF et al., editors: *Pediatric pain management and sedation handbook*, St. Louis, 1997, Mosby.

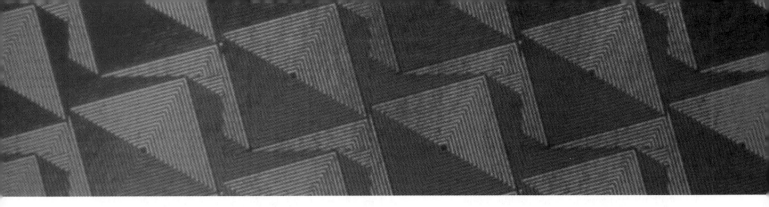

chapter six
OPIOID ANALGESICS

Chris Pasero, Russell K. Portenoy, and Margo McCaffery
Reviewers: Terry Dimaggio, Jane Faries, Betty R. Ferrell, Debra B. Gordon, Lex Hubbard, Terry Karapas, Pamela Kedziera, Janice Rae, Susan L. Schroeder, Georgeanne V. Stilley, Barbara Vanderveer, and Linda Vanni

CHAPTER OUTLINE

TERMINOLOGY

Addiction: A pattern of compulsive drug use characterized by a continued craving for an opioid and the need to use the opioid for effects other than pain relief.

Adjuvant analgesic: A drug that has a primary indication other than pain (e.g., local anesthetics and muscle relaxants) but is analgesic for some painful conditions.

Agonist-antagonist: A type of opioid (e.g., nalbuphine and butorphanol) that binds to the kappa opioid receptor site acting as an agonist (capable of producing analgesia) and simultaneously to the mu opioid receptor site acting as an antagonist (reversing agonist effects).

Analgesic ceiling: A dose beyond which further increases in dose do not provide additional analgesia.

Antagonist: Drug that competes with agonists for opioid receptor binding sites; can displace agonists, thereby inhibiting their action. Examples include naloxone, naltrexone, and nalmefene.

Balanced analgesia: Also referred to as continuous, multimodal analgesia.

Blood-brain barrier: A barrier that exists between circulating blood and brain, preventing damaging substances from reaching brain tissue and cerebrospinal fluid.

Bioavailability: The extent to which a dose of a drug reaches its site of action.

Breakthrough pain: Pain that increases above the pain addressed by the ongoing analgesics. Includes incident pain and end of dose failure.

Ceiling effect: A dose above which further dose increments produce no change in effect.

Efficacy: The maximal effect that can be produced by a given dose of a drug.

Half-life: The time it takes for the plasma concentration (amount of drug in the body) to be reduced by 50%. Four to five half-lives are required for a drug to be eliminated from the body.

Hydrophilic: Readily absorbed in aqueous solution.

Intraspinal: "Within the spine"; term referring to the spaces or potential spaces surrounding the spinal cord into which medications can be administered. Most often, the term is used when referring to the epidural and intrathecal routes of administration. Sometimes used interchangeably with the term neuraxial.

Lipophilic: Readily absorbed in fatty tissues.

Metabolite: The product of biochemical reactions during drug metabolism.

Mu-agonist: A type of opioid. Includes morphine and other opioids that relieve pain by binding to the mu receptor sites in the nervous system. Used interchangeably with the terms full agonist, pure agonist, and morphine-like drug.

Narcotic: See "Opioid." Obsolete term for "opioid," in part because the government and media use the term loosely to refer to a variety of substances of potential abuse. Legally, controlled substances classified as narcotics include opioids, cocaine, and various other substances.

Neuropathic pain: Pain initiated or caused by a primary lesion or dysfunction in the nervous system.

Nociceptor: A receptor preferentially sensitive to a noxious stimulus or to a stimulus that would be noxious if prolonged.

Opioid: Preferred to "narcotic." Refers to natural, semi-synthetic, and synthetic drugs that relieve pain by binding to opioid receptors in the nervous system. The term "opioid" is preferred to "opiate" because it includes all agonists and antagonists with morphine-like activity, as well as naturally occurring and synthetic opioid peptides.

Paresthesia: Abnormal anesthetic sensation (e.g., numbness, tingling).

Physical dependence: Physical reliance on an opioid evidenced by withdrawal symptoms if the opioid is abruptly stopped or an antagonist is administered.

Potency: The dose required to produce a specified effect.

Preemptive analgesia: Preinjury pain treatments (e.g., preoperative epidural analgesia and preincision local anesthetic infiltration) to prevent the establishment of peripheral and central sensitization of pain.

Primary afferent neuron: See definition of "nociceptor."

Sequential trials: One drug is tried and if the results are unfavorable, it is discontinued and another drug is tried. A trial and error approach in which one drug after another is tried until the desired effects occur.

Supraspinal: Outside the level of the spinal cord.

Tolerance: A process characterized by decreasing effects of a drug at its previous dose or the need for a higher dose of drug to maintain an effect.

TABLE 6.1 ● ● ● ● ●

Misconceptions | Opioid Analgesics

MISCONCEPTION	CORRECTION
1. Taking opioids for pain relief leads to addiction.	Addiction occurring as a result of taking opioids for pain relief is rare ($<1\%$).
2. How much analgesia opioids can produce is limited.	The dose and the analgesic effect of mu agonist opioids have no ceiling.
3. Not all pain responds to opioids.	All pain responds to opioids, but some types of pain are more responsive than others. Opioids are particularly effective in relieving visceral and somatic pain and less effective in relieving neuropathic pain. Although a number of factors can affect opioid responsiveness, no evidence exists that any characteristic of the pain or the patient causes uniform opioid resistance.
4. Opioid treatment should be withheld in the early stages of disease to prevent the development of tolerance and lack of analgesia in the later stages.	Tolerance should be expected after several days of opioid treatment, but thereafter the dose usually stabilizes if pain is stable. In addition, tolerance is treatable, usually by increasing the opioid dose; no ceiling to the analgesia of opioids exists, and patients develop tolerance to respiratory depression. Clinicians should not withhold opioid treatment from patients with long life expectancies or delay initiating opioid therapy for fear of encountering unmanageable tolerance.
5. The more potent opioids are the more therapeutically superior opioids.	Potency does not determine efficacy. Potency can be viewed as the ratio of the dose of two analgesics required to produce the same analgesic effect. All mu agonist opioids are capable of producing the same degree of analgesia when given at equianalgesic doses. Increased potency alone does not provide any advantage because the more potent drugs also exhibit a parallel increase in their ability to produce undesirable effects.
6. When pain is no longer relieved by a given opioid dose, the opioid should be discontinued to allow the receptors to "reset" and become more sensitive to opioids.	Continued stimulation of opioid receptors does not result in desensitization. Stopping the opioid will not make the receptors more sensitive to opioids. When a given dose is safe but ineffective, the dose should be increased by appropriate percentages, keeping in mind that no ceiling to the analgesia of mu agonist opioids exists.
7. Opioids frequently cause clinically significant respiratory depression.	Opioid-induced respiratory depression is rare if opioid doses are titrated slowly and decreased when increased sedation is detected. Clinically significant opioid-induced respiratory depression can be avoided in opioid-naive patients by careful nurse monitoring of sedation levels. Tolerance to the respiratory depressant effect of opioids develops within 72 hours of administration. Therefore in patients who have been taking opioids on a long-term basis a wider margin of safety exists. The fear of causing death from respiratory depression by administering opioids to the terminally ill also is exaggerated. Large doses of opioids given to relieve pain during the withholding and withdrawal of life support in terminally ill patients does not hasten death.
8. Agonist-antagonist opioid analgesics are safer than other opioids because they do not produce respiratory depression and will prevent addiction and discourage drug-seeking behavior.	At equianalgesic doses all opioids cause equal respiratory depression. The agonist-antagonist opioid drugs have a ceiling for the amount of analgesia and respiratory depression they cause (i.e., beyond a certain dose no further respiratory depression or analgesia is produced), but this is usually above recommended doses. Furthermore, respiratory depression is not readily reversed by naloxone in buprenorphine. Agonist-antagonist opioids can produce significant sedation and extremely unpleasant dysphoria. Addiction is no less likely with agonist-antagonist drugs than with other opioids. Finally, the practice of administering agonist-antagonist opioid analgesics to known drug abusers to discourage drug-seeking behavior is not appropriate because it may precipitate withdrawal. Because agonist-antagonist drugs antagonize at the mu opioid receptor site, they should be avoided in patients who are physically dependent on opioid drugs.

Continued.

TABLE 6.1—cont'd ● ● ● ● ●

Misconceptions | Opioid Analgesics

MISCONCEPTION	CORRECTION
9. Endorphins and enkephalins are effective analgesics.	Endorphins and enkephalins bind to opioid receptor sites and prevent the release of the neurotransmitters, thereby inhibiting the transmission of pain impulses. Unfortunately, endogenous opioids degrade too quickly to be considered useful analgesics. Although administering morphine and other opioids probably temporarily decreases production of endogenous opioids, belief that use of opioids, such as morphine, should be avoided for this reason is unfounded.

May be duplicated for use in clinical practice. From McCaffery M, Pasero C: *Pain: Clinical manual,* pp. 163-164. Copyright © 1999, Mosby, Inc. See text for references.

Some of the most persistent barriers to the effective treatment of pain come from clinician and patient fears and misconceptions surrounding the use of opioid analgesics (Table 6.1). Abundant research shows that physicians underprescribe opioid analgesics, nurses give inadequate doses (often less than physicians prescribe), and patients take too little to control their pain (AHCPR, 1992; Hitchcock, Ferrell, McCaffery, 1994; Jacox, Carr, Payne et al., 1994; Marks, Sacher, 1973; Oden, 1989; Ward, Goldberg, Miller-McCauley, 1993; Weis, Sriwatanakul, Alloza, 1983). (See Chapter 1 for more on the undertreatment of pain.)

In the past the use of opioid analgesics to control patients' pain was thought to be strictly the domain of the physician. Typically one opioid dose was prescribed for a wide range of patients. It is now known that opioid doses must be individualized to meet each patient's unique analgesic needs. To accomplish this, a collaborative approach to managing pain is recommended (AHCPR, 1992; Jacox, Carr, Payne et al., 1994).

Physicians begin the collaborative process by discussing pain and its consequences with their patients, then prescribing appropriate therapies for its management. Pharmacists provide expert information on the pharmacology and pharmacokinetics of analgesics and facilitate the clinician's acquisition of them. Nurses, whether they are providing care in the home, hospital, or other setting, are in a unique position to meet the patients' pain management needs and are increasingly recognized as the patients' primary pain managers (Pasero, 1994; Pasero, McCaffery, 1996a).

A collaborative approach to high-quality pain control requires patients with pain and the health care team members who care for them to share common goals, a common knowledge base, and a common language with regard to the use of opioid drugs in managing pain. These elements must be expressed in practical terms. A common language includes use of a pain rating scale. A shared common goal may be determined by discussion between the patient and caregivers and might be as simple as a pain level of 3/10 or better to enable the patient to get out of bed and walk down the hall. An example of important knowledge shared by patient and caregivers is that opioids can be used safely and effectively for these painful events.

This chapter is based on the assumption that pain is best managed with a collaborative approach and that nurses have an active and pivotal role in the daily, ongoing use of opioid analgesics. For the nurse to fulfill this role, it is essential that institutional policies, physicians' orders, and regulatory agencies support the nurses' role in teaching patients about pain and in assessing and managing it. This is especially critical with regard to titrating opioid doses and treating side effects (Pasero, 1994; Pasero, McCaffery, 1996a).

Facts about opioid analgesics support the need for nurses to work with flexible analgesic doses and intervals. For example, no set dose of opioid analgesic is safe and effective. The physician who prescribes the opioid analgesic usually is not present for its onset, peak effect, and duration. These are times when titration may be needed. Although suggesting that nurses titrate opioid analgesics may seem to be a novel idea to some, remember that patient-controlled analgesia (PCA) allows patients to titrate (e.g., administer an additional amount and determine the frequency of dosing). Surely the nurse should be able to do this for a patient who is unable to perform this activity (Pasero, McCaffery, 1996a).

This chapter presents the underlying mechanisms of opioid analgesics and their side effects. Relevant pharmacologic concepts are explained. The indications for opioid analgesic use and guidelines and strategies for administering them are discussed, including how to determine the right opioid drug, dose, interval, and route for patients. The differences in using opioid analgesics for acute, cancer, and chronic nonmalignant pain are delineated throughout the chapter. Important points to include in patient and family teaching are presented, including guidelines for discussing addiction. The controversies and conclusions regarding withholding opioid analgesic treatment are discussed. Misconceptions related to the use of opioid analgesics are presented and corrected in Table 6.1. Selected terms and definitions are listed at the beginning of this chapter to facilitate an understanding of the chapter content.

BASIC PHYSIOLOGY AND PHARMACOLOGY OF OPIOID ANALGESICS

Groups of Opioids

Opioids are divided into two major groups. The largest group is the morphine-like agonists. The terms morphine-like drugs, mu agonists, pure agonists, and full agonists are used interchangeably. Throughout this chapter, the term mu agonist will be used when referring to opioid drugs in this group. The other group of opioids is the agonist-antagonist group and is further divided into the mixed agonist-antagonists and the partial agonists.

Underlying Mechanisms of Opioid Analgesia and Side Effects

Endogenous opioid system

It is thought that opioids activate endogenous (internal) pain-modulating systems (Portenoy, 1996a) and produce analgesia and other effects by mimicking the action of endogenous opioid compounds (Portenoy, 1996b). Endogenous opioids are composed of three distinct families of peptides (naturally occurring compounds of two or more amino acids), all pharmacologically related to morphine: enkephalins, dynorphins, and β-endorphins.

Endogenous opioids appear to function as neurotransmitters and modulators of neurotransmission, but not everything about their physiologic role is known (Reisine, Pasternak, 1996). It is known that they are associated with the systems that regulate homeostasis and the stress response and that they have a role in producing analgesia. Little is known about their function in chronic pain states. Endorphin levels have been found to be lower in some patients with chronic pain (Portenoy, 1996a).

Opioid receptors

Drugs exert their effects on the body by interacting with specialized macromolecular components in cells called drug receptors. Drug receptors usually are cellular proteins, but can be enzymes, carbohydrate residues, and lipids. The binding of drug molecules to their specific receptor molecules often is described as similar to a key fitting a lock (Figure 6.1). Binding affinity refers to the strength of attachment of a drug to the receptor site, and drugs bind with varying strength (Ferrante, 1996). The electromagnetic forces produced by the bond between a drug and receptor distort the configuration of the recep-

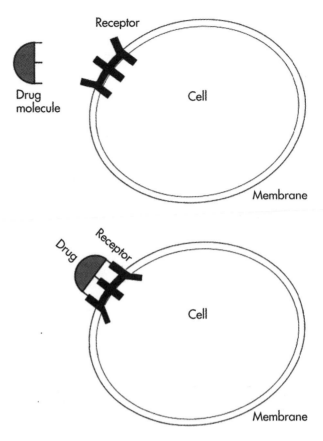

May be duplicated for use in clinical practice. As appears in McCaffery M, Pasero C: *Pain: Clinical manual*, p. 165, 1999, Mosby, Inc.

● ● ● ● ●

FIGURE 6.1. **Drug and receptor interaction.** Figure 6.1 Illustrates the binding of drug molecules to their specific receptor molecules, often described as similar to a key fitting a lock. The electromagnetic forces produced by the bond between a drug and receptor distort the configuration of the receptor molecule, changing its biochemical properties and functions. The body's responses to the drug are a result of these changes.

From Spencer RT: Pharmacodynamics and pharmacokinetics. In *Clinical pharmacology and nursing management*, ed 4, p 64 , Philadelphia, 1993, JB Lippincott Company.

tor molecule, changing its biochemical properties and functions. The body's responses to the drug are a result of these changes (Ross, 1996; Spencer, 1993).

Researchers think that receptors evolved for the purpose of interacting with endogenous compounds. The endogenous opioid system is an excellent example of this interaction (Spencer, 1993). Opioid receptors are located in the CNS, pituitary gland, and the GI tract. They are particularly abundant in the periacqueductal gray (PAG) and dorsal horn of the spinal cord. Nociceptors carrying information about noxious stimuli from the periphery terminate in the dorsal horn of the spinal cord. These cells release neurotransmitters, such as adenosine triphosphate, glutamate, and substance P. It is at this site that endogenous and exogenous opioids play an important role in pain control by locking onto opioid receptors and blocking the release of neurotransmitters, principally

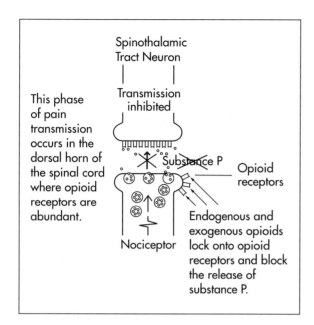

This phase of pain transmission occurs in the dorsal horn of the spinal cord where opioid receptors are abundant.

Spinothalamic Tract Neuron

Transmission inhibited

Substance P

Opioid receptors

Nociceptor

Endogenous and exogenous opioids lock onto opioid receptors and block the release of substance P.

May be duplicated for use in clinical practice. From McCaffery M, Pasero C: *Pain: Clinical manual*, p. 166. Copyright © 1999, Mosby, Inc.

● ● ● ● ●

FIGURE 6.2.   Opioid receptors. Figure 6.2 shows how pain transmission is blocked when endogenous and exogenous opioids lock onto opioid receptors located in the dorsal horn of the spinal cord and inhibit the release of the neurotransmitter, substance P.

substance P (Portenoy, 1996a) (Figure 6.2). (For more on pain transmission, refer to Chapter 2.)

Traditionally, opioid analgesics were thought to produce analgesia only through the CNS as described. However, opioid receptors have been found also on peripheral terminals of sensory nerves and cells of the immune system. Current research shows that opioid analgesics also block substance P peripherally by binding to the opioid receptors in peripheral nerve cells (Portenoy, 1996a). This may account for the antiinflammatory actions of opioid drugs on peripheral tissues (Stein, Yassouridis, 1997).

Classes of Opioid Receptor Sites

Three major classes or types of opioid receptor sites are involved in analgesia: mu, delta, and kappa. When a drug binds to any of these receptor sites as an agonist, it produces analgesia. Antagonists are drugs that also bind to opioid receptors but produce no analgesia. If an antagonist is present, it competes with opioid molecules for binding sites on the receptors. When a drug binds to any of the opioid receptor sites as an antagonist, analgesia and other effects are blocked. For example, naloxone, an opioid antagonist, can bind to the mu site and reverse analgesia and other opioid side effects, such as respiratory depression and sedation (Portenoy, 1996a) (see Table 6.2 for summary of actions at opioid receptor type).

Opioid drugs that produce analgesia all have agonist effects at one or more of the opioid receptor site types

(Portenoy, 1996b). Most of the clinically useful opioid analgesics bind primarily to mu opioid receptor sites. These are the mu agonist opioid analgesics, which are considered the mainstay of analgesia for acute and cancer pain. Examples of mu agonist opioid analgesics are morphine, hydromorphone (Dilaudid), fentanyl, oxycodone, hydrocodone, codeine, methadone (Dolophine), and meperidine (Demerol). Mu agonists can be administered by numerous routes, and onset of analgesia is within minutes by some routes. They can be combined with almost any of the nonopioid and adjuvant analgesics.

The mixed agonist-antagonist opioid analgesics are designated as mixed because they bind to more than one opioid receptor site. They bind as agonists, producing analgesia at the kappa opioid receptor sites, and as weak antagonists at the mu opioid receptor sites. Mixed agonist-antagonists opioid analgesics include butorphanol (Stadol), nalbuphine (Nubain), pentazocine (Talwin), and dezocine (Dalgan). Compared with mu agonists, the mixed agonist-antagonists produce more dysphoria and psychotomimetic effects and less intense respiratory depression (Reisine, Pasternak, 1996).

The only partial agonist opioid drug available in the United States is buprenorphine (Buprenex). It is referred to as partial because it binds as an agonist at the mu and kappa opioid receptors but has limited intrinsic efficacy (Portenoy, 1996b; Reisine, Pasternak, 1996). In the clinical setting this means that analgesia plateaus as the dose is increased.

Opioid Receptors and Side Effects

The type of opioid receptor site and its location determine the effects an opioid drug produces. In addition to producing analgesia, opioid drugs produce a number of other effects, including constipation, nausea and vomiting, sedation, respiratory depression, and urinary retention (Reisine, Pasternak, 1996) (see Table 6.2).

The main GI effect of opioid drugs is decreased intestinal propulsive motility and delayed gastric emptying, leading to constipation (Lipman, Gauthier, 1997). Constipation, which is the most common of the opioid side effects, occurs from opioid binding to receptors located in the GI tract and the CNS (Chaney, 1995). Nausea and vomiting are the result of opioid binding to receptors located in the fourth ventricle of the brain; urinary retention occurs from binding in the spinal cord; respiratory depression from binding in the ventral medulla of the brain stem; and sedation from binding in the brain (Chaney, 1995).

Pharmacologic Concepts

After systemic administration, an opioid drug is absorbed into the vascular system. For the drug to produce a pharmacologic effect, it must leave the plasma, diffuse into the tissues, reach the opioid receptors, and activate

● ● ● ● ●

TABLE 6.2 Summary of Actions at Opioid Receptor Sites

OPIOID RECEPTOR SITE	ACTIVITY	OPIOIDS WITH AGONIST ACTION	OPIOIDS WITH ANTAGONIST ACTION
Mu (μ)	Spinal and supraspinal analgesia, respiratory depression, cardiovascular effects, physical dependence, tolerance, ↓ GI motility, urinary retention, pruritis, euphoria	Pure: e.g., morphine, methadone, codeine, fentanyl, sufentanil, alfentanil, oxycodone, levorphanol, oxymorphone, hydromorphone (Dilaudid), meperidine (Demerol)	Pure: naloxone (Narcan), naltrexone (Trexan), nalmefene (Revex), butorphanol (Stadol), nalbuphine (Nubain), pentazocine (Talwin), dezocine (Dalgan) Partial: buprenorphine, (Buprenex)
Kappa (κ)	Spinal and supraspinal analgesia, miosis, psychotomimetic effects (dysphoria, agitation), and sedation without pronounced respiratory depression, euphoria, or GI effects.	Butorphanol, nalbuphine, pentazocine, buprenorphine, sufentanil (weak affinity)	Pure: naloxone, naltrexone, nalmefene
Delta (δ)	Spinal and supraspinal analgesia without respiratory compromise. (Effects are under investigation.)	Levorphanol, dezocine, sufentanil (weak affinity), morphine (weak affinity)	Naloxone, naltrexone, nalmefene, pentazocine

May be duplicated for use in clinical practice. From McCaffery M, Pasero C: *Pain: Clinical manual*, p. 167. Copyright © 1999, Mosby, Inc.

The effects (activity) a drug produces depends on the type(s) of opioid receptor(s) to which the drug binds and whether the drug acts as an agonist or an antagonist at that opioid receptor type. When a drug binds to any of these receptor sites as an agonist, it produces analgesia and other effects. When a drug binds to any of the opioid receptor sites as an antagonist, analgesia and other effects are blocked. Table 6.2 summarizes the activity of drugs when they bind to any of three opioid receptor types that are involved in analgesia.

GI, gastrointestinal.

Information from Ferrante M: Principles of opioid pharmacotherapy: Practical implications of basic mechanisms, *J Pain Symptom Manage* 11(5):265-273, 1996; Foley KM: Misconceptions and controversies regarding the use of opioids in cancer pain, *Anti-Cancer Drugs* 6(Suppl 3):4-13, 1995; Markley HG: Chronic head-ache: Appropriate use of opiate analgesics, *Neurology* 44(Suppl 3):S18-S24, May 1994; Reisine T, Pasternak G: Opioid analgesics and antagonists. In Hardman JG, Limbird LE, editors: *Goodman and Gilman's the pharmacological basis of therapeutics*, ed 9, pp 521-555, New York, 1996, McGraw-Hill; Twycross RG: Opioids. In Wall PD, Melzack R, editors: *Textbook of pain*, ed 3, pp 943-962, New York, 1994, Churchill Livingstone.

---

them (Benedetti, 1990). Appropriate use of opioid analgesics requires an understanding of these processes and some important pharmacologic concepts. The following is a discussion of pharmacokinetics (what the body does to a drug) and pharmacodynamics (what the drug does to the body) (Benet, 1996). Tolerance, cross-tolerance, physical dependence, addiction, pseudoaddiction, and equianalgesia also are discussed.

Pharmacokinetics

Absorption, Bioavailability, First Pass Effect, Solubility

Absorption is the rate and extent to which a drug leaves its site of administration. A more clinically important concept than absorption is bioavailability, which is the extent to which a dose of a drug reaches its site of action (Benet, Kroetz, Sheiner, 1996) or how much drug is available in the plasma for therapeutic effect. It is thought that opioid drugs are 100% bioavailable when administered intravenously because they are introduced directly into the systemic circulation. However, bioavailability is reduced when they are administered by the oral route (Coyle, Cherny, Portenoy, 1995).

When administered orally, opioids are absorbed from the GI tract and are transported by the portal vein to the liver, the primary site of drug metabolism, before they reach systemic circulation. Bioavailability depends on how much of the drug is absorbed in the GI tract and inactivated as it passes through the liver. This is called the first pass effect. First pass effect is why the dose of an opioid drug by the oral route must be much larger than by the parenteral route to produce equal analgesia (Coyle, Cherny, Portenoy, 1995; Spencer, 1993). For example, the bioavailability of morphine when given orally is between 15% and 64% because of first pass losses (Ferrante, 1996) (Figure 6.3).

Many factors influence a drug's absorption and bioavailability besides route of administration. The site of absorption, including its surface area and quality of

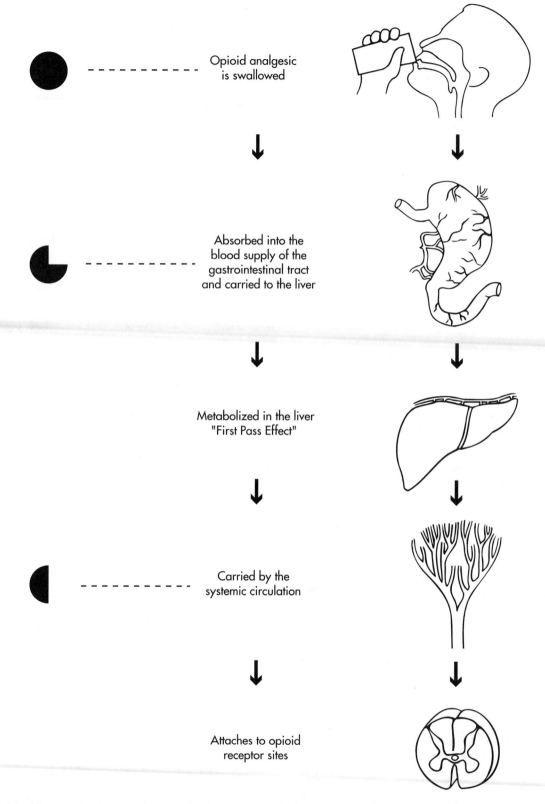

Opioid analgesic
is swallowed

Absorbed into the
blood supply of the
gastrointestinal tract
and carried to the liver

Metabolized in the liver
"First Pass Effect"

Carried by the
systemic circulation

Attaches to opioid
receptor sites

FIGURE 6.3.   **Drug absorption and metabolism by the oral route.** The solid sphere represents an opioid analgesic pill. Decreasing size of the pill represents loss through absorption in the gastrointestinal tract and metabolism in the liver. The half sphere represents the dose of opioid available for analgesia at the opioid receptor sites (bioavailability) after it has been diminished by absorption and metabolism.

blood circulation, is important. Drugs are absorbed rapidly from large surface areas, such as the intestinal mucosa, and when there is increased blood flow at the site. A high concentration of drug in a small volume leads to faster absorption compared with a low concentration in a large volume (Benedetti, Butler, 1990). The presence of a pathologic condition also affects bioavailability (Benet, Kroetz, Sheiner, 1996). For example, bioavailability is increased in hepatic dysfunction because the liver cannot metabolize and excrete the drug efficiently (Reisine, Pasternak, 1996).

Characteristics of the drug itself also help to determine its bioavailability. A drug's bioavailability will be decreased if it is a drug for which the liver has a great capacity to metabolize and excrete (Benet, Kroetz, Sheiner, 1996), such as hydromorphone. When given intravenously, hydromorphone is 100% bioavailable and the recommended dose is 1.5 mg; when given orally, which subjects the drug to significant liver metabolism and first pass effect, the equianalgesic dose is five times greater at 7.5 mg.

A drug's solubility also influences its bioavailability. The more lipid soluble (also referred to as lipophilic, meaning readily dissolved into fatty tissues) the drug, the more readily it moves through membranes; thus the faster and greater its absorption. When administered by the IV route, most opioid drugs act promptly, but when administered by the SC and intraspinal routes, the more lipid soluble drugs act more rapidly than those that are less lipid soluble (Reisine, Pasternak, 1996). For example, opioids, such as fentanyl and sufentanil are highly lipid soluble and have a rapid onset of action and short duration; morphine and hydromorphone are not lipid soluble but are hydrophilic (readily dissolved in aqueous solution) and have a slower onset of action and longer duration; meperidine is intermediate between these drugs. Lipophilicity and all the other factors discussed in this section can affect the efficacy and toxicity of a drug and therefore must be considered when establishing an opioid analgesic regimen (Benet, Kroetz, Sheiner, 1996).

Protein Binding

Many drugs are bound to plasma proteins, primarily albumin. Plasma protein binding can be viewed as a transport mechanism that delivers drugs to their sites of metabolism. Plasma protein binding limits a drug's concentration in tissues and at its site of action because only unbound drug is in equilibrium across membranes and can move freely. Bound drug is devoid of pharmacologic activity; drug responses, whether efficacious or toxic, are a function of unbound concentrations (Benet, Kroetz, Sheiner, 1996; Spencer, 1993).

Metabolites

As discussed, when a drug passes through the liver, it is subjected to multiple biochemical processes and reactions (metabolism) that change part of the drug into different compounds. Enzymes mediate most of these processes and reactions. The resulting products are called metabolites (Spencer, 1993). Many opioid analgesics have metabolites, including morphine (morphine-6-glucuronide [M6G] and morphine-3-glucuronide [M3G]), meperidine (normeperidine), and propoxyphene (norpropoxyphene). Metabolites are referred to as being active, having pharmacologic action, or inactive, having no pharmacologic action.

Metabolites often have properties and characteristics different from their parent drug. Sometimes their pharmacologic actions are indistinguishable from the parent drug (Reisine, Pasternak, 1996), but their biologic activity may be increased, decreased, or eliminated (Spencer, 1993). For example, the major metabolite of morphine, M6G, is analgesic like its parent but is significantly more potent (Foley, 1995; Reisine, Pasternak, 1996).

Half-life, Clearance, Steady State, and Cumulation

Drugs are eliminated from the body either unchanged or as metabolites. The kidney is the primary organ for elimination of drugs and metabolites. Drugs are also excreted in the feces, breast milk, sweat, saliva, tears, hair, and skin. The pulmonary route of excretion is important mainly for anesthetic gases and vapors (Benet, Kroetz, Sheiner, 1996).

Terminal half-life provides an estimate of how fast a drug leaves the body. By definition half-life is the time it takes for the amount of drug in the body to be reduced by 50% (Spencer, 1993). Half-life varies significantly from one drug to another. For example, the half-life of morphine is 2 to 4 hours, whereas the half-life of levorphanol is 12 to 15 hours. Terminal half-life is different from, but sometimes confused with, distribution half-life, which reflects the time necessary for a drug to move from the blood and plasma to other tissues (Willens, Myslinski, 1993).

Clearance is also a measure of the body's ability to eliminate a drug from the body. Clearance depends on the organs of elimination coming in contact with the blood or plasma containing the drug (Reisine, Pasternak, 1996). Box 6.1 illustrates the formula to calculate creatinine clearance.

A drug's half-life changes according to the body's ability to clear the drug; therefore both half-life and clearance are important to consider when developing a regimen for long-term opioid analgesic administration. Because they are interrelated, both are influenced by age, gender, disease, and body composition. For example, because clearance decreases with age, half-life can be expected to increase (Benet, Kroetz, Sheiner, 1996; Foley, 1995).

A concept closely related to half-life is steady state. A steady state is approached when the rate of excretion of a drug equals the rate at which the drug enters the system. Long-term opioid analgesic treatment is designed to maintain a steady state of opioid within the therapeutic

● ● ● ● ●

> **BOX 6.1** **Creatinine Values and Formula for Calculating Creatinine Clearance**
>
> Serum creatinine
> Newborn: 0.3-1.0 mg/dl
> Infant: 0.2-0.4 mg/dl
> Child: 0.3-0.7 mg/dl
> Adolescent: 0.5-1.0 mg/dl
> Adult male: 0.6-1.5 mg/dl
> Adult female: 0.5-1.2 mg/dl
> Elderly: may be normal but creatinine clearance may be decreased
> Creatinine clearance
> Newborn: 40-65 ml/min
> Male <40 years old: 97-137 ml/min
> Female <40 years old: 88-128 ml/min
> Adult male: 85-125 ml/min
> Adult female: 75-115 ml/min
> Elderly: decreased
> Creatinine clearance can be easily estimated using the following formula:
> Creatine clearance (ml/min) =
> (140 − age) × (Weight in kg) ÷ (serum creatinine [mg/dl] × 72)
> (For women, multiply by 0.85)

May be duplicated for use in clinical practice. From McCaffery M, Pasero C: *Pain: Clinical manual,* p. 170. Copyright © 1999, Mosby, Inc.

Box 6.1 provides serum creatinine and creatinine clearance values for all age groups and the formula for calculating creatinine clearance.

dL, deciliter; *kg,* kilogram; *mg,* milligram; *min,* minute; *ml,* milliliter; ×, times.

range. Half-life is taken into account when estimating how long it will take for a given opioid drug to reach steady state. For example, the full effects of a change in dose of an opioid drug will not be seen until the time equal to four to five times the half-life of the opioid drug has passed (Benet, Kroetz, Sheiner, 1996; Coyle, Cherny, Portenoy, 1995). When steady state is reached by continuous infusion, the various opioids differ little in terms of duration.

If a drug is excreted slower than it is absorbed, serum drug levels rise. This phenomenon is called cumulation (Spencer, 1993). With long-term opioid analgesic administration the opioid drug and/or its metabolites, especially those with long half-life, can cumulate and produce toxic effects. Meperidine's metabolite, normeperidine, has a long half-life (15 to 20 hours) compared with the half-life of its parent, meperidine (2 to 3 hours). Long after meperidine is discontinued, even after short-term use, patients are at risk for the toxic effects of normeperidine, which include irritability, tremors, and seizures (AHCPR, 1992; APS, 1992).

Pharmacodynamics
Opioid Responsiveness: Potency and Efficacy

Clinicians confuse a number of terms when discussing opioid analgesics and their patients' responses to opioid analgesic treatment. Commonly confused and misused terms include efficacy, potency, responsiveness, and resistance.

The meaning of efficacy varies, depending on the context in which it is used. Intrinsic efficacy is a pharmacology term defined as the proportion of opioid receptors that must be occupied by a drug to produce a given effect. The receptor occupancy required for an agonist to produce a response is inversely proportional to its intrinsic efficacy (Portenoy, 1996b).

In the clinical setting, efficacy (sometimes called maximal efficacy) refers to the maximal effect that can be produced by a drug (Portenoy, 1996b). Simply put, it is the level or degree of analgesia that can be achieved by increasing the dose of the drug to the point of limiting side effects. By this definition, the true maximal effect of a drug may not be achieved in some instances until unacceptable side effects are optimally treated (Foley, Inturrisi, 1992; Nies, Spielberg, 1996; Portenoy, 1996b).

The term efficacy often is contrasted and confused with the term potency, which refers to the dose of a drug required to produce a specified effect. Relative potency is the dose of two analgesics required to produce the same analgesic effect (Foley, Inturrisi, 1992). For example, parenteral hydromorphone is more potent than parenteral morphine because the dose of hydromorphone required to achieve the same analgesia as morphine is about one sixth that of the morphine dose. On the basis of single dose studies, the relative potency of parenteral hydromorphone and parenteral morphine is 1.5:10.

A common misconception is that the more potent a drug is, the more therapeutically superior it is. In reality, all opioid analgesics are capable of producing the same degree of analgesia if doses are appropriately adjusted (Hill, Chapman, Saeger et al., 1990; Nies, Spielberg, 1996; Portenoy, 1996b). Increased potency alone does not provide any advantage because the more potent drugs also exhibit a parallel increase in their ability to produce undesirable effects (Foley, Inturrisi, 1992).

The clinical relevance of efficacy and potency and why potency is less important than efficacy in the clinical setting is better understood by comparing the differences between butorphanol, a mixed agonist-antagonist opioid analgesic, and morphine, a mu agonist opioid analgesic. Although butorphanol is five times more potent than morphine (2 mg of butorphanol produces analgesia comparable to 10 mg of morphine), it has a maximal efficacy far lower than that of morphine. That is, butorphanol's analgesic effect plateaus as the dose is increased, and further dose increases for unrelieved pain will produce no increase in analgesia (analgesic ceiling). On the other hand, morphine, like other mu agonist opioid analgesics, has no analgesic ceiling, and the only limiting factor in increasing its dose is the incidence and severity of side effects (Portenoy, 1996b).

The term efficacy often is used when clinicians discuss the patient's response to opioid analgesic treatment. A better term to describe clinical response is the term opioid responsiveness. Opioid responsiveness refers to the probability that adequate analgesia (tolerable and manageable side effects and satisfactory pain relief) can be achieved during dose titration (Foley, 1995; Portenoy, 1996b).

Opioid responsiveness is influenced by patient characteristics and the particular type of pain or pain syndrome being treated. However, it is a common misconception that certain patient characteristics, such as age, or types of pain, such as neuropathic, are opioid resistant. No evidence exists that either of these factors cause uniform opioid resistance. In fact, all individuals and types of pain are opioid responsive, but they vary in the degree to which they respond. It is best to view opioid responsiveness on a continuum rather than an all-or-none phenomenon (Cherny, Thaler, Friedlander-Klar, 1994; Foley, 1995; Portenoy, 1996b).

Opioid analgesics should be considered for the treatment of all types of pain, remembering that some types respond better than others. For example, opioid responsiveness is reduced in neuropathic pain states compared with visceral or somatic pain (Cherny, Thaler, Friedlander-Klar, 1994; Foley, 1995; Portenoy, 1996b). The opioid doses that might be needed to control neuropathic pain may be more likely to cause intolerable side effects (Weissman, 1996). Opioid responsiveness is affected also by any factor that increases the risk of dose-limiting toxicity, such as advanced age and cumulation of metabolites (Portenoy, 1996b).

Significant variation exists in patients' responsiveness to opioid analgesics. With the same opioid, one patient may achieve excellent analgesia with few side effects, whereas another patient experiences intolerable side effects with minimal or no analgesia (interindividual differences). Patients can vary also in their individual responsiveness to different opioid analgesics (intraindividual differences). For example, a patient may experience unacceptable nausea and poor analgesia with one opioid analgesic and no nausea but unacceptable somnolence and lesser, equal, or better analgesia with another (Galer, Coyle, Pasternak, 1992; Portenoy, 1996b).

Tolerance

Tolerance refers to a process characterized by decreasing effects of a drug at a constant dose of the drug or, conversely, the need for a higher dose of drug to maintain an effect. Tolerance should be viewed as a descriptive label that indicates a change in the relationship between dose and response (Portenoy, 1996b). Continued exposure to the drug is the primary cause of tolerance. In terms of tolerance to opioid drugs, it is a physiologic response that should be expected when an individual takes an opioid drug for several days or longer. Tolerance should not be confused with addiction, and it is not a predictor of abuse (Reisine, Pasternak, 1996). It occurs regardless of why the opioid is used. Both persons abusing opioids and those taking opioids for pain relief will likely develop tolerance to some drug effects. The term does not apply when a decrease in a drug's effect can be attributed to increasing physical pathologic conditions or psychologic reasons rather than to drug exposure (Foley, 1995; Portenoy, 1996b).

Tolerance to analgesia may be evident after a few days of treatment. The first indication of tolerance is most commonly a decrease in the duration of analgesia for a given opioid dose (Jacox, Carr, Payne et al., 1994) followed by a decrease in analgesic effect. This can be treated easily, usually by increasing the opioid dose or decreasing the interval between doses.

Clinicians often incorrectly conclude that patients with chronic disease who experience diminished analgesia after a period of stable dosing have developed tolerance. Although tolerance could be the cause, it should not be assumed to be the "driving force" behind the need for dose escalation in a patient with chronic pain. If dose escalation is required, recurrence of disease or development of new pathology is the most likely cause (Collin, Poulain, Gauvain-Piquard et al., 1993; Foley, 1995; Portenoy, 1996b). Therefore whenever dose escalation is necessary, it is recommended that a differential diagnosis be made to rule out new or recurrent pathology or psychologic processes (Portenoy, 1996b) (Box 6.2).

After the opioid is titrated to an acceptable dose, the dose stabilizes if the pain is stable. Further dose escalation in patients with stable pain syndromes is unusual. If analgesia declines (because of tolerance or worsening disease), it is handled easily, usually by increasing the dose. For these reasons, clinicians should not withhold opioid analgesia from patients with long life expectancies or delay initiating opioid analgesic treatment for fear of producing tolerance or reaching a dose beyond which no further analgesia can be obtained.

It is important to reinforce information about tolerance and ceiling effect to patients and families because they frequently are reluctant to begin opioid analgesic treatment. Often, they are concerned that the effectiveness of opioid analgesics will diminish over time and that the patient will be subjected to severe pain in later stages of disease if the opioid is started in the early stages (Portenoy, 1996b).

Tolerance to the nonanalgesic effects of an opioid drug (i.e., side effects) occurs and can be beneficial in achieving a balance between analgesia and side effects (Portenoy, 1996b). The rate of developing tolerance to each of the nonanalgesic effects of opioid drugs varies. For example, patients usually develop tolerance to mental clouding and nausea within days or weeks (Foley, 1995;

● ● ● ● ●

BOX 6.2	**Differential Diagnosis for Declining Analgesic Effect**

INCREASED ACTIVITY IN NOCICEPTIVE PATHWAYS

Increasing activation of nociceptors in the periphery
    Due to mechanical factors (e.g., tumor growth)
    Due to biochemical changes (e.g., inflammation)
    Due to peripheral neuropathic processes (e.g., neuroma formation)
Increased activity in the central nociceptive pathways
    Due to central neuropathic processes (e.g., sensitization, shift in receptive fields, change in modulatory processes)

PSYCHOLOGIC PROCESSES[1]

Increasing psychologic distress (e.g., anxiety or depression)
Change in cognitive state leading to altered pain perception or reporting (e.g., delirium)
Conditioned pain behavior independent of the drug

TOLERANCE

Due to pharmacodynamic processes
Due to pharmacokinetic processes
Due to psychologic processes

May be duplicated for use in clinical practice. As appears in McCaffery M, Pasero C: *Pain: Clinical manual*, p. 172, 1999, Mosby, Inc.

Box 6.2 provides possible explanations for declining analgesic effect. Whenever dose escalation is necessary, it is recommended that a differential diagnosis be made to rule out new or recurrent pathologic or psychologic processes.

[1]Other than conditioned responses to the drug.

From Portenoy RK: Opioid analgesics. In Portenoy RK, Kanner RM, editors: *Pain management: Theory and practice*, p 255, Philadelphia, 1996, FA Davis.

Portenoy, 1996b), but they rarely if ever develop tolerance to constipation. This is why a bowel management regimen should be routinely implemented in patients receiving long-term opioid analgesics (Coyle, Cherny, Portenoy, 1995) (see pp. 261-270 for management of opioid side effects).

Tolerance to respiratory depression also develops rapidly, usually within a few days of opioid administration. Tolerance to this effect allows dose escalation to whatever dose is required for analgesia. Studies have shown that patients with cancer pain may require doses ranging from 30 to 7000 mg of morphine (or equivalent) (Foley, 1995). Although there appears to be no limit to the degree of tolerance to respiratory depression that may develop, there is always a lethal dose for the individual.

Pain itself may diminish the side effects of opioids. Evidence exists that patients thought to be tolerant to the adverse effects of an opioid drug can experience a return of side effects if the pain is lessened or eliminated. Consider a patient who is tolerant to opioid-induced sedation and nausea associated with high doses of morphine taken for pain associated with a malignant lesion. The patient may experience anew all of the adverse effects of morphine, including respiratory depression, if an intervention, such as cordotomy, suddenly eliminates the pain. Under these circumstances patients may develop signs and symptoms of overdose if the opioid dose is not reduced promptly after the intervention (Jacox, Carr, Payne, 1994; Portenoy, 1996b).

Cross-Tolerance

As mentioned, tolerance to analgesic effects is managed by increasing the opioid dose; however, when an increased dose brings with it intolerable and unmanageable side effects, another option is to switch to an alternative opioid drug. When switching to another opioid analgesic, the clinical implications of a phenomenon called cross-tolerance must be considered.

Cross-tolerance is the development of tolerance to the effects of other pharmacologically related drugs, particularly those that act at the same receptor site. In other words a patient who is tolerant to morphine may be tolerant to other mu agonist opioids, such as hydromorphone, fentanyl, or meperidine. However, when switching to another opioid, it is extremely important for clinicians to assume that cross-tolerance will be incomplete (Foley, 1995). This means that the starting dose of the new opioid must be reduced by at least 50% of the calculated equianalgesic dose to prevent overdosing. Then the dose is gradually increased as needed to the point of pain relief and tolerable and manageable side effects (Coyle, Cherny, Portenoy, 1995; Levy, 1993).

Another important point to remember about cross-tolerance is that it may not develop equally to all of the drug effects (Nies, Spielberg, 1996). The clinical implication is that a patient receiving morphine may have developed tolerance to nausea, but when switched to the new opioid drug may experience severe nausea. Thus surveillance of all of the opioid's effects is warranted when switching to an alternative opioid (see pp. 253-261 for more on switching to an alternative opioid).

Opioid Tolerant Versus Opioid Naive

The terms opioid-tolerant and opioid-naive are used to distinguish between patients who have, or have not, respectively, been taking opioid drugs regularly. By convention, most clinicians will consider a patient who has used opioids regularly for approximately 7 days or more to be opioid-tolerant. The clinical importance is that such individuals are assumed to have developed tolerance to most of the opioid side effects. Most importantly, the occurrence of respiratory depression is rare in opioid-tolerant individuals whose doses are carefully titrated. The fear of producing respiratory depression in these individuals usually is overstated. This fear should not interfere with adequate opioid dosing. In addition, compared with opioid-naive individuals, opioid-tolerant individuals are generally able to tolerate faster escalation in larger doses of opioid drugs without experiencing life-threatening side effects (Foley, 1995; Jacox, Carr, Payne et al., 1994).

Failing to appreciate the differences between opioid-tolerant and opioid-naive individuals can lead to overdosing opioid-naive patients and underdosing opioid-tolerant patients. This is especially evident with the use of IV PCA. Many clinicians have discovered that the doses of opioid analgesics tolerated well by opioid-tolerant patients can produce significant side effects in opioid-naive postoperative patients (Parker, Holtmann, White, 1991). For example, opioid-naive postoperative patients are more likely to experience significant opioid-induced sedation with a continuous infusion than opioid tolerant patients with cancer pain who often receive the major portion of their opioid requirement as a continuous infusion without experiencing side effects such as sedation.

Likewise, clinicians who are accustomed to caring for opioid-naive patients may prescribe too small of an opioid analgesic dose for an opioid-tolerant patient. In one study the maximum doses required for acceptable analgesia were 80 mg/h of morphine, 50 mg/h of meperidine (use of this drug is not recommended), and 60 mg/h of hydromorphone. Side effects and safety profiles were acceptable (Kerr, Sone, DeAngelis et al., 1988). Some cancer patients have required as much as 40,000 mg of IV morphine per 24 hours to achieve adequate analgesia (Weinstein, 1994). These findings reinforce that no ceiling on analgesia exists when mu agonist opioid analgesics are used, and "high" doses are safe and appropriate in many opioid-tolerant individuals.

Physical Dependence

Physical dependence is a physiologic phenomenon manifested by the development of withdrawal syndrome after abrupt discontinuation of therapy, substantial dose reduction, or administration of an antagonist drug such as naloxone (Portenoy, 1996b). It is most commonly seen in individuals who have taken large doses of opioid analgesics for a long period of time; however, it has been observed also in individuals who have taken low doses or who have taken opioid analgesics for a short period of time (Compton, 1997). Therefore physical dependence should be expected in individuals after repeated doses of an opioid drug for more than 2 or 3 days.

Physical dependence requires no treatment unless withdrawal symptoms occur or are anticipated. Withdrawal can be suppressed with gradual reduction in dose over 7 to 10 days (Coyle, Cherny, Portenoy, 1995). One recommendation for weaning adults is to give half the previous dose for the first 2 days and then reduce the dose by 25% every 2 days. When the dose reaches the equivalent of approximately 30 mg/day of oral morphine, this dose may be given for 2 days and then discontinued (APS, 1992).

Confusion regarding the differences between physical dependence and addiction presents a persistent barrier to effective pain management. Physical dependence indicates neither the presence nor absence of addiction, and addiction may exist with or without the capacity for withdrawal that defines physical dependence. The fear of addiction continues to prevent patients and families from seeking appropriate pain management and caregivers from providing it. It is important that caregivers understand and reinforce to patients and families the differences between the two phenomena.

Addiction (Psychologic Dependence) and Pseudoaddiction

Addiction is a type of psychologic dependence as contrasted with physical dependence. The American Pain Society (APS, 1992) defines addiction as "a pattern of compulsive drug use characterized by a continued craving for an opioid and the need to use the opioid for effects other than pain relief" (p. 26). An important message in this definition is that taking opioids for pain relief is not addiction, no matter how long a person takes opioids or at what doses. Individuals taking opioid drugs for relief of pain are using them therapeutically; they do not seek psychic effects from opioid drugs as do individuals who are addicted (Compton, 1997). Addiction is further defined as a psychologic and behavioral syndrome with three distinguishing characteristics: (1) loss of control over drug use, (2) compulsive drug use, and (3) continued use despite harm (Portenoy, 1996b) (see Chapter 10 for more on addiction).

How likely is it that addiction will occur as a result of using opioids for pain relief? In a classic study of nearly 12,000 hospitalized patients with no history of drug abuse who received opioid analgesics during hospitalization, only four developed an addiction disorder. Only one of these was defined as major (Porter, Jick, 1980). In retrospective reviews of more than 24,000 patients who received opioids for pain relief, only 7 could be identified as having an addiction disorder develop (Friedman, 1990). Thus research indicates that the medical use of opioid drugs for pain relief is rarely associated with the development of addiction. Other surveys have produced similar results (see p. 50).

Behaviors indicative of uncontrolled pain or fear of uncontrolled pain often are misinterpreted as addiction. For example, patients who receive opioid doses that are too low or at intervals greater than the opioid's duration of action may understandably try to manipulate the staff into giving them more analgesic. They may respond with demanding behavior, "clock-watching," hoarding of opioid analgesics during periods of reduced symptoms, or requesting an extra opioid analgesic prescription for fear of running out and experiencing severe pain (see Table 3.3, pp. 52-53). These behaviors are commonly referred to as pseudoaddiction (Weissman, Haddox, 1989). Pain relief, usually accomplished by increasing opioid doses or providing an extra prescription in case it is needed, typically eliminates these behaviors.

Equianalgesia

The term equianalgesia means approximately equal analgesia and is used when referring to the doses of various opioid analgesics that provide approximately the same pain relief. An equianalgesic chart (see Table 6.12, pp. 241-243) provides a list of analgesic doses, both oral and parenteral, that are approximately equal to each other in ability to provide pain relief. These doses are also referred to as equianalgesic dose units. Most of the doses in equianalgesic charts are based on single dose studies, often conducted with opioid-naive surgical patients, using morphine, 10 mg IM, for comparison. The parenteral doses listed are typical of IM doses given approximately every 3 to 4 hours (see pp. 240-261 for practical application of the equianalgesic chart).

Equianalgesic dose calculation provides a basis for selecting the appropriate starting dose when changing from one opioid drug or route of administration to another. However, these calculations are just estimates and vary with repeated dosing and opioid rotation (see pp. 253-257). The optimal dose for the patient is determined always by titration (Dunbar, Chapman, Buckley et al., 1996; Foley, Inturrisi, 1992; Lawlor, Turner, Hanson et al., 1997).

Conversion Charts

Conversion charts for opioid analgesics are provided by drug manufacturers to assist clinicians in converting from various other opioids to the opioid being marketed. They usually provide a conservative estimate of the dose of the new opioid that will be required. The charts often assume that the switch to the new opioid is likely to be taking place in an opioid-tolerant patient. The reasoning behind using conversion charts is that cross-tolerance is not complete and patients respond differently to different opioids. Side effects and overdosing can be more readily avoided by using conservative estimates of the dose of the new drug. Thus conversion charts are not the same as equianalgesic charts. Rather they take into consideration equianalgesic doses and reduce that estimate.

Because conversion charts are conservative in their estimate of what the initial dose of the new drug should be, many patients require titration upward to achieve satisfactory analgesia. For example, the manufacturer of transdermal fentanyl cautions that when using the estimates from its conversion chart, 50% of the patients switched from other opioids by other routes to transdermal fentanyl will require an increase in dose after the initial dose of transdermal fentanyl (Janssen, 1996).

Conservative conversion charts should be used to make conversions in one direction only. If the same conversion chart is used to convert in the opposite direction, the patient very likely would be overdosed. In other words, care must be taken to be sure the conversion chart is used to calculate doses in the desired direction. For example, a current conversion chart for OxyContin (manufacturer, 1996) recommends that a patient taking 200 mg of MS Contin every 12 hours be converted to 80 mg of Oxy-Contin every 12 hours, probably a safe and conservative estimate. However, if this same chart were used to convert a patient from 80 mg of OxyContin every 12 hours to 200 mg of MS Contin every 12 hours, the MS Contin dose would probably be considerably more than the patient requires (see pp. 253-257).

When studies that clarify equianalgesic dosing are lacking, such as is the case with fentanyl, various conversion formulas evolve. These formulas, and even the ones used in this text, are not necessarily comparable; different formulas lead to different answers.

KEY CONCEPTS IN ANALGESIC THERAPY
Balanced Analgesia

As discussed in Chapter 4, a continuous multimodal approach, commonly called "balanced analgesia," is considered by some experts to be the ideal for treating pain that is of a continuous nature (APS, 1997; Coyle, Cherny, Portenoy, 1995; Kehlet, 1997a). Balanced analgesia uses combined analgesic regimens, thereby reducing the likelihood of significant side effects from a single agent or method. It may include several different drugs, such as NSAIDs, opioids, and local anesthetics or other adjuvant analgesics. Drug choices and routes of administration must be carefully determined, along with establishing the lowest possible effective doses. With the exception of neuropathic pain syndromes such as diabetic neuropathy and postherpetic neuralgia that respond best to adjuvant analgesics, opioid drugs are commonly the mainstay analgesic in a balanced analgesia approach.

Preemptive analgesia

Preemptive analgesia involves an intervention implemented before noxious stimuli are experienced, which is designed to reduce the impact of these stimuli on the CNS. Balanced analgesia administered preemptively, as well as after the noxious event occurs, is considered by some experts to be the ideal. In a review of the clinical trials of preemptive analgesia, Woolf and Chong (1993) state that ideal preoperative, intraoperative, and postoperative treatment would include "NSAIDs to reduce the activation/centralization of nociceptors, local anesthetics to block sensory inflow, and centrally acting drugs such as opiates" (p. 367).

Although some studies have shown impressive preemptive effects by combining opioids with NSAIDs and local anesthetics by a variety of routes (Liu, Carpenter, Neal, 1995; Woolf, Chong, 1993), the results have not been definitive, and the role of opioid drugs is not clear.

Less emphasis on the use of opioid drugs and more on the use of local anesthetics, primarily by sufficiently long regional blockade, appears to be indicated for effective and sustained preemptive analgesia (Kehlet, 1997a, b). Preemptive analgesia should be considered before surgery, painful procedures, and whenever pain management is expected to be difficult (Portenoy, 1992).

Around the Clock (ATC) Dosing

Two basic principles of providing effective pain management are preventing pain and maintaining a pain rating that is satisfactory to the patient. These may require that the mainstay analgesic be administered on a scheduled ATC basis, rather than as needed (PRN), to maintain stable analgesic blood levels. This preventive approach to pain management is based on the knowledge that less drug is needed to prevent the recurrence of pain than to relieve it (Reisine, Pasternak, 1996).

To prevent recurrence of pain, ATC dosing is indicated whenever pain is predicted to be present for more than 12 out of 24 hours. In other words, ATC dosing should be considered when pain itself is ATC or present 12 or more hours out of 24. The use of continuous analgesia prevents the undertreatment of pain in patients who are hesitant to request pain medication and eliminates delays patients encounter waiting for caregivers to prepare and administer pain medication.

ATC dosing for continuous pain should be accompanied by provision of additional analgesic doses (called supplemental doses, breakthrough doses, or rescue doses) to relieve pain that exceeds, or breaks through, the ongoing pain (see the following). For example, when analgesia is provided orally, ATC dosing often is accomplished with a combination of controlled-release opioid given at scheduled times with rescue doses of immediate-release opioid given when pain breaks through. When invasive routes are used to manage pain, a continuous infusion with PCA boluses or clinician-administered rescue doses accomplishes the same objectives as this oral approach.

Breakthrough pain

Breakthrough pain is defined as transient moderate to severe pain that increases above the pain addressed by the ongoing analgesics. The term is used most often in reference to patients with continuous cancer or chronic nonmalignant pain. Breakthrough pain in patients with cancer pain is a common occurrence, reported by two thirds of individuals with continuous chronic pain (Portenoy, Hager, 1990).

Breakthrough pain can have a sudden or gradual onset. It can be brief or prolonged; some episodes are spontaneous and others are associated with an identifiable precipitant, such as stress or a change in the weather. When pain is brief and precipitated by a voluntary action, such as movement, it is referred to as incident pain. Another

type of breakthrough pain is called end of dose failure. End of dose failure is characterized by a return of pain before the next dose is due and often is amenable to increasing the dose of the analgesic. If not, the intervals between doses must be shortened (Portenoy, Kanner, 1996).

Breakthrough pain should be expected and planned for when managing chronic pain. Short-acting mu agonist opioid analgesics are recommended to provide rescue doses when breakthrough pain occurs. It is recommended that the same route and opioid that is used ATC for the management of a patient's continuous pain be used to manage the breakthrough pain. For example, immediate-release oral morphine is appropriate for breakthrough pain in patients taking controlled-release morphine. A short half-life opioid drug, such as fentanyl or morphine, is recommended when methadone or transdermal fentanyl is the mainstay analgesic (Coyle, Cherny, Portenoy, 1995).

PRN Dosing

PRN dosing ordinarily requires patients to request analgesia. Effective PRN dosing requires the patient's active participation. Patient teaching must include reminding patients to "stay on top of pain" and request analgesia before pain is severe and out of control. Obviously crucial to the effective use of PRN dosing is a rapid response to reports of pain and to requests for an analgesic.

PRN dosing of opioid analgesics is appropriate for certain types of pain, such as intermittent pain. It is useful when initiating opioid analgesic therapy in opioid-naive patients with moderate to severe chronic pain, especially when pain is escalating rapidly. In these cases, PRN dosing allows for a rapid response to the patient's need for pain relief while minimizing the chance of over-dose. PRN dosing is also helpful when pain is decreasing rapidly (Coyle, Cherny, Portenoy, 1995). Because patients with acute pain recover and pain resolves, ATC dosing may be replaced with PRN dosing (Pasero, McCaffery, 1996a).

Patient-Controlled Analgesia (PCA)

PCA is an interactive method of pain management that permits patients to treat their pain by self-administering doses of analgesics. The PCA approach recognizes that only the patient can feel the pain and only the patient knows how much analgesic will relieve it (Pasero, McCaffery, 1993). By allowing patients to determine dosing, PCA addresses the significant variations in analgesic requirements between individuals. PCA is similar to responsive PRN dosing in that it requires patients to recognize that they are experiencing pain and request analgesia (e.g., by pressing a button on a pump to deliver a PCA bolus). The difference between PRN and PCA is that with PCA the patient rather than a caregiver administers the analgesic, so the delay in waiting for a caregiver's response to the request for analgesia is eliminated. Just as with effective PRN dosing, patients are reminded to "stay on top of the pain" to maintain a steady analgesic level and administer doses before pain is severe and out of control.

PCA has been used to manage all types of pain. It is used most commonly to manage acute pain and less often for cancer pain because most cancer pain can be managed with oral opioid analgesics. Although patients with pain often self-administer their oral analgesics (see Inpatient Oral PCA, p. 199), the term PCA is applied usually when dosing opioids by the SC, IV, and epidural routes. Typically, a special infusion pump is used to deliver PCA by these routes of administration. In this context, PCA refers to the bolus dose the patient controls when pressing a button on or attached to the pump. PCA can be delivered by two modes: PCA bolus doses with a continuous infusion (also called a basal rate) or

PCA bolus doses alone (see p. 220 for PCEA and pp. 248-253 for clinical use of PCA).

Mu agonist opioid analgesics, specifically morphine, meperidine, hydromorphone, and fentanyl, are the most common analgesics administered by PCA. Frequently, local anesthetics and sometimes the alpha$_2$-adrenergic drug clonidine are added to the opioid drug for epidural PCA (see pp. 227-231).

Appropriateness of PCA

A number of factors need to be considered in determining whether a patient is a candidate for PCA (Box 6.3). Great care must be taken to ensure that PCA is appropriate, especially the additional cost of a PCA pump and the risks of an invasive route of administration.

Frequently age is used inappropriately as a criterion for determining whether a patient is a candidate for PCA.

BOX 6.3

GUIDELINES

USE OF IV PCA

Patient Selection
- For patients with chronic pain, oral and other noninvasive routes produce unmanageable and intolerable side effects.
- For patients with acute pain (e.g., surgery, trauma), the oral and other noninvasive routes have been considered and are not an option because they would produce unmanageable and intolerable side effects at the anticipated doses required for adequate analgesia.
- In the patient with chronic pain or who is terminally ill, the patient's need for parenteral administration of an opioid analgesic is expected to be longer than 1 or 2 days.
- Patient is able to understand the relationship between pain, pushing the PCA button, and pain relief, and can physically self-administer a PCA dose using the available equipment.

Other Considerations
Pumps are available.
Cost is not prohibitive.
Staff (or family) is trained to explain, assess, manage, and document IV PCA.

Surgical Procedures for Which IV PCA Is Commonly Prescribed
Cesarean section when epidural anesthesia/analgesia is not used
Abdominal, vaginal hysterectomy
Anterior and posterior repair
Bladder surgery

Surgical Procedures—cont'd
Ureteral reimplantation
Penile implant
Radical prostatectomy
Mastectomy
Gastroplasty
Abdominoplasty
Inpatient rectal surgeries
Major plastic surgeries and skin grafts
Major hand, ankle, or foot repair
Joint replacement
Long bone surgery
Laminectomy
Shoulder repair
Radical neck

Medical Conditions for Which IV PCA Is Commonly Prescribed
Cancer pain
Sickle cell pain
Burn pain
HIV pain
Fractures
Pancreatitis
Nephrolithiasis

HIV, human immunodeficiency virus (AIDS); *IV*, intravenous; *PCA*, patient-controlled analgesia

Information from Agency for Health Care Policy and Research (AHCPR): *Acute pain management: Operations or medical procedures and trauma. Clinical practice guideline.* AHCPR Publication No. 92-0032, Rockville, MD, U.S. Public Health Service, AHCPR, February, 1992; Ferrell BR, Griffith H: Cost issues related to pain management: Report from the cancer pain panel of the Agency for Health Care Policy and Research, *J Pain Symptom Manage* 9(4):221-234, 1994; Levy MH: Pharmacologic management of cancer pain, *Sem Oncol* 21(6):718-739, 1994; Pasero C: *Acute pain management service policy and procedure manual*, Rolling Hills Estates, CA, 1994, Academy Medical Systems, Inc; Pasero C, McCaffery M: Unconventional PCA: Making it work for your patient, *Am J Nurs* 93(9):38-41, 1993.

This has presented a barrier to its use in children and the elderly. Clinicians often hesitate to prescribe PCA for children believing that they are too young to understand the concept of PCA and how to use the pump appropriately. However, PCA has been used effectively and safely in developmentally normal children as young as 5 years old (APS, 1992). Although IV PCA has been shown to be safe in elderly patients (Egbert, Parks, Short et al., 1990), clinicians often do not prescribe it for fear of producing confusion in these patients. However, research shows that a number of factors other than opioid drugs cause mental confusion (Duggleby, Lander, 1994; Rosenberg, Kehlet, 1993; Rosenberg, Rosenberg-Adamsen; Rosenberg, Kehlet, 1995; Simpson, Lee, Cameron, 1996).

To be considered a candidate for PCA, patients must be able to understand the relationship between pain, pushing the PCA button, and pain relief (APS, 1992). In cases when PCA is warranted, patients should not be denied access to this modality simply because of their age. Instead, they should be carefully screened for their cognitive and physical ability to manage their pain by PCA.

Unconventional use of the PCA pump

In situations in which patients are unable or unwilling to self-administer analgesics, creative ways have been found to use PCA technology safely and effectively, such as family-controlled analgesia and nurse-activated dosing. With family-controlled analgesia, one family member or significant other is designated to be the patient's primary pain manager and has the responsibility of pressing the PCA button (Pasero, McCaffery, 1993; Pasero, 1994). With nurse-activated dosing, the patient's primary nurse has that responsibility. Some institutions have even adapted their PCA equipment for patients who are cognitively able to use PCA but are physically unable to press the button, such as patients with rheumatoid arthritis (Pasero, McCaffery, 1993; Pasero, 1994) (Box 6.4).

GUIDELINES FOR OPIOID ANALGESIC ADMINISTRATION

Safe and effective use of opioid analgesics requires the development of an individualized treatment plan. This begins with a comprehensive pain assessment, which includes clarifying the goals of treatment and discussing options with the patient and family. The need for periodic reevaluation of the goals is common and should be expected as disease progresses or, in the case of acute pain, as pain resolves (Portenoy, 1996b).

Goals are stated as simply as possible and shared among the patient, family, and caregivers. Goals ordinarily include the patient's desired pain rating and the activities that accompany this pain level. For example, a postoperative patient may identify a comfort goal of 3/10 to enable regular use of the incentive spirometer and

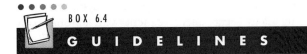

BOX 6.4

G U I D E L I N E S

UNCONVENTIONAL USE OF THE PCA PUMP[1]

Patient Selection

Patient is unable to understand the relationship between pain, pushing the PCA button, and pain relief, and/or cannot physically self-administer a PCA dose using the available equipment.[2]

Family-Controlled Analgesia

One family member or significant other is designated to be the patient's primary pain manager and has the responsibility of pressing the PCA button.

Guidelines for selecting a primary pain manager for family-controlled analgesia:

1. Spends a significant amount of time with the patient.
2. Is willing to assume responsibility of being primary pain manager.
3. Is willing to accept and respect patient's reports of pain (if able to provide) as the best indicator of how much pain the patient is experiencing; knows how to use and interpret a pain rating scale.
4. Understands the purpose and goals of the patient's pain management plan.
5. Understands the concept of maintaining a steady analgesic blood level.
6. Recognizes the signs of pain and side effects and adverse reactions to the opioid.

Nurse-Activated Dosing

1. The patient's primary nurse is designated to be the patient's primary pain manager (the primary nurse is the only person who presses the PCA button during that nurse's shift).
2. The guidelines for selecting a primary pain manager for family-controlled analgesia apply to nurse-activated dosing.
3. This method may be used:
   • In addition to a basal rate as a means of managing breakthrough pain with bolus doses. Patients are assessed q30 minutes for the need for a bolus dose.
   • Without a basal rate as a means of maintaining analgesia with ATC bolus doses.

May be duplicated for use in clinical practice. From McCaffery M, Pasero C: *Pain: Clinical manual,* p. 177. Copyright © 1999, Mosby, Inc.

q, every.

[1]Before variations of conventional PCA are used, institutional policies and procedures should be approved and staff (and patients and families when indicated) trained to assess and manage the therapies.

[2]In all cases of unconventional use of PCA the control of analgesia is returned to patients as soon as they are able to assume it.

Information from Pasero C: *Acute pain management service policy and procedure manual,* Rolling Hills Estates, CA, 1994, Academy Medical Systems, Inc; Pasero C, McCaffery M: Unconventional PCA: Making it work for your patient, *Am J Nurs* 93(9):38-41, 1993.

may state that the mild sedation accompanying this level of analgesia is acceptable. A patient with chronic pain may identify a comfort goal of 2/10 as necessary for engaging in employment and may state that sedation is not compatible with this goal.

Opioid Drug Selection

Many factors are considered when determining the appropriate opioid analgesic for the patient with pain

(Box 6.5). These include the unique characteristics of the various opioids and patient characteristics, such as pain intensity, patient age, coexisting disease, current drug regimen and potential drug interactions, prior treatment outcomes, and patient preference.

Characteristics of selected mu agonist opioids

As discussed previously in this chapter, the mu agonist opioid analgesics are capable of managing all pain

• • • • •

BOX 6.5

G U I D E L I N E S

USE OF OPIOIDS FOR ACUTE AND CHRONIC PAIN

1. Develop an individualized treatment plan that includes specific goals related to pain intensity, activities, and side effects (e.g., pain rating of 3/10 to ambulate) accompanied by minimal or no sedation and other side effects tolerable or manageable.
2. Consider using multimodality balanced analgesia.
3. Consider preemptive analgesia before surgery or painful procedures.
4. Drug selection
   a. Consider diagnosis, condition, or surgical procedure, current or expected pain intensity, age, whether major organ failure is present (especially renal, hepatic, or respiratory), and presence of coexisting disease.
   b. Consider pharmacologic issues (e.g., accumulation of metabolites and effects of concurrent drugs and possible interactions).
   c. Consider individual differences (note prior treatment outcomes) and patient preference.
   d. Be aware of available routes of administration (e.g., oral, IV, SC, intraspinal) and formulation (e.g., controlled-release or immediate-release).
   e. Be aware of cost differences.
5. Route selection
   a. Use least invasive route possible.
   b. Consider convenience and patient's ability to adhere to the regimen.
   c. Consider staff's (or family's, patient's) ability to monitor and provide care required (e.g., intraspinal routes).
6. Dosing and dose titration
   a. Consider previous dosing requirement and relative analgesic potencies when initiating therapy.
   b. Use pain intensity and equianalgesic chart to determine starting dose then titrate until adequate analgesia is achieved or dose-limiting side effects are encountered.
   c. Use appropriate dosing schedule (e.g., ATC or PRN).
   d. When a dose is safe but additional analgesia is desired, titrate upward by 25% for mild increase, 50% for

moderate increase, and 100% for considerable increase in analgesia.
   e. Provide rescue doses for breakthrough pain.
   f. Consider PCA.
   g. Recognize that for chronic pain, tolerance is rarely the "driving force" for dose escalation; consider disease progression when increasing dose requirements occur.
7. Trials of alternative opioids
   a. Trial of another opioid should be done only after the first opioid has been titrated upward to determine whether adequate analgesia can be obtained without intolerable side effects.
   b. Be aware of incomplete cross-tolerance and start the new opioid at about 50% of the estimated equianalgesic dose.
8. Treatment of side effects
   a. Be aware of the prevalence and impact of opioid side effects.
   b. Use a preventive approach in the management of constipation, including for patients receiving short-term opioid treatment (e.g., postoperative patients).
   c. Prevent respiratory depression by monitoring sedation levels in opioids-naive patients.
   d. Advise patient/family which side effects are likely to subside.
9. Monitoring
   a. Evaluate the treatment plan on the basis of the specific goals identified at the outset and including pain intensity, side effects, and activity levels on an ongoing basis.
   b. Make necessary modifications to treatment plan.
10. Tapering and cessation of treatment
   a. Decrease in accordance with decreased pain ratings.
   b. Be aware of potential for withdrawal syndrome and need for tapering schedule in patients who have been receiving opioid therapy for more than a few days.
   c. Use equianalgesic dosing to determine appropriate decreases in doses.

May be duplicated for use in clinical practice. As appears in McCaffery M, Pasero C: *Pain: Clinical manual*, p. 178, 1999, Mosby, Inc.

ATC, around-the-clock; *IV*, intravenous; *PCA*, patient-controlled analgesia.

Modified from Coyle N, Cherny N, Portenoy RK: Pharmacologic management of cancer pain. In McGuire D, Yarbro CH, Ferrell BR, editors: *Cancer pain management*, ed 2, pp 89-130, Boston, 1995, Jones and Bartlett Publishers.

intensities and are effective for many different painful conditions. They are the most common analgesics used to manage moderate to severe pain. Mu agonists are also recommended for the management of breakthrough pain. See Table 6.3 for a summary of information on selected mu opioid analgesics. For more detail about the characteristics of the various opioid analgesics as they relate to route of administration, see pp. 194-239. The equianalgesic chart in Table 6.12 on pp. 241-243 contains dosing and pharmacokinetic information on the various opioid analgesics.

The previously used classification of opioid analgesics as "weak" or "strong" is outdated. Instead, opioid analgesics are conventionally labeled as being appropriate for the treatment of mild, moderate, or severe pain. In reality, however, all the various mu agonists are capable of producing comparable analgesia if the dose is adjusted appropriately.

● ● ● ● ● ●
TABLE 6.3

CHARACTERISTICS OF SELECTED MU OPIOID AGONIST DRUGS[1]

Mu Opioid Agonist Drug	Routes Administered	Comments
Morphine	PO (IR and CR), SL, R, IV, IM, SC, EA, IA	Standard for comparison. Multiple routes of administration. Three controlled-release formulations available, but they are not therapeutically equivalent. Begin with lower doses in elderly. Active metabolite M6G can accumulate with repeated dosing in renal failure.
Codeine	PO, IM, SC	IM has unpredictable absorption and high side effect profile; used orally for mild to moderate pain. Usually compounded with nonopioid (e.g., Tylenol No. 3).
Fentanyl	OTFC, IV, IM, TD, EA, IA	Fast-acting; short half-life. At steady state, slow elimination from tissues can lead to a prolonged half-life (up to 12 h). On the basis of clinical experience, fentanyl, 1 μg/h transdermally, is roughly equivalent to morphine, 2 mg/24 h orally, and fentanyl, 100 μg/h parenterally and transdermally, is roughly equivalent to 4 mg/h morphine parenterally. Opioid-naive patients should be started on no more than 25 μg/h transdermally. Transdermal fentanyl NR for acute pain management. OTFC awaiting FDA approval for management of breakthrough pain.
Hydrocodone	PO	Used for mild to moderate pain; available in nonopioid combination only (e.g., Vicodin, Lortab).
Hydromorphone (Dilaudid)	PO, R, IV, IM, SC, EA, IA	Useful alternative to morphine. No evidence that active metabolites are clinically relevant. Available in high-potency parenteral formulation (10 mg/ml) useful for SC infusion; 3 mg R roughly equivalent to 650 mg aspirin; oral controlled-release available in Canada, soon to be available in the United States.
Levorphanol (Levo-Dromoran)	PO, IV, IM, SC	Long half-life can lead to accumulation within 2-3 days of repetitive dosing.
Meperidine (Demerol)	PO, IV, IM, SC, EA, IA	No longer preferred for the management of acute or chronic pain because of potential toxicity from accumulation of metabolite, normeperidine. Half-life of normeperidine = 15-20 h; NR in elderly or patients with impaired renal function; continuous IV infusion NR. The most appropriate candidates for meperidine use are patients with acute pain who are otherwise healthy and are allergic to other opioids, such as morphine and hydromorphone, or have demonstrated a more favorable outcome with meperidine than other opioid drugs.
Methadone (Dolophine)	PO, SL, R, IV, SC, IM, EA, IA	Long half-life can lead to delayed toxicity from accumulation at start of therapy and with each dose increment; as a result, treatment should be started with PRN dosing.

Continued.

CHARACTERISTICS OF SELECTED MU OPIOID AGONIST DRUGS[1]

Mu Opioid Agonist Drug	Routes Administered	Comments
Oxycodone	PO (IR and CR), R	Used for moderate pain combined with a nonopioid (e.g., Percocet, Tylox). As single entity, can be used like oral morphine for severe pain. Rectal and parenteral formulation not available in the United States.
Oxymorphone (Numorphan)	IV, IM, SC, R	Used for moderate to severe pain. No oral preparation. Available in 5 mg rectal suppositories.
Propoxyphene (Darvon)	PO	Long half-life. Accumulation of toxic metabolite norpropoxyphene with repetitive dosing. Inappropriate for use in elderly. Used in combination with acetaminophen (Darvocet) and aspirin (Darvon Compound).

May be duplicated for use in clinical practice. From McCaffery M, Pasero C: *Pain: Clinical manual*, pp. 179-180. Copyright © 1999, Mosby, Inc.

Table 6.3 summarizes characteristics of selected mu opioid agonist analgesics.

[1]See Table 6.12, pp. 241-243, for dosing and pharmacokinetic information.

CR, controlled-release; *EA*, epidural analgesia; *h*, hour; *IM*, intramuscular; *IR*, immediate-release; *IA*, intrathecal analgesia; *IV*, intravenous; μg, microgram; *mg*, milligram; *ml*, milliliter; *M6G*, morphine-6-glucuronide; *NR*, not recommended; *OTFC*, oral transmucosal fentanyl citrate; *PO*, oral; *q*, every; *R*, rectal; *SC*, subcutaneous; *SL*, sublingual; *TD*, transdermal; *UK*, unknown.

Information from Agency for Health Care Policy and Research (AHCPR): *Acute pain management: Operations or medical procedures and trauma: Clinical practice guideline.* AHCPR Publication No. 92-0032, Rockville, MD, U.S. Public Health Service, February, 1992, AHCPR; American Pain Society (APS): *Principles of analgesic use in the treatment of acute and cancer pain*, ed 3, pp 41, Glenview, IL, 1992, APS; Austin KL, Stapleton JV, Mather LE: Multiple intramuscular injections: A major source of variability in analgesic response to meperidine, *Pain* 8:47-62, 1980; Beaver WT, Frise GA: A comparison of the analgesic effect of oxymorphone by rectal suppository and intramuscular injection in patients with postoperative pain, *J Clin Pharmacol* 17:276-291, 1977; Beaver WT, Wallenstein SL, Rogers A et al.: Analgesic studies of codeine and oxycodone in patients with cancer. I & II. Comparisons of oral with intramuscular codeine and of oral with intramuscular oxycodone, *J Pharmacol Exp Ther* 207:92-100, 1978; Beers MH, Ouslander JG, Rollingher I et al.: Explicit criteria for determining inappropriate medication use in nursing home residents, *Arch Intern Med* 151:1825-1832, 1991; Deglin JH, Vallerand AH: *Davis' drug guide*, ed 5, Philadelphia, 1995, FA Davis; *Drug facts and comparisons*, St. Louis, 1996, Wolters Kluwer; Hunt RF, Abbott Laboratories, Hospital Products Division: Letter communication to Malcolm Cohen, MD, Mt. Sinai Medical Center, Miami Beach, FL, July 11, 1989; Jacox A, Carr DB, Payne R et al.: *Management of cancer pain: Clinical practice guideline* No. 9. AHCPR Publication No. 94-0592, Rockville, MD, U.S. Public Health Service, March 1994, AHCPR; Kealey GP: Opioids and analgesia, *J Burn Care Rehabil* 16(3):363-364, May/June 1995; Leow KP, Cramond T, Smith MT: Pharmacokinetics and pharmacodynamics of oxycodone when given intravenously and rectally to adult patients with cancer pain, *Anesth Analg* 80:296-302, 1995; Portenoy RK: Opioid analgesics. In Portenoy RK, Kanner RM, editors: *Pain management: Theory and practice*, pp 249-276, Philadelphia, 1996, FA Davis; Reisine T, Pasternak G: Opioid analgesics and antagonists. In Hardman JG, Limbird LE, editors: *Goodman and Gilman's the pharmacological basis of therapeutics*, ed 9, pp 521-555, New York, 1996, McGraw-Hill; Willens JS, Myslinski NR: Pharmacodynamics, pharmacokinetics, and clinical uses of fentanyl, sufentanil, and alfentanil, *Heart Lung* 22(3):239-251, 1993.

The characteristics of opioid analgesics vary widely. Understanding the unique characteristics of each helps to determine the optimal opioid analgesic for the individual patient. The following is a general overview of selected mu agonists that are commonly used for pain management.

Morphine

The mu agonist opioid morphine is the standard with which all other opioid drugs are compared. It is the most commonly used drug for cancer pain because of extensive research, clinical experience with its use, and early development of controlled-release formulations. In 1982 the World Health Organization (WHO, 1986) designated morphine as the preferred drug for cancer pain management. However, since that time, much has been learned about morphine and its pharmacologic actions, causing many clinicians to reassess it as the first choice opioid for some patients requiring long-term opioid treatment (Foley, 1995; Portenoy, 1996b; Portenoy, 1997).

Morphine has two main metabolites, morphine–3–glucuronide (M3G) and morphine-6-glucuronide (M6G). M3G is the primary metabolite of morphine but it is not active at the opioid receptor; M6G is active at the opioid receptor. The effects (both analgesia and side effects) of morphine are due in part to M6G (Portenoy, 1992; Portenoy, Thaler, Inturrisi, 1992).

With chronic oral morphine dosing, such as for cancer pain treatment, blood levels of M6G typically exceed those of morphine (Reisine, Pasternak, 1996). Unanticipated opioid toxicity and such adverse effects as pronounced nausea and respiratory depression are attributed to accumulation and high blood concentrations of M6G and are especially likely in patients with renal failure (Foley, 1995; Portenoy, 1996b). The various factors that influence blood levels of morphine, M6G, and M3G are listed in Table 6.4.

Morphine is hydrophilic (soluble in aqueous solution), which contributes to its relatively slow onset and long

●●●●○

TABLE 6.4 **Factors That Influence Blood Levels of Morphine, M6G, and M3G**

FACTOR	MORPHINE	M6G	M3G
Oral route		↑	
Age >70 years		↑	↑
Male sex	↓	↓	
Concurrent use of rifampin	↓	↓	↓
Concurrent use of tricyclic antidepressants			↑
Concurrent use of rantidine	↑		
Renal failure		↑	

May be duplicated for use in clinical practice. From McCaffery M, Pasero C: *Pain: Clinical manual*, p. 181. Copyright © 1999, Mosby, Inc.

Morphine has two main metabolites, morphine-3-glucuronide (M3G) and morphine-6-glucuronide (M6G). M3G is the primary metabolite of morphine, but it is not active at the opioid receptor, M6G is active at the opioid receptor. With chronic oral morphine dosing, blood levels of M6G typically exceed those of morphine. Unanticipated opioid toxicity and adverse effects are attributed to accumulation and high blood concentrations of M6G. Table 6.4 lists the various factors that influence blood levels of morphine, M6G, and M3G.

↑, increased blood level; ↓, decreased blood level; *M3G*, morphine-3-glucuronide; *M6G*, morphine-6-glucuronide.

Information from Babul N, Darke AC: Disposition of morphine and its glucuronide metabolites after oral and rectal administration: Evidence of route specificity, *Clin Pharmacol Ther* 54(3):286-292, 1993; Foley KM: Misconceptions and controversies regarding the use of opioids in cancer pain, *Anti-Cancer Drugs* 6(Suppl 3):4-13, 1995; Fromm MF, Eckhardt K, Li S et al.: Loss of analgesic effect of morphine due to coadministration of rifampin, *Pain* 72(1, 2):261-267, 1997; Portenoy RK, Kanner RM, editors: *Pain management: Theory and practice*, pp 249-276, Philadelphia, 1996, FA Davis; Reisine T, Pasternak G: Opioid analgesics and antagonists. In Hardman JG, Limbird LE, editors: *Goodman and Gilman's the pharmacological basis of therapeutics*, ed 9, pp 521-555, New York, 1996, McGraw-Hill.

duration of action compared with the more lipophilic (soluble in fatty tisssue) opioid drugs. This is not relevant during continuous dosing but may be important when intermittent boluses are used systemically or intraspinally (Gianino, York, Paice, 1996). Morphine has a short half-life of 2 to 4 hours; the half-life of M6G is slightly longer (Foley, 1995; Reisine, Pasternak, 1996). Morphine does not persist in tissues; 24 hours after the last dose, tissue concentrations are low (Reisine, Pasternak, 1996). It is estimated that approximately 40% of the given dose of oral morphine is available for therapeutic effect because of first pass effect. This is why the recommended dose of morphine by the oral route is higher than that by the parenteral route (Ferrante, 1996; Jacox, Carr, Payne et al., 1994) (see Tables 6.3 on pp. 179-180 and 6.12 on pp. 241-243).

Codeine

Codeine has limited use in the management of severe pain (Cousins, Umedaly, 1996; Levy, 1994). At the customary doses used, codeine provides analgesia for mild pain only. The recommended maximum oral dose of 60 mg of codeine produces analgesia equal to 600 mg of aspirin (less than two 325 mg tablets) (Reisine, Pasternak, 1996). Combination preparations of codeine and acetaminophen also are not appropriate for moderate to severe or escalating pain. The ceiling on the maximum safe daily doses of acetaminophen and aspirin limits dose increases for inadequate pain control (refer to Chapter 4, p. 116.)

Unlike morphine, codeine is approximately 60% as effective orally as it is parenterally. This is because codeine, like levorphanol, oxycodone, and methadone, undergoes less first pass metabolism than morphine. Once absorbed, codeine is metabolized in the liver to morphine, its active form[1] (Reisine, Pasternak, 1996).

As with other opioids, extremely wide variations exist between individuals in terms of absorption and analgesic requirements of codeine. As much as a fivefold difference exists in peak blood levels, with peak at approximately 30 to 60 minutes after IM administration. Ninefold differences in minimum effective analgesic concentration have been found by this route. Late respiratory depression also can occur. Thus by the IM route codeine is unpredictable, making it unfavorable for use in postoperative pain management (Cousins, Umedaly, 1996).

Fentanyl

Fentanyl has been used extensively in anesthesia and administered IV and epidurally (see p. 225) for the treatment of acute pain. It is frequently combined with benzodiazepines to produce analgesia and sedation during painful procedures (see Chapter 8). With the development of the transdermal patch (see p. 206) and oral transmucosal fentanyl citrate (see p. 202) it has found wider acceptance in the treatment of cancer pain and some chronic nonmalignant pain than in the past.

Fentanyl is metabolized in the liver and has no active metabolites (Foley, 1995). It differs from morphine in terms of onset and duration of action. When given as a single IV bolus, its onset is faster (within 1 to 5 minutes) and its duration is shorter at less than 1 hour as the drug moves from blood to muscle to fat. After repetitive dosing

---

[1]The metabolism of codeine to its active form depends on the presence of the enzyme P4502D6. Two genotypes of cytochrome P4502D6 exist, rendering patients extensive metabolizers or poor metabolizers. Extensive metabolizers are able to perform catalyzed biotransformation of codeine (and other drugs). However, approximately 8% of Caucasians and 2% of African-Americans are poor metabolizers, making them unresponsive to codeine's analgesic effect (Kroemer, Eichelbaum, 1995). Certain drugs, such as paroxetine (Paxil) and fluoxetine (Prozac), may inhibit cytochrome P4502D6, and therefore, could potentially interfere with the metabolism of codeine, but the clinical significance of this is not clear.

or continuous infusion of fentanyl, a steady state is approached. Although fentanyl is reported to have a terminal half-life of approximately 3 to 4 hours, at steady state, slow removal of fentanyl from storage sites can result in a longer terminal half-life (up to 12 hours) (Mather, Denson, 1992; Willens, Myslinski, 1993). This can lead to accumulation and late and prolonged duration of sedation and respiratory depression (Marshall, Longnecker, 1996; Mather, Denson, 1992; Willens, Myslinski, 1993). Elderly patients, in particular, may be subject to this effect (Willens, Myslinski, 1993). When given transdermally, continued absorption from skin depots occurs as the drug is eliminated, and half-life lengthens to 13 to 24 hours.

Fentanyl has minimal hemodynamic effects. Bradycardia and chest wall rigidity occur with high-dose fentanyl anesthesia (Cook, Davis, Lerman, 1996). Respiratory depression and apnea can occur with rapid IV administration of fentanyl. Because of its fast onset, this occurs usually within minutes of administration.

Hydrocodone

Hydrocodone is available combined with acetaminophen and should be considered for the management of mild to moderate pain only. It has a peak time of 60 minutes and a half-life of 3.8 hours. It may have fewer side effects (Levy, 1994) and has been shown to provide better analgesia and greater patient acceptability than codeine (Condra, 1997).

The fixed combinations of hydrocodone and acetaminophen (Lortab, Vicodin, Lorcet, Hydrocet) and aspirin (Lortab ASA) provide several choices in terms of the amount of hydrocodone per dose. Hydrocodone is available in combination with 500 mg of acetaminophen in 2.5, 5, 7.5, and 10 mg strengths. It is also available in 10 mg strength with 650 mg of acetaminophen. A 7.5 mg hydrocodone and 500 mg acetaminophen elixir also is available.

Regardless of available strengths, combination preparations of hydrocodone and acetaminophen are not appropriate for moderate to severe pain or escalating pain. The ceiling on the maximum safe daily doses of acetaminophen limits dose increases for inadequate pain control (see Chapter 4). Hydrocodone is not available as a single entity (without acetaminophen) and potential value of this is not known.

Hydromorphone

Hydromorphone is considered another first line opioid analgesic for postoperative pain management and is appropriate for some cancer pain treatment. By the IV route, hydromorphone has a rapid onset (within 5 minutes), short time to peak effect (10 to 20 minutes), and short duration (3 to 4 hours) (Coda, Tanaka, Jacobson et al., 1997) (see Tables 6.3 on pp. 179-180 and 6.12 on pp. 241-243).

No evidence exists that hydromorphone's major metabolites are clinically relevant (Rapp, Egan, Ross et al., 1996), but all of their effects have not been clearly defined. Because hydromorphone has a short half-life (2 to 3 hours) and no clinically relevant metabolites, it may be a better drug than morphine for patients with renal insufficiency, particularly the elderly (Foley, 1995; *Management of cancer pain,* 1993).

Hydromorphone can be given by a variety of routes, including oral, rectal, SC, IM, IV, epidural, and intrathecal. When given orally, hydromorphone is 30% to 40% bioavailable and has an oral to parenteral ratio of 5:1 (Foley, 1995). Repeated dosing does not change this oral parenteral ratio because it has no analgesic metabolites that accumulate (*Management of cancer pain,* 1993).

Hydromorphone is more potent than morphine, meaning that equal analgesia is provided with fewer milligrams of hydromorphone than morphine. The exact morphine to hydromorphone potency equivalence ratio is uncertain. Most equianalgesic charts list the ratio of morphine to hydromorphone as 7:1 (10 mg = 1.5 mg); however, equianalgesic chart estimates were established on single dose studies. Some clinicians believe the ratio to be 4:1 (Levy, 1996) or 5:1 (Coda, O'Sullivan, Donaldson et al., 1997; Coda, Tanaka, Jacobson et al., 1997; Foley, 1995; Houde, Wallenstein, Beaver, 1986) with single doses and repeated dosing. A study using IV PCA demonstrated the ratio to be 3:1 (Dunbar, Chapman, Buckley et al., 1996).

With repeated dosing of hydromorphone, it is most likely that 2 to 3 mg of parenteral hydromorphone is equal to 10 mg of parenteral morphine. One group of researchers found hydromorphone to be five times more potent than morphine when given second, but only 3.7 times more potent when given first (Lawlor, Turner, Hanson et al., 1997). In other words, these researchers recommended a ratio of 5:1 (10 mg morphine = 2 mg hydromorphone) when converting from morphine to hydromorphone and a ratio of 3.7:1 (10 mg morphine = 2.7 mg hydromorphone) when converting from hydromorphone to morphine. As mentioned before, when switching from one opioid analgesic to another, conservative estimates must be used and the optimal dose determined by titration.

Although available in oral form (2, 4, and 8 mg tablets) and rectal suppositories (3 mg), hydromorphone does not come in a controlled-release formulation in the United States, which has limited its use in the management of cancer and chronic nonmalignant pain. Controlled-release formulations of hydromorphone are available in Canada and are currently being investigated for use in the United States (Foley, 1995; Portenoy, 1996b).

One advantage of hydromorphone over morphine is that hydromorphone is commercially available in a high-potency parenteral formulation (10 mg/ml) that allows for smaller injection or infusion volumes in patients who require opioid analgesics by parenteral administration. This is especially important when opioids are delivered by the SC route (Levy, 1996). Hydromorphone has been used extensively for SC intermittent bolusing and continuous infusions with or without PCA capability for the treatment of cancer pain (Bruera, Brennels, Michaud et al., 1987; Coyle, 1996; Coyle, Mauskop, Maggard et al., 1986; Moulin, Johnson, Murray-Parsons et al., 1992) (see pp. 210-211 for more on SC infusions).

Many institutions have made hydromorphone the first or second choice opioid analgesic next to morphine for postoperative IV PCA. This is logical because the two are pharmacokinetically and pharmacodynamically similar. A study comparing hydromorphone to morphine by IV PCA in opioid-naive patients (mostly female, mean age 48) after lower abdominal surgery showed that both drugs provided adequate and comparable analgesia with no difference in side effects (Rapp, Egan, Ross et al., 1996). Cognitive performance was poorer, but mood elevations were better in patients receiving hydromorphone compared with those receiving morphine. Hydromorphone, however, was generally more expensive than morphine, and cost is a consideration when establishing a primary IV PCA drug or in choosing one for SC or IV infusion for chronic cancer pain.

Levorphanol

Like methadone, levorphanol (Levo-Dromoran) is considered a second line drug for cancer pain, indicated for patients who cannot tolerate morphine because of inadequate analgesia and excessive side effects (Foley, 1995). Levorphanol's pharmacologic effects are similar to morphine. It is available for oral and parenteral administration (Reisine, Pasternak, 1996) and has a parenteral to oral ratio of 1:2 (Foley, 1995). It is available orally only in 2 mg tablets, which can make titration difficult. Although it produces analgesia for just 4 to 6 hours, levorphanol has a long half-life, varying between 12 and 15 hours (Foley, 1995; Levy, 1994). Despite a long half-life, clinical problems with levorphanol are fewer than with methadone (Fainsinger, Schoeller, Bruera, 1993) (see Tables 6.3 on pp. 179-180 and 6.12 on pp. 241-243).

Meperidine

Meperidine (Demerol) continues to be the most widely used opioid analgesic for the management of pain in spite of sufficient evidence that it is not appropriate as a first-line opioid analgesic for the management of any type of pain (AHCPR, 1992; Jacox, Carr, Payne et al., 1994; Levy, 1994). Numerous misconceptions about meperidine persist (Table 6.5). The appeal of meperidine may be in its rapid onset of action and peak effect and short duration of action (Reisine, Pasternak, 1996). However, other opioids, such as hydromorphone, have comparable features and no toxic metabolites.

When given orally, the analgesic effects of meperidine are felt within 30 minutes. Its peak effect is within 1 to 2 hours and its duration of action approximately 3 hours (Reisine, Pasternak, 1996). Meperidine is one-fourth as effective when given orally as when given parenterally (APS, 1992). It has a half-life of 2 to 3 hours. By the SC and IM routes, onset of action is 10 minutes and peak effect is 30 minutes with a duration of up to 4 hours. Although absorbed by all routes of administration, the rate of absorption is erratic after IM injection, with a wide range of peak plasma concentrations (Austin, Stapleton, Mather, 1980; Reisine, Pasternak, 1996) (see Tables 6.3 on pp. 179-180 and 6.12 on pp. 241-243).

A major drawback to the use of meperidine is its active metabolite, normeperidine. Normeperidine is a CNS stimulant and can produce irritability, tremors, muscle twitching, jerking, agitation, and seizures (AHCPR, 1992; Jacox, Carr, Payne et al., 1994). Normeperidine has a half-life of 15 to 20 hours compared with meperidine's half-life of 3 hours (Reisine, Pasternak, 1996).

Because normeperidine is eliminated by the kidneys, meperidine should not be used in patients with decreased renal function (Reisine, Pasternak, 1996). Although commonly used, it is a particularly poor choice in the elderly and patients with sickle cell disease because most have some degree of renal insufficiency. Because repeated dosing increases the risk of accumulation of normeperidine, meperidine should not be prescribed for patients requiring long-term opioid treatment, such as those with cancer or chronic nonmalignant pain (Jacox, Carr, Payne et al., 1994; Levy, 1994). It is rarely indicated for use in children (Antonopolous, Bollinger, Goshman, 1996). The effects of normeperidine have been observed even in young, otherwise healthy patients given sufficiently high doses of meperidine postoperatively (Hinnant, 1996).

Meperidine is contraindicated in patients receiving monoamine oxidase (MAO) inhibitors and in patients with untreated hypothyroidism, Addison's disease, benign prostatic hypertrophy, or urethral stricture. It should be used with extreme caution in patients with preexisting convulsive disorders and in patients with atrial flutter or other supraventricular tachycardias (Antonopolous, Bollinger, Goshman, 1996).

Research shows that meperidine is more likely than other opioid drugs to cause delirium in postoperative patients of all ages. In one study meperidine more than doubled the risk of delirium when given either epidurally or IV (Marcantonio, Juarez, Goldman et al., 1994).

The most appropriate candidates for meperidine use are patients with acute pain who are otherwise healthy and are allergic to other opioids, such as morphine and hydromorphone (AHCPR, 1992; Jacox, Carr, Payne et al., 1994), or have demonstrated a more favorable outcome with meperidine than other opioid drugs. If meperidine is used in these patients, frequent high doses should be

TABLE 6.5 ● ● ● ● ●

Misconceptions | Meperidine

MISCONCEPTION	CORRECTION
1. Meperidine causes less respiratory depression than morphine.	At equianalgesic doses opioid analgesics produce equal respiratory depression.
2. Meperidine is less likely than morphine to cause addiction.	The abuse liability for meperidine is comparable to that of morphine. In other words people addicted to opioids find morphine and meperidine equally attractive.
3. Meperidine causes less constriction of the sphincter of Oddi and the biliary tract than does morphine.	Both meperidine and morphine cause constriction of the sphincter of Oddi and the biliary tract. Laboratory studies show that morphine may cause more constriction in animals, but this has never been shown to be clinically relevant in humans. In humans, morphine and meperidine caused a rise in bile duct pressure of 52.7% and 61.3%, respectively.
4. Meperidine is less constipating than morphine.	Meperidine may be less constipating but only when used chronically, and chronic use is not recommended.
5. Long-term clinical experience with meperidine proves it is safe and effective.	Although meperidine has been the most frequently prescribed opioid for several decades, therapeutic doses (e.g., 75-100 mg IM for adults) were seldom used, and studies show that during these years many patients were undertreated for pain. Furthermore, problems may have gone unnoticed because the existence of the metabolite normeperidine was not known and patients were not assessed for signs of neurotoxicity. Meperidine cannot be used safely if pain is treated aggressively.

May be duplicated for use in clinical practice. From McCaffery M, Pasero C: *Pain: Clinical manual*, p. 184. Copyright © 1999, Mosby, Inc.

Meperidine (Demerol) continues to be the most widely used opioid analgesic for the management of pain despite sufficient evidence that it is not appropriate as a first-line opioid analgesic for the management of any type of pain. Table 6.5 corrects some of the many persistent misconceptions about meperidine.

IM, intramuscular; *mg*, milligram.

Information from Coelho JCU, Runkel N, Herfarth C et al.: Effect of analgesic drugs on electromyographic activity of the gastrointestinal tract and sphincter of oddi and on biliary pressure, *Ann Surg* 204(1):53-58, 1986; Jacox A, Carr DB, Payne R et al.: *Management of cancer pain: Clinical practice guideline* No. 9, AHCPR Publication No. 94-0592, Rockville, MD, U.S. Public Health Service, March 1994, AHCPR; Jaffe JH, Martin WR: Opioid analgesics and antagonists. In Goodman AG, Rall TW, Nies AS, Taylor P, editors: *Goodman and Gilman's the pharmacological basis of therapeutics*, pp 485-521, New York, 1990, Pergamon Press; Radnay PA, Brodman E, Mankikar D et al.: The effect of equianalgesic doses of fentanyl, morphine, meperidine, and pentazocine on common bile duct pressure, *Anaesthesist* 29: 26-29, 1980.

---

avoided. The course of treatment with meperidine should be restricted to no more than a few days with the dosage limited to 600 mg within a 24-hour period (APS, 1992).

Patients who are taking meperidine should be evaluated frequently, probably every 8 to 12 hours, for signs of CNS irritability, specifically restlessness, shakiness, tremors, twitching, and jerking. Tremors are assessed by asking patients to stretch out their arms in front and noting a tremor in the hands that cannot be controlled. Patients are also questioned about being awakened at night by twitching or jerking. If the symptoms are present and have occurred after the initiation of meperidine doses, they may be due to normeperidine accumulation. The patient should be switched immediately to another mu agonist opioid analgesic, such as morphine or hydromorphone. Further accumulation of normeperidine may result in seizures (Kaiko, Foley, Grabinski, 1983).

Because the half-life of the stimulant normeperidine is much longer than that of the depressant meperidine and the latter drug may be partially suppressing the effects of the former, symptoms of toxicity may worsen as the dose of meperidine is decreased. Therefore, if the dose is suddenly lowered in a patient with these symptoms of normeperidine accumulation, a depressant or an anticonvulsant should be considered. Naloxone should never be used for these patients because it does not reverse the action of normeperidine and may even exacerbate the CNS hyperexcitability by decreasing the level of the depressant meperidine (Kaiko, Foley, Grabinski, 1983).

Meperidine is frequently underprescribed, which may be one of the reasons it continues to be considered a safe drug. The initial optimal dose of meperidine recommended for adults with moderate to severe pain is 75 to 100 mg, with some adults requiring 150 mg. The interval between doses ranges from 2 to 4 hours, with 3 hours as the average (Reisine, Pasternak, 1996). These doses would quickly exceed the 600 mg/24 hours recommended by APS and produce numerous adverse effects.

As mentioned, meperidine can be administered by the oral route, but just as with the parenteral route, it is rarely dosed appropriately. Meperidine is less than one-fourth as effective when administered orally as when administered parenterally. This means that if a patient is receiving 75 mg of meperidine by the IV or IM routes over a 3 to 4 hour period, 300 mg orally will be required to produce equianalgesia. Even if the patient's pain had decreased by 50% at the time the switch was made from parenteral to oral, 150 mg would be required orally. Obviously, doses required for analgesia by the oral route produce a significant risk of accumulation of normeperidine, making oral meperidine inappropriate for any type of pain management.

By any route of administration, the logic of using meperidine for any type of pain management should be questioned. There clearly are safer opioid choices.

Methadone

Methadone was commonly used for cancer pain management before the introduction of controlled-release products. The WHO guidelines suggest that methadone be used as a second line opioid analgesic in patients with prior exposure to opioid drugs (Foley, 1995; WHO, 1986). Some clinicians limit the use of methadone to the treatment of advanced cancer pain in patients for whom cost and access to prescription opioids are real obstacles and to those who exhibit a true allergy to morphine (Levy, 1994).

Methadone can be administered by multiple routes, including oral (tablets or solution), rectal, SC, IV, epidural, and intrathecal. It is inexpensive (less expensive than morphine and hydromorphone) (Thomas, Bruera, 1995; Watanabe, Belzile, Kuehn et al., 1996) and has a lower abuse potential (Levy, 1994). However, methadone is used in drug abuse detoxification programs and has a negative connotation for many patients because it is perceived as a drug for addicts (Foley, 1995).

After administration, methadone is well absorbed and redistributes extensively into muscle and fat. It has a similar onset of analgesia compared with morphine, and plasma concentrations peak at approximately 2 hours after oral administration (Crews, Sweeney, Denson, 1993; Reisine, Pasternak, 1996). It is extensively metabolized in the liver and its oral bioavailability is 85%, which is significantly higher than morphine. This is reflected in a lower parenteral/oral potency ratio of 1:2 compared with 1:6 for morphine. The half-life of methadone is long and highly variable (12 to 190 hours) (Portenoy, 1996b). Studies examining methadone's duration of analgesia have produced conflicting results (Gourlay, Willis, Lamberty, 1986; Grochow, Scheidler, Grossman et al., 1989). It is generally believed to be 4 to 8 hours (Foley, 1995). Wide interindividual variability exists in the clearance of methadone, but it is much lower than that of other opioid drugs (Mather, Denson, 1993) (see Tables 6.3 on pp. 179-180 and 6.12 on pp. 241-243).

An opioid with a short half-life is desirable for the treatment of severe cancer pain because the safety is rel-

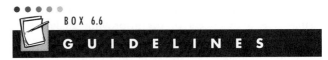

BOX 6.6

GUIDELINES

ORAL METHADONE DOSING

One method to minimize the risk of drug accumulation during initial dosing with methadone is to use a PRN regimen, allowing the patient to determine the interval between doses. Alternately, a fixed schedule (e.g., q6h) can be used. Start with 10% to 25% of the equianalgesic dose of methadone. Provide a second short acting drug (e.g., morphine or hydromorphone) for rescue doses.

May be duplicated for use in clinical practice. From McCaffery M, Pasero C: *Pain: Clinical manual*, p. 185. Copyright © 1999, Mosby, Inc.

The traditional equianalgesic estimates (e.g., 20 mg of methadone orally being equal to 30 mg of morphine orally) are based on single doses of opioids for opioid-naive patients and are inappropriate in providing starting doses of oral methadone for opioid-tolerant patients. In switching these patients to methadone, individual titration is crucial because traditional conversion ratios underestimate the potency of methadone. Box 6.6 presents suggestions for initial oral methadone dosing.

h, hour; PRN, as needed; *q*, every.

Information from Coyle N, Cherny N, Portenoy RK: Pharmacologic management of cancer pain. In McGuire D, Yarbro CH, Ferrell BR, editors: *Cancer pain management*, ed 2, pp 89-130, Boston, 1995, Jones and Bartlett Publishers; Inturrisi CE, Colburn WA: Pharmacokinetics of methadone. In Foley KM, Inturrisi CE, editors: *Advances in pain research and therapy*, vol 8, pp 191-198, New York, 1986, Raven Press; Inturrisi CE, Portenoy RK, Max MB et al.: Pharmacokinetic-pharmacodynamic relationships of methadone infusions in patients with cancer pain, *Clin Pharmacol Ther* 47:565, 1990; Portenoy RK: Opioid analgesics. In Portenoy RK, Kanner RM, editors: *Pain management: Theory and practice*, pp 249-276, Philadelphia, 1996, FA Davis.

atively greater as the dose is titrated up quickly. An opioid drug with a long half-life, such as methadone, will take a long time to reach steady state after dosing is initiated or changed. The maximum analgesic effect of the dosing regimen cannot be determined until steady state is achieved (Foley, 1995; Portenoy, 1996b). Therefore days or weeks of drug accumulation may occur after a period of rapid dose titration. In some cases this may lead to a delayed onset of adverse effects. For these reasons, methadone is considered a poor choice for patients who are difficult to monitor or are predisposed to opioid side effects, such as the elderly, noncompliant patients, and those with major organ failure (Portenoy, 1996b).

One method to minimize the risk of drug accumulation during initial dosing with methadone is to use a PRN regimen, allowing the patient to determine the interval between doses (Inturrisi, Colburn, 1986). A second short-acting drug, such as morphine or hydromorphone, is provided for rescue doses. The frequency of rescue doses should decrease as the patient reaches steady state (see Box 6.6 for suggestions for oral methadone dosing).

In opioid-tolerant patients, cross-tolerance is incomplete with methadone (Inturrisi, Portenoy, Max et al., 1990; Ivarsson, Neil, 1989), so switching to methadone may be an option for treatment of intolerable and unmanageable side effects or for improving analgesia in cases of escalating dose requirements with other mu agonist opioid analgesics. The traditional equianalgesic estimates (e.g., 20 mg of methadone orally being equal to 30 mg of morphine orally) are based on single doses of opioids for opioid-naive patients and are inappropriate in providing starting doses of oral methadone for opioid-tolerant patients.

In switching these patients to methadone, clinicians have found that very close attention to individual titration is crucial because traditional conversion ratios underestimate the potency of methadone (Bruera, Watanabe, Fainsinger et al., 1995; Crews, Sweeney, Denson, 1993; Manfredi, Borsook, Chandler et al., 1997; Mercante, 1997; Vigano, Fan, Bruera, 1996). Some researchers propose that methadone is almost 10 times more potent than suggested in equianalgesic charts (Bruera, Pereira, Watanabe et al., 1996; Bruera, Watanabe, Fainsinger et al., 1995). Therefore it is recommended that initial methadone dosing begin with 10% to 25% of the equianalgesic dose (Coyle, Cherny, Portenoy, 1995; Portenoy, 1996b) (see Box 6.6).

As mentioned, the exact duration of methadone's action is variable. Whether IV doses of methadone can provide a longer duration of analgesia than comparable IV doses of morphine is unclear. Studying patients with chronic cancer pain over a 5- to 6-day period, the dosing intervals for both drugs given as IV boluses remained the same, approximately 4 hours (Grochow, Scheidler, Grossman et al., 1989).

By contrast, although no data are provided, Berde and Kain (1996) report that a constant analgesic effect can be achieved by intermittent IV boluses every 4 to 6 hours or oral doses of methadone every 4 to 8 hours. Thus methadone IV boluses may be a suitable alternative to PCA or continuous IV infusion of morphine when these methods of administration are not available.

A long duration of action by the IV route is also suggested in a study showing that a single IV bolus of methadone (0.2 mg/kg) given before major surgery to 15 children and adolescents provided sustained analgesia postoperatively. Methadone had a very prolonged elimination and low clearance rate in the patient sample. This was found to be independent of age and weight (Berde, Sethna, Holtzman et al., 1987). However, it is unclear whether or how pain was assessed in this study, although the authors reported that patients were comfortable and required no analgesia for 12 to 36 hours after surgery. It is also unclear whether the children and adolescents were offered and refused analgesics or whether they simply did not request analgesics, which is common behavior in this age group. If the children in this study thought that analgesics would be administered by the IM route, they may have preferred to endure pain rather than an injection.

In adults who were given a single IV bolus of 20 mg of methadone intraoperatively, more than half required no more than acetaminophen during the postoperative period. Those who required opioid analgesics did not request supplemental analgesia until 18 hours after surgery. The mean duration of analgesia from the 20 mg of methadone in this study was 27 hours (Gourlay, Wilson, Glynn, 1982).

Significant differences in duration of pain relief were found in adults who were given either 20 mg of IV morphine or 20 mg of IV methadone intraoperatively followed by 5 mg doses of the same opioid in response to reports of pain in the recovery room and on the surgical ward. No differences were found between the two groups in the amount of opioid required in the recovery room, but the time to first supplemental dose on the surgical ward was approximately 6 hours for patients who had received morphine compared with almost 21 hours for patients who had received methadone. Quality of pain relief, as assessed by VAS, was the same for both groups, with a mean score between 1/10 and 2/10, but significantly less supplemental methadone (11.5 mg) than morphine (41 mg) was required on the surgical ward (Gourlay, Willis, Lamberty, 1986).

The only study comparing duration of action of IV morphine and methadone that described systematic assessment of pain in children is a study of children 3 to 7 years old undergoing major surgery (Berde, Beyer, Bournaki et al., 1991). The duration of analgesia obtained from IV boluses of methadone and morphine given intraoperatively were compared by assessing pain ratings and supplemental doses required postoperatively. During the first 36 hours after surgery, fewer supplemental doses of analgesic were required in those who received methadone than in those who received morphine. Those who received methadone intraoperatively also reported lower pain scores. No major adverse events occurred in either group. Recommended doses of perioperative methadone for children include a loading dose of 0.1 to 0.2 mg/kg with a 0.05 mg/kg supplemental dose every 4 to 12 hours (Cook, Davis, Lerman, 1996).

Methadone can be administered by the rectal route, although rectal preparations are not available in the United States. Custom-made suppositories are sometimes prepared for use in cancer pain management (Bruera, Schoeller, Fainsinger et al., 1992). In a Canadian study, improved pain relief and substantial cost savings were demonstrated when cancer patients were switched from hydromorphone subcutaneously by continuous infusion to methadone suppositories (Watanabe, Belzile, Kuehn et al., 1996).

Oxycodone

Oxycodone is commonly used to treat acute, cancer, and chronic nonmalignant pain of mild to severe intensity. For many years oral oxycodone was available only compounded with a nonopioid, such as acetaminophen, restricting its use to mild to moderate pain. Now it is available orally as a single entity drug in both immediate-release and controlled-release formulations.

Oxycodone is metabolized in the liver to its active metabolite, oxymorphone.[1] After administration, oxycodone's bioavailability is 50% to 80% and its half-life is short (3 to 4 hours). Twice the amount of oxycodone is required orally than intramuscularly (Beaver, Wallenstein, Rogers et al., 1978). Oxycodone has been found to be less toxic than equianalgesic doses of codeine (Levy, 1994).

Oxycodone is not available in the United States in suppository form for rectal administration; however, oral preparations are administered rectally. Absorption and peak blood levels by the rectal route appear to be comparable to that of the oral route, but maximum blood concentration is prolonged. Bioavailability by the rectal route is estimated to be 45% to 60% (Leow, Cramond, Smith, 1995; Warren, 1996).

Single-dose rectal and IV oxycodone were compared in opioid-naive patients with cancer pain. IV oxycodone produced rapid analgesia in 5 to 8 minutes compared with 30 to 60 minutes after rectal administration; however, duration of analgesia was more than twice as long by the rectal route (8 to 12 hours) compared with the IV route (4 hours). The marked interindividual variation in the pharmacokinetics and pharmacodynamics of oxycodone emphasize the need for individualized dosing regimens. (Leow, Cramond, Smith, 1995) (see Tables 6.3 on pp. 179-180 and 6.12 on pp. 241-243).

Oxymorphone

Oxymorphone is indicated for moderate to severe pain. When given IV, it has a quick onset (5 to 10 minutes). Its peak time is 15 minutes with a duration of 3 to 6 hours and half-life of 2 to 3 hours. It sometimes is used as a preoperative medication and a supplement for balanced anesthesia.

Oxymorphone is well absorbed by the IM, SC, and IV routes. Besides morphine and hydromorphone, oxymorphone is the only other opioid analgesic commercially available in the United States as a rectal suppository (Numorphan). By the rectal route, its onset of action is 15 to 30 minutes, with a peak time of 120 minutes. In one study rectal oxymorphone was found to be one-tenth as potent as IM oxymorphone but one twentieth as potent in terms of peak effect (Beaver, Frise, 1977). The lack of an oral preparation of oxymorphone limits its use in pain management, especially for cancer and chronic nonmalignant pain (see Tables 6.3 on pp. 179-180 and 6.12 on pp. 241-243).

Propoxyphene

Propoxyphene (Darvon) is one of the most widely prescribed analgesics for mild to moderate pain. It often is used in combination with acetaminophen (Darvocet) or aspirin (Darvon Compound). Propoxyphene is one-half to one-third as potent as codeine. Its recommended dose of 100 mg is equal in analgesic effect to 60 mg of codeine, which is known to be equal to 600 mg (less than two 325 mg tablets) of aspirin. At equianalgesic doses, propoxyphene has the same incidence of side effects as codeine. It has a longer half-life (6 to 12 hours) than codeine and can accumulate and produce toxicity with repeated doses. In addition, propoxyphene has an active metabolite, norpropoxyphene, with a half-life of 30 to 36 hours. With repeated dosing, it too can accumulate (see Tables 6.3 on pp. 179-180 and 6.12 on pp. 241-243).

Norpropoxyphene produces less CNS depression than propoxyphene, but with repeated dosing can produce pulmonary edema and cardiotoxicity (Reisine, Pasternak, 1996). Apnea, cardiac arrest, and death have been reported. In addition, naloxone may not reverse norpropoxyphene and it is poorly dialyzed (Barkin, Lubenow, Bruehl et al., 1996; McQuay, 1989). Overdose of propoxyphene may be prominently associated with seizures (Barkin, Lubenow, Bruehl et al., 1996).

Because of the limitations imposed by the toxicity of propoxyphene and norpropoxyphene, propoxyphene is appropriate only for short-term mild, intermittent pain. It is not recommended for the treatment of continuous cancer and chronic nonmalignant pain. Propoxyphene is an especially poor choice for use in the elderly because most have some degree of renal insufficiency and both propoxyphene and norpropoxyphene are eliminated by the kidneys. Unfortunately, despite its inappropriateness, propoxyphene is one of the most common analgesics prescribed for this population group. It remains one of the most commonly prescribed drugs for patients in nursing homes (Beers, Ouslander, Rollingher, 1991; Ferrell, 1995; Wilcox, Himmelstein, Woolhandler, 1994).

A further problem is that propoxyphene is commonly prescribed in combination with diazepam (Valium), greatly increasing adverse effects, such as respiratory depression, sedation, and cognitive impairment. This may

---

[1]The metabolism of oxycodone to its active form depends on the presence of the enzyme P4502D6. Two genotypes of cytochrome P4502D6 exist, rendering patients extensive metabolizers or poor metabolizers. Extensive metabolizers are able to perform catalyzed biotransformation of oxycodone (and other drugs). However, approximately 8% of Caucasians and 2% of African-Americans are poor metabolizers, making them unresponsive to oxycodone's analgesic effect (Kroemer, Eichelbaum, 1995). Certain drugs, such as paroxetine (Paxil) and fluoxetine (Prozac), may inhibit cytochrome P4502D6 and therefore could potentially interfere with the metabolism of oxycodone, but the clinical significance of this is not clear.

increase the likelihood of falls (Wilcox, Himmelstein, Woolhandler, 1994). In addition to being a poor choice of analgesia, it is more costly than other analgesics such as codeine (Benedetti, 1995).

Characteristics of selected agonist-antagonist opioids

Agonist-antagonists are not recommended as first-line drugs for any type of pain (APS, 1992; AHCPR, 1992; Jacox, Carr, Payne et al., 1994). A major limitation is that they have a ceiling to analgesia. Another problem is limited routes of administration. All are available parenterally, but only pentazocine is available orally and butorphanol is available by nasal spray. The agonist-antagonists are subdivided into partial agonists (buprenorphine [Buprenex]) and mixed agonist-antagonists (butorphanol [Stadol], dezocine [Dalgan], nalbuphine [Nubain], and pentazocine [Talwin]).

Some clinicians use agonist-antagonist opioid analgesics believing that they cause no respiratory depression or less than the mu agonists (see Table 6.1). At equianalgesic doses all opioids produce equal respiratory depression. Agonist-antagonists do have a ceiling on the respiratory depression they produce but they also have a ceiling on their analgesia. When the analgesic ceiling is reached, any increase in dose will not produce an increase in analgesia (APS, 1992). This is why they are especially inappropriate for severe, escalating pain. In addition, because these drugs are antagonists at the mu opioid receptor site, patients receiving mu agonist opioid analgesics should not be given an agonist-antagonist because this can precipitate reversal of opioid effects and withdrawal syndrome (AHCPR, 1992; APS, 1992; Jacox, Carr, Payne et al., 1994).

Buprenorphine

Buprenorphine (Buprenex) is the only partial agonist opioid drug. It can be given parenterally and is absorbed by the oral mucosa, but because of significant first pass metabolism it is not available in an oral formulation (Barkin, Lubenow, Bruehl, 1996).

Buprenorphine has been used for postoperative pain and as an adjunct to anesthesia. In contrast to butorphanol and pentazocine, buprenorphine does not produce adverse cardiac effects, so it is acceptable for use when myocardial infarction is suspected (Benedetti, 1995; Reisine, Pasternak, 1996).

Sedation, nausea, vomiting, dizziness, sweating, and headache are the most common side effects of parenteral buprenorphine (Reisine, Pasternak, 1996). Patients often cite a desire to discontinue the drug more because of side effects than because of inadequate analgesia (Benedetti, 1995), although nausea and vomiting appear to be less than with morphine (Barkin, Lubenow, Bruehl, 1995;

Benedetti, 1995). It lacks dysphoric and psychomimetic effects (Barkin, Lubenow, Bruehl, 1996).

Respiratory depression usually is not a problem with the administration of buprenorphine; however, it is unclear whether this is due to a ceiling effect as seen with nalbuphine and pentazocine. Once they occur, respiratory depression and other side effects are not readily reversed by naloxone (Reisine, Pasternak, 1996); very high doses (10 to 12 mg) of naloxone may be required (Foley, Inturrisi, 1992). Its use for labor pain should be avoided (APS, 1992).

A sublingual preparation of buprenorphine is available in some countries and may provide relief of mild to moderate pain. Sublingual buprenorphine absorption occurs within 5 minutes. Bioavailability is 55% with peak plasma concentrations occurring generally at approximately 2 hours (Foley, Inturrisi, 1992; Weinberg, Inturrisi, Reidenberg et al., 1988). Side effects of sublingual buprenorphine are minor (bitter taste, burning sensation, light-headedness) and incidence is rare (Weinberg, Inturrisi, Reidenberg et al., 1988).

Butorphanol

Butorphanol (Stadol) is available for administration parenterally and intranasally. The onset of action after IM administration is 10 to 20 minutes, and peak effect occurs in 30 to 60 minutes with a duration of 3 to 4 hours. After IV administration, onset is within 5 minutes, peak effect in 10 minutes, and duration is 3 hours (Vogelsang, Hayes, 1991). Bioavailability after transnasal absorption is 60% to 70%. By this route, the onset of action is 5 to 15 minutes, peak effect is at 1 hour, and duration is up to 4 hours. Butorphanol does not have active metabolites (Vogelsang, Hayes, 1991). Its half-life is short (3 to 4 hours) and is increased in the elderly and persons with decreased creatinine clearance (Barkin, Lubenow, Bruehl, 1996; Reisine, Pasternak, 1996).

Butorphanol nasal spray is available in the United States and may be useful in opioid-naive patients who cannot tolerate oral opioids (Portenoy, 1996b; 1993; Levy, 1996). It has been used intranasally for pain after cesarean section (Abboud, Zhu, Gangolly et al., 1991; Benedetti, 1995) and may be appropriate for outpatient treatment of moderate to severe acute headache pain (Diamond, Diamond, 1997; Markley, 1994). Intranasal butorphanol (5, 15, and 25 µg/kg) has been shown to reduce the requirement for supplemental analgesia after bilateral myringotomy and tube placement in children 6 months of age and older (Means, Bennie, Dierdorf et al., 1997).

In opioid-naive patients who are taking occasional mu agonists, such as codeine or oxycodone, the addition of butorphanol nasal spray may provide additive analgesia. However, in opioid-tolerant patients, such as those receiving ATC morphine, the addition of butorphanol spray should be avoided because it may reverse analgesia and precipitate withdrawal.

Parenteral butorphanol has been used for labor and postpartum pain, as a preanesthesia sedative and analgesic, and as an anesthetic supplement. Postanesthesia and post-delivery shivering have been treated with parenteral butorphanol (Vogelsang, Hayes, 1991), but its use for shivering always should be questioned if mu agonist opioids have been given (AHCPR, 1992). Butorphanol has been added to morphine for epidural bolus administration for the purpose of preventing pruritis and nausea. Although relief of pruritis has been reported, profound sedation, respiratory depression, and reversal of analgesia can occur (Abboud, Moore, Zhu et al., 1987; Hunt, Naulty, Malinow et al., 1989; Lawhorn, McNitt, Fibuch et al., 1991).

Adverse effects of butorphanol include headache, vertigo, lethargy, a feeling of floating, confusion, and light-headedness. Psychomimetic effects are possible and include hallucinations, unusual dreams, and depersonalization (Barkin, Lubenow, Bruehl et al., 1996; Reisine, Pasternak, 1996). Parenteral butorphanol is associated with a high degree of sedation (40%) (Benedetti, 1995; Vogelsang, Hayes, 1991). Therapeutic doses of butorphanol can produce levels of respiratory depression equal to mu opioid agonist drugs. Its ceiling for respiratory depression is reached at doses of 30 to 60 μg/kg (Vogelsang, Hayes, 1991). Butorphanol by any route is not recommended for use in the treatment of myocardial infarction or patients with hypertension because it produces multiple adverse effects on cardiac function, including increased pulmonary arterial pressure and cardiac workload (Barkin, Lubenow, Bruehl et al., 1996; Nagashima, Karamanian, Malovany et al., 1976; Vogelsang, Hayes, 1991).

Dezocine

Although dezocine (Dalgan) is classified as an agonist-antagonist opioid, some researchers question the existence of antagonist properties. It has been administered with mu opioid agonists and other agonist–antagonists without precipitating withdrawal symptoms (Barkin Lubenow, Bruehl et al., 1996; Wilson, Cohen, Kezer et al., 1995). Dezocine undergoes extensive first pass hepatic metabolism and is without active metabolites. It is recommended that doses be reduced if used in patients with hepatic or renal dysfunction. No evidence of changes exist in pressure within the common bile duct or ampulla of Vater in patients after biliary surgery. Mental status changes and delirium have been reported with use of dezocine in elderly patients (Barkin, Lubenow, Bruehl et al., 1996).

Nalbuphine

Nalbuphine (Nubain) is available only by the parenteral route; it is well absorbed intramuscularly, subcutaneously, and intravenously. Analgesic effect is felt 15 minutes after IM injection (Benedetti, 1995). Nalbuphine is metabolized in the liver and has a half-life of 5 hours (Reisine, Pasternak, 1996). In contrast to butorphanol and pentazocine, nalbuphine does not produce adverse cardiac effects so it is acceptable for use when myocardial infarction is suspected (Benedetti, 1995; Reisine, Pasternak, 1996).

Nalbuphine frequently is used for managing labor pain. It has been delivered by IV PCA in the first stage of labor. However, IV PCA nalbuphine is limited to use only up to late in the first stage of labor because it produces significant maternal sedation, and PCA alone does not provide sufficient analgesia for the later stages of labor (Wittels, Sevarino, 1992).

At equianalgesic doses, nalbuphine and morphine produce a similar degree of respiratory depression. The ceiling for respiratory depression is reached at doses of greater than 30 mg of nalbuphine (Benedetti, 1995); however, no increase in analgesia beyond 30 mg occurs. In general, nalbuphine, like other agonist-antagonists does not provide any safeguard against respiratory depression and produces excessive sedation while providing minimal amounts of pain relief as doses are increased above the ceiling dose. The mu agonist opioids are better choices for all types of pain.

Single dose (2.5 to 5 mg) and continuous infusions of parenteral nalbuphine sometimes are used to prevent or treat side effects, primarily pruritis, associated with mu agonist opioid epidural analgesia; however, reversal of analgesia can occur (Benedetti, 1995; Kendrick, Woods, Daly et al., 1996). Preservative-free nalbuphine has been added to single epidural bolus doses, epidural analgesic infusions, and patient-controlled epidural analgesia for the prevention of opioid side effects (James, Nelson, Langevin et al., 1997; Parker, Holtmann, White, 1997). Overall the results have been unimpressive. The risk of inadvertently reversing analgesia and the aftermath of reestablishing pain control must be weighed against the benefit of a small reduction in severity of relatively minor side effects, especially when other methods of control have not been tried (see pp. 261-270).

Pentazocine

Pentazocine (Talwin) is of little value in the management of pain. It was originally introduced as an opioid analgesic with little or no abuse potential because it lacks euphoric effects (Benedetti, 1995; Levy, 1994; Reisine, Pasternak, 1996). It has since been recognized as a drug with abuse potential.

Pentazocine can be given orally or parenterally. It has a short duration of action and a very high side effect profile. The most common side effects are sedation, sweating, nausea, and dizziness. Respiratory depression occurs at high doses and is reversible with naloxone. Pentazocine causes dysphoria, anxiety, nightmares, depersonalization, and hallucinations. After prolonged use, abrupt discontinuation causes worse withdrawal symptoms than morphine and other opioids (Barkin, Lubenow, Bruehl et al., 1996; Benedetti, 1995; Reisine, Pasternak, 1996).

Other opioid analgesics

A number of new opioid drugs are currently being used or investigated for use in pain management. The following are examples of these analgesics.

Pentamorphone

Pentamorphone is an opioid currently under investigation. It has been found to produce unusual analgesic effects. With PCA to establish efficacy and potency, pentamorphone was found to be more efficacious than morphine in the first hour after surgery because significantly more patients achieved a VAS (0 to 100 mm) of 30 mm with pentamorphone. Thereafter pentamorphone and morphine were found to be equally efficacious. Under conditions of equal analgesia the potency ratio between pentamorphone and morphine was found to be 252:1 (Ginsberg, Grichnik, Muir et al., 1996).

Remifentanil

Remifentanil is a new mu agonist opioid analgesic used for general anesthesia and during monitored anesthesia care. It is mentioned here because it also has been administered by continuous IV infusion to treat pain in the critically ill (Evans, Park, 1997). The pharmacokinetic characteristics of remifentanil are unlike any other opioid analgesic. It is highly lipophilic and has an extremely rapid clearance of 3.1 minutes with a terminal half-life of less than 10 minutes. The time necessary for the plasma concentration of remifentanil to decrease by 50% after infusion, regardless of the duration of the infusion, is just 3 to 4 minutes (Sabapathy, 1997; Smith, Morgan, 1997).

Because remifentanil is an ultrashort-acting opioid, it must be given by continuous infusion when used for analgesia. Recommended infusion rate for safe and effective postoperative analgesia in the immediate postextubation period is 0.05 to 0.23 μg/kg per minute (Yarmush, D'Angelo, Kirkhart et al., 1997). Remifentanil's short duration of action has both advantages and disadvantages. Reducing or stopping the infusion results in rapid dissolution of adverse effects; however, rapid elimination results in the patients having no analgesia "on board" when infusion is stopped (Smith, Morgan, 1997).

Recommended dosing for analgesia in the postanesthesia care unit (PACU) and intensive care unit (ICU) is 0.1 μg/kg per minute by continuous IV infusion (Sabapathy, 1997). Rapid IV administration results in a high incidence of muscle rigidity, respiratory depression, and apnea. Its postoperative use should be limited to areas where it can be supervised by trained anesthesia personnel and very closely monitored (Sabapathy, 1997; Smith, Morgan, 1997).

Remifentanil has a metabolite, GR90291, which is 1/4600th the potency of remifentanil. It is excreted unchanged in the urine with a half-life of approximately 2 hours. In one study of patients with renal failure, the pharmacokinetics and pharmacodynamics of remifentanil were not altered, but the elimination of GR90291 was markedly reduced; the half-life of the metabolite increased to more than 26 hours. However, during a typical surgical procedure in these patients, metabolite accumulation did not produce significant opioid effect (Hoke, Shlugman, Dershwitz et al., 1997). Further research and clinical experience is needed in the use of remifentanil.

Tramadol

Tramadol (Ultram) is a relatively new opioid analgesic in the United States marketed for moderate to moderately severe pain. It has been the most prescribed analgesic for years in Germany (Stubhaug, Grimstad, Breivik, 1995). Tramadol is unique in that it has both opioid and nonopioid analgesic mechanisms. It is not a NSAID. Although its mode of action is not completely understood, tramadol and its main metabolite, o-demethyl tramadol (M1), exert an analgesic effect through two mechanisms: they bind to the mu opioid receptors as agonists (opioid effect) and weakly inhibit the reuptake of serotonin and norepinephrine (nonopioid effect), similar to the effect of tricyclic antidepressants (Barnung, Treschow, Borgbjerg, 1997; Dayer, Collart, Desmeules, 1994; Stubhaug, Grimstad, Breivik, 1995) (see Chapter 7 for more on tricyclic antidepressants).

Tramadol is available in the United States for oral administration, and in other countries it has been administered by the IV route. The recommended dose of tramadol is 50 to 100 mg every 4 to 6 hours. After oral administration, it is rapidly and well absorbed. It is metabolized by the liver and excreted by the kidneys. The formation of M1 depends on cytochrome P4502D6, so effectiveness may be reduced in some individuals (see footnote, p. 187). Analgesic effect is felt within 60 minutes, with a peak effect at 2 to 3 hours. Its bioavailability is 75%. The half-lives of tramadol and M1 are 5 to 6 hours and 7 to 9 hours, respectively (Barnung, Treschow, Borgbjerg, 1997).

According to one study of elderly patients with chronic pain, 50 mg of tramadol was equal to acetaminophen, 300 mg, and codeine, 30 mg (Rauck, Ruoff, McMillen, 1994). Studies on the effectiveness of oral tramadol for postoperative pain management have produced mixed results. Some studies have shown that it produces good postoperative analgesia (Houmes, Voets, Verkaaik et al., 1992; Vickers, O'Flaherty, Szekely et al., 1992); however, the study designs have been questioned (Stubhaug, Grimstad, Breivik, 1995). Researchers comparing oral tramadol (50 and 100 mg), acetaminophen (1000 mg) plus codeine (60 mg), and placebo after orthopedic surgery found acetaminophen plus codeine to be significantly superior to placebo and both strengths of tramadol. Side effects, especially vomiting, were more common in the tramadol groups and appeared to be unrelated to the dose of tramadol (Stubhaug, Grimstad, Breivik, 1995). When administered by the IV route preoperatively, tramadol did not produce a preemptive analgesic effect (Koprulu, Dogruer, Karpat, 1997).

Side effects of tramadol include dizziness, constipation, headache, nausea, vomiting, sedation, and orthostatic hypotension. Tramadol has been reported to produce significant nausea and vomiting (Grond, Meuser, Zech et al., 1995; Stubhaug, Grimstad, Breivik, 1995). For this reason, it is recommended that tramadol therapy be initiated at a dose of 25 to 50 mg daily for the first 2 or 3 days to reduce the incidence of nausea (Katz, 1995).

The risk of respiratory depression with tramadol appears to be low. However, caution is recommended when multiple doses are administered to patients with hepatic or renal impairment. In these patients the elimination half-life of tramadol is increased twofold; therefore the interval of administration should be increased if administered in multiple doses (Lee, McTavish, Sorkin, 1993). Dose reduction is recommended in patients with creatinine clearances of less than 30 ml/minute and in patients with cirrhosis of the liver. Daily doses of tramadol should not exceed 300 mg in elderly patients older than 75 because they experience a longer half-life and higher serum concentrations than younger adults.

A case was reported of a patient with chronic renal impairment who was taking 100 mg of tramadol three times a day for 14 days. Approximately 72 hours after the dose was increased to four times a day, the patient demonstrated symptoms of opioid overdose. The symptoms of respiratory depression disappeared after administration of naloxone (Barnung, Treschow, Borgbjerg, 1997).

Seizures have been identified as a risk associated with the use of tramadol. Seizures have occurred with recommended doses and most often with higher doses. The risk of seizures is enhanced in patients with epilepsy, those with a history of seizures, those identified to be at risk for a seizure (head trauma, CNS infection), and patients taking tricyclic antidepressants, MAO inhibitors, neuroleptics, and/or other drugs that reduce the seizure threshold. Tramadol should not be used in patients with increased intracranial pressure or head injury.

Because tramadol is not a scheduled drug, clinicians may not be aware that it has opioid effects. Like other opioids, it should be used cautiously in persons who are recovering from substance abuse disorders.

Patient characteristics

Other important factors to consider when selecting the optimum opioid analgesic are intrinsic to the patient. These factors include pain intensity, patient age, coexisting disease, current drug regimen and potential drug interactions, prior treatment outcomes, patient preference and convenience, and cost.

Pain Intensity

Evaluation of the patient's report of pain intensity is critical to the development of an individualized opioid analgesic treatment plan. A variety of pain rating scales exist for the purpose of assessing pain intensity (see Chapter 3). Overall, pain intensity may be discussed in terms of mild, moderate, and severe. For all intensities of pain, the preferred route is oral and the preferred opioids are the mu agonists. Some exceptions are noted in the following.

Mild pain may not require an opioid. A nonopioid such as ibuprofen may be sufficient. If an opioid is appropriate, mild pain theoretically could be treated with any of the opioids, even morphine if the dose is kept low. However, it is far more customary to use an opioid-nonopioid combination, such as codeine or oxycodone compounded with a nonopioid such as acetaminophen.

Pain of moderate intensity may also be satisfactorily relieved with a nonopioid. If an opioid is required, an opioid-nonopioid combination may be selected. However, as mentioned previously, the dose of the opioid will be restricted by the dose of the nonopioid with which it is compounded. Therefore, for many patients with moderate pain, a single entity opioid will be a wiser choice because it will allow the opioid dose to be titrated upward without concern about exceeding the recommended total daily dose of a nonopioid.

For mild or moderate pain, the agonist-antagonist pentazocine (Talwin) may be appropriate orally for some patients. Another agonist-antagonist that may be appropriate for moderate pain is intranasal butorphanol (Stadol nasal spray). The other agonist-antagonists are available only by the parenteral route. For severe pain, mu agonists are preferred. As discussed, numerous options exist, including the prototypical drug, morphine.

In addition to providing valuable information needed to select the correct analgesic for a patient, evaluating the severity of pain may suggest the underlying mechanism and pain syndrome. For example, the pain associated with radiation-induced nerve injury usually is not severe. The occurrence of severe pain in a previously irradiated area suggests recurrent or new pathology in the patient with cancer (Coyle, Cherny, Portenoy, 1995; Portenoy, 1996b).

In the case of postoperative pain management research and clinical experience determine the expected or usual pain intensity associated with surgical procedures and are used as guides for opioid selection and determining appropriate starting doses for pain relief. For example, pain associated with a thoracotomy is expected to be severe. Preplanning for severe postthoracotomy pain includes the placement of an epidural catheter for intraoperative and postoperative pain management using a mu agonist opioid analgesic.

Patient Age

For the younger patient with no major organ failure, any of the available mu agonist opioids can be selected. For the elderly and those with major organ failure, changes in metabolism and elimination of drugs must be considered. Opioids with a short half-life are recommended, such as morphine, hydromorphone, and oxycodone. These drugs will achieve stable plasma concentrations within 24 hours (four to five half-lives) and are therefore simpler to titrate and monitor (Coyle, Cherny, Portenoy, 1995). Mu agonists with a long half-life, such as methadone and levorphanol, are avoided in elderly patients. Drugs with active metabolites, such as meperidine and propoxyphene, are also avoided in elderly patients and in all patients with renal dysfunction.

Coexisting Disease

Major organ failure, particularly cardiac, hepatic, and renal failure, influences the distribution, clearance, and excretion of opioids. Opioids also decrease the cough reflex, release histamine leading to bronchial constriction, and dry secretions (Lipman, Gauthier, 1997). Because of their respiratory depressive effects, opioids must be used with caution in patients with compromised respiratory function (AHCPR, 1992; Reisine, Pasternak, 1996). Caution in using opioids is exercised in patients with major organ failure by starting with less than the usual recommended doses and titrating upward gradually.

All opioid drugs are metabolized to some extent by the liver. In patients with liver disease, clearance is decreased and bioavailability and half-life of opioids are increased. This can lead to adverse effects from higher than expected plasma concentrations of these drugs (AHCPR, 1992). The metabolism of morphine and methadone is not significantly altered in liver disease, so these drugs are well tolerated by patients with liver disease (Coyle, Cherny, Portenoy, 1995; Foley, Inturrisi, 1992; Twycross, 1994); however, methadone is considered a second-line drug for these patients (Portenoy, 1996b). Doses of propoxyphene should be reduced (Barkin, Lubenow, Bruehl et al., 1996) or avoided altogether in patients with liver disease.

Patients with renal disease may accumulate the active metabolites of meperidine (normeperidine), propoxyphene (norpropoxyphene), and morphine (M6G). Metabolite accumulation has been most problematic with meperidine. Normeperidine may accumulate regardless of the route of administration (AHCPR, 1992; Marcantonio, Juarez, Goldman et al., 1994). Because normeperidine is eliminated by the kidneys, meperidine is contraindicated in patients with compromised renal function (AHCPR,

1992; APS, 1992; Foley, Inturrisi, 1992). Morphine and propoxyphene should be avoided in patients with end-stage renal disease (Barkin, Lubenow, Bruehl et al., 1996).

Although morphine elimination is unimpaired in patients with renal disease, the metabolite M6G has decreased clearance and increased elimination half-life in these patients. This can lead to cumulation of this metabolite, which produces increased and prolonged effects typical of mu agonists (Twycross, 1994). Therefore, caution and close monitoring is recommended when using morphine on a long-term basis in patients with renal insufficiency (AHCPR, 1992; Coyle, Cherny, Portenoy, 1995; Foley, 1995; Portenoy, 1996b; Reisine, Pasternak, 1996). A trial of an alternative opioid, such as hydromorphone, is recommended if morphine toxicity occurs in a patient with renal disease (Portenoy, 1996b).

Other opioid choices for patients with renal or hepatic failure include hydromorphone, oxymorphone, and fentanyl. Sinatra (1992b) recommends IV fentanyl as the optimal agent for patients with hepatorenal dysfunction. He reasons that fentanyl's analgesic effect is achieved with a relatively small number of drug molecules, thus the metabolic load is minimized.

Remifentanil is independent of liver and kidney function, and accumulation does not occur. It has an extremely short duration of action and rapid recovery, unaffected by either the duration of IV infusion or the total dose given. It has been used for sedation and analgesia in critically ill patients, such as in patients after organ transplant (Evans, Park, 1997). The elimination of its metabolite, GR90291, is markedly reduced in patients with renal failure, increasing the half-life of GR90291 from 2 hours to 26 hours. However, accumulation of GR90291 has not been shown to produce adverse effects (Hoke, Shlugman, Dershwitz et al., 1997). Further research and clinical experience with this opioid is needed.

When indicated by the type and severity of pain, the use of alternative routes may be a solution for some patients with major organ failure. Opioids can be given in lower doses by the epidural and intrathecal routes compared with the doses needed when given by the oral and parenteral routes. Because of this, patients with major organ failure sometimes are able to tolerate opioids by an intraspinal route that they were unable to tolerate by the oral or parenteral routes. Lipophilic drugs, such as fentanyl and sufentanil, can accumulate; morphine and hydromorphone may be better choices by the epidural route in patients with hepatic dysfunction and CNS depression (Sinatra, 1992b).

Current Drug Regimen and Potential Drug Interactions

Many patients with pain, especially those with coexisting disease and chronic pain, take several medications. Coadministration of two or more drugs often can result in a change in the metabolism, clearance, or both of the drugs (Benet, Kroetz, Sheiner, 1996). It is extremely important when developing an opioid treatment plan to know all the medications the patient is taking and how they will interact with the opioid and to monitor on an ongoing basis for drug interactions.

Phenobarbital and phenytoin increase the metabolism of meperidine, and phenytoin and the antitubercular drug, rifampin, increase the metabolism of methadone. This can result in decreased plasma levels of these opioids. The tricyclic antidepressants, clomipramine and amitriptyline, may increase the bioavailability and half-life of morphine. This would cause a rise in plasma morphine levels (APS, 1992; Coyle, Cherny, Portenoy, 1995). Treatment with rifampin can result in complete loss of the analgesic effects of morphine (Fromm, Eckhardt, Li et al., 1997). In the presence of MAO inhibitors, meperidine can precipitate excitation, hyperpyrexia, convulsions, and death (Coyle, Cherny, Portenoy, 1995).

When drugs with anticholinergic effects, such as antihistamines, phenothiazines, tricyclic antidepressants, and antiparkinsonian drugs, are administered with opioids, constipation may increase. It is therefore very important to emphasize a bowel management regimen in patients taking any of these drugs with opioids (Coyle, Cherny, Portenoy, 1995). (See Table 6.17 on pp. 262-264.)

Seizures have been identified as a risk associated with the use of tramadol. This risk is enhanced when patients are taking tricyclic antidepressants, MAO inhibitors, neuroleptics, and other drugs that reduce the seizure threshold.

In a recent study the benzodiazepine antagonist, flumazenil, was found to enhance postoperative morphine analgesia. The researchers state that these findings support their hypothesis that benzodiazepines given for preoperative sedation antagonize the analgesic effects of opioids given postoperatively (Gear, Miaskowski, Heller et al., 1997).

Additive effects when opioid drugs are combined with other drugs also must be considered when implementing a pain treatment plan. Close monitoring of sedation is indicated when opioids are combined with antidepressants, phenothiazines, benzodiazepines, or neuroleptics. Because of their sedative and respiratory depressive effects, the amount of opioid that can be safely administered may be limited (APS, 1992; Coyle, Cherny, Portenoy, 1995; Reisine, Pasternak, 1996).

Combining drugs can have a positive effect on analgesia and side effects. Coadministration of amphetamine has been reported to enhance the analgesic effects while counteracting the sedative effects of both morphine and meperidine (APS, 1992; Reisine, Pasternak, 1996) (See Chapter 7 for more on the effects of adjuvant drugs.)

Prior Treatment Outcomes

The patient's response to an opioid analgesic cannot be predicted except on the basis of the patient's previous experience with the drug. If a patient reports having pre-

viously experienced unmanageable side effects with an opioid, explore with the patient the occurrence, severity, and management of the side effects. An attempt should be made to determine whether the side effects were really unmanageable (e.g., nausea unresponsive to antiemetics) or simply unmanaged (e.g., no attempt made to relieve nausea).

A true allergy to an opioid is extremely rare (Kaplan, Krishnamurthy, Nori, 1994). Often, patients erroneously report being "allergic" to an opioid after experiencing side effects from it in the past. For example, patients commonly mistake nausea and vomiting after an opioid bolus dose as an allergy to the opioid.

In case of intolerable and unmanageable side effects, switching to another opioid may be indicated. Sequential trials of different opioids are necessary to find the optimal balance between analgesia and side effects (Benedetti, 1990; Galer, Boyle, Pasternak et al., 1992) (See pp. 253-261 for more on switching to another opioid).

Patient Preferences and Convenience

Often, patients have preferences when it comes to the choice of opioid, route of administration, and scheduling of doses, especially patients with prior opioid experience. Respecting patients' preferences whenever feasible and making the opioid treatment regimen as convenient as possible may help the patient adhere better to the plan. Occasionally preferences are based on myths and misconceptions that can be corrected by providing factual information. During the initial interview with the patient, time can be taken to determine whether this is the case and ensure that the patient has an accurate understanding of pain management.

Although the oral route is the preferred route of administration for chronic pain management, it may not be optimal for all patients. Although the rectal route is safe and effective, some patients with family caregivers are uncomfortable with the thought of a family member administering rectal medications to them. Occasionally patients who can self-administer their medications object to doing so by the rectal route. In these cases, alternative opioid delivery systems, such as the fentanyl transdermal patch, may provide a solution.

Complying with the established opioid treatment regimen can become a problem for some patients, especially if the regimen requires the patient to take several pills several times a day. Elderly patients in particular may forget to take their pills at the prescribed intervals or object to taking so many pills. For these patients, a controlled-release preparation of the opioid may be ideal. This will allow the patient to take pills as few times as twice daily instead of several times a day required by immediate-release preparations. Scheduling doses along with other medications the patient is already accustomed to taking also is recommended. For example, individuals can take their morning opioid dose with their daily vitamin. The fentanyl transdermal patch, which is changed only every 3 days in most individuals, can be considered also for patients who are unreliable in taking oral medications.

Cost

The cost of an opioid is an important consideration in selecting the optimal opioid for the pain treatment plan, especially for long-term opioid therapy. The cost of medications can vary greatly. For example, a survey in 1994 revealed that generic oxycodone with acetaminophen ranged from $9.00 to $25.69 for 100 tablets. Analysis of equianalgesic doses of opioids revealed a 19-fold price difference among opioid prescriptions (Ferrell, Griffith, 1994).

A number of factors influence the cost of drugs, including packaging of the drug, wholesale prices, and pharmacy dispensing fees. As a rule, morphine and especially methadone are significantly less expensive than other opioids, bulk containers of drugs are less expensive than prefilled syringes and unit dose or blister packs, and large hospitals or urban chain pharmacies that can purchase drugs in large quantities are likely to charge less than small independent pharmacies (Kunz, 1994).

The use of multiple prescriptions (polypharmacy) to manage pain is more costly than single prescriptions. Although combined modalities are recommended (see p. 174 for more on balanced analgesia), single opioids in sufficient doses may provide adequate pain control and certainly should be tried before adding adjuvant analgesics (Ferrell, Griffith, 1994).

Today, most individuals assume all or at least part of the cost of their medications. The insured patient's ability to pay depends on the amount of their copayment. Great care should be taken to ensure cost savings for patients with end-stage disease so that appropriate pain management is not prohibitive and does not overburden patients and families with excessive costs. Physicians can assist patients in obtaining free prescriptions for pain medications. Application can be made to the patient assistance programs offered by several of the pharmaceutical companies (see Box 6.7).

Routes of Administration

Regardless of the type of pain being treated, opioids should be administered by the least invasive and safest route capable of producing satisfactory analgesia, and generally only one route of administration at a time should be used. The oral route is the preferred route of administration for opioids and should always be considered before other routes because it is relatively safe, convenient, and inexpensive (AHCPR, 1992; Coyle, Cherny, Portenoy, 1995; Jacox, Carr, Payne et al., 1994). However, as a general rule, if rapid onset of analgesia is desired, the IV route is used. Then the patient is transitioned to the oral route when pain is under control and the patient is able to retain oral medication.

Over the course of time, more than one route of administration usually is necessary. For example, in a postoperative patient, the process of transitioning from IV to oral may require the use of both the old and the new routes to ensure continuous analgesia. The patient may receive PRN boluses by the IV route and the oral analgesic until the appropriate dose of the oral analgesic is determined. Nevertheless, the length of time such patients receive analgesics by more than one route should be as short as possible.

In a survey of patients with progressive cancer pain more than half required more than one route of administration to maintain pain control during the last 4 weeks of life. This occurred usually when patients were unable to swallow. The routes used included rectal, SC, IV, and epidural. Sometimes patients required more than one route at a time (Coyle, Adelhardt, Foley et al., 1990).

For many patients, satisfactory analgesia may be accomplished with either the oral or the IV route. However, other routes of administration are available and are indicated in certain situations. For patients unable or unwilling to take medications by the oral route, noninvasive alternatives are available, such as the rectal and transdermal routes. For major thoracic, abdominal, and joint surgeries, which are associated with severe postoperative pain, intraspinal opioids are indicated. Table 6.6 summarizes the advantages and disadvantages to some of the routes of opioid administration.

Oral

The oral route usually is preferred for administering opioids to patients with chronic pain. It allows for flexibility in dosing and is capable of producing steady analgesic blood levels. Another advantage of the oral route is that it can provide adequate relief for a wide range of pain intensities, from mild to severe pain; the most common reason for failure to achieve analgesia by the oral route is insufficient dose administration (Coyle, Portenoy, 1996).

• • • • •

TABLE 6.6 **Routes of Opioid Administration**

ROUTE	COMMENTS
Oral	Inexpensive, simple, noninvasive; should be considered before all other routes. Preferred in cancer and chronic nonmalignant pain management. Opioids are subject to extensive hepatic metabolism; slow onset but just as effective as other routes if doses are high enough and given ATC.
Oral transmucosal	Oral transmucosal fentanyl citrate (OTFC) is approved for conscious sedation and use as an anesthetic premedication administered by trained personnel in a monitored setting. A new OTFC has been shown to be effective and convenient in managing breakthrough pain in patients with cancer; awaiting FDA approval. Opioid bypasses significant hepatic metabolism.
Buccal	Supporting data meager; suitable preparations generally unavailable and impractical.
Sublingual	Buprenorphine, fentanyl, and methadone absorbed well; currently only buprenorphine is available in the United States. Morphine is commonly used by the sublingual route, but research is limited.
Rectal	Currently morphine, oxymorphone, and hydromorphone are commercially available in the United States. Alternative for patients unable or unwilling to take analgesics orally. Considerable variation in dose required to produce effect and time to reach effect. Starting dose usually is same dose as oral dose. Any opioid may be compounded by pharmacy for rectal administration or given in an aqueous solution, unmodified tablet, or crushed and placed in gelatin capsule; controlled-release formulations should not be crushed or dissolved.
Vaginal	No commercially available formulations; research lacking, but absorption does occur by this route.
Transdermal	Available in fentanyl citrate drug delivery system incorporated within an adhesive patch. Can provide analgesia for 48-72 h by continuous drug release into the skin. Slow onset, gradual decline after patch is removed. Difficult to titrate; must use IR opioid until analgesia is achieved. Alternative for patients unable or unwilling to take analgesics orally or have failed other opioids and could benefit from a trial. Not suitable for acute pain or severe escalating pain.
Intranasal	Butorphanol is available in the United States but not recommended for cancer or chronic nonmalignant pain. Sufentanil is currently being studied for use as a preanesthetic. Major drawback, especially in children, is burning and stinging on instillation. Bypasses significant hepatic metabolism.
Nebulized	Nebulization is not recommended as a route for analgesia, primarily because current administration techniques result in very small amounts of analgesic being absorbed. However, nebulized morphine is used for management of dyspnea in end-stage terminal illness (e.g., chronic lung disease, heart failure).
Subcutaneous • Single or repetitive bolus • CI with or without PCA	Morphine and hydromorphone most common opioids administered subcutaneously. Alternative when patient is unable to take opioid orally or parenteral route is indicated but venous access is limited. Easy to access, but technique and care require more skill and expertise than oral or rectal administration. Infusion pumps add expense, but are more convenient and allow for CI; newer pumps allow PCA capability.
Intravenous • Single or repetitive bolus • CI with or without PCA	Indicated when rapid titration is required. Provides steady blood levels. Opioids with short half-life recommended. Boluses or PCA commonly used for postoperative pain management. Duration is dose dependent. When steady state is reached by continuous infusion, the various opioids differ little in terms of duration. For long-term CI, permanent venous access is recommended; indicated for cancer and chronic nonmalignant pain when patient has dose-limiting side effects from other systemic routes.
Intraarterial	Direct injection into artery is rarely used; most common use with neonates by indwelling umbilical artery catheter. Requires great care and expertise; first pass is avoided, cleansing effects of lung are not available by this route.
Epidural • Single or repetitive bolus • CI with or without PCA • Chronic: Implanted for CI with side port for bolus injections	Indicated for major abdominal, thoracic, and joint surgeries when severe acute pain is anticipated; rarely indicated for cancer and chronic nonmalignant pain management (e.g., may be alternative for patients with dose-limiting side effects from systemic opioid analgesics). Infusion pumps add expense, but are more convenient and allow for continuous infusion and PCA capability. Duration is dose dependent. When steady state is reached by continuous infusion, the various opioids differ little in terms of duration. May be cost-effective for patients with cancer or chronic nonmalignant pain and long life expectancy; may be administered by external catheter and pump or by implanted infusion pump. Local anesthetics frequently added to opioids by this route.

May be duplicated for use in clinical practice. From McCaffery M, Pasero C: *Pain: Clinical manual*, pp. 195-196. Copyright © 1999, Mosby, Inc.   *Continued.*

● ● ● ● ●

TABLE 6.6	Routes of Opioid Administration—cont'd
ROUTE	**COMMENTS**
Intrathecal • Acute: Single bolus • Chronic: Implanted for CI with side port for bolus injections	Indicated for some acute pain (single bolus most commonly used because temporary indwelling catheters are difficult to maintain); rarely indicated for cancer and chronic nonmalignant pain management (e.g., may be alternative for patients with dose-limiting side effects from systemic opioid analgesics). May be cost-effective for patients with cancer or chronic nonmalignant pain and long life expectancy; usually administered by implanted infusion pump.
Intraarticular (joint)	Shown to produce adequate analgesia for joint surgeries, but further studies are needed to establish best opioids and local anesthetics to use by this route.
Intracerebroventricular	Rarely indicated. Should be considered investigational.

May be duplicated for use in clinical practice. From McCaffery M, Pasero C: *Pain: Clinical manual*, pp. 195-196. Copyright © 1999, Mosby, Inc.

Opioid analgesics can be administered by a wide variety of routes. Table 6.6 summarizes the advantages and disadvantages to some of these.

ATC, around-the-clock; *CI*, continuous infusion; *FDA*, Food and Drug Administration; *IR*, immediate-release; *PCA*, patient-controlled analgesia.

Information from Benet LZ, Kroetz DL, Sheiner LB: Pharmacokinetics. In Hardman JG, Limbird LE, editors: *Goodman and Gilman's the pharmacological basis of therapeutics*, ed 9, pp. 3-27, New York, 1996, McGraw-Hill; Biddle C, Gilliland C: Transdermal and transmucosal administration of pain-relieving and anxiolytic drugs: A primer for the critical care practitioner, *Heart Lung* 12:115-124, 1992; Coyle N, Cherny N, Portenoy RK: Pharmacologic management of cancer pain. In McGuire D, Yarbro CH, Ferrell BR, editors: *Cancer pain management*, ed 2, pp. 89-130, Boston, 1995, Jones and Bartlett; Foley KM, Inturrisi CE: Opioid therapy: General principles, advances, controversies, alternative routes and methods of administration, *Syllabus of the Postgraduate Course*, Memorial Sloan-Kettering Cancer Center, New York, NY, April 2-3, 1992; Joshi GP, McCarroll SM, O'Brien TM et al.: Intraarticular analgesia following knee arthroscopy, *Anesth Analg* 76:333-336, 1993; Kalso E, Tramer MR, Carroll D et al.: Pain relief from intra-articular morphine after knee surgery: A qualitative systemic review, *Pain* 71:127-134, 1997; Portenoy RK: Opioid analgesics. In Portenoy RK, Kanner RM, editors: *Pain management: Theory and practice*, pp 249-276, Philadelphia, 1996, FA Davis; Reuben SS, Connelly NR: Postarthroscopic meniscus repair analgesia with intraarticular ketorolac or morphine, *Anesth Analg* 82:1036-1039, 1996; Stanley TH, Ashburn MA: Novel delivery systems: Oral transmucosal and intranasal transmucosal, *J Pain Symptom Manage* 7(3):163-171, 1992; Vranken J, Vissers K, Oosterbosch J et al.: Intra-articular sufentanil analgesia after arthroscopic knee surgery, *Br J Anaesth* 8(1):A400, 1997.

Most mu agonists are available in oral form. Of the agonist–antagonist opioids, only pentazocine is available orally. Oral opioids in tablet form can be taken by most patients. For those who cannot take tablets, many are available in liquid formulation. For those that are not, tablets can be crushed and put into concentrated suspensions (APS, 1992). Controlled-release formulations, however, should not be crushed because this destroys the release mechanisms.

Disadvantages of the Oral Route

Two major disadvantages of the oral route are that it has a slow onset of action and a relatively delayed peak time (90 to 120 minutes after ingestion and longer in the case of controlled-release tablets), making it inappropriate for severe, escalating pain. Its use is limited when it is imperative to get severe pain under control quickly, such as for pain related to surgery or myocardial infarction.

Although opioids tend to have a longer duration of action orally than parenterally, intervals between doses of immediate-release preparations remain short, commonly 4 hours. This requires the patient to take six doses a day and interferes with patient activities, such as sleeping. The patient must also remember to take all doses to maintain a constant level of analgesia. Another disadvantage is that oral dosing may be associated with higher levels of metabolites, such as M6G, than by other routes of administration (Babul, Darke, 1993; Foley, Inturrisi, 1992).

The oral route is not an option for patients who are NPO (nothing by mouth), such as immediately after surgery. Some patients cannot tolerate the oral route because of GI obstruction or difficulty swallowing (APS, 1992; Benet, Kroetz, Sheiner, 1996; Coyle, Cherny, Portenoy, 1995). Absorption by the oral route can be altered by a number of factors, including presence of food, gastric emptying time, and GI motility (Coyle, Portenoy, 1996). Controlled-release preparations appear to be less affected by the presence of food than immediate-release preparations.

The effectiveness of the oral route depends on patient compliance. Patients who must self-administer but cannot remember or are remiss in taking medications are not good candidates for the oral route unless they are able to take formulations designed for once a day dosing.

Finally, some oral medications, such as methadone, have a bitter taste, to which most patients object. After administration, "chasers" of applesauce or lemon drops may be helpful in reducing the bitterness (Gardner-Nix, 1996).

Oral Opioid Formulations

The relatively new controlled-release opioid preparations have rendered the oral route more convenient than in the past by requiring only once or twice a day dosing. These preparations allow for slow, uniform absorption of the opioid for 12 to 24 hours, making them ideal for the management of continuous cancer pain and some chronic nonmalignant pain (APS, 1992; Coyle, Cherny, Portenoy, 1995). Opioids available in oral controlled-release formulation in the United States include morphine (MS Contin, Oramorph SR, Kadian) and oxycodone (OxyContin). In other countries (and probably shortly in the United States) other opioids are available in controlled-release formulation, including codeine (Dhaliwal, Sloan, Arkistall et al., 1995) and hydromorphone (Hagen, Babul, 1997).

Oral Morphine

MS Contin and Oramorph SR, controlled-release formulations of morphine, are available in 15, 30, 60, and 100 mg tablets; MS Contin also is available in a 200 mg tablet. The recommended dosing interval is every 12 hours and no less than every 8 hours. Steady state with ATC dosing of controlled-release morphine may not be reached for 1 to 2 days, so these preparations alone are not appropriate if rapid titration is required (Portenoy, 1996b). Supplemental doses of immediate-release opioid are necessary for rapid control of pain by the oral route.

Although both MS Contin and Oramorph SR are controlled-release formulations, they are not bioequivalent, which means they should not be used interchangeably. The Food and Drug Administration (FDA) does not consider any controlled-release dosage forms to be therapeutically equivalent unless bioequivalent data have been submitted. The FDA assigns a "BC" code to controlled-release products for which bioequivalence data have not been submitted. The FDA has assigned a "BC" code to MS Contin and Oramorph SR because bioequivalence data have produced conflicting results (McCaffery, Lochman, 1996).

Drugs can be pharmaceutically equivalent without being therapeutically equivalent. MS Contin and Oramorph SR are pharmaceutically equivalent because they contain the same drug, have the same dosage form, can deliver the same amount of drug, are both available in 15, 30, 60, and 100 mg strengths, and are given by the same route. However, the two are not necessarily therapeutically equivalent because they use different controlled-release mechanisms. This means that the same dose of each product may not affect the patient in the same way (McCaffery, Lochman, 1996).

Although Oramorph SR and MS Contin do not meet FDA requirements for therapeutic equivalence, the FDA and some state laws have allowed pharmacists, physicians, institutions, and health care plans to consider them therapeutically equivalent. Consequently, patients are sometimes switched from one to the other (McCaffery, Lochman, 1996) (see Box 6.8 for recommendations when switching from one pharmaceutically equivalent product to another).

Another controlled-release formulation of morphine, Kadian, is available in 20, 50, and 100 mg capsules and can be given every 12 to 24 hours. Some researchers believe Kadian has an improved controlled-release profile over other formulations. The fluctuation of plasma concentrations of Kadian at steady state have been found to be less than immediate-release morphine and MS Contin (Broomhead, Kerr, Tester et al., 1997; Gourlay, Cherry, Li et al., 1997).

Kadian has been compared with MS Contin in patients with cancer pain (Broomhead, Kerr, Tester et al.,

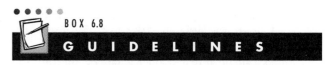

BOX 6.8

G U I D E L I N E S

SWITCHING FROM ONE PHARMACEUTICALLY EQUIVALENT PRODUCT TO ANOTHER

- Examples of pharmaceutically equivalent products are MS Contin, Oramorph SR, and Kadian at 100 mg each.
- Assume that some difference may exist in therapeutic effects between the products.
- Completely switch from one product to the other. Avoid having patients take more than one product at a time (except during the transition phase) and avoid switching back and forth between products. The same formulation should be used if the patient is moved from hospital to home and vice versa.
- Advise the patient and family that the new drug may not have the same effect as the previous drug and that the dose may need to be adjusted.
- Monitor pain and sedation. Use a flow sheet for documentation so that problems can be detected early.
- Instruct the patient and family about the different products (e.g., Oramorph SR tablets are white and about the size of an aspirin; MS Contin tablets are smaller and each strength is a different color). Tell the patient to question anyone who attempts to substitute one brand for another.

May be duplicated for use in clinical practice. From McCaffery M, Pasero C: *Pain: Clinical manual*, p. 197. Copyright © 1999, Mosby, Inc.

Drugs can be pharmaceutically equivalent without being therapeutically equivalent. This is because the drugs use different controlled-release mechanisms. This means that the same dose of each product may not affect the patient in the same way. Box 6.8 lists examples of drugs that are pharmaceutically equivalent but not therapeutically equivalent and guidelines for switching from one to another. *mg*, milligram.

Information from McCaffery M, Lochman C: Controlled release morphine products, *Am J Nurs* 96(4):65, 1996.

1997). Patients received treatment according to the random assignment to one of three groups: (1) Kadian every 12 hours, (2) Kadian every 24 hours, or (3) MS Contin every 12 hours. All patients were titrated to adequate analgesia with immediate-release morphine solution before treatment. Immediate-release morphine was used during the study for breakthrough pain. The time before the need for remedication in group 1 patients was 16.1 hours, group 2 was 9.1 hours, and group 3 was 8.7 hours. Kadian doses either every 12 hours or every 24 hours resulted in similar pain control (measured by VAS and verbal report) to MS Contin every 12 hours. Kadian given every 24 hours provided adequate pain control in more than 50% of the patients throughout the 24-hour dosing period. No significant differences were found in side effects between the groups, and patients preferred Kadian over the other two preparations.

In another study Kadian once daily and MS Contin every 12 hours provided equivalent pain relief and side effects. Although more patients indicated a preference for MS Contin, the difference was not statistically significant (Gourlay, Cherry, Li et al., 1997).

Patients can be initiated on Kadian by splitting the dose in half and administering it every 12 hours or by taking the full dose once daily. It is recommended that the dose be titrated every other day. Opioid-naive patients should be started on 20 mg and increased by no more than 20 mg every other day.

Of the controlled-release preparations, MS Contin has the smallest tablet, which is an important consideration in patients who have difficulty swallowing. MS Contin tablets are also color coded according to dose, which may help prevent errors in dosing.

Oral Oxycodone

Oxycodone is used extensively by the oral route and is available in both immediate-release and controlled-release formulations. It is available alone or in combination with varying amounts of acetaminophen (Percocet, Tylox, Roxicet, Endocet) or aspirin (Percodan, Roxiprin, Endodan). The amount of oxycodone in any capsule or tablet is 5 mg. The acetaminophen dose is 325 mg except for Tylox, which has 500 mg of acetaminophen per capsule. The difference produced by the additional acetaminophen does not appear to have analgesic significance (Levy, 1994).

A major drawback to the use of oxycodone combinations is that the dose of acetaminophen makes titration difficult. Increases in the dose of oxycodone for inadequate pain relief are limited by acetaminophen's and aspirin's recommended maximum daily dose of 4 g (see Chapters 4 and 5). Therefore combination preparations of oxycodone and acetaminophen or aspirin are appropriate for mild to moderate pain only.

Other preparations have allowed broader use of oxycodone. Oxycodone is the only opioid analgesic besides morphine that is available in the United States in 12-hour controlled-release form (OxyContin) for twice daily dosing. OxyContin is available in 10, 20, 40, and 80 mg tablets. These are small tablets and are colored coded according to dose. Analgesic onset occurs in most patients within 1 hour of administration of controlled-release oxycodone (Rust, 1997). The release mechanism of OxyContin differs from that of MS Contin. OxyContin exhibits a biphasic absorption pattern with an initial release of oxycodone at 0.6 hours and a prolonged release at 6.9 hours. The rationale for this formulation is to provide an extended duration of analgesia without significantly compromising the brisk onset of analgesia inherent in conventional immediate-release products (Patt, 1996).

Immediate-release oxycodone (OxyIR), a single entity formulation, with 5 mg per tablet, is available for breakthrough pain. Although a ratio of 1:1 has been recommended when switching patients from oral morphine to single entity oral oxycodone (Glare, Walsh, 1993), many clinicians have used a more cautious morphine/oxycodone ratio of 1.5:1 or 2.2:1 (Beaver, Wallenstein, Rogers et al., 1978; Foley, 1985). When converting to oral oxycodone from oral morphine, an appropriate conservative estimate is 15 to 20 mg of oxycodone per 30 mg of morphine; however, when converting to oral morphine from oral oxycodone, an appropriate conservative estimate is 30 mg of morphine per 30 mg of oxycodone. A concentrated oral solution of 20 mg/ml of plain oxycodone (Intensol) also is available with a calibrated dropper for measuring doses of 5, 10, 15, or 20 mg.

Controlled-release oxycodone has been found to be safe and effective for cancer pain management (Kaplan, Parris, Citron et al., 1995). It also has been studied for use in postoperative pain management. Controlled-release morphine and controlled-release oxycodone were compared for relative potency and onset of analgesia in patients after abdominal hysterectomy. Onset of action for both was 45 minutes in nearly all of the patients, with higher doses providing faster onset than lower doses. A 2:1 dose ratio (morphine/oxycodone) produced equianalgesic effects (Kaiko, Lacouture, Hopf et al., 1996; Patt, 1996).

After abdominal or gynecologic surgery, 182 patients experiencing moderate to severe pain were given a single dose of either controlled-release oxycodone (10, 20, and 30 mg), immediate-release oxycodone (15 mg), immediate-release oxycodone (10 mg) plus acetaminophen (650 mg), or placebo (Sunshine, Olson, Colon et al, 1996). All active treatments were superior to placebo for all pain measurements. Patients responded differently among the three levels of controlled-release oxycodone with 20 and 30 mg being significantly better than 10 mg for pain relief. The median time to onset of relief was shortest (32 minutes) for oxycodone plus acetaminophen and longest (46 minutes) for 30 mg controlled-release oxycodone. For all active treatments, peak pain intensity differences and peak pain relief occurred approximately 2 to 4 hours after administration. At 1 hour, oxycodone plus acetaminophen and immediate-release oxycodone were significantly better than controlled-release oxycodone, but as expected, controlled-release oxycodone provided better relief at 9 through 12 hours. The controlled-release oxycodone preparations had durations of pain relief of 10 to 12 hours. The most common side effect was somnolence, followed by dizziness and headache.

In one study of patients with moderate to severe pain from chronic osteoarthritis, a 20 mg dose of controlled-release oxycodone every 12 hours reduced pain over the 2-week study period (Purdue Pharma LP, 1996). Therapy at this dose improved quality of life with significant weekly reductions in the negative impact of pain on enjoyment of life, mood, and sleep pattern. In one long-term trial, patients with osteoarthritis received a daily dose of 40 mg of oral oxycodone. Adverse effects, such as sleepiness, pruritis, and dizziness, declined over time. Acceptability of treatment was high in these patients (Purdue Pharma LP, 1996).

The findings of these studies show that controlled-release oxycodone formulations are safe and effective for moderate to severe pain. Because of the lag time of approximately 45 minutes before meaningful pain relief, they are suitable for previous ATC dosing only with supplemental doses of immediate-release PRN.

Inpatient Oral PCA

A major advantage of using PCA is the elimination of the delay period between the patient's request for analgesia and the nurse administering it. The use of PCA in the hospital is administered most often by the IV, SC, or epidural routes. Although patients commonly self-administer oral pain medications in the home setting, oral PCA in the hospital setting is a new concept. However, it has been used safely and effectively in this setting for the treatment of all types of pain. One pioneering hospital's pain care quality improvement team reports that not one incident of patient noncompliance or loss or diversion of analgesics has occurred with its oral PCA program (Faries, 1997). With the use of oral PCA, this hospital has seen a 10% increase in patient satisfaction with oral analgesics (see Box 6.9 and Form 6.1).

BOX 6.9

GUIDELINES

INPATIENT ORAL PCA

Patient Selection

1. Patient has no contraindications to using the oral route of administration.
2. Patient appears to be cognitively able to self-administer oral analgesia: Understands the relationship between pain, taking a dose of pain medication, and pain relief.
3. Can cognitively understand how and physically use the necessary supplies (e.g., open the wrist pouch and document appropriately in the pain relief diary).

Other Considerations

Supplies are available.
Staff is trained to explain to patient, and assess, manage, and document oral PCA.

Equipment Provided to Patient

Pain relief diary (kept in patient's room) (see Form 6.1)
Wrist pouch for storage of analgesic doses

Patient Teaching

1. Review prescription.
2. Explain that one dose at a time will be given to store in wrist pouch and any doses left over when oral PCA is discontinued must be returned to nurse.
3. Remind patients to keep pain medication with them in wrist pouch at all times.
4. Tell patients to "stay on top of pain" by taking dose before pain becomes severe.
5. Show patients how and what to document in diary:
   • Time and amount of dose taken
   • Pain rating
   • Side effects

6. Tell patients why, when, and what information needs to be reported to nurse:
   • After taking a dose so that nurse can provide the next dose to keep in pouch
   • Inadequate pain relief so that nurse can perform assessment and take appropriate action
   • Side effects so that nurse can perform assessment and take appropriate action
   • Inability to perform recovery activities at expected level of function
   • Loss of medication
7. Explain to patient that because of substance control regulations, noncompliance with oral PCA policy and procedure (e.g., loss of controlled substance) will necessitate discontinuing oral PCA; staff will administer analgesics.
8. Provide written prescription and instructions.

Nursing Responsibilities Related to Assessment, Documentation, Substance Control

   • Respond promptly to patient needs (i.e., replace used doses, assess inadequate pain relief, side effects, adverse reactions).
   • Report to physician and document adverse effects, lack of pain relief, patient noncompliance, inability to perform responsibilities, and if oral PCA is discontinued for any reason other than patient discharge.
   • Document assessments, interventions, discontinuation of oral PCA.
   • Document doses in controlled substance record when they are dispensed to patient.
   • Count and document amount remaining in patients' pouches at end of shift.
   • Count, waste, and document unused medication.
   • Report unaccounted for doses.

May be duplicated for use in clinical practice. As appears in McCaffery M, Pasero C: *Pain: Clinical manual*, p. 199. Copyright © 1999, Mosby, Inc.

Although patients commonly self-administer oral pain medications in the home setting, oral PCA in the hospital setting is a relatively new concept. Box 6.9 provides considerations and guidelines for providing oral PCA in the inpatient hospital setting.

PCA, patient-controlled analgesia.

Courtesy Wellmont Health System, Holston Valley Medical Center, Pain Care Quality Improvement Team, Kingsport, TN, 1997.

FORM 6.1 **PATIENT PAIN RELIEF DIARY**

PATIENT INFORMATION

Take 1 or 2 _____ Every _____ Hour(s)
if Needed for Pain

My goals include:
- ☐ A pain rating of _____
- ☐ Take ____ deep breaths and cough every hour
- ☐ Walk____ times per day
- ☐ _____

COMMENTS
_____
_____
_____
_____
_____

DATE	TIME	HOW MANY PILLS I TOOK?	RATE YOUR PAIN 1 HOUR AFTER TAKING YOUR PAIN PILLS ← PAIN RATING → None Mod. Severe	ARE YOU MEETING YOUR RECOVERY GOALS?	REVIEWED & ACTION TAKEN, IF ANY	DATE TIME	NURSE SIGNATURE
			0 1 2 3 4 5 6 7 8 9 10	YES NO			
			0 1 2 3 4 5 6 7 8 9 10	YES NO			
			0 1 2 3 4 5 6 7 8 9 10	YES NO			
			0 1 2 3 4 5 6 7 8 9 10	YES NO			
			0 1 2 3 4 5 6 7 8 9 10	YES NO			
			0 1 2 3 4 5 6 7 8 9 10	YES NO			
			0 1 2 3 4 5 6 7 8 9 10	YES NO			
			0 1 2 3 4 5 6 7 8 9 10	YES NO			
			0 1 2 3 4 5 6 7 8 9 10	YES NO			
			0 1 2 3 4 5 6 7 8 9 10	YES NO			
			0 1 2 3 4 5 6 7 8 9 10	YES NO			
			0 1 2 3 4 5 6 7 8 9 10	YES NO			
			0 1 2 3 4 5 6 7 8 9 10	YES NO			

I understand and agree to follow the instructions as written on the back of this form

Patient Signature _____ Date _____

Pills not recorded as taken by the patient in the hospital must be returned.

_____ # of pills returned

nurse initials   date/time

Trend in Oral Analgesics for Postoperative Pain

With the current trend toward early discharge of patients after relatively major surgical procedures, consideration must be given to more aggressive pain treatment in the home setting than is possible with the traditional fixed combination opioid/nonopioid analgesics. The fixed dose of the nonopioid limits the number of tablets that patients may take in a 24-hour period without exceeding the recommended total daily dose of, for example, 4000 mg of acetaminophen. Single entity opioids, such as morphine or oxycodone, may be ideal alternatives. As in Canada, clinicians in the United States can expect to have more choices in oral formulations in the future, making the oral route more applicable in all care settings.

Oral transmucosal

The oral mucosa functions, like the skin, as a barrier to dangerous substances. It differs from the skin in that it is significantly more vascular, more permeable to drugs with similar properties, and has a lower drug depot (storage) effect than the skin. Absorption from the oral transmucosa is optimized with drugs that are lipid soluble, such as fentanyl, buprenorphine, and methadone (Stanley, Ashburn, 1992; Weinberg, Inturrisi, Reidenberg et al., 1988). Three areas within the mouth can be used for oral transmucosal drug delivery: the sublingual, buccal, and gingival areas. These areas usually are regarded as separate routes of administration and are studied and discussed separately.

Sublingual

Use of the sublingual route involves placing the drug under the tongue for absorption through the oral mucosa into the systemic circulation. Because the drug is absorbed directly into systemic circulation, first pass effect is avoided (Weinberg, Inturrisi, Reidenberg et al., 1988). Of all the areas within the mouth for oral transmucosal drug administration, the sublingual area appears to be the highest in drug permeability (Stanley, Ashburn, 1992).

Few opioids have been administered by the sublingual route. Hospice nurses report success with morphine by the sublingual route (Robinson, Wilkie, Campbell, 1995), but it is thought that this is related to the fact that the drug is eventually swallowed because sublingual absorption of morphine is poor (Foley, Inturrisi, 1992; Weinberg, Inturrisi, Reidenberg et al., 1988).

The effects of lipid solubility, oral cavity pH, and drug contact time on sublingual absorption of various opioids and naloxone have been studied. It was found that drugs with high lipid solubility and in an alkaline environment improved absorption. Compared with morphine at pH 6.5 (18% absorption), the more lipophilic opioids, buprenorphine (55%), fentanyl (51%), and methadone (34%), were absorbed to a significantly greater extent, whereas levorphanol, hydromorphone, oxycodone, heroin, and the opioid antagonist naloxone were

not. At a pH of 8.5, methadone absorption increased to 75%. Drug absorption was not affected by concentration, but was affected by contact time. Sixty percent of the maximum methadone and fentanyl absorption at 10 minutes was seen at 2.5 minutes of contact time; maximum buprenorphine absorption was complete by 2.5 minutes of contact time. Side effects were minor (bitter taste, burning sensation, light-headedness), and fentanyl and buprenorphine were associated with the lowest incidence (Weinberg, Inturrisi, Reidenberg et al., 1988).

Although fentanyl and methadone are well absorbed sublingually, no preparations are commercially available (Weinberg, Inturrisi, Reidenberg et al., 1988) (see following discussion on oral transmucosal fentanyl). A sublingual preparation of buprenorphine is available in other countries and may provide relief of mild to moderate pain. Sublingual buprenorphine absorption occurs within 3 to 5 minutes, bioavailability is 55%, and peak plasma concentrations generally occur at approximately 3 hours (Foley, Inturrisi, 1992).

An advantage of the sublingual route is that it requires little expertise, preparation, or supervision to administer a drug by this route (Weinberg, Inturrisi, Reidenberg et al., 1988). Unfortunately, the sublingual route has limited value for the administration of opioids because formulations are lacking, absorption is poor, and high doses cannot be given (Coyle, Cherny, Portenoy, 1995; Foley, Inturrisi, 1992). In addition, proper administration is seldom possible because the drug must be in contact with the oral mucosa at least 5 minutes, a length of time most patients find intolerable.

Buccal, Gingival

The buccal route of administration involves placement of the drug, usually in tablet form, inside the mouth between the mucosal surface of the cheek and the gum of the upper molars. The gingival route involves placing the tablet form between the upper lip and the gum of the incisors. Of all of the areas in the mouth for oral transmucosal drug administration, the gingival route appears to be the lowest in drug permeability (Stanley, Ashburn, 1992).

Evidence exists that morphine is absorbed by the buccal and gingival routes; however, research findings vary significantly and patients complain of an extremely unpleasant bitter taste. Furthermore, these routes require that the tablet remain in contact with the gum for a long period of time, sometimes up to six hours, which makes this approach uncomfortable and impractical for most patients (Foley, Inturrisi, 1992; Stanley, Ashburn, 1992).

If the buccal or gingival routes must be used, the site should be rinsed with water to remove residues of the drug after absorption. If these routes are used repeatedly, the site should be rotated because irritation of the mucous membrane can occur (Spencer, 1993).

Oral Transmucosal Fentanyl Citrate (OTFC)

Fentanyl has been incorporated within a sweetened matrix and placed on a stick (OTFC). To administer OTFC, patients are instructed to suck on the matrix and, holding onto the stick, move it around the inside of the mouth and gums and above and below the tongue so that it dissolves in the saliva. A portion of the fentanyl diffuses across the oral mucosa (25%) and the rest is swallowed and partially absorbed through the stomach and the intestine (75%) (Berryman, 1997; Streisand, Varvel, Stanski, 1991) (Figure 6.4).

Compared with oral fentanyl administration, OTFC yields higher and more rapidly attained plasma concentrations and greater bioavailability. These characteristics provide evidence that OTFC passes by mucosal transport directly into the systemic circulation without undergoing first pass metabolism in the liver. In addition, a fentanyl depot in the oral mucosa does not appear to exist because elimination of OTFC is similar to single doses of IV fentanyl (Streisand, Varvel, Stanski, 1991). The clinical implications of this are that the onset of analgesia will be more consistent and rapid than by the oral route of administration and side effects will dissipate quickly when administration is discontinued.

Because OTFC has a rapid onset (5 minutes) and peak effect (within 15 minutes) and a short duration of action (2.5 to 5 hours) with single dosing (Berryman, 1997), it is ideal for providing conscious sedation and as a premedication for surgery and procedures. OTFC (Oralet) is approved by the FDA for these purposes in adults and children weighing more than 15 kg (33 lb). It has the benefits of providing analgesia, sedation, and anxiolysis rapidly, noninvasively, and painlessly (Streisand, Varvel, Stanski, 1991), so it is especially appealing for use with children. Because these patients usually are opioid naive, the manufacturer recommends that OTFC be administered only by trained personnel in an anesthesia-monitored setting (Abbott Laboratories, 1995). It is also used on opioid-naive patients in areas such as the emergency department (Stanley, Ashburn, 1992).

OTFC for Breakthrough Pain

Initial use of OTFC was in opioid-naive individuals, and a relatively high incidence of side effects, such as nausea (17%), vomiting (34%), and hypoventilation (11%) but no deaths, occurred (Abbott Laboratories, 1995; Berryman, 1997). Unfortunately, the incidence of side effects, especially respiratory depression, caused some clinicians to hesitate to use OTFC. However, an analgesic that is rapidly absorbed, easily administered, and potent, such as OTFC, may be ideal for the management of breakthrough cancer and chronic nonmalignant pain in patients who are opioid-tolerant. The developers of OTFC have conducted new clinical trials for this purpose and, pending FDA approval, plan to

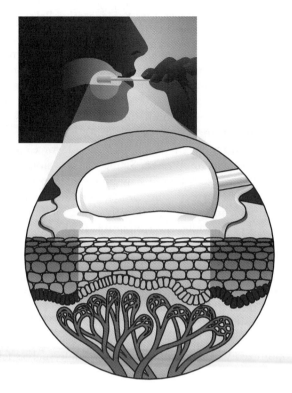

May be duplicated for use in clinical practice. As appears in McCaffery M, Pasero C: *Pain: Clinical manual,* p. 202, 1999, Mosby, Inc.

● ● ● ● ●
FIGURE 6.4.   Oral transmucosal fentanyl citrate (OTFC). Oral transmucosal fentanyl citrate is incorporated within a sweetened matrix and placed on a stick. Patients are instructed to suck on the matrix and, holding onto the stick, move it around the inside of the mouth and gums and above and below the tongue so that it dissolves in the saliva. Approximately 25% of the fentanyl diffuses across the oral mucosa, and the rest is swallowed and partially absorbed through the stomach and the intestine.

Courtesy Anesta Corporation, Salt Lake City, UT, 1998.

make a new OTFC product (Actiq) available early in 1999 (Berryman, 1997).

Breakthrough pain, reported by two thirds of individuals with continuous chronic pain, is transient moderate to severe pain that increases above the pain addressed by the ongoing analgesics. Relatively brief breakthrough pain precipitated by a voluntary action, such as movement (incident pain), would be most amenable to treatment with OTFC (Portenoy, 1996b).

Ashburn, Fine, and Stanley (1989) first reported effectiveness in the use of OTFC to manage breakthrough pain in a patient with metastatic carcinoma of the lung. They cited fentanyl's short duration, considered a drawback in the management of continuous pain, as an advantage in treating breakthrough pain because it allowed their patients to avoid excessive sedation and other side effects associated with the longer acting oral opioids typically used for breakthrough cancer pain.

Researchers who have conducted clinical trials of OTFC for the management of breakthrough cancer pain found that it provided very good to excellent analgesia with minimal side effects with patient-titrated dose ranges of 200 to 1600 μg (American Society of Clinical Oncology, 1997; Fine, Marcus, De Boer, 1991) (see Box 6.23, p. 245). In many cases patients reported improved analgesia compared with the relief obtained from their previous regimen for managing breakthrough pain. In addition, patients found OTFC easy to titrate. A trend toward decreased effectiveness over time was not found, suggesting that significant tolerance to the beneficial effects does not develop with long-term exposure to OTFC. Somnolence, dizziness, and nausea were cited as the most common side effects, and these were found to be dose-dependent (American Society of Clinical Oncology, 1997). Mild itching was another common side effect of OTFC. The fact that side effects were minimal may be due to the tolerance to opioids common in this patient population (Streisand, 1994). Chest muscle rigidity and apnea, which are life-threatening adverse effects of IV fentanyl, are not reported when OTFC is used according to directions (Streisand, Varvel, Stanski, 1991).

As mentioned above, OTFC is contained in a sweetened matrix form. The use of a sugar base preparation on a stick, similar to a lollipop, to administer an opioid has created some controversy (Coyle, Cherny, Portenoy, 1995; Yaster, 1995). Some clinicians believe that linking candy and opioids might encourage drug abuse, especially when used with children. As has been explained previously in this chapter and throughout this manual, the potential for addiction as a result of taking opioids for pain relief is extremely low. Yaster (1995) appropriately points out that drugs have long been sweetened to make them more palatable to both children and adults and that it is ludicrous to think that experiencing humane pain treatment as a child will lead to drug abuse later in life.

Intranasal

The intranasal route has been used for centuries to administer a number of different drugs. Like the oral transmucosal route, the intranasal route with a rich blood supply has easy access to systemic circulation and bypasses significant hepatic metabolism (Stanley, Ashburn, 1992).

The mixed agonist-antagonist opioid butorphanol has been used intranasally. A small aerosol device calibrated to deliver a set dose of drug is placed in the nostril for drug delivery. Intranasal butorphanol is easy for patients to use, has a consistent absorption pattern, and has been shown to provide adequate analgesia for some types of postoperative pain. However, because it is an agonist-antagonist and patients with cancer pain usually are receiving mu agonists for pain, it is unlikely to be used substantially for treatment of pain in this population (Coyle, Cherny, Portenoy, 1995; Foley, Inturrisi, 1992) (see p. 188).

Intranasal sufentanil has been found to be not only analgesic and sedative with minimal side effects when used as a preanesthetic agent but it also allows for easier separation of children from their parents before surgery. When administered to children (1.5 to 4.0 μg/kg), intranasal sufentanil produced sedation within 10 minutes. However, doses higher than 3.0 μg/kg were found to produce decreases in chest wall compliance and a significant incidence of postoperative vomiting (Henderson, Brodsky, Fisher et al., 1988). Single doses of intranasal sufentanil (15 μg) have been effective in producing sedation in adults (Helmers, Noorduin, Van Peer et al., 1989).

Sufentanil can be instilled intranasally in droplet form, using parenteral formulation, or with a swab. A major drawback, especially in children, is that nasal instillation can cause burning and stinging (Biddle, Gilliland, 1992; Stanley, Ashburn, 1992). Also, some children object to any form of nose drops probably because it is similar to a sensation of drowning.

Nebulized

Up to 70% of terminally ill patients experience dyspnea, a particularly distressing symptom. Morphine is the drug of choice, usually given orally or sublingually, for relief of dyspnea. For the opioid-naive patient, 5 mg SC or 15 mg PO or sublingually is recommended; for opioid-tolerant patients, their usual dose must be increased by 100% to 150% (Bruera, MacMillan, Pither et al., 1990).

Morphine also can be nebulized for the treatment of dyspnea. Nebulized morphine has been reported to be safe and effective in treating dyspnea associated with end-stage chronic obstructive pulmonary disease (COPD), congestive heart failure, and lung cancer (Fancombe, Chater, 1993; Fancombe, Chater, 1994).

As yet no controlled trials have been done on patients with cancer-related dyspnea, and the mode of action, if indeed nebulized morphine is effective, is unknown. It is thought to work either centrally on respiration and perception, or locally in opioid receptors in the lungs. It provides the additional benefits of reducing and loosening mucous secretions (Howe, 1995).

Several opioids besides morphine (e.g., fentanyl, hydromorphone, codeine) have been nebulized, but controlled studies are lacking. Use of morphine is the most widely reported. To administer, preservative-free parenteral morphine is diluted to 2 ml to 5 ml with sterile water or normal saline and nebulized by face mask over a 15-minute period. Morphine doses range from 5 mg to 25 mg every 4 hours. Nebulized morphine has a variable bioavailability of 9% to 35%. Maximum serum concentrations are reached within 10 to 45 minutes (Chrubasik, Wust, Friedrich et al., 1988; Davis, Lam, Butcher et al., 1992; Fancombe, Chater, 1994). Nebulization is not recommended as a route for analgesia, primarily because current administration techniques result in very small amounts of analgesic being absorbed.

Rectal

The rectal route offers an excellent, but frequently overlooked, alternative to the oral route. Hospice nurses caring for the terminally ill often use the rectal route to administer medications. It is inexpensive and does not involve technical equipment or expertise to the extent that is required for parenteral administration. When patients are unable to take oral medications, the parenteral routes may be avoided by administering analgesics rectally.

The rectal route is most commonly used when patients have persistent or temporary nausea and vomiting, GI tract obstruction, or mental status changes (Allen, 1997; Warren, 1996). It is particularly useful when other routes are unavailable and a delay is expected before the patient can be assessed for alternative treatment (Warren, 1996). The rectal route may be contraindicated in patients who are neutropenic or thrombopenic (platelet count of 50 or less) because of potential rectal bleeding from insertion of the suppository (Coyle, Cherny, Portenoy, 1995; Coyle, Portenoy, 1996).

Theoretically, all opioid analgesics may be administered rectally. Those commercially available as rectal suppositories in the United States are morphine, methadone, hydromorphone, and oxymorphone. Other opioids, including oxycodone, codeine, meperidine, and buprenorphine, also can be absorbed rectally (McCaffery, Martin, Ferrell, 1992; Watanabe, Kondo, Asakura et al., 1994).

All opioids may be compounded for rectal administration. This may be done by a pharmacy or in the home by following simple directions (see Box 6.10). Because of the lack of commercially available rectal preparations of opioids in various strengths, oral tablets, oral solutions and suspensions, and injectable products have been administered, sometimes without further alteration of the medication (Allen, 1997; Benet, Kroetz, Sheiner, 1996; Coyle, Cherny, Portenoy, 1995; Warren, 1996).

Rectal Anatomy and Drug Absorption

Understanding the anatomy of the rectum is important for effective use of the rectal route. The rectum makes up the last 15 to 19 cm of the large intestine. Minimal migration of rectal preparations occur through the length of the rectum. Thus, the total surface area for drug absorption consists of a region approximately 6 to 8 cm long with no digestive enzymes. Three veins are responsible for blood return in the rectum. The middle and inferior rectal veins drain the remainder of the rectum into the inferior vena cava, bypassing the liver. The superior rectal vein drains the upper rectum into the portal vein, which transports the drug to the liver for metabolism (first pass effect) (Warren, 1996). Approximately 50% of the drug absorbed from the rectum bypasses the liver (Benet, Kroetz, Sheiner, 1996; Warren, 1996).

The clinical implication of the rectal anatomy is that extensive hepatic metabolism can be avoided by administering the drug into the lower part of the rectum. Insertion of the drug into the upper portion of the rectum (15 to 20 cm high) would negate one of the primary advantages of rectal administration (reduced first pass effect) (Warren, 1996).

In addition to placement of the suppository, a number of other factors influence rectal absorption of drugs, including the condition of the rectal mucosa, blood flow to the rectal area, use of lubricants, and presence of feces (Coyle, Cherny, Portenoy, 1995; Warren, 1996). Dehydration can slow dissolution of the drug form, and constipation may prevent contact of the drug with the rectal mucosa. Drugs administered in an aqueous solution are absorbed faster than those in an oil-based solution (McCaffery, Martin, Ferrell, 1992; Warren, 1996). Suspensions and suppositories absorb slowly and continuously. When administering a solution or suspension, the likelihood of spontaneous expulsion by the patient before the drug is absorbed can be prevented by administering volumes no greater than 60 ml (Warren, 1996).

Rectal administration can cause irritation of the rectal mucosa, especially with repetitive administration, although lubricants are helpful in preventing this (Allen, 1997; Benet, Kroetz, Sheiner, 1996). It is best to use water-soluble lubricants or plain tap water to facilitate insertion of suppositories (McCaffery, Martin, Ferrell, 1992; Warren, 1996). See Box 6.10 for guidelines on maximizing the rate and amount of drug absorption by the rectal route of administration.

Rectal Dosing

The effective dose of opioids by the rectal route is approximately equal to oral dosing (Coyle, Cherny, Portenoy, 1995; McCaffery, Martin, Ferrell, 1992), but there is reason to consider reducing the starting dose by approximately 25%. In one study, 39 patients who were receiving MS Contin orally were switched to the same dose by the rectal route (Maloney, Kesner, Klein, 1989). All but one patient achieved adequate analgesia, but 28% required a decrease in the rectal dose because of excessive drowsiness.

A major disadvantage of the rectal route is that many individuals find it objectionable and are reluctant to use it. This can be especially problematic when family members must administer rectal medications and when medications must be administered several times a day. Controlled-release formulations of rectal opioids are currently in development, which should improve acceptance of this route of administration (Coyle, Cherny, Portenoy, 1995).

Studies support the efficacy of rectal administration of oral controlled-release opioids. By the rectal route, these formulations demonstrate good absorption and slow steady release compared with the rapid absorption and high peak effect of immediate-release preparations. Compared with controlled-release opioids given orally, studies show either equal or greater systemic absorption, lower

G U I D E L I N E S

RECTAL ADMINISTRATION OF OPIOID ANALGESICS

1. Position the patient on the left side with the upper leg flexed or in knee-chest position.
2. Lubricate the dosage form with a water-soluble lubricant or a small amount of water. If rectum is dry, instill 5 to 10 ml warm water with a syringe attached to a catheter before inserting tablets or capsules.
3. Do not crush controlled-release preparations.
4. Gently insert the dosage form approximately a finger's length into the rectum at an angle toward the umbilicus so that the medication is placed against the rectal wall. If a suppository is used, the blunted end should be introduced first.
5. Keep liquid volumes of drug preparations at less than 60 ml to prevent spontaneous expulsion. Amounts of 25 ml are usually retained without difficulty. These may be injected into the rectal cavity with a lubricated rubber-tipped syringe or large-bore Foley catheter and balloon. Inflating the balloon may assist in retention.
6. Minimize the number of insertions. When administering multiple tablets for a single dose, enclose them in a single gelatin capsule.
7. Do not split or halve a suppository as this can cause errors in dosing. If it must be halved, cut it lengthwise.
8. After the finger is withdrawn, hold the buttocks together until the urge to expel has ceased.
9. Although rectal irritation is a concern, it need not be a limiting factor when administering commercially prepared suppositories, tablets, or capsules. Irritation may be avoided or treated with lubrication, gentle insertion, and appropriate topical medications, such as cortisone ointment.

10. Prevent chronic rectal irritation. Avoid repeated rectal instillation of solutions of drugs with alcoholic vehicles or drugs that use glycols as solubilizing agents (parenteral forms of lorazepam, diazepam, chlordiazepoxide, and phenytoin).
11. Avoid rectal administration of enteric-coated tablets. The pH of the colon is alkaline and these preparations require an acidic environment to be dissolved and the active drug to be released. The active drug would likely be expelled with the coating intact.

Pediatric Considerations

1. In syringe, combine drug and smallest amount of diluent possible for adequate mixture and for administration using a syringe and catheter.
2. Cut the distal 5 to 10 cm of a 14 F catheter.
3. Attach the syringe of medication solution to the distal end of the catheter.
4. Carefully flush air from catheter without losing medication solution.
5. Lubricate the tip of the catheter.
6. Gently insert catheter tip well into the rectum:
   • Infant: 1 inch (2.5 cm)
   • 2 to 4 years old: 2 inches (5 cm)
   • 4 to 10 years old: 3 inches (7.5 cm)
   • 11 years old: 4 inches (10 cm)
7. Smoothly inject medication solution.
8. Hold buttocks together for 5 to 10 minutes to prevent expulsion.

May be duplicated for use in clinical practice. From McCaffery M, Pasero C: *Pain: Clinical manual,* p. 205. Copyright © 1999, Mosby, Inc.

Box 6.10 presents guidelines for maximizing absorption when administering analgesics by the rectal route. Pediatric considerations are included.

cm, centimeter; *F,* French; *ml,* milliliter.

Information from Abd-El-Maeboud K et al.: Rectal suppository: Common-sense and mode of insertion, *Lancet* 338(8770):798-800, 1991; McCaffery M, Martin L, Ferrell BR: Analgesic administration via rectum or stoma, *J Enterostomal Therapy Nurs* 19(4):114-121, 1992; Warren DE: Practical use of rectal medications in palliative care, *J Pain Symptom Manage* 11(6):378-387, 1996; Wong, D: *Wong and Whaley's clinical manual of pediatric nursing,* ed 4, St. Louis, 1996, Mosby.

peak concentration, and a more prolonged time to peak by the rectal route (Babul, Darke, Anslow et al., 1992; Cronin, Kaiko, Goldenheim, 1991; Kaiko, Fitzmartin, Thomas et al., 1992). Controlled-release oral formulations must not be crushed or dissolved.

Controlled-release morphine tablets (Oramorph SR) were found to be safe and effective when administered every 12 hours by the rectal or vaginal routes to eight patients with cancer pain. No consistent changes were found from the oral route in the frequency of adverse experiences, morphine requirements, or pain intensity ratings. Three of the eight patients reported better pain relief and five reported the same relief as achieved with the oral route (Grauer, Bass, Wenzel et al., 1992).

Just as with the oral route, underdosing can occur with the rectal route. The most common reason for failure to achieve adequate analgesia is insufficient dose administration. It is best to control severe escalating pain rapidly with parenteral opioids, then switch to rectal administration with scheduled ATC doses. Even severe pain that is stable can be managed by the rectal route if the principles of good pain management are followed (McCaffery, Martin, Ferrell, 1992).

Stomal

Treatment of a variety of cancers may include creation of an ostomy. Sigmoid colostomies (left-sided), which produce formed stool, are more likely than other ostomies to be an effective alternative route for administering opioids. Ostomies that are constructed of jejunum, ileum, ascending, transverse, and high descending colon (produce wet, liquid, or semisolid effluent) generally have rapid transit times. The constant pressure of the watery effluent from these ostomies will push out the drug form before it can be dissolved and absorbed (McCaffery, Martin, Ferrell, 1992).

Colostomies usually are created in areas of the colon that are drained by vessels that go directly to the portal vein, subjecting drugs that are present to hepatic metabolism. Thus ostomy administration cannot be equated to rectal administration because it does not avoid first pass effect (Benet, Kroetz, Sheiner, 1996; Warren, 1996). However, the starting dose usually is the same as that for oral or rectal administration. Very limited information is available about the efficacy of stomal administration of opioids. However, this route may be an effective alternative for some patients, at least temporarily. Box 6.11 presents guidelines for the administration of medications through a stoma.

Vaginal

Although opioid preparations for vaginal administration are not commercially available, opioids are absorbed by this route. Anecdotally, many patients have reported using the vaginal route for opioid administration. As mentioned in the discussion on rectal administra-tion, controlled-release morphine (Oramorph SR) was found to be safe and effective when administered every 12 hours by the vaginal route to patients with cancer pain. Patients in this study reported no consistent changes from the oral route in the frequency of adverse experiences, morphine requirements, or pain intensity ratings (Grauer, Bass, Wenzel et al., 1992). As with any route or drug that has not been fully researched, other routes known to be safe and effective are preferred and recommended.

Transdermal

Fentanyl (Duragesic) is the first opioid available by the transdermal route. The high lipophilicity of fentanyl makes it ideal for absorption into the skin. The skin under the drug reservoir (Figure 6.5) absorbs fentanyl, and depots of the drug concentrate in the upper skin layers, fat, and skeletal muscles. From these depots, fentanyl is gradually released into systemic circulation (Figure 6.6). Once in place, the transdermal system is capable of providing continuous release of fentanyl at a nearly constant rate for 72 hours (Janssen, 1996).

The fentanyl transdermal system is incorporated within an adhesive patch that is available in 25, 50, 75, and 100 μg/h doses. In opioid-naive patients the initial dose of transdermal fentanyl should not exceed 25 μg/h; initial doses of 50, 75, and 100 μg/h should only be used in opioid-tolerant individuals after calculating the appropriate dose on the basis of previous opioid exposure (see Box 6.12, p. 208). Multiple patches may be applied to

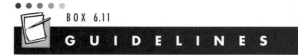

BOX 6.11

GUIDELINES

ADMINISTERING MEDICATIONS THROUGH A STOMA

1. Consider appropriateness of stoma (i.e., does it produce a formed stool?).
2. Ensure adequate hydration of the stomal mucosa. If it is dry, instill 10 ml warm water with a syringe attached to a catheter.
3. Determine bowel direction and insert the drug form a finger's depth into the stoma.
4. Insert a foam colostomy plug (Conseal Colostomy Plug, Coloplast, Tampa, FL). The plug may be left in place until bowel function occurs or until it is time for the next dose.
5. Ask the patient to recline for 15 to 30 minutes to prevent expulsion or loss as a result of gravity.

May be duplicated for use in clinical practice. From McCaffery M, Pasero C: *Pain: Clinical manual,* p. 206. Copyright © 1999, Mosby, Inc.

Information about the efficacy of stomal administration of opioids is limited. However, this route may be an effective alternative for some patients, at least temporarily. Box 6.11 provides guidelines for the administration of medications through a stoma.

ml, milliliter.

Information from McCaffery M, Martin L, Ferrell BR: Analgesic administration via rectum or stoma, *J Enterostomal Therapy Nurs* 19(4):114-121, 1992.

achieve a desired dose. The number of patches is generally limited, not so much by a maximum dose as by the available skin area because sites must be rotated every 2 to 3 days when the patch is changed. As mentioned above, the life of the transdermal fentanyl patch is approximately 72 hours, although some patients may require a new patch every 48 hours (Coyle, Portenoy, 1996).

Indications

Transdermal fentanyl is recommended for use in the management of moderate to severe cancer and some chronic nonmalignant pain with a stable pain pattern that requires continuous opioid treatment and cannot be managed by the oral route of administration (Coyle, Portenoy, 1996; Payne, Chandler, Einhaus, 1995). The convenience of the transdermal route of administration may help patients adhere to the treatment plan more easily than the oral route, which entails remembering to take medication at least once a day, if not more often (Coyle, Portenoy, 1996). It may also be a suitable alternative for patients who are allergic to morphine or hydromorphone because fentanyl is in a different chemical category (Jaffe, Martin, 1990).

Although transdermal fentanyl is recommended for stable chronic pain only (Coyle, Portenoy, 1996; Lipman, Ashburn, 1994; Payne, Chandler, Einhaus, 1995), it has been studied for use in titrating patients with uncon-

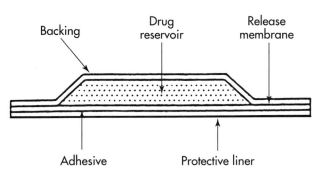

(Not to Scale)

● ● ● ● ●

F I G U R E 6.5. Transdermal fentanyl drug delivery system. Figure 6.5 illustrates the transdermal fentanyl drug delivery system. The skin under the drug reservoir absorbs fentanyl, and depots of the drug concentrate in the upper skin layers, fat, and skeletal muscles. From these depots, fentanyl is gradually released into systemic circulation. Once in place, the transdermal system is capable of providing continuous release of fentanyl at a nearly constant rate for 72 hours.

From Duragesic (fentanyl transdermal system) CII Package Insert (revised June 1994). Janssen Pharmaceutical, Titusville, NJ 08560.

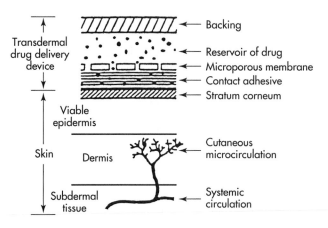

● ● ● ● ●

F I G U R E 6.6. Pathway of absorption from transdermal fentanyl. Figure 6.6 illustrates the pathway of absorption from transdermal fentanyl. The skin under the drug reservoir absorbs fentanyl, and depots of the drugs concentrate in the upper skin layers, fat, and skeletal muscles. From these depots, fentanyl is gradually released into systemic circulation.

Modified from Varuel JR, Shafer SL, Hwang SS, Coen PA, Stanski DR: Absorption characteristics of transdermally administered fentanyl, *Anesthesiology,* 1989 in Duragesic (fentanyl transdermal system) CII Package Insert (revised June 1994). Janssen Pharmaceutical, Titusville, NJ 08560.

trolled cancer pain. The initial recommended dose of transdermal fentanyl was increased by 150% and, rather than waiting 3 days after application to titrate as the manufacturer recommends, doses were titrated on a day-to-day basis. This approach was found to be safe and effective with the use of immediate-release oral morphine for breakthrough pain in opioid-tolerant patients. The researchers caution that careful monitoring of patient response is essential when this approach is used (Korte, 1994; Korte, de Stoutz, Morant, 1996).

A high number of patients in open-label studies comparing transdermal fentanyl to oral morphine have stated a preference for transdermal fentanyl and continued to use it after study completion. Several factors may account for this preference, including much longer intervals between doses (every 48 to 72 hours), improved sleep, and less sedation and constipation (Donner, Zenz, Tryba et al., 1996; Hammack, Mailliard, Loprinzi, 1996; Korte, de Stoutz, Morant, 1996).

Evidence exists that the incidence of constipation (Donner, Zenz, Tryba et al., 1996; Korte, de Stoutz, Morant, 1996) and sedation (Ahmedzai, Brooks, 1997) is lower with transdermal fentanyl than with oral morphine. The lower incidence of constipation does not appear to be dose-related because higher fentanyl doses yielded comparable decreases in constipation. No obvious explanation exists for the reduced incidence of sedation, and this observation remains to be confirmed. A lesser constipating effect may be because the transdermal route is not an enteral route and the opioid does not come into direct contact with the bowel. Despite the effect on con-

stipation, a bowel management regimen usually is recommended during long-term therapy (see p. 261).

Compared with other racial groups, Oriental patients may react differently to transdermal fentanyl. One group of researchers reported acute severe dizziness and nausea within the first hours of transdermal fentanyl application in their Oriental patient sample. The researchers suggested that this may be unique to Oriental patients because they generally have less subcutaneous fat than Caucasians (Yeo, Lam, Chan et al., 1997).

A common misconception is that patients who have minimal body fat, such as cachetic patients, will not be able to absorb fentanyl by the transdermal route. However, no studies demonstrate that the pharmacokinetics of transdermal fentanyl change depending on the amount of a patient's body fat.

Transdermal fentanyl can cause any opioid-related side effects, including respiratory depression (Grond, Zech, Lehmann et al., 1997). Mild erythema, itching, and rash at the site of application are fairly common and resolve at the next scheduled patch change (Ahmedzai, Brooks, 1997; Donner, Zenz, Tryba et al., 1996; Korte, de Stoutz, Morant, 1996).

Transdermal Patch Application

To correctly apply the fentanyl patch it must be placed on nonirritated and nonirradiated skin, usually on the flat surface of the chest, back, flank, or upper arm. Before application, the site is prepared by clipping (not shaving) the hair, cleaning with water, and drying. Soap, oil, lotion, and alcohol should be avoided. Patches should not be cut or altered in any way and should be applied as soon as they are removed from their packaging. The patch is pressed firmly in place with the palm of the hand for 30 seconds (Janssen, 1996). At 72 hours when it is time to replace the fentanyl patch, the application site should be rotated to prevent chronic local irritation (Calis, Kohler, Corso, 1992). Because some residual drug may be left on used patches, it is recommended that they be disposed of by flushing down the toilet immediately after removal (Janssen, 1996).

The transdermal fentanyl patch is a sealed system that poses little risk of the caregiver coming into contact with the drug when applying it to the patient. However, if the gel from the reservoir accidentally contacts the caregiver's skin, the area should be washed with copious amounts of water. Again, soap, alcohol, and other solvents are not used because these may enhance the drug's ability to penetrate the skin (Janssen, 1996).

Disadvantages of Transdermal Fentanyl

A major drawback to the use of transdermal fentanyl is that it takes 12 to 16 hours (4 to 5 hours for newer formulations not yet on the market) for substantial analgesic effect to be experienced by the patient once dosing begins, and titration to an effective dose may require days, necessitating the addition of an opioid by an alternate route during this period. Occasionally, patients are in a setting that allows for titration with parenteral fentanyl while converting to the transdermal fentanyl system (Coyle, Cherny, Portenoy, 1995; Lehmann, DeSio, Radvany et al., 1997; Zech, Grond, Lynch et al., 1992). More often, immediate-release preparations of oral opioids, such as morphine, are administered PRN during the transition (Dahl, 1996).

Another disadvantage of the transdermal system is that it does not allow for easy dose adjustment in the management of side effects. If the patch is removed because of adverse effects, a depot of fentanyl remains and serum concentrations decline very slowly, falling about 50% in approximately 17 hours. If naloxone is indicated, it may be necessary to administer it by slow infusion over a period of hours (Coyle, Cherny, Portenoy, 1995; Coyle, Portenoy, 1996; Janssen, 1996).

Transdermal fentanyl absorption also may be increased by either external or internal sources of heat. Care must be taken when using the transdermal route in febrile patients. Drug absorption by the transdermal route is influenced by elevated temperature; a temperature of 104° F can cause serum fentanyl concentration to increase by one-third, necessitating monitoring for side effects and adjustment of dose (Janssen, 1996). Patients should also be cautioned against taking excessively hot showers (Korte, de Stoutz, Morant, 1996). Sleeping in a heated waterbed or putting a heating pad over the patch will also increase the amount of fentanyl being absorbed.

Switching Between Transdermal Fentanyl and Another Opioid

For patients who are already taking opioids and will be switching to transdermal fentanyl, it is necessary to convert the current opioid dose to a dose of transdermal fentanyl estimated to be equivalent. Dose conversion is done to prevent withdrawal symptoms during transition, maintain adequate analgesia, and allow for dose adjustment. However, with fentanyl no universally accepted guidelines exist for equianalgesic dosing.

As with all opioids, significant interindividual variability exists in fentanyl metabolism and doses must be titrated according to patient response (Ahmedzai, Brooks, 1997; Coyle, Cherny, Portenoy, 1995). The manufacturer of transdermal fentanyl cautions that 50% of patients converted to transdermal fentanyl using their conversion chart will require an increased dose after initial application of the patch (Janssen, 1996). See p. 174 for more on conversion charts and Box 6.12 for the formula most clinicians use to switch from oral morphine to transdermal fentanyl.

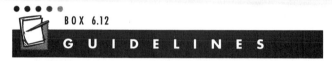

BOX 6.12

G U I D E L I N E S

SWITCHING FROM ORAL MORPHINE TO TRANSDERMAL FENTANYL

To convert controlled-release morphine dose to starting transdermal fentanyl dose using morphine 2 mg/24 h PO approximately equal to fentanyl 1 μg/h transdermally:[1]
1. Calculate the 24 h morphine dose (e.g., if the patient is receiving 200 mg of morphine by oral controlled-release formulation q12h, the total 24 h dose is 200 mg × 2 = 400 mg).
2. To determine the initial dose of fentanyl, divide the 24 h morphine dose by 2 (e.g., 400 mg of morphine ÷ 2 = 200 μg/h of transdermal fentanyl).
3. Apply the first patch at the time the patient takes the last dose of slow-release morphine.

Rescue doses should be provided along with ATC doses, especially when a long-acting formulation is used. See Box 6.23, p. 245.

May be duplicated for use in clinical practice. From McCaffery M, Pasero C: *Pain: Clinical manual,* p. 208. Copyright © 1999, Mosby, Inc.

[1] When studies that clarify equianalgesic dosing are lacking, such as is the case with fentanyl, various conversion formulas evolve. These formulas, and even the ones used in this text, are not necessarily comparable; different formulas lead to different answers. This conversion formula may be used to convert the patient from oral morphine to transdermal fentanyl and vice versa. The current recommendation by the manufacturer may be used only to convert from oral morphine to transdermal fentanyl, not vice versa, and the clinician should expect that approximately 50% of the patients will require additional analgesia.

h, hour; *μg,* microgram; *mg,* milligram.

Information from Dahl J: Fentanyl postscript, *Cancer Pain Update* (41):6, Fall 1996; Donner B, Zenz M, Tryba M et al.: Direct conversion from oral morphine to transdermal fentanyl: A multicenter study in patients with cancer pain, *Pain* 64:527-534, 1996; McCaffery M: How to calculate a rescue dose, *Am J Nurs* 96(4):65-66, 1996.

After patients are stabilized on the transdermal patch, later reports of inadequate pain control and an increase in the dose requirement of immediate-release opioid used for breakthrough pain may be an indication that it is necessary to increase the dose of transdermal fentanyl. See Table 6.7 for the amounts of various immediate-release opioids and the doses at which an increase in the transdermal fentanyl dose is recommended.

Clearly, more research is needed to determine more accurate initial doses of transdermal fentanyl when converting from various opioids administered by other routes. Admission to a care setting where parenteral titration can be provided is costly and not feasible for most patients with cancer who prefer to stay home, remaining as independent as possible. A multicenter study of nearly 100 patients with "stable and low-level" cancer pain was conducted to examine the feasibility of a conversion chart with much higher initial dose estimates than current charts recommend. Findings revealed that initial conversion from oral morphine to transdermal fentanyl with a ratio of 100:1 is safe and effective. For example, according to this study's conversion, a patient taking approximately 120 mg of oral morphine per day would require 1.2 mg/ day of fentanyl and a 50 μg/h fentanyl patch would be appropriate for such a patient (Donner, Zenz, Tryba et al., 1996).

Not for Acute Pain Management

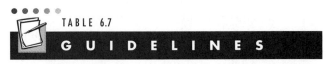

Transdermal fentanyl is not recommended for use in managing acute or postoperative pain, including in the outpatient setting. It also is not recommended for use in opioid-naive children less than 12 years of age or patients less than 18 years of age who weigh less than 50 kg (110 lb). Deaths have occurred as a result of transdermal fentanyl being used to manage acute pain in children in the outpatient setting (Lehmann, DeSio, Radvany et al., 1997). It also is not indicated for mild or intermittent pain that is responsive to "as needed" opioids or non-opioids (Janssen, 1996).

Some studies have been done on the use of transdermal fentanyl for postoperative pain (Caplan, Ready, Oden et al., 1989; Gourlay, Kowalski, Plummer et al., 1989, 1990; Miguel, Kreitzer, Reinhart et al., 1992). The incidence of side effects when used for postoperative pain management is quite high. For example, respiratory depression occurred in 14% of the patients in two studies (Caplan, Ready, Oden et al., 1989; Plezia, Linford, Kramer et al., 1988) and in 23% in another study (Gourlay, Kowalski, Plummer et al., 1989).

A recent study examined a transdermal fentanyl patch with an analgesic onset of 4 to 5 hours (not available in the United States) or placebo patch applied to patients 60 minutes before induction for abdominal surgery (Lehmann, DeSio, Radvany et al., 1997). All patients received IM ketorolac 30 minutes before the end of surgery. As would be expected, significantly better pain relief occurred in the fentanyl group than the placebo group. However, the value of pain relief in this study is questionable because it is recommended that pain be assessed with activity in postoperative patients (Kehlet, 1997a,b), and this study defined pain relief as a VAS of <5 (on 0 to 10 VAS) at rest. Most patients in both groups required PRN analgesia, with more administered to the placebo group. A very high percentage (71%) of patients in the fentanyl group experienced nausea. This study reinforces that the limitations imposed by the transdermal route of administration and current available preparations (difficult titration, slow onset of analgesia) make transdermal fentanyl inappropriate for postoperative pain management.

Parenteral

The parenteral route includes the IM, SC, and IV routes of administration.

Intramuscular (IM)

Although commonly used, the IM route of administration is not recommended for pain management. The IM route has numerous disadvantages and essentially no advantages. Disadvantages include painful administration, unreliable absorption with a 30 to 60 minute lag time to peak effect, and a rapid drop in action compared with oral administration. Chronic IM administration can result in sterile abscess and fibrosis of muscle and soft tissue. The IM route is a particularly poor choice for the elderly, who have decreased muscle mass, and children, who will endure severe pain rather than accept an IM injection (AHCPR, 1992; APS, 1992).

TABLE 6.7

GUIDELINES

DETERMINING THE NEED FOR A 25 μg/h INCREASE IN THE DOSE OF TRANSDERMAL FENTANYL

Opioid (PO formulation)	Amount
Morphine	90 mg/24 h
Oxycodone	45 mg/24 h
Hydromorphone	12 mg/24 h
Codeine	300 mg/24 h

May be duplicated for use in clinical practice. As appears in McCaffery M, Pasero C: *Pain: Clinical manual,* p. 209, 1999, Mosby, Inc.

After patients are stabilized on transdermal fentanyl, later reports of inadequate pain control and an increase in the dose requirement of immediate-release opioid used for breakthrough pain may be an indication that it is necessary to increase the dose of transdermal fentanyl. Table 6.7 shows the amounts of various immediate-release opioids and the doses at which an increase in the transdermal fentanyl dose is recommended.

h, hour; PO, oral.

Modified from Duragesic (fentanyl transdermal system) CII Package Insert (revised June 1994). Janssen Pharmaceutical, Titusville, NJ 08560.

The effects of IM meperidine vary considerably in different individuals and within the same individual. IM administration of meperidine has been shown to produce as much as a fivefold difference between individuals in the time to reach peak concentration. Any one patient given meperidine at different times of the day demonstrated a twofold difference in time to peak concentration. Pain control was poor during the first 4-hour dosing interval, and satisfactory pain control did not occur until the third or fourth dose. Pain control after an injection usually was not achieved until 45 minutes had passed, lasted only 75 to 90 minutes, and increased steadily to severe levels by the fourth hour after injection (Austin, Stapleton, Mather, 1980). Presumably, these results apply to any opioid given by the IM route.

In addition to being ineffective, the IM route of administration is dangerous, especially for opioid-naive patients. Unreliable absorption makes it difficult to predict peak times of the opioid administered. As noted previously, IM meperidine doses do not result in satisfactory pain control until the third or fourth dose. This may reflect the fact that absorption was very slow and that the first dose was still being absorbed 8 to 12 hours later. Poor pain relief because of slow absorption is likely to result in additional doses being administered, leading to more opioid accumulation in the tissues. If circulation improves, the speed of absorption increases. Should side effects, such as respiratory depression occur, the severity may be worsened and duration quite prolonged.

The unpredictability of the IM route warrants much closer monitoring of patients receiving opioids by this route than is customarily practiced. Careful nurse monitoring of respiratory status and sedation is critical to help ensure that clinically significant respiratory depression does not go undetected (see pp. 267–270 for more on sedation and respiratory depression). Many institutions have established monitoring protocols for patients receiving IM opioids that are similar to those developed for IV PCA and epidural analgesia. For example, for postoperative patients, respiratory status and sedation level are assessed every 1 to 2 hours during the first 24 hours after surgery (Pasero, McCaffery, 1994).

If the IM route must be used, the site of the IM injection can influence the onset of analgesia and the analgesic plasma level. Injection into the deltoid muscle, which is well-perfused, will provide a faster and higher plasma level than an injection into a less well-perfused muscle like the gluteal muscle (Benedetti, 1990). Because of the small size of the deltoid muscle and the proximity of major nerves and blood vessels, this site is appropriate only for small volumes of medications (see Chapter 8 for injection sites and how to reduce the discomfort of IM injections).

Subcutaneous (SC)

The SC route of administration for the continuous infusion (CI) of opioids as opposed to intermittent in-

jections is gaining in popularity as an alternative route for patients with chronic cancer pain who are unable to take oral medications and who do not have central venous access. The SC route obviates the need for normal GI function. It is appropriate also for patients who experience dose-limiting side effects with oral opioids or require parenteral opioids because of bowel obstruction but have limited venous access (Benedetti, Butler, 1990).

 The SC route is rarely used for acute pain management because onset is slow; however, indwelling cannulas have been placed subcutaneously in children while under general anesthesia for intermittent morphine bolusing after surgery. This technique caused minimal distress to the children and was preferred over IM injections by 95% of staff (Lamacraft, Cooper, Cavalletto, 1997).

The most common opioid analgesics administered by SCCI are hydromorphone and morphine. Oxymorphone and levorphanol also have been administered subcutaneously. Methadone is not recommended because it can cause irritation by this route (Coyle, 1996; Foley, 1995).

Absorption and distribution vary depending on the placement of the needle and the patient's adipose tissue (Benedetti, Butler, 1990). However, cachexia is not a contraindication to SC analgesia. For conversion from oral morphine to SC morphine, a relative equivalency ratio of 3:1 is used, the same ratio used to calculate doses for the IV route (Coyle, Mauskop, Maggard et al., 1986; Moulin, Johnson, Murray-Parsons, 1992).

Patients show a preference for SC continuous infusion over IV infusion. They cite greater and easier mobility and better pain control among the reasons for this preference (Bruera, Brennels, Michaud et al., 1987).

 Although better absorbed than IM, SCCI administration still has the disadvantages of being painful, time consuming, and often disliked by patients, especially children. The technique of administration is relatively simple to master, but it does require a greater expertise than the oral route. Additional drawbacks are that sterile technique must be used, and the patient and caregivers must become familiar and skilled in the use of needles, syringes, an infusion pump, and other equipment. The SC injection site must be changed at least weekly and as mentioned, the amount that can be infused or bolused must be limited to prevent irritation, pain, necrosis, and sloughing at the site.

High-concentration opioid formulations are used for SCCI infusion because infusion volumes must be limited. Infusion pumps with the capability of delivering in tenths of a milliliter are necessary to accommodate the high-concentration/low-volume infusions. Most patients can absorb 2 or 3 ml/h, and some can absorb as much as 5 ml/h (Coyle, 1996). When necessary, some patients can even tolerate an infusion up to 8 ml/h for a few hours. Rescue doses are provided as SC PCA boluses. In patients requiring high infusion volumes, two sites can be used to deliver the required amount. For example, one site can be used for the infusion and one for rescue boluses. A four-way stopcock can be used to branch an infusion from one infusion pump to two sites (Stevenson, Gordon, 1996) (see Figure 6.7 and Box 6.13 for guidelines on SC administration).

Successful SCCI administration in the home depends on the ability of the family and community health care system to manage the technology in the home. The cost and insurance coverage must be considered (Coyle, Cherny, Portenoy, 1995). Because an infusion device and supplies are necessary, SCCI administration usually is more expensive than oral administration. Programmable portable pumps and disposable pumps are available; disposable infusion devices have been found to be more expensive than the programmable infusion pumps (Moulin, Johnson, Murray-Parsons, 1992).

Important points to address when establishing a plan for parenteral opioid analgesic infusion in the home include determining who will assume primary responsibility for the technologic aspects of the infusion, educating the patient and family regarding the infusion and pain and side effect assessment, and ensuring appropriate monitoring and follow-up (Coyle, Cherny, Portenoy, 1995) (see Box 6.13).

Intravenous (IV)

The IV route is most efficient when an immediate analgesic effect is required, such as for acute, severe escalating pain. It allows for rapid titration. The IV route is most commonly used for short courses of therapy in a hospitalized setting where patients can be closely monitored because many who benefit from IV analgesia are opioid naive, such as surgical patients (Benedetti, Butler, 1990).

Methods of IV administration include bolus, continuous infusion, and PCA. A steady state is better maintained with a continuous infusion compared with the bolus method. When steady state is reached by continuous infusion, the various opioids differ little in terms of duration.

Duration of analgesia by bolus administration is dose dependent; the higher the dose, usually the longer the duration. IV boluses may be used to produce analgesia that lasts approximately as long as IM or SC doses. For example, a single 10 mg IV bolus of morphine may produce analgesia for 3 hours. However, of all routes of administration, IV produces the highest peak concentration of the drug, and the peak concentration is associated with the highest level of toxicity (e.g., sedation, nausea). To decrease the peak effect and lower the level of toxicity, IV boluses may be administered more slowly (e.g., 10 mg of morphine over a 15-minute period) or smaller doses administered more often (e.g., 5 mg of morphine every 60 to 90 minutes).

The IV route may be used temporarily for patients with cancer pain or chronic nonmalignant pain who require rapid titration. It is an alternative for patients with cancer and chronic nonmalignant pain who are unable to

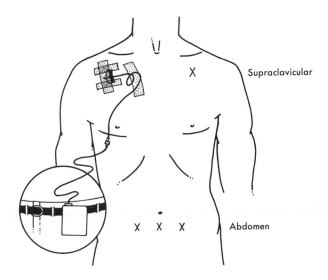

May be duplicated for use in clinical practice. From McCaffery M, Pasero C: *Pain: Clinical manual*, p. 211. Copyright © 1999, Mosby, Inc.

● ● ● ● ● ○
F I G U R E   6.7.   Subcutaneous infusion needle placement. Figure 6.7 shows sites for SC infusion needle placement, which may be attached to an ambulatory infusion pump. X marks sites that interfere with mobility. Other sites to consider include upper arms and thighs. Sites should be rotated.

take oral opioid analgesics. In the terminally ill patient, bowel obstruction and dose-limiting side effects with other systemic opioids are common reasons for long-term IV infusion (Coyle, Cherny, Portenoy, 1995). Central lines are placed whenever possible for long-term IV infusion.

When patients are switched from oral dosing to parenteral administration, they typically report greater effectiveness with the IV route, but this should not be misconstrued. Opioids are not more effective when given by the IV route than by other routes, they are simply more bioavailable (100%) because first pass hepatic metabolism is avoided (Benet, Kroetz, Sheiner, 1996; Levy, 1994). A patient may very well feel less pain and fewer side effects, but this only reflects relatively higher plasma concentrations of the drug. The IV route may avoid certain side effects, such as nausea, caused when the drug was taken orally.

There are drawbacks to the use of the IV route. Use of this route depends on venous availability and ability to maintain patency. Sterile technique is required to prevent systemic infection. The IV route is generally more expensive and requires more expertise to use than the oral route. If continuous IV infusion or IV PCA is used, equipment and tubings are required. Patients accustomed to the independence of oral analgesics may find adjusting to the IV route difficult.

Special Considerations About the Use of the IV Route in Pediatric Patients

It is well documented that children will endure severe pain rather than receive a painful and frightening IM injection. In addition, the disadvantages of the IM route of administration, such as fluctuating analgesic levels and

BOX 6.13

GUIDELINES

SUBCUTANEOUS CONTINUOUS INFUSION (SCCI)

Before Initiating SC Therapy

- Convert current opioid dose to equianalgesic parenteral opioid dose; calculate rescue dose (see pp. 244-246).

Placing SC Needle and Initiating Infusion

⇒ A single SC infusion site can usually accept up to 2 to 3 ml/h.

⇒ Highly concentrated solutions (e.g., hydromorphone 10 mg/ml or morphine 10 mg or more/ml are used for SC infusion). (The pharmacy can prepare a parenteral morphine formulation by dissolving 50 mg in 1 ml of liquid.)

- Sites: Any area with a layer of SC fat is acceptable. Select the site that least interferes with mobility (ask patient about preferred sites and lying positions). Primary sites: left or right subclavicular anterior chest wall; left, right, or center abdomen. Other sites: upper arms, thighs, or buttocks. (Document why alternative sites are used.)

- Skin prep: Shave excessive hair. Scrub with 2% tincture of iodine swabsticks in circular motion from center outward. After 30 seconds, wipe with alcohol swab. If patient is iodine sensitive, scrub area for 1 minute with alcohol and allow to air dry. If iodophor solution is used, apply liberally and allow to air dry.

- Needle insertion: Use a 27-gauge butterfly needle placed at a 45-degree angle or use a Minimed Sof-set. (Be sure to remove introducer needle by grasping tip protruding from top of disk and pulling it straight out. The plastic catheter that surrounded the introducer needle is left in place.)

- Dressing: Keep site as visible as possible; cover with a moisture-responsive transparent adhesive dressing, such as Op-Site. Tape may be used if patient prefers or is allergic to transparent dressing. Make a loose loop of infusion tubing and anchor with tape. Write date and time on small piece of adhesive tape and place on edge of dressing.

- Pump: Infusion pump must be able to deliver in tenths of a milliliter (0.1 ml/h). Pumps used to deliver continuous infusions or PCA are usually acceptable. Ideally, the pump should be portable and lightweight. Portable disposable infusion devices (Travenol, Baxter; Graseby) also are used for SC infusion.

- Documentation: Site, solution, including concentration and additives, biomedical number on pump if nondisposable pump is used (for risk management tracking purposes), initial infusion rate and PCA dose, delay, and hour limit if prescribed. If PCA is not used, document immediate-release opioid prescription for management of breakthrough pain.

Maintaining SC Infusion

- Site should be checked at least twice daily (q4h if the infusion rate is >1.5 ml/h). Family can be instructed to check the site in the morning before the patient dresses and in the evening after undressing.

- Site inflammation, erythema, leakage, bruising, swelling, and burning indicate the need for a site change.
- Infusion site should be changed q7d or sooner if inflammation, leakage, or swelling occurs.
- Change tubings and drug reservoirs according to institutional policy and procedure.

Troubleshooting

- Because the SC route has a slow onset, it is not acceptable for uncontrolled, severe escalating pain. The IV route must be used to control pain if necessary before SC infusion is initiated. Before discontinuing IV access, give an IV bolus dose equal to the hourly opioid dose the patient has been receiving to allow time for opioid absorption by the SC route and to prevent loss of pain control during the transition.
- If breakthrough pain occurs despite dose adjustments, poor absorption at the site may be the problem. Changing the infusion site may reestablish analgesia without increasing the dosage.
- If possible, increase the concentration of the infusion solution when the required dosage nears 2 ml/h.
- If the infusion is >2 ml/h, a four-way stopcock and two SC infusion sets can be used to branch the infusion from one infusion pump to two SC sites. The sites can be as close as 2 inches apart. In extreme cases (when switching to another route is not possible or death is imminent) this double-site method can be used to provide the mainstay opioid and a third site used for PCA bolus doses for management of breakthrough pain; however, the more sites used to deliver opioid, the fewer available sites for rotation. When multiple sites are used, more frequent assessment of sites is necessary (at least q4h).

Preparing for Discharge From the Hospital

- As soon as possible before discharge, determine whether SC infusion will be continued at home.
- If so, determine family's willingness to maintain SC infusion in the home because this is vital to successful therapy (see Patient Teaching).
- Make necessary referrals and contacts (e.g., home health, hospice, home infusion company, insurance company) to arrange for appropriate level of home care after discharge.
- Make arrangements with local pharmacy for preparation of drug reservoirs so that the family can pick up drug reservoirs and other supplies weekly.

Patient Teaching

- Provide demonstrations and verbal and written instructions on needle placement, site care, pain and side effect assessment, management of breakthrough pain, pump management, and documentation.

Continued.

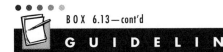

BOX 6.13—cont'd

G U I D E L I N E S

SUBCUTANEOUS CONTINUOUS INFUSION (SCCI)

- Allow patient and family time to practice working with supplies and pump under the guidance of a clinician.
- Remind family to keep extra batteries for portable pump at home. Routine battery changes can be done once the typical battery life for the patient is determined (battery life depends on infusion rate and PCA demands).
- Provide instructions on how to obtain and store extra drug reservoirs.
- Provide family with name and number of 24 h contact person.
- Reassure patient and family that another route can be substituted at any time if the SC route does not work.

Discontinuing SC Administration

1. Determine need for alternative analgesia. If patient will receive short-acting oral opioids, give the first scheduled dose 1 hour before stopping the SC infusion. If the patient will receive a controlled-release opioid, give the first scheduled dose 2 hours before stopping the SC infusion.
2. Turn off pump.
3. Loosen dressing and pull infusion set straight out with a swift motion. Apply pressure for 30 seconds. If the skin is intact, a dressing is not needed. If the site is excoriated, dress with triple antibiotic cream and gauze until healed.
4. Discard unused opioid solution according to institutional policy and procedure.

May be duplicated for use in clinical practice. From McCaffery M, Pasero C: *Pain: Clinical manual,* pp. 212-213. Copyright © 1999, Mosby, Inc.

The SC route of administration for the continuous infusion of opioids as opposed to intermittent injections is an alternative route for patients with chronic cancer pain who are unable to take oral medications and who do not have central venous access and for patients who experience dose-limiting side effects with oral opioids.

d, day; *h,* hour; *mg,* milligram; *ml,* milliliter; *q,* every; *SC,* subcutaneous.

Information from Bruera E, Brennels C, Michaud M et al.: Continuous SC infusion of narcotics using a portable disposable device in patients with advanced cancer, *Cancer Treatment Rep* 71(6):635-637, 1987; Capes D, Martin K, Underwood R: Performance of a restrictive flow device and an electronic syringe driver for continuous subcutaneous infusion, *J Pain Symptom Manage* 14(4):210-217, 1997; Coyle N: Cancer patients and subcutaneous infusions, *Am J Nurs* 96(3):61, 1996; Coyle N, Mauskop A, Maggard J et al.: Continuous subcutaneous infusions of opiates in cancer patients with pain, *Oncol Nurs Forum* 13(4):53-57, 1986; Stevenson KK, Gordon DB: Policy and procedure: Continuous subcutaneous opioid infusion, Madison, Wis, 1996, University of Wisconsin Hospitals & Clinics.

---

unpredictable absorption, that exist for adults exist also for children (Houck, 1998). Therefore, the IV route is especially appealing for use in children.

IV bolus doses of opioid analgesics are acceptable for severe, escalating pain (see Table 8.4 on p. 379 for pediatric dosing guidelines). Continuous IV infusions provide a steady analgesic level and are highly effective for use in children, especially those who are not candidates for IV PCA (see p. 253 and Table 6.15, p. 255, for pediatric IV PCA dosing guidelines). Initial loading doses of 0.05 to 0.1 mg/ kg of IV morphine followed by maintenance infusion of 0.025 to 0.03 mg/kg per hour are recommended for children (Houck, 1998) (see Chapter 14 for neonatal and infant dosing recommendations).

Intraspinal (epidural and intrathecal)

The term "intraspinal" refers to the spaces or potential spaces surrounding the spinal cord into which medications can be administered. Most often, the term is used when referring to the epidural and intrathecal routes of administration. The word "neuraxial" also is used to describe intraspinal analgesia. The word "spinal" is used interchangeably with the word "intrathecal" when referring to route of administration (see following on spinal anatomy). Table 6.8 discusses some of the persistent misconceptions related to epidural analgesia.

Box 6.14 on p. 215 presents patient selection guidelines and considerations for intraspinal analgesia. For information on selecting a starting dose for epidural and intrathecal analgesia in opioid-tolerant patients, see p. 260. See Chapter 13 for intraspinal analgesia in obstetrics.

Spinal Anatomy

The human spinal column consists of 33 individual vertebra referred to by their location: (1) 7 cervical, (2) 12 thoracic, (3) 5 lumbar, (4) 5 caudal or sacral (fused into one bone, the sacrum), and (5) 4 coccygeal (fused into one bone, the coccyx) (Figure 6.8, p. 216). Vertebrae consist of an anterior body, the laminae that protect the lateral spinal cord, and spinous processes that project outwardly and posteriorly from the laminae. The vertebrae become larger as they descend in the vertebral column. The bones of the laminae are bound together by a number of ligaments (e.g., the dense ligamentum flavum) (Figure 6.9, p. 216).

The spinal cord is located within and protected by the bony vertebral column and connective tissue (meninges). It is a continuous structure extending from the foramen magnum to approximately the first or second lumbar (L1-L2) vertebral interspace. The subarachnoid space (also called the intrathecal space in the caudal part of the spine) surrounds the spinal cord, separated by the pia mater. The

TABLE 6.8 ● ● ● ● ●

Misconceptions   Epidural Analgesia

MISCONCEPTION	CORRECTION
1. Compared with traditional routes of administration, the incidence of respiratory depression is higher when opioids are administered by the epidural route.	Clinically significant opioid-induced respiratory depression occurs less often when opioids are administered by the epidural route (0.07%–0.4%) than by the IM route (0.9%). The incidence of respiratory depression by the epidural route is closer in comparison to the incidence by IV PCA (0.1%–0.23%). Clinically significant opioid-induced respiratory depression can be avoided in opioid-naive patients by slow titration, careful nurse monitoring of sedation levels and respiratory status, and decreases in the opioid dose when increased sedation is detected.
2. Patients receiving epidural analgesia must be cared for in intensive care settings where their respiratory status can be mechanically monitored.	Patients receiving epidural analgesia have been cared for safely outside of the intensive care setting for many years. Nurse monitoring is the best and most common method for monitoring respiratory status in patients receiving epidural analgesia.
3. Epidural local anesthetics cause excessive and disabling sensory and motor blockade.	Local anesthetics are administered in low (subanesthetic) doses (e.g., 0.0625%–0.125% bupivacaine) for epidural analgesia. Higher doses are required to produce significant motor and sensory blockade (0.5%–0.75%). Patients receiving epidural analgesia are able to ambulate and perform all the routine recovery activities expected of them to the extent their medical or surgical condition allows. The occasional occurrence of minor temporary numbness of lower extremities is resolved easily by decreasing the dose or removing the local anesthetic from the epidural analgesic solution.

In spite of widespread use, misconceptions related to epidural analgesia persist. Table 6.8 corrects some of these misconceptions.

IM, intramuscular; *IV,* intravenous; *PCA,* patient-controlled analgesia.

Information from Ashburn MA, Love G, Pace NL: Respiratory-related critical events with intravenous patient-controlled analgesia, *Clin J Pain* 10:52-56, 1994; Pasero C, McCaffery M: Preventing and managing opioid induced respiratory depression, *Am J Nurs* 94(4):25-31, 1994; Ready LB, Loper KA, Nessly M et al.: Postoperative epidural morphine is safe on surgical wards, *Anesthesiology* 75:452-456, 1991; Scott DA, Beilby DSN, McClymont C: Postoperative analgesia using epidural infusions of fentanyl with bupivacaine, *Anesthesiology,* 83:727-737, 1995; Sidebotham D, Dijkhuizen RJ et al.: The safety and utilization of patient-controlled analgesia, *J Pain Symptom Manage* 14:202-209, 1997; St. Marie B, Williams A: *Management of cancer pain with epidural morphine* (independent study module), St. Paul, MN, 1994, Sims Deltec Inc; Sullivan F, Muir M, Ginsberg B: A survey on the clinical use of epidural catheters for acute pain management, *J Pain Symptom Manage* 9:303-307, 1994.

subarachnoid space is filled with clear, colorless, cerebrospinal fluid (CSF) that continually circulates and bathes the spinal cord. The dura is composed of the arachnoid and dura mater membranes and separates the epidural space from the subarachnoid space. The epidural space is a potential space filled with vasculature, fat, and a network of nerve extensions. No fluid is in the epidural space; a true space is created when volume or air is injected into it (Bridenbaugh, Greene, Brull, 1998) (see Figure 6.9).

The fact that the epidural space is a potential space has clinical implications for nurses. Although injecting large amounts of air is not recommended, small amounts, such as tiny bubbles within the infusion tubing when therapy is initiated, are not considered dangerous. In addition, because the epidural catheter is in a space and not a blood vessel, a continuous epidural infusion may be stopped for hours and restarted without concern that the catheter has become occluded. However, crystallization of the saline within the epidural catheter can occur when catheters are unused for prolonged periods. In these

cases, weekly or biweekly irrigation is recommended (DuPen, DuPen, 1998).

At each vertebral body level, nerve roots exit from the spinal cord bilaterally. Specific skin surface areas are innervated by a single spinal nerve or group of spinal nerves. These skin areas are called dermatomes (Figure 6.10, p. 217). Dermatome assessment is done most often by anesthesiologists to determine the level of spinal anesthesia for surgical procedures and postoperative analgesia when epidural local anesthetics are used.

Delivery of Intraspinal Analgesics

Delivery of analgesics by the intraspinal routes can be accomplished by inserting a needle into the subarachnoid space (for intrathecal analgesia) or the epidural space and injecting the analgesic, or threading a catheter through the needle and taping it in place temporarily for bolus dosing or continuous administration (Figures 6.11 to 6.13 on p. 218). Temporary catheters are used primarily for short-term acute pain management and are usu-

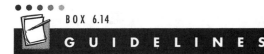

BOX 6.14

GUIDELINES

USE OF INTRASPINAL ANALGESIA

Patient Selection

- Absence of contraindications to epidural needle or catheter placement (e.g., coagulopathies, abnormal clotting studies, sepsis, history of multiple abscesses).
- For patients with chronic pain, systemic opioid therapy produces unmanageable and intolerable side effects.
- For patients with acute pain (e.g., surgery, trauma), the systemic routes have been considered and are not an option because they would produce unmanageable and intolerable side effects at the anticipated doses required for adequate analgesia.
- Patient has a painful condition or surgical procedure for which reduced morbidity and mortality is important but impractical or unattainable with other routes of administration. Such conditions include major thoracic, abdominal, and orthopedic surgery; intractable myocardial infarction.
- Intraspinal preemptive analgesia could prevent or reduce the severity of a chronic pain syndrome (e.g., elective amputation).
- Intraspinal route will be used to deliver anesthesia for surgery and a single bolus dose before removal of needle or catheter will produce acceptable postoperative analgesia (e.g., cesarean section).
- Patient has a pain syndrome that may be responsive to a specific intraspinal therapy such as local anesthetics, clonidine, or steroids (e.g., neuropathic pain unresponsive to oral adjuvant analgesics).[1]
- In the patient with cancer or chronic nonmalignant pain who will receive long-term intraspinal opioid therapy, a reduction in pain in response to a trial dose of an intraspinally administered opioid has been experienced.[1]

Other Considerations

- Appropriate equipment and supplies are available for therapy.
- Staff (or family) are trained to assess and manage epidural analgesia.
- Clinical support systems available ATC if needed.

Surgical Procedures for Which Intraspinal Analgesia Is Commonly Prescribed

Cesarean section
Thoracotomy
Aortic surgery
Vascular surgery of the lower extremities
Major joint replacement
Limb amputation
Whipple procedure
Large open upper abdominal surgery (e.g., open cholecystectomy, pancreatectomy, nephrectomy, liver surgery, stomach surgery)
Large open lower abdominal surgery (e.g., small bowel, mesentery, colon, radical prostate, total abdominal hysterectomy)
Major breast reconstruction

Medical Conditions for Which Intraspinal Analgesia Is Commonly Prescribed

Intractable cancer pain
Intractable neuropathic pain
Myocardial ischemia unresponsive to conventional treatment

May be duplicated for use in clinical practice. From McCaffery M, Pasero C: *Pain: Clinical manual*, p. 215. Copyright © 1999, Mosby, Inc.

[1]The variables that are used to select patients and evaluate efficacy for long-term intraspinal analgesia for the treatment of chronic nonmalignant pain need further research.

ATC, around the clock.

Information from Agency for Health Care Policy and Research (AHCPR): *Acute pain management: Operations or medical procedures and trauma. Clinical practice guideline.* AHCPR Publication No. 92-0032, Rockville, MD, U.S. Public Health Service, AHCPR, February, 1992; Ferrell BR, Griffith H: Cost issues related to pain management: Report from the cancer pain panel of the Agency for Health Care Policy and Research, *J Pain Symptom Manage* 9(4):221-234, 1994; Levy MH: Pharmacologic management of cancer pain, *Semin Oncol* 21(6):718-739, 1994; Pasero C: *Acute pain management service policy and procedure manual*, Rolling Hills Estates, CA, 1994, Academy Medical Systems, Inc; St. Marie B, Williams A: *Management of cancer pain with epidural morphine* (independent study module), St. Paul, MN, 1994, Sims Deltec Inc.

---

ally removed after 2 to 4 days. Temporary indwelling intrathecal catheters raise concerns about CNS infection (risk of infection is thought to be less with epidural catheters) and present technical difficulties associated with the necessary use of microcatheters. As a result, they are used less often than temporary indwelling epidural catheters (Brownridge, Cohen, Ward, 1998; DuPen, DuPen, 1998; Gwirtz, 1992; Hurley, 1992). Intrathecal catheters for acute pain management are used more often for providing anesthesia and/or a single analgesic bolus dose.

For severe intractable chronic pain, a long-term epidural catheter can be inserted, then tunneled subcutaneously for intermittent bolusing or continuous infusion by an external ambulatory pump. Tunneled epidural catheters can be used for weeks to months to deliver analgesics. The tunneling is done to decrease the incidence of infection and accidental displacement (see Figure 6.14, p. 219).

Long-term epidural and intrathecal catheters also can be placed surgically (implanted) and tunneled subcutaneously to an implanted port in the subcutaneous tissue in the lower rib area or an implanted pump in a

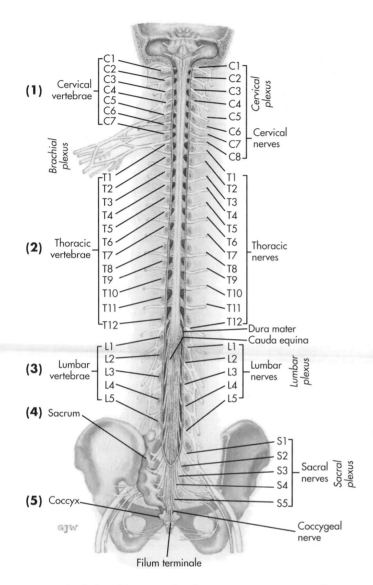

● ● ● ● ●
F I G U R E 6.8 **Vertebral column.** The human spinal column consists of 33 individual vertebra referred to by their location: (1) 7 cervical, (2) 12 thoracic, (3) 5 lumbar, (4) 5 caudal or sacral (fused into one bone, the sacrum), and (5) 4 coccygeal (fused into one bone, the coccyx). At each vertebral body level, nerve roots exit from the spinal cord bilaterally. Specific skin surface areas are innervated by a single spinal nerve or group of spinal nerves.

From Thibodeau GA, Patton KT: *Anatomy & physiology,* p. 463, ed 3, St. Louis, 1996, Mosby.

subcutaneous pocket in the abdomen (DuPen, DuPen, 1998; St. Marie, Williams, 1994) (Figure 6.14, p. 219). When indwelling intrathecal catheters are used for chronic pain management, they usually are implanted because they are easier to maintain and risk of infection is thought to be less (Bedder, 1996).

The level of nociceptive input (e.g., surgical site, site of injury, tumor location) and the characteristics of the opioid being administered are most important in determining the vertebral level at which the catheter is placed. Long-

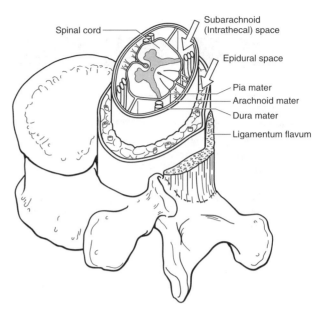

● ● ● ● ●
F I G U R E 6.9 **Spinal anatomy.** The spinal cord is a continuous structure extending from the foramen magnum to approximately the first or second lumbar (L1-L2) vertebral interspace. The subarachnoid space (also called the intrathecal space in the caudal part of the spine) surrounds the spinal cord, separated by the pia mater. The subarachnoid space is filled with cerebrospinal fluid (CSF) that continually circulates and bathes the spinal cord. The dura is composed of the arachnoid and dura mater membranes and separates the epidural space from the subarachnoid space. The epidural space is a potential space filled with vasculature, fat, and a network of nerve extensions.

From Salerno E, Willens J: *Pain management handbook,* p. 441, St. Louis, 1996, Mosby.

term catheters for treatment of cancer pain associated with spinal lesions can be placed in a location that avoids the tumor while providing necessary analgesia (DuPen, DuPen, 1998). Temporary epidural catheters for acute pain management usually are placed at the lumbar or thoracic vertebral level (see pp. 221–222).

Intraspinal Catheterization

Intraspinal needle and catheter insertion is performed usually by an anesthesiologist or certified registered nurse anesthetist. Nurses often assist with the procedure by preparing supplies and monitoring and supporting the patient during the procedure. Informed consent is obtained before the procedure.

The technique for placing a temporary percutaneous epidural catheter varies among physicians; however, the points made in the following patient teaching example can be generalized to epidural catheter placement in all patients and may be helpful in reinforcing the physician's explanation of the procedure to patients. The same principles apply to intrathecal needle and catheter placement.

Patient Example

Mr. R. and his wife want to know everything about the epidural catheter placement procedure he is

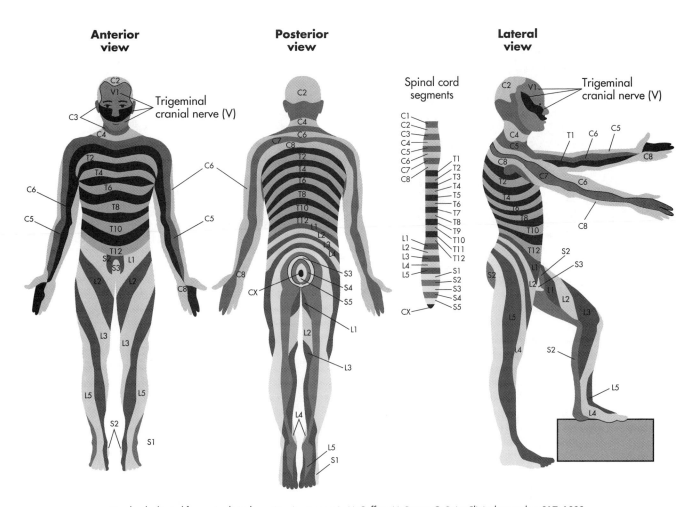

Anterior view

Posterior view

Lateral view

Trigeminal cranial nerve (V)

Spinal cord segments

Trigeminal cranial nerve (V)

May be duplicated for use in clinical practice. As appears in McCaffery M, Pasero C: *Pain: Clinical manual,* p. 217, 1999, Mosby, Inc.

● ● ● ● ●
FIGURE 6.10 **Dermatomes.** Segmental dermatome distribution of spinal nerves to the front, back, and side of the body. *C,* Cervical segments; *T,* thoracic segments; *L,* lumbar segments; *S,* sacral segments; *CX,* coccygeal segment. Dermatomes are specific skin surface areas innervated by a single spinal nerve or group of spinal nerves. Dermatome assessment is done to determine the level of spinal anesthesia for surgical procedures and postoperative analgesia when epidural local anesthetics are used.

From Thibodeau GA, Patton KT: *Anatomy & physiology,* ed 3, p. 468, St. Louis, 1996, Mosby.

going to receive later today. His nurse reinforces the physician's explanation by providing the following information:

"You'll either be in a sitting position or lying on your side for the procedure. The doctor will be behind you facing your back. First he'll wash a small area on your back with a sponge. This may feel cool. Then he'll put drapes on your back to keep the area as clean as possible. You'll need to roll your shoulders inward and push your back out slightly. The doctor will use a local anesthetic to numb the place where the catheter will go. Sometimes injecting the local anesthetic produces a burning, stinging sensation that lasts less than a minute. It usually takes the doctor about 2 or 3 minutes to insert the needle into the epidural space. This will feel like dull pressure against your back. Next the doctor inserts the catheter through the needle into the epidural space, which usually takes less than a minute. As he inserts the catheter you may feel some sparklike sensations in your legs and feet. These will go away very quickly. The doctor will remove the epidural needle and tape the catheter in place up your back to your shoulder. After the catheter is taped in place you'll be able to move and turn and lie on your back like you did before the procedure. The whole procedure usually takes less than 30 minutes. You may feel a very slight irritation for an hour or two after the procedure just at the site where the catheter goes into your back. If you feel any more discomfort in your back than that at any time while the catheter is in place, you'll need to let us know. Can I answer any questions?"

During intraspinal needle placement, most anesthesiologists are able to recognize when the point of the needle penetrates the dense ligamentum flavum (see Figure 6.9).

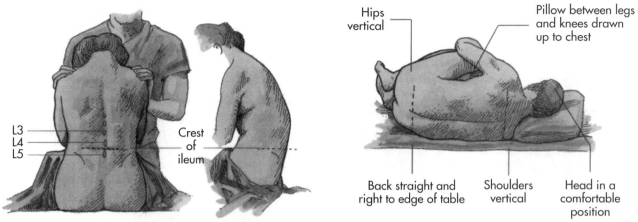

FIGURE 6.11 **Patient positioned for catheter placement.** Figure 6.11 shows two positions patients can assume for the epidural catheter placement procedure.

Courtesy Astra Pharmaceuticals, L.P., 50 Otis Street, Westborough, MA 01581-4500.

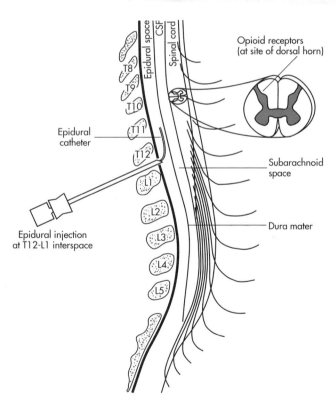

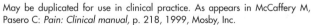

May be duplicated for use in clinical practice. As appears in McCaffery M, Pasero C: *Pain: Clinical manual*, p. 218, 1999, Mosby, Inc.

● ● ● ● ● ●
FIGURE 6.12 **Epidural needle and catheter placement.** Delivery of analgesics by the intraspinal routes can be accomplished by inserting a needle into the epidural space *(shown)* for epidural analgesia or the subarachnoid space for intrathecal analgesia and injecting the analgesic or threading a catheter through the needle and taping it in place temporarily for bolus dosing or continuous administration.

Modified from Sinatra R: Spinal opioid analgesia: An overview. In Sinatra RS, Hord AH, Ginsberg B, Preble LM, editors: *Acute pain: Mechanisms and management*, p 107, St. Louis, 1992, Mosby.

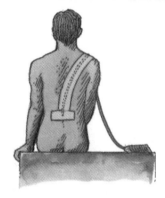

FIGURE 6.13 **Epidural catheter taped in place.** Figure 6.13 shows the catheter taped in place for continuous epidural infusion, patient-controlled epidural analgesia, or intermittent epidural bolusing.

Courtesy Astra Pharmaceuticals, L.P., 50 Otis Street, Westborough, MA 01581-4500.

In addition, entry into the epidural space exerts a negative pressure, which is registered by a loss of resistance in the syringe attached to the needle (Chadwick, Bonica, 1995). If the epidural space is the desired location, the anesthesiologist does not advance the needle further. If advanced further, the needle will penetrate the dura and enter the subarachnoid space. When in the subarachnoid space, free-flowing CSF can be aspirated. If a blood vessel is entered during placement, blood often can be aspirated.

Even when neither CSF nor blood is aspirated, many anesthesiologists confirm epidural needle placement by injecting a test dose of lidocaine with epinephrine when thought to be in the epidural space (use is controversial in pregnant patients; see Chadwick, Bonica, 1995; Mulroy, Norris, Liu, 1997). If the needle is in a blood

**External catheter and ambulatory
infusion pump**

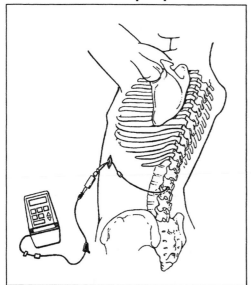

**Implantable port and an ambulatory
infusion pump**

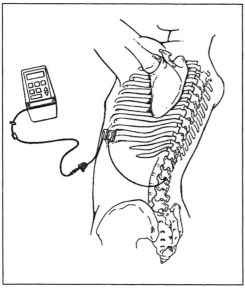

Implantable pump

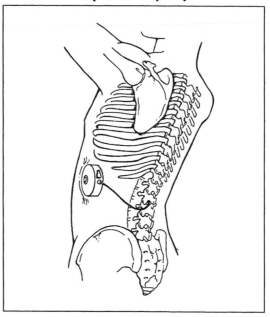

May be duplicated for use in clinical practice. As appears in McCaffery M, Pasero C: *Pain: Clinical manual,* p. 219, 1999, Mosby, Inc.

● ● ● ● ●
FIGURE 6.14 **Intraspinal delivery systems for chronic pain.** Figure 6.14 shows three intraspinal opioid delivery systems for the treatment of chronic pain.

From St. Marie B, Williams A: *Management of cancer pain with epidural morphine* [independent study module], St. Paul, MN, 1994, Sims Deltec Inc.

vessel, the epinephrine will cause the patient's heart rate and blood pressure to increase suddenly and significantly; if in the subarachnoid space, the lidocaine will produce sensory anesthesia within 5 minutes. If the patient exhibits neither of these changes, the needle is thought to be in the epidural space and the catheter is threaded through the needle (Covino, Wildsmith, 1998; Mulroy, Norris, Liu, 1997).

Anesthesiologists turn the bevel of the intraspinal needle upward to facilitate threading the catheter in an cephalad (toward the head) direction. Although rarely necessary for routine temporary intraspinal catheter placement, the only way to confirm conclusively the exact location of an intraspinal catheter is radiographically using contrast dye. When percutaneous catheters are to be used in the home setting, some clinicians recommend an epiduragram to confirm catheter position before patient discharge (DuPen, DuPen, 1998).

Methods for Administering Intraspinal Analgesia

The three methods for administering intraspinal analgesia are: (1) bolus (administered by the clinician), (2) continuous infusion (administered by a pump), and (3) patient-controlled epidural analgesia (administered by the patient usually using a pump).

Clinician-administered bolus method. Clinicians can provide analgesia by administering a single intrathecal or epidural bolus injection or the catheter can be left in place for intermittent bolus injections. The duration of the patient's pain usually determines which bolus method is used.

For some surgical procedures a single intraspinal bolus provides sufficient pain control for several hours. For example, an epidural or intrathecal bolus of morphine often is administered after cesarean section (see Chapter 13) and some gynecologic and urologic procedures. This single intraspinal dose is capable of providing analgesia for up to 24 hours. After this period of time, pain usually can be controlled with oral or IV analgesics.

When moderate to severe pain is expected to be constant for more than 24 hours, the epidural catheter can be left in place to provide intermittent analgesic bolus doses. As mentioned, when the intrathecal route is used for acute pain, analgesia is administered most often by single bolus; however, implanted ports can be accessed to deliver intermittent boluses for long-term intraspinal pain management. When an intrathecal catheter is implanted for long-term pain control, analgesia usually is provided by continuous infusion.

The major drawback of the intermittent epidural bolus method is that a steady analgesic level is difficult to maintain, especially when bolus doses are administered PRN. Relatively large doses of the opioid are given and a "peak and trough" effect occurs. Patients experience side effects at the peak (highest analgesic concentration level) and pain at the trough (lowest analgesic concentration level). Rather than a PRN approach to epidural dosing it may be preferable to consider smaller scheduled ATC doses. A dosing frequency of less than every 6 hours is not recommended (DuPen, DuPen, 1998) (see Box 6.15 for guidelines for administering intermittent boluses through a temporary epidural catheter).

Continuous infusion. The principle of providing continuous pain control with intraspinal analgesia can be accomplished by using an external (for acute and chronic pain) or implanted (for chronic pain) infusion pump to deliver a continuous infusion (also called basal rate) of an analgesic solution. Supplemental bolus doses are prescribed for breakthrough pain and can be administered using the clinician-administered bolus mode available on most external infusion pumps or as outlined in Box 6.15. When implanted ports are used to deliver continuous infusion and/or intermittent boluses, meticulous aseptic precautions

should be taken to protect the port from bacterial contamination (See DuPen, DuPen, 1998; St. Marie, Williams, 1994).

Patient-controlled epidural analgesia (PCEA). PCEA permits patients to treat their pain by self-administering doses of epidural analgesics to meet their individual analgesic requirements. When PCEA is used, a basal rate usually provides most of the patient's analgesic requirement and the PCEA bolus doses are used to manage breakthrough pain. If a basal rate is not provided, it is especially important to remind patients to "stay on top of the pain" to maintain a steady neuraxial analgesic level and self-administer bolus doses before pain is severe and out of control.

Drug Bioavailability by the Intraspinal Routes

In contrast to drugs administered systemically, drugs administered intraspinally are extremely potent (i.e., very small doses are effective) because distribution of the drug brings it close to the action site (opioid receptors in the dorsal horn of the spinal cord). This is particularly true when opioids are delivered by the intrathecal route where they are carried by the CSF directly to the receptors in the dorsal horn of the spinal cord. After epidural administration, drugs are distributed by three main pathways: (1) diffusion through the dura into the CSF then into the spinal cord directly to the receptors, (2) vascular uptake by the vessels in the epidural space into systemic circulation, and (3) uptake by the fat in the epidural space; a drug depot is created from which drug can eventually enter the systemic circulation (Gianino, York, Paice, 1996).

Direct delivery of opioids to the site of analgesic action explains why the dose of an opioid by the intraspinal routes is much smaller than required by the parenteral route to produce equal analgesia (i.e., the closer the opioid is delivered to the opioid receptors, the lower the required analgesic dose). For example, when converting opioid-tolerant patients from one route to another, the required dose of morphine is approximately three times less by the epidural route than by the IV route (ratio may vary for other opioids), and the dose required by the intrathecal route is approximately 10 times less than by the epidural route to produce equal analgesia (DuPen, DuPen, 1998) (see pp. 257-261 for information on switching to and from the intraspinal routes).

Solubility

One of the most important factors influencing drug absorption and bioavailability by the intraspinal routes is drug solubility. The more lipid soluble (readily dissolved in fatty tissue) the drug, the more readily it moves through membranes, resulting in faster and greater absorption. For example, when administered epidurally, lipid soluble opioids, such as fentanyl, rapidly traverse the dura into the CSF, then exit the aqueous CSF and easily penetrate the lipid-rich spinal tissue. This contributes to

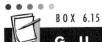

BOX 6.15

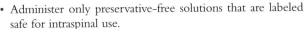

INTERMITTENT BOLUSES VIA A TEMPORARY SHORT-TERM EPIDURAL CATHETER

- Administer only preservative-free solutions that are labeled safe for intraspinal use.
- Before injecting, verify with another RN that the preservative-free drug, dosage, and volume is in accordance with physician's order.
- Before injecting, verify that the catheter to be injected is the epidural catheter. This is best accomplished by tracing the catheter from the port cap to the catheter insertion site in the patient's back.
- To prevent exerting too much pressure on injection, administer analgesic in at least a 5 ml syringe.
- The use of indwelling epidural filters depends on institutional policy; however, solutions drawn unfiltered from glass ampules always should be injected through a 0.22 μm filter.
- Maintain sterility of the epidural system when removing catheter port cap, attaching syringes, and replacing port cap. (Some institutions require disinfecting connection before removing port cap. Use only nonneurotoxic agents [e.g., Betadine] to disinfect intraspinal catheter connections or ports [alcohol often is used to cleanse skin of secretions, but should not be used to disinfect catheter connections or ports].)

- Before injecting analgesic, use an empty syringe to gently aspirate catheter; allow time for fluid to travel up catheter:
  - Minimal fluid return (e.g., <0.5 ml) indicates catheter is in the epidural space.
  ⇒ Steadily (speed of injection depends on resistance met during injection) inject analgesic through catheter filter (if filter is used).
  - Free-flowing clear fluid (CSF) return indicates catheter may be in the intrathecal space.
  ⇒ Do not administer analgesic; notify anesthesiologist.
  - Bloody aspirate indicates catheter may be in a blood vessel.
  ⇒ Do not administer analgesic; notify anesthesiologist.
- Do not inject analgesic if patient reports pain on steady injection; notify anesthesiologist.
- Some resistance during injection is normal, but if strong resistance is met during injection, reposition the patient so that the spine is flexed. If resistance continues, stop and notify anesthesiologist.
- Do not flush epidural catheter after injecting analgesic unless specifically ordered to do so.

May be duplicated for use in clinical practice. From McCaffery M, Pasero C: *Pain: Clinical manual*, p. 221. Copyright © 1999, Mosby, Inc.

When moderate to severe pain is expected to be constant for more than 24 hours, the epidural catheter can be left in place to provide intermittent analgesic bolus doses. A frequency of less than every 6 hour boluses is not recommended. Box 6.15 presents guidelines for intermittent bolus administration through a temporary epidural catheter.

CSF, cerebrospinal fluid; *mg*, milligram; *ml*, milliliter.

Information from DuPen SL, DuPen AR: Spinal analgesia. In Ashburn MA, Rice LJ, editors: *The management of pain*, pp. 171-186, New York, 1998, Churchill Livingstone; St. Anthony Medical Center: Peridural analgesia: Administering the intermittent bolus, Rockford, IL, 1997, the Center; University Hospital, University of Utah Health Science Center, Department of Nursing: Clinical standard: Pain management: Epidural narcotic administration by intermittent bolus, Salt Lake City, UT, 1992, University Hospital.

---

fentanyl's fast onset of action (5 minutes). However, hydrophilic opioids (readily dissolved in aqueous solution), such as morphine, have difficulty traversing the dura to reach the aqueous CSF. By either the epidural or intrathecal route, once in the aqueous CSF, hydrophilic drugs prefer to remain there. Eventually high enough concentrations of morphine are reached in the CSF, and the drug moves into the spinal cord to the opioid receptors. This helps to explain intraspinal morphine's slow onset of action (30 to 90 minutes) (Sinatra, 1992a; Sinatra, 1998).

An opioid's duration of action when administered by the intraspinal routes is determined in large part by the amount of the drug that remains in the CSF. Because morphine is hydrophilic and tends to remain within the aqueous CSF, a depot of drug molecules is created there. This ensures continued opioid receptor binding by replenishing molecules that dissociate and are cleared from

the spinal action sites. This helps to explain morphine's exceptionally long duration of analgesia from a single intraspinal bolus dose (up to 24 hours). On the other hand, the highly lipid soluble opioids like fentanyl traverse membranes readily and are easily removed by vasculature or remain trapped within the fat of the epidural space. This causes a rapid decline in drug concentration at spinal action sites and results in a short duration of analgesia (2 hours). With the exception of lofentanil, which dissociates slowly and has a longer duration, the highly lipid soluble opioids are best administered by continuous infusion to prolong their limited duration of activity (Sinatra, 1992a; Sinatra, 1998). When steady state is reached by continuous infusion, the various opioids differ little in terms of duration.

Dermatomal spread. Because hydrophilic drugs like morphine dissolve readily into the CSF, they are carried rostrally (toward the brain) through the circulating CSF. This results in a broad spread of analgesia across many dermatomes. The opposite is true of lipophilic opioids, like fentanyl and sufentanil, which produce what is called "segmental" analgesia. As discussed, lipophilic opioids do not remain in the CSF but are redistributed to other tissues (e.g., spinal cord tissue, epidural fat, and vasculature), so there is very little rostral spread. The dermatomal levels obtained with lipophilic opioids are related to the surface area in contact with the drug (Gourlay, Cherry, Plummer et al., 1987; Gourlay, Murphy, Plummer et al., 1989). Postmortem studies confirm that the largest concentration of lipophilic opioid is found near the tip of the catheter (Boersma, Heykants, ten Kate et al., 1991).

Placing the epidural catheter close enough to the opioid receptors and to the level of nociceptive input (e.g., surgical site) is critical, especially when lipophilic opioids are administered (Hansdottir, Bake, Nordberg, 1996; Hansdottir, Woestenborghs, Nordberg, 1995; Hubbard, 1992a,b; Nicholson, Rowlingson, 1992). In addition, numerous studies support optimal catheter placement at the thoracic level rather than the lumbar level, when administering lipophilic opioids for acute pain (Bodily, Chamberlain, Ramsey et al., 1989; Chisakuta, George, Hawthorne, 1995; Sawchuk, Ong, Unruh et al., 1993; Scott, Beilby, McClymont, 1995; Wiebalck, Brodner, Van Aken, 1997).

Studies have shown that lumbar epidural fentanyl infusions are equivalent to IV fentanyl infusions and that the mode of action of a lumbar epidural fentanyl infusion is primarily through systemic absorption (Glass, Estok, Ginsberg et al., 1992; Sandler, Stringer, Panos et al., 1992). Even lumbar administration of dilute lipophilic solutions at high infusion rates may result in plasma concentration levels equal to parenterally administered opioids (Lubenow, 1992). However, a number of studies have shown that administration of lipophilic opioids at the appropriate dermatomal level for acute pain (e.g., thoracic for abdominal and thoracic surgeries) affords excellent pain control and other benefits, such as earlier extubation, fewer systemic side effects, and attenuation of stress hormones, compared with IV opioids (Dogra, Blau, Lucas et al., 1997; Harukuni, Yamaguchi, Sato et al., 1995; Salomaki, Laitinen, Nuutinen, 1991); For practitioners choosing lumbar placement of epidural catheters, especially to treat upper abdominal and thoracic nociceptive input, morphine is the best choice of drug.

For certain types of surgery, thoracic epidural anesthesia and analgesia clearly have more advantages than lumbar epidural anesthesia and analgesia. Thoracic anesthesia and analgesia has been shown to improve intraoperative and postoperative ventilation, lower blood loss, reduce metabolic load, reduce surgical stress response, lower the incidence of thromboembolism, and maintain renal function at lower local anesthetic and opioid doses

than lumbar anesthesia and analgesia (Lema, Sinha, 1994; Liu, Carpenter, Neal, 1995) (see Chapter 2 for more on the effects of epidural analgesia on patient outcome).

Many physicians are reluctant to attempt thoracic catheter placement (Lema, Sinha, 1994). They prefer the lumbar over the thoracic level because the spinal cord becomes smaller as it progresses distally and the lumbar spinous processes are angulated posteriorly and farther apart making epidural catheter placement easier in the lumbar area. When placed below the spinal cord, the risk of trauma to the spinal cord is eliminated.

It is a common misconception that thoracic epidural catheter placement is technically difficult and causes more neurologic damage than lumbar catheter placement. A review of surveys of more than 18,000 epidural anesthetics performed in university hospitals revealed that placement of epidural catheters at thoracic vertebral levels does not confer higher risk than placement at lumbar levels (Liu, Carpenter, Neal, 1995). In fact, studies show that thoracic epidural anesthesia and analgesia is associated with a low risk of neurologic complications and may even be safer than lumbar catheters (Liu, Carpenter, Neal, 1995; Tanaka, Watanabe, Hurada et al., 1993).

Selected Analgesics Administered by the Intraspinal Routes

The two main types of drugs administered intraspinally to treat pain are opioids and local anesthetics. The alpha$_2$-adrenergic agonist clonidine is used for cancer pain and is gaining in popularity for managing acute pain. Baclofen (Lioresal), a muscle relaxant and antispastic agent, is administered intraspinally for treatment of spasticity (see Chapter 7 for discussion of Baclofen). These drugs can be administered alone or in combination with each other. The rationale for combining drugs is that they work synergistically to provide better analgesia and fewer side effects at lower doses.

Opioids

For most patients receiving intraspinal analgesia, the opioid provides the mainstay analgesia. The mu agonist opioids, morphine and fentanyl, are the most common opioids administered by the epidural route; sufentanil, alfentanil, hydromorphone (Dilaudid), and meperidine (Demerol) are administered less often. The primary opioid administered by the intrathecal route is morphine. Table 6.9 provides a summary of the characteristics of selected opioids administered intraspinally.

Morphine.   Morphine was the first opioid to be administered intraspinally for the relief of pain in humans (Wang, Nauss, Thomas, 1979) and the first to receive FDA approval for intraspinal administration (de Leon-Casasola, Lema, 1996). Morphine is an excellent choice of opioid for intraspinal analgesia because it can be given by all of the intraspinal delivery methods. It is ideal for single bolus dose intraspinal administration because it has

TABLE 6.9

SUMMARY OF CHARACTERISTICS OF SELECTED INTRASPINAL OPIOIDS

Analgesic	Onset[1] (min)	Peak[1] (min)	Duration[1-3] (h)	Half-life (h)	Solubility	Spread	Comments
Morphine	30-90 (EA); 30-60 (IA)	90-120 (EA); 60 (IA)	Up to 24 (EA); up to 24 (IA)	2-3	Hydrophilic (soluble in aqueous solution)	Wide	Standard for comparison; can be administered by all intraspinal methods of delivery; ideal for large single bolus dose but with risk of late respiratory depression (6-12 h); drug of choice if lumbar placement.
Fentanyl	5-15 (EA); 5 (IA)	10-20 (EA); 10 (IA)	1-3 (EA); 2-4 (IA)	3-4	High lipid (soluble in fat)	Narrow; segmental	Because of short duration, continuous infusion preferred to intermittent boluses; catheter location important. At steady state, slow elimination from tissues can result in a long half-life (up to 12 h) and accumulation leading to late and prolonged sedation and respiratory depression.
Hydromorphone (Dilaudid)	15-30 (EA)	45-60 (EA)	Up to 18 (EA)	2-3	More lipid soluble (10 times) than morphine; less lipid soluble than meperidine and fentanyl	Less than morphine; more than meperidine and fentanyl	Similar to morphine in analgesia and side effects; no evidence that active metabolites are clinically relevant.
Meperidine (Demerol)	5-30 (EA); 10 (IA)	30 (EA); 15 (IA)	6-8 (EA); 6-16 (IA)	2-3	More lipid soluble than morphine and hydromorphone; less lipid soluble than fentanyl	Less than morphine and hydromorphone; more than fentanyl	Toxic metabolite, normeperidine, can cause CNS irritability, seizures regardless of route of administration; metabolite half-life is 15-20 h. Contraindicated in elderly and patients with impaired renal function.

May be duplicated for use in clinical practice. From McCaffery M, Pasero C: *Pain: Clinical manual*, pp. 223-224. Copyright © 1999, Mosby, Inc.   *Continued.*

● ● ● ● ●
TABLE 6.9—cont'd

SUMMARY OF CHARACTERISTICS OF SELECTED INTRASPINAL OPIOIDS

Analgesic	Onset[1] (min)	Peak[1] (min)	Duration[1-3] (h)	Half-life (h)	Solubility	Spread	Comments
Sufentanil	5-10 (EA); 5 (IA)	10 (EA); 15-20 (IA)	2-3 (EA); 2-3 (IA)	2-4	Very high lipid (2 times more lipid soluble than fentanyl)	Narrow; segmental	Because of short duration, continuous infusion is preferred to intermittent boluses; catheter location important; analgesia and side effects similar to fentanyl but less likely to accumulate; more sedating than other opioids.

May be duplicated for use in clinical practice. From McCaffery M, Pasero C: *Pain: Clinical manual*, pp. 223-224. Copyright © 1999, Mosby, Inc.

Table 6.9 summarizes characteristics of selected intraspinal opioids.

[1]Onset, peak, and duration are based on single bolus administration.

[2]Duration of analgesia is dose dependent; the higher the dose, usually the longer the duration.

[3]When steady state is reached by continuous infusion, the various opioids differ little in terms of duration.

EA, epidural analgesia (single bolus dose); *h*, hour; *IA*, intrathecal (single bolus dose); *min*, minutes.

Information from Baraka A, Noueihid R, Hajj S: Intrathecal injection of morphine for obstetric analgesia, *Anesthesiology* 54:136-140, 1981; Graf G, Frasca A, Sinatra RS: Optimizing postoperative analgesia with a rapidly acting epidural anesthetic, *Anesthesiology* 69:A338, 1988; Gwirtz KH: Single-dose intrathecal opioids in the management of acute postoperative pain. In Sinatra R, Hord AH, Ginsberg B, Preble LM, editors: *Acute pain: Mechanisms and management*, pp 253-268, St. Louis, 1992, Mosby; Lubenow TR: Epidural analgesia: Considerations and delivery methods. In Sinatra R, Hord AH, Ginsberg B, Preble LM, editors: *Acute pain: mechanisms and management*, pp 233-242, St. Louis, 1992, Mosby; McQuay HJ: Opioid clinical pharmacology and routes of administration, *Br Med Bull* 47(3):703-717, 1991; Turner JL, Sibert KS, Sinatra RS: Epidural and spinal analgesia in the post-cesarean delivery patient. In Sinatra R, Hord AH, Ginsberg B, Preble LM, editors: *Acute pain: Mechanisms and management*, pp 269-278, St. Louis, 1992, Mosby; Van der Auwera D, Verborgh C, Camu F: Analgesic and cardiorespiratory effects of epidural sufentanil and morphine, *Anesth Analg* 66:999-1003, 1987; Willens JS, Myslinski NR: Pharmacodynamics, pharmacokinetics, and clinical uses of fentanyl, sufentanil, and alfentanil, *Heart Lung* 22(3):239-251, 1993.

a particularly long duration of action (up to 24 hours). It is administered also by continuous infusion and PCEA. Table 6.10 contains common PCEA prescription ranges for opioid-naive patients.

With bolus injection in the opioid-naive patient, intraspinal morphine has a slow onset of analgesia (30 to 90 minutes) and a peak effect of approximately 90 minutes. Additional analgesia usually is required until morphine takes effect. For example, some clinicians administer an epidural dose of a faster acting lipophilic opioid analgesic, such as fentanyl (onset 5 minutes), at the time of the single epidural morphine bolus or initiation of infusion therapy to provide analgesia until morphine takes effect (Sinatra, 1998; Sinatra, Sevarino, Chung, 1991; Turner, Sibert, Sinatra, 1992).

Morphine's ability to spread rostrally makes the vertebral location of intraspinal administration less critical than when administering lipophilic opioids for acute postoperative pain. For example, intraspinal morphine can be administered in the lumbar region to produce analgesia after thoracic surgery (Chaney, Furry, Fluder et al., 1997) and in the thoracic region for oral and facial pain treatment (Sakuramoto, Kanai, Matoba et al., 1996).

Because of its slow onset and rostral spread allowing binding with opioid receptors in the ventral medulla, large volume bolus doses (>5 mg) of epidural morphine have been known to produce late respiratory depression (approximately 2 to 12 hours after lumbar injection). Earlier respiratory depression at 5 to 10 minutes and before 2 hours also can occur due to vascular uptake of morphine (Chaney, 1995; St. Marie, Williams, 1994). Monitoring the opioid-naive patient's level of sedation and respiratory status at least every 2 hours for 12 to 24 hours after a clinician-administered intraspinal bolus of morphine is recommended (Gwirtz, 1992; Vanderveer, 1997).

Fear of late respiratory depression has caused some clinicians to avoid using epidural morphine in opioid-naive patients. However, rostral spread and late respiratory depression are uncommon when epidural morphine is administered in smaller more frequent bolus doses and by continuous infusion (deLeon-Casasola, Lema, 1996). Continuous administration leads to steady state, with little variation in drug levels near the respiratory centers (Gianino, York, Paice, 1996). PCEA with continuous infusion has been found to be a highly effective and safe

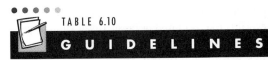

TABLE 6.10

G U I D E L I N E S

COMMON PCEA PRESCRIPTION RANGES FOR OPIOID-NAIVE ADULTS

Drug	Loading Dose	PCEA Dose	Delay	Basal
Morphine	2-6 mg	0.2-0.5 mg	10 min	0-0.8/h
Hydromorphone (Dilaudid)	0.8-1.5 mg	0.15-0.3 mg	10 min	0.15-0.3 mg/h
Fentanyl	25-100 μg	10-50 μg	10 min	0.40 μg/h
Sufentanil	0.3-0.7 μg/kg	5-7 μg	10 min	0.1-0.2 μg/kg/h

May be duplicated for use in clinical practice. From McCaffery M, Pasero C: *Pain: Clinical manual,* p. 225. Copyright © 1999, Mosby, Inc.

Table 6.10 provides common PCEA prescription ranges for opioid-naive adults.

h, hour; *kg,* kilogram; *μg,* microgram; *mg,* milligram; *min,* minute, *PCEA,* patient-controlled epidural analgesia.

Information from de Leon-Casasola OA, Lema MJ: Postoperative epidural opioid analgesia: What are the choices? *Anesth Analg* 83:867-875, 1996; Vanderveer B, Clinical Coordinator, Acute and Cancer Pain Service, University Hospital, University of Kentucky, Lexington, KY: Personal communication with author Chris Pasero, November 20, 1997; Walmsley PNH: Patient-controlled epidural analgesia. In Sinatra RS, Hord AH, Ginsberg B, Preble LM, editors: *Acute pain: Mechanisms and management,* pp 312-320, St. Louis, 1992, Mosby.

method of administering morphine to opioid-naive patients (Walmsley, 1992).

As with more lipophilic drugs, when a continuous epidural infusion of morphine is discontinued, concentrations of opioid decline because there is no opioid drug depot in the CSF to replenish the dissociating molecules at the receptor sites. Because side effects (e.g., sedation, respiratory depression) will decrease, not increase, after continuous epidural morphine and PCEA are discontinued, IV lines, if otherwise unnecessary, can be removed and routine monitoring (e.g., every shift) of level of sedation and respiratory status is customary (Vanderveer, 1997).

As would be expected, continuous epidural infusion of morphine was found to produce better analgesia than intermittent epidural bolusing of morphine (Rauk, Raj, Knarr et al., 1994). This, plus a lower incidence of respiratory depression, may make epidural morphine administered by continuous infusion preferable to intermittent bolusing for postoperative pain management (de Leon-Casasola, Lema, 1996).

Fentanyl. Fentanyl has been used extensively in anesthesia and is used widely for epidural analgesia, especially for acute pain. Single intraspinal doses of fentanyl provide analgesia for just 2 to 3 hours (Grass, Sakima, Schmidt et al., 1997), making this method of administration appropriate only for very short-term pain control, such as following ambulatory surgery. Because lipid soluble opioids like fentanyl have such a short duration, administration by continuous infusion or PCEA, rather than intermittent bolus dosing, is preferred for extended pain control.

As discussed, after repetitive dosing or continuous infusion of fentanyl, a steady state is approached. In this condition, the terminal half-life of fentanyl depends on how much is taken into tissue for storage and how quickly it is released. Although fentanyl is reported to have a terminal

half-life of approximately 3 to 4 hours, at steady state, slow removal of fentanyl from storage sites can result in a longer terminal half-life (up to 12 hours) (Mather, Denson, 1992; Willens, Myslinski, 1993). This can lead to accumulation and late and prolonged duration of sedation and respiratory depression (Marshall, Longnecker, 1996; Mather, Denson, 1992; Willens, Myslinski, 1993). Elderly patients and obese patients, in particular, may be subject to this effect (Willens, Myslinski, 1993). As a rule, however, early onset respiratory depression is more common than delayed with epidural fentanyl. This reflects vascular uptake of the opioid and occurs most often within an hour of initial injection (Chaney, 1995; St. Marie, Williams, 1994).

Hydromorphone. Hydromorphone (Dilaudid) is used less often than morphine and fentanyl for epidural analgesia. Its lipid solubility is intermediate between morphine and fentanyl. Because it is 10 times more lipophilic than morphine, its onset of analgesia (15 to 30 minutes) is faster and its duration of action (up to 18 hours) is shorter. Hydromorphone is capable of spreading rostrally and can produce delayed respiratory depression after large bolus administration (de Leon-Casasola, Lema, 1996; Turner, Sibert, Sinatra, 1992). The incidence of pruritis may be less with epidural hydromorphone than with epidural morphine (de Leon-Casasola, Lema, 1996).

Hydromorphone by PCEA after cesarean section provided satisfactory pain relief with three to four times less hydromorphone than when given by IV PCA (Parker, White, 1992). In another study (Parker, Sawaki, White, 1992) postcesarean section patients received either (1) hydromorphone by PCEA; (2) hydromorphone by PCEA plus continuous infusion; (3) hydromorphone and bupivacaine by PCEA; or (4) hydromorphone and bupivacaine by PCEA plus continuous infusion. The authors reported that the addition of bupivacaine did not improve pain relief or reduce side effects. This may be due, in large part, to problems related to administering epidural bupivacaine at the lumbar level, especially by continuous infusion. Patients in groups 3 and 4 experienced a higher incidence of urinary retention than groups 1 and 2; however, the reported 22% incidence of lower extremity numbness occurred only in patients in group 4 who were receiving continuous bupivacaine. The incidence of pruritis was high in all four groups (55% to 72%); nausea requiring treatment also was relatively high in all groups (9% to 20%) except group 1 (0%).

The 0% incidence of nausea in patients who received hydromorphone by PCEA without bupivacaine and without a continuous infusion in the above study is impressive and contributed to the lower overall incidence of side effects in groups 1 and 2 compared with groups 3 and 4. However, this finding is inconsistent with other studies conducted by two of these researchers (Parker, White, 1992; Parker, Holtmann, White, 1997). In one study (Parker, White, 1992) 17% of patients receiving hydromorphone by PCEA without bupivacaine and without a continuous infusion required treatment for nausea, and in a later study (Parker, Holtmann, White, 1997) 20% experienced nausea.

One study compared epidural hydromorphone by various delivery methods with epidural morphine by PRN intermittent bolus doses for treatment of pain after major orthopedic surgeries (Gan, Ginsberg, Perno et al., 1997). Patients received either (1) hydromorphone by PRN intermittent epidural bolus doses, (2) hydromorphone by PCEA alone, (3) hydromorphone by PCEA with a basal rate, or (4) morphine by PRN intermittent epidural bolus doses. No differences were noted in pain scores, sedation scores, and side effects between the treatment groups. Patients in group 3 (PCEA with a basal rate) received two and a half to three times the amount of hydromorphone as those in groups 1 and 2, and one patient in group 3 was withdrawn from the study because of respiratory depression. The authors recommended PCEA hydromorphone without a basal rate as an alternative to intermittent epidural boluses of morphine.

Hydromorphone has metabolites, and although all of their effects have not been clearly defined, they are not believed to be clinically relevant. Because hydromorphone has a short half-life (2 to 3 hours) and no active metabolites, it may be a better drug than morphine for patients with renal insufficiency (Portenoy, 1996b). Hydromorphone is a good alternative to morphine also when high concentrations of drug are required, because the epidural hydromorphone/epidural morphine conversion ratio is 1:5 (i.e., 10 mg/ml of epidural hydromorphone is approximately equal to 50 mg/ml of epidural morphine) (Gianino, York, Paice, 1996).

Meperidine. Meperidine (Demerol) is administered by the epidural route less often than fentanyl and morphine. Clinicians who prefer meperidine by this route cite the potential advantages of less vascular uptake than more lipophilic opioids like fentanyl, a faster onset of analgesia (5 to 30 minutes) than less lipophilic opioids like morphine (Etches, Gammer, Cornish, 1996), and an intermediate dermatomal spread that allows lumbar administration regardless of the site of nociceptive input (Slinger, Shennib, Wilson, 1995). Meperidine also has been shown to produce local anesthetic effects (Armstrong, Morton, Nimmo, 1993).

The primary disadvantage of using meperidine epidurally is its toxic metabolite, normeperidine (see also pp. 183-185). Meperidine plasma levels >350 ng/ml and normeperidine plasma levels of >400 ng/ml are reported to cause CNS irritability (Kaiko, Foley, Grabinski et al., 1983). Research shows that meperidine is more likely than other opioid drugs to cause delirium in postoperative patients of all ages. In one study meperidine more than doubled the risk of delirium when given either epidurally or IV (Marcantonio, Juarez, Goldman et al., 1994).

Like IV meperidine, studies have not shown clear advantages to using meperidine over other opioids by the epidural route (Cox, Serpell, Bannister et al., 1996). Often, researchers who suggest that meperidine may be a preferred choice of epidural opioid have failed to analyze normeperidine plasma levels and assess for CNS toxicity (Etches, Gammer, Cornish, 1996; Ngan Kee, Lam, Chen, 1997; St. Onge, Fugere, Girard, 1997). One study failed to assess for signs of CNS toxicity and collected normeperidine plasma levels for only 24 hours (Paech, Moore, Evans, 1994).

In a study comparing epidural to IV meperidine (Slinger, Shennib, Wilson, 1995), plasma normeperidine levels were the same for both routes, despite the fact that the total meperidine dosage was much less by the epidural route. CNS irritability (shakiness and tremors) was noted when normeperidine plasma levels reached >300 ng/ml, and the peak mean normeperidine plasma level after 72 hours of continuous epidural meperidine infusion was 573 ng/ml. No patients had seizures in this study, but 40% experienced CNS irritability.

Use of epidural meperidine during labor may present an increased risk of normeperidine toxicity to both the mother and fetus, which can extend into the postpartum period (Kuhnert, Kuhnert, Philipson et al., 1985; Kuhnert, Philipson, Kuhnert et al., 1985). Epidural meperidine is used often for pain after cesarean section. Breast feeding infants of mothers receiving meperidine in the postpartum period are at higher risk for neurobehavioral depression than breast feeding infants of mothers who receive other opioids (Wittels, Glosten, Faure, 1997). Further research is needed to determine the extent of the effects of meperidine and normeperidine on these populations of patients (see Chapter 13 for more on effects of meperidine and normeperidine in obstetric patients and neonates).

If meperidine is used epidurally, administering it by PCEA without a continuous infusion rather than by continuous infusion alone has been shown to reduce total meperidine consumption (Etches, Gammer, Cornish, 1996) and lower normeperidine plasma levels (Paech, Moore, Evans, 1994). The addition of bupivacaine may improve pain relief and allow a reduced dose and lower serum concentrations of meperidine (St. Onge, Fugere, Girard, 1997), but this combination can cause significant hypotension, oliguria, or excessive motor or sensory blockade (Etches, Gammer, Cornish, 1996). Dilution and volume of epidural meperidine injectate were found to have no effect on the systemic uptake of meperidine (Ngan Kee, Lam, Chen, 1997). Clearly, better opioid choices than meperidine exist for epidural administration.

Methadone. Methadone is a lipophilic opioid and, like other lipophilic opioids, produces less rostral spread than morphine. Because it is cleared rapidly from the CSF, it has a relatively short duration (4 hours) by the intraspinal routes (Mercante, 1997). Methadone may be an option for patients with cancer pain that require continuous intraspinal pain treatment, but the concerns discussed earlier in this chapter about its long half-life (12 to 190 hours) and accumulation with repetitive dosing and continuous infusion apply (see p. 185).

Although rarely used for postoperative pain management, intermittent lumbar epidural boluses of 4 to 5 mg methadone in 20 ml of saline produced 4 to 6 hours of good postoperative pain relief for upper abdominal and thoracic surgery (Welch, Hrynaszkiewicz, 1981). Intrathecal bolus doses of methadone were administered to patients after total knee or hip replacement (Jacobson, Chabal, Brody et al., 1990). Morphine, 0.5 mg intrathecally, was found to produce prolonged analgesia compared with 5, 10, and 20 mg intrathecal doses of methadone. All doses of methadone produced excellent analgesia for 4 hours, but 20 mg doses produced unacceptable side effects.

Sufentanil. Sufentanil is used less frequently than fentanyl for epidural analgesia. It is two times more lipid soluble than fentanyl. Pain relief by the epidural route is detected within 3 minutes of injection and duration is similar to fentanyl. A single epidural dose of 40 to 55 μg (12.5 μg intrathecal) of sufentanil produced effective analgesia for approximately 3 hours (Graf, Sinatra, Chung, et al., 1991; Lu, Schafer, Gardner, et al., 1997), so it may be ideal for some ambulatory surgical procedures and often is used to treat pain after cesarean section. Larger single doses can produce profound respiratory depression and are not recommended (Graf, Sinatra, Chung et al., 1991; Lu, Schafer, Gardner et al., 1997).

For extended pain relief, sufentanil administered by continuous infusion, rather than intermittent bolusing, is recommended (de Leon-Casasola, Lema, 1996). Sufentanil has a shorter half-life (2 to 3 hours) and less risk of accumulation than fentanyl because it is eliminated from storage sites faster (Willens, Myslinski, 1993).

The incidence of most side effects and quality of analgesia with epidural sufentanil is comparable to fentanyl at equianalgesic doses (Grass, Sakima, Schmidt et al., 1997). However, of all the opioids administered epidurally, sufentanil is associated with the highest incidence of sedation (Chaney, 1995), and late respiratory depression can occur (Broekema, Gielen, Hennis, 1996).

Sufentanil has been suggested as a better choice than morphine when epidural analgesia is used in postoperative cancer patients who are receiving chronic opioid treatment (de Leon-Casasola, Lema, 1993). Opioid-tolerant cancer patients who were well controlled on 250 mg/day oral morphine achieved significantly better postoperative pain control with epidural sufentanil than with epidural morphine. Full pain control was achieved in these patients with smaller equianalgesic doses of sufentanil than morphine.

Studies show that sufentanil analgesia is optimal when combined with local anesthetic (Hansdottir, Bake, Nordberg, 1996; Wiebalck, Brodner, Van Aken, 1997). Because of its high lipid solubility, placement of the epidural catheter close to the nociceptive input (e.g., surgical site) is especially important when sufentanil is used (Hansdottir, Bake, Nordberg, 1996; Hansdottir, Woestenborghs, Nordberg, 1995; Wiebalck, Brodner, Van Aken, 1997).

Intraspinal opioid side effects. Opioid side effects are discussed at length later in this chapter. The effect of the intraspinal routes of administration on the various opioid side effects is addressed (see pp. 261-270).

Local Anesthetics

Local anesthetics frequently are combined with epidural opioids for the treatment of acute or chronic pain. Although the use of local anesthetics by the epidural route is widespread for short- and long-term pain management, their long-term intrathecal use is controversial because of the potential for neurotoxicity. As a result, they are administered less often by the intrathecal route (DuPen, DuPen, 1998; Liu, 1998).

Low ("subanesthetic") doses of local anesthetics work synergistically with intraspinal opioids to provide better analgesia at lower doses than would be possible with the opioid alone. A reduction in doses results in a lower incidence of adverse effects of both opioids and local anesthetics (de Leon-Casasola, Lema, 1996). In addition to improved analgesia and fewer side effects, adding local anesthetics to epidural opioids has been shown to improve GI function and reduce cardiovascular, pulmonary, and infectious complications in postoperative patients (Liu, Neal, Carpenter, 1995) (see Chapter 2).

Low concentrations of the lipid soluble amide-type local anesthetics bupivacaine (Marcaine) (0.0625-0.125%) and ropivacaine (Naropin) (0.2%) are used most often for epidural analgesia. Compared with other local anesthetics, these are better able to block nerve fibers that carry pain with minimal effect on sensory and motor fibers ("differential sensory and motor blockade") (Covino, Wildsmith, 1998; Gianino, York, Paice, 1996). Bupivacaine and ropivacaine are moderate to fast acting (onset within 5 to 20 minutes) and have a long duration of action (bupivacaine epidural block up to 12 hours; ropivacaine has a slightly shorter duration) (Covino, Wildsmith, 1998). Ropivacaine appears to have less CNS and cardiac toxicity than equipotent doses of bupivacaine (Covino, Wildsmith, 1998; Scott, Emanuelsson, Mooney et al., 1997).

For spinal anesthesia and analgesia, bupivacaine, lidocaine, and mepivacaine are administered most often. Local anesthetics administered intrathecally act faster than when administered epidurally because they are delivered in the immediate vicinity of the spinal cord; because such minute amounts are used when drugs are administered intrathecally, they also have a shorter duration of action (Covino, Wildsmith, 1998).

Bupivacaine, lidocaine, and tetracaine have been administered by implanted intrathecal pump (Gianino, York, Paice, 1996). Concern has been raised about lidocaine's inherently higher potential for intrathecal neurotoxicity (Liu, 1998). However, there appear to be multiple factors involved in producing intraspinal neurotoxicity, and this complication warrants further research.

Action of intraspinal local anesthetics. The sites of action of intraspinal local anesthetics are in the spinal cord and at the level of the spinal nerve roots (Cousins, Bromage, 1998). Intraspinal local anesthetics decrease the influx of sodium and efflux of potassium at the neuron level, thereby blocking the generation and the conduction of nerve impulses and slowing or stopping pain transmission (Gianino, York, Paice, 1996). They also may inhibit the release of substance P by inhibiting calcium channels (Liu, 1998).

The size of a nerve fiber influences its sensitivity to local anesthetics. There are three categories of nerve fibers: (1) A fibers are myelinated somatic nerves, (2) B fibers are myelinated autonomic nerves, and (3) C fibers are unmyelinated nerves. A fibers are further divided into alpha, beta, gamma, and delta fibers. The smallest of the A fibers are in the fast-conducting delta (δ) group. The B and C fibers also are small in diameter. Fortunately, the smaller diameter Aδ and C nerve fibers carry pain impulses. This is fortuitous because local anesthetics block nerve conduction in small nerve fibers faster and at lower concentrations than in large fibers. Therefore it is possible to give very low doses intraspinally to block the impulses on the Aδ and C fibers without blocking the larger fibers that dramatically affect sensory and motor function (Gianino, York, Paice, 1996; Paice, Williams, 1995).

Epidural local anesthetics are carried in the CSF to the dorsal root ganglion of the spinal nerve fibers immediately adjacent to their site of administration. This accounts for their rapid onset of action, especially by the

intrathecal route (Covino, Wildsmith, 1998). The catheter is placed as close as possible to the dermatomes that, when blocked, will produce the most effective spread of analgesia for the site of nociceptive input (e.g., surgical site, site of injury, tumor location) (Broekema, Gielen, Hennis, 1996; Lubenow, 1992; Sinatra, 1998).

Absorption, distribution, and clearance of intraspinal local anesthetics. Bupivacaine and ropivacaine plasma concentrations increase and eventually plateau with continuous epidural infusion (Emanuelsson, Zaric, Nydahl, 1995). The larger the total dose of local anesthetic injected, the higher the blood level of local anesthetic. Local tissue binding also affects local anesthetic absorption. Because both bupivacaine and ropivacaine have high lipid solubility, they tend to bind to fat within the epidural space, resulting in fewer free drug molecules to diffuse into the vascular space than less lipid soluble local anesthetics.

Once in the blood, bupivacaine and ropivacaine are widely distributed to highly perfused organs; first to the lungs, then the heart, brain, liver, kidney, uterus (all local anesthetics cross the placenta). Lesser amounts are simultaneously distributed to muscle, fat, and connective tissue (Woods, DiFazio, 1995).

Bupivacaine and ropivacaine are metabolized primarily by the liver, so hepatic blood flow and function make an impact on their rates of metabolism. Because only a small amount is cleared by the kidneys, renal function has minimal impact on the use of these local anesthetics (Woods, DiFazio, 1995). The half-life of epidural bupivacaine and ropivacaine is approximately 5 hours and 3 hours, respectively (Emanuelsson, Zaric, Nydahl, 1995).

Adverse reactions. Allergy to local anesthetics is uncommon, and the doses of local anesthetic used for intraspinal analgesia rarely result in blood concentrations sufficient to cause systemic effects. However, vascular uptake or injection or infusion of local anesthetic directly into the systemic circulation can result in adverse reactions related to high blood levels of local anesthetic. CNS signs of systemic toxicity include ringing in ears, metallic taste, slow speech, irritability, twitching, and seizures. Signs of cardiotoxicity include circumoral tingling and numbness, bradycardia, cardiac dysrhythmias, acidosis, and cardiovascular collapse.

Unwanted local anesthetic effects. The goal of adding low-dose local anesthetics to epidural opioids for pain management is to provide analgesia, not to produce anesthesia. Patients should be able to ambulate if their condition allows, and epidural analgesia should not hamper this important recovery activity. However, many factors, including location of the epidural catheter, local anesthetic dose, and variability in patient response, can result in patients experiencing motor and sensory deficits and other unwanted local anesthetic effects.

Because epidural local anesthetics produce a sympathetic blockade, vasodilation occurs. Minor hypotension, including orthostatic hypotension, is relatively common. Studies show that thoracic placement of epidural catheters for administration of local anesthetics is associated with less sympathetic block of the lower extremities than lumbar-placed catheters and may reduce complications resulting from postoperative epidural analgesia with local anesthetics, such as difficulty ambulating, urinary retention, and orthostatic hypotension (Liu, Carpenter, Neal, 1995). Thoracic, rather than lumbar, epidural administration of local anesthetics is recommended, especially when early postoperative ambulation is expected to be a priority (Wiebalck, Brodner, Van Aken, 1997).

Unwanted local anesthetic effects often can be corrected with simple treatment. For example, hypotension frequently is corrected with hydration, and a change in position may relieve temporary sensory loss in an extremity. Treatment of urinary retention and minor extremity weakness usually includes decreasing the epidural infusion rate slightly. Patients are asked to remain in bed until muscle weakness resolves. A nonopioid can be given ATC to provide additional pain relief while the epidural analgesic is decreased.

Sometimes removing the local anesthetic from the analgesic solution is necessary, such as when signs of local anesthetic toxicity are detected or simple treatment of hypotension or motor and sensory deficits has been unsuccessful. In any case, care of the patient receiving epidural analgesia includes taking safety precautions and reporting all unwanted effects of epidural local anesthetics to an anesthesiologist. Table 6.11 describes the assessment of some of the effects of epidural local anesthetics.

Clonidine

Clonidine is an alpha₂-agonist commonly used to treat chronic neuropathic pain. It is also useful for acute pain (see also Chapter 7). Clonidine is thought to produce analgesia by binding to alpha₂-receptors located in the dorsal horn near the location of opioid receptors. Here it inhibits substance P, thereby blocking the generation of an action potential (Coyle, Cherny, Portenoy, 1995).

When added to epidural local anesthetics, clonidine can prolong and intensify anesthesia; it acts synergistically when combined with epidural opioids, allowing a lower dose of opioid with correspondingly fewer side effects (Eisenach, De Kock, Klimscha, 1996). Coadministration of clonidine with meperidine intrathecally was found to enhance the duration and degree of meperidine spinal anesthesia and prolong the duration of postoperative analgesia (Acalovschi, Bodolea, Manoiu, 1997). Increased sedation and a tendency toward bradycardia and a decrease in mean arterial pressure in patients in this study were thought to be potentiated by the clonidine.

The perioperative course of more than 200 patients who underwent coronary artery bypass surgery over a 9-month period were studied retrospectively (Turfrey, Sutcliffe, Ray et al., 1997). All patients received general anesthesia maintained with propofol and alfentanil. Half of the patients continued with the alfentanil infusion after surgery until they were able to use IV PCA alfentanil. After 24 hours, this was changed to IV PCA morphine of 1 mg boluses with a delay interval of 5 minutes and no basal rate (group 1). The other half of the patients in this study received a thoracic epidural anesthesia block with 0.5% bupivacaine followed by a continuous infusion of bupivacaine, 0.125%, and clonidine, 0.6 μg/ml, during and after surgery (group 2). The infusion rate was adjusted to maintain a block between the first and second thoracic dermatomes after surgery. New dysrhythmias occurred in 32% of the patients in group 1 compared with 18% in group 2. A trend toward reduced incidence of respiratory complications was noted in group 2. The time to tracheal extubation was decreased in group 2, with 21% of the patients being extubated immediately after surgery compared with 2% of patients in group 1 being extubated immediately after surgery. No neurologic problems resulted from the use of thoracic epidural analgesia in this study.

The use of epidural clonidine as the sole analgesic agent during and after major abdominal surgery was studied for analgesic potency (De Kock, Wiederkher, Laghmiche et al., 1997). Patients were given clonidine epidurally with an initial dose of either 2 μg/kg followed by an infusion of 0.5 μg/kg per hour (group 1; n = 10), or 4 μg/kg followed by an infusion of 1 μg/kg per hour (group 2; n = 20), or 8 μg/kg followed by an infusion of 2 μg/kg per hour (group 3; n = 20). All patients were given general anesthesia with propofol concomitantly with the epidural clonidine infusion during surgery. The epidural clonidine infusions were continued for the study period of 12 hours after surgery. A high number of patients (26%) were withdrawn during surgery (most from groups 1 and 2), which the authors attribute to the strict criteria assigned for adequate anesthesia. During the first 12 hours after surgery, epidural clonidine was the only analgesic agent required by only four patients, all in group 3. The authors caution that the high number of patients removed from this study limits the value of statistical analysis, but that the results show that epidural clonidine provided dose-dependent control of hypertension and tachycardia during surgery and dose-dependent postoperative analgesia without major side effects.

Because clonidine is not an opioid, it does not produce respiratory depression, nausea, or pruritus (Eisenach, De Kock, Klimscha, 1996). As mentioned, sedation can occur with clonidine, although less by the intraspinal routes than by the IV route (Bernard, Kick, Bonnet, 1995). Other side effects include dry mouth, bradycardia, and hypotension. These appear to be minimized when clonidine is given in low doses and by continuous infusion rather than bolus dosing (Rockemann, Seeling,

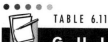

TABLE 6.11

G U I D E L I N E S

ASSESSMENT OF UNWANTED EFFECTS OF EPIDURAL LOCAL ANESTHETICS

Unwanted Effect	Cause and Comments	Assessment	What to Report
Sensory and/or motor deficit	Many factors, including vertebral location of the epidural catheter, local anesthetic dose, and variability in patient response, can result in patients experiencing unwanted sensory and/or motor deficit. The lower the level of intraspinal catheter placement, the lower the affected dermatome.	Sensory deficit: Every shift, ask patients to point to numb and tingling skin areas (numbness and tingling at the incision site is common and usually normal). Motor deficit: Every shift, ask patients to bend their knees and lift the buttocks off the mattress. Most are able to do this without difficulty. Determine patients' ability to bear weight and ambulate. Ask patients to remain in bed if they are unable to bear weight. Provide assisted ambulation PRN.	• Complete loss of sensation in a skin area • Muscle weakness, inability to move extremities or bear weight • Numbness and tingling in areas distant to the nociceptive site • Changes in sensory or motor deficit from last assessment (e.g., a lower location or increased intensity) • Unresolved deficits after changes in therapy have been made
Urinary retention	Epidural analgesics are delivered close to the micturation center, located in the lower segments of the spinal cord. The combination of epidural local anesthetics and opioids can cause relaxation of the detrusor muscle. An opioid-induced increase in sphincter tone can make urination difficult. The central effects of opioids and motor and sensory blockade can interfere with perception of bladder fullness and the patient's attention to bladder stimuli.	Regularly assess for bladder distention; in and out or Foley catheterization if needed.	• Persistent urinary retention
Local anesthetic toxicity	Toxicity can result from vascular uptake or injection or infusion of local anesthetic directly into the systemic circulation. Elderly patients may be at higher risk for toxicity from accumulation because most have a decreased ability to clear local anesthetics.	Every shift, assess for and ask patients about signs of local anesthetic toxicity: circumoral tingling and numbness, ringing in ears, metallic taste, slow speech, irritability, twitching, seizures, cardiac dysrhythmias. Stop local anesthetic administration if signs are present.	• Signs of local anesthetic toxicity

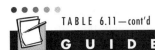

TABLE 6.11—cont'd

GUIDELINES

ASSESSMENT OF UNWANTED EFFECTS OF EPIDURAL LOCAL ANESTHETICS

Unwanted Effect	Cause and Comments	Assessment	What to Report
Adverse hemo-dynamic effects	Because local anesthetics block nerve fibers, they affect the sympathetic nervous system and cause vasodilation. Mild hypotension is common. Some patients receiving intraspinal local anesthetics experience significant hypotension and bradycardia, especially when rising from a prone position or after large dose increases or boluses. Thoracic placement of the epidural catheter is associated with fewer hemodynamic disturbances.	Regular assessment of HR and BP, including orthostatic blood pressure before ambulation until dose is stabilized and it is clear that bradycardia and hypotension are not problems.	• Symptomatic hypotension and/or bradycardia • Persistent hypotension and/or bradycardia • Symptomatic orthostatic hypotension

Epidural local anesthetics can produce some unwanted effects. Table 6.11 lists the causes of some of these effects, as well as how to assess and when to report them. *BP,* blood pressure; *HR,* heart rate.

Information from de Leon-Casasola OA, Lema MJ: Postoperative epidural opioid analgesia: What are the choices? *Anesth Analg* 83:867-875, 1996; Gianino JM, York MM, Paice JA: *Intrathecal drug therapy for spasticity and pain,* New York, 1996, Springer; Liu SS: Local anesthetics and analgesia. In Ashburn MA, Rice LJ, editors: *The management of pain,* pp 141-169, New York, 1998, Churchill Livingstone; Liu SS, Carpenter RL, Neal J: Epidural anesthesia and analgesia, *Anesthesiology* 82:1474-1506, 1995; Paice JA, Williams AR: Intraspinal drugs for pain. In McGuire D, Yarbro CH, Ferrell BR, editors: *Cancer pain management,* ed 2, pp 131-158, Boston, 1995, Jones and Bartlett Publishers.

Duschek et al., 1997). Regular assessment of sedation, blood pressure, and pulse is warranted when clonidine is administered by any route (see Chapter 7 and Box 7.2 on pp. 313-315 for guidelines on clonidine use for chronic pain).

Combined Spinal-Epidural Anesthesia (CSEA)

"Combined spinal-epidural anesthesia" (CSEA) for labor and delivery, during cesarean section, after cesarean section, and other postoperative pain relief is used primarily to minimize the shortcomings of both intrathecal and epidural analgesia while taking advantage of their benefits (Cousins, Veering, 1998). CSEA involves placing an epidural needle (typically, 16- or 18-gauge Touhy) into the epidural space then passing a much smaller gauge and longer spinal needle (e.g., 29-gauge Quincke needle) through the epidural needle into the subarachnoid space. Subarachnoid placement is confirmed by aspiration of CSF. Opioid or local anesthetic is injected into the subarachnoid space, producing rapid and profound analgesia. The subarachnoid needle is removed and an epidural catheter is inserted to administer supplemental anesthetic doses as needed during surgery to prolong the block, or supplemental analgesic doses during labor, or to provide analgesia after cesarean section (Cousins, Veering, 1998; Gautier, Debry, Fanard et al., 1997).

A major concern about the CSEA technique is inadvertent passage of the epidural catheter through the hole in the dura made by the spinal needle and the possibility of extensive subarachnoid effects from epidurally injected local anesthetics. Precautions such as use of fine-gauge spinal needles and routine aspiration and test dose administration are recommended (Brownridge, Cohen, Ward, 1998; Cousins, Veering, 1998). Further clinical use of this method to perfect materials and technique is warranted.

Because the CSEA technique uses the intrathecal route to use lower doses of local anesthetic for laboring patients, less motor block is produced. The epidural route is used for supplemental boluses. With appropriate assessment, CSEA has allowed patients to safely and comfortably ambulate during labor (Brownridge, Cohen, Ward, 1998; Gautier, Debry, Fanard et al., 1997).

Complications Associated With the Intraspinal Routes of Administration

Although extremely effective routes for administering analgesics, the epidural and intrathecal routes are not without potential for complications. These include postdural puncture headache, intraspinal catheter migration, and neurologic complications from trauma to neural tissue, injection or infusion of neurotoxic agents, infection, and hematoma.

Dural Puncture

Obviously the dura is punctured when intrathecal analgesia is administered. Very small gauge needles and microcatheters (e.g., 32-gauge) are used to help prevent postdural puncture headache (PDPH) after intrathecal analgesia (Chadwick, Bonica, 1995). Inadvertent dural puncture, often referred to as "wet tap," can occur during placement of an epidural catheter. It is the most common complication from epidural catheter placement with an incidence between 0.61% and 10.9% (Mulroy, Norris, Liu, 1997), most often in young women (Chadwick, Bonica, 1995). The anesthesiologist usually knows when a dural puncture has occurred and will attempt needle placement at a higher vertebral interspace.

In some patients a dural puncture poses no problems. However, in many patients, the leakage of CSF through the hole created in the dura causes a dull, aching, or throbbing headache. The headache may be frontal, occipital, or diffuse in location. It usually is moderate to severe in intensity and may be accompanied by neck stiffness, photophobia, visual disturbances, nausea, and vomiting. Patients routinely report that the headache worsens when they move into a sitting or standing position and improves when they lie down (Chadwick, Bonica, 1995).

After a dural puncture, the anesthesiologist usually alerts the staff to assess the patient for headache. Sometimes the headache appears during epidural analgesia after a decrease in the epidural continuous infusion rate or when the epidural catheter is removed. Most commonly, the headache occurs 1 to 5 days after the dural puncture and persists for 3 to 5 days. On rare occasions, a PDPH lasts for months (Chadwick, Bonica, 1995).

Treatment of PDPH usually is symptomatic and conservative, consisting of administering oral opioid and nonopioid analgesics and reassuring the patient that the headache will most likely resolve within a week. Concentrated CSF can worsen symptoms, so to foster production of CSF, fluid intake is encouraged. Some clinicians use caffeine, which is thought to relieve symptoms by producing cerebral vasoconstriction (Chadwick, Bonica, 1995).

Blood patch.

The most effective and aggressive treatment of PDPH is to stop the leakage of CSF by injecting the patient's blood (typically 10 to 15 ml drawn from the antecubital vein) into the epidural space (Chadwick, Bonica, 1995). This is called a "blood patch" and works similar to plugging a hole with a cork. Results are dramatic with almost immediate headache relief in 95% of patients undergoing blood patch. Patients may report a minor backache after the injection of blood into the epidural space. Complications from this procedure are very rare and include epidural infection and nerve root compression (Chadwick, Bonica, 1995).

Injecting Dextran 40 in saline (Rheomacrodex) epidurally, rather than blood, may be an alternative treatment for PDPH. In Sweden, a patient was treated with Dextran 40 when a PDPH persisted despite two consecutive blood patches (Reynvoet, Cosaert, Desmet et al., 1997). Symptoms were relieved after 25 ml of Dextran 40 was injected into the epidural space and followed by a 3 ml/h infusion of Dextran 40 in saline through an epidural catheter. Informed consent is recommended because Dextran 40 in saline is not approved for epidural administration.

Another novel treatment for PDPH is the IV infusion of adenocorticotropic hormone (ACTH). Patients with PDPH unresponsive to conservative treatment were given a single IV infusion of ACTH, 1.5 units/kg in 250 ml normal saline over a 30-minute period (Kshatri, Foster, 1997). Headache resolved within 2 to 6 hours. The exact mechanism of action of ACTH in patients with PDPH is unknown, but it is thought to result from its adrenal (release of hormones) or extraadrenal (metabolic) physiologic actions.

Catheter Displacement

Displacement of temporary catheters during analgesic therapy is a relatively common occurrence and often caused by patients accidentally pulling catheters out during activity. Proper taping of the catheter and teaching patients to avoid tugging on the catheter helps to minimize the incidence of displacement. Catheter displacement of permanent catheters used for chronic pain is reported to be approximately 7% (Bedder, 1996) (see Box 6.16 and p. 248 for checking for optimal epidural catheter location).

Catheter Migration

Catheter migration can occur at any time during epidural analgesia therapy and despite correct catheter placement. Epidural catheters can migrate out of the epidural space through the dura into the subarachnoid space or into the vascular system through an epidural blood vessel. The incidence of intrathecal migration during epidural analgesia therapy is 0.26% to 0.6%. The reported incidence of vessel entry, which includes those occurring during placement and during therapy is 0.2% to 11% (Mulroy, Norris, Liu, 1997).

Early signs of epidural catheter migration during continuous infusion or PCEA are likely to be subtle and noted most often by a change in the patient's pain control or side effects since the last assessment. Signs and symptoms of epidural catheter migration are more pro-

BOX 6.16 Intraspinal Catheter Displacement and Migration

Immediately report any of the following to an anesthesiologist:

INDICATIONS OF A DISPLACED
INTRATHECAL CATHETER
• Inadequate pain relief (e.g., a previously comfortable patient reports loss of pain control).
• No pain reduction with increase in opioid dose.
⇒ Confirmed by no CSF aspirant from catheter.

INDICATIONS OF A DISPLACED EPIDURAL CATHETER
• Inadequate pain relief (e.g., a previously comfortable patient reports loss of pain control).
• No pain reduction with increase in opioid dose.

INDICATIONS OF AN INTRATHECAL MIGRATION OF
AN EPIDURAL CATHETER
• Unexplained increase in opioid-induced side effects (e.g., a previously alert patient is excessively sedated or nauseated).
• Sensory and/or motor block (possible if solution contains local anesthetics).
⇒ Confirmed by aspiration of CSF from epidural catheter.

INDICATIONS OF AN INTRAVASCULAR MIGRATION
• Inadequate pain relief (e.g., a previously comfortable patient reports loss of pain control).
• Unexplained increase in opioid-induced side effects (e.g., a previously alert patient is sedated or nauseated [increase in side effects is possible even though the patient is being underdosed after intravascular migration because the opioid is being delivered systemically]).
• Signs and symptoms of local anesthetic toxicity (e.g., metallic taste, ringing ears, circumoral numbness, slow speech, irritability [possible if solution contains local anesthetics]).
⇒ Confirmed by aspiration of free-flowing blood from catheter.

May be duplicated for use in clinical practice. From McCaffery M, Pasero C: *Pain: Clinical manual,* p. 233. Copyright © 1999, Mosby, Inc.

Displacement of temporary intraspinal catheters during analgesic therapy is a common occurrence and often caused by patients accidentally pulling them out. Catheter migration can occur at any time during epidural analgesia therapy and despite correct catheter placement. Epidural catheters can migrate out of the epidural space through the dura into the subarachnoid space or into the vascular system through an epidural blood vessel. Box 6.16 provides indications of intraspinal catheter displacement and migration.

CSF, cerebrospinal fluid

Information from Pasero C: *Acute pain management service policy and procedure manual.* Rolling Hills Estates, CA, 1994, Academy Medical Systems, Inc.

nounced when analgesia is administered by the bolus method (Box 6.16).

Patient Example

Mr. E. had a nephrectomy yesterday morning and is receiving a continuous epidural infusion of morphine and bupivacaine for his postoperative pain. During previous assessments, Mr. E. has been alert, comfortable with a pain rating no higher than 4 on a scale of 0 to 10, and ambulating without assistance. This time, Mr. E. rates his pain as 0. He is oriented but very drowsy with a respiratory rate of 18 breaths/min. The nurse knows that the only sedating medication Mr. E. is receiving is the epidural morphine, and Mr. E. confirms that he has taken only the medications the nurse has given him. The nurse checks the epidural infusion pump and finds it is programmed correctly and functioning properly. Mr. E. tells the nurse that he cannot ambulate because his "legs are numb." The nurse suspects the epidural catheter has migrated into the subarachnoid space. (Intrathecal infusion of an epidural dose of opioid would explain the change in Mr. E.'s sedation level, and intrathecal infusion of an epidural dose of bupivacaine would explain Mr. E's report of lower extremity sensory loss.) The nurse stops the epidural infusion and takes Mr. E.'s blood pressure, which is 120/70, only slightly lower than his baseline. The nurse assigns a nursing assistant to stay with Mr. E. and take vital signs every 5 minutes (the high dose of opioid could cause respiratory depression and the high dose of bupivacaine could cause adverse hemodynamic effects) while she notifies an anesthesiologist. The anesthesiologist easily aspirates 5 ml CSF from the catheter confirming that it is in the subarachnoid space. The catheter is removed, and Mr. E. recovers without difficulty.

Direct Needle or Catheter Trauma

Trauma to neural tissue from intraspinal needles and catheters is extremely rare. Nerve root trauma usually is indicated by patient reports of pain that is severe, sharp, and radiating along a nerve when the needle is placed. Trauma from the indwelling intraspinal catheter is more common with long-term intraspinal analgesic treatment for chronic pain than with short-term intraspinal analgesia for acute pain management. For example, tissue fibrosis around the indwelling epidural catheter tip can occur with long-term use. This can lead to spinal cord compression producing neurologic impairment of varying degrees (Chadwick, Bonica, 1995). Tissue fibrosis rarely occurs in intrathecal catheters (Bedder, 1996).

Injection or Infusion of Neurotoxic Agents

A number of agents can cause intraspinal neurotoxicity. Preservatives and antitoxins, including alcohol, phenol, formaldehyde, and sodium metabisulfite, are toxic to the CNS (Paice, Williams, 1995). High concentrations of local anesthetics also can cause neurotoxicity (Chadwick, Bonica, 1995). Other agents that have resulted in significant neurologic damage after accidental epidural infusion include antibiotics, potassium chloride, and total parenteral nutrition (Paice, Williams, 1995). All agents and solutions injected or infused intraspinally must be sterile, preservative-free, and regarded safe for intraspinal administration (Box 6.17).

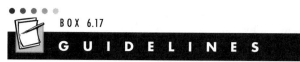

• • • • •

BOX 6.17

GUIDELINES

PREVENTION OF INTRASPINAL NEUROTOXICITY

The following measures may be helpful in preventing inadvertent intraspinal injection or infusion of neurotoxic agents:

- Do not use agents from a multiple-dose vial; it is wise to assume that all multiple-dose vials contain preservatives.
- Use only nonneurotoxic agents to disinfect intraspinal catheter connections and ports (e.g., alcohol often is used to cleanse skin of secretions, but should not be used to disinfect catheter connections or ports).
- Boldly label indwelling epidural catheters used for intermittent analgesic bolusing.
- Avoid using infusion lines with injection ports for epidural analgesia; if such tubing must be used, tape over every injection port.
- Use color-coded infusion lines made specifically for epidural analgesia.
- Label infusion lines when patients have several.
- Double check the labels of epidural analgesia drug reservoirs for wording that indicates the solution is both preservative-free and prepared for intraspinal use.
- Return to the pharmacy drug reservoirs and agents that are unclearly labeled, cloudy, or contain particulate matter.

May be duplicated for use in clinical practice. From McCaffery M, Pasero C: *Pain: Clinical manual,* p. 234. Copyright © 1999, Mosby, Inc.

Neurologic complications can result from injection or infusion of neurotoxic agents. Box 6.17 lists precautions that can be taken to prevent this from happening.

Infection

A very rare (<0.0015%) but serious complication of intraspinal analgesia is infection in the epidural space (Chadwick, Bonica, 1995). Formation of an intraspinal abscess can cause spinal cord compression or sepsis and, in extreme cases, paralysis. Intraspinal infection is thought to be more common when intraspinal catheters are left in place for a prolonged time, such as to treat chronic pain (Chadwick, Bonica, 1995). The incidence of infection with externalized tunneled epidural systems may be higher than with totally implanted drug delivery systems (DuPen, DuPen, 1998). Theoretically, the risk of meningitis is less with epidural catheterization than intrathecal catheterization (Bedder, 1996).

Causes of intraspinal infection include spontaneous infection, hematogenous spread during episodes of bacteremia, and infection as a result of poor aseptic technique. Localized skin infection at the intraspinal needle or catheter entry site also can occur. This can result in infection tracking down the catheter from the skin entry site to the epidural or intrathecal space. Contamination of the intrathecal or epidural system can occur during drug reservoir preparation, catheter placement, refilling

implanted reservoirs, or administration of the analgesic. When an external infusion pump is used to deliver intraspinal analgesia, contamination can occur while loading the pump, connecting the catheter to the infusion tubing, or changing the drug reservoir.

Early signs and symptoms of an intraspinal infection can be difficult to detect. Skin site infection and fever are not always present (DuPen, DuPen, 1998). The cardinal signs of intraspinal infection are increasing diffuse back pain or tenderness and/or pain and/or paresthesia on intraspinal injection. Bowel and/or bladder dysfunction may also be present.

Although practice varies, intraspinal catheters usually are removed when signs of infection are detected and the catheter tip cultured. (To decrease the risk of hematogenous spread to the subarachnoid or epidural space, anesthesiologists also usually remove intraspinal catheters when infection occurs outside the intrathecal or epidural space.) Removal of implanted catheter systems sometimes can be avoided when superficial infections are treated early and aggressively with local wound care and antibiotics (DuPen, DuPen, 1998).

Intraspinal infection is confirmed by magnetic resonance imaging (MRI) or computed tomography (CT). Usually a neurology or neurosurgery consultation is requested. Treatment of a confirmed intraspinal abscess ranges from antibiotics to surgical removal of the abscess.

Certain precautions to prevent intraspinal infection and regular assessment for signs of infection are necessary in patients who receive a single intraspinal analgesic bolus or are receiving continuous intraspinal analgesia or PCEA (Box 6.18).

Epidural Hematoma

Puncture of epidural blood vessels during intraspinal needle or catheter placement occurs in approximately 3% to 12% of patients. These rarely cause problems. However, epidural hematoma can occur as a result of this trauma or spontaneously in patients taking anticoagulants and in those with blood clotting disorders (Chadwick, Bonica, 1995). Symptomatic epidural hematomas are extremely rare; the exact incidence is unknown (Liu, Carpenter, Neal, 1995).

Like epidural infection, early detection of epidural hematoma is difficult because symptoms often are obscure. Patients may report inadequate or uneven (better on one side than the other) pain relief. The cardinal signs of epidural hematoma are increasing diffuse back pain or tenderness and/or pain and/or paresthesia on epidural injection. Bowel and/or bladder dysfunction may also be present. As the hematoma increases in size, sensory or motor deficit may develop. Although paraplegia is extremely rare with intraspinal analgesia, when it does occur, it is most often caused by epidural hematoma (Liu, Carpenter, Neal, 1995).

Epidural hematoma is confirmed by MRI or CT, and a neurology or neurosurgery consultation is requested.

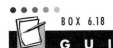

BOX 6.18

GUIDELINES

PREVENTION OF INTRASPINAL INFECTION

- Minimize the number of times the intraspinal infusion system is entered (e.g., limit frequent and unnecessary drug reservoir changes).
- Use strict aseptic technique when handling supplies used for intraspinal catheter placement and when connecting drug reservoir to infusion tubing, administering supplemental boluses, and refilling reservoirs. (Use only nonneurotoxic agents to disinfect intraspinal catheter connections or ports [e.g., alcohol often is used to cleanse skin of secretions, but should not be used to disinfect catheter connections or ports].)
- Report intraspinal system disconnects immediately to anesthesiologist:
⇒ Wrap the free end of the epidural catheter with a sterile 4 × 4 and contact the anesthesiologist who will determine whether the catheter is to be removed or repaired and the infusion continued.
⇒ Obtain a physician's order for interim analgesia.
- Regularly assess intraspinal catheter entry site, implanted port, or pump site (usually as often as IV sites are assessed).
- Monitor patient's temperature (usually q4h).
- Immediately report to an anesthesiologist signs and symptoms of infection, including infection thought to be unrelated to intraspinal catheterization (e.g., wound, urinary, and pulmonary infections).
- Immediately report unexplained changes in sensory and/or motor deficit since last assessment, particularly

increases in spite of decreases in the analgesic infusion rate.

Signs and Symptoms of Infection
Skin infection at intraspinal catheter entry site, implanted port, or pump site
- Inflammation, edema, drainage, warmth at intraspinal catheter entry site, implanted port or pump site.
- Patient reports soreness around intraspinal catheter entry site, implanted port, or pump site.

Epidural or intrathecal space infection
- Patient reports constant diffuse back pain or tenderness.
- Patient reports pain and/or paresthesia during bolus injection.
- Inadequate pain relief.
- Sensory and/or motor deficit (particularly unexplained changes since last assessment).
- Skin infection of intraspinal catheter entry site may or may not be present.
- Fever may or may not be present.

Signs of Acute Bacterial Infection
- Fever
- Headache
- Nuchal rigidity
- Brudzinski's and Kernig's signs
- Altered mental status
- Convulsions

May be duplicated for use in clinical practice. From McCaffery M, Pasero C: *Pain: Clinical manual*, p. 235. Copyright © 1999, Mosby, Inc.

Intraspinal infection is rare, and early signs and symptoms can be difficult to detect. Box 6.18 lists the signs and symptoms of intraspinal infection and precautions that can be taken to prevent intraspinal infection in patients who receive intraspinal analgesia.

h, hour; *q*, every.

Information from Pasero C: *Acute pain management service policy and procedure manual*, Rolling Hills Estates, CA, 1994, Academy Medical Systems.

Epidural hematomas usually are treated by immediate surgical removal of the hematoma (Chadwick, Bonica, 1995).

As with intraspinal infection, patient recovery without neurologic injury depends on early recognition and aggressive treatment. Regular patient assessment and reporting to an anesthesiologist abnormal blood clotting studies and physicians' orders for anticoagulants before and during intraspinal analgesia may help to prevent epidural hematoma (see also Box 6.19).

Patient Example

Mrs. U. has been receiving a continuous epidural infusion of fentanyl and bupivacaine for the last 36 hours for her postoperative hysterectomy pain. Her epidural site is clean and dry without edema, redness, or drainage. Mrs. U. says that the area around the epidural site in her back is "tender."

She also reports numbness and tingling of her thighs. She has been afebrile and all of her vital signs have been stable since surgery. Her pain rating is 2 on a scale of 0 to 10. Mrs. U.'s nurse knows that early signs of an epidural abscess or hematoma often are subtle. The cardinal sign of both of these complications is diffuse back pain or tenderness. Although lumbar epidural administration of bupivacaine can cause temporary numbness and tingling of the lower extremities, they could be signs of neurocompression caused by an epidural abscess or hematoma. The nurse asks an anesthesiologist to assess Mrs. U. as soon as possible. The anesthesiologist's examination is negative. Mrs. U.'s back tenderness resolves without treatment and her thigh numbness and tingling resolves with a slight decrease in the epidural infusion rate.

BOX 6.19

GUIDELINES

REMOVAL OF SHORT-TERM EPIDURAL CATHETERS

Requirements of Nurse Removal of an Epidural Catheter

- Institutional policy and procedure that supports removal of epidural catheters by the registered nurse.
- Knowledge and skills necessary to remove an epidural catheter gained by completing institutional competency requirements.
- An anesthesiologist's order to remove the epidural catheter.

Considerations Before Removal of an Epidural Catheter

- If warranted (e.g., if patient is receiving or received anticoagulants during epidural therapy), blood clotting studies have been checked and abnormal findings reported to anesthesiologist.
- Signs of infection have been reported to anesthesiologist.
- Pain is under control.
- Adequate oral analgesia has been given to the patient who is receiving epidural analgesia from short duration opioid (e.g., fentanyl, sufentanil) so that pain control is maintained when epidural analgesia is discontinued.
- The procedure has been explained to the patient, including the oral analgesic regimen that will replace the epidural analgesia.

Considerations Related to Removing an Epidural Catheter

- Epidural catheters are considered hazardous waste so universal precautions are warranted.

- Removal of the epidural catheter is facilitated when the patient assumes a position similar to the one suggested for catheter placement (i.e., sitting or side-lying with the back arched out toward the nurse). This position helps to spread the vertebrae apart.
- Although gentle traction is necessary to remove the catheter, it should come out easily and painlessly. If resistance is met or the patient reports pain or unusual sensations (e.g., tingling or a "catch in the back"), the procedure is terminated and the anesthesiologist or pain nurse is notified.
- After the catheter is removed, the catheter tip is checked for the presence of a black or blue mark. This indicates that the catheter was removed intact. If the tip has no mark, the anesthesiologist is notified.
- After cleaning the entry site and surrounding skin with the institution's recommended solution (usually mild soap and water), some nurses cover the epidural catheter site with a Band-Aid, others leave it open to air.
- Signs of catheter entry site infection are reported to the anesthesiologist.
- Documentation includes patient tolerance of the procedure, presence of mark on catheter tip, condition of epidural catheter entry site and surrounding area, and specifics of a difficult or unusual removal.

May be duplicated for use in clinical practice. From McCaffery M, Pasero C: *Pain: Clinical manual*, p. 236. Copyright © 1999, Mosby, Inc.

Removing short-term epidural catheters is within the scope of practice for registered nurses in most states in the United States. Box 6.19 lists important steps and considerations regarding the removal of temporary epidural catheters.

cm, centimeter.

Information from Pasero C: *Acute pain management service policy and procedure manual*, Rolling Hills Estates, CA, 1994, Academy Medical Systems, Inc.

It is important to teach patients and families about what to expect during intraspinal analgesia therapy, including that the signs of intraspinal infection and hematoma can develop after the epidural catheter is removed and can occur even if the course of intraspinal analgesia was short and uneventful. They should be told to immediately report diffuse back pain or tenderness and signs of infection. They should know that it may be necessary to remind the primary physician that they received intraspinal analgesia during hospitalization as this sometimes is overlooked as a possible cause of symptoms.

Epidural Catheter Removal

Removing short-term epidural catheters is within the scope of practice for registered nurses in most states in the United States. Most state boards of nursing have approved this activity by registered nurses who possess the knowledge and skill to do so and where institutional policy and

procedure support it. The procedure for removing epidural catheters varies, but Box 6.19 lists important steps and considerations that can be generalized to all situations.

Special Considerations About the Use of Epidural Analgesia in Pediatric Patients

Improved technology, the increased use of epidural anesthesia and analgesia in adults, and high parental acceptance of regional techniques has led to an increased use of epidural analgesia in pediatric patients (Broadman, Rice, 1998). Epidural analgesia is used for pain management in children of all ages, from the premature infant to the adolescent, and for many types of surgery. Intrathecal analgesia is used infrequently in children and will not be discussed here.

It is important for clinicians and other caregivers to be familiar with the particulars of caring for children receiving epidural analgesia before providing this method of analgesic delivery. The same analgesics are administered epidurally to children as are administered to adults, and children are subject to the same side effects and complications related to epidural analgesia as adults. Following are dosing recommendations and comments about various aspects of care as they relate to infants and children receiving epidural analgesia.

Epidural Catheter Placement

As with other aspects of pediatric care, epidural needles and catheters should be placed by anesthesiologists who are experienced in performing these procedures in pediatric patients. It is important that the clinician understand the anatomic, physiologic, pharmacologic, and psychologic differences related to the child's size and stage of development. Meticulous attention to detail in selection and preparation of the site for epidural needle placement and careful aspiration before drug injection is critical in children (Broadman, Rice, 1998; Houck, 1998).

Epidural catheters often are placed in children after induction of general anesthesia; light sedation may be sufficient in older children. EMLA cream can be applied to the site 2 hours before needle placement to reduce the pain of needle insertion for subcutaneous local anesthetic infiltration before placing the epidural needle (Broadman, Rice, 1998).

Although epidural analgesia may be administered at any vertebral level, a lumbar or caudal approach is used most often in children. The depth of the epidural space increases as a child grows, which is a primary reason why caudal analgesia is used more often than lumbar epidural analgesia in infants and toddlers. Placement at the thoracic epidural level is more challenging than at the caudal and lumbar levels (Broadman, Rice, 1998) and usually is reserved for older children having upper abdominal and thoracic procedures (Houck, 1998).

Caudal analgesia has been used extensively in pediatric patients. It is popular because of the ease of needle placement, reliability, and safety of the technique (Broadman, Rice, 1998; Houck, 1998). It is easier to thread the catheter in the cephalad direction using a caudal approach, and there may be a reduced chance of causing direct damage to the spinal cord at this level in this age group (Broadman, Rice, 1998).

Caudal analgesia is ideal for lower body procedures. By threading the catheter rostrally or using larger doses of local anesthetic, the caudal approach can be used to provide analgesia also for procedures affecting higher dermatomes (e.g., sacral [S5] to thoracic [T10]) (Broadman, Rice, 1998; Houck, 1998).

Dressing and securing the caudal catheter.

Properly dressing and securing the caudal catheter is extremely important to reduce the possibility of the infant soiling the dressing and the active toddler inadvertently pulling the catheter out. One clear occlusive dressing can be placed below the catheter over the gluteal crease to prevent upward spread of urine and feces. A second clear occlusive dressing is placed on the upper edge of the first clear dressing and in such a fashion as to cover the catheter about 2.0 cm in all directions (Broadman, Rice, 1998).

Caregivers must inspect the epidural catheter dressing frequently (e.g., every 4 hours). The anesthesiologist should be notified if the dressing becomes excessively soiled or loosened. Loosened dressings can be reinforced with tape until the anesthesiologist can perform a dressing change.

Method of Delivery

All three methods of epidural analgesic delivery previously discussed (bolus, continuous infusion, patient-controlled epidural analgesia [PCEA]) are used in pediatric patients. Use of PCEA requires that the child understand the relationship between pain, pressing the PCEA button, and pain relief, and be physically able to administer a PCEA dose using the available equipment. It is extremely important to remind parents and caregivers not to press the PCEA button for the child unless they have been designated as the child's primary pain manager (see Box 6.4 on p. 177).

Analgesic Agents

As with adults, a combination of opioid and local anesthetic is customarily administered epidurally to infants and children. Typically, a mu agonist opioid, such as fentanyl, morphine, or hydromorphone (Dilaudid), is combined with subanesthetic doses of a local anesthetic without epinephrine, such as lidocaine (0.1% to 0.5%), bupivacaine (Marcaine) (0.0625% to 0.1%), or ropivacaine (Naropin) (0.05% to 0.1%). As discussed, combining analgesics produces a synergistic effect, resulting in improved analgesia at lower doses of each than would be possible with either analgesic alone. Lower doses reduce the incidence and severity of side effects. Box 6.20 provides pediatric epidural analgesia dosing guidelines.

Drug solubility and the location of the epidural catheter tip are important considerations in selecting the best opioid for epidural analgesia. When the tip of the epidural catheter is placed at the spinal levels innervating the site of injury (tumor location, surgical site), lipophilic opioids, such as fentanyl and sufentanil, are commonly used. However, when the surgery is extensive, covering many dermatomal levels, or when the catheter tip is placed at the lumbar or caudal level for upper abdominal or thoracic procedures, hydrophilic opioids, such as morphine and hydromorphone, are recommended because they are capable of spreading rostrally (Houck, 1998).

Side effects and complications.

Epidural analgesia can be administered safely outside of a monitored setting if the nursing staff is educated in observing and managing pediatric epidural analgesia (Houck, 1998). Children are subject to the same complications as adults, including epidural catheter migration, infection, and hematoma, and to the same opioid-induced side effects as adults, including constipation, nausea and vomiting, pruritus,

BOX 6.20

G U I D E L I N E S

PEDIATRIC EPIDURAL ANALGESIA DOSING[1]

Continuous Infusions

- Fentanyl, 2 μg/ml, and bupivacaine, 0.1%, at 0.15 to 0.2 ml/kg per hour for infants <6 mo.
- Fentanyl, 2 μg/ml, and bupivacaine, 0.1%, at 0.3 to 0.4 ml/kg per hour for children.
- Fentanyl, 1 μg/ml, and lidocaine, 0.3%, at 0.5 ml/kg per hour for children <20 kg.
- Fentanyl, 1.5 μg/ml, and lidocaine, 0.5%, at 0.3 ml/kg per hour for children >20 kg (maximum dose: 14 to 16 ml/h).
- Hydromorphone (Dilaudid), 10 μg/ml, and bupivacaine, 0.1%, at 0.05 to 0.1 ml/kg per hour for infants <6 mo.
- Hydromorphone (Dilaudid), 10 μg/ml, and bupivacaine, 0.1%, at 0.1 to 0.2 ml/kg per hour for children.
- Morphine, 20 μg/ml, and bupivacaine 0.1%, at 0.2 to 0.4 ml/kg per hour.
- Lidocaine, 0.1%, at 1 ml/kg per hour for infants <4 kg.

Patient-Controlled Epidural Analgesia (PCEA)

- Fentanyl, 2 μg/ml, and bupivacaine, 0.1%, at 0.2 ml/kg per hour basal rate (continuous infusion) and 0.1 ml PCEA dose every 15 to 30 min.
- Hydromorphone (Dilaudid), 10 μg/ml, and bupivacaine, 0.1%, at 0.2 ml/kg per hour basal rate (continuous infusion) and 0.1 ml PCEA dose every 15 to 30 min.
- Morphine, 20 μg/ml, and bupivacaine, 0.1%, at 0.2 ml/kg per hour basal rate (continuous infusion) and 0.1 ml PCEA dose every 15 to 30 min.

May be duplicated for use in clinical practice. From McCaffery M, Pasero C: *Pain: Clinical manual*, p. 238. Copyright © 1999, Mosby, Inc.

Box 6.20 provides dosing guidelines for continuous epidural analgesic infusions and PCEA.

h, hour; *μg,* microgram; *ml,* milliliter; *PCEA,* patient-controlled epidural analgesia.

[1] Dose required for analgesia will depend on vertebral location of the epidural catheter; lower doses are possible when opioids are administered close to the nociceptive site (e.g., surgical incision). This is especially true of the lipid-soluble opioids.

Information from Berde CB, Kain ZN: Pain management in infants and children. In Motoyama EK, Davis PJ, editors: *Smith's anesthesia for infants and children,* pp 385-402, St. Louis, 1996, Mosby; Yaster M, Andresini J, Krane EJ: Epidural analgesia. In Yaster M, Krane EJ, Kaplan RF et al., editors: *Pediatric pain management and sedation handbook,* pp 113-145, St. Louis, 1997, Mosby.

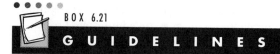

BOX 6.21

G U I D E L I N E S

CARE OF THE PEDIATRIC PATIENT RECEIVING EPIDURAL ANALGESIA

- Only physicians who are experienced in providing pediatric epidural analgesia should prescribe and supervise the care of infants and children receiving epidural analgesia.
- Ongoing didactic education should be provided to nurses regarding their role in monitoring and caring for infants and children receiving epidural analgesia.
- 24 h in-hospital anesthesia coverage should be available.
- The patient should be evaluated by the anesthesiologist or pain service at least daily.
- Level of sedation and respiratory rates and quality should be monitored and recorded every hour for at least the first 24 h postoperatively.
- Pain should be assessed q1-2h for at least the first 24 h.
- Heart rate and blood pressure should be recorded q4h.
- Infants <6 mo old having severe neurologic deficits, receiving hydrophilic opioids, or at an otherwise increased risk for respiratory depression should be placed on a cardiorespiratory monitor.
- Presence of sensory deficit and motor weakness should be determined q4h.
- Changes in vital signs and sensory deficit and/or motor weakness should be reported promptly to an anesthesiologist or a member of the pain service.
- In inactive children, position should be changed and skin assessed frequently for breakdown. Heels should be padded to prevent pressure necrosis.
- If their condition allows, children may ambulate during epidural analgesia. Ability to bear weight and walk should be confirmed before ambulation; assisted ambulation is required until the ability to ambulate independently is firmly established.
- Before administration, an anesthesiologist or a member of the pain service should approve the concurrent administration of any medications that produce sedation.

May be duplicated for use in clinical practice. From McCaffery M, Pasero C: *Pain: Clinical manual,* p. 238. Copyright © 1999, Mosby, Inc.

Box 6.21 lists guidelines and recommendations for caring for the pediatric patient receiving epidural analgesia.

Information from Houck CS: The management of acute pain in the child. In Ashburn MA, Rice LF, editors: *The management of pain,* ed 3, pp 651-666, New York, 1998, Churchill Livingstone.

sedation, and respiratory depression. Medications for the treatment of side effects should be prescribed and opioid doses decreased whenever possible to reduce or eliminate a side effect. Box 6.21 outlines important aspects of caring for children receiving epidural analgesia.

As discussed later in this chapter, nurse monitoring of sedation level and respiratory status is critical to preventing clinically significant opioid-induced respiratory de-

pression (see pp. 267-270). When excessive sedation is detected, epidural opioid doses must be decreased. Adding a nonopioid, such as acetaminophen, ibuprofen, or ketorolac, to the treatment plan may facilitate decreasing doses. Infants less than 6 months old are at higher risk than others for clinically significant opioid-induced respiratory depression (Pasero, McCaffery, 1994), and many clinicians recommend mechanical monitoring during epidural analgesia in this age group (see Box 6.21). Late respiratory depression from slow onset and rostral spread of large single bolus doses of hydrophilic opioids is a concern; however, when steady state is reached with small bolus doses and continuous infusion, late respiratory depression is uncommon (Gianino, York, Paice, 1996).

Severe pruritus from epidural analgesia can be a problem with children as they may excoriate their skin with excessive scratching. Although pruritis can occur with all epidural opioids, it is most common with morphine. Using hydromorphone, rather than morphine, when a hydrophilic opioid is indicated may be helpful in reducing the incidence and severity of pruritus (Houck, 1998). In addition, the child's nails should be short and smooth. An elbow restraint (or "welcome sleeve") can be used or the shirt sleeve can be pinned to cover the hands. Diphenhydramine (Benadryl) or hydroxyzine (Atarax) may be helpful in relieving symptoms; however, it is important to remember that these agents can produce sedation.

 Unwanted local anesthetic effects. Infants and young children may be frightened if they experience sensory deficit or motor weakness from the epidural local anesthetic. Assessment for these common and unwanted effects includes asking children if their legs feel heavy and if they can wiggle their toes and lift their legs off the bed or bend their knees and lift their buttocks off the bed. Sensory response can be assessed by tickling the bottom of the feet and asking children if they feel any numb or tingling areas on their skin. Ability to bear weight and walk is confirmed before ambulation; assisted ambulation is imperative until the ability to ambulate independently is firmly established. The presence of sensory deficit and/ or motor weakness should be reported promptly to an anesthesiologist or member of the pain service and is usually treated with a decrease in the epidural analgesic dose.

Regular skin assessment and care are warranted in children receiving epidural analgesia. Children who are inactive and too young to communicate sensory loss and motor weakness are at particularly high risk for skin breakdown and should be assessed frequently. Position should be changed often in these children. In the child with a cast, sensory deficit from epidural local anesthetics may make it difficult for the child to sense cast tightness; sometimes it is necessary to split the cast.

Bradycardia, hypotension, and orthostatic hypotension may occur with epidural local anesthetics. Heart rate and blood pressure should be assessed regularly and significant changes reported to an anesthesiologist.

Urinary retention is another unwanted side effect of both epidural opioids and local anesthetics. Often, reducing the analgesic dose can resolve urinary retention. However, urinary catheterization may be necessary (see Box 8.3 on p. 372 regarding atraumatic urinary catheterization).

It is a misconception that children are more resistant to systemic local anesthetic toxicity than adults. The metabolism of local anesthetics in neonates is greatly reduced. Children eliminate local anesthetics faster than neonates and infants, but slower than adults (Rice, 1996). The early CNS manifestations of local anesthetic toxicity discussed earlier in this chapter may not be apparent in children. The first signs of toxicity in children may be dysrhythmias or cardiovascular collapse (Broadman, Rice, 1998).

Selecting an Analgesic and Route of Administration

Using more than one opioid and route of administration to manage pain is confusing, costly, and usually not necessary. With some exceptions (see following discussion), the preferred opioids are mu agonists and the preferred route is oral. Of course, the fact that the oral route is preferred does not mean it is always possible or appropriate.

As a rule, treatment of moderate to severe cancer and chronic nonmalignant pain is started with just one analgesic at a time by one route of administration and only one analgesic at a time is added. For example, patients who have no contraindication to opioid therapy should not receive an adjuvant analgesic until opioid therapy has been optimized. When therapy is initiated with more than one drug, it is more difficult to determine the cause and therefore the management of adverse effects. A higher probability of additive toxicity also exists (Portenoy, 1997).

Occasionally initiating opioid therapy in addition to an adjuvant analgesic for chronic pain is warranted. For example, it may be necessary to use an IV opioid initially to control moderate to severe pain associated with a chronic nonmalignant pain syndrome for which the appropriate mainstay analgesic is an adjuvant that requires gradual titration over days or weeks before becoming effective (see Chapter 7). In this case, it would be inhumane to expect the patient to endure severe pain while the adjuvant analgesic takes effect. As soon as the moderate to severe pain is resolved, the opioid can be discontinued.

As opposed to chronic pain, managing acute pain often requires beginning with more than one route and more than one analgesic. This is because there is not enough time to evaluate the patient's response to one analgesic at a time. Therefore decisions about postoperative analgesics are made on the basis of research findings and clinical experience. The intensity of pain is anticipated, and combined analgesic regimens are planned preoperatively whenever possible. For example, in addition to an ATC oral or IV NSAID, for some major surgeries, an epidural catheter is placed preoperatively for continuous infusion of opioid and local anesthetic to control anticipated severe postoperative pain.

The practice of using two different parenteral routes of administration at the same time or parenteral and intraspinal routes at the same time to administer opioids is rarely necessary and can be dangerous (Ready, Loper, Nessly et al., 1991). In particular, the administration of IM opioids to opioid-naive patients receiving IV or epidural analgesia can result in excessive sedation and clinically significant respiratory depression (see pp. 267-270).

Selecting a Starting Opioid Dose

Traditionally, age and weight have been used to determine starting opioid dose. However, studies have shown that there is no correlation between weight and analgesic requirements (Burns, Hodsman, McLintock et al., 1989; Ginsberg, Cohen, Ossey et al., 1989; Monk, Parker, White, 1990). Age, on the other hand, is a valid consideration. Starting doses should be adjusted for patients at the extremes of the age spectrum, such as neonates and infants, who have incomplete organ development, and the elderly, who have increased sensitivity to drug effects. For both the very young and the very old, initial doses are adjusted downward and a longer interval between doses is anticipated. For example, a common recommendation is to lower the recommended adult starting dose in the elderly (>70 years) by 25% to 50% (AHCPR, 1992). No matter what method is used to predict analgesic requirements, the starting dose for opioid treatment is merely an estimate. When a starting dose is given, it is titrated up or down according to patient response.

Using the equianalgesic chart

The term equianalgesia means approximately equal analgesia and is used when referring to the doses of various opioid analgesics that provide approximately the same pain relief. Using the equianalgesic chart in Table 6.12 as an example, note that the chart provides a list of analgesics at doses, both oral and parenteral, that are approximately equal to each other in the ability to provide pain relief. In other words, all of the doses are theoretically interchangeable for providing pain relief. These doses are also referred to as equianalgesic dose units. Most of the doses in equianalgesic charts are made on the basis of single dose studies, often conducted with surgical patients, using morphine, 10 mg IM, for comparison. The parenteral doses listed are typical of IM doses given approximately every 3 to 4 hours.

A patient's pain intensity and the equianalgesic chart are practical tools to use to determine an appropriate opioid starting dose for an opioid-naive patient. To become familiar with the equianalgesic chart, note that it has several columns. The first column lists the common opioid analgesics. Morphine is listed first because it has been the standard for comparison, and the others follow in alphabetical order. The second column lists the equianalgesic doses of opioids by the parenteral (IM, SC, IV) route. The third column lists the equianalgesic doses

of opioids by the oral route. The last four columns provide pharmacokinetic information about the specific opioids.

All the opioid doses listed in the equianalgesic chart are appropriate starting doses given about every 4 hours for adults with severe pain. Percentages of these doses are used to determine the appropriate starting dose for moderate and mild pain. As discussed previously, mild pain may not require an opioid. A nonopioid, such as ibuprofen or acetaminophen, may be appropriate. If an opioid is indicated, mild pain can be treated with a low dose of any of the opioids or an opioid-nonopioid combination, such as codeine or oxycodone compounded with acetaminophen.

To demonstrate the use of pain intensity and the equianalgesic chart to determine an appropriate starting dose, consider a patient with severe pain who is to receive parenteral morphine. The appropriate starting dose for such a patient is 10 mg of morphine parenterally every 4 hours. If instead of severe pain the patient has moderate pain, the starting dose would be 50% of 10 mg (5 mg) of morphine, and for mild pain, 25% of 10 mg (2.5 mg) (Box 6.22, p. 244). When given by the IV route, the total 4-hour dose is given by smaller boluses over the 4-hour interval.

Patient Example

Three opioid-naive patients have just been admitted to the PACU. All three will be managed with IV boluses of hydromorphone (Dilaudid). Pain intensity and the equianalgesic chart are used to determine appropriate starting doses for each patient. Pain intensity is assessed by using a 0 to 10 numerical pain rating scale. The following steps are taken to determine appropriate starting doses:

Patient No. 1

1. **Hydromorphone is located in the first column of the equianalgesic chart.**
2. **Moving horizontally from hydromorphone to column number two (parenteral route), the appropriate dose for severe pain is located (1.5 mg).**
3. **Patient No. 1 reports a pain rating of 8/10 or severe pain.**
4. **The appropriate starting dose for patient No. 1 is 1.5 mg of IV hydromorphone over 4 hours.**
5. **The calculation for the first bolus is 1.5 mg ÷ 4 (1/4 of the 4 h dose) = approximately 0.4 mg (0.375 mg), titrating up or down using larger or smaller doses depending on patient response (pain intensity and side effects).**

Patient No. 2

1. **Steps 1 to 2 outlined for patient No. 1 are followed.**
2. **Patient No. 2 reports a pain rating of 5/10 or moderate pain.**

Text continued on p. 243.

TABLE 6.12

EQUIANALGESIC DOSE CHART

A Guide to Using Equianalgesic Dose Charts
- Equianalgesic means approximately the same pain relief.
- The equianalgesic chart is a guideline. Doses and intervals between doses are titrated according to individual's response.
- The equianalgesic chart is helpful when switching from one drug to another or switching from one route of administration to another.
- Dosages in this equianalgesic chart are not necessarily starting doses. They suggest a ratio for comparing the analgesia of one drug to another.
- The longer the patient has been receiving opioids, the more conservative the starting doses of a new opioid. (See discussion on conversion charts p. 174.)

Opioid Mu Agonists	Parenteral (IM/SC/IV) (over ~ 4 h)	Oral (PO) (over ~ 4 h)	Onset (min)	Peak (min)	Duration[1] (h)	Half-life (h)
Morphine	10 mg	30 mg	30-60 (PO)	60-90 (PO)	3-6 (PO)	2-4
			30-60 (CR)[2]	90-180 (CR)[2]	8-12 (CR)[2]	
			30-60 (R)	60-90 (R)	4-5 (R)	
			5-10 (IV)	15-30 (IV)	3-4 (IV)[1,3]	
			10-20 (SC)	30-60 (SC)	3-4 (SC)	
			10-20 (IM)	30-60 (IM)	3-4 (IM)	
Codeine	130 mg	200 mg NR	30-60 (PO)	60-90 (PO)	3-4 (PO)	2-4
			10-20 (SC)	UK (SC)	3-4 (SC)	
			10-20 (IM)	30-60 (IM)	3-4 (IM)	
Fentanyl	100 μg/h parenterally and trans-dermally ≅ 4 mg/h morphine parenterally; 1 μg/h transder-mally ≅ morphine 2 mg/24 h orally	—	5 (OT)	15 (OT)	2-5 (OT)	3-4[4];
			1-5 (IV)	3-5 (IV)	0.5-4 (IV)[1,3]	
			7-15 (IM)	10-20 (IM)	0.5-4 (IM)	
			12-16 h (TD)	24 h (TD)	48-72 (TD)	13-24 (TD)
Hydrocodone (as in Vicodin, Lortab)	—	30 mg[5] NR	30-60 (PO)	60-90 (PO)	4-6 (PO)	4
Hydromorphone (Dilaudid)	1.5 mg[6]	7.5 mg	15-30 (PO)	30-90 (PO)	3-4 (PO)	2-3
			15-30 (R)	30-90 (R)	3-4 (R)	
			5 (IV)	10-20 (IV)	3-4 (IV)[1,3]	
			10-20 (SC)	30-90 (SC)	3-4 (SC)	
			10-20 (IM)	30-90 (IM)	3-4 (IM)	
Levorphanol (Levo-Dromoran)	2 mg	4 mg	30-60 (PO)	60-90 (PO)	4-6 (PO)	12-15
			10 (IV)	15-30 (IV)	4-6 (IV)[1,3]	
			10-20 (SC)	60-90 (SC)	4-6 (SC)	
			10-20 (IM)	60-90 (IM)	4-6 (IM)	
Meperidine (Demerol)	75 mg	300 mg NR	30-60 (PO)	60-90 (PO)	2-4 (PO)	2-3
			5-10 (IV)	10-15 (IV)	2-4 (IV)[1,3]	
			10-20 (SC)	15-30 (SC)	2-4 (SC)	
			10-20 (IM)	15-30 (IM)	2-4 (IM)	

Continued.

● ● ● ● ●
TABLE 6.12—cont'd

EQUIANALGESIC DOSE CHART—cont'd

Opioid *Mu Agonists*	Parenteral (IM/SC/IV) (over ~ 4 h)	Oral (PO) (over ~ 4 h)	Onset (min)	Peak (min)	Duration[1] (h)	Half-life (h)
Methadone (Dolophine)	10 mg[7]	20 mg[8]	30-60 (PO) UK (SL) 10 (IV) 10-20 (SC) 10-20 (IM)	60-120 (PO) 10 (SL) UK (IV) 60-120 (SC) 60-120 (IM)	4-8 (PO) UK (SL) 4-8 (IV)[1,3] 4-8 (SC) 4-8 (IM)	12-190
Oxycodone (as in Percocet, Tylox)	—	20 mg	30-60 (PO) 30-60 (CR)[9] 30-60 (R)	60-90 (PO) 90-180 (CR)[9] 30-60 (R)	3-4 (PO) 8-12 (CR)[9] 3-6 (R)	2-3 4.5 (CR)
Oxymorphone (Numorphan)	1 mg	(10 mg R)	15-30 (R) 5-10 (IV) 10-20 (SC) 10-20 (IM)	120 (R) 15-30 (IV) UK (SC) 30-90 (IM)	3-6 (R) 3-4 (IV)[1,3] 3-6 (SC) 3-6 (IM)	2-3
Propoxyphene[10] (Darvon)	—	—	30-60 (PO)	60-90 (PO)	4-6 (PO)	6-12
Agonist- *antagonists*						
Buprenorphine[11] (Buprenex)	0.4 mg	—	5 (SL) 5 (IV) 10-20 (IM)	30-60 (SL) 10-20 (IV) 30-60 (IM)	UK (SL) 3-4 (IV)[1,3] 3-6 (IM)	2-3
Butorphanol[11] (Stadol)	2 mg	—	5-15 (NS)[12] 5 (IV) 10-20 (IM)	60-90 (NS) 10-20 (IV) 30-60 (IM)	3-4 (NS) 3-4 (IV)[1,3] 3-4 (IM)	3-4
Dezocine (Dalgan)	10 mg	—	5 (IV) 10-20 (IM)	UK (IV) 30-60 (IM)	3-4 (IV)[1,3] 3-4 (IM)	2-3
Nalbuphine[11] (Nubain)	10 mg	—	5 (IV) <15 (SC) <15 (IM)	10-20 (IV) UK (SC) 30-60 (IM)	3-4 (IV)[1,3] 3-4 (SC) 3-4 (IM)	5
Pentazocine[11] (Talwin)	60 mg	180 mg	15-30 (PO) 5 (IV) 15-20 (SC) 15-20 (IM)	60-180 (PO) 15 (IV) 60 (SC) 60 (IM)	3-4 (PO) 3-4 (IV)[1,3] 3-4 (SC) 3-4 (IM)	2-3

May be duplicated for use in clinical practice. From McCaffery M, Pasero C: *Pain: Clinical manual*, pp. 241-243. Copyright © 1999, Mosby, Inc. *Continued.*

Table 6.12 provides equianalgesic doses and pharmacokinetic information about selected opioid drugs. Characteristics and comments about selected mu opioid agonist drugs can be found in Table 6.3, pp. 179-180.

ATC, around-the-clock; *CR,* oral controlled-release; *h,* hour; *IM,* intramuscular; *IV,* intravenous; *μg,* microgram; *mg,* milligram; *min,* minute; *NR,* not recommended; *NS,* nasal spray; *OT,* oral transmucosal; *PO,* oral; *R,* rectal; *SC,* subcutaneous; *SL,* sublingual; *TD,* transdermal; *UK,* unknown.

[1]Duration of analgesia is dose dependent; the higher the dose, usually the longer the duration.

[2]As in, e.g., MS Contin.

[3]IV boluses may be used to produce analgesia that lasts approximately as long as IM or SC doses. However, of all routes of administration, IV produces the highest peak concentration of the drug, and the peak concentration is associated with the highest level of toxicity (e.g., sedation). To decrease the peak effect and lower the level of toxicity, IV boluses may be administered more slowly (e.g., 10 mg of morphine over a 15-minute period) or smaller doses may be administered more often (e.g., 5 mg of morphine every 1-1.5 hours).

[4]At steady state, slow release of fentanyl from storage in tissues can result in a prolonged half-life of up to 12 h.

[5]Equianalgesic data not available.

[6]The recommendation that 1.5 mg of parenteral hydromorphone is approximately equal to 10 mg of parenteral morphine is based on single dose studies. With repeated dosing of hydromorphone (e.g., PCA), it is more likely that 2-3 mg of parenteral hydromorphone is equal to 10 mg of parenteral morphine.

● ● ● ● ●
TABLE 6.12—cont'd

EQUIANALGESIC DOSE CHART—cont'd

May be duplicated for use in clinical practice. From McCaffery M, Pasero C: *Pain: Clinical manual*, pp. 241-243. Copyright © 1999, Mosby, Inc.

[7] In opioid-tolerant patients converted from continuous IV hydromorphone to continuous IV methadone, start with 10%-25% of the equianalgesic dose.

[8] In opioid-tolerant patients converted to methadone, start PO dosing PRN with 10%-25% of equianalgesic dose.

[9] As in, e.g., OxyContin.

[10] 65-130 mg = approximately 1/6th of all doses listed in this chart.

[11] Used in combination with mu agonists, may reverse analgesia and precipitate withdrawal in opioid-dependent patients.

[12] In opioid-naive patients who are taking occasional mu agonists, such as codeine or oxycodone, the addition of butorphanol nasal spray may provide additive analgesia. However, in opioid-tolerant patients, such as those receiving ATC morphine, the addition of butorphanol nasal spray should be avoided because it may reverse analgesia and precipitate withdrawal.

NOTE: This equianalgesic chart is based on the clinical experience of the chapter authors and the following references:

Information from American Pain Society (APS): *Principles of analgesic use in the treatment of acute and cancer pain*, ed 3, Glenview, IL, 1992, APS; Berryman D, Marketing Manager, Anesta Corp, Salt Lake City, UT: Personal communication by telephone with Chris Pasero, August 21, 1997; Bruera E, Pereira J, Watanabe S et al.: Opioid rotation in patients with cancer pain, *Cancer* 78(4):857, 1996; Coda BA, O'Sullivan B, Donaldson G et al.: Comparative efficacy of patient-controlled administration of morphine, hydromorphone, or sufentanil for the treatment of oral mucositis pain after bone marrow transplantation, *Pain* 72:333-346, 1997; Coda BA, Tanaka A, Jacobson RC et al.: Hydromorphone analgesia after intravenous bolus administration, *Pain* 71(1):41-48, 1997; Deglin JH, Vallerand AH: *Davis' drug guide*, ed 5, Philadelphia, 1995, FA Davis; *Drug facts and comparisons*, St. Louis, 1996, Wolters Kluwer Co; Dunbar PJ, Chapman CR, Buckley FP et al.: Clinical analgesic equivalence for morphine and hydromorphone with prolonged PCA, *Pain* 68:226-270, 1996; Glare PA, Walsh TD: Dose-ranging study of oxycodone for chronic pain in advanced cancer, *J Clin Oncol* 11(5):973-978, 1993; Foley KM: The treatment of cancer pain, *N Engl J Med* 313:84-95, 1985; Foley KM, Inturrisi CE: Opioid therapy: General principles, advances, controversies, alternative routes and methods of administration, *Syllabus of the Postgraduate Course*, Memorial Sloan-Kettering Cancer Center, New York, NY, April 2-3, 1992; Kaiko RF, Lacouture P, Hopf K et al.: Analgesic onset and potency of oral controlled release (CR) oxycodone CR and morphine, *Clin Pharmacol Ther* 59(2):130-133, 1996; Lawlor P, Turner K, Hanson J et al.: Dose ratio between morphine and hydromorphone in patients with cancer pain: A retrospective study, *Pain* 72(1,2):79-85, 1997; Manfredi PL, Borsook D, Chandler SW et al.: Intravenous methadone for cancer pain unrelieved by morphine and hydromorphone: Clinical observations, *Pain* 70:99-101, 1997; Portenoy RK: Opioid analgesics. In Portenoy RK, Kanner RM, editors: *Pain management: Theory and practice*, pp 249-276, Philadelphia, 1996, FA Davis; Reisine T, Pasternak G: Opioid analgesics and antagonists. In Hardman JG, Limbird LE, editors: *Goodman and Gilman's the pharmacological basis of therapeutics*, ed 9, pp 521-555, New York, 1996, McGraw-Hill; Vogelsang J, Hayes SR: Butorphanol tartrate (Stadol): A review, *J Post Anesthesia Nurs* 6(2):129-135, 1991; Weinberg DS, Inturrisi CE, Reidenberg B et al.: Sublingual absorption of selected opioid analgesics, *Clin Pharmacol Ther* 44:335-342, 1988; Wilson JM, Cohen RI, Kezer EA et al.: Single and multiple-dose pharmacokinetics of dezocine in patients with acute and chronic pain, *J Clin Pharmacol* 35:395-403, 1995.

---

3. **The appropriate starting dose for moderate pain is 50% of the starting dose for severe pain. The calculation is 1.5 mg × 50% (or 1.5 mg ÷ 2) = 0.75 mg.**

4. **The appropriate starting dose for patient No. 2 is 0.75 mg of hydromorphone by the IV route over 4 h.**

5. **The calculation for the first bolus is 0.75 mg ÷ 4 (1/4 of the 4 h dose) = approximately 0.2 mg, titrating up or down using larger or smaller boluses depending on patient response (pain intensity and side effects).**

Patient No. 3

1. **Steps 1 to 2 outlined for patient No. 1 are followed.**

2. **Patient No. 3 reports a pain rating of 3/10 or mild pain.**

3. **The appropriate starting dose for mild pain is 25% of the starting dose for severe pain. The calculation is 1.5 mg × 25% (or 1.5 mg ÷ 4) = 0.375 mg.**

4. **The appropriate starting dose for patient No. 3 is approximately 0.4 mg of hydromorphone by the IV route over 4 h.**

5. **The calculation for the first bolus is 0.4 mg ÷ 4 (1/4 of the 4 h dose) = approximately 0.1 mg, titrating up or down using larger or smaller boluses depending on patient response (pain intensity and side effects).**

As mentioned, the doses in the equianalgesic chart are made on the basis of a 4-hour dosing schedule. To determine the appropriate starting dose when the dosing schedule is other than every 4 hours, other calculations are necessary.

Patient Example

Mr. H. has cancer pain. Until now he has been controlling his pain with two Percocet (oxycodone, 5 mg, plus acetaminophen, 325 mg, per tablet) q4h ATC. He reports that his pain has been increasing. He rates his pain as 6/10. The decision is made to begin treatment with oral controlled-release oxycodone. The clinician calculates Mr. H.'s starting dose as follows:

1. **10 mg oxycodone (2 Percocet) × 6 doses/day = 60 mg/day.**

2. **60 mg ÷ 2 (number of doses/24 h with 12 h dosing) = 30 mg.**

Mr. H. is started on 30 mg controlled-release oxycodone q12h. Acetaminophen 650 mg is continued ATC. This will provide the same analgesia at more convenient dosing intervals for the opioid.

NOTE: **This approach for managing Mr. H.'s pain is logical and conservative. Other approaches may be used (e.g., starting at a higher dose [40 mg] of controlled-release oxycodone).**

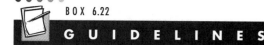

• • • • •
BOX 6.22

GUIDELINES

SELECTION OF AN OPIOID STARTING DOSE

1. Use an equianalgesic chart and your patient's pain intensity to determine an appropriate opioid starting dose.
2. Locate the prescribed opioid in column one in the equianalgesic chart (e.g., morphine).
3. Move horizontally from column one to column two if the opioid is to be given by the parenteral route or to column three if by the oral route.
4. This is the appropriate starting dose for an opioid-naive patient with severe pain (e.g., 30 mg of PO morphine).

- If the patient has moderate pain, calculate a dose that is 50% of the dose for severe pain: Severe pain dose ÷ 2 (50%) = Appropriate starting dose for patient with moderate pain (e.g., 15 mg of PO morphine).
- If the patient has mild pain, calculate a dose that is 25% of the dose for severe pain: Severe pain dose ÷ 4 (25%) = Appropriate starting dose for patient with mild pain (e.g., 7.5 mg of PO morphine).

May be duplicated for use in clinical practice. From McCaffery M, Pasero C: Pain: Clinical manual, p. 244. Copyright © 1999, Mosby, Inc.

mg, milligram; PO, oral.

A patient's pain intensity and the equianalgesic chart are practical tools to use to determine an appropriate opioid starting dose for an opioid-naive patient. Box 6.22 demonstrates how to combine these two tools to determine an appropriate starting dose for opioid-naive patients with mild, moderate, or severe pain intensity.

Continuous infusions

In patients with cancer pain or opioid-naive postoperative or trauma patients in the ICU who will require parenteral opioids, a maintenance continuous infusion is initiated after pain is controlled with IV or SC boluses (Coyle, Cherny, Portenoy, 1995). As mentioned, additional boluses offered every 15 to 30 minutes are prescribed for the management of breakthrough pain (see Rescue doses in the next section and pp. 251-252 for continuous infusions in opioid-naive patients outside of the ICU).

Patient Example

Ms. A. has been admitted directly to the ICU after an automobile accident and emergency abdominal surgery. She is on a ventilator and is somewhat disoriented and restless. She is unable to provide self-reports of pain yet. Her pain is to be controlled with a continuous IV infusion of morphine. The following calculation of the starting dose is necessary:

1. **Morphine is located in the first column of the equianalgesic chart.**
2. **Moving horizontally from morphine to column number two (parenteral route), the ap-**

propriate starting dose for severe pain is located (10 mg over a 4 h period).

3. **Because Ms. A. is expected to have moderate to severe pain, an appropriate conservative starting dose for her is 5 mg (50% of 10 mg) of morphine IV over a 4 h period.**
4. **Ms. A. is to receive a continuous IV infusion, so an hourly dose must be calculated: 5 mg ÷ 4 h = approximately 1.3 mg/h.**

The nurse suspects that Ms. A.'s restlessness may be related to unrelieved pain, so she administers a loading IV bolus equal to the starting hourly dose (1.3 mg) and begins the opioid infusion immediately. Within 45 minutes, Ms. A. is no longer restless and her vital signs are stable.

Rescue doses

The term rescue dose is used interchangeably with supplemental or breakthrough dose. All patients who receive ATC opioid analgesics should have access to rescue doses of an immediate-release mu agonist opioid analgesic to treat breakthrough pain (see p. 175 for more on breakthrough pain). They should be offered every 1 to 2 hours for patients taking oral opioids and every 15 to 30 minutes for patients taking parenteral opioids. Rescue doses may be taken at anytime, even at the same time as the ATC opioid (APS, 1992).

For patients taking oral opioids, the recommended amount of opioid for rescue doses is between one tenth and one sixth (a range of approximately 10% to 15%) of the total daily dose of the ATC opioid analgesic (Box 6.23). This calculation is used consistently, regardless of the total daily dose of opioid. For example, the range of a given rescue dose for a patient receiving a total daily dose of 8000 mg of controlled-release morphine would be 800 mg (one tenth) to 1333 mg (one sixth) (APS, 1992; McCaffery, 1996).

Patient Example

Mr. H. is receiving 30 mg of PO controlled-release oxycodone twice daily. The rescue dose range is determined by calculating one-tenth and one-sixth of the total daily dose.

The calculation is a follows:

$$30 \text{ mg} \times 2 = 60 \text{ mg/day}$$

$$60 \text{ mg} \div 10 \ (1/10) = 6 \text{ mg}$$

$$60 \text{ mg} \div 6 \ (1/6) = 10 \text{ mg}$$

Mr. H.'s rescue dose range is approximately 5 to 10 mg of immediate release oxycodone q 1 to 2 h PRN for breakthrough pain.

The recommended rescue dose for patients receiving continuous parenteral opioid infusions is 25% to 50% of the hourly opioid dose (see Box 6.23). (Although one

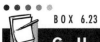

BOX 6.23

GUIDELINES

CALCULATION OF RESCUE DOSES

The formula for calculating rescue doses usually is one tenth (1/10) to one sixth (1/6) (10% to 15%[1]) of the total daily dose. Whenever possible, rescue doses should be the same opioid and route as the ATC drug (e.g., use oral immediate-release morphine as rescue for controlled-release morphine).

- Immediate-release and controlled-release morphine or oxycodone. Example: 180 mg/24 h PO morphine.

  Total daily dose ÷ 10 (1/10 or 10%), e.g., 180 mg ÷ 10 = 18 mg

  Total daily dose ÷ 6 (1/6 or 15%[1]), e.g., 180 mg ÷ 6 = 30 mg = The range of the rescue dose of immediate release morphine or oxycodone that can be taken q1-2h, e.g., 18 (20) to 30 mg PO immediate-release morphine

- Transdermal fentanyl

  Immediate-release oral morphine usually is recommended for controlled-release opioid formulations that do not have an immediate-release formulation of the same opioid available. To use oral immediate release morphine, it is necessary to convert the other opioid to morphine equivalents. Example: 200 μg transdermal fentanyl.

  Total μg/h of fentanyl × 2 = approximate equianalgesic total daily dose of oral morphine,[2] e.g., 200 μg × 2 = 400 mg PO morphine

  Approximate equianalgesic total daily dose of oral morphine ÷ 10 (1/10 or 10%), e.g., 400 mg ÷ 10 = 40 mg PO morphine.

  Approximate equianalgesic total daily dose of oral morphine ÷ 6 (1/6 or 15%[1]), e.g., 400 mg ÷ 6 = Approximately 70 mg PO morphine = The range of the rescue dose of immediate release morphine that can be taken q1-2h, e.g., 40 to 70 mg PO morphine

- Oral transmucosal fentanyl citrate (OTFC)[3]

  The customary method of calculating rescue doses made on the basis of patients' total daily opioid requirements is not recommended by the manufacturer of OTFC when using OTFC to manage breakthrough pain. Instead, the manufacturer recommends that patients who are using OTFC for the first time be instructed to start with a single 200 μg unit of OTFC and finish it within 15 minutes. If this dose is not sufficient, they should wait another 15 minutes then finish a second 200 μg unit of OTFC over a 15-minute period. If this dose is not sufficient, this process can be repeated one more time (a maximum of three 200 μg OTFC units or 600 μg). For the next episode of breakthrough pain, patients who achieved satisfactory pain relief and tolerable side effects with 2 or more OTFC units (400 μg) should begin with 400 μg taken over a 15-minute period. The same titration process is used (i.e., if after another 15 minutes the first 400 μg is not sufficient, another 400 μg should be taken over a 15-minute period). If this dose is not sufficient, this process can be repeated two more times (a maximum of four 400 μg OTFC units or 1600 μg).

- Parenteral opioid infusions[4]

  The recommended rescue dose for patients receiving continuous parenteral or epidural opioid infusions is 25% to 50% of the hourly opioid dose. Rescue doses should be offered at least q30min to patients receiving continuous parenteral infusions without PCA (e.g., for an opioid tolerant patient: morphine, 10 mg/h IV, with IV bolus doses of morphine, 2.5 to 5 mg q30min PRN).

All patients who receive ATC opioid analgesics should have access to rescue (supplemental) doses of an immediate-release mu agonist opioid analgesic to treat break-through pain. Box 6.23 provides guidelines for calculating rescue doses for various opioid formulations and routes of administration.

[1]One-sixth is equal to 17%. The assignment of 15% to one-sixth is done to simplify calculation for those who prefer to use percentages.

[2]When studies that clarify equianalgesic dosing are lacking, such as is the case with fentanyl, various conversion formulas evolve. These formulas, and even the ones used in this text, are not necessarily comparable; different formulas lead to different answers. This conversion formula may be used to convert the patient from oral morphine to transdermal fentanyl and vice versa. The current recommendation by the manufacturer may be used only to convert from oral morphine to transdermal fentanyl, not vice versa, and the clinician should expect that approximately 50% of the patients will require additional analgesia.

[3]OTFC is expected to be available early 1999.

[4]Although one tenth to one sixth of the 24-hour dose can be used to calculate rescue doses for parenteral opioid treatment, hourly percentages are simpler and the results are essentially the same.

ATC, around-the-clock; h, hour; IV, intravenous; μg, microgram; mg, milligram; min, minute; PO, oral; q, every.

Information from Berryman D, Marketing Manager, Anesta Corp., Salt Lake City, UT: Personal communication by telephone with Chris Pasero, August 21, 1997; Dahl J: Fentanyl postscript, *Cancer Pain Update* (41):6, Fall 1996; McCaffery M: How to calculate a rescue dose, *Am J Nurs* 96(4):65-66, 1996.

tenth to one sixth of the 24-hour dose can be used to calculate rescue doses for parenteral opioid treatment, hourly percentages are simpler with continuous parenteral opioid infusions and the results are essentially the same.) The total amount of the parenteral rescue doses given in 1 hour may be equal to but ordinarily do not exceed the hourly opioid dose. The need for rescue doses greater than the hourly opioid dose indicates a need to increase the hourly opioid dose. For example, an opioid-tolerant patient receiving 6 mg/h of IV morphine could be given a 3 mg rescue dose but ordinarily should not repeatedly be given more than two 3 mg boluses in an hour. If more than two boluses are required, the continuous infusion should be increased.

Patient Example

Ms. A. is receiving a continuous IV infusion of morphine at 1.3 mg/h after an automobile accident and abdominal surgery. The IV rescue dose range is calculated as follows:

$$1.3 \text{ mg} \times 25\% \text{ (or } 1.3 \text{ mg} \div 4) =$$
$$\text{approximately } 0.3 \text{ mg}$$

$$1.3 \text{ mg} \times 50\% \text{ (or } 1.3 \text{ mg} \div 2) =$$
$$\text{approximately } 0.7 \text{ mg}$$

Ms. A.'s rescue dose range is 0.3 mg to 0.7 mg (not to exceed 1.3 mg total in rescue doses in one hour) of IV morphine provided q 15 to 30 minutes PRN for breakthrough pain.

Dose Titration

Titration of the opioid dose usually is required at the beginning of therapy and repeatedly during the course of treatment. Whereas patients with cancer pain most often are titrated upward over time for progressive pain, patients with acute pain, particularly postoperative pain, are eventually titrated downward as pain resolves (see also discussion of opioid side effects on pp. 261-270 and tapering of opioid doses on p. 270).

Considerable variation exists in the amount of opioid individuals require for comfort (APS, 1992). For example, as much as a 10-fold difference exists among patients in opioid requirements during the postoperative period (Benedetti, 1990). This wide variability reinforces the need for prompt and individualized attention to unrelieved pain. At all times, inadequate pain relief is addressed with gradual escalation of the opioid dose until adequate analgesia is reported or intolerable and unmanageable side effects occur. The absolute opioid dose is unimportant as long as the balance between pain relief and side effects is favorable (Coyle, Portenoy, 1996). The goal of titration is to use the smallest dose that provides satisfactory pain relief with the fewest side effects.

Dose titration in selected clinical areas

Providing effective pain control while minimizing opioid-induced side effects presents a special challenge for nurses who work in outpatient surgery settings, PACUs, and ICUs, who must deal also with the additional CNS depression caused by the sedative and anesthetic agents that are administered intraoperatively and sometimes throughout care in the ICU. Furthermore, many of these patients are opioid naive. Less difficulty is experienced when a multimodality approach is used. If a NSAID was not given preoperatively, it may be started in the PACU or ICU or epidural opioids may be combined with a long-acting local anesthetic (see Chapter 4 for more) (Pasero, McCaffery, 1996a).

Before a trauma or postoperative patient becomes oriented enough to provide self-reports of pain, the nurse should assume that pain is present by the fact that sufficient noxious stimuli is present and as soon as it is safe administer IV boluses of opioids. The presence of other signs of pain, such as moaning, facial grimacing, or elevated vital signs, may be considered in the assessment of pain, but they are not reliable indicators of pain and their absence does not necessarily mean the absence of pain.

If IV PCA is used for postoperative pain control, the clinician-administered bolus mode on the infusion pump can be used in the PACU to titrate patients to comfort. This eliminates the time-consuming task of signing out, drawing up, and administering opioid boluses from a separate syringe.

For patients receiving epidural analgesia, epidural boluses may be administered and titrated to comfort. This avoids the sedation produced from administering IV opioid boluses. Administration of epidural opioid bolus doses seems to be within the scope of practice for nurses in most states in the United States. In 1993, one of the authors (Pasero) requested from state boards of nursing a statement of their positions on this matter. Of those who responded (48), most had approved the administration of epidural bolus doses by registered nurses who possess the knowledge and skill to do so. A protocol can be developed for selecting opioid doses for epidural bolusing on the basis of pain intensity and the maintenance opioid dose (Box 6.24).

Patient Example

Mr. L. is awake, responding, and knows where he is when admitted to the PACU after a right total knee replacement. He has an epidural catheter in place with a continuous infusion of 50 μg/h fentanyl and 0.125% bupivacaine. He reports moderate to severe right knee pain (6/10). He is oriented, has no nausea, and his respiratory rate is 16. The anesthesiologist's order calls for titration with epidural boluses of 50% to 100% of the hourly opioid dose for patients with moderate to severe pain. At 10:30 Mr. L.'s nurse administers one epidural bolus of 25 μg (50 μg × 50% [or 50 μg ÷ 2] = 25 μg) using the clinician-administered bolus mode on the pump. At 10:45 Mr. L. reports that his pain is somewhat relieved but continues to be moderate (5/10). He is more alert now and his vital signs are stable. The nurse administers another epidural bolus of 25 μg. At 10:55 Mr. L. reports a pain rating of 3/10. Mr. L. is transferred to the nursing unit at 11:15 with his epidural continuous infusion at 50 μg/h fentanyl and 0.125% bupivacaine and a pain rating of 2/10.

Pain control should be included in the criteria for discharge from one area of care to another. For example, many short stay units, outpatient surgery units, and

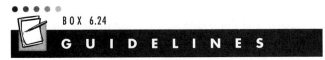

G U I D E L I N E S

TITRATION WITH CLINICIAN-ADMINISTERED EPIDURAL BOLUSES

The total opioid dose provided by clinician-administered supplemental epidural bolus(es) within a 1-hour period should not exceed the maximum 1-hour epidural opioid dose prescribed for the patient:

- Patients receiving basal rate (continuous infusion) only: Total opioid dose provided by clinician-administered supplemental epidural bolus(es) within a 1-hour period should not exceed the epidural opioid dose provided by the basal rate (e.g., if basal rate is 40 μg/h of fentanyl, the total opioid dose provided by clinician-administered bolus[es] should not exceed 40 μg of fentanyl in a 1-hour period).
- Patients receiving PCEA: Total opioid dose provided by clinician-administered supplemental epidural bolus(es) within a 1-hour period should not exceed the maximum 1-hour limit (e.g., if the 1-hour limit for PCEA morphine is 1.6 mg, the total opioid dose provided by clinician-administered bolus[es] should not exceed 1.6 mg of morphine in a 1-hour period).

NOTE: If frequent administration of supplemental bolus doses is necessary or if more than the prescribed maximum hourly opioid dose is required, the patient should be reevaluated and an increase in the mainstay opioid dose considered.

May be duplicated for use in clinical practice. From McCaffery M, Pasero C: *Pain: Clinical manual,* p. 247. Copyright © 1999, Mosby, Inc.

Administration of epidural opioid bolus doses is within the scope of practice for nurses in most states in the United States. Box 6.24 presents a protocol for titrating patients with epidural boluses.

h, hour; *μg,* microgram; *mg,* milligram; *PCEA,* patient-controlled epidural analgesia.

PACUs establish a comfort goal of at least 4/10 before discharge (Pasero, 1994).

Identifying the need for an opioid dose increase

The first sign that an increase in opioid dose is needed is most commonly a decrease in the duration of analgesia for a given opioid dose. For example, a patient receiving IV PCA may self-administer the maximum hourly amount of opioid prescribed in less than 1 hour (see pp. 248-253 for more on PCA) or a patient taking a controlled-release opioid may report breakthrough pain occurring invariably toward the end of the continuous analgesic dosing interval, such as in the 11th hour of a 12-hour dosing schedule.

Patients also may report the need for an increased number of rescue doses. As a rule of thumb, two or more rescue doses during a 12-hour period (four to six daily) should alert the clinician that the opioid regimen for cancer or chronic nonmalignant pain needs to be reevaluated (Jacox, Carr, Payne et al., 1994; Levy, 1996) (see Table 6.7 on p. 209 for guide to increasing the dose of transdermal fentanyl).

When an increase in the opioid dose is necessary, it can be done by percentages. When a slight improvement in analgesia is needed, a 25% increase in opioid dose may be sufficient; for a moderate effect, a 50% increase, and for a strong effect, such as for the treatment of severe pain, a 100% increase may be indicated (Levy, 1996). The time at which the dose should be increased is typically determined by considering the onset or peak effect of the opioid. For example, titration of IV opioid doses may occur as often as every 5 to 15 minutes (depending on the lipid solubility of the drug), whereas titration of oral controlled-release opioids may occur every 24 to 48 hours. Increases in the ATC analgesia must be accompanied by proportional increases in the rescue dose, so that the size of rescue doses remains an effective percentage of the fixed dose (Coyle, Portenoy, 1996).

Patient Example

Ms. L. is in outpatient recovery after a laparoscopy. Her pain is 6/10. She has an order for titration to comfort with IV morphine boluses of up to 4 mg/bolus. Ten minutes after a 2 mg bolus she reports her pain as 5/10. Her nurse gives another bolus, this time of 3 mg (50% increase in the dose of the last bolus). Within 15 minutes Ms. L. says she is comfortable with a pain rating of 3/10. At that time she is given 2 Vicodin (5 mg hydrocodone and 500 mg acetaminophen), which is prescribed for her pain control at home. She is discharged 2 hours later with a pain rating of 3/10.

Another method of increasing opioid doses is possible when the patient is receiving ATC opioids and taking rescue doses. If the combination of the ATC dose and the rescue doses provides satisfactory pain relief, the ATC dose can be increased to the amount of opioid provided by the current ATC dose and rescue doses. This may allow elimination or a considerable decrease in the number of rescue doses required.

Patient Example

Mr. K. has been receiving a continuous SC infusion of 1 mg/h of hydromorphone at home. He has required SC rescue doses of 0.5 mg of hydromorphone q 30 to 45 minutes with a total of 18 boluses required per 24 h period to maintain an acceptable comfort level (4/10). The decision is made to increase the dose of hydromorphone provided by continuous infusion on the basis of his total 24-hour requirement.

1 mg/h × 24 h = 24 mg/day (continuous infusion)

0.5 mg × 18 = 9 mg/day (bolus doses)

24 mg + 9 mg = 33 mg

33 mg ÷ 24 = 1.4 mg/h

Mr. K.'s hydromorphone dose by continuous SC infusion is increased to 1.4 mg/h.

The new rescue dose range is calculated (see Box 6.23 on p. 245):

1.4 mg × 25% (or 1.4 mg ÷ 4) = approximately 0.4 mg

1.4 mg × 50% (or 1.4 mg ÷ 2) = 0.7 mg

Mr. K.'s rescue dose range is approximately 0.4 mg to 0.7 mg of SC morphine q 15 to 30 minutes PRN for breakthrough pain.

The next day Mr. K. reports that his comfort level is 2/10 and he has required only 2 rescue doses since the increase in his continuous infusion.

Patient Example

Mrs. R. is reporting inadequate relief of her cancer pain after a period of stable dosing with 30 mg of PO immediate-release morphine q4h. She reports taking an increased number of rescue doses (about 5 doses of 10 mg immediate release morphine/day). Most of the time the rescue doses are required during the last hour of the dosing interval. She is finding it increasingly difficult to work and sleep. She rates her pain as moderate (5/10) most of the day. Mrs. R. would like to try controlled-release morphine with a 25% increase in the opioid dose.

30 mg × 6 doses = 180 mg/day (ATC dose)

10 mg × 5 = 50 mg/day (rescue doses)

180 mg + 50 mg = 230 mg/day

230 mg × 25% (or 230 mg ÷ 4) = approximately 60 mg

230 mg + 60 mg = 290 mg (25% increase in opioid dose)

290 mg ÷ 2 (q12h doses) = 145 mg controlled release morphine q12h

Controlled-release morphine is available in 15, 30, 60, 100, and 200 mg tablets. Mrs. R. will take one 15, one 30, and one 100 mg tablet q 12 h.

The new rescue dose is calculated (see Box 6.23):

290 mg ÷ 10 (1/10) = 30 mg

290 mg ÷ 6 (1/6) = 50 mg

Mrs. R.'s new rescue dose range is 30 to 50 mg q1-2h PRN for breakthrough pain. Because a lag period occurs before the onset of controlled-release morphine, Mrs. R. takes 30 mg of immediate-release morphine when she takes the first dose of controlled-release morphine. Two days later Mrs. R. reports that she is able to work and sleep better and has a pain rating of 2/10 most of the day without the need for rescue doses.

Patients should be involved in the decision to increase the opioid dose. Valuable information is obtained by asking patients to describe the pattern of pain they are experiencing. For example, patients commonly take more rescue doses during the times when they are active than when they are resting. Patients with cancer pain or chronic nonmalignant pain who work or are particularly active frequently take more than two rescue doses during a 12-hour period. Many patients would prefer to administer additional boluses during these periods of activity rather than risk increased sedation that can accompany an increase in the ATC opioid dose. Some postoperative patients receiving PCA prefer less than complete pain relief rather than risk nausea with an increased dose.

Checking for optimal epidural catheter location

When patients report inadequate pain relief during epidural analgesic continuous infusion or PCEA, the entire epidural line from the infusion pump to the epidural catheter site should be checked. Inadequate pain relief may be due to a number of mechanical and technical factors, including incorrect loading of the pump, a disconnection of the catheter from the infusion pump tubing, an empty drug reservoir, a disconnected PCEA button, a malfunctioning pump or tubing, or the epidural catheter may have been inadvertently pulled out.

When bolus doses and increases in the epidural analgesic dose do not yield satisfactory pain control or produce "patchy" (e.g., one-sided) analgesia and the epidural catheter appears to be in place, the infusion line connected, and the infusion pump infusing correctly, the anesthesiologist is notified. Anesthesiologists can check to see whether the epidural catheter is in the optimal location by administering a concentrated dose of local anesthetic through the catheter. Optimal catheter placement would produce a bilateral sensory block of the desired dermatomes; lack of such a block would indicate that the catheter location is not optimal. If location is less than optimal, the epidural catheter should be removed and alternatives considered. The patient selection considerations listed in Box 6.14 on p. 215 can be used to determine whether the epidural catheter should be replaced.

Patient-Controlled Analgesia

PCA pumps may be used to administer opioids by the SC, IV, or epidural routes. Use of a PCA pump requires prescribing a number of parameters, many of which are safety features to help prevent overdosing (see Box 6.25).

BOX 6.25   PCA Pump Features

- Drug concentration: Concentration of drug per milliliter solution in the drug reservoir.
- Drug reservoir volume: Amount of solution in drug reservoir.
- PCA bolus dose: Amount patient will receive each time a bolus is self-administered.
- Delay interval (lockout): Amount of time that must elapse between PCA doses administered.
- Basal rate: Amount of the continuous infusion. This feature is optional.
- Hour limit: The total amount the patient can receive in one hour by PCA bolus doses and basal rate.
- Important history available in most PCA pumps:
  - PCA attempts: Number of times patient presses the PCA button.
  - PCA injections: Number of times patient successfully self-administers a PCA dose.
  - Volume given.
  - Volume remaining in drug reservoir.

May be duplicated for use in clinical practice. From McCaffery M, Pasero C: *Pain: Clinical manual*, p. 249. Copyright © 1999, Mosby, Inc.

Box 6.25 defines PCA pump features.

PCA, patient-controlled analgesia.

For example, the amount of opioid a patient receives each time a PCA bolus is self-administered and the total amount the patient can receive in 1 hour can be limited.

For patients with cancer pain receiving continuous infusions, PCA offers an independent means of managing breakthrough pain. In these opioid-tolerant patients, the continuous infusion provides most of the opioid requirement (APS, 1992) and the PCA bolus dose is larger and given at longer intervals than with opioid-naive patients. For example, a bolus dose usually is 25% to 50% of the hourly continuous infusion dose, and the delay interval usually is set at 15 to 30 minutes.

Patient Example

Mrs. S. has been receiving a SC infusion of morphine 30 mg/h to control her cancer pain. While in the hospital, the nurses offer her SC rescue bolus doses q2h. Often, Mrs. S. tolerated pain rather than ask the nurses for a rescue dose. Her family is concerned that this pattern will continue at home. Her nurse discusses the concept of PCA with Mrs. S. and her family. They are receptive to the idea of using SC PCA to control Mrs. S.'s breakthrough pain. Her PCA bolus dose is calculated at 8 mg (approximately 25% of the hourly morphine dose) with a delay interval of 15 minutes. Mrs. S. uses the PCA button readily, reports better pain control, and is significantly more satisfied with her pain treatment plan.

Like other methods for controlling pain, the starting PCA prescription for opioid-naive patients is selected by

using the patient's pain intensity and the equianalgesic chart (see Table 6.12 on pp. 241-243). The starting PCA prescription is just an estimate of a patient's opioid requirement, which is titrated according to how the patient responds. The following is a discussion of the clinical implications of using the patient's pain intensity and the equianalgesic chart to select the starting IV PCA prescription for an opioid-naive patient.

To a great extent, the success of IV PCA depends on prescribing PCA bolus doses that can be self-administered frequently enough for patients to manage their pain effectively. Large PCA bolus doses at delay intervals (lockout) of 15 to 30 minutes often are required and well tolerated by opioid-tolerant patients with cancer or chronic nonmalignant pain. Smaller PCA doses at shorter delay intervals are best for opioid-naive patients to prevent excessive sedation at peaks (highest opioid blood level) and breakthrough pain at troughs (lowest opioid blood level).

The length of the delay interval should allow for adequate analgesic coverage during times when patients need the most opioid. For example, postoperative patients should be able to activate PCA before and frequently during potentially painful activities, such as ambulation, self-care, and physical therapy or respiratory therapy treatments (Pasero, McCaffery, 1996a). The characteristics of the opioid, such as the onset and peak times, also influence the length of the delay interval. The American Pain Society (1992) recommends a delay interval between 5 and 10 minutes for most IV opioids. For example, the delay interval is most commonly 5 to 6 minutes for IV fentanyl and 8 minutes for IV morphine and hydromorphone (unpublished data, Chris Pasero). The delay interval often is increased to 8 and 10 minutes, respectively, for opioid-naive elderly patients to ensure that titration upward is done slowly.

The American Pain Society (1992) recommends that the 1 hour limit be set at three to five times the projected hourly IV requirement for at least the first 24 hours. Key to this is assessing the patient's pain and observing the actual hourly opioid consumption over time and adjusting the hour limit up or down as necessary (see Box 6.26 for how to select a starting IV PCA prescription.)

Most PCA pumps allow for programming of a 1 hour limit, some offer a 4 hour limit, and some pumps allow bypassing this parameter altogether. The practice of bypassing the hour limit is not recommended in opioid-naive patients. The purpose of the hour limit is not only to help prevent overdosing but also to alert the caregiver when an increased opioid dose is necessary. Use of a 1 hour limit is preferable to a 4 hour limit for at least two reasons: (1) the caregiver is alerted to the need for an increase in the opioid dose sooner (i.e., within 1 hour instead of within 4 hours); (2) it avoids the scenario of neglecting to increase the dose in patients who use the

BOX 6.26

GUIDELINES

CALCULATION OF THE STARTING PRESCRIPTION FOR IV PCA FOR OPIOID-NAIVE PATIENTS

1. Use an equianalgesic chart and your patient's pain intensity prior to titration to determine a starting maintenance prescription for PCA.
2. Locate the prescribed opioid in column one in the equianalgesic chart. (Example: morphine.)
3. Move horizontally from column one to column two, the parenteral route. The dose in column two is the appropriate starting opioid dose given over 4 hours for an opioid-naive patient with severe pain, e.g., morphine, 10 mg *(starting opioid dose over 4 h period)*.
    - If your patient has moderate pain, calculate a dose that is 50% of the dose for severe pain: Severe pain dose ÷ 2 (50%) = appropriate starting dose, e.g., 10 mg ÷ 2 = 5 mg *(starting opioid dose over 4 h period for moderate pain)*.
    - If your patient has mild pain, calculate a dose that is 25% of the dose for severe pain: Severe pain dose ÷ 4 (25%) = appropriate starting dose, e.g., 10 mg ÷ 4 = 2.5 mg *(Starting opioid dose over 4 h period for mild pain)*.
4. Determine the projected hourly requirement (This is not the hour limit):
    - Starting dose (from step 3 above) ÷ 4 h = projected hourly requirement, e.g., for severe pain: 10 mg ÷ 4 = 2.5 mg *(projected hourly requirement)*.
5. The American Pain Society (APS) recommends that the hour limit be 3 to 5 times the patient's projected hourly requirement. This range can be used to determine an appropriate hour limit. Most often the mid range (average) is prescribed.
    - Projected hourly requirement × 3 = Low end of hour limit range, e.g., 2.5 mg × 3 = 7.5 mg.
    - Projected hourly requirement × 5 = high end of hour limit range, e.g., 2.5 mg × 5 = 12.5 mg.
    - Low end of range + High end of range ÷ 2 = Mid range of hour limit, e.g., 7.5 mg + 12.5 mg = 20 ÷ 2 = 10 mg *(average hour limit)*.
6. Delay interval (lockout) is selected by considering the prescribed opioid's pharmacologic characteristics and APS recommendations. Most often the mid range (average) is prescribed.
    - Morphine, hydromorphone, meperidine: range 5 to 10 minutes, e.g., 8 minutes *(average delay interval)*.
    - Fentanyl: range 4 to 8 minutes.
7. Determine the number of times the patient can self-administer PCA bolus doses in 1 hour by dividing 60 minutes by the selected delay interval, e.g., 60 ÷ 8 = Approximately 7.
8. PCA bolus dose is determined by dividing the hour limit by the number of times the patient can self-administer PCA bolus doses in 1 hour, e.g., 10 mg ÷ 7 = approximately 1.4 mg *(PCA bolus dose without basal)*.
9. Basal rate is optional. If a basal rate is prescribed, it should be no more than one half of the projected hourly requirement (see step 4), e.g., 2.5 mg ÷ 2 = 1.25 mg. The amount of the basal rate is included as part of the hour limit amount. When a basal rate is prescribed, the PCA bolus dose should be decreased or the hour limit increased accordingly. Basal rate should be ≤ the PCA bolus dose.
10. For loading and when needed during therapy, clinician-administered bolus doses are usually equal to the projected hourly requirement (see step 4), e.g., 2.5 mg *(loading dose)*.

    Example of a starting IV PCA prescription for an opioid-naive patient with severe pain using morphine: PCA bolus dose = 1.0 mg; delay = 8 min; basal rate = up to 1.0 mg; hour limit = 8 mg; loading dose = 2.5 mg.

May be duplicated for use in clinical practice. From McCaffery M, Pasero C: *Pain: Clinical manual*, p. 250. Copyright © 1999, Mosby, Inc.

A patient's pain intensity and the equianalgesic chart are practical tools to use to determine an appropriate starting IV PCA prescription for an opioid-naive patient. Box 6.26 demonstrates how to combine these two tools to determine an appropriate starting IV PCA prescription for opioid-naive patients with mild, moderate, or severe pain intensity. Prescription ranges can be calculated in advance and included in prewritten physician orders to standardize and facilitate the prescribing of IV PCA. (See also Table 6.13, p. 252.)

h, hour; *mg*, milligram; *min*, minute; *PCA*, patient-controlled analgesia.

Information from American Pain Society (APS): *Principles of analgesic use in the treatment of acute and cancer pain*, ed 3, Glenview, IL, 1992, APS.

---

4 hour amount in less than 4 hours (e.g., if a patient uses the 4 hour amount in 2 hours and is left for 2 hours without analgesia).

Patient Example

Mrs. B. is in the PACU after a total abdominal hysterectomy. She will be managing her postoperative pain with IV PCA morphine. Mrs. B.'s nurse has attached the PCA pump to Mrs. B.'s IV line and will use the clinician-administered bolus mode on the pump to deliver IV boluses of morphine until Mrs. B. can manage her own pain. By use of the equianalgesic chart, the calculation for the clinician-administered IV boluses for titration in the PACU is as follows:

1. Morphine is located in the first column of the equianalgesic chart.
2. Moving horizontally from morphine to column number two (parenteral route), the appropriate dose for severe pain is located (10 mg).

3. Mrs. B. reports a pain rating of 9/10 or severe pain, so the appropriate starting dose for her is 10 mg of morphine IV over a 4 h period (approximately 2.5 mg/h).

4. The nurse decides to administer the starting hourly dose and titrate up or down by use of larger or smaller boluses, depending on patient response (pain intensity and side effects).

Mrs. B. required three boluses of 2.5 mg within a 45-minute period to reduce her pain to 4/10, which is acceptable to her. She is reporting mild nausea requiring no treatment and is ready to manage her own pain. Because Mrs. B. is opioid naive, her starting PCA prescription is selected with the equianalgesic chart and her pain intensity before titration, which was 9/10 or severe:

1. The amount of morphine appropriate for Mrs. B. is 10 mg over a 4-hour period.

2. The projected hourly requirement for Mrs. B. is 10 mg ÷ 4 h = 2.5 mg.

3. The range of doses that is appropriate for the hour limit is determined by increasing the projected hourly requirement by 3 to 5:

   • 2.5 mg × 3 = 7.5 mg (low end of range)

   • 2.5 mg × 5 = 12.5 mg (high end of range)

   • Mid (average) range is 7.5 mg + 12.5 mg = 20 mg ÷ 2 = 10 mg.

   • The average starting hour limit is approximately 10 mg.

4. The average delay interval for morphine is approximately 8 minutes.

5. The number of times Mrs. B. can self-administer a PCA dose in 1 hour is 60 minutes ÷ 8 = approximately 7 times.

6. The PCA dose is 10 mg ÷ 7 times/h = approximately 1.4 mg/PCA dose.

Because Mrs. B. is reporting mild nausea, the decision is made to start with a slightly lower PCA dose and no basal rate. Her starting IV PCA prescription is: PCA dose = 1 mg; delay interval = 8 minutes; basal rate = 0; hour limit = 7 mg.

The nurse reviews with Mrs. B. how to use the PCA pump to manage her pain. Mrs. B. is discharged from the PACU mildly sedated, comfortable with a pain rating of 3/10, and self-administering PCA without difficulty.

To save time and prevent errors, tables with PCA prescription ranges commonly used for opioid-naive patients with severe, moderate, and mild pain can be developed in advance (see Table 6.13 for an example of PCA prescription ranges for severe pain). These can be posted in areas where physicians prescribe PCA. Preprinted physician orders with the appropriate starting IV PCA prescriptions for the most commonly used opioids guide physicians to select individualized doses on the basis of their patients' pain intensity.

Patient-only PCA

Sometimes family members, friends, and even staff members, who may think they are helping, decide to activate PCA for the patient. This can produce life-threatening sedation and respiratory depression. The dangers of this action must be explained to patients, family, and friends. As alternatives, family and friends are encouraged to remind the patient to press the PCA button or contact a staff member if they think the patient is experiencing uncontrolled pain (Pasero, 1996).

Adding a continuous infusion to IV PCA in opioid-naive patients

The purpose of a continuous infusion (basal rate) is to help maintain a stable analgesic level. It has the advantage of letting the patient sleep without frequent interruptions by pain (APS, 1992). If a continuous infusion is not added, patients must self-administer the PCA dose often enough to maintain a stable analgesic level. Although a continuous infusion is recommended and commonplace for opioid-tolerant patients, the addition of a continuous infusion to IV PCA bolus doses for opioid-naive patients outside of the ICU is controversial.

Studies have produced mixed findings in terms of the effectiveness and safety of adding continuous infusions to IV PCA in opioid-naive patients. Some researchers report that the addition of a continuous infusion does not improve analgesia, produces excessive side effects, and results in consumption of higher amounts of opioid drug (Parker, Holtmann, White, 1991; Smythe, Zak, O'Donnell, 1996). Others find less fluctuation in sedation and better pain control and recommend the addition of a continuous infusion to IV PCA for some patients (Hansen, Noyes, Lehman, 1991; Rayburn, Smith, Woods, 1989).

Although the studies yield conflicting results, clinical experience indicates that the addition of a continuous infusion to IV PCA for opioid-naive patients can be done safely and produce excellent results. Some clinicians initiate IV PCA therapy with a continuous infusion routinely for patients with severe acute pain; others add it if pain is uncontrolled with PCA alone; still others use a continuous infusion only at night to help maintain steady analgesic blood levels while patients sleep (unpublished data, Chris Pasero). The decision to add a continuous infusion to IV PCA for opioid-naive children and elderly patients should be made on the basis of patient response rather than a preconceived notion that they cannot tolerate continuous infusions.

As mentioned, when IV PCA is used to manage pain in opioid-tolerant patients, the continuous infusion usually

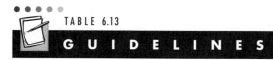

TABLE 6.13

GUIDELINES

STARTING IV PCA PRESCRIPTION RANGES FOR OPIOID-NAIVE ADULTS[1]

Drug	Typical Concentration	Loading Dose	PCA Dose	Delay	Basal Rate	Hour Limit
Morphine	1 mg/ml	2.5 mg repeat PRN	0.6–2.0 mg	5–10 min	0–1.25 mg/h	7.5–12.5 mg/h
Hydromor-phone	0.2 mg/ml	0.4 mg repeat PRN	0.1–0.3 mg	5–10 min	0–0.2 mg/h	1.2–2.0 mg/h
Fentanyl	10 μg/ml	25 μg repeat PRN	5–20 μg	4–8 min	0–10 μg	75–125 μg/h
Meperidine[2]	10 mg/ml	20 mg repeat PRN	5–20 mg	5–10 min	0–10 mg/h[3] NR	50–100 mg/h

May be duplicated for use in clinical practice. From McCaffery M, Pasero C: *Pain: Clinical manual*, p. 252. Copyright © 1999, Mosby, Inc.

To save time and prevent errors, tables with PCA prescription ranges commonly used for opioid-naive patients with severe, moderate, and mild pain can be developed in advance. Table 6.13 is an example of one for severe pain.

[1]Prescription ranges in this table are calculated for severe pain. Ranges for moderate pain are 50% of those for severe pain, for mild pain 25%.

[2]Should be used for very brief course, in patients who are allergic to the other opioids listed in this chart.

[3]Accumulation of normeperidine can cause toxic CNS effects and is more likely to occur when meperidine is administered by continuous infusion.

h, hour; *μg,* microgram; *mg,* milligram; *min,* minute; *ml,* milliliter; *NR,* not recommended; *PRN,* as needed.

Information from American Pain Society (APS): *Principles of analgesic use in the treatment of acute and cancer pain,* ed 3, Glenview, IL, 1992, APS; Hunt RF, Abbott Laboratories, Hospital Products Division: Letter communication to Malcolm Cohen, MD, Mt. Sinai Medical Center, Miami Beach, FL, July 11, 1989.

---

provides the larger part of the patient's total opioid requirement, with PCA doses being used as rescue doses (APS, 1992). The opposite is true for opioid-naive patients receiving IV PCA. When a continuous infusion is added to IV PCA for these patients, it should not exceed one half the projected hourly requirement (APS, 1992). It is important to note that projected hourly requirement is not the hour limit (see Box 6.26).

Key to the safe use of continuous infusions in opioid-naive patients is close nurse monitoring of sedation and respiratory status (see pp. 267-270 for more on monitoring sedation and respiratory depression) and decreasing the opioid dose if increased sedation is detected (Eige, 1992; Pasero, McCaffery, 1994; Sinatra, 1998). For postoperative patients, it also is important to consider decreasing the opioid dose, beginning with a 25% to 50% decrease in the continuous infusion, each day after the day of surgery as the patient recovers and experiences less pain (see also Tapering on p. 270).

Patient Example

Mrs. G. is managing her pain after total hip replacement with IV PCA hydromorphone. She has been stable since surgery 4 hours ago. She is mildly sedated with a respiratory rate of 16 breaths/minute. She has self-administered an average of 4 PCA doses every hour since PCA was started in the PACU. She rates her pain 4/10 and says that she is unable to fall asleep and is afraid that if she does, her pain will get out of control. Adding a basal rate to her PCA therapy may provide a solution. Mrs. G. self-administers a PCA dose of 0.2 mg about 4 times/h. Her hourly requirement is 0.2 mg × 4 = 0.8 mg/h. The American Pain Society (1992) recommends that the basal rate be no more than one half of the projected hourly requirement: 0.8 mg ÷ 2 = 0.4 mg. Because Mrs. G. is elderly (78 years old), a conservative basal rate of 0.1 mg is started. Later that day Mrs. G. reports that she is able to rest much better, is no longer worried about losing pain control, and does not have to "work so hard" to keep her pain under control. (She now averages 1 to 2 PCA doses/h.) She notes that her present pain rating of 2/10 is better than before the basal rate was added. She is mildly sedated with a respiratory rate of 16 breaths/minute.

Initiating PCA in the PACU

When IV PCA is prescribed for postoperative patients, it should be initiated when patients arrive in the PACU postoperatively. Initiating IV PCA in the PACU rather than on the nursing unit allows the health care team to evaluate patient response to the therapy early in the postoperative course and prevents delays in analgesia on the nursing unit. A particularly dangerous scenario to avoid is that of patients receiving IM opioid injections on the nursing unit while waiting for IV PCA to be initiated (Pasero, McCaffery, 1996a).

After pain is under control in the PACU, pain management plans can be reviewed with patients, including what action to take when pain relief is inadequate. The PCA button should be given to patients as soon as they are awake and alert enough to manage their own pain. PACU nurses can review the safety mechanisms of the infusion pump and how to correctly use the PCA button, reminding patients that it is for their use only. As mentioned, many PACUs establish discharge goals that include acceptable pain ratings for patients, usually 4/10 or less (Pasero, McCaffery, 1996a).

PCA titration

PCA starting prescriptions are estimates of what patients will require. It is crucial that patients be evaluated regularly and titrated when necessary to maintain adequate analgesia along with tolerable and manageable side effects. Patients reporting inadequate pain relief with the use of PCA require prompt evaluation. The need for readjustment of PCA parameters is signaled by pain ratings above the identified comfort goal or by unmanageable or intolerable side effects. Pain ratings and incidence of side effects, in addition to the patient's account and the PCA history retained in the pump's memory, provide valuable information about the pain and should be used to guide the various approaches to titration. For example, approaches differ between patients who are not activating PCA before painful activity (incident pain) and those who reach their maximum hour limit of opioid (see Table 6.14 for interventions).

The use of PCA does not absolve nurses from their role as the patient's primary pain manager. Simply telling a patient to "press the PCA button" does not constitute acceptable pain management. Likewise, concluding that a patient is "using too much" opioid or "pressing the PCA button too much" (e.g., when a patient self-administers the maximum programmed amount [hour limit] in less than 1 hour) has no scientific basis and creates an adversarial relationship between patient and caregiver. More important, it presents a tremendous barrier to providing acceptable pain treatment and improving patient outcome.

Special considerations about the use of IV PCA in pediatric patients

PCA is safe, effective, and used commonly in children older than 5 years of age (Berde, Kain, 1996). The same patient selection guidelines and considerations for the use of PCA in adults apply to children (see Box 6.3 on p. 176). It is extremely important to remind parents and caregivers not to press the PCA button for the child unless they have been designated as the child's primary pain manager. For example, parents can be the primary pain manager for a child who is unable to understand the relationship between pain, pushing the PCA button, and pain relief (see Box 6.4 on p. 177, Unconventional Use of the PCA Pump). Table 6.15 provides IV PCA dosing guidelines for pediatric patients. The principles regarding starting dose estimates and titration for adults apply also to children.

Switching to Another Opioid Analgesic

Very little difference exists in the ability of mu agonist opioid drugs to relieve pain. Analgesia is dose related rather than opioid related. Thus unrelieved pain per se usually is not a sound reason for switching to another opioid. Other options for improving analgesia should be tried, such as increasing the opioid dose, providing a NSAID ATC, or adding local anesthetic to epidural opioids. Side effects that are intolerable and unmanageable are more likely to be an appropriate reason to switch to another opioid (see Table 6.16 on p. 256 for options when analgesia from opioids is limited by side effects). Because of great interindividual variability, even opioids that bind to the same receptor site can produce side effects of different intensities in patients.

Patient difficulty in adhering to an analgesic regimen may also be a sound reason to switch to another opioid (Levy, 1993). Sometimes another opioid allows a reduction in pills or liquid volume needed for pain relief. Fewer or smaller doses may be possible, making it easier for some patients to comply with the pain treatment regimen.

Occasionally switching from one opioid or route to another opioid or route is done to reduce the cost of long-term opioid treatment. For example, in one case the cost of opioid treatment was reduced from $1000 per day to less than $25 per day when a patient was switched from parenteral hydromorphone to oral methadone. However, the cost of the 10-day hospital stay required during the conversion process was not included in the cost analysis (Thomas, Bruera, 1995). Thus several factors must be considered when switching opioids is done to reduce costs.

When switching an opioid-tolerant patient to an alternative opioid drug, it is wise to assume that cross-tolerance will be incomplete (Foley, 1995). This means that a patient who has developed tolerance to one opioid analgesic may not be equally tolerant to another. Therefore when switching to a new opioid, opioid-tolerant patients should be started on one half (50%) to two thirds (66%) of the equianalgesic dose of the new opioid (Coyle, Cherny, Portenoy, 1995; Levy, 1993) (see pp. 172-174 for more on cross-tolerance and use of conversion charts and Box 6.6 on p. 185 on guidelines for switching to methadone).

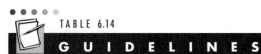

TABLE 6.14

G U I D E L I N E S

IMPROVEMENT OF PAIN CONTROL AND REDUCTION OF SIDE EFFECTS ASSOCIATED WITH IV PCA AND EPIDURAL ANALGESIA

Problem	Intervention
No pain relief with no side effect(s)	1. ✓ infusion system is patent and functioning from pump to patient access site. 2. ✓ pump is loaded and programmed correctly. 3. ✓ PCA (PCEA) button is attached to pump. Review PCA (PCEA) history (see disproportionate injection/attempt ratio below). 4. ✓ delay interval is appropriate (see Table 6.10 on p. 225 or Box 6.26 on p. 250 and Table 6.13 on p. 252). 5. Relieve pain by administering supplemental boluses (see Box 6.24 on p. 247 or Box 6.26 on p. 250). 6. Increase the opioid dose 25%–100%: For patient with basal rate only, increase basal rate; for opioid-tolerant patient, increase the basal rate with a proportional increase in the PCA (PCEA) bolus dose; for opioid-naive postoperative patient who is receiving a basal rate in addition to PCA (PCEA), first try increasing the basal rate. If this is ineffective, increase PCA (PCEA) bolus dose. 7. Increase hour limit proportionately.
No pain relief with side effect(s)	1. Treat with side effect medication. 2. Add or increase nonopioid or appropriate adjuvant. 3. Decrease opioid dose 25% (basal rate first).
Pain relief with side effect(s)	1. Treat with side effect medication. 2. Decrease opioid dose by 25%–50%; larger decrease may be necessary to treat excessive sedation and/or respiratory depression.
Pain relief with side effect(s) occurring just after PCA (PCEA) dose administration (e.g., excessive sedation after self-administration of PCA [PCEA] dose)	1. Treat with side effect medication. 2. To decrease the peak effect and lower the level of toxicity, give smaller doses more often (i.e., decrease the PCA [PCEA] bolus dose 25%–50% and shorten the delay interval).
Pain relief except during activity; no side effects	Remind patient to self-administer PCA (PCEA) before activity (e.g., 2–3 minutes IV PCA; 5–10 minutes PCEA), then continue to self-administer as needed during activity.

Maximum programmed amount used (hour limit reached)	In this situation, the infusion pump will not allow the patient to self-administer anymore PCA (PCEA) bolus doses until the PCA hour elapses. Patients may or may not be in pain, but the need to increase the dose is the same for all who reach their hour limit. The hour limit should be 3–5 times the estimated hourly requirement (see Box 6.26 on p. 250).
	  • If patient is in pain, relieve pain by administering supplemental boluses (see Box 6.24 on p. 247 or Box 6.26 on p. 250).
	  • All patients:
	1. ✓ delay is appropriate and hour limit is calculated (see Table 6.10 on p. 225 or Box 6.26 on p. 250 and Table 6.13 on p. 252) and programmed correctly.
	2. Increase the opioid dose 25%–100%: For opioid-tolerant patient, increase the basal rate with a proportional increase in the PCA (PCEA) bolus dose and hour limit; for opioid-naive patient, add or increase basal rate and/or increase PCA (PCEA) bolus dose.
	3. Increase hour limit proportionately.

Somnolence, respiratory depression	1. In opioid-naive patient, stop opioid; in opioid-tolerant patient, consider decreasing opioid dose by 75%, instead of stopping opioid, to maintain enough opioid to prevent withdrawal. 2. Consider administering naloxone (see Box 6.29 on p. 270). 3. Add nonsedating nonopioid. 4. Resume opioid with 50% reduction in opioid dose when sedation level and respiratory status acceptable.

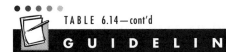

TABLE 6.14—cont'd

GUIDELINES

IMPROVEMENT OF PAIN CONTROL AND REDUCTION OF SIDE EFFECTS ASSOCIATED WITH IV PCA AND EPIDURAL ANALGESIA

Problem	Intervention

Disproportionate number of injections and attempts (injection/attempt ratio)	1. ✓ patient is only one pressing PCA (PCEA) button (often when another person is activating PCA [PCEA] for the patient, a disproportionate injection/attempt ratio is found).
	2. Determine ratio of injections to attempts (number of attempts ÷ number of injections).
	  • If ratio is <1 injection to 2 or 3 attempts and patient has no pain, do nothing.
	  • If ratio is <1 injection to 2 or 3 attempts and patient has pain, relieve pain by administering supplemental boluses (see Box 6.24 on p. 247 or Box 6.26 on p. 250) and increase opioid dose 25%-100%.
	  • If ratio is >1 injection to 3 attempts and patient has no pain relief, establish pain relief with supplemental boluses (see Box 6.24) and remind patient to "press the button to give yourself a dose of pain medicine before pain is severe, then put the button down and wait long enough (2 or 3 minutes for IV PCA; 5-10 minutes for PCEA) to evaluate the effect of the dose before pressing the button again."

May be duplicated for use in clinical practice. From McCaffery M, Pasero C: *Pain: Clinical manual,* pp. 254-255. Copyright © 1999, Mosby, Inc.

PCA starting prescriptions are estimates of what patients will require. Patients reporting inadequate pain relief or side effects with the use of PCA require prompt evaluation. The need for titration of PCA is signaled by pain ratings above the identified comfort goal or by unmanageable or intolerable side effects.

PCA, patient-controlled analgesia; *PCEA,* patient-controlled epidural analgesia.

Information from Pasero C: *Acute pain management service policy and procedure manual,* Rolling Hills Estates, CA, 1994, Academy Medical Systems, Inc.

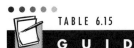

TABLE 6.15

GUIDELINES

PEDIATRIC IV PCA DOSING

Opioid Analgesic	PCA Dose	Delay (Lock-out)	Basal Rate
Morphine	10-30 μg/kg/dose	6-10 minutes	0-30 μg/kg/h
Fentanyl	0.5-1.0 μg/kg/dose	6-10 minutes	0-1.0 μg/kg/h
Hydromorphone (Dilaudid)	3-5 μg/kg/dose	6-10 minutes	0-5 μg/kg/h

May be duplicated for use in clinical practice. From McCaffery M, Pasero C: *Pain: Clinical manual,* p. 255. Copyright © 1999, Mosby, Inc.

Table 6.15 presents pediatric IV PCA dosing guidelines.

h, hour; *kg,* kilogram; *μg,* microgram.

Information from Houck CS: The management of acute pain in the child. In Ashburn MA, Rice LF, editors: *The management of pain,* ed 3, pp 651-666, New York, 1998, Churchill Livingstone; Yaster M, Krane EJ, Kaplan RF et al., editors: *Pediatric pain management and sedation handbook,* Formulary, St. Louis, 1997, Mosby.

Patient Example

Mr. T. has been receiving a continuous IV infusion of meperidine, 20 mg/h, with 5 mg rescue bolus doses PRN since his admission to ICU 15 days ago after an automobile accident. Hand tremors and twitching are noted during assessment and thought to be due to normeperidine accumulation. He is to be switched immediately to an equianalgesic continuous IV infusion of morphine. The following calculation is necessary:

1. Determine the total daily dose of meperidine from continuous infusion and rescue bolus doses:

  • 20 mg × 24 h = 480 mg

  • 5 mg × 3 rescue boluses in the last 24 h = 15 mg

  • 480 mg + 15 mg = 495 mg

2. Locate the dose of IV meperidine listed in the equianalgesic chart (75 mg).

●●●●●

TABLE 6.16   **Options When Analgesia From Opioids is Limited by Side Effects**

OPTION	APPROACHES
Reduce systemic opioid requirement	
Pharmacologic techniques	Adjuvant analgesics
	Spinal opioids
Nonpharmacologic techniques	Cognitive-behavioral methods
	Physical methods (ice, TENS)
	Exercise programs
	Rehabilitation programs
	Anesthetic therapies (e.g., blocks)
	Surgical treatment (e.g., cordotomy)
Identify an opioid with a more favorable balance between analgesia and side effects	Sequential opioid trials
Improve the tolerability of the opioid regimen to allow further dose escalation	More aggressive side effect management (e.g., psychostimulant for somnolence)

May be duplicated for use in clinical practice. As appears in McCaffery M, Pasero C: *Pain: Clinical manual,* p. 256, 1999, Mosby, Inc.

Table 6.16 lists some of the options to consider when analgesia from opioids is limited by side effects.

TENS, transcutaneous electrical nerve stimulation.

Modified from Portenoy RK: Adjuvant analgesics in pain management. In Doyle D, Hanks GWC, MacDonald N, editors: *Oxford textbook of palliative medicine,* ed 2, pp. 361-390, New York, 1998, Oxford University Press.

---

3. **Determine the number of equianalgesic dose units**
   in the 24 h meperidine dose: 495 mg ÷ 75 mg = 6.6 units.
4. **Locate the dose of IV morphine listed in the equi-analgesic chart that is approximately equal to 75 mg of meperidine (10 mg).**
5. **Determine the 24 h equianalgesic dose of IV morphine:**
   10 mg × 6.6 units = 66 mg of morphine/24 h.
6. **Determine the hourly morphine dose: 66 mg ÷ 24 hours = 2.8 mg/h.**
7. **Because Mr. T. has been receiving meperidine for several days, he may have developed tolerance to the analgesia of meperidine. However, he may not be equally tolerant to morphine. Therefore Mr. T. will be started on two thirds (66%) of the equianalgesic dose of morphine: 2.8 mg × 66% (or 2.8 mg × 0.66) = approximately 1.8 mg.**

Rescue doses of 0.5 mg (approximately 25% of the hourly opioid dose) IV morphine PRN are prescribed for breakthrough pain (see Box 6.23 on p. 245).

If the opioid-tolerant patient has been taking a high dose of opioid, it is best not to abruptly discontinue the present opioid and convert to the new in one step. This could cause a significant overdose that precipitates undesirable side effects or an underdose that precipitates severe pain. Instead, it is best to make the transition with 50% of the current opioid dose combined with 50% of the projected dose for the new opioid for several days.

From this starting point, gradual increases in the new opioid drug and decreases in the old can be made until the switch is complete. The higher the dose of the current opioid, the more important it is to make the transition using 50/50 dosing (see Box 6.27 for guidelines when switching from one opioid to another).

Patient Example

For the last 2 months Mrs. Q. has been receiving a continuous SC infusion of morphine, 25 mg/h, with 5 mg rescue bolus doses PRN. She has developed unmanageable sedation and confusion. Her physician would like her to be switched to an equianalgesic continuous SC infusion of hydromorphone. The following calculation is necessary:

1. **Determine the total daily dose of morphine from continuous infusion and rescue bolus doses:**

   - 25 mg × 24 h = 600 mg

   - 5 mg × 4 rescue boluses in the last 24 h = 20 mg

   - 600 mg + 20 mg = 620 mg

2. **Locate the dose of parenteral morphine listed in the equianalgesic chart (10 mg).**
3. **Determine the number of equianalgesic dose units in the 24 h morphine dose: 620 mg ÷ 10 mg = 62 units.**
4. **Locate the dose of parenteral hydromorphone listed in the equianalgesic chart that**

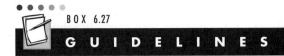

GUIDELINES

SWITCHING FROM ONE OPIOID TO ANOTHER

1. Determine the total daily dose of the present opioid (e.g., morphine, 30 mg, taken q4h PO: 30 mg × 6 doses/day = 180 mg/24 h).
2. Locate the dose of the present opioid by the present route listed in the equianalgesic chart (e.g., 30 mg).
3. Determine the number of equianalgesic dose units in the 24 h dose (No. 1) by dividing the 24 h dose by the equianalgesic dose (step 2) (e.g., 180 mg ÷ 30 mg = 6 units).
4. Locate the dose of the new opioid by the present (or new) route listed on the equianalgesic chart (e.g., hydromorphone, 7.5 mg).
5. Determine the 24 h dose of the new opioid by multiplying the equianalgesic dose of the new opioid (step 4) by the equianalgesic dose units of the present opioid (step 3) (e.g., 7.5 mg × 6 units = 45 mg/24 h).
6. Divide the 24 h dose of the new drug by the number of doses to be given each 24 h (e.g., 45 mg/24 h ÷ 6 doses = 7.5 mg q4h).
7. If the patient is opioid tolerant and has been taking a high dose of opioid, it is best not to abruptly discontinue the present opioid and convert to the new in one step. This could lead to an overdose, causing undesirable side effects, or an underdose, precipitating severe pain. Instead, in these cases, make the transition starting with 50% of the current opioid dose combined with 50% of the projected dose for the new opioid. Gradual increases in the new opioid drug and decreases in the old can be made until the switch is complete over a period of several days (e.g., hydromorphone: 7.5 mg × 50% [or 7.5 mg ÷ 2]) = 3.75 mg; morphine: 30 mg × 50% [or 3.75 mg ÷ 2]) = 15 mg. Start by giving hydromorphone 3.75 mg PO q4h and morphine 15 mg PO q4h. It may be necessary to adjust the dose of the new opioid (i.e., maintain the 50% dose of the old opioid and increase the new opioid for insufficient pain relief). Once the combined doses provide good pain control, drop the old opioid and double the new.

Occasionally, during opioid treatment it is necessary to switch from one opioid to another. Calculating the equianalgesic dose of the new opioid increases the likelihood that patients will tolerate the switch to a new opioid without loss of pain control or excessive side effects. Box 6.27 provides calculations for equianalgesic dosing.

h, hour; *hs*, at sleep; *mg*, milligram; *PO*, oral; *q*, every.

is approximately equal to 10 mg of morphine (1.5 mg).
5. Determine the 24 h equianalgesic dose of parenteral hydromorphone: 1.5 mg × 62 units = 93 mg of hydromorphone/24 h.
6. Determine the hourly hydromorphone dose: 93 mg ÷ 24 hours = approximately 4 mg/h.

7. Because Mrs. Q. has been receiving morphine for several days, she may have developed tolerance to the analgesia of morphine. However, she may not be equally tolerant to hydromorphone. Therefore Mrs. Q. will be started on two thirds (66%) of the equianalgesic dose of hydromorphone: 4 mg × 66% (or 4 mg × 0.66) = approximately 3 mg.
8. Rescue doses of 1 mg parenteral hydromorphone PRN are prescribed for breakthrough pain (see Box 6.23 on p. 245).
9. Because Mrs. Q has been receiving a high dose of opioid for a long period of time, it is best to make the transition to the new opioid slowly. To do this, she is started on 50% of the new opioid dose (hydromorphone 3 mg/h ÷ 2 = 1.5 mg/h) while taking 50% of the old opioid dose (morphine 25 mg/h ÷ 2 = 12.5 mg/h) for several days. Gradual increases in the hydromorphone dose and decreases in the morphine dose are made until the switch to hydromorphone is complete. Inadequate pain relief is treated with rescue doses and increases in the hourly hydromorphone dose. Within 9 days, the switch to hydromorphone is complete without loss of pain control, and Mrs. Q. is much less sedated and confused.

Switching From Epidural to IV Opioid Analgesia

Occasionally, a patient must be switched from epidural opioids to IV opioids before the transition to oral analgesia can be made (e.g., when the epidural catheter is accidentally pulled out or analgesia is unsatisfactory because the epidural catheter location is less than optimal). When this happens, conversion ratios usually are used as guidelines for selecting starting IV doses. Studies are lacking and controversy exists over the correct ratios to use when switching opioid-naive patients from the various epidural opioids to parenteral opioids (see pp. 260-261 for selecting starting epidural opioid doses in opioid tolerant individuals). Most often, a conversion ratio of 1:10 is used to determine a starting dose when switching opioid-naive patients from epidural morphine to IV morphine (Sinatra, 1992). Many clinicians use ratio of 1:5 for switching from epidural hydromorphone to IV hydromorphone and a ratio of 1:3 for switching patients from epidural fentanyl to IV fentanyl.

Patient Example

Mr. O. received an above-the-knee amputation 2 days ago. A continuous epidural infusion of fentanyl and bupivacaine was initiated 36 hours before surgery to provide preemptive analgesia and keep

Mr. O. pain free (see Chapter 4 and p. 174 for more on preemptive analgesia). The epidural analgesic infusion was continued to control his postoperative pain. His current epidural analgesic dose is fentanyl 40 μg/h and bupivacaine 0.125%. His preoperative and postoperative pain ratings have been consistently <1/10. Mr. O. has a fever and possible wound infection. Because of the possible infection, the anesthesiologist wants to remove the epidural catheter and switch Mr. O. to IV PCA morphine. To determine the equianalgesic IV PCA morphine prescription, Mr. O.'s 24 h epidural fentanyl dose must first be converted to an equianalgesic 24 h IV fentanyl dose, then the 24 h IV fentanyl dose can be used to determine an equianalgesic 24 h IV morphine dose. From this, the IV PCA morphine prescription can be calculated.

1. Determine Mr. O.'s 24 h epidural fentanyl dose: 24 × 40 μg = 960 μg/24 h.
2. Use the conversion ratio of 1:3 to determine the 24 h equianalgesic IV fentanyl dose: 960 μg × 3 = 2880 μg/24 h.
3. Determine the hourly IV fentanyl dose: 2880 μg ÷ 24 h = 120 μg/h.
4. Locate the dose of fentanyl by the IV route in the equianalgesic chart (100 μg/h ≅ 4 mg/h morphine or 25 μg/h ≅ 1 mg/h morphine).
5. Determine the hourly equianalgesic dose of IV morphine by dividing the hourly fentanyl dose by the equianalgesic fentanyl dose: 120 μg ÷ 25 μg = 4.8 mg/h.

The following calculations are used to determine the appropriate starting IV PCA prescription for Mr. O. (see Box 6.26 on p. 250):

1. The projected hourly requirement for Mr. O. is 4.8 mg.
2. An appropriate conservative starting hour limit is three times the projected hourly requirement: 4.8 mg × 3 = approximately 14 mg.
3. The usual delay interval for morphine is 8 minutes.
4. The number of times Mr. O. can self-administer a PCA dose in 1 hour is: 60 minutes ÷ 8 = approximately 7 times.
5. The PCA dose is: 14 mg ÷ 7 = approximately 2 mg/ PCA dose.

Mr. O.'s physician would like him to have a small basal rate. His starting IV PCA prescription is: PCA dose = 1.5 mg; delay interval = 8 minutes; basal rate = 0.5 mg/h; hour limit (adjusted for basal rate) = 11 mg.

IV PCA is initiated as soon as the epidural fentanyl is discontinued. Mr. O. tolerated the transition to IV PCA without needing clinician-administered boluses or losing pain control.

Patient Example

Mrs. J. had a Whipple procedure 3 days ago. Her postoperative pain has been well controlled (3/10)

with PCEA morphine (basal rate = 0.1 mg/h; PCEA dose = 0.1 mg; delay interval = 10 minutes; hour limit = 0.7 mg). While ambulating this morning, Mrs. J.'s epidural catheter was accidentally pulled out. Mrs. J. is NPO with an NG tube, so she is unable to take oral analgesia and will be given IV PCA morphine instead. Because Mrs. J. will continue with the same opioid (morphine) and the same method of administration (PCA), the calculation for determining an equianalgesic starting prescription for the IV route is relatively simple. The ratio of 1:10 is used to calculate starting doses when changing from the epidural morphine to IV morphine:

1. Determine the equianalgesic IV PCA dose: 0.1 mg (PCEA dose) × 10 = 1 mg.
2. Determine the equianalgesic IV basal rate: 0.1 mg (basal rate) × 10 = 1 mg.
3. The delay interval of 10 minutes is acceptable for both IV PCA and PCEA morphine.
4. The equianalgesic hour limit is 0.7 mg × 10 = 7 mg.

An appropriate starting IV PCA morphine prescription for Mrs. J. would be: PCA dose = 1 mg; delay interval = 10 minutes; basal rate = 1 mg; hour limit = 7 mg.

Switching From IV to Oral Opioid Analgesia

Most often switching to another route of administration is done when acute pain subsides and the opioid-naive patient is switched from IV opioids to oral opioids. Equianalgesic doses increase the likelihood that the transition to the oral route will be done without loss of pain control.

Patient Example

Mrs. J. had a Whipple procedure 5 days ago. She has been managing her postoperative pain using IV PCA morphine for the last 2 days; the first 3 days were managed with epidural analgesia. Her condition has improved to the point that her basal rate was discontinued yesterday and today she presses her PCA button once or twice an hour. She is tolerating oral fluids. Her physician wants to discontinue PCA and has prescribed 1 Percocet (oxycodone, 5 mg, plus acetaminophen, 325 mg per tablet) q4h PRN for pain. To be sure this prescription is comparable to what Mrs. J. has been taking to control her pain with IV PCA, her nurse calculates Mrs. J.'s analgesic requirements:

1. Determine Mrs. J.'s current total 24 h dose of morphine by adding up the number of times she self-administered morphine during the last 24 h (29 times) and multiplying it by the PCA dose (1 mg). The total 24 h dose of morphine is: 1 mg × 29 times =

29 mg. (Although Mrs. J. received a basal rate for the first 2 hours of the last 24 hours, this amount is not added to the calculation because she no longer requires it.)

2. Locate the equianalgesic dose of morphine by the IV route in the equianalgesic chart (10 mg).
3. Determine the number of equianalgesic dose units in the 24 h dose of morphine by dividing the total 24 h dose (29 mg) by the equianalgesic dose (10 mg): 29 mg ÷ 10 = 2.9 dose units.
4. Locate the equianalgesic dose of PO oxycodone in the equianalgesic chart (20 mg).
5. Determine the 24 h dose of PO oxycodone that will be required by multiplying the equianalgesic dose of oxycodone (20 mg) by the equianalgesic dose units of morphine (2.9 units): 20 mg × 2.9 = 58 mg of PO oxycodone.
6. Determine the number of doses of oxycodone that may be taken as prescribed each 24 h: 1 dose q4h each 24 h = 6 doses.
7. Determine the number of doses that would be equianalgesic to what Mrs. J. is currently taking by dividing the total 24 h dose of oxycodone (58 mg) by the number of doses that may be taken as prescribed each 24 h (6 doses): 58 mg ÷ 6 doses = approximately 9.7 mg oxycodone/ dose.
8. Determine whether the prescription the physician has written is equianalgesic: Because Percocet has just 5 mg of oxycodone per tablet, Mrs. J. would need to take 2 tablets, not 1, q4h to achieve the level of pain relief provided by IV PCA morphine. The acetaminophen (325 mg/tablet) will provide some additional analgesia, but not enough. The prescription the physician has written is not equianalgesic to the previous dose. Rather, it is about one half the previous dose and probably will not provide adequate relief for Mrs. J.
9. Mrs. J.'s nurse first faxes her calculations to the physician and follows with a telephone call to discuss her calculations. The physician agrees that the prescription needs to be changed to 2 Percocet q4h.

Switching From One Opioid and Route to Another Opioid and Route

Switching to another route also occurs in opioid-tolerant patients with cancer pain when they are no longer able to take oral medications and require other routes, such as rectal, transdermal, SC, IV, or epidural. Sometimes a change from one route to another requires a change from one opioid to another.

Patient Example

Mr. S., previously at home, had satisfactory pain control with 120 mg of PO controlled-release oxycodone twice daily and did not require rescue doses. He has been admitted for initiation of a hydromorphone SC infusion because he can no longer swallow. He finds the rectal route of administration objectionable and the transdermal route is not considered appropriate because his pain is expected to escalate rapidly as his disease begins to progress. To determine the dose of SC hydromorphone that is approximately equal to the dose of PO oxycodone Mr. S. is taking, the following calculations are necessary:

1. Determine the total 24 h dose of oxycodone: 120 mg × 2 doses/24 h = 240 mg/24 h.
2. Locate the equianalgesic dose of PO oxycodone in the equianalgesic chart (20 mg).
3. Determine the number of equianalgesic dose units in the 24 h dose by dividing the 24 h dose of oxycodone by the equianalgesic dose of PO oxycodone: 240 mg ÷ 20 mg = 12 units.
4. Locate the dose of SC hydromorphone listed in the equianalgesic chart that is approximately equal to 20 mg of PO oxycodone (1.5 mg).
5. Determine the 24 h dose of SC hydromorphone by multiplying the dose of SC hydromorphone by the equianalgesic dose units of oxycodone: 1.5 mg × 12 units = 18 mg/24 h.
6. Divide the 24 h dose of hydromorphone by the number of doses to be given each 24 h: 18 mg ÷ 24 doses = approximately 0.8 mg/h.
7. Because Mr. S. is opioid tolerant, he is started on two thirds (66%) of the equianalgesic dose of hydromorphone: 0.8 mg × 66% (or 0.8 mg × 0.66) = 0.5 mg.
8. In Mr. S.'s situation it is not possible to make the transition using a combination of 50% oxycodone and 50% hydromorphone. Therefore when the oxycodone is discontinued and the hydromorphone is started, he is watched closely for side effects and rescue bolus doses of 0.2 mg of SC hydromorphone PRN (see Box 6.23 on p. 245) are offered at least q 30 minutes for breakthrough pain. He tolerates the transition without difficulty.

Switching From Multiple Opioids and Routes to One Opioid and Route

Sometimes patients are taking multiple opioid prescriptions by more than one route to control their pain. For example, they may be taking an IM opioid to control their ongoing pain and using a combination opioid and nonopioid, such as Percocet, for breakthrough pain. To switch a patient from multiple opioids and routes to one opioid and one route, the total daily dose of all of the opioids must be calculated.

Patient Example

Mr. C. has been admitted from a skilled nursing facility for diagnostic tests and evaluation of his osteoarthritis pain. His current prescription for pain control is 50 mg IM meperidine q4h PRN and 1 to 2 Vicodin (hydrocodone, 5 mg, and acetaminophen, 500 mg/tablet) PO q4h PRN. He has required an average of 6 doses of meperidine and 12 Vicodin per day for the last 5 days when his pain began to worsen. He rates his pain as 4/10 most of the day, which is acceptable for him. His physician would like to discontinue the meperidine and Vicodin and switch Mr. C. to controlled-release oxycodone. The total 24 h dose of opioid is calculated as follows:

1. Determine the 24 h dose of meperidine: 50 mg × 6 doses = 300 mg.
2. Determine the equianalgesic dose units of meperidine: 300 mg ÷ 75 = 4 units.
3. Determine the 24 h dose of hydrocodone: 5 mg × 12 = 60 mg.
4. Determine the equianalgesic dose units of hydrocodone (although equianalgesic data are unavailable for hydrocodone, 30 mg is used as an amount approximately equal to the other opioid doses listed in the equianalgesic chart): 60 mg ÷ 30 = 2 units.
5. Determine the 24 h total equianalgesic dose units: 4 + 2 = 6 units/24 h.
6. Determine the 24 h dose of oxycodone by multiplying the dose units/24 h (6) by the equianalgesic dose of oral oxycodone (20 mg): 20 mg × 6 = 120 mg.
7. Because Mr. C is opioid tolerant, he is started on two thirds (66%) of the equianalgesic dose of oxycodone: 120 mg × 66% (or 120 mg × 0.66) = approximately 80 mg/24 h.
8. Determine the q12h starting dose of controlled-release oxycodone: 80 mg ÷ 2 = 40 mg.

In Mr. C.'s case, combining the old with the new opioid during transition is not feasible. Therefore, when the pervious opioids are discontinued and the controlled-release oxycodone is started, he is watched closely for side effects, and rescue doses of PO immediate-release oxycodone are used for breakthrough pain (see Box 6.23 on p. 245):

- 80 mg ÷ 10 (1/10) = approximately 10 mg.

- 80 mg ÷ 6 (1/6) = approximately 15 mg.

Mr. C. is given 10 mg of immediate-release oxycodone with the first dose of controlled-release oxycodone. Rescue doses are offered hourly. Ibuprofen is administered q8h ATC. During the first 24 h of the transition to controlled-release oxycodone, Mr. C. required just two rescue doses and rated his pain 2/10 most of the day. He reported being able to sleep through the night for the first time in a week. No changes were made in his starting oxycodone dose. He was discharged to the skilled nursing unit 72 hours later with a pain rating of 2/10.

Initiating Epidural Analgesia in Opioid-Tolerant Patients

Initiating epidural analgesia in opioid-tolerant patients involves initial opioid dose conversion followed by titration. Studies are lacking and controversy exists over the correct conversion ratio to use when switching opioid-tolerant patients from oral or parenteral opioids to epidural opioids. When switching from parenteral morphine to epidural morphine, a conversion ratio of 3:1 is recommended (DuPen, DuPen, 1998). The 3:1 parenteral/epidural ratio is found by the use of a conversion tool that considers the influence of pain severity, patient's age, previous systemic opioid dose, and the presence of neuropathic pain (DuPen, Williams, 1994; DuPen, DuPen, 1998). A 10:1 ratio is used to switch from an epidural to intrathecal opioid dose (DuPen, DuPen, 1998).

As discussed previously, ratios are used only for calculating starting doses, then the dose is titrated to achieve acceptable analgesia and tolerable side effects. It is recommended that epidural analgesia in opioid-tolerant patients be initiated in a setting where the patient can be observed closely for side effects until the opioid dose is stabilized (DuPen, DuPen, 1998). The conversion begins with calculating the total 24-hour dose of oral or parenteral opioid.

Patient Example

Mrs. W. has cancer pain and has experienced intolerable and unmanageable side effects with oral morphine, SC hydromorphone, and oral oxycodone. She currently is taking 160 mg of controlled-release oxycodone q12h and has not required any rescue doses for several days. She will have an epidural morphine delivery system implanted tomorrow. What epidural morphine starting dose would be appropriate for Mrs. W.?

1. Determine the total 24 h dose of oxycodone: 160 mg × 2 doses/24 h = 320 mg/24 h.
2. Locate the PO dose of oxycodone in the equianalgesic chart (20 mg).
3. Determine the number of equianalgesic dose units in the 24 h dose of oxycodone by dividing the 24 h dose by the equianalgesic dose: 320 mg ÷ 20 mg = 16 units.
4. Locate the dose of parenteral morphine listed in the equianalgesic chart that is ap-

proximately equal to 20 mg of PO oxy-codone (10 mg).

5. Determine the 24 h dose of parenteral morphine by multiplying the equianalgesic dose of parenteral morphine by the equi-analgesic dose units: 10 mg × 16 units = 160 mg/24 h.

6. Use the 3:1 ratio to determine the 24 h epidural morphine dose by dividing the 24 h parenteral dose of morphine by 3: 160 mg ÷ 3 = approximately 53 mg/24 h.

7. Determine the hourly epidural morphine dose by dividing the total 24 h epidural morphine dose by 24 hours: 53 mg ÷ 24 = approximately 2 mg/h.

Mrs. W. may have developed tolerance to oxycodone, but she may not be equally tolerant to morphine. Therefore she is started on 50% of the calculated starting epidural morphine dose (1 mg/h) while taking 50% of the previous oxycodone dose (80 mg q12h) for several days. Gradual increases in the epidural morphine dose and decreases in the oral oxycodone dose are made until the switch to epidural morphine is complete. Inadequate pain relief is treated with increases in the hourly epidural morphine dose. Within 5 days, Mrs. W. is completely comfortable without side effects on 1.5 mg/h of epidural morphine.

Managing Side Effects

In opioid-naive patients common opioid side effects include constipation, nausea and vomiting, sedation, respiratory depression, pruritus, and mental confusion and clouding. As the patient becomes opioid tolerant, these side effects, except for constipation, tend to subside. Other less common opioid side effects include urinary retention, delirium, myoclonic jerks, and seizures. There is great individual variation in the development of opioid-induced side effects. Most can be managed by using an individualized approach.

Prevention rather than treatment of opioid side effects is an important principle of pain management. Most side effects are dose dependent (Chaney, 1995). Therefore a practical approach is to include the use of nonsedating analgesics that have an opioid dose–sparing effect, such as nonopioids and local anesthetics, so that the lowest effective opioid dose can be given. For some patients, particularly postoperative patients, simply decreasing the opioid dose is sufficient to eliminate or make a side effect tolerable (Pasero, McCaffery, 1994). Decreases in opioid doses can be accomplished by percentages. If the side effect is mild, 25% may be appropriate; for more effect, 50% to 100% may be appropriate.

The following is a discussion of many of the opioid side effects. Table 6.17 is a guide to preventing and managing the common ones. See p. 167 for information on

the specific opioid receptor binding sites of each side effect.

GI dysfunction

Opioids can delay gastric emptying, slow bowel motility, and decrease peristalsis. They also may reduce secretions from the colonic mucosa. The result is slow moving, hard stool that is difficult to pass. At its worst, GI dysfunction can result in ileus, fecal impaction, and obstruction (Levy, 1994; Lipman, Gauthier, 1997).

Constipation is the most common opioid side effect and the only one for which individuals do not develop tolerance. Thus it requires a preventive approach, regular assessment, and aggressive management if symptoms are detected. Factors contributing to the problem of constipation in patients taking opioids include advanced age, immobility, abdominal disease, and concurrent medications. All patients placed on ATC opioid analgesics should be directed to take laxatives regularly. Treatment continues as long as the patient takes opioids (Levy, 1994).

Attention to diet and exercise in addition to providing for privacy and convenience for patients are important aspects of bowel management but are insufficient alone to prevent opioid-induced constipation. Bulk laxatives, natural roughage, and large amounts of fluid are sometimes unpalatable and ineffective. In addition, if fluid intake is inadequate, bulk laxatives, such as psyllium (Metamucil), can cause fecal impaction and obstruction. Stool softeners alone are inadequate. Starting with a combination of stool softener and mild peristaltic stimulant, such as Senokot-S, is recommended (Levy, 1994; Sykes, 1996). Other tips on managing constipation are listed in Table 6.17.

Thoracic epidural analgesia of opioids and bupivacaine is associated with faster recovery from postoperative ileus, earlier discharge from the hospital, and lower cost of care compared with traditional methods of a pain control. In fact, epidural local anesthetics are recommended for the treatment of paralytic ileus (Liu, Carpenter, Neal, 1995).

Nausea and Vomiting

Initiating or increasing opioid therapy may cause nausea by stimulating the chemoreceptor trigger zone in the brain, slowing GI mobility, and sensitizing the labyrinths-vestibular system (needed for balance and equilibrium) (Dean, 1994; Lindley, Dalton, Fields, 1990; Storey, 1994). Nausea is most common with the initial opioid dose and usually subsides within weeks of opioid therapy (Coyle, Cherny, Portenoy, 1995).

Prophylactic treatment of nausea is not recommended because the antiemetics customarily used to treat nausea produce sedation and other undesirable effects (Levy, 1994; Pasero, McCaffery, 1994). However, patients should

Text continued on p. 264.

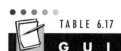

TABLE 6.17

GUIDELINES

PREVENTING AND MANAGING OPIOID-INDUCED SIDE EFFECTS

Side Effect	Management

Constipation	1. Begin all patients on ATC opioids with *one* of the combined stool softener and mild peristaltic stimulants (start on postoperative patients as soon as permissible)
	   • Docusate sodium sulfosuccinate 100 mg + casanthranol 30 mg (Pericolace) 1 cap qd to 2 caps tid
	   • Docusate sodium 50 mg + senna 8.6 mg (Senokot-S) 1 tab qd to 4 tabs tid
	2. If no BM in any 48 h period, add *one to two* of the following:
	   • Senna (Senokot) 187 mg 2 tabs hs to 4 tabs tid
	   • Bisacodyl (Dulcolax) 5 mg PO hs to 15 mg PO tid
	   • Milk of magnesia 30 to 60 ml qd or bid
	   • Lactulose (Chronulac: 10g/15 ml) 15 to 60 ml qd or bid
	3. If no BM by 72 h, perform rectal examination to rule out impaction. If not impacted, go to step 4. If impacted, go to step 5.
	4. If not impacted, try *one* of the following:
	   • Bisacodyl (Dulcolax) suppository 10 mg
	   • Magnesium citrate 8 oz PO
	   • Senna extract (X-prep liquid) 2.5 oz PO
	   • Mineral oil 30 to 60 ml PO
	   • Milk of magnesia 25 ml + cascara 5 ml suspension
	   • Fleet enema
	5. If impacted:
	   • Administer rescue analgesic or tranquilizer if indicated before disimpaction.
	   • Manually disimpact if stool is soft enough.
	   • If not, soften with glycerin suppository or oil retention enema, then disimpact manually.
	   • Follow up with enema (tap water, soapsuds) until clear.
	   • Increase daily bowel regimen.
	6. In patients with refractory constipation consider use of:
	   • A prokinetic agent to improve colonic transit (cisapride or metoclopramide [Reglan]).
	   • Oral administration of naloxone to produce "bowel withdrawal" without concurrent systemic withdrawal. Treatment should incorporate starting at a dose of 0.8 mg bid and doubling the dose q 2 to 3 days until a favorable response, increased pain, or signs of withdrawal occur.
	
	Pediatric Consideration: Begin all patients on ATC opioids with *one* of the combined pediatric stool softener and mild peristaltic stimulants (start on postoperative patients as soon as permissible)

Nausea, vomiting	1. Titrate opioid doses slowly and steadily.
	2. Because many of the drugs used to treat nausea are sedating, before initiating drug treatment of nausea:
	   • Add or increase nonopioid or adjuvant for additional pain relief so that the opioid dose can be reduced.
	   • If analgesia is satisfactory, reduce opioid dose by 25%.
	3. Drug treatment of nausea and vomiting differs according to the cause.
	   • If caused by stimulation of the chemoreceptor trigger zone (common cause of vomiting), ondansetron (Zofran), prochlorperazine (Compazine), thiethylperazine (Torecan), or haloperidol (Haldol) may be helpful.
	   • If caused by slowed GI motility, metoclopramide may be helpful.
	   • For nausea associated with motion (often accompanied by vertigo), dimenhydrinate (Dramamine) may be helpful. Scopolamine patches are sometimes used but may cause confusion and should be removed after 72 h.

Continued.

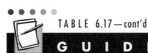

TABLE 6.17—cont'd

GUIDELINES

PREVENTING AND MANAGING OPIOID-INDUCED SIDE EFFECTS

Side Effect	Management

Nausea, vomiting—*cont'd*	4. For chronic nausea in advanced cancer:
	  • Give metoclopramide 10 mg q 4 h SC or PO.
	  • If nausea persists, add dexamethasone 10 mg bid.
	  • If nausea persists, add other antiemetics.
	5. Other suggestions:
	  • Haloperidol 0.5 mg tid up to 15 mg/day + antihistamine (hydroxyzine or cyclizine) + dexamethasone, and/or ondansetron.
	  • Switch to another opioid.
	  • Switch to an intraspinal route.
	  • Use of an anesthetic or neurosurgical technique to allow drug reduction.
	6. Support use of relaxation techniques.
	Pediatric Considerations
	1. If analgesia is satisfactory, reduce opioid dose by 10%-25%.
	2. Add or increase nonopioid or nonsedating adjuvant for additional pain relief so that the opioid dose can be reduced.
	3. Ondansetron 0.1 mg/kg IV or metoclopramide 0.1-0.2 mg/kg IV or droperidol 0.03-0.075 mg/kg IV.

Pruritus	1. If analgesia is satisfactory, reduce opioid by 25%. 2. Add or increase nonopioid or nonsedating adjuvant for additional pain relief so that the opioid dose can be reduced. 3. Diphenhydramine (Benadryl) 12.5-25 mg IV or 25-50 mg PO may be given to alleviate symptoms, but is sedating; nalbuphine (Nubain) 2.5-5 mg SC or IV, or butorphanol (Stadol) 1 mg IV may eliminate itching but frequently reverse analgesia. 4. Naloxone (0.8 mg/1000 ml) IV infusion titrated to effect is generally used only after steps 1-3 have failed. Pediatric Considerations 1. If analgesia is satisfactory, reduce opioid dose by 10%-25%. 2. Add or increase nonopioid or nonsedating adjuvant for additional pain relief so that the opioid dose can be reduced. 3. Diphenhydramine 1 mg/kg IV or butorphanol 0.03-0.05 mg/kg IV. 4. Naloxone 0.5 μg/kg/h by IV infusion only after steps 1-3 have failed.

Mental confusion, clouded consciousness, delirium, hallucinations, paranoia	1. Evaluate underlying cause; consider role of primary therapy.
	2. Eliminate nonessential CNS acting medications, e.g., steroids.
	3. If analgesia is satisfactory, reduce opioid by 25%.
	4. Reevaluate and treat underlying process if appropriate.
	5. If delirium persists, consider:
	  • Trial of neuroleptic (e.g., haloperidol 0.5-1 mg PO bid or tid or 0.25-0.5 mg IV or IM)
	  • Switch to another opioid.
	  • Switch to an intraspinal route.
	6. Use of an anesthetic or neurosurgical technique to allow drug reduction.
	Avoid using naloxone, even if delirium is thought to be due to the opioid.

Sedation	1. Determine whether sedation is due to the opioid. It is most likely due to the opioid if opioid therapy has just started or if there has been a recent increase in dose. 2. Eliminate nonessential CNS depressant medications. 3. If analgesia is satisfactory, reduce opioid dose by 10%-25%. 4. Add or increase nonopioid or nonsedating adjuvant for additional pain relief so that the opioid dose can be reduced. 5. Add simple stimulants during the day, e.g., caffeine. 6. Consider giving a lower opioid dose more frequently to decrease peak concentration.

May be duplicated for use in clinical practice. From McCaffery M, Pasero C: *Pain: Clinical manual*, pp. 262-264. Copyright © 1999, Mosby, Inc.　　*Continued.*

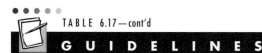

TABLE 6.17—cont'd

GUIDELINES

PREVENTING AND MANAGING OPIOID-INDUCED SIDE EFFECTS

Side Effect	Management
Sedation—*cont'd*	7. If analgesia is unsatisfactory or dose reduction is not viable, consider adding a psychostimulant, e.g., methylphenidate (Ritalin) or pemoline (Cylert).
	8. If excessive sedation persists, consider:
	• Switch to another opioid.
	• Switch to an intraspinal route.
	• Use of an anesthetic or neurosurgical technique to allow drug reduction.
	See also respiratory depression below and Box 6.28 on p. 267 and 6.29 on p. 270.
Respiratory depression	1. Nurse monitor sedation level and respiratory status q1–2h during the first 24 h in opioid-naive patients treated for moderate to severe pain (see Box 6.28 on p. 267).
	2. Add or increase nonopioid or of nonsedating adjuvants so that the opioid dose can be reduced.
	3. Decrease opioid dose by 25% when excessive sedation is detected.
	4. If patient is minimally responsive or unresponsive to stimulation, stop opioid administration and consider administering naloxone (Narcan).
	Box 6.29 on p. 270 outlines naloxone administration technique for adults and children.

May be duplicated for use in clinical practice. From McCaffery M, Pasero C: *Pain: Clinical manual*, pp. 262-264. Copyright © 1999, Mosby, Inc.

Table 6.17 is a guide to preventing and managing some of the common opioid-induced side effects. Pediatric considerations are included.

bid, twice daily; *BM*, bowel movement; *cap*, capsule; *GI*, gastrointestinal; *hs*, at sleep; *IM*, intramuscular; *IV*, intravenous; *μg*, microgram; *mg*, milligram; *ml*, milliliter; *oz*, ounce; *PO*, oral; *q*, every; *qd*, once daily; *SC*, subcutaneous; *tab*, tablet; *tid*, three times daily.

Information from Coyle N, Director, Supportive Care Program, Memorial Sloan-Kettering Cancer Center, New York, NY: Personal communication by telephone with Chris Pasero, Sept. 8, 1997; Coyle N, Cherny N, Portenoy, RK: Pharmacologic management of cancer pain. In McGuire D, Yarbro CH, Ferrell BR, editors: *Cancer pain management*, ed 2, pp 89-130, Boston, 1995, Jones and Bartlett Publishers; Levy MH: Pain management in advanced cancer, *Semin Oncol* 12:404, 1985; Portenoy RK: Opioid analgesics. In Portenoy RK, Kanner RM, editors: *Pain management: Theory and practice*, pp 249-276, Philadelphia, 1996, FA Davis; Storey P: *Primer of palliative care*, Gainesville, FL, 1994, Academy of Hospice Physicians; Yaster M, Billett C, Monitto C: Intravenous patient-controlled analgesia. In Yaster M, Krane EJ, Kaplan RF, et al., editors: *Pediatric pain management and sedation handbook*, pp 89-111, St. Louis, 1997, Mosby.

---

have access to an antiemetic should the need for one occur. In some patients nausea is a consistent problem. In these cases an antiemetic should be used preventively and perhaps ATC.

Slow and steady opioid titration helps to reduce nausea. Adjustments in diet and activity plus the use of relaxation techniques also may be helpful in the management of nausea (Coyle, Cherny, Portenoy, 1995). Table 6.17 outlines approaches commonly used to treat opioid-induced nausea and vomiting.

Postoperative Nausea and Vomiting

Opioids are among a number of factors that increase the incidence of postoperative nausea and vomiting (PONV), including general anesthesia and long duration of surgery (Koivuranta, Laara, Snare et al., 1997). Many patients consider PONV to be as debilitating as the pain associated with the surgery. It also is associated with detrimental effects, including aspiration of vomitus, tension on sutures, increased intracranial and intraocular pressure, and fluid and electrolyte imbalance. PONV has been described as the "big little problem" by clinicians who manage it (Watcha, White, 1995).

The drugs traditionally used to manage PONV produce many unwanted side effects. For example, droperidol and the phenothiazines, such as promethazine (Phenergan), are sedative, dysphoric, and can produce tachycardia, bradycardia, and increases and decreases in blood pressure; high doses of metoclopramide (Reglan) can produce extrapyramidal side effects (McGee, Alexander, 1979). IM hydroxyzine (Vistaril) is especially irritating to the muscle and soft tissue and can produce sterile abscesses.

No scientific basis exists for the belief that drugs such as promethazine enhance the analgesic effects of opioids. In addition to producing sedation, some studies show that promethazine increases sensitivity to pain and increases the amount of opioid required to produce satisfactory pain relief (McGee, Alexander, 1979). The doses of hydroxyzine that would be required to produce analgesia create significant risk of respiratory depression that is not reversible by naloxone (Gordon, 1995). Thus the common practice of routinely administering these drugs regardless of whether the patient is nauseated should be discouraged.

Ondansetron (Zofran), an antiserotonin drug, appears to be an excellent choice for managing PONV (Watcha, White, 1995). Compared with metoclopramide, ondansetron has been shown to be superior for both prevention when administered as a premedicant (Alexander, Fennelly, 1997) and for postoperative treatment of PONV (Polati, Verlato, Finco et al., 1997). Side effects of ondansetron are minor (headache, light-headedness, constipation), adding to its appeal. It does not produce sedation, delay emergence, or prolong the stay in the PACU because of drowsiness (Bodner, Poler, White, 1991). Cost has been shown to be more than droperidol but less than metoclopramide (Watcha, Smith, 1994). Many clinicians believe the additional cost of ondansetron is justified when weighed against the cost of treating the effects of poorly managed PONV.

The IV sedative hypnotic propofol (Diprivan) is gaining popularity in the postoperative setting for symptom control. At subhypnotic doses (5 to 10 mg IV push q4-6h or 0.5 to 1 mg/kg per hour continuous infusion) propofol has been shown to be effective in reducing the overall incidence of PONV in patients at high risk for PONV without untoward sedative or cardiovascular effects compared with placebo (Elias, 1997; Ewalenko, Janny, Dejonckheere et al., 1996).

Patient Example

Mr. F. is receiving IV PCA hydromorphone for management of his pain after radical prostatectomy. His prescription is: PCA dose = 0.2 mg; delay interval = 8 minutes; basal rate = 0.1 mg. His pain rating is 0. He reports feeling nauseated for a few minutes after he presses his PCA button. He has been given an antiemetic twice without relief and dislikes feeling "sleepy" after the antiemetic is given. The anesthesiologist has left orders to decrease the opioid dose 25% to 50% for minor side effects. Because Mr. F. is completely comfortable and slightly drowsy, his nurse decides to decrease his PCA dose by 50%: 0.2 mg × 50% (or 0.2 mg ÷ 2) = 0.1 mg. (Mr. F.'s report that nausea occurs only after he administers a PCA dose means he is experiencing toxicity at the peak concentration of the PCA dose. The best treatment for this is smaller PCA doses and/or shorter delay intervals. If reducing the PCA dose is ineffective, the delay interval can be shortened to 6 minutes. Had Mr. F. reported constant nausea, it would be appropriate to decrease the basal rate and consider also decreasing the PCA dose [see Table 6.14 on p. 254].) Within an hour, Mr. F. is less drowsy and reports that nausea no longer occurs when he administers PCA.

Biliary spasm

Opioids increase smooth muscle tone in the biliary tract, especially in the sphincter of Oddi, which regulates the flow of bile and pancreatic fluids. This can result in a decrease in biliary and pancreatic secretions and a rise in bile duct pressure that can last up to 12 hours. Patients may experience epigastric distress and occasionally biliary spasm (Benedetti, Butler, 1990; Lindley, Dalton, Fields, 1990).

All opioids are capable of causing constricture of the sphincter of Oddi and the biliary tract. One laboratory study showed that morphine may cause more biliary constricture in animals (Coelho, Runkel, Herfarth et al., 1986) than other opioids, but this has never been shown to be clinically relevant in humans. Fentanyl, morphine, meperidine, and pentazocine caused a rise in bile duct pressure of 99.5%, 52.7%, 61.3%, and 15.1%, respectively in humans (Radnay, Brodman, Mankikar et al, 1980). Although pentazocine produced the smallest rise in this study, it causes dysphoria, anxiety, nightmares, depersonalization, and hallucinations, has an analgesic ceiling, and is not recommended for the management of any type of pain (Barkin, Lubenow, Bruehl et al., 1996; Reisine, Pasternak, 1996).

Pruritus

Pruritus (itching) is a side effect of opioids and the most common side effect when opioids are delivered by the intraspinal routes. Although opioids release histamine from mast cells, this does not appear to be the underlying mechanism of pruritus. Instead it is thought to be due to cephalad migration of the opioid in CSF and subsequent interaction in the medulla. A higher incidence of pruritus occurs with intraspinal morphine than other opioids because morphine ascends in a cephalad direction through the CSF. Pruritus also is more common in obstetric patients than other patients as a result of an interaction of estrogen with the opioid receptors (Chaney, 1995).

Pruritus is sometimes generalized all over the body but usually is localized to the face, neck, or upper thorax. It rarely is accompanied by a rash. When the opioid is given by continuous epidural infusion or PCEA, the most effective and efficient treatment for pruritus is to decrease the opioid dose. Decreasing the opioid dose is facilitated by adding or increasing a nonopioid and adding a local anesthetic to the epidural opioid solution to provide additional pain relief. Ironically, antihistamines may relieve the symptoms of pruritus, probably as a result of their sedative effects (Chaney, 1995). When antihistamines are combined with intraspinal analgesia, it is particularly important to monitor sedation (see Table 6.17).

Use of Antagonists and Agonist-Antagonists to Treat Opioid Side Effects

Low-dose opioid antagonists, such as naloxone (Narcan) and nalmefene (Revex), and agonist-antagonist opioids, such as nalbuphine and butorphanol sometimes are used to prevent or treat minor opioid side effects, especially pruritus. Preservative-free nalbuphine has been added to hydromorphone PCEA for the prevention of "bothersome" side effects in patients after cesarean section (Parker, Holtmann, White, 1997). Patients received hydromorphone by PCEA either (1) without nalbuphine, (2) with 0.02 mg/ml nalbuphine, (3) with 0.04 mg/ml nalbuphine, or (4) with 0.08 mg/ml nalbuphine. The overall incidences of nausea and pruritus in all four groups were similar; the need for bladder catheterization was reduced by the addition of nalbuphine. Pain relief and patient satisfaction was not improved by the addition of nalbuphine, and the highest concentration of nalbuphine resulted in increased PCA demands.

In another study epidural butorphanol failed to reduce the side effects of epidural morphine (Gambling, Howell, Huber et al., 1994). In addition, patients who received epidural butorphanol reported significantly higher levels of somnolence compared with those who did not receive epidural butorphanol.

The risk of adding side effects and inadvertently reversing analgesia with an antagonist or agonist-antagonist opioid plus the aftermath of reestablishing pain control must be weighed against the benefit of a small reduction in severity of relatively minor side effects. The reasoning that additional analgesia is provided when agonist-antagonist opioids are used for reversal of side effects is faulty because the doses used to treat the side effects are one fourth to one half those recommended for analgesia. Especially when given by infusion, antagonist and agonist-antagonist treatment increases nursing time and cost of care and ties the patient to another infusion pump. For these reasons, treatment with opioid antagonists and agonist-antagonist opioids usually are reserved for severe cases of side effects (Sinatra, 1998). Other methods for managing opioid side effects, such as decreasing the opioid dose and providing antihistamines, always should be tried first.

Treatment of pruritus in patients who have received a single epidural or intrathecal bolus of morphine is difficult because the opioid dose cannot be reduced once it is given. Pruritus in these patients is commonly treated preventively with a single oral dose of 6 mg of the opioid antagonist naltrexone at the time of the epidural or intrathecal injection. This dose has been shown to prevent pruritus without reversing analgesia (Abboud, Afrasiabi, Davidson et al., 1990; Abboud, Lee, Zhu et al., 1990).

Although further study is needed to determine optimal dosing for prophylactic treatment of pruritus with nalmefene, single IV doses of 20 μg to 40 μg given after skin closure have been effective in treating pruritus associated with single epidural boluses of 4 mg of morphine without reversing analgesia (Stuart, McDavid, 1997). Another group of researchers found 0.395 μg/kg to be the average dose of nalmefene required to stop itching without reversing analgesia from single-dose epidural morphine (Brown, Paige, Berger, 1997). When antagonists are used in this manner to treat side effects, patients should be assessed frequently for maintenance of pain control. This is especially important when nalmefene is used because its duration (10 hours) is close to that of epidural morphine (12 hours).

Urinary retention

Opioids increase smooth muscle tone in the bladder and ureters and can cause bladder spasm and urgency. An opioid-induced increase in sphincter tone can make urination difficult. The central effects of opioids may reduce a patient's attention to bladder stimuli, which can result in urinary retention (Lindley, Dalton, Fields, 1990). Urinary retention is most common in elderly men. Tolerance to urinary retention does develop. As with the other opioid-induced side effects, decreasing the opioid dose is the most effective treatment of urinary retention. In and out catheterization once or twice may be sufficient to relieve urinary retention in postoperative patients. For persistent urinary retention and for urinary retention in patients with chronic pain, Foley catheterization is recommended rather than repeated catheterizations if the opioid dose cannot be reduced (Coyle, Cherny, Portenoy, 1995; Levy, 1994) (see Table 6.17).

Myoclonus

Myoclonic jerks usually are experienced only by patients receiving high doses of opioids for types of pain, which are the least responsive to opioids such as incident pain from bony metastasis or neuropathic pain (Levy, 1994). Although all opioids can produce myoclonus, the effect is most prominent with meperidine, presumably from normeperidine accumulation. Mild myoclonus is common and may resolve as tolerance develops (Coyle, Cherny, Portenoy, 1995). Clonazepam (Klonopin), 0.25 mg to 0.5 mg orally two or three times daily, helps to control jerking but is sedating. Attempts should be made to control pain with lower opioid doses and by adding or increasing adjuvant analgesics and considering the use of anesthetic procedures (Coyle, Cherny, Portenoy, 1995; Levy, 1994).

Mental status changes

Confusion, disorientation, and cognitive impairment are among the most feared of opioid-induced side effects for patients and families. Mild cognitive impairment and occasional hallucinations may occur when opioid therapy is initiated and with significant dose increases. Patients can be reassured that these are transient and will resolve within days to a couple of weeks (Coyle, Cherny, Portenoy, 1995; Levy, 1994).

Delirium in the terminally ill has a variety of manifestations, including hallucinations, disorientation, clouding consciousness, fear, and paranoia. Opioids usually are not a cause but may be a contributing factor. Potential causes of delirium are major organ failure, neoplastic involvement of the CNS, sepsis, hypoxia, and electrolyte disorders, such as hypercalcemia (Coyle, Cherny, Portenoy, 1995; Levy, 1994). Table 6.17 outlines treatment options.

In the postoperative setting opioids are often blamed for the occurrence of confusion. The common reaction of many clinicians is to abruptly discontinue the opioid. However, in many cases a better approach is to add or increase a nonopioid or nonsedating adjuvant and decrease the opioid dose (Pasero, McCaffery, 1994).

Little supports the assertion that opioids usually are the major cause of cognitive impairment. In fact, pain and other factors, such as sleep disturbance, type of surgery, choice of opioid, and method of administering opioids, have been directly linked to postoperative cognitive impairment.

Decline in mental status was linked to poor pain control in patients aged 50 to 80 in one study. Pain, not analgesic intake, predicted mental decline (Duggleby, Lander, 1994). This study suggests that improving pain management practices, including administering appropriate doses of opioids, is one way to reduce confusion after surgery.

The choice of method used to provide postoperative pain control may influence the incidence of mental confusion in opioid-naive patients. Fewer complications, including mental confusion, were found in elderly men receiving IV PCA morphine compared with those receiving IM morphine (Egbert, Parks, Short et al., 1990).

The choice of opioid used to control pain also may influence the incidence of mental confusion. In a study comparing IV PCA morphine and IV PCA fentanyl in postoperative patients, fentanyl produced less depression of postoperative cognitive function (Herrick, Ganapathy, Komar et al., 1996). IV PCA morphine and IV PCA hydromorphone were compared for analgesic efficacy, side effects, mood, and cognitive function. Both medications provided adequate analgesia without difference in side effects. Although the patients receiving hydromorphone experienced improved mood, they also demonstrated poorer cognitive performance than the morphine group (Rapp, Egan, Ross et al., 1996). The research regarding the differences in cognitive effects produced by the various opioids is not definitive. Further investigation is warranted.

Unfortunately, it is quite common for practitioners to deny epidural analgesia to cognitively impaired or confused patients, but for some types of surgery the epidural route may actually be preferable to others. Liu, Carpenter, and Neal (1995) point out that, ". . . previous studies have demonstrated less sedation in patients receiving epidural analgesia (local anesthetic or opioid) than those receiving parenteral opioid . . . these data suggest potential for reduction in postoperative cognitive dysfunction from use of epidural analgesia" (p. 1492).

Sedation

Most patients experience sedation at the beginning of opioid therapy and whenever the opioid dose is increased significantly (Coyle, Portenoy, 1996). Although a disturbing side effect, especially for patients on long-term opioid therapy, they can be reassured that tolerance to sedation usually develops over a period of days to weeks. If significantly sedated, patients should be discouraged from performing dangerous activities, such as driving or operating complicated mechanical equipment, until sedation subsides. Care must be taken not to confuse sedation with exhaustion and the need to "catch up" on sleep when poorly controlled pain is finally controlled (Coyle, Cherny, Portenoy, 1995).

Unfortunately, for patients receiving short-term opioid therapy, time does not allow for development of tolerance to sedation. In addition to affecting the patient's ability to participate in the recovery process, if left untreated, excessive sedation progresses to clinically significant opioid-induced respiratory depression in opioid-naive patients. Excessive sedation in patients receiving short-term opioid treatment is treated by decreasing the opioid dose (Pasero, McCaffery, 1994).

Because of the relationship between sedation and respiratory depression, sedation is monitored every 1 to 2 hours during the first 12 to 24 hours after surgery in opioid-naive patients who receive opioids for moderate to severe pain (Pasero, McCaffery, 1994). Catheter migration to either the intravascular or intrathecal space should be ruled out in patients receiving epidural analgesia who have a sudden change in sedation level. An example of a sedation scale that can be used to monitor patients receiving opioids can be found in Box 6.28.

● ● ● ● ●

BOX 6.28 Sedation Scale

S = Sleep, easy to arouse
1 = Awake and alert
2 = Slightly drowsy, easily aroused
3 = Frequently drowsy, arousable, drifts off to sleep during conversation
4 = Somnolent, minimal or no response to physical stimulation

---

May be duplicated for use in clinical practice. From McCaffery M, Pasero C: *Pain: Clinical manual,* p. 267. Copyright © 1999, Mosby, Inc.

Box 6.28 illustrates a scale that can be used to assess sedation levels in patients receiving opioid analgesia.

Patient Example

Mrs. P. is 4 hours after abdominal hysterectomy. She is receiving a continuous epidural infusion of fentanyl 40 μg/h with bupivacaine 0.0625% for management of her postoperative pain. Mrs. P. rates her pain as 1/10. She has a sedation level of 3 on a scale of 1 to 4 and drifts off to sleep before completing a sentence. Over the last 2 hours, the depth of her respirations has become shallower and her hourly respiratory rate has decreased from 16 to 12 breaths/minute. The anesthesiologist has written an order to decrease Mrs. P.'s epidural opioid dose by 25-50% for a sedation level of 3. Since Mrs. P. has good pain control, her nurse decides to decrease the dose by 50%: 40 μg/h $\times$ 50% (or 40 μg/h $\div$ 2) = 20 μg/h. Mrs. P.'s nurse asks the nursing assistant to check Mrs. P.'s sedation and respiratory rate and to ask Mrs. P. to deep breathe every 30 minutes. Within two hours, Mrs. P. has a sedation level of 2 and is able to carry on a conversation without falling asleep. Her respiratory rate is 16 breaths/minute and her pain rating is stable at 1/10.

Sometimes patients experience persistent sedation during long term opioid treatment, particularly if other sedating drugs are taken or there are underlying conditions that cause sedation, such as metabolic disturbances (Coyle, Cherny, Portenoy, 1995). Table 6.17 outlines a step-by-step approach that can be taken to treat sedation that begins with determining if the cause of the sedation is the opioid. The opioid is likely to be the cause if opioid therapy has just started or the dose has recently been increased.

If possible, the opioid dose is decreased to treat sedation also in patients receiving long term opioid treatment. Giving less opioid more frequently helps to decrease peak concentration and may be effective in some cases. For example, large PCA doses and long delay intervals can be reduced in patients who report excessive sedation following PCA injection. If opioid dose reduction is unsuccessful, adding a psychostimulant is an option. Methylphenidate (Ritalin) or dextroamphetamine are typically started at 2.5 mg to 5 mg in the morning and repeated midday. Doses can be titrated upward; few patients require more than 40 mg. If unacceptable sedation persists in spite of these measures, the patient can be switched to another opioid. Intraspinal opioids and/or local anesthetics or neurolysis are considered when all other approaches fail or are not possible (Coyle, Cherny, Portenoy, 1995).

Coadministration of Other Sedating Drugs

As mentioned, the administration of IM opioids to opioid naive patients receiving IV or epidural analgesia is unnecessary and can result in excessive sedation and clin-

ically significant respiratory depression. Instead, patients who are receiving IV or epidural opioid analgesia and experiencing uncontrolled pain should be carefully re-evaluated. Clinician-administered IV or epidural supplemental doses and increases in the dose of the mainstay opioid usually are indicated (Pasero, McCaffery, 1996a).

Although not necessarily contraindicated with parenteral and intraspinal analgesia, muscle relaxants and anxiolytics can produce sedation. Therefore, prior to administering them, it is best to obtain approval for their administration from the physician responsible for the pain management plan (e.g., anesthesiologist with postoperative epidural analgesia). When these drugs are administered, close monitoring of sedation is warranted.

Respiratory depression

Respiratory depression is assessed on the basis of what is normal for a particular individual. Respiratory depression associated with opioid use usually is described as clinically significant when there is a decrease in rate and depth of respirations from baseline, rather than just by a specific number of respirations per minute. This means that in some cases even patients breathing less than 10 breaths per minute may not have respiratory depression if they are breathing deeply (Pasero. McCaffery, 1994).

Clinically significant respiratory depression is the most feared of the opioid-induced side effects. Like sedation, tolerance to respiratory depression develops over a period of days to weeks. The longer the patient receives opioids, the wider the margin of safety. Therefore, fear of respiratory depression in patients who have been receiving opioids for more than a week should not pose a barrier to administering adequate opioid doses.

There is no set dose of an opioid that is safe for all patients. All opioid naive patients are at risk for clinically significant respiratory depression when they receive their first dose of an opioid. IV access for naloxone administration usually is maintained for 24 to 48 hours after a stable epidural opioid dose has been achieved. After that time, naloxone rarely is needed because most patients are alert and, in many cases, are ready for a decrease in the epidural opioid dose.

Patients at higher risk than others for opioid-induced respiratory depression are infants less than 6 months old, opioid-naive patients who are elderly, and those who have coexisting conditions such as chronic pulmonary disease or major organ failure (Pasero, McCaffery, 1994). Because pain stimulates respiration (Borgbjerg, Nielsen, Franks, 1996), patients in whom pain is controlled after a period of poor control are at risk for respiratory depression and should be watched closely until steady state is reached.

Clinically significant opioid-induced respiratory depression in opioid-naive patients can be prevented by careful opioid titration and close nurse monitoring of sedation (see Box 6.28) and respiratory status (Levy,

1994; Pasero, McCaffery, 1994). Nursing observation is the best method for monitoring sedation level and respiratory status. Mechanical monitoring, such as pulse oximetry, usually is warranted only if patients have preexisting conditions that require it (de Leon-Casasola, Parker et al., 1994; Ready, Loper, Nessly et al., 1991; Scherer, Schmutzler, Geibler et al, 1993; Sinatra, 1998; Sullivan, Muir, Ginsberg, 1994).

The importance of monitoring sedation to prevent clinically significant respiratory depression cannot be overemphasized. As the American Pain Society (1992) succinctly states, "No patient has succumbed to (opioid-induced) respiratory depression while awake" (p. 23). This is because more opioid is required to produce respiratory depression than to produce sedation. Prevention of clinically significant respiratory depression involves decreasing the opioid dose when excessive sedation is detected. Nonsedating opioid-sparing analgesics can be given to provide additional analgesia (Pasero, McCaffery, 1994) (see Table 6.17).

Subacute Overdose

In patients receiving regular doses of opioids for several days or longer, subacute overdose is far more common than acute respiratory depression. Subacute overdose is manifested by progressive (hours to days) somnolence and respiratory depression and pinpoint pupils. The risk of this occurring is much higher during titration of opioids with long half-lives, such as methadone and levorphanol. The treatment for subacute overdose is merely withholding one or two opioid doses until the symptoms have resolved, then reducing the ongoing opioid dose by 25% (Jacox, Carr, Payne et al., 1994).

Reversing Respiratory Depression

If it is necessary to use naloxone to reverse clinically significant respiratory depression, it should be titrated very carefully. Sometimes more than one dose of naloxone is necessary because naloxone has a shorter duration (1 hour) than most opioids. However giving too much naloxone or giving it too fast can precipitate severe pain that is extremely difficult to control and increase sympathetic activity leading to hypertension, tachycardia, ventricular dysrhythmias, pulmonary edema, and cardiac arrest (Brimacombe, Archdeacon, Newell et al., 1991). In physically dependent patients withdrawal syndrome can be precipitated; patients who have been receiving opioids for more than 1 week may be exquisitely sensitive to antagonists (APS, 1992). Box 6.29 outlines the procedure for correctly administering naloxone to an adult.

Patient Example

Ms. V. is receiving a continuous epidural infusion of fentanyl, 50 µg/h, with bupivacaine, 0.1%, for her postoperative pain after a colon resection. She is found with a sedation level of 4 on a scale of 1 to 4, but she arouses with physical stimulation. Her respirations are shallow and her respiratory rate is 6 breaths/minute. The first action the nurse who finds Ms. V. takes is to stop the epidural infusion. The nurse continues to arouse Ms. V. and asks a coworker to bring a syringe of diluted naloxone (0.4 mg naloxone/10 ml saline). When the naloxone arrives, the nurse slowly administers it while observing Ms. V.'s response. After about 3 ml (0.12 mg), Ms. V. has a sedation level of 3, arouses easily, and is able to follow the nurse's instructions to deep breathe. The nurse stops administering naloxone after 0.12 mg because the desired effect is a reversal of Ms. V.'s sedation and respiratory depression without loss of pain control. The physician is notified and alternative analgesia (ketorolac, 15 mg IV) is given because the epidural analgesia is stopped. Ms. V.'s sedation and vital signs are monitored closely until her sedation level is stable at <3. When Ms. V.'s sedation level is <3 and her respiratory depth returns to baseline and respiratory rate is >9 breaths/minute, the epidural analgesia is restarted at 25 µg/h with bupivacaine 0.1% (50% reduction). The ketorolac is continued q6h ATC.

As mentioned, nalmefene also is used for reversal of opioid side effects. Parenteral nalmefene, 0.5 µg/kg, is comparable in safety and efficacy to 1.0 µg/kg of parenteral naloxone. A 1 mg parenteral dose of nalmefene is capable of blocking 80% of the opioid receptors within 5 minutes of administration (Ohmeda, 1995). A single IV dose of 0.25 µg/kg can reportedly reverse opioid-induced respiratory depression (Stuart, McDavid, 1997).

The recommendations and precautions for naloxone apply to nalmefene, particularly careful titration to effect. The half-life of nalmefene (approximately 10 hours) is much longer than that of naloxone (1 hour), so reversal effects will last much longer with nalmefene than naloxone. Repeated doses of naloxone are sometimes necessary to maintain reversal because the duration of most opioids is longer than the duration of naloxone. This would not be the case with nalmefene. A single dose of nalmefene may be sufficient to reverse opioid-induced sedation and respiratory depression, but maintaining pain control may be difficult because its duration is much longer than most opioids. More research is needed to address these issues.

Inappropriate Use of Opioid Antagonists

More often than clinically significant respiratory depression, cancer patients receiving long-term opioid treatment may develop confusion and be somewhat sedated but remain easily aroused with an acceptable respiratory rate and depth. Great care must be taken to prevent the administration of an opioid antagonist drug to patients exhibiting such symptoms because the symptoms may be

● ● ● ● ●

BOX 6.29

G U I D E L I N E S

NALOXONE ADMINISTRATION

1. Patients who require naloxone (Narcan) usually meet all of the following criteria:
   - Unresponsive to physical stimulation
   - Shallow respirations or respiratory rate <8 breaths/min
   - Pinpoint pupils
2. Stop the administration of the opioid and any other sedative drugs. If given IV, maintain IV access.
3. Summon help. Ask a coworker to prepare naloxone (see No. 4) and bring it to you. Remain with the patient and continue to attempt to arouse him/her.
4. Mix 0.4 mg (1 ampule) of naloxone and 10 ml of normal saline in a syringe for IV administration.[3]
5. Administer the dilute naloxone solution IV[4] very slowly (0.5 ml over 2 min)[5] while you observe the patient's response (titrate to effect).
6. The patient should open his/her eyes and talk to you within 1 to 2 minutes. If not, continue IV naloxone at the same rate up to a total of 0.8 mg or 20 ml of dilute

naloxone. If no response, begin looking for other causes of sedation and respiratory depression.

7. Discontinue the naloxone administration as soon as the patient is responsive to physical stimulation and able to take deep breaths when told to do so. Keep the syringe nearby. Another dose of naloxone may be needed as early as 30 minutes after the first dose because the duration of naloxone is shorter than the duration of most opioids.
8. Assign a staff member to monitor sedation and respiratory status and to remind the patient to deep breathe every 1 to 2 minutes until the patient becomes more alert.
9. Notify the primary physician and pain service. Document your actions.
10. Provide a nonopioid for pain relief.
11. Resume opioid administration at one half the original dose when the patient is easily aroused and respiratory rate is >9 breaths/min.

May be duplicated for use in clinical practice. From McCaffery M, Pasero C: *Pain: Clinical manual,* p. 270. Copyright © 1999, Mosby, Inc.

Box 6.29 provides the recommended titrate-to-effect procedure for administering naloxone (Narcan) to reverse clinically significant respiratory depression. Giving too much naloxone or giving it too fast can precipitate severe pain, which is extremely difficult to control, and increase sympathetic activity leading to hypertension, tachycardia, ventricular dysrhythmias, pulmonary edema, and cardiac arrest. In physically dependent patients withdrawal syndrome can be precipitated; patients who have been receiving opioids for more than 1 week may be exquisitely sensitive to antagonists.

[1]For infants and children, follow the same procedure outlined in Box 6.29 with the following exceptions: (1) Respiratory rate that requires naloxone will vary according to infant's/child's usual rate; (2) Naloxone dose for children weighing >40 kg, follow dosing recommendations in Box 6.29; for children weighing <40 kg, dilute 0.1 mg naloxone in 10 ml of saline to make a 10 μg/ml solution. Administer IV at 0.5 μg/kg every 2 minutes until desired effect is achieved.

[2]Physicians' orders for opioids should include an order for naloxone administration according to APS recommendations, or a protocol incorporating the APS recommendations can be adopted for use by any nurse who suspects a patient is experiencing clinically significant opioid-induced respiratory depression.

[3]If naloxone is available only in a prefilled syringe, 10 ml of saline can be drawn into a 12 ml syringe, leaving enough room to accept the transfer of naloxone from the prefilled syringe. This procedure would ensure correct dilution.

[4]If IV route is inaccessible, administer undiluted naloxone, 0.4 mg, subcutaneously or intramuscularly. The patient should respond within 5 minutes. If not, repeat dose up to a total of 2 mg.

[5]This is the recommended amount and rate for administering naloxone to reverse opioid-induced respiratory depression. Administering a larger amount in a shorter period of time than this risks reversing more than opioid-induced respiratory depression (e.g., analgesia).

μg, microgram; *mg,* milligram; *ml,* milliliter; *min,* minute; *IV,* intravenous.

Information from American Pain Society (APS); *Principles of analgesic use in the treatment of acute and cancer pain,* ed 3, Glenview, IL, 1992, APS; Brimacombe J, Archdeacon J, Newell S et al.: Two cases of naloxone-induced pulmonary oedema: The possible use of phentolamine in management, *Anesth Intens Care* 19(4):578-580, 1991; Deglin JH, Vallerand AH: *Davis' drug guide,* ed 5, Philadelphia, 1995, FA Davis Company; Pasero C, McCaffery M: Preventing and managing opioid induced respiratory depression, *Am J Nurs* 94(4):25-31, 1994; Reisine T, Pasternak G: Opioid analgesics and antagonists. In Hardman JG, Limbird LE, editors: *Goodman & Gilman's the pharmacological basis of therapeutics,* ed 9, pp 521-555, New York, 1996, McGraw-Hill.

---

caused by disease progression rather than opioid overdose. This is not an emergency situation, and observation for a few hours is the best diagnostic and therapeutic approach (Manfredi, Ribeiro, Chandler et al., 1997). If a terminally ill patient cannot be aroused and an opioid overdose is suspected, an opioid antagonist drug is warranted only if it is clear that this is not a natural progression of the disease.

Tapering and Cessation of Therapy

For patients with acute pain who are receiving parenteral or epidural analgesia, plans are necessary for

smoothly weaning the patient as pain decreases or the patient is able to use a less invasive route of administration. Although most patients experience less pain as the days pass after surgery, it should not be assumed that all patients will follow this pattern. For example, the duration of postoperative pain tends to be longer in the elderly (Melzack, Abbott, Zackon et al., 1987). It is best to evaluate patients individually and taper starting analgesic doses on the basis of the patient's reports of pain and ability to perform recovery activities rather than a preconceived notion of when parenteral or epidural analgesics should be discontinued.

In preparation for discharge transition to oral analgesia should be started as soon as the patient is able to retain fluids and pain is well controlled. As function returns and pain lessens, the parenteral or epidural opioid dose can be reduced 25% once or twice daily.

To make the transition from epidural analgesia to oral analgesia as smooth as possible, the characteristics of the epidural opioid are considered before discontinuing it. When patients are receiving lipophilic epidural opioids (short duration; e.g., fentanyl, sufentanil), the oral analgesic can be administered before discontinuing epidural analgesia so that patients remain comfortable during the transition. Because analgesia tends to last longer after discontinuing hydrophilic epidural opioids (e.g., morphine, hydromorphone), these patients can be informed of the availability of oral analgesia and reminded to ask for it as soon as they feel pain return and before it becomes severe. Many nurses encourage patients to take their oral analgesic before sleep on the evening that epidural analgesia is discontinued to prevent them from waking up in severe pain. In all cases, patients should be comfortable before epidural analgesia is discontinued. Frequent pain assessment (every 1 to 2 hours) during the transition provides an opportunity to evaluate and adjust as needed the new analgesic regimen.

Analgesic doses other than the usual prescriptions for oral codeine or oxycodone should be considered to manage moderate to severe pain during and after the transition and at home. When opioids are compounded with acetaminophen or aspirin, the total daily dose is limited by the maximum recommended dose of nonopioid. A better choice may be to switch the patient from parenteral or epidural analgesia to oral hydromorphone, morphine, or single entity oxycodone. Oral morphine, 15 to 30 mg, or oral hydromorphone, 4 to 8 mg, would provide more pain relief than the customary opioid/nonopioid analgesics.

UNWARRANTED WITHHOLDING OF OPIOIDS

Long-Term Opioid Treatment for Chronic Nonmalignant Pain

When opioids are used to treat chronic nonmalignant pain, the principles are the same as for other types of pain. The controversies about whether opioids should be used in individuals with chronic nonmalignant pain will be discussed in Chapter 11.

Opioids During Weaning From Mechanical Ventilation

Critically ill patients who require tracheal intubation and mechanical ventilation usually require opioids for pain relief. Opioids are commonly indicated to treat the pain associated with a critically ill patient's underlying condition or disease process. They are warranted also because tracheal intubation, mechanical ventilation, and the aftermath of care, such as chest physiotherapy and suctioning, are reported to be extremely painful (Carroll, Magruder, 1993; Murray, Plevak, 1994; Puntillo, 1990; Ryan, Luer, 1991).

When critically ill patients show improvement, they are gradually weaned from mechanical ventilation. Unfortunately, many physicians discontinue all opioids before beginning the weaning process. This practice has grown out of a fear that opioids will produce adverse respiratory effects and impede weaning. However, the fear of respiratory depression, cited as the main reason for stopping opioids before weaning, usually is unfounded in critically ill patients. Most critically ill patients will receive opioids long enough for some tolerance to develop. Therefore fear of respiratory depression should not be a barrier to continuing opioids for patients who have been receiving them for several days or longer (APS, 1992; Jacox, Carr, Payne et al., 1994).

In addition, loss of pain control can cause weaning to fail. Unrelieved pain can result in respiratory dysfunction. Even when the source of pain is remote from the thoracic and abdominal region, respiratory dysfunction can occur (de Leon-Casasola, Lema, 1992). Involuntary responses to pain cause reflex muscle spasm at the site of tissue damage and in muscle groups above and below the site. Patients with pain also voluntarily limit their thoracic and abdominal muscle movement in an effort to reduce the pain they are experiencing (Cousins, 1994).

The measurable respiratory effects of severe pain are small tidal volumes and high inspiratory and expiratory pressures, as well as decreases in vital capacity, functional residual capacity, and alveolar ventilation. If adequate pain relief is not provided, these effects can progress to significant pulmonary complications, such as atelectasis and pneumonia (Cousins, 1994). In addition, hypoxemia from decreased oxygen saturation can result in cardiac and wound complications and mental dysfunction (Rosenberg, Kehlet, 1993). (See Chapter 2 for more on the harmful effects of unrelieved pain.)

Abrupt discontinuation of opioids can have other undesirable consequences besides loss of pain control. At the time of weaning, many critically ill patients have been receiving opioids long enough to have developed physical dependence. If the opioid is stopped abruptly for weaning, physically dependent patients will experience withdrawal syndrome. Signs of withdrawal include restlessness and agitation and may be confused with failed weaning or "ICU psychosis." The practice of abrupt discontinuation of opioids can result in inaccurate assessment of the patient's response and inappropriate treatment (e.g., benzodiazepines to sedate the patient).

If a reduced opioid dose is required for successful weaning, using a multimodality, balanced analgesia approach may make it easier to do so without compromising good pain control (Murray, Plevak, 1994). If a nonopioid is not being administered ATC already, one can be added before weaning to allow a reduced opioid dose. Other appropriate nonsedating adjuvants, such as local anesthetics added to epidural opioids, should be considered.

The intraspinal routes are frequently used to deliver opioids to the critically ill (see pp. 213-239). One of the benefits of intraspinal analgesia in mechanically ventilated patients is excellent analgesia with less threat of respiratory depression during weaning. In addition, a number of studies have demonstrated improved pulmonary function with intraspinal analgesia (Liu, Carpenter, Neal, 1995) (see Chapter 2).

Managing Pain in the Terminally Ill

The Council on Ethical and Judicial Affairs of the American Medical Association maintains its 1988 position that "the administration of a drug necessary to ease the pain of a patient who is terminally ill and suffering excruciating pain may be appropriate medical treatment even though the effect of the drug may shorten life" (AMA, 1992). Despite this, a study of more than 9000 terminally ill hospitalized patients revealed that 50% of conscious seriously ill patients who died in the hospital experienced moderate to severe pain at least half of the time (SUPPORT, 1995). Four in 10 experienced severe pain; 59% preferred a treatment plan that focused on comfort, but 10% received care contrary to this (Lynn, Teno, Phillips, 1997).

The underdosing of terminally ill patients is particularly tragic because it is usually made on the basis of the unfounded fear that the opioid will produce adverse respiratory effect and hasten death. However, most terminally ill patients have been receiving opioids long enough to have developed tolerance to the opioid's respiratory depressant effects. In fact, in a study of patients from whom life support had been withdrawn or withheld, those who received analgesics and sedatives lived longer (2.2 hours) than those who did not receive analgesics and sedatives (Wilson, Smedira, Fink et al., 1992). This study suggests that the underlying disease, not the analgesics and sedatives, usually determines death (Brody, Campbell, Faber-Langendoen et al., 1997).

The enormous tolerance that patients develop to the respiratory depressant effects of opioids is illustrated by numerous accounts of opioid doses that have escalated over time. One group of clinicians reported that in patients surveyed with advanced cancer almost 40% required increases in their opioid requirements by 25% during the last 4 weeks of the life. Total daily opioid doses in these patients ranged from 7 to 35, 164 IM morphine equivalents. Five percent used an opioid dose of >900 IM morphine equivalents per day 4 weeks before death, and within 24 hours of death, this proportion increased to 9%. Even pa-

tients receiving the highest doses were titrated in the home setting. These findings reinforce that "high" doses of opioids are both appropriate and safe in terminally ill patients with pain (Coyle, Adelhardt, Foley et al., 1990).

Most patients with advanced cancer lose the ability to communicate during the final days of life. This loss of communication should not be interpreted as loss of pain. Pain often increases as death approaches. Patients who are confused, grimacing, moaning, agitated, or restless most likely are experiencing unrelieved pain and require an increase in the opioid dose (Levy, 1985, 1994).

DOCUMENTING PAIN MANAGEMENT

Documentation is a means for communicating pain assessments (e.g., pain ratings), interventions to manage the pain, and the patient's response (e.g., pain ratings and side effects). The more severe the pain, the more often it is assessed and documented. The use of opioid analgesics requires documentation, not only as an intervention but also for substance control purposes. When invasive therapies are used, such as epidural analgesia and PCA, special flow sheets are useful for ensuring that the patient's pain assessments, side effects, and use of opioids during therapy are documented. Use of a flow sheet helps to centralize and standardize documentation, avoid duplication of documentation, save time, meet substance control requirements, and provide an overall picture of the patient's pain experience during treatment. Chapter 3 discusses documentation of pain in depth and offers examples of a variety of flow sheets.

Patient and family teaching about pain and the pain management plan also must be documented. Many institutions use a checklist format for ensuring that important teaching is done before therapies are initiated (see Form 6.2). The form is shared by everyone who teaches the patient about the pain management plan. For example, when used for teaching surgical patients about the pain management plan, the checklist is initiated during the preoperative testing appointment and included as part of the patient's admitting record. The checklist communicates to the admitting nurse important information about the patient's pain history, current medication use, and what patient teaching needs to be done or reinforced before therapy is initiated.

PATIENT AND FAMILY TEACHING

Ensuring that patients obtain the maximum benefit from opioid analgesics requires education of the patient and family. Numerous educational pamphlets have been developed to address dosing schedules, routes of administration, side effects, and common misconceptions. Readers are encouraged to identify these publications, review them, and select those that meet the needs of their patient population. Many of these are excellent and can be obtained in bulk free of charge or for a small fee

● ● ● ● ●

FORM 6.2 **Pain Management Plan Patient Teaching Checklist**

( ) The goals of the pain management plan are:

_____

_____

( ) Indicators of pain, use of pain rating tool: _____ Comfort goal: _____

( ) Effects and management of unrelieved pain

( ) Pain management options discussed; patient will receive:

    ( ) Intrathecal analgesia

    ( ) Continuous epidural analgesia   ( ) Epidural patient-controlled analgesia

    ( ) IV patient-controlled analgesia   ( ) SC patient-controlled analgesia

    ( ) Parent-controlled analgesia

        ( ) Primary pain manager _____

        ( ) Secondary pain manager _____

    ( ) Oral patient-controlled analgesia

    ( ) Nurse-activated dosing

    ( ) Other _____

( ) Use of equipment and/or supplies

    ( ) Demonstrated   ( ) Return demonstrated

( ) Safety features and precautions

( ) Initiation procedure

( ) Possible side effects and complications

( ) Expected course of treatment, discontinuation procedure, postinfusion analgesia

( ) Nondrug methods for managing pain _____

( ) Daily milestones

( ) Current medications discussed, including OTC drugs _____

_____

_____

( ) Additional discussion: _____

_____

_____

_____

( ) Written materials issued

_____   _____

Clinician   Date

● ● ● ● ●
BOX 6.30

Resources for Obtaining Patient Education Materials

- Agency for Health Care Policy and Research (AHCPR) Clearinghouse: (800) 358-9295
  AHCPR Acute Pain Management Patient Guide
  AHCPR Management of Cancer Pain Patient Guide
- City of Hope Medical Center (626) 359-8111, ext. 3829
  1500 E. Duarte Rd., Duarte, CA 91010
  Prescription for Life (patient handbook for cancer pain management)
  Will It Hurt? Helping Your Child Cope With Surgery
  Will It Hurt? Helping Your Child Cope With Medical Procedures
  Will It Hurt? Helping Your Infant or Young Child in the Hospital
- Fox Chase Cancer Center
  Pain Management Center
  7701 Burholme Ave.
  Philadelphia, PA 19111
  No More Pain (information booklet for patients)
- National Institutes of Health National Cancer Information Service: (800) 4-CANCER or American Cancer Society: (800) 227-2345
  Get Relief From Cancer Pain (patient information booklet)
- Wisconsin Cancer Pain Initiative (608) 262-0978
  1300 University Ave., Room 3671 MSC
  Madison, WI 53706
  Children's Cancer Pain **Can** *Be Relieved* (information booklet for parents)

May be duplicated for use in clinical practice. From McCaffery M, Pasero C: *Pain: Clinical manual*, p. 274. Copyright © 1999, Mosby, Inc.

Box 6.30 lists resources for obtaining patient and family teaching materials. The materials are free or may be purchased for a small fee.

(e.g., from the Agency for Health Care Policy and Research or from pharmaceutical companies). Box 6.30 lists some resources for patient education materials.

Rather than address all of these issues again, we have chosen to focus on what we believe is the single most significant barrier to achieving pain relief with opioid analgesics—fear of addiction. This appears to be the most challenging area of patient and family education, and indeed of education of health care professionals. Therefore we offer a variety of approaches and encourage the reader to use them liberally and critically examine their effectiveness with each patient and family. Research is needed to identify the most effective ways of educating all of us about addiction.

Patients who are taking opioids and their families usually worry about addiction and often confuse the definitions of addiction, tolerance, and dependence. Lack of knowledge, misconceptions, and fears about addiction may prevent patients from requesting or taking their pain medication, cause them to take less pain medication than they need to control their pain, or to "hold of" as long as possible between doses until pain is severe and out of control. Patients tend to worry more about addiction the longer they take opioids. As time passes, friends and family express concerns about extended opioid use, and the patient may become more sensitive to media messages to "just say no to drugs."

A national telephone survey of 1000 Americans revealed that 85% were fearful of becoming overreliant on pain medication, and 82% were concerned about becoming addicted. They were particularly alarmed by the word "narcotic." Furthermore, findings in the study revealed that only 41% of the respondents believed that all or almost all pain can be relieved (The Mayday Fund, 1993).

These misconceptions have an impact on pain control. A survey of 270 patients with cancer revealed that concern about addiction resulted in a reluctance to report pain and to use analgesics (Ward, Goldberg, Miller-McCauley et al., 1993).

With the current trend toward outpatient care, family members are assuming the roles of caregiver and pain manager in the home setting. Research shows that family caregivers undermedicate their loved one's pain on the basis of "extreme" fears of addiction, respiratory depression, and drug tolerance (Ferrell, Grant, Chan et al., 1995). This makes teaching patients and their families about these phenomena a priority when long-term opioid treatment begins and throughout the course of treatment.

Unfortunately, teaching the facts about addiction, tolerance, and physical dependence often fails to allay fears and change attitudes. Efforts to present the facts about such emotionally charged issues frequently are overshadowed by fiercely held beliefs. No proven method exists for breaking down such strong barriers to achieving effective pain control. Where one method may work with one patient, it may fail with the next. Giving consistent and confident explanations about addiction and repeating information frequently during treatment provides reassurance to patients. Table 6.18 provides considerations and examples of responses to the concerns patients and families express about addiction. We recommend using a variety of these approaches at the start and during the course of opioid treatment.

In addition to talking with patients about opioids and their side effects, providing written information reinforces explanations about the method of opioid delivery, dosage, dosing schedules, and other important points the patient will need to remember. Boxes 6.31 to 6.37 provide examples of patient information forms. Often, patient information is provided in the form of a brochure or pamphlet. Boxes 6.38 and 6.39 provide examples of patient information brochures that describe IV PCA and epidural analgesia, respectively.

● ● ● ● ●

TABLE 6.18 **Discussing Addiction With Patients and Their Families**

ISSUE	APPROACH
Concern about addiction. Patient is thinking, "I don't want to get hooked."	• Assume all patients who take opioids and their families will have some concern about addiction. Don't wait for them to express concern. Initiate discussion with comments such as, "This pain medicine is sometimes called a narcotic, and lots of people wonder if taking a narcotic will cause addiction. This hardly ever happens. Do you have any concerns about this?" (Be sure to ask family caregivers this question.) • To encourage discussion, ask, "What do you know about addiction? Have you known people with drug or alcohol problems?" • Assume that health care providers have expressed to patients and their families concerns about addiction. Ask, "What have other nurses and doctors said to you about addiction?" • If the patient has no questions, simply say, "There's no need to worry about addiction being caused by taking pain medicine to be comfortable. Taking pain medicine for pain relief is not the same thing as addiction. If you think of any questions, please let us know."
The word "narcotic" has a negative connotation. Patient may say, "Narcotics are what drug addicts take."	• Reinforce that pain medicines are "good" drugs by linking adequate pain control to achieving goals or improving quality of life. For example, equate an activity the patient values, such as walking the dog, with taking pain medicine to achieve a comfort goal of 3 on a 0 to 10 scale. • Avoid the words "narcotics" or "drugs." • Use the words "pain medicine" or "pain medication." • Refer to the analgesics by brand names, e.g., MS Contin rather than morphine. • "It's true that many addicts take narcotics, but that is a case of using medicine for the wrong reason. Taking a narcotic for pain relief is the right reason to use pain medicine. Any medicine can be used in the wrong way or the right way."
Confusion about addiction, tolerance, and physical dependence. Patient may say, "I don't want to be like those street addicts who get sick and crazy whenever they can't get a dose."	• "It's easy to confuse addiction with tolerance and physical dependence. Addiction to pain medicine would mean that your pain has gone away, but you still take the medicine regularly when you don't need it, maybe just to 'escape from your problems.' I don't know any patients who do this. If the pain decreases, they take less pain medicine. If the pain stops, they stop taking pain medicine." • "Physical dependence means that you would go into withdrawal if you suddenly stopped taking the medicine. Physical dependence occurs with many medicines, such as cortisone, after they are taken regularly for weeks. Even caffeine can cause physical dependence. For example, if everyday you consume several caffeine-containing beverages, such as coffee or soft drinks, and one day you don't drink any, you would probably experience withdrawal in the form of a headache. That's why we tell you not to suddenly stop taking your pain medication. If you take pain medicine regularly and you suddenly stop, you could develop withdrawal symptoms, like sweating, tearing, and diarrhea. To avoid withdrawal, the dose is decreased gradually over a few days so that your body can adjust to lower doses. Physical dependence is not the same thing as addiction and does not cause addiction." • "Tolerance to pain medicine means that the dose no longer relieves as much pain. When this happens, it is easily handled by raising the dose. This is not the same thing as addiction and does not cause addiction." (see below)
Reluctance to begin opioid treatment for fear that the effectiveness of opioid analgesics will diminish over time. Patient may say, "If I take too much medicine, it will stop working." Or, "It won't work when I really need it later."	• "You don't need to save your pain medicine until your pain gets bad and you really need it. Pain medicine will not stop working. You can start taking pain medicine regularly every day when you only hurt a little. If you hurt more, the dose can be increased or other medicine can be added. Don't deny yourself pain relief now." • "Many people 'save' pain medicine for later, but you don't need to. There is no limit to the amount of pain medicine we can give you for pain relief." • "Although larger doses may be needed over time, the pain medicine does not stop working." • "It's not possible to 'use up' the pain-relieving effect of pain medicine." • Use patient examples by drawing similarities when appropriate, e.g., "I am taking care of someone who, like you, wanted to hold off taking pain medicine. But he did start taking it after we assured him it would keep working. Last week his pain increased, and we were able to double his dose of pain medication and relieve his pain without any difficulty."

May be duplicated for use in clinical practice. From McCaffery M, Pasero C: *Pain: Clinical manual*, pp. 275-276. Copyright © 1999, Mosby, Inc.   *Continued.*

● ● ● ● ●

TABLE 6.18   **Discussing Addiction With Patients and Their Families—cont'd**

ISSUE	APPROACH
Misconception that the risk of addiction is high. Patient may say, "Look at all the people on television who get addicted."	• Use descriptors, e.g., "Addiction **very rarely** happens in people who are taking pain medicine to relieve pain." • Use graphics, e.g., pie charts, bar graphs, to show that addiction is rare. Simply draw a large circle and put a small dot in it to represent those who become addicted. • Use research, e.g., "A survey of more than 11,000 people taking opioids for pain relief found only 4 people became addicted." • Whenever possible, draw parallels to the patient's response to previous dose reduction, e.g., "Do you remember when you reduced the dose of your pain medicine after surgery without any problems? That proves that you can stop taking the medicine when the pain stops." • Use patient examples, e.g., "I am caring for a woman right now who took the same pain medicine you are taking for several weeks. Because of successful surgery, her pain is gone. Now that she has no need for her pain medicine, she has found that she doesn't want it at all." or "I am taking care of several patients who are taking the same pain medicine you are and not one is addicted to it." • "Headlines sometimes report that a movie star or a rock star is addicted to pain relievers. This makes it sound like taking pain medicine causes addiction. Chances are that the star had problems with drugs in the past. Or, the person may have had a pain problem and was wrongly labeled an addict. Remember, thousands of people take pain medicine everyday without becoming addicted."
Persistent fear that "If anybody gets addicted, it will probably be me."	• "Ask yourself, 'If I had no pain, would I still want to take this pain medicine? If I stopped hurting, would I lie to my doctor to get more pain medicine? Would I try to buy it on the streets?' If the answer is no, then you would be able to stop taking the medication if the pain stopped." • "I take care of many people who take pain medicine to stay comfortable, and none of them has become addicted." • Draw similarities to a specific patient similar to this patient. An example for a patient with chronic pain might be, "Not too long ago I cared for a man about your age. He had a tumor somewhat like yours and his pain was right here over his chest, just like yours. We started him on the same pain medicine you're taking and he did very well. It took us a week or so to hit exactly the right dose, but then he took it around the clock every day. He didn't get addicted. He started playing golf again and actually took a trip to visit his children." • For a patient with short-term pain, a patient example might be, "Last week I cared for a man who had his knee replaced. He was afraid of addiction and was reluctant to take his pain medicine after surgery. Because of this, he was in pain and not able to perform his exercises with the physical therapist. He ended up with a very stiff knee because he didn't control his pain effectively."
Misconception that ATC dosing will lead to addiction; belief that pain medicine should be taken only when pain is present. Patient may say, "If I take it when I don't need it, it's like being addicted."	• "Certainly you need pain medicine when you feel pain, but you also need it to prevent pain." • "Pain needs to be kept under control just like we control diseases like high blood pressure. We don't wait until a person with high blood pressure has a stroke before we give medicine to control his blood pressure. We ask the person to take blood pressure medicine at regular times everyday to keep the blood pressure under control. The same logic applies to pain. We don't want to wait for the pain to return and become severe before giving pain medicine. We want you to take it regularly to keep pain under control." • "Remember, we will be working with you and watching your doses carefully to be sure that what you are taking is safe and right for you." • "The purpose of pain medicine is to put you back in control of your life rather than let pain control your life. Right now, pain controls what you do. We want to put you back in charge. Taking pain medicine regularly in the right doses is how you get control again." • "People think that, like John Wayne, they should bite the bullet with pain. This makes a good movie, but it doesn't make a good life." • "Pain is harmful to your health. Sometimes we get so concerned about the possible harm from pain medicine that we forget that pain is also dangerous. Research shows that pain increases cancer growth and decreases your immune function so that you are more prone to other diseases and infections." • "Addiction **very rarely** occurs from taking pain medicine. Whether you take pain medicine regularly or occasionally does not change this."

Information from Jacox A, Carr DB, Payne R et al.: *Managing cancer pain: Consumer version.* Clinical practice guideline No. 9. AHCPR Publication No. 94-0595, Rockville, MD, U.S. Public Health Service, AHCPR, March 1994; Lang SL, Patt RB: *You don't have to suffer,* New York, 1994, Oxford University Press.

BOX 6.31

PATIENT MEDICATION INFORMATION

Fentanyl Patch (generic name)

BRAND NAME: Duragesic (Fentanyl Transdermal System)

TYPE OF PAIN MEDICINE: Opioid (narcotic)

DESCRIPTION:
A thin adhesive (sticky) patch that comes in four sizes:
  25 μg/hr (micrograms/hour)
  50 μg/hr
  75 μg/hr
  100 μg/hr

USES:
Relieves pain.

DOSAGE AND ADMINISTRATION:
- Take only as directed.
- These directions may change.
- There is no maximum dose or number of patches your doctor can prescribe for you.
- Doses are prescribed in micrograms/hour (μg/hr).
- The patch releases medicine slowly. It takes 12 to 18 hours to feel relief when starting the patch or increasing the dose.
- Short-acting pain medicines will be ordered to use in between patch changes if needed to control pain.
- Usually patches are changed every 72 hours. Call your doctor or nurse if pain relief does not last 72 hours.
- Do not cut or alter the patch in any way.

HOW TO APPLY DURAGESIC:
- Place the patch on skin above the waist. Front or back of body can be used.
- If skin has body hair, clip hair close to skin. DO NOT SHAVE SKIN.
- Do not place patch on cut or irritated skin.
- Make sure skin is dry. Do not use soap, oils, lotions, or alcohol on skin where patch will be placed.
- Steps
  1. Take patch out of protective pouch.
  2. Pull protective backing off sticky side of patch by using tab that sticks out. Discard backing.
  3. Apply patch immediately to dry, nonhairy area of skin.
  4. Press patch firmly on skin with the palm of your hand for 30 seconds.
  5. Wash hands.
  6. After 72 hours, remove all patches and apply new ones on different places.
  7. If patch should fall off of skin, replace with a new patch.

May be duplicated for use in clinical practice. As appears in McCaffery M, Pasero C: *Pain: Clinical manual*, pp. 277-278, 1999, Mosby, Inc.   *Continued.*

BOX 6.31—cont'd

PATIENT MEDICATION INFORMATION—cont'd

Fentanyl Patch (generic name)

BRAND NAME: Duragesic (Fentanyl Transdermal System)

DISPOSAL:
Fold used patch in half so sticky side sticks to itself. Flush used patches down the toilet immediately.

POSSIBLE SIDE EFFECTS:
- Constipation: Fentanyl and other opioids block pain and block bowels. Constipation can be controlled with daily laxatives.
- Nausea and vomiting: Less common than constipation. Can be controlled with other medicines. If this occurs, call your doctor or nurse.
- Drowsiness: May occur when starting opioids or increasing dose. This usually goes away in 48 to 72 hours. Rest as needed.
- Confusion: This is less common than drowsiness. If this happens, call your doctor or nurse.

PRECAUTIONS:
- Be careful driving or using machinery such as lawn mowers, power tools, or saws.
- Be careful when drinking alcohol. Alcohol will increase drowsiness.
- Call your doctor or nurse if pain increases, if you do not get pain relief, or if pain relief does not last 72 hours.
- Do not apply heat, such as a heating pad or a prolonged hot shower, over the patch. This may increase your dose and cause side effects.

STOPPING MEDICATIONS: Do not suddenly stop using your patch. Fentanyl and other opioids must be stopped gradually. Call your doctor or nurse for directions.

REMEMBER!
- Don't run out of patches.
- Keep count of your patches.
- Get a **new** prescription filled a few days before you run out of patches. This prescription cannot be **re**filled or phoned into your pharmacy or drug store.

COMMENTS:

WARNING: Keep this and all medicines out of the reach of children.

BOX 6.32

PATIENT MEDICATION INFORMATION

Hydromorphone (generic name)

BRAND NAME: Dilaudid

TYPE OF PAIN MEDICINE: Opioid (narcotic)

DESCRIPTION:
Dilaudid tablets come in four strengths:
  2 mg: orange
  4 mg: yellow
  8 mg: white (triangle shape)

USES:
Relieves pain.
Sometimes used to control cough.

DOSAGE AND ADMINISTRATION:
- Take only as directed. You should feel pain relief in 30 to 60 minutes.
- These directions may change.
- There is no maximum dose or number of tablets your doctor can prescribe for you.
- Usually taken every 2 to 4 hours.
- You may need to adjust your schedule.
- May be taken alone or in addition to other pain medications.
- May be taken with other medications.
- May be taken with or without food.
- If you miss a dose of your medicine, take it as soon as possible. If it is almost time for the next dose, skip the missed dose. Do not take two doses at one time to make up for your missed dose.
- Inform your doctor before you begin taking any new medicine, either prescribed or over-the-counter.

POSSIBLE SIDE EFFECTS:
- Constipation: Dilaudid and other opioids block pain and block bowels. Constipation can be controlled with daily laxatives.
- Nausea and vomiting: Less common than constipation. Can be controlled with other medicines. If this occurs, call your doctor or nurse.
- Drowsiness: May occur when starting Dilaudid or increasing dose. This usually goes away in 48 to 72 hours. Rest as needed.
- Confusion: This is less common than drowsiness. If this happens, call your doctor or nurse.

PRECAUTIONS:
- Be careful driving or using machinery such as lawn mowers, power tools, or saws.
- Be careful when drinking alcohol. Alcohol will increase drowsiness.
- Call your doctor or nurse if pain increases or if you do not get pain relief.

May be duplicated for use in clinical practice. As appears in McCaffery M, Pasero C: *Pain: Clinical manual*, pp. 279-280, 1999, Mosby, Inc.   *Continued.*

PATIENT MEDICATION INFORMATION—cont'd

Hydromorphone (generic name)

BRAND NAME: Dilaudid

STOPPING MEDICATIONS: Do not suddenly stop taking this medicine. Dilaudid and other opioids must be stopped gradually. Call your doctor or nurse for directions.

REMEMBER!
- Don't run out of pills.
- Keep count of your pills.
- Get a **new** prescription filled a few days before you run out of pills. This prescription cannot be **re**filled or phoned into your pharmacy or drug store.

COMMENTS:

WARNING: Keep this and all medicines out of the reach of children.

May be duplicated for use in clinical practice. As appears in McCaffery M, Pasero C: *Pain: Clinical manual,* pp. 279-280, 1999, Mosby, Inc.
Courtesy Fox Chase Cancer Center/Pain Management, Philadelphia, PA, 1997.

BOX 6.33

PATIENT MEDICATION INFORMATION

Morphine Sulfate (generic name)
Immediate-Release Tablets or Capsules

BRAND NAMES:
Morphine Sulfate Tablets
MSIR (Morphine Sulfate Immediate-Release)

TYPE OF PAIN MEDICINE: Opioid (narcotic)

DESCRIPTION:
MSIR comes in two strengths:
   15 mg tablet: white round
   30 mg tablet: white oblong
   15 mg capsule: white and blue
   30 mg capsule: gray and purple
Generics may look different.

USES:
Relieves pain.
Sometimes used to control cough and/or shortness of breath.

DOSAGE AND ADMINISTRATION:
- Take only as directed. You should feel pain relief in 30 to 60 minutes.
- These directions may change.
- There is no maximum dose or number of tablets your doctor can prescribe for you.
- Usually taken every 3 to 4 hours.
- You may need to adjust your schedule.
- May be taken alone or in addition to other pain medications.
- May be taken with other medications.
- May be taken with or without food.
- If you miss a dose of your medicine, take it as soon as possible. If it is almost time for the next dose, skip the missed dose. Do not take two doses at one time to make up for your missed dose.
- Inform your doctor before you begin taking any new medicine, either prescribed or over-the-counter.
- Capsule contents can be sprinkled over soft food, added to liquids, or given in gastric or NG tubes.

POSSIBLE SIDE EFFECTS:
- Constipation: Morphine and other opioids block pain and block bowels. Constipation can be controlled with daily laxatives.
- Nausea and vomiting: Less common than constipation. Can be controlled with other medicines. If this occurs, call your doctor or nurse.
- Drowsiness: May occur when starting morphine or increasing dose. This usually goes away in 48 to 72 hours. Rest as needed.
- Confusion: This is less common than drowsiness. If this happens, call your doctor or nurse.

May be duplicated for use in clinical practice. As appears in McCaffery M, Pasero C: *Pain: Clinical manual*, pp. 281-282, 1999, Mosby, Inc.   *Continued.*

● ● ● ● ●
BOX 6.33—cont'd

PATIENT MEDICATION INFORMATION—cont'd

Morphine Sulfate (generic name)
Immediate-Release Tablets or Capsules

BRAND NAMES:
Morphine Sulfate Tablets
MSIR (Morphine Sulfate Immediate-Release)

PRECAUTIONS:
- Be careful driving or using machinery such as lawn mowers, power tools, or saws.
- Be careful when drinking alcohol. Alcohol will increase drowsiness.
- Call your doctor or nurse if pain increases or if you do not get pain relief.

STOPPING MEDICATIONS: Do not suddenly stop taking this medicine. Morphine and other opioids must be stopped gradually. Call your doctor or nurse for directions.

REMEMBER!
- Don't run out of pills.
- Keep count of your pills.
- Get a **new** prescription filled a few days before you run out of pills. This prescription cannot be **re**filled or phoned into your pharmacy or drug store.

COMMENTS:

WARNING: Keep this and all medicines out of the reach of children.

May be duplicated for use in clinical practice. As appears in McCaffery M, Pasero C: *Pain: Clinical manual*, pp. 281-282, 1999, Mosby, Inc.
Courtesy Fox Chase Cancer Center/Pain Management, Philadelphia, PA, 1997.

BOX 6.34

PATIENT MEDICATION INFORMATION

Controlled-Release Morphine (generic name)

BRAND NAME: MS Contin

TYPE OF PAIN MEDICINE: Opioid (narcotic)

DESCRIPTION:
MS Contin tablets come in five strengths:
    15 mg: blue
    30 mg: purple
    60 mg: orange
    100 mg: gray
    200 mg: green

USES:
Relieves pain.
Sometimes used to control cough and shortness of breath.

DOSAGE AND ADMINISTRATION:
- Take only as directed. It will take 2 hours to feel relief.
- These directions may change.
- There is no maximum dose or number of tablets your doctor can prescribe for you.
- The morphine in MS Contin is slowly released. Pain relief should last 12 hours.
- Usually taken every 12 hours.
- You may need to adjust your schedule.
- Take at the same time every day.
- Short-acting pain medicines will be ordered to use in between doses if needed to control pain.
- May be taken alone or in addition to other pain medications.
- May be taken with other medications.
- May be taken with or without food.
- If you miss a dose of your medicine, take it as soon as possible. If it is almost time for the next dose, skip the missed dose. Do not take two doses at one time to make up for your missed dose. If you miss your dose by 4 or more hours, take your short-acting pain medicine for pain relief until the next dose of MS Contin is due.
- Inform your doctor before you begin taking any new medicine, either prescribed or over-the-counter.

POSSIBLE SIDE EFFECTS:
- Constipation: Morphine and other opioids block pain and block bowels. Constipation can be controlled with daily laxatives.
- Nausea and vomiting: Less common than constipation. Can be controlled with other medicines. If this occurs, call your doctor or nurse.
- Drowsiness: May occur when starting morphine or increasing dose. This usually goes away in 48 to 72 hours. Rest as needed.
- Confusion. This is less common than drowsiness. If this happens, call your doctor or nurse.

May be duplicated for use in clinical practice. As appears in McCaffery M, Pasero C: *Pain: Clinical manual,* pp. 283-284, 1999, Mosby, Inc.   *Continued.*

BOX 6.34—cont'd

PATIENT MEDICATION INFORMATION—cont'd

Controlled-Release Morphine (generic name)

BRAND NAME: MS Contin

PRECAUTIONS:
- Do not break, crush, or chew tablets.
- Be careful driving or using machinery such as lawn mowers, power tools, or saws.
- Be careful when drinking alcohol. Alcohol will increase drowsiness.
- Call your doctor or nurse if pain increases or if you do not get pain relief.

STOPPING MEDICATIONS: Do not suddenly stop taking this medicine. Morphine and other opioids must be stopped gradually. Call your doctor or nurse for directions.

REMEMBER!
- Don't run out of pills.
- Keep count of your pills.
- Get a *new* prescription filled a few days before you run out of pills. This prescription cannot be *re*filled or phoned into your pharmacy or drug store.

COMMENTS:

WARNING: Keep this and all medicines out of the reach of children.

● ● ● ● ●
BOX 6.35

PATIENT MEDICATION INFORMATION

Morphine Liquid Concentrate (generic name)

BRAND NAMES:
Roxanol (Morphine Sulfate Immediate Release, Concentrated Oral Solution)
MSIR Oral Solution Concentrate

TYPE OF PAIN MEDICINE: Opioid (narcotic)

DESCRIPTION:
A colorless liquid (20 mg morphine per ml)

USES:
Relieves pain.
Sometimes used to control cough and shortness of breath.

DOSAGE AND ADMINISTRATION:
- Take only as directed. You should feel pain relief in 30 to 60 minutes.
- These directions may change.
- There is no maximum dose or amount of medicine your doctor can prescribe for you.
- Doses are prescribed in ml (milliliters), cc (cubic centimeters), or mg (milligrams).
- May be mixed with juice or water.
- One drop of blue food coloring may be added to the bottle if you have trouble seeing how to measure the liquid.
- Usually taken every 3 to 4 hours.
- You may need to adjust your schedule.
- May be taken alone or in addition to other pain medications.
- May be taken with other medications.
- May be taken with or without food.
- If you miss a dose of your medicine, take it as soon as possible. If it is almost time for the next dose, skip the missed dose. Do not take two doses at one time to make up for your missed dose.
- Inform your doctor before you begin taking any new medicine, either prescribed or over-the-counter.

POSSIBLE SIDE EFFECTS:
- Constipation: Morphine and other opioids block pain and block bowels. Constipation can be controlled with daily laxatives.
- Nausea and vomiting: Less common than constipation. Can be controlled with other medicines. If this occurs, call your doctor or nurse.
- Drowsiness: May occur when starting morphine or increasing dose. This usually goes away in 48 to 72 hours. Rest as needed.
- Confusion: This is less common than drowsiness. If this happens, call your doctor or nurse.

May be duplicated for use in clinical practice. As appears in McCaffery M, Pasero C: *Pain: Clinical manual*, pp. 285-286, 1999, Mosby, Inc.   *Continued.*

BOX 6.35—cont'd

PATIENT MEDICATION INFORMATION—cont'd

Morphine Liquid Concentrate (generic name)

BRAND NAMES:
Roxanol (Morphine Sulfate Immediate Release, Concentrated Oral Solution)
MSIR Oral Solution Concentrate

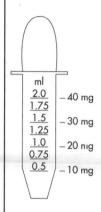

PRECAUTIONS:
- Measure your dose with a dropper, medicine cup, or syringe. Do not use a teaspoon or tablespoon. Remember mg (milligrams) do not equal ml (milliliters). (1 cc = 1 ml = 20 mg)
- Be careful driving or using machinery such as lawn mowers, power tools, or saws.
- Be careful when drinking alcohol. Alcohol will increase drowsiness.
- Call your doctor or nurse if pain increases or if you do not get pain relief.

STOPPING MEDICATIONS: Do not suddenly stop taking this medicine. Morphine and other opioids must be stopped gradually. Call your doctor or nurse for directions.

REMEMBER!
- Don't run out of medicine.
- Keep count of how many doses you have left.
- Get a **new** prescription filled a few days before you run out of medicine. This prescription cannot be **re**filled or phoned into your pharmacy or drug store.

COMMENTS:

WARNING: Keep this and all medicines out of the reach of children.

May be duplicated for use in clinical practice. As appears in McCaffery M, Pasero C: *Pain: Clinical manual*, pp. 285-286, 1999, Mosby, Inc.
Courtesy Fox Chase Cancer Center/Pain Management, Philadelphia, PA, 1997.

● ● ● ● ●
BOX 6.36

PATIENT MEDICATION INFORMATION

Oxycodone (generic name)
Immediate-Release Liquid or Tablets

BRAND NAMES:
OxyIR
Roxicodone
Roxicodone Intensol

TYPE OF PAIN MEDICINE: Opioid (narcotic)

DESCRIPTION:
OxyIR: 5 mg beige/orange capsules.
Roxicodone tablets come in one strength: 5 mg white scored (line down the center) tablet
Roxicodone liquid comes in 5 mg per 5 ml (1 tsp) cherry flavor (red color)
Roxicodone Intensol solution comes in 20 mg per ml (colorless).
Generics (nonbrand names): may look different.

USES:
Relieves pain.

DOSAGE AND ADMINISTRATION:
- Take only as directed. You should feel pain relief in 30 to 60 minutes.
- These directions may change.
- There is no maximum dose or amount of medicine your doctor can prescribe for you.
- Doses are prescribed in ml (milliliters), cc (cubic centimeters), or mg (milligrams).
- May be mixed with juice or water.
- Usually taken every 3 to 4 hours.
- You may need to adjust your schedule.
- May be taken alone or in addition to other pain medications.
- May be taken with other medications.
- May be taken with or without food.
- If you miss a dose of your medicine, take it as soon as possible. If it is almost time for the next dose, skip the missed dose. Do not take two doses at one time to make up for your missed dose.
- Inform your doctor before you begin taking any new medicine, either prescribed or over-the-counter.

POSSIBLE SIDE EFFECTS:
- Constipation: Oxycodone and other opioids block pain and block bowels. Constipation can be controlled with daily laxatives.
- Nausea and vomiting: Less common than constipation. Can be controlled with other medicines. If this occurs, call your doctor or nurse.
- Drowsiness: May occur when starting oxycodone or increasing dose. This usually goes away in 48 to 72 hours. Rest as needed.
- Confusion: This less common than drowsiness. If this happens, call your doctor or nurse.

May be duplicated for use in clinical practice. As appears in McCaffery M, Pasero C: *Pain: Clinical manual*, pp. 287-288, 1999, Mosby, Inc.

Continued.

PATIENT MEDICATION INFORMATION—cont'd

Oxycodone (generic name)
Immediate-Release Liquid or Tablets

BRAND NAMES:
OxyIR
Roxicodone
Roxicodone Intensol

PRECAUTIONS:
- If you are taking the liquid form, measure your dose with a dropper, medicine cup, or syringe. Do not use a teaspoon or tablespoon. Remember mg (milligrams) do not equal ml (milliliters).
- Be careful driving or using machinery such as lawn mowers, power tools, or saws.
- Be careful when drinking alcohol. Alcohol will increase drowsiness.
- Call your doctor or nurse if pain increases or if you do not get pain relief.

STOPPING MEDICATIONS: Do not suddenly stop taking this medicine. Oxycodone and other opioids must be stopped gradually. Call your doctor or nurse for directions.

REMEMBER!
- Don't run out of medicine.
- Keep count of how many doses you have left.
- Get a *new* prescription filled a few days before you run out of medicine. This prescription cannot be *re*filled or phoned into your pharmacy or drug store.

COMMENTS:

WARNING: Keep this and all medicines out of the reach of children.

May be duplicated for use in clinical practice. As appears in McCaffery M, Pasero C: *Pain: Clinical manual*, pp. 287-288, 1999, Mosby, Inc. Courtesy Fox Chase Cancer Center/Pain Management, Philadelphia, PA, 1997.

● ● ● ● ●
BOX 6.37

PATIENT MEDICATION INFORMATION

Controlled-Release Oxycodone (generic name)

BRAND NAME: OxyContin (Oxycodone HCl Controlled-Release Tablets)

TYPE OF PAIN MEDICINE: Opioid (narcotic)

DESCRIPTION:
OxyContin tablets come in four strengths:
    10 mg: white #10 on pill
    20 mg: pink #20 on pill
    40 mg: yellow #40 on pill
    80 mg: green #80 on pill

USES:
Relieves pain.

DOSAGE AND ADMINISTRATION:
- Take only as directed. You should feel pain relief in 1 hour.
- These directions may change.
- There is no maximum number of tablets your doctor can prescribe for you.
- The oxycodone in OxyContin is slowly released. Pain relief usually lasts 12 hours.
- Usually taken every 12 hours.
- You may need to adjust your schedule.
- Take at the same time every day.
- Short-acting pain medicines will be ordered to use in between doses if needed to control pain.
- May be taken alone or in addition to other pain medications.
- May be taken with other medications.
- May be taken with or without food.
- If you miss a dose of your medicine, take it as soon as possible. If it is almost time for the next dose, skip the missed dose. Do not take two doses at one time to make up for your missed dose. If you miss your dose by 4 or more hours, take your short-acting pain medicine for pain relief until the next dose of OxyContin is due.
- Inform your doctor before you begin taking any new medicine, either prescribed or over-the-counter.

POSSIBLE SIDE EFFECTS:
- Constipation: Oxycodone and other opioids block pain and block bowels. Constipation can be controlled with daily laxatives.
- Nausea and vomiting: Less common than constipation. Can be controlled with other medicines. If this occurs, call your doctor or nurse.
- Drowsiness: May occur when starting oxycodone or increasing dose. This usually goes away in 48 to 72 hours. Rest as needed.
- Confusion: This is less common than drowsiness. If this happens, call your doctor or nurse.

May be duplicated for use in clinical practice. As appears in McCaffery M, Pasero C: *Pain: Clinical manual*, pp. 289-290, 1999, Mosby, Inc.

Continued.

PATIENT MEDICATION INFORMATION—cont'd

Controlled-Release Oxycodone (generic name)

BRAND NAME: OxyContin (Oxycodone HCl Controlled-Release Tablets)

PRECAUTIONS:
- Do not break, crush, or chew tablets.
- Be careful driving or using machinery such as lawn mowers, power tools, or saws.
- Be careful when drinking alcohol. Alcohol will increase drowsiness.
- Call your doctor or nurse if pain increases or if you do not get pain relief.

STOPPING MEDICATIONS: Do not suddenly stop taking this medicine. Oxycodone and other opioids must be stopped gradually. Call your doctor or nurse for directions.

REMEMBER!
- Don't run out of pills.
- Keep count of your pills.
- Get a *new* prescription filled a few days before you run out of pills. This prescription cannot be *re*filled or phoned into your pharmacy or drug store.

COMMENTS:

WARNING: Keep this and all medicines out of the reach of children.

May be duplicated for use in clinical practice. As appears in McCaffery M, Pasero C: *Pain: Clinical manual,* pp. 289-290, 1999, Mosby, Inc. Courtesy Fox Chase Cancer Center/Pain Management, Philadelphia, PA, 1997.

• • • • •

| BOX 6.38 | *Patient Information Brochure: Intravenous Patient-Controlled Analgesia (IV PCA)* |

HOW DOES PAIN AFFECT THE BODY?

When you are injured, pain warns you to protect yourself and avoid further injury. However, unrelieved pain can be harmful, especially when you are sick or after surgery. Pain can make it difficult to take a deep breath and interferes with your ability to move and walk. This can result in complications and a long stay in the hospital.

HOW WILL OTHERS KNOW HOW MUCH PAIN YOU HAVE?

• Your nurses will check you often while you are receiving IV PCA. They will ask you to rate your pain on a 0 to 10 scale. A rating of 0 means you feel no pain at all, 5 means you feel a moderate amount of pain, and 10 means you feel the worst pain you can imagine.

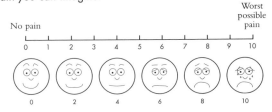

• Your comfort goal is _____ . If you are unable to maintain this level of comfort, especially during activities such as deep breathing and walking, let your nurse know. The dose of pain medicine usually can be increased to keep you as comfortable as possible.

WHAT ARE SOME OF THE GOALS OF PAIN MANAGEMENT WITH IV PCA?

• To keep pain from becoming severe and out of control.
• To keep comfortable so that you can sleep, deep breathe, walk, and visit with others.
• To decrease the length of time spent in the hospital.

HOW DOES IV PCA WORK?

• Pain medicine will be given by a small pump through your IV line. If you have surgery, the pump will be attached to your IV in the recovery room.
• You will have a PCA button that is attached to the pump. You can press the button to give yourself a dose of pain medicine when you hurt.
• You also may be given a small amount of pain medicine continuously.
• The recovery room nurse will manage your pain for you when you arrive in the recovery room, then give you the PCA button as soon as you are awake enough to manage the pain yourself.

• It is difficult to treat pain when it is severe, so it is important to "stay on top" of your pain. When you begin to feel some discomfort, press the PCA button, then wait a few minutes to see if the dose helped to relieve the pain. If the pain has not been relieved, press the PCA button again.

IS IV PCA SAFE?

• The pump will be programmed to give you an amount of pain medicine that is typically safe for someone your sex, size, age, and diagnosis or type of surgery. If this is too much, the dose of the pain medicine can be reduced.
• The pump will be programmed with a safe hourly limit and safe time between doses so you cannot give yourself too much pain medicine too often.
• You are the only person who will know when you are hurting and when it is necessary and safe to have a dose of pain medicine. Therefore **you are the only person who should press the PCA button.** Your family, visitors, physicians, and hospital personnel are not to press the PCA button.
• Let the nurse know before you take any other medicines, including the ones you usually take at home.

WHAT ARE THE SIDE EFFECTS OF IV PCA?

• Itching is not an allergic reaction but is a fairly common side effect of pain medicine. Ask the nurse for medicine to relieve the itching when necessary.
• Nausea can occur from pain medicine, and it also can be treated with medicine that has been prescribed.
• Some patients have difficulty urinating while taking pain medicine. Reducing the dose of pain medicine helps relieve this side effect, and it usually resolves on its own within 48 hours.
• Pain medicine slows the bowel and can cause constipation. If your condition allows, the nurse will give you medicine to prevent constipation.
• Excessive drowsiness and respiratory depression are the most serious but least common side effects of pain medicine. Less than 1% of our patients experience these effects. These two side effects develop slowly. Nurses will be checking your sedation and breathing frequently. If detected, both are easily treated and corrected by decreasing the dose of pain medicine.

HOW LONG WILL IV PCA BE USED?

• As your condition improves, your pain will decrease. You will find that you need to press the PCA button less often as you improve.
• The dose of pain medicine will be decreased gradually until the pump is no longer necessary and you are able to use a different method for taking pain medicine.

May be duplicated for use in clinical practice. As appears in McCaffery M, Pasero C: *Pain: Clinical manual,* p. 291, 1999, Mosby, Inc.

In addition to talking with patients about opioids and their side effects, providing written information reinforces explanations about the method of opioid delivery and other important points the patient will need to remember. Box 6.38 provides an example of a patient information brochure on IV PCA.

From Pasero C: *Acute pain management service policy and procedure manual,* Rolling Hills Estates, CA, 1994, Academy Medical Systems, Inc.

Faces pain rating scale modified from Wong DL: *Whaley & Wong's essentials of pediatric nursing,* ed 5, pp. 1215-1216, St. Louis, 1997, Mosby.

BOX 6.39 Patient Information Brochure: Patient Controlled Epidural Analgesia (PCEA)

HOW DOES PAIN AFFECT THE BODY?

When you are injured, pain warns you to protect yourself and avoid further injury. However, unrelieved pain can be harmful, especially when you are sick or after surgery. Pain can make it difficult to take a deep breath and interferes with your ability to move and walk. This can result in complications and a long stay in the hospital.

HOW WILL OTHERS KNOW HOW MUCH PAIN YOU HAVE?

- Your nurses will check you often while you are receiving PCEA. They will ask you to rate your pain on a 0 to 10 scale. A rating of 0 means you feel no pain at all, 5 means you feel a moderate amount of pain, and 10 means you feel the worst pain you can imagine.

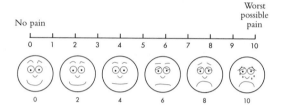

- Your comfort goal is _____ . If you are unable to maintain this level of comfort, especially during activities such as deep breathing and walking, let your nurse know. The dose of pain medicine usually can be increased to keep you as comfortable as possible.

WHAT ARE SOME OF THE GOALS OF PAIN MANAGEMENT WITH PCEA?

- To keep pain from becoming severe and out of control.
- To keep comfortable so that you can sleep, deep breathe, walk, and visit with others.
- To decrease the length of time spent in the hospital.

HOW DOES PCEA WORK?

- Pain medicine will be given by a small pump through an epidural catheter, which is a tiny tubing the anesthesiologist will put in your back before surgery.
- The pump will give you a small amount of pain medicine continuously.
- You also will have a PCEA button that is attached to the pump. You can press the PCEA button to give yourself a dose of pain medicine when you hurt.
- The recovery room nurse will manage your pain for you when you arrive in the recovery room, then give you the PCEA button as soon as you are awake enough to manage the pain yourself.
- It is difficult to treat pain when it is severe, so it is important to "stay on top" of your pain. When you begin to feel some discomfort, press the PCEA button, then wait a few minutes to see if the dose helped to relieve the pain. If the pain has not been relieved, press the PCEA button again.

HOW IS THE EPIDURAL CATHETER PLACED?

- You will be positioned on your side or sitting up with your back arched out to the anesthesiologist.
- Your back will be washed with a cool soap solution.
- The anesthesiologist will inject local anesthetic to numb the area where the catheter will go. This will sting like a bee bite.

- You will feel pressure against your back while the anesthesiologist finds the epidural space.
- A very small catheter will be inserted through the needle into the epidural space, and then the needle will be removed.
- The catheter will be taped to your back and up to your shoulder where it will be connected to the pump.
- While the catheter is in place, you may lie on your back, turn, walk, and perform any activities your physician approves.

IS PCEA SAFE?

- The pump will be programmed to give you an amount of pain medicine that is typically safe for someone your sex, size, age, and diagnosis or type of surgery. If this is too much, the dose of the pain medicine can be reduced.
- The pump will be programmed with a safe hourly limit and safe time between doses so you cannot give yourself too much pain medicine too often.
- You are the only person who will know when you are hurting and when it is necessary and safe to have a dose of pain medicine. Therefore **you are the only person who should press the PCEA button.** Your family, visitors, physicians, and hospital personnel are not to press the PCEA button.
- Let the nurse know before you take any other medicines, including the ones you usually take at home.

WHAT ARE THE SIDE EFFECTS OF PCEA?

- Itching is not an allergic reaction but is a fairly common side effect of pain medicine. Ask the nurse for medicine to relieve the itching when necessary.
- Nausea can occur from pain medicine, and it also can be treated with medicine that has been prescribed.
- Some patients have difficulty urinating while taking pain medicine. Reducing the dose of pain medicine helps relieve this side effect, and it usually resolves on its own within 48 hours.
- Pain medicine slows the bowel and can cause constipation. If your condition allows, the nurse will give you medicine to prevent constipation.
- Excessive drowsiness and respiratory depression are the most serious but least common side effects of pain medicine. Less than 1% of our patients experience these effects. These two side effects develop slowly. Nurses will be checking your sedation and breathing frequently. If detected, both are easily treated and corrected by decreasing the dose of pain medicine.
- Numbness and tingling from the epidural local anesthetic is normal in and around the surgery incision area. Let your nurse know if numbness or tingling occurs in other areas. If you have difficulty feeling or moving your legs, stay in bed and call your nurse. This usually can be corrected by reducing the dose of pain medicine. Be sure to ask someone to help you up the first few times you walk.

HOW LONG WILL PCEA BE USED?

- As your condition improves, your pain will decrease. You will find that you need to press the PCEA button less often as you improve.
- The dose of pain medicine will be decreased gradually until the pump is no longer necessary and you are able to use a different method for taking pain medicine.
- Your nurse will remove the epidural catheter. This is a simple and painless procedure.

May be duplicated for use in clinical practice. As appears in McCaffery M, Pasero C: *Pain: Clinical manual*, p. 292, 1999, Mosby, Inc.

In addition to talking with patients about opioids and their side effects, providing written information reinforces explanations about the method of opioid delivery and other important points the patient will need to remember. Box 6.39 provides an example of a patient information brochure on PCEA.

From Pasero C: *Acute pain management service policy and procedure manual*, Rolling Hills Estates, CA, 1994, Academy Medical Systems, Inc.

Faces pain rating scale modified from Wong DL: *Whaley & Wong's essentials of pediatric nursing*, ed 5, pp. 1215-1216, St. Louis, 1997, Mosby.

References

Abbott Laboratories: Fentanyl Oralet (oral transmucosal fentanyl citrate) package insert, Abbott Park, IL, 1995, Abbott Laboratories.

Abboud TK, Afrasiabi A, Davidson J et al: Prophylactic oral naltrexone with epidural morphine: effect on adverse reactions and ventilatory responses to carbon dioxide, *Anesthesiology* 72:233-237, 1990.

Abboud TK, Lee K, Zhu J et al: Prophylactic oral naltrexone with intrathecal morphine for cesarean section: effects on adverse reactions and analgesia, *Anesth Analg* 71:367-370, 1990.

Abboud TK, Moore M, Zhu J et al: Epidural butorphanol or morphine for the relief of post-cesarean section pain: ventilatory responses to carbon dioxide, *Anesth Analg* 66:887-893, 1987.

Abboud TK, Zhu J, Gangolly J et al: Transnasal butorphanol: a new method for pain relief in postcesarean section pain, *Acta Anaesthesiol Scand* 35:14-18, 1991.

Acalovschi I, Bodolea C, Manoiu C: Spinal anesthesia with meperidine: effects of added α-adrenergic agonists: epinephrine versus clonidine, *Anesth Analg* 84:1333-1339, 1997.

Agency for Health Care Policy and Research (AHCPR): *Acute pain management: operations or medical procedures and trauma. Clinical practice guideline,* AHCPR Publication 92-0032, Rockville, MD, February, 1992, U.S. Public Health Service, AHCPR.

Ahmedzai S, Brooks D: Transdermal fentanyl versus sustained-release oral morphine in cancer pain: preference, efficacy, and quality of life, *J Pain Symptom Manage* 13(5):254-261, 1997.

Alexander R, Fennelly M: Comparison of ondansetron, metoclopramide and placebo as premedicants to reduce nausea and vomiting after major surgery, *Anesthesia* 52:695-703, 1997.

Allen LV: Suppositories as drug delivery systems, *J Pharmaceutic Care Pain Symptom Control* 5(2):17-26, 1997.

American Medical Association (AMA) Council on Ethical and Judicial Affairs: Decisions near the end of life, *JAMA* 267(16):2229-2233, 1992.

American Pain Society (APS): *Principles of analgesic use in the treatment of acute and cancer pain,* ed 3, Glenview, IL, 1992, APS.

American Pain Society (APS): *Perioperative analgesia: approaching the 21st century, Study guide,* Glenview, IL, 1997, APS.

American Society of Clinical Oncology (ASCO): *Proceedings of ASCO Thirty-third Annual Meeting,* 16:41a, 52a, May 17-20, 1997.

Antonopolous J, Bollinger K, Goshman L: Guidelines for use of meperidine, *Drug Policy Perspect* 2(3):25-27, 1996.

Armstrong PJ, Morton CPJ, Nimmo AF: Pethidine has local anesthetic action on peripheral nerves in vivo, *Anaesthesia* 48:382-386, 1993.

Ashburn MA, Fine PC, Stanley TH: Oral transmucosal fentanyl citrate for the treatment of breakthrough cancer pain: a case report, *Anesthesiology* 71(4): 615-617, 1989.

Austin KL, Stapleton JV, Mather LE: Multiple intramuscular injections: a major source of variability in analgesic response to meperidine, *Pain* 8:47-62, 1980.

Babul N, Darke AC, Anslow JA et al: Pharmacokinetics of two novel rectal controlled-release morphine formulations, *J Pain Symptom Manage* 7:400-405, 1992.

Babul N, Darke AC: Disposition of morphine and its glucuronide metabolites after oral and rectal administration: evidence of route specificity, *Clin Pharmacol Ther* 54(3):286-292, 1993.

Barkin RL, Lubenow TR, Bruehl S et al: Management of chronic pain, *Disease-A-Month* 42(7):389-454, 1996.

Barnung SK, Treschow M, Borgbjerg, FM: Respiratory depression following oral tramadol in a patient with impaired renal function, *Pain* 71:111-112, 1997.

Beaver WT, Frise GA: A comparison of the analgesic effect of oxymorphone by rectal suppository and intramuscular injection in patients with postoperative pain, *J of Clin Pharm* 17:276-291, 1977.

Beaver WT, Wallenstein SL, Rogers A et al: Analgesic studies of codeine and oxycodone in patients with cancer. I & II. Comparisons of oral with intramuscular codeine and of oral with intramuscular oxycodone, *J Pharmacol Exp Ther* 207:92-100, 1978.

Bedder MD: Epidural opioid therapy for chronic nonmalignant pain: critique of current experience, *J Pain Symptom Manage* 11:353-356, 1996.

Beers MH, Ouslander JG, Rollingher I et al: Explicit criteria for determining inappropriate medication use in nursing home residents, *Arch Intern Med* 151:1825-1832, 1991.

Benet LZ: Introduction. In Hardman JG, Limbird LE, editors: *Goodman & Gilman's the pharmacological basis of therapeutics,* ed 9, pp 1-2, New York, 1996, McGraw-Hill.

Benet LZ, Kroetz DL, Sheiner LB: Pharmacokinetics. In Hardman JG, Limbird LE, editors: *Goodman & Gilman's the pharmacological basis of therapeutics,* ed 9, pp 3-27, New York, 1996, McGraw-Hill.

Benedetti C: Acute pain: a review of its effects and therapy with systemic opioids. In Benedetti C, Chapman CR, Giron G, editors: Opioid analgesia: recent advances in systemic administration, *Advances in pain research and therapy,* Vol 14, pp 367-424, New York, 1990, Raven Press.

Benedetti C: Opioids, sedatives, hypnotics, ataractics. In Bonica JJ, McDonald JS, editors: *Principles and practice of obstetric analgesia and anesthesia,* ed 2, pp 575-614, Baltimore, 1995, Williams & Wilkins.

Benedetti C, Butler SH: Systemic analgesics. In Bonica JJ, editor: *The management of pain,* ed 2, pp 1640-1675, Philadelphia, 1990, Lea & Febiger.

Berde CB, Beyer JE, Bournaki MC et al: Comparison of morphine and methadone for the prevention of pain in 3 to 7-year-old children, *J Pediatr* 119:136-141, 1991.

Berde CB, Kain ZN: Pain management in infants and children. In Motoyama EK, Davis PJ, editors: *Smith's anesthesia for infants and children,* ed 6, pp 385-402, St. Louis, 1996, Mosby.

Berde CB, Sethna NF, Holtzman RS et al: Pharmacokinetics of methadone in children and adolescents in the perioperative period, *Anesthesiology* 67:A519, 1987 (abstract).

Bernard J-M, Kick O, Bonnet F: Comparison of intravenous and epidural clonidine for postoperative patient-controlled analgesia, *Anesth Analg* 81:706-712, 1995.

Berryman D, Marketing manager: Anesta Corp., Salt Lake City, UT: Personal communication by telephone with Chris Pasero, August 21, 1997.

Biddle C, Gilliland C: Transdermal and transmucosal administration of pain-relieving and anxiolytic drugs: a primer for the critical care practitioner, *Heart Lung* 12:115-124, 1992.

Bodily MN, Chamberlain DP, Ramsey MD et al: Lumbar versus thoracic epidural catheter for post-thoracotomy analgesia, *Anesthesiology* 71(3A):A1146, 1989 (abstract).

Bodner M, Poler SM, White PF: Antiemetic efficacy of ondansetron after ambulatory surgery, *Anesth Analg* 73:250-254, 1991.

Boersma FP, Heykants J, ten Kate A et al: Sufentanil concentration in the human spinal cord after long-term epidural infusion, *Pain Clin* 4:199-203, 1991.

Borgbjerg FM, Nielsen K, Franks J: Experimental pain stimulates respiration and attenuates morphine-induced respiratory depression: a controlled study in human volunteers, *Pain* 64:123-128, 1996.

Bridenbaugh PO, Green NM, Brull SJ: Spinal (subarachnoid) neural blockade. In Cousins MJ, Bridenbaugh PO, editors: *Neural blockade in clinical anesthesia and management of pain,* pp 203-241, Philadelphia, 1998, Lippincott.

Brimacombe J, Archdeacon J, Newell S et al: Two cases of naloxone-induced pulmonary oedema: the possible use of phentolamine in management, *Anesthesia Intens Care* 19(4):578-580, 1991.

Broadman LM, Rice LJ: Neural blockade for pediatric surgery. In Cousins MJ, Bridenbaugh PO, editors: *Neural blockade in clinical anesthesia and management of pain,* ed 3, pp 615-637, Philadelphia, 1998, Lippincott-Raven.

Brody H, Campbell ML, Faber-Langendoen K et al: Withdrawing intensive life-sustaining treatment: recommendations for compassionate clinical management, *N Engl J Med* 336(9):652-657, 1997, (sounding board).

Broekema AA, Gielen MJM, Hennis PJ: Postoperative analgesia with continuous epidural sufentanil and bupivacaine: a prospective study in 614 patients, *Anesth Analg* 82:754-759, 1996.

Broomhead A, Kerr R, Tester W et al: Comparison of once-a-day sustained-release morphine formulation with standard oral morphine treatment for cancer pain, *J Pain Symptom Manage* 14(2):63-73, 1997.

Brown MM, Paige GB, Berger JJ: Nalmefene reverses pruritus caused by neuraxial morphine longer than naloxone, *Reg Anesth* 22(2S):48, 1997.

Brownridge P, Cohen SE, Ward ME: Neural blockade for obstetrics and gynecologic surgery. In Cousins MJ, Bridenbaugh PO, editors: *Neural blockade in clinical anesthesia and management of pain,* ed 3, pp 557-604, Philadelphia, 1998, Lippincott-Raven.

Bruera E, Brennels C, Michaud M et al: Continuous SC infusion of narcotics using a portable disposable device in patients with advanced cancer, *Cancer Treatment Rep* 71(6):635-637, 1987.

Bruera E, MacMillan K, Pither J et al: Effects of morphine on the dyspnea of terminal cancer patients, *J Pain Symptom Manage* 5(6):341-344, 1990.

Bruera E, Schoeller T, Fainsinger RL et al: Custom-made suppositories of methadone for severe cancer pain, *J Pain Symptom Manage* 7:372-374, 1992.

Bruera E, Watanabe S, Fainsinger RL et al: Custom-made capsules and suppositories of methadone for patients on high-dose opioids for cancer pain, *Pain* 62:141-146, 1995.

Bruera E, Pereira J, Watanabe S et al: Opioid rotation in patients with cancer pain, *Cancer* 78(4):857, 1996.

Burns JW, Hodsman NBA, McLintock TTC et al: The influence of patient characteristics on the requirements for postoperative analgesia, *Anaesthesia* 44:2-6, 1989.

Calis KA, Kohler DR, Corso DM: Transdermally administered fentanyl for pain management, *Clin Pharmacol* 99:22-36, 1992.

Caplan RA, Ready LB, Oden RV et al: Transdermal fentanyl for postoperative pain management, *JAMA* 261:1036-1039, 1989.

Carroll KC, Magruder CC: The role of analgesics and sedatives in the management of pain and agitation during weaning from mechanical ventilation, *Crit Care Nurs Q* 15(4):68-77, 1993.

Chadwick HS, Bonica JJ: Complications of regional anesthesia. In Bonica JJ, McDonald JS, editors: *Principles and practice of obstetric analgesia and anesthesia*, ed 2, pp 538-572, Baltimore, 1995, Williams & Wilkins.

Chaney MA: Side effects of intrathecal and epidural opioids, *Can J Anaesth* 42(10):891-903, 1995.

Chaney MA, Furry PA, Fluder EM et al: Intrathecal morphine for coronary artery bypass grafting and early extubation, *Anesth Analg* 84:241-248, 1997.

Cherny NI, Portenoy RK: Practical issues in the management of cancer pain. In Wall PD, Melzack R, editors: *Textbook of pain*, ed 3, pp 1437-1467, Edinburgh, 1994, Churchill Livingstone.

Cherny NI, Thaler HT, Friedlander-Klar H: Opioid responsiveness of cancer pain syndromes caused by neuropathic or nociceptive mechanisms: a combined analysis of controlled, single-dose studies, *Neurology* 44:857-861, 1994.

Chisakuta AM, George KA, Hawthorne CT: Postoperative epidural infusion of a mixture of bupivacaine 0.2% with fentanyl for upper abdominal surgery, *Anaesthesia* 50:72-75, 1995.

Chrubasik J, Wust H, Friedrich G et al: Absorption and bioavailability of nebulised morphine, *Br J Anesth* 61:228-230, 1988.

Coda BA, O'Sullivan B, Donaldson G et al: Comparative efficacy of patient-controlled administration of morphine, hydromorphone, or sufentanil for the treatment of oral mucositis pain following bone marrow transplantation, *Pain* 72:333-346, 1997.

Coda BA, Tanaka A, Jacobson RC et al: Hydromorphone analgesia after intravenous bolus administration, *Pain* 71(1):41-48, 1997.

Coelho JCU, Runkel N, Herfarth C et al: Effect of analgesic drugs on electromyographic activity of the gastrointestinal tract and sphincter of Oddi and on biliary pressure, *Ann Surg* 204(1):53-58, 1986.

Collin E, Poulain P, Gauvain-Piquard A et al: Is disease progression the major factor in morphine "tolerance" in cancer pain treatment? *Pain* 55:319-326, 1993.

Condra LJ: Hydrocodone/acetaminophen: another alternative for postoperative pain management, *Drug Policy Perspect* 3(7):147-150, 1997.

Cook DR, Davis PJ, Lerman J: Pharmacology of pediatric anesthesia. In Motoyama EK, Davis PJ, editors: *Smith's anesthesia for infants and children*, ed 6, pp 159-209, St. Louis, 1996, Mosby.

Cousins MJ: Acute postoperative pain. In Wall PD, Melzack R, editors: *Textbook of pain*, ed 3, pp 357-385, New York, 1994, Churchill Livingstone.

Cousins MJ, Umedaly HS: Postoperative pain management in the neurosurgical patient, *Int Anesthesiol Clin* 34:179-193, 1996.

Cousins MJ, Veering BT: Epidural neural blockade. In Cousins MJ, Bridenbaugh PO, editors: *Neural blockade in clinical anesthesia and management of pain*, pp 243-321, Philadelphia, 1998, Lippincott.

Covino BG, Wildsmith JAW: Clinical pharmacology of local anesthetic agents. In Cousins MJ, Bridenbaugh PO, editors: *Neural blockade in clinical anesthesia and management of pain*, pp 97-128, Philadelphia, 1998, Lippincott.

Cox CR, Serpell MG, Bannister J et al: A comparison of epidural infusions of fentanyl or pethidine with bupivacaine in the management of postoperative pain, *Anaesthesia* 51:695-698, 1996.

Coyle N: Cancer patients and subcutaneous infusions, *Am J Nurs* 96(3):61, 1996.

Coyle N, Adelhardt J, Foley KM et al: Character of terminal illness in the advanced cancer patient: pain and other symptoms during the last four weeks of life, *J Pain Symptom Manage* 5(2):83-93, 1990.

Coyle N, Cherny N, Portenoy, RK: Pharmacologic management of cancer pain. In McGuire D, Yarbro CH, Ferrell BR, editors: *Cancer pain management*, ed 2, pp 89-130, Boston, 1995, Jones & Bartlett Publishers.

Coyle N, Mauskop A, Maggard J et al: Continuous subcutaneous infusions of opiates in cancer patients with pain, *Oncol Nurs Forum* 13(4):53-57, 1986.

Coyle N, Portenoy RK: Pharmacologic management of cancer pain. In *Cancer nursing*, ed 2, pp 1035-1055, Philadelphia, 1996, WB Saunders.

Crews JC, Sweeney NJ, Denson DD: Clinical evidence of decreased cross-tolerance of methadone in patients refractory to high dose μ-opioid receptor agonist analgesics for management of terminal cancer pain, *Cancer* 72: 2266-2272, 1993.

Cronin CM, Kaiko RF, Goldenheim PD: Bioavailability of oral MS Contin tablets, *Clin J Pain* 7:41-66, 1991 (abstract).

Compton P: When does "drug-seeking" behavior signal addiction, *Am J Nurs* 97(5):17-18, May 1997.

Dahl J: Fentanyl postscript, *Cancer Pain Update* (41):6, Fall 1996.

Davis C, Lam W, Butcher M et al: Low systemic bioavailability of nebulised morphine: therapeutic role for the relief of dyspnea, *Br J Cancer* 65 (Suppl 16):12, 1992.

Dayer P, Collart L, Desmeules J: The pharmacology of tramadol, *Drugs* 47 (Suppl 1):3-7, 1994.

Dean GE: Managing nausea, *Nursing* 24(11):25, 1994.

De Kock M, Wiederkher P, Laghmiche JA et al: Epidural clonidine used as the sole analgesic agent, *Anesthesiology* 86:285-292, 1997.

de Leon-Casasola OA, Lema MJ: Spinal opioid analgesia; influence on clinical outcome. In Sinatra RS, Hord AH, Ginsberg B et al., editors: *Acute pain: mechanisms and management*, pp 293-303, St. Louis, 1992, Mosby.

de Leon-Casasola OA, Lema MJ: Epidural bupivacaine/sufentanil therapy for postoperative pain control in patients tolerant and unresponsive to epidural bupivacaine/morphine, *Anesthesiology* 80:303-309, 1993.

de Leon-Casasola OA, Lema MJ: Postoperative epidural opioid analgesia: What are the choices? *Anesth Analg* 83:867-875, 1996.

de Leon-Casasola OA, Parker B, Lema MJ et al: Postoperative epidural bupivacaine-morphine therapy, *Anesthesiology* 81:368-375, 1994.

Dhaliwal HS, Sloan P, Arkistall WW et al: Randomized evaluation of controlled-release codeine and placebo in chronic cancer pain, *J Pain Symptom Manage* 19(8):612-623, 1995.

Diamond S, Diamond ML: Emergency treatment of migraine: insights into current options, *Postgrad Med* 101(1):169-179, January 1997.

Dogra S, Blau WS, Lucas W et al: Epidural analgesia compared with IV PCA in lung transplant patients, *Reg Anesth* 22(2S):107, 1997 (scientific poster).

Donner B, Zenz M, Tryba M et al: Direct conversion from oral morphine to transdermal fentanyl: a multicenter study in patients with cancer pain, *Pain* 64: 527-534, 1996.

Drug facts and comparisons, St. Louis, 1996, Wolters Kluwer.

Duggleby W, Lander J: Cognitive status and postoperative pain: older adults, *J Pain Symptom Manage* 9(1):19-27, 1994.

Dunbar PJ, Chapman CR, Buckley FP et al: Clinical analgesic equivalence for morphine and hydromorphone with prolonged PCA, *Pain* 68:226-270, 1996.

DuPen SL, DuPen AR: Spinal analgesia. In Ashburn MA, Rice LJ, editors: *The management of pain*, pp 171-186, New York, 1998, Churchill Livingstone.

DuPen SL, Williams AR: The dilemma of conversion from systemic to epidural morphine: a proposed conversion tool for treatment of cancer pain, *Pain* 56:113-118, 1994.

Egbert AM, Parks LH, short LM et al: Randomized trial postoperative patient-controlled analgesia vs. Intramuscular narcotics in frail elderly men, *Arch Intern Med* 150:1897-1903, 1990.

Eige S: PCA opioids: common side effects and their treatment. In Sinatra RS, Hord AH, Ginsberg B, et al., editors: *Acute pain: mechanisms and management*, pp 182-193, St. Louis, 1992, Mosby.

Eisenach JC, De Kock M, Klimscha W: α_2-Adrenergic agonists for regional anesthesia, *Anesthesiology* 85:655-674, 1996.

Elias M: Propofol for opioid-induced side effects, *Reg Anesth* 22(5):483-489, 1997 (letter to the editor).

Emanuelsson B-M, Zaric D, Nydahl P-A: Pharmacokinetics of ropivacaine and bupivacaine during 21 hours of continuous epidural infusion in healthy male volunteers, *Ansth Analg* 81:1163-1168, 1995.

Etches RC, Gammer T-L, Cornish R: Patient-controlled epidural analgesia after thoracotomy: a comparison of meperidine with and without bupivacaine, *Anesth Analg* 83:81-86, 1996.

Evans TN, park GR: Remifentanil in the critically ill, *Anaesthesia* 52(8):797-811, 1997.

Ewalenko P, Janny S, Dejonckheere M et al: Antiemetic effect of subhypnotic doses of propofol after thyroidectomy, *Br J Anaesth* 77:463-467, 1996.

Fainsinger R, Schoeller T, Bruera E: Methadone in the management of cancer pain: a review, *Pain* 52:137-147, 1993.

Fancombe M, Chater S: Case studies outlining use of nebulized morphine for patients with end-stage chronic lung and cardiac disease, *J Pain Symptom Manage* 8:221-226, 1993.

Fancombe M, Chater S: Clinical application of nebulized opioids for treatment of dyspnea in patients with malignant disease, *Support Care Cancer* 2:184-187, 1994.

Faries J, Pain management coordinator, Wellmont Health System, Holston Valley Medical Center, Kingsport, TN: Personal telephone communication with Chris Pasero, Aug. 1, 1997.

Ferrante M: Principles of opioid pharmacotherapy: practical implications of basic mechanisms, *J Pain Symptom Manage* 11(5):265-273, 1996.

Ferrell BA: Pain evaluation and management in the nursing home, *Ann Intern Med* 123:681-687, 1995.

Ferrell BR, Grant M, Chan J et al: The impact of cancer pain education on family caregivers of elderly patients, *Oncol Nurs Forum* 22(8):1211-1218, 1995.

Ferrell BR, Griffith H: Cost issues related to pain management: report from the cancer pain panel of the Agency for Health Care Policy and Research, *J Pain Symptom Manage* 9(4):221-234, 1994.

Fine PG, Marcus M, De Boer AJ et al: An open label study of oral transmucosal fentanyl citrate (OFTC) for the treatment of breakthrough cancer pain, *Pain* 45(2):149-153, 1991.

Foley KM: The treatment of cancer pain, *N Engl J Med* 313:84-95, 1985.

Foley KM: Misconceptions and controversies regarding the use of opioids in cancer pain, *Anti-Cancer Drugs* 6(Suppl 3):4-13, 1995.

Foley KM, Inturrisi CE: Opioid therapy: general principles, advances, controversies, alternative routes and methods of administration, *Syllabus of the Postgraduate Course*, Memorial Sloan-Kettering Cancer Center, New York, NY, April 2-3, 1992.

Friedman DP: Perspectives on the medical use of drugs of abuse, *J Pain Symptom Manage* 5(Suppl 1):S2-S5, 1990.

Fromm MF, Eckhardt K, Li S et al: Loss of analgesic effect of morphine due to coadministration of rifampin, *Pain* 72(1, 2):261-267, 1997.

Galer BS, Coyle N, Pasternak GW et al: Individual variability in response to different opioids: report of five cases, *Pain* 49(1):87-91, 1992.

Gambling DR, Howell P, Huber C et al: Epidural butorphanol does not reduce side effects from epidural morphine after cesarean birth, *Anesth Analg* 78:1099-1104, 1994.

Gan TJ, Ginsberg B, Perno R et al: Is postoperative patient-controlled epidural analgesia with hydromorphone better than epidural morphine? *Anesth Analg* 84:S293, 1997.

Gardner-Nix J: Oral methadone for managing chronic nonmalignant pain, *J Pain Symptom Manage* 11(5):321-328, 1996.

Gautier PE, Debry F, Fanard L et al: Ambulatory combined spinal-epidural analgesia for labor: influence of epinephrine on bupivacaine-sufentanil combination, *Reg Anesth* 22(2):143-149, 1997.

Gear RW, Miaskowski C, Heller PH et al: Benzodiazepine mediated antagonism of opioid analgesia, *Pain* 71(1):25-29, 1997.

Gianino JM, York MM, Paice JA: *Intrathecal drug therapy for spasticity and pain*, New York, 1996, Springer.

Ginsberg B, Cohen NA, Ossey KD et al: The use of PCA to assess the influence of demographic factors on analgesic requirements, *Anesthesiology* 71:A688, 1989 (abstract).

Ginsberg B, Grichnik KP, Muir M et al: Patient controlled analgesia used to assess the efficacy and potency of a new opioid, *Pain Res Manage* 1(4):227-231, 1996.

Glare PA, Walsh TD: Dose-ranging study of oxycodone for chronic pain in advanced cancer, *J Clin Oncol* 11(5):973-978, 1993.

Glass PSA, Estok P, Ginsberg B et al: Use of patient-controlled analgesia to compare the efficacy of epidural to intravenous fentanyl administration, *Anesta Analg* 74:345-351, 1992.

Gordon D: Hydroxyzine doesn't "help" opioids, *Am J Nurs* 95(8):20, 1995.

Gourlay GK, Cherry DA, Li S et al: Pharmacokinetics and pharmacodynamics of twenty-four-hourly Kapanol compared to twelve-hourly MS Contin in the treatment of severe cancer pain, *Pain* 69(3):295-302, 1997.

Gourlay GK, Cherry DA, Plummer JL et al: The influence of drug polarity on the absorption of opioid drugs into CSF and subsequent cephalad migration following lumbar epidural administration: application to morphine and pethidine, *Pain* 31:297-305, 1987.

Gourlay GK, Kowalski SR, Plummer JL et al: The transdermal administration of fentanyl in the treatment of postoperative pain: pharmacokinetics and pharmacodynamic effects. *Pain* 37:193-202, 1989.

Gourlay GK, Kowalski SR, Plummer JL et al: The efficiency of transdermal fentanyl in the treatment of postoperative pain: a double-blind comparison of fentanyl and placebo systems, *Pain* 40:21-28, 1990.

Gourlay GK, Murphy TM, Plummer JL et al: Pharmacokinetics of fentanyl in lumbar and cervical CSF following lumbar epidural and intravenous administration, *Pain* 38:253-295, 1989.

Gourlay GK, Willis RJ, Lamberty J: A double-blind comparison of the efficacy of methadone and morphine in postoperative pain control, *Anesthesiology* 64:322-327, 1986.

Gourlay GK, Wilson PR, Glynn CJ, Pharmacodynamics and pharmacokinetics of methadone during the perioperative period, *Anesthesiology* 57:458-467, 1982.

Graf G, Sinatra RS, Chung J et al: Epidural sufentanil for postoperative analgesia: dose-response in patients recovering from major surgery, *Anesth Analg* 73:405-409, 1991.

Grass JA, Sakima NT, Schmidt R et al: A randomized, double-blind, dose-response comparison of epidural fentanyl versus sufentanil after cesarean section, *Anesth Analg* 85:365-371, 1997.

Grauer PA, Bass J, Wenzel E et al: A feasibility study of the rectal and vaginal administration of sustained-release morphine sulfate tablets (Oramorph SR™) for the treatment of cancer-related pain, *Abstracts, 49th American Society of Hospital Pharmacists (ASHP) annual meeting*, p 68, 1992 ASHP.

Grochow L, Scheidler V, Grossman S et al: Dose intravenous methadone provide longer lasting analgesia than intravenous morphine? *Pain* 38:151, 1989.

Grond S, Meuser T, Zech D et al: Analgesic efficacy and safety of tramadol enantiomers in comparison with racemate: a randomized, double-blind study with gynaecological patients using intravenous patient-controlled analgesia, *Pain* 62:313-320, 1995.

Grond S, Zech D, Lehmann KA et al: Transdermal fentanyl in long-term treatment of cancer pain: a prospective study of 50 patients with advanced cancer of the gastrointestinal tract or the head and neck region, *Pain* 69(1, 2):191-198, 1997.

Gwirtz KH: Single-dose intrathecal opioids in the management of acute postoperative pain. In Sinatra RS, Hord AH, Ginsberg B, et al., editors: *Acute pain: mechanisms and management*, pp 253-268, St. Louis, 1992, Mosby.

Hagen NA, Babul N: Comparative clinical efficacy and safety of a novel controlled-release oxycodone formulation and controlled-release hydromorphone in the treatment of cancer pain, *Cancer* 79(7):1428-1437, 1997.

Hammack JE, Mailliard JA, Loprinzi CL: Transdermal fentanyl in the management of cancer pain in ambulatory patients: an open label pilot study, *J Pain Symptom Manage* 12(4):234-240, 1996.

Hansdottir V, Bake B, Nordberg G: The analgesic efficacy and adverse effects of continuous sufentanil and bupivacaine infusion after thoracotomy, *Anesth Analg* 83:394-400, 1996.

Hansdottir V, Woestenborghs R, Nordberg G: The cerebrospinal fluid and plasma pharmacokinetics of sufentanil after thoracic or lumbar epidural administration, *Anesth Analg* 80:724-729, 1995.

Hansen LA, Noyes MA, Lehman ME: Evaluation of patient-controlled analgesia (PCA) versus PCA plus continuous infusion in postoperative cancer patients, *J Pain Symptom Manage* 6(1):4-14, 1991.

Harukuni I, Yamaguchi H, Sato S et al: The comparison of epidural fentanyl, epidural lidocaine, and intravenous fentanyl in patients undergoing gastrectomy, *Anesth Analg* 81:1169-1174, 1995.

Helmers JH, Noorduin H, Van Peer A et al: Comparison of intravenous and intranasal sufentanil absorption and sedation, *Can J Anaesth* 36:494, 1989.

Henderson JM, Brodsky DA, Fisher DM et al: Pre-induction of anesthesia in pediatric patients with nasally administered sufentanil, *Anesthesiology* 68:671, 1988.

Herrick IA, Ganapathy S, Komar W et al: Postoperative cognitive impairment in the elderly, *Anaesthesia* 51:356-360, 1996.

Hill HF, Chapman CR, Saeger LS et al: Steady-state infusions of opioids in human. II. Concentration-effect relationships and therapeutic margins, *Pain* 43(1):69-79, 1990.

Hinnant D: Minimizing meperidine use, *Am J Nurs* 96(8):18, 1996.

Hitchcock LS, Ferrell BR, McCaffery M: The experience of chronic nonmalignant pain, *J Pain Symptom Manage* 9:312-318, 1994.

Hoke JF, Shlugman D, Dershwitz M et al.: Pharmacokinetics and pharmacodynamics of remifentanil in persons with renal failure compared with healthy volunteers, *Anesthesiology* 87:533-541, 1997.

Houck CS: The management of acute pain in the child. In Ashburn MA, Rice LF, editors: *The management of pain*, ed 3, pp 651-666, New York, 1998, Churchill Livingstone.

Houde RW, Wallenstein SL, Beaver WT: Evaluation of analgesics in patients with cancer pain. In Lasagna I, editor: *International encyclopedia of pharmacology and therapeutics*, vol 1, pp 59-67, New York, 1986, Pergamon Press.

Houmes RJ, Voets MA, Verkaaik A et al: Efficacy and safety of tramadol versus morphine for moderate and severe postoperative pain with special regard to respiratory depression, *Anesth Analg* 74:510-514, 1992.

Howe JL: Nebulized morphine for hospice patients, *Am J Hospice Palliative Care* 12(5):6, 1995.

Hubbard L: Community-based pain service. In Sinatra RS, Hord AH, Ginsberg B, et al., editors: *Acute pain: mechanisms and management*, pp 539-559, St. Louis, 1992a, Mosby.

Hubbard L: More on epidural fentanyl analgesia (letter to the editor), *Anesth Analg* 75:865-866, 1992b.

Hunt CO, Naulty JS, Malinow AM et al: Epidural butorphanol-bupivacaine for analgesia during labor and delivery, *Anesth Analg* 68:323-327, 1989.

Hurley RJ: Continuous spinal analgesia. In: Sinatra RS, Hord AH, Ginsberg B, et al., editors: *Acute pain: mechanisms and management*, pp 321-325, St. Louis 1992, Mosby.

Inturrisi CE, Colburn WA: Pharmacokinetics of methadone. In Foley KM, Inturrisi CE, editors: *Advances in pain research and therapy*, vol 8, pp 191-198, New York, 1986, Raven Press.

Inturrisi CE, Portenoy RK, Max MB et al: Pharmacokinetic-pharmacodynamic relationships of methadone infusions in patients with cancer pain, *Clin Pharmacol Ther* 47:565, 1990.

Ivarsson M, Neil A: Differences in efficacies between morphine and methadone demonstrated in the guinea pig ileum: a possible explanation for previous observations on incomplete opioid cross-tolerance, *Pharm Toxicol* 65:368, 1989.

Jacobson L, Chabal C, Brody MC et al: Intrathecal methadone: a dose-response study and comparison with morphine 0.5 mg, *Pain* 43:141-148, 1990.

Jacox A, Carr DB, Payne R et al: *Management of cancer pain: clinical practice guideline* No. 9., AHCPR Publication No. 94-0592, Rockville, MD, U.S. Public Health Service, AHCPR, March 1994.

Jaffe JH, Martin WR: Opioid analgesics and antagonists. In Goodman AG, Rall TW, Nies AS, et al., editors: *Goodman and Gilman's the pharmacological basis of therapeutics*, pp 485-521, New York, 1990, Pergamon Press.

James CF, Nelson EO, Langevin PB et al: Adding low doses of epidural nalbuphine to morphine for postcesarean analgesia, *Anesth Analg* 84:S391, 1997.

Janssen Pharmaceutica, Duragesic® (fentanyl transdermal system) package insert, Titusville, NJ, 1996, Janssen Pharmaceutica.

Kaiko RF, Fitzmartin RD, Thomas GB et al: The bioavailability of morphine in controlled-release 30 mg tablets per rectum compared with immediate release 30 mg rectal suppositories and controlled-release 30 mg oral tablets, *Pharmacotherapy* 12:107-113, 1992.

Kaiko RF, Foley KM, Grabinski PY et al: Central nervous system excitatory effects of meperidine in cancer patients, *Ann Neurol* 13:180-185, 1983.

Kaiko RF, Lacourture P, Hofp K et al: Analgesic onset and potency of oral controlled-release (CR) oxycodone CR and morphine, *Clin Pharmacol Ther* 59(2):130-133, 1996.

Kaplan BZ, Krishnamurthy U, Nori D: Opiate desensitization in a terminally ill cancer patient with pain: physician assisted succor, *Am J Hospice Palliative Care*, pp 34-39, January/February 1994.

Kaplan R, Parris W, Citron M et al: Decrease in opioid-related adverse events during chronic therapy with controlled-release oxycodone in cancer pain patients (abstract), *American Pain Society (APS) Program Book*, Glenview, IL, 1995, APS.

Katz WA: The role of tramadol in the management of musculoskeletal pain, *Today's Therapeutic Trends* 13(3):177-186, 1995.

Kehlet H: Regional anesthesia and outcomes: the second round will require a change in tactics, *live presentation at American Society of Regional Anesthesiologists (ASRA) 22nd Annual Meeting*, Atlanta, GA, April 12, 1997a.

Kehlet H: Multimodal approach to control postoperative pathophysiology and rehabilitation, *Br J Anaesth* 78(5):606-617, May 1997b.

Kendrick WD, Woods AM, Daly MY et al: Naloxone versus nalbuphine infusion for prophylaxis of epidural morphine-induced pruritis, *Anesth Analg* 82:641-647, 1996.

Kerr IG, Sone M, DeAngelis C et al: Continuous narcotic infusion with patient-controlled analgesia for chronic cancer pain in outpatients, *Ann Intern Med* 108(4):554-557, 1988.

Koprulu AS, Dogruer K, Karpat H: Preoperative tramadol for pain relief after abdominal hysterectomy: Does tramadol have a pre-emptive analgesic effect? *Br J Anaesth* 78(1):A409, 1997 (abstract).

Korte W: Titration with TTS fentanyl systems for previously uncontrolled cancer pain *Anesth Analg* 79(3):612-613, 1994 (letter to editor).

Korte W, de Stoutz N, Morant R: Day-to-day titration to initiate transdermal fentanyl in patients with cancer pain: short- and long-term experiences in a prospective study of 39 patients, *J Pain Symptom Manage* 11(3):139-146, 1996.

Koivuranta M, Laara E, Snare L et al: A survey of postoperative nausea and vomiting, *Anaesthesia* 52:443-449, 1997.

Kroemer HK, Eichelbaum HK: "It's the genes, stupid: molecular bases and clinical consequences of genetic cytochrome P450 2D6 polymorphism, *Life Sciences* 46(26):2285-2298, 1995.

Kshatri AM, Foster PA: Adrenocorticotropic hormone infusion as a novel treatment for postdural puncture headache, *Reg Anesth* 22(5):432-434, 1997.

Kuhnert BR, Philipson EH, Kuhnert EH et al: Disposition of meperidine and normeperidine following multiple doses in labor, I, *Am J Obstet Gynecol* 151:406-409, 1985.

Kuhnert BR, Kuhnert PA, Philipson EH et al: Disposition of meperidine and normeperidine following multiple doses in labor, II, *Am J Obstet Gynecol* 151:410-415, 1985.

Kunz K: Opioid cost factors, *Cancer Pain Update*, p 3, Fall 1994.

Lamacraft G, Cooper Mg, Cavalletto BP: Subcutaneous cannulae for morphine boluses in children: assessment of a technique, *J Pain Symptom Manage* 13:43-49, 1997.

Lawhorn CD, McNitt JD, Fibuch EE et al: Epidural morphine with butorphanol for postoperative analgesia after cesarean section, *Anesth Analg* 72:53-57, 1991.

Lawlor P, Turner K, Hanson J et al: Dose ratio between morphine and hydromorphone in patients with cancer pain: a retrospective study, *Pain* 72(1,2):79-85, 1997.

Lee CR, McTavish D, Sorkin EM: Tramadol, *Drugs* 46:313-340, 1993.

Lehmann LJ, DeSio JM, Radvany T et al: Transdermal fentanyl in postoperative pain, *Reg Anesth* 22(1):24-28, 1997.

Lema MJ, Sinha I: Thoracic epidural anesthesia and analgesia, *Pain Digest* 4:3-11, 1994.

Leow KP, Cramond T, Smith MT: Pharmacokinetics and pharmacodynamics of oxycodone when given intravenously and rectally to adult patients with cancer pain, *Anesth Analg* 80:296-302, 1995.

Levy MH: Pain management in advanced cancer, *Sem Oncol* 12:404, 1985.

Levy MH: Medical management of cancer pain. In Warfield C, editor: *Principles and practice of pain management*, pp 235-250, New York, 1993, McGraw-Hill.

Levy MH: Pharmacologic management of cancer pain, *Semin Oncol* 21(6):718-739, 1994.

Levy MH: Pharmacologic treatment of cancer pain, *N Engl J Med* 335(15):1124-1132, 1996.

Lindley CM, Dalton JA, Fields SM: Narcotic analgesics, *Cancer Nurs* 13(1):28-38, 1990.

Lipman AG, Ashburn MA: Titration with TTS fentanyl systems for previously uncontrolled cancer pain, *Anesth Analg* 79(3):612-613, 1994 (response to letter to editor).

Lipman AG, Gauthier ME: Pharmacology of opioid drugs: basic principles. In Portenoy RK, Bruera E, editors: *topics in palliative care*, vol 1, pp 137-161, New York, 1997, Oxford University Press.

Liu SS: Local anesthetics and analgesia. In Ashburn MA, Rice LJ, editors: *The management of pain*, pp 141-169, New York, 1998, Churchill Livingstone.

Liu SS, Carpenter RL, Neal J: Epidural anesthesia and analgesia, *Anesthesiology* 82:1474-1506, 1995.

Lu JK, Schafer PG, Gardner TL et al: The dose-response pharmacology of intrathecal sufentanil in female volunteers, *Anesth Analg* 85:372-379, 1997.

Lubenow TR: Epidural analgesia: considerations and delivery methods. In Sinatra RS, Hord AH, Ginsberg B, et al, editors: *Acute pain: mechanisms and management*, pp 233-242, St. Louis, 1992, Mosby.

Lynn J, Teno JM, Phillips RS: Perceptions by family members of the dying experience of older and seriously ill patients, *Ann Intern Med* 126(2):97-106, 1997.

Maloney CM, Kesner RK, Klein G: The rectal administration of MS Contin: clinical implications of use in end stage cancer, *Am J Hospice Care* 6:34-35, 1989.

Management of cancer pain: proceedings of a roundtable, Mont Sainte-Anne, Quebec, Canada, February 1993, Toronto, Canada, 1993, Remtulla and Associates.

Manfredi PL, Borsook D, Chandler S et al: Intravenous methadone for cancer pain unrelieved by morphine and hydromorphone: clinical observations, *Pain* 70:99-101, 1997.

Marcantonio ER, Juarez G, Goldman L et al: The relationship of postoperative delirium with psychoactive medications, *JAMA* 272(19):1518-1522, 1994.

Markley HG: Chronic headache: appropriate use of opiate analgesics, *Neurology* 44(Suppl 3):S18-S24, May 1994.

Marks RM, Sacher EJ: Undertreatment of medical inpatients with narcotic analgesics, *Ann Intern Med* 78(2):173-181, 1973.

Marshall BE, Longnecker DE: General anesthetics. In Hardman RG, Limbird LE, editors: *Goodman and Gilman's the pharmacological basis of therapeutics*, ed 9, pp 307-330, New York, 1996, McGraw-Hill.

Mather LE, Denson DD: Pharmacokinetics of systemic opioids for the management of pain. In Sinatra RS, Hord AH, Ginsberg B, et al., editors: *Acute pain: mechanisms and management*, pp 78-92, St. Louis, 1992, Mosby.

The Mayday Fund 1993 pain survey, New York, 1993, The Mayday Fund.

McCaffery M: How to calculate a rescue dose, *Am J Nurs* 96(4):65-66, 1996.

McCaffery M, Martin L, Ferrell BR: Analgesic administration via rectum or stoma, *J Enterostom Ther Nurs* 19(4):114-121, 1992.

McCaffery M. Lochman C: Extended release morphine products, *Am J Nurs* 96(4):65, 1996.

McGee JL, Alexander MR: Phenothiazine analgesia: fact or fantasy? *Am J Hosp Pharm* 36:633-640, May 1979.

McQuay HJ: Opioids in chronic pain, *Br J Anaesth* 63:213, 1989.

McQuay HJ: Opioid clinical pharmacology and routes of administration, *Br Med Bull* 47(3):703-717, 1991.

Means L, Bennie R, Dierdorf S et al: Transnasal butorphanol is effective for postoperative pain relief in children undergoing myringotomy, *Anesth Analg* 84:S443, 1997.

Melzack R, Abbott FV, Zackon W et al: Pain on a surgical ward: a survey of the duration and intensity of pain and the effectiveness of medication, *Pain* 29:67-72, 1987.

Mercante S: Methadone in cancer pain, *Eur J Pain* 1:77-85, 1997.

Miguel R, Kreitzer J, Reinhart D et al: Utility of a new transdermal fentanyl delivery system for postoperative pain control: a multicenter trial, *Anesthesiology* 77:A886, 1992 (abstract).

Monk TG, Parker RK, White PF: Use of PCA in geriatric patients: effect of aging on the postoperative analgesic requirement, *Anesth Analg* 70:S272, 1990.

Moulin DE, Johnson NG, Murray-Parsons N et al: Subcutaneous narcotic infusions for cancer pain: treatment outcome and guidelines for use, *Can Med Assoc J* 146(6):891-897, 1992.

Mulroy MF, Norris MC, Lieu SS: Safety steps for epidural injection of local anesthetics: review of the literature and recommendations, *Anesth Analg* 85:1346-1356, 1997.

Murray MJ, Plevak DJ: Analgesia in the critically ill patient, *New Horizons* 2(1):56-63, 1994.

Nagashima H, Karamanian A, Malovany R et al: Respiratory and circulatory effects of intravenous butorphanol and morphine, *Clin Pharmacol Ther* 19:738-745, 1976.

Ngan Kee WD, Lam KK, Chen PP: Epidural meperidine after cesarean section: the effect of diluent volume, *Anesth Analg* 85:380-384, 1997.

Nicholson BD, Rowlingson J: More on epidural fentanyl analgesia, *Anesth Analg* 75:866, 1992 (letter to the editor).

Nies AS, Spielberg SP: Principles of therapeutics. In Hardman JG, Limbird LE, editors: *Goodman & Gilman's the pharmacological basis of therapeutics*, ed 9, pp 43-62, New York, 1996, McGraw-Hill.

Oden RV: Acute postoperative pain: incidence, severity, and the etiology of inadequate treatment, *Anesthesiol Clin North Am* 7(1):1-15, 1989.

Ohmeda Pharmaceutical Products Division, Inc: Revex (nalmefene HCL injection) package insert, Liberty Corner, NJ, 1995.

Paech MJ, Moore JS, Evans SF: Meperidine for patient-controlled analgesia after cesarean section, *Anesthesiology* 80:1268-1276, 1994.

Paice JA, Williams AR: Intraspinal drugs for pain. In McGuire D, Yarbro CH, Ferrell BR, editors: *Cancer pain management*, ed 2, pp 131-158, Boston, 1995, Jones & Bartlett Publishers.

Parker RK, Holtmann B, White PF: Patient-controlled analgesia: Does a concurrent opioid infusion improve pain management after surgery? *JAMA* 266(14):1947-1952, 1991.

Parker RK, Holtmann B, White PF: Patient-controlled epidural analgesia: interactions between nalbuphine and hydromorphone, *Anesth Analg* 84:757-763, 1997.

Parker RK, White PF: Epidural patient-controlled analgesia: an alternative to intravenous patient-controlled analgesia for pain relief after cesarean section, *Anesth Analg* 75:245-251, 1992.

Parker RK, Sawaki Y, White PF: Epidural patient-controlled analgesia: influence of bupivacaine and hydromorphone basal infusion on pain control after cesarean section, *Anesth Analg* 75:740-746, 1992.

Pasero C: *Acute pain management service policy and procedure manual*, Rolling Hills Estates, CA, 1994, Academy Medical Systems.

Pasero C: PCA: For patients only, *Am J Nurs* 96(9):22-23, 1996.

Pasero C, McCaffery M: Unconventional PCA: making it work for your patient, *Am J Nurs* 93(9):38-41, 1993.

Pasero C, McCaffery M: Preventing and managing opioid induced respiratory depression, *Am J Nurs* 94(4):25-31, 1994.

Pasero C, McCaffery M: Postoperative pain management in the elderly. In Ferrell BR, Ferrell BA, editors: *Pain in the elderly*, pp 45-68, Seattle, 1996a, International Association for the Study of Pain (IASP).

Pasero C, McCaffery M: Alternative use of PCA, *Am J Nurs* 96(10):66-68, 1996b.

Patt RB: Using controlled-release oxycodone for the management of chronic cancer and noncancer pain, *American Pain Society (APS) Bulletin* 6(4):1-6, 1996.

Payne R, Chandler S, Einhaus M: Guidelines for the clinical use of transdermal fentanyl, *Anti-Cancer Drugs* 6(Suppl 3):50-53, 1005, 1995.

Plezia PM, Linford J, Kramer TH et al: Transdermally administered fentanyl for postoperative pain: randomized double-blind placebo controlled trial, *Anesthesiology* 69:A364, 1988 (abstract).

Polati E, Verlato G, Finco G et al: Ondansetron versus metoclopramide in the treatment of postoperative nausea and vomiting, *Anesth Analg* 85:395-399, 1997.

Portenoy RK: Clinical application of opioid analgesics. In Sinatra RS, Hord AH, Ginsberg B, et al., editors: *Acute pain: mechanisms and management*, pp 93-101, St. Louis, 1992, Mosby.

Portenoy RK: Basic mechanisms. In Portenoy RK, Kanner RM, editors: *Pain management: theory and practice,* pp 19-39, Philadelphia, 1996a, FA Davis.

Portenoy RK: Opioid analgesics. In Portenoy RK, Kanner RM, editors: *Pain management: theory and practice,* pp 249-276, Philadelphia, 1996b, FA Davis.

Portenoy RK, editor: *Real patients, real problems: optimal assessment and management of cancer pain. A monograph for continuing medical education,* Glenview, Ill, 1997, American Pain Society (APS).

Portenoy RK, Hagen NA: Breakthrough pain: definition, prevalence and characteristics, *Pain* 41:273-281, 1990.

Portenoy RK, Kanner RM: Definition and assessment of pain. In Portenoy RK, Kanner RM, editors: *Pain management: theory and practice,* pp 3-18, Philadelphia, 1996, FA Davis.

Portenoy RK, Thaler HT, Inturrisi CE: The metabolite morphine-6-glucuronide contributes to the analgesia produced by morphine infusion in patients with pain and normal renal function. *Clin Pharmacol Ther* 51(4):422-431, 1992.

Porter J, Jick J: Addiction rare in patients treated with narcotics, *N Engl J Med* 302:123, 1980.

Puntillo KA: Pain experiences of intensive care unit patients, *Heart Lung* 19:526-533, 1990.

Purdue Pharma LP: Product insert for oxycontin CII, Purdue Pharma LP, Norwalk, CT, 1996.

Radnay PA, Brodman E, Mankikar D et al: The effect of equianalgesic doses of fentanyl, morphine, meperidine, and pentazocine on common bile duct pressure, *Anaesthetist* 29:26-29, 1980.

Rapp SE, Egan KJ, Ross BK et al: A multidimensional comparison of morphine and hydromorphone patient-controlled analgesia, *Anesth Analg* 82:1043-1048, 1996.

Rauck RL, Raj PP, Knarr DC et al: Comparison of the efficacy of epidural morphine given by intermittent injection or continuous infusion for the management of postoperative pain, *Reg Anesth* 19:316-324, 1994.

Rauck RL, Ruoff GE, McMillen JI: Comparison of tramadol and acetaminophen with codeine for long-term pain management in elderly patients, *Curr Therap Res* 55(12):1417-1431, 1994.

Rayburn WF, Smith CV, Woods MP: Combined continuous and demand narcotic dosing for patient-controlled analgesia after cesarean section, *Anesthesiol Rev* 17(5):58-62, 1989.

Ready LB, Loper KA, Nessly M et al: Postoperative epidural morphine is safe on surgical wards, *Anesthesiology* 75:452-456, 1991.

Reisine T, Pasternak G: Opioid analgesics and antagonists. In Hardman JG, Limbird LM, editors: *Goodman & Gilman's the pharmacological basis of therapeutics,* ed 9, pp 521-555, New York, 1996, McGraw-Hill.

Reynvoet MEJ, Cosaert PAJM, Desmet MFR et al: Epidural dextran 40 patch for postdural puncture headache, *Anaesthesia* 52:886-888, 1997.

Rice L: Regional anesthesia and analgesia. In Motoyama EK, Davis PJ, editors: *Smith's anesthesia for infants and children,* ed 6, pp 403-442, St. Louis, 1996, Mosby.

Robinson JM, Wilkie DJ, Campbell B: Sublingual and oral morphine administration. In Wilkie DJ, editor: Relieving cancer pain, *Nurs Clin North Am* 30(4):725-743, Philadelphia, Saunders, December 1995.

Rockemann MG, Seeling W, Duschek S et al: Epidural bolus clonidine/morphine versus epidural patient-controlled bupivacaine/sufentanil: quality of postoperative analgesia and cost-identification analysis, *Anesth Analg* 85:864-849, 1997.

Rosenberg J, Kehlet H: Postoperative mental confusion: association with postoperative hypoxemia, *Surgery* 114(1):76-81, 1993.

Rosenberg J, Rosenberg-Adamsen S, Kehlet H: Post-operative sleep disturbance: causes, factors, and effects on outcome, *Eur J Anaesthesiol* 12(Suppl 10):28-30, 1995.

Ross EM: Pharmacodynamics. In Hardman RG, Limbird LE, editors: *Goodman & Gilman's the pharmacological basis of therapeutics,* ed 9, pp 29-41, New York, 1996, McGraw-Hill.

Rust D: Controlled-release tablets now available in 80 mg strength to relieve persistent pain, *Oncol Nurs Forum* 24(5):919, 1997.

Ryan B, Luer JM: Respiratory pharmacology and the weaning patient: implications for critical care nursing, *AACN Clin Issues Crit Care Nurs* 2(5):361-371, 1991.

Sabapathy M: Remifentanil: an ultra-short acting analgesia for anesthesia, *Drug Policy Perspect* 3(3):33-38, 1997.

Sakuramoto C, Kanai I, Matoba M et al: Treatment of postoperative pain with thoracic epidural morphine in oral malignant tumor patients, *Clin J Pain* 12:142-144, 1996.

Salomaki T, Laitinen J, Nuutinen L: A randomized, double-blind comparison of epidural versus intravenous fentanyl infusion for analgesia after thoracotomy, *Anesthesiology* 75:790-795, 1991.

Sandler AN, Stringer D, Panos L et al: A randomized, double-blind comparison of lumbar epidural and intravenous fentanyl infusions for postthoracotomy pain relief, *Anesthesiology* 77:626-634, 1992.

Sawchuk CWT, Ong B, Unruh HW et al: Thoracic versus lumbar epidural fentanyl for postthoracotomy pain, *Ann Thorac Surg* 55:1472-1476, 1993.

Scherer C, Schmutzler M, Geibler R et al: Complications related to thoracic epidural analgesia: a prospective study in 1071 surgical patients, *Acta Anaesthesiol Scand* 37:370-374, 1993.

Scott DA, Beilby DSN, McClymont C: Postoperative analgesia using epidural infusions of fentanyl with bupivacaine, *Anesthesiology* 83:727-737, 1995.

Scott DA, Emanuelsson B-M, Mooney PH et al: Pharmacokinetics and efficacy of long-term epidural ropivacaine infusion for postoperative analgesia, *Anesth Analg* 85:1322-1330, 1997.

Simpson T, Lee ER, Cameron C: Patients' perceptions of environmental factors that disturb sleep after cardiac surgery, *Am J Crit Care* 5(3):173-181, 1996.

Sinatra RS: Spinal opioid analgesia: an overview. In: Sinatra RS, Hord AH, Ginsberg B, et al., editors: *Acute pain: mechanisms and management,* pp 225-232, St. Louis, 1992a, Mosby.

Sinatra RS: Pain management in patients suffering from major organ failure. In Sinatra RS, Hord AH, Ginsberg B, et al., editors: *Acute pain: mechanisms and management,* pp 399-411, St. Louis, 1992b, Mosby.

Sinatra RS: Acute pain management and acute pain services. In Cousins MJ, Bridenbaugh PO, editors: *Neural blockade in clinical anesthesia and management of pain,* pp 793-835, Philadelphia, 1998, Lippincott.

Sinatra RS, Sevarino FB, Chung JH et al: Comparison of epidurally administered sufentanil, morphine, and sufentanil-morphine combination for postoperative analgesia, *Anesth Analg* 72:522-527, 1991.

Slinger P, Shennib H, Wilson S: Postthoracotomy pulmonary function: a comparison of epidural versus intravenous meperidine infusions, *J Cardiothorac Vasc Anesth* 9(2):128-134, 1995.

Smith MA, Morgan M: Remifentanil, *Anaesthesia* 52:291-293, 1997 (editorial).

Smythe MA, Zak MB, O'Donnell MP: Patient-controlled analgesia versus patient-controlled analgesia plus continuous infusion after hip replacement surgery, *Ann Pharmacother* 30:224-227, March 1996.

Spencer RT: Pharmacodynamics and pharmacokinetics. In *Clinical pharmacology and nursing management,* ed 4, pp 62-81, Philadelphia, 1993, JB Lippincott.

Stanley TH, Ashburn MA: Novel delivery systems: oral transmucosal and intranasal transmucosal, *J Pain Symptom Manage* 7(3):163-171, 1992.

Stein C, Yassouridis A: Peripheral morphine analgesia, *Pain* 71:119-121, 1997 (editorial).

Stevenson KK, Gordon D: *Policy and procedure: continuous subcutaneous opioid infusion,* Madison, Wis, 1996, University of Wisconsin Hospital and Clinics.

St. Marie B, Williams A: *Management of cancer pain with epidural morphine* (independent study module), St. Paul, Minn, 1994, Sims Deltec Inc.

St. Onge S, Fugere F, Girard M: Bupivacaine decreases epidural meperidine requirements after abdominal surgery, *Can J Anaesth* 44(4):360-366, 1997.

Storey P: *Primer of palliative care,* Gainesville, Fla, 1994, Academy of Hospice Physicians.

Streisand JB: OTFC: a new opioid delivery system, *APS Bull* 4(2):1-3, 21, 1994.

Streisand JB, Varvel JR, Stanski DR: Absorption and bioavailability of oral transmucosal fentanyl citrate, *Anesthesiology* 75(2):223-229, 1991.

Stuart AL, McDavid AJ: Nalmefene, an intravenous alternative to naltrexone for extradural morphine prophylaxis, *Reg Anesth* 22(3):291, 1997 (letter to the editor).

Stubhaug A, Grimstad J, Breivik H: Lack of analgesic effect of 50 and 100 mg oral tramadol after orthopaedic surgery: a randomized, double-blind, placebo and standard active drug comparison, *Pain* 62:111-118, 1995.

Sullivan F, Muir M, Ginsberg B: A survey on the clinical use of epidural catheters for acute pain management, *J Pain Symptom Manage* 9:303-307, 1994.

Sunshine A, Olson NZ, Colon A et al: Analgesic efficacy of controlled-release oxycodone in postoperative pain, *J Clin Pharmacol* 36(7): 595-603, 1996.

SUPPORT Principle Investigators: A controlled trial to improve care for seriously ill hospitalized patients, *JAMA* 274(20):1591-1598, 1995.

Sykes NP: A volunteer model for comparison of laxatives in opioid-related constipation, *J Pain Symptom Manage* 11(6):363-369, 1996.

Tanaka K, Watanabe R, Hurada T et al: Extensive application of epidural anesthesia and analgesia in a university hospital: incidence of complications related to technique, *Reg Anesth* 18:34-38, 1993.

Thomas Z, Bruera E: Use of methadone in a highly tolerant patient receiving parenteral hydromorphone, *J Pain Symptom Manage* 10(4): 315-317, 1995.

Turfrey DJ, Ray DAA, Sutcliffe NP et al: Thoracic epidural anaesthesia for coronary artery bypass graft surgery, *Anaesthesia* 52:1090-1095, 1997.

Turner JL, Sibert KS, Sinatra RS: Epidural and spinal analgesia in the post-cesarean delivery patient. In Sinatra RS, Hord AH, Ginsberg B, et al., editors: *Acute pain: mechanisms and management,* pp. 269-278, St. Louis, 1992, Mosby.

Twycross RG: Opioids. In Wall PD, Melzack R, editors: *Textbook of pain,*? ed 3, pp 943-962, New York, 1994, Churchill Livingstone.

Vanderveer B, Clinical Coordinator, Acute and Cancer Pain Service, University Hospital, University of Kentucky, Lexington, KY: Personal communication with author Chris Pasero, November 20, 1997.

Vickers MD, O'Flaherty D, Szekely SM, et al: Tramadol: pain relief by an opioid without depression of respiration, *Anaesthesia* 47:291-296, 1992.

Vigano A, Fan D, Bruera E: Individualized use of methadone and opioid rotation in the comprehensive management of cancer pain associated with poor prognostic indicators, *Pain* 67:115-119, 1996.

Vogelsang J, Hayes SR: Butorphanol tartrate (Stadol): a review, *J Post Anesthesia Nurs* 6(2):129-135, 1991.

Walmsley PNH: Patient-controlled epidural analgesia. In Sinatra RS, Hord AH, Ginsberg B, et al., editors: *Acute pain: mechanisms and management,* pp 312-320, St. Louis, 1992, Mosby.

Wang JK, Nauss LA, Thomas JE: Pain relief by intrathecally applied morphine in man, *Anesthesiology* 50:149-150, 1979.

Ward SE, Goldberg N, Miller-McCauley V et al: Patient-related barriers to management of cancer pain, *Pain* 52:319-324, 1993.

Warren DE: Practical use of rectal medications in palliative care, *J Pain Symptom Manage* 11(6):378-387, 1996.

Watcha MF, Smith I: Cost effectiveness analysis of antiemetic therapy for ambulatory surgery, *J Clin Anesth* 6:370-377, 1994.

Watcha MF, White PF: Post-operative nausea and vomiting: Do they matter? *Eur J Anaesthesiol* 12 (Suppl 10):18-23, 1995.

Watanabe S, Belzile M, Kuehn N et al: Capsules and suppositories of methadone for patients on high-dose opioids for cancer pain: clinical and economic con siderations, *Cancer Treat Rev* 22:131-136, 1996.

Watanabe S, Kondo T, Asakura N et al: Intraoperative combined administration of indomethacin and buprenorphine suppositories as prophylactic therapy for post-open-cholecystectomy pain, *Anesth Analg* 79:85-88, 1994.

Weinberg DS, Inturrisi CE, Reidenberg B et al: Sublingual absorption of selected opioid analgesics, *Clin Pharmacol Ther* 44:335-342, 1988.

Weinstein SM: In patients with chronic pain, what is the suggested maximum doe of sustained-release morphine? *Primary Care Cancer* 14(1):15, 1994.

Weis OF, Sriwatanakul K, Alloza JL et al: Attitudes of patients, housestaff, and nurses toward postoperative analgesic care, *Anesth Analg* 62:70-74, 1983.

Weissman D: Assessment of the patient with non-opioid responsive pain, *Cancer Pain Update* 41:3, Fall 1996.

Weissman DE, Haddox JD: Opioid pseudoaddiction: an iatrogenic syndrome, *Pain* 36:363-366, 1989.

Welch DB, Hrynaszkiewicz A: Postoperative analgesia using epidural methadone: administration by the lumbar route for thoracic pain relief, *Anaesthesia* 36:1051-1054, 1981.

Wiebalck A, Brodner G, Van Aken H: The effects of adding sufentanil to bupivacaine for postoperative patient-controlled epidural analgesia, *Anesth Analg* 85:124-129, 1997.

Wilcox SM, Himmelstein DU, Woolhandler S: Inappropriate drug prescribing for the community-dwelling elderly, *JAMA* 272(4):292-296, 1994.

Willens JS, Myslinski NR: Pharmacodynamics, pharmacokinetics, and clinical uses of fentanyl, sufentanil, and alfentanil, *Heart Lung* 22(3): 239-251, 1993.

Wilson JM, Cohen RI, Kezer EA et al: Single and multiple-dose pharmacokinetics of dezocine in patients with acute and chronic pain, *J Clin Pharmacol* 35:395-403, 1995.

Wilson WC, Smedira NG, Fink C et al: Ordering and administration of sedatives and analgesics during the withholding and withdrawal of life support from critically ill patients, *JAMA* 267(1):949-953, 1992.

Wittels B, Glosten B, Faure EAM: Postcesarean analgesia with both epidural morphine and intravenous patient-controlled analgesia: neurobehavioral outcomes among nursing neonates, *Anesth Analg* 85:600-606, 1997.

Wittels B, Severino FB: PCA in the obstetric patient. In Sinatra RS, Hord AH, Ginsberg B, et al., editors: *Acute pain: mechanisms and management,* pp 175-181, St. Louis, 1992, Mosby.

Woods AM, DiFazio CA: Pharmacology of local anesthetics and related drugs. In Bonica JJ, McDonald JS, editors: *Principles and practice of obstetric analgesia and anesthesia,* ed 2, pp 297-323, Baltimore, 1995, Williams & Wilkins.

Woolf CJ, Chong MS: Preemptive analgesia: treating postoperative pain by preventing the establishment of central sensitization, *Anesth Analg* 77:362-379, 1993.

Wong D: *Wong and Whaley's clinical manual of pediatric nursing,* ed 4, St. Louis, 1996, Mosby.

World Health Organization (WHO): *Cancer pain relief,* Geneva, 1986, WHO.

Yarmush J, D'Angelo R, Kirkhart B et al: A comparison of remifentanil and morphine sulfate for acute postoperative analgesia after total intravenous anesthesia with remifentanil and propofol, *Anesthesiology* 87:235-243, 1997.

Yaster M: Pain Relief, *Pediatrics* 95(3):427-428, 1995 (commentaries).

Yeo W, Lam KK, Chan ATC et al: Transdermal fentanyl for severe cancer-related pain, *Palliative Med* 11:233-239, 1997.

Zech DFJ, Grond SUA, Lynch J et al: Transdermal fentanyl and initial dose-finding with patient-controlled analgesia in cancer pain: a pilot study with 20 terminally ill cancer patients, *Pain* 50:293-301, 1992.

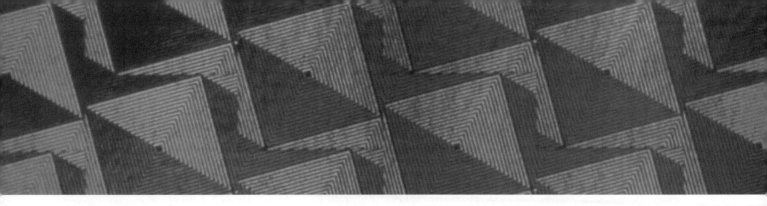

chapter seven
ADJUVANT ANALGESICS

Russell K. Portenoy and Margo McCaffery

TERMINOLOGY

TERMS RELATED TO PAIN MANAGEMENT

Allodynia: A nonpainful stimulus is felt as painful in spite of the tissues appearing normal; common in many neuropathic pain conditions.

Continuous dysesthesias: In this chapter this is used interchangeably with continuous neuropathic pain.

Crescendo pain: A period of rapid pain escalation often associated with increasing distress and functional impairment.

Deafferentation pain: Pain after injury to nerve root or peripheral nerve and inferred to have a predominating central mechanism. A nonspecific term.

Dysesthesia: An unpleasant abnormal sensation, including allodynia. Commonly described as pins and needles, such as a limb "falling asleep." Paresthesia, by comparison, is abnormal but not painful. Burning, electrical, tingling, hypersensitive to stimuli, may include area of sensory loss.

Lancinating: Stabbing, knifelike.

Medically ill patients: Patients with other debilitating pathologic condition/illness in addition to pain, as opposed to those who have only the symptom of pain and are otherwise healthy.

Neuralgia: Pain in the distribution of a nerve (e.g., sciatica, trigeminal neuralgia). Often felt as an electrical shock-like pain.

NMDA: *N*-Methyl-D-aspartate. In this chapter the term is used in conjunction with drugs that are NMDA receptor blockers, such as ketamine or dextromethorphan.

Paresthesia: Includes sensations of numbness, prickling, tingling, and heightened sensitivity.

Paroxysmal: Sudden periodic attack or recurrence.

Refractory: Resistant to ordinary treatment.

Sequential trials: One drug is tried, and if the results are unfavorable, it is discontinued and another drug is tried. A trial-and-error approach in which one drug after another is tried until the desired effects occur.

Systemic drug treatment; systemic administration: Administration of a drug by a route that allows it to be absorbed into the general circulation. Such routes include oral, parenteral (IV, IM, SC), rectal, vaginal, topical application, and transdermal. By contrast, the spinal route of administration deposits the drug directly into the central nervous system, minimizing the amount of drug that reaches the general circulation.

Tabetic pain: Sharp, lightning type of pain; also called lancinating pain.

TERMS RELATED TO RESEARCH

Anecdotal evidence: Clinical observations or case reports.

Case reports: Published reports of one or more patients in situations that are not representative of controlled trials.

Controlled studies/trials: A group of studies that control for various effects by using placebo comparison, single- or double-blind design, or random assignment of subjects.

Double blind: Neither the subjects nor the administrators/evaluators of the treatment know who is receiving what. For the sake of safety, someone not directly involved in the investigation (often the pharmacy) holds the code to what is being administered, and this code can be broken at any time if deemed necessary.

Meta-analysis: A systematic review of all research reported during a given period of time that meets certain criteria for inclusion in the analysis.

Open-label: Both the investigators and the subjects know what treatment the subjects are receiving. An investigator administers an analgesic to a sample of patients and follows them through treatment, observing the effects. Disadvantage is the potential for patient selection bias and observer bias. Tentative conclusions may be drawn.

Placebo controlled: The effects of a drug are compared with a those of a placebo and the study is either single or double blinded. Results may be stated with much more confidence than those findings from studies in which the drug is not compared with a placebo.

Randomized: Patients are randomly assigned to different groups, assigned by chance alone. Each group receives a different treatment, including one group with placebo or no treatment.

Single blind study: The investigators know what treatments the subjects are receiving, but the subjects are "blinded" (i.e., they do not know what they are receiving).

The term *adjuvant analgesic* describes any drug that has a primary indication other than pain but is analgesic in some painful conditions. This terminology is widely accepted but can be problematic. Adjuvant analgesics may be used both as "add-on" therapy to an opioid regimen or as distinct primary therapy in certain painful disorders.

In the palliative care literature adjuvant analgesics are also called *coanalgesics,* a term that includes nonopioid analgesics such as acetaminophen. In the palliative care setting adjuvant analgesics are typically coadministered with an opioid to enhance pain relief, treat pain that is refractory to the analgesic, or allow reduction of the opioid dose for the purpose of limiting side effects.

For chronic pain unrelated to cancer or other progressive medical diseases, the adjuvant analgesics are often used alone—not as adjuvant to any other therapy. Some adjuvant analgesics are used alone as nonspecific multipurpose analgesics, and others are used in selected disorders as primary analgesics. The use of adjuvants as primary analgesics is expanding rapidly.

Initial clinical experience with adjuvant analgesics was mostly in the treatment of chronic pain of neuropathic origin. The role of adjuvant analgesics has expanded now to include other types of chronic pain and acute pain such as postoperative or burn pain.

Considerable research is currently underway to explain the role of adjuvant analgesics. Much of what is covered in this chapter will be modified over the next few years. Thus throughout the chapter an effort is made to stipulate the type of evidence that supports various suggestions and findings and to note when research is lacking.

Various research terms are used to designate types of research support. Some of these terms are explained at the beginning of this chapter (Terminology) to enable the clinician to evaluate the relative worthiness of the evidence available currently and in the future. For example, clinical observations of astute clinicians, often referred to as anecdotal evidence, are a valuable contribution, especially when research is lacking. However, when findings are derived from a placebo-controlled double-blind study, they are far more convincing. The adjuvant analgesics comprise an extraordinarily diverse group of drug classes. A generally useful, broad classification distinguishes those that may be considered nonspecific, multipurpose analgesics from those used for more specific indications (Box 7.1). Major classes of adjuvant analgesics, along with examples, are listed in Table 7.2.

GENERAL CONSIDERATIONS

The use of adjuvant analgesics in the management of pain is a "labor-intensive" endeavor that requires frequent contact with the patient. The selection of an adjuvant

TABLE 7.1 ● ● ● ● ●

Misconceptions	Adjuvant Analgesics
MISCONCEPTION	CORRECTION
1. Adjuvant analgesics are as reliable in producing pain relief as are opioids or nonopioids.	Fewer patients respond adequately to adjuvant analgesics than to opioids and nonopioids. Furthermore, adjuvants tend to have a much slower onset of analgesia and more side effects.
2. Adjuvants are only effective for chronic neuropathic pain.	Some adjuvant analgesics such as tricyclic antidepressants, corticosteroids, and psychostimulants are multipurpose analgesics that may be useful for both neuropathic and nociceptive pain.
3. Adjuvant analgesics are appropriate only for chronic, not acute, pain.	Some adjuvant analgesics such as clonidine are useful for both acute and chronic pain.
4. Use of adjuvant analgesics is usually no more time consuming than use of other analgesic groups.	Drug selection and dose titration of adjuvants is more difficult and "labor intensive" than with opioids and nonopioids.
5. Pain relief from antidepressants depends on their ability to relieve depression in the patient with pain.	The analgesic effect of antidepressants is not dependent on their antidepressant activity. Both depressed and nondepressed patients with pain report analgesia. Furthermore, the analgesic dose is often lower than that required to treat depression, and the onset of analgesia typically occurs much sooner, usually within 1 week.
6. Antidepressants are more appropriate analgesics for burning neuropathic pain than for stabbing and knifelike neuropathic pain.	Research shows that antidepressants may be effective for both lancinating (knifelike) and continuous neuropathic pain.
7. Drugs marketed as muscle relaxants, such as methocarbamol (Robaxin), relieve muscle pain by relaxing the muscle.	No evidence exists that "muscle relaxants" relax skeletal muscle in humans. Although these drugs can relieve musculoskeletal pain, this may not be due to relaxation of skeletal muscle.

May be duplicated for use in clinical practice. From McCaffery M, Pasero C: *Pain: Clinical manual*, p. 303. Copyright © 1999, Mosby, Inc.
See text for references.

● ● ● ● ●

BOX 7.1	**Broad Classification of Adjuvant Analgesics**

Role of adjuvants in analgesic therapy: Adjuvants may be used in addition to other analgesics or alone as distinct primary therapy for certain painful conditions. Most experience with adjuvant analgesics has been in the treatment of chronic pain, but use of adjuvants is now expanding to include treatment of acute pain.

Two classes:

I. Multipurpose adjuvant analgesics. Some of these (e.g., clonidine) are useful for both acute and chronic pain.
Examples of drugs:
 A. Antidepressants
 B. Corticosteroids
 C. Clonidine (alpha$_2$-adrenergic agonist)
 D. Psychostimulants

II. Adjuvant analgesics for specific types of pain
Examples of pain conditions and recommended adjuvant analgesics:
 A. Continuous chronic neuropathic pain (e.g., antidepressants)
 B. Lancinating chronic neuropathic pain (e.g., anticonvulsants)
 C. Chronic bone pain such as bony metastasis or osteoporosis (e.g., calcitonin)
 D. Malignant bowel obstruction (e.g., octreotide)
 E. Chronic musculoskeletal pain (e.g., muscle relaxants) (Although these are traditionally used, evidence of specific usefulness is minimal.)
 F. Postoperative pain (e.g., epidural clonidine)

drug and an optimal dosing regimen necessitates a systematic assessment of the patient both initially and throughout the course of therapy with the adjuvant drug. Over time, changes in pain, side effects, or any quality-of-life concerns may necessitate a change in therapeutic strategy.

Drug Selection

The selection of a specific adjuvant analgesic is usually determined by the characteristics of the pain such as continuous burning neuropathic pain versus sharp and shooting pain. In many situations multiple drug options exist. The initial choice is made on the basis of comprehensive assessment of the patient and one's best clinical judgment.

Dosing

Low initial doses and gradual dose escalation may avoid early side effects or allow tolerance or adjustment to the side effects. In medically ill patients this precaution is especially appropriate when adjuvant analgesics are initiated. When low doses and slow titration are used to optimize the balance between pain relief and adverse effects, patients must be forewarned that onset of analgesia is likely to be delayed. Otherwise, patients may become discouraged and stop taking the drug.

Variability in Response

For all the adjuvant analgesics, responses will vary considerably from one patient to another. Although specific patient characteristics, such as advanced age or coexistent major organ failure, may increase the likelihood of some adverse responses, neither favorable effects nor specific side effects can be reliably predicted in the individual patient.

For these reasons, sequential trials of adjuvant analgesics are often useful. That is, one drug is tried and if the results are unfavorable, it is discontinued and another

drug is tried. The possibility and potential benefit of trying one adjuvant analgesic after another should be explained to the patient at the start of therapy to enhance compliance and reduce the distress that may occur as treatments fail.

Polypharmacy

In patients with chronic nonmalignant pain who are not medically ill, an adjuvant analgesic may be the only drug taken by the patient on a regular basis. However, in the palliative care setting, adjuvant analgesics are typically administered to patients who are receiving multiple drugs. Although this is widely regarded as appropriate in the care of terminally ill patients, the potential for additive side effects and unpredictable adverse effects must be anticipated whenever an adjuvant is added to an existing drug regimen.

When the patient is receiving opioid and nonopioid analgesics, the decision to add, or continue, an adjuvant analgesic must be made on the basis of a careful assessment of outcomes and a clear understanding of the goals of care. If the adjuvant yields demonstrable benefit without serious risk or side effects that impair quality of life, ample justification exists for continuing them. Additional pain relief at the price of sedation or mental clouding is not acceptable for patients whose goals include restoration of function but may be completely appropriate for those who seek comfort as the only goal.

Positioning of Treatment

For almost all patients with acute pain and for patients with persistent moderate or severe pain caused by advanced incurable disease, opioids should be initiated and titrated to maximum effect before an adjuvant analgesic is added. Opioids are almost always the mainstay of analgesia for these patients, and they should not receive an adjuvant analgesic until opioid therapy has been optimized.

●●●●●
TABLE 7.2

ADJUVANT ANALGESICS: MAJOR CLASSES WITH EXAMPLES

Generic Name	Brand Name	Generic Name	Brand Name
Anticonvulsants		*Neuroleptics*	
Carbamazepine	Tegretol	Fluphenazine	Prolixin
Clonazepam	Klonopin	Methotrimeprazine	Levoprome
Divalproex sodium	Depakote	Pimozide	Orap
Gabapentin	Neurontin	*NMDA Blockers*	
Lamotrigine	Lamictal	Dextromethorphan	
Phenytoin	Dilantin	Ketamine	
Valproic acid	Depakene (valproates include divalproex sodium and valproic acid)	*Alpha₂-adrenergic Agonists*	
		Clonidine	Catapres
Antidepressants		Tizanidine	Zanaflex
Amitriptyline	Elavil	Dexmedetomidine	Currently being developed
Clomipramine	Anafranil	*Topical Agents*	
Desipramine	Norpramin	Capsaicin	Zostrix
Doxepin	Sinequan	Local anesthetics	e.g., EMLA
Fluoxetine	Prozac	*Drugs for Sympathetically Maintained Pain*	
Imipramine	Tofranil	Phenoxybenzamine	Dibenzyline
Maprotiline	Ludiomil	Nifedipine	Procardia
Nefazodone	Serzone	Prazosin	Minipress
Nortriptyline	Aventyl, Pamelor	Propranolol	Inderal
Paroxetine	Paxil	*Psychostimulants*	
Sertraline	Zoloft	Dextroamphetamine	Dexedrine
Trazodone	Desyrel	Methylphenidate	Ritalin
Venlafaxine	Effexor	Pemoline	Cylert
Oral Local Anesthetics		*"Muscle Relaxants"*	
Mexiletine	Mexitil	Orphenadrine	Norflex
Tocainide	Tonocard	Cyclobenzaprine	Flexeril
GABAergic		Carisoprodol	Soma
Baclofen	Lioresal	Chlorzoxazone	Parafon Forte DSC
Corticosteroids		Methocarbamol	Robaxin
Dexamethasone	Decadron		
Methylprednisolone	Medrol		
Prednisone	Deltasone, Meticorten		

May be duplicated for use in clinical practice. From McCaffery M, Pasero C: *Pain: Clinical manual*, p. 305. Copyright © 1999, Mosby, Inc.

In the palliative care setting, usually the safest and most efficient approach is to add an adjuvant analgesic to an opioid regimen after it is clear that the opioid produces inadequate analgesia despite dose escalation to limiting side effects. Although some clinicians attempt to improve patient response by initiating therapy with an opioid and an adjuvant analgesic concurrently, this approach increases the risk of additive toxicity and may make it difficult to determine which drug is responsible for the resulting analgesia or side effects.

In the palliative care setting, one of the reasons for initiating analgesic therapy with opioids rather than adjuvants is that the adjuvant analgesics are, as a group, less re-liable analgesics. For example, 70% to 90% of cancer patients who receive opioid therapy are likely to achieve satisfactory pain relief in a few days (Portenoy, 1989; Schug, Zech, Dorr, 1990; Schug, Zech, Grond et al., 1992; Ventafridda, Tamburini, Caraceni et al., 1990; World Health Organization, 1990). By contrast, studies of the tricyclic antidepressants show that these drugs require treatment for weeks to obtain optimal results. They provide greater than 50% pain relief for only 50% to 75% of patients with neuropathic pain (Kishore-Kumar, Max, Schafer et al., 1990; Max, Culnane, Schafer et al., 1987).

Thus fewer patients respond adequately to adjuvants than to opioids, and most adjuvants have a slower onset of analgesic effect, either because the adjuvant must accumulate before it becomes analgesic or because therapy is initiated at low doses to avoid side effects. Many of the adjuvant drugs are more likely than opioids to produce troublesome side effects.

Chronic noncancer pain is highly variable, and the therapeutic goals often emphasize function as much as comfort. The use of long-term opioid therapy is controversial in many such populations and, in some, nondrug therapies are preferred. When analgesics are considered appropriate, nonopioids are often the first choice, followed by the addition of adjuvants when indicated. In some cases of moderate to severe chronic nonmalignant pain in which immediate comfort is the overriding goal, nonopioid analgesia may be insufficient, and the delayed onset of analgesia from an adjuvant may be unacceptable. In this instance an opioid may be used initially for more rapid pain control, and the adjuvant may be initiated soon thereafter with the intention of decreasing the opioid as the adjuvant becomes effective.

MULTIPURPOSE ADJUVANT ANALGESICS FOR CHRONIC PAIN

Studies have shown that some adjuvant analgesics are effective for many different pain syndromes, suggesting that they be used as multipurpose analgesics as are the opioids and nonopioid analgesics. For chronic pain those multipurpose adjuvant analgesics that are currently considered to be among the more useful in clinical practice include antidepressants, corticosteroids, and alpha$_2$-adrenergic agonists (e.g., clonidine). Except for the antidepressants, these drugs may be used in both acute and chronic pain. Antidepressants are not well suited for acute pain for a variety of reasons such as the fact that analgesia is often delayed for days and sometimes weeks.

Antidepressant Drugs

Antidepressant adjuvant analgesics are typically divided into two major groups: the tricyclics and the "newer" antidepressants. See Table 7.3 for a more detailed listing by class with examples.

Evidence is compelling that the tricyclic antidepressants are analgesic in a variety of chronic pain syndromes (Egbunike, Chaffee, 1990; Getto, Sorkness, Howell, 1987; Magni, 1991; Monks, 1994; Onghena, Van houdenhove, 1992). The efficacy of the tertiary amine compounds such as amitriptyline (Elavil) has been demonstrated in a large number of controlled and uncontrolled trials. Although research is more limited with the secondary amines such as desipramine (Norpramin), they too have been shown to be useful with a variety of neuropathic pains. Following is a list of tricyclic antidepressants, along with types of pain for which they have been shown to be effective.

ANTIDEPRESSANT ADJUVANT ANALGESICS: CLASSES WITH EXAMPLES	
Classes	Examples
Tricyclic Antidepressants	
Tertiary amines	Amitriptyline (Elavil)
	Clomipramine (Anafranil)
	Doxepin (Sinequan)
	Imipramine (Tofranil)
Secondary amines	Desipramine (Norpramin)
	Nortriptyline (Aventyl, Pamelor)
"Newer" Antidepressants	
Phenethylamine	Venlafaxine (Effexor)
Triazolopyridine	Trazodone (Desyrel)
	Nefazodone (Serzone)
Selective serotonin reuptake inhibitors (SSRIs)	Fluoxetine (Prozac)
	Paroxetine (Paxil)
	Sertraline (Zoloft)
Tetracyclic	Maprotiline (Ludiomil)
Aminoketone	Bupropion (Wellbutrin)

May be duplicated for use in clinical practice. From McCaffery M, Pasero C: Pain: Clinical manual, p. 306. Copyright © 1999, Mosby, Inc.

Overview of specific antidepressants
Amitriptyline (Elavil)

This drug has been shown to be effective for:
- Migraine and other types of headache (Couch, Ziegler, Hassanein, 1976; Diamond, Baltes, 1971; Gobel, Hamouz, Hansen et al., 1994; Gomersall, Stuart, 1973; Indaco, Carrieri, 1988; Okasha, Ghaleb, Sadek, 1973)
- Arthritis (Frank, Kashini, Parker et al., 1988)
- Chronic low back pain (Ward, 1986)
- Postherpetic neuralgia (Watson, Chipman, Reed et al., 1992; Watson, Evans, Reed et al., 1982)
- Fibromyalgia (Carrette, McCain, Bell et al., 1986; Dinerman, Felsen, Goldenberg, 1985)
- Painful diabetic polyneuropathy (Max, Culnane, Schafer et al., 1987; Max, Lynch, Muir et al., 1992; Turkington, 1980)
- Central pain (Leijon, Boivie, 1989)
- Chronic facial pain (Sharav, Singer, Schmidt et al., 1987)
- Cancer pain (Ventafridda, Bonezzi, Caraceni et al., 1987)

Imipramine (Tofranil)

This drug has been shown to be effective for:
- Arthritis (Glick, Fowler, 1979; Gringas, 1976; McDonald-Scott, 1969)

- Headache (Lance, Curran, 1964)
- Painful diabetic neuropathy (Kvinesdal, Molin, Froland et al., 1984; Sindrup, Ejlertsen, Froland et al., 1989; Sindrup, Gram, Skjold et al., 1990, Turkington, 1980)
- Low back pain (Alcoff, Jones, Rust et al., 1982)
- Idiopathic chest pain (Cannon, Quyyumi, Mincemoyer et al., 1994)

Doxepin (Sinequan)

This drug was effective in:
- Coexistent pain and depression (Evans, Gensler, Blackwell et al., 1973; Ward, Bloom, Friedel, 1979)
- Headache (Morland, Storli, Mogstad, 1979; Okasha, Ghaleb, Sadek, 1973)
- Low back pain (Hameroff, Cork, Scherer et al., 1982)

Clomipramine (Anafranil)

This drug has been shown to be effective in:
- Varied neuropathic pains and idiopathic pain (Eberhard, Von Knorring, Nilsson et al., 1988; Langohr, Stohr, Petruch, 1982; Panerai, Monza, Movillia et al., 1990; Sindrup, Gram, Skjold et al., 1990)

Desipramine (Norpramin)

This drug was effective in:
- Postherpetic neuralgia and painful diabetic neuropathy (Kishore-Kumar, Max, Schafer et al., 1990; Max, Lynch, Muir et al., 1992; Sindrup, Gram, Skjold et al., 1990)

Nortriptyline (Aventyl, Pamelor)

This drug was effective in:
- Mixed neuropathic pains (Panerai, Monza, Movillia et al., 1990)

Nortriptyline Combined With Fluphenazine

This drug was effective in:
- Painful diabetic polyneuropathy (Gomez-Perez, Riell, Dies et al., 1985)

Newer Antidepressants

The "newer" antidepressants have also been studied, with somewhat less definitive results. The analgesic efficacy of maprotiline (Ludiomil) has been established in controlled comparisons against clomipramine in idiopathic pain (Eberhard, von Knorring, Nilsson et al., 1988) and against amitriptyline in postherpetic neuralgia (Watson, Chipman, Reed et al., 1992). Although a trial of trazodone (Desyrel) for dysesthetic pains in patients with traumatic myelopathy did not demonstrate a favorable effect (Davidoff, Guarracini, Roth et al., 1987), benefits were suggested in another controlled trial performed in patients with cancer pain (Ventafridda, Bonezzi, Caraceni et al., 1987).

With regard to the analgesic effectiveness of selective serotonin reuptake inhibitors (SSRIs), paroxetine (Paxil) was effective for diabetic neuropathy (Sindrup, Gram, Brosen et al., 1990). Although case reports suggested that fluoxetine (Prozac) has analgesic effects (Diamond, Frietag, 1989; Geller, 1989; Walsh, 1986), a controlled trial in patients with diabetic neuropathy failed to demonstrate benefit from this drug (Max, Lynch, Muir et al., 1992).

On the other hand, a more recent double-blind comparison of fluoxetine, desipramine, and amitriptyline in postherpetic neuralgia revealed that all three have the potential to relieve pain (Davies, Reisner-Keller, Rowbotham, 1996). In this study no significant difference was found in their analgesic effect. Fluoxetine had few side effects but, interestingly, had the highest dropout rate. Another controlled study of 59 patients with rheumatic pain revealed that both amitriptyline, 25 mg, and fluoxetine, 20 mg, given over a 4-week period produced significant pain relief compared with placebo (Rani, Naidu, Prasad et al., 1996). Fluoxetine was considered superior to amitriptyline because of fewer side effects. Other SSRIs have not been systematically studied as analgesics in patient populations.

An open-label survey of patients treated with alprazolam, a benzodiazepine with antidepressant effects, suggested that this drug may also be analgesic in patients with neuropathic pain caused by cancer (Fernandez, Adams, Homes, 1987).

Fewer clinical trials have specifically evaluated the efficacy of antidepressants as analgesics for cancer pain. Nonetheless, several partially controlled trials (Breivik, Rennemo, 1982; Ventafridda, Bianchi, Ripamonti et al., 1990; Ventafridda, Bonezzi, Caraceni et al., 1987) and other reports (Magni, Arsie, DeLeo, 1987) generally confirm the analgesic potential of the tricyclic antidepressants in the cancer population.

Summary

Substantial evidence exists that antidepressant drugs have analgesic effects in diverse types of chronic pain. Given the range of pain syndromes that are potentially responsive, it is appropriate to classify these drugs as nonspecific, multipurpose analgesics. The strongest evidence of analgesic efficacy is found in the numerous controlled trials of the tertiary amine drugs, the best studied of which has been amitriptyline. Although less abundant data support the efficacy of the secondary amine tricyclic drugs, desipramine has been carefully studied and has clear analgesic potential.

Antidepressants with more selective actions are also analgesic, and clinical interest is particularly strong in the SSRIs because of their relatively good side effect profile (Boyer, Blumhardt, 1992; Cooper, 1988; Kerr,

Fairweather, Mahendran et al., 1992). Among the SSRIs, some evidence supports the analgesic efficacy of paroxetine and fluoxetine, but data are equivocal or absent for the others. The SSRIs appear to be weaker analgesics than the tricyclics, a finding confirmed in one controlled comparison (Sindrup, Gram, Brosen et al., 1990).

A systematic review of controlled trials of antidepressants in neuropathic pain supports the effectiveness of antidepressants in relieving neuropathic pain (McQuay, Tramer, Nye et al., 1996). Comparisons of tricyclic antidepressants do not show any significant difference between them. Paroxetine is less effective than imipramine. A comparison of this review with a similar review of anticonvulsants (McQuay, Carroll, Jadad et al., 1995) suggests that analgesia and side effects with antidepressants are comparable with those of anticonvulsants, and evidence does not support the common impression that burning pain should be treated with antidepressants and lancinating pain with anticonvulsants. Both anticonvulsants and antidepressants were effective in diabetic neuropathy, with 50% to 85% achieving greater than 50% pain relief.

Mechanism of action

The analgesic effect of these drugs does not depend on their antidepressant activity. Controlled studies have demonstrated that the analgesic dose is often lower than that required to treat depression, and the onset of analgesia typically occurs much sooner, usually within 1 week (Kvinesdal, Molin, Froland et al., 1984; Langohr, Stohr, Petruch, 1982; Leijon, Boivie, 1989; Panerai, Monza, Movillia et al., 1990; Sindrup, Gram, Brosen et al., 1990; Sindrup, Gram, Skjold et al., 1990; Watson, Evans, Reed et al., 1982). Moreover, nondepressed patients can experience analgesia and depressed patients can report pain relief without a change in mood (Alcoff, Jones, Rust et al., 1982; Kishore-Kumar, Max, Schafer et al., 1990; Max, Culnane, Schafer et al., 1987; Max, Lynch, Muir et al., 1992; Sindrup, Gram, Brosen et al., 1990).

Several hypotheses have been proposed to explain the analgesia produced by the antidepressants. The most widely accepted postulates that their ability to block the reuptake of neurotransmitters such as serotonin and norepinephrine in the central nervous system increases activity in endogenous pain-modulating pathways (Basbaum, Fields, 1984; Besson, Chaouch, 1987; Yaksh, 1979). Neurons originating in the brain stem descend to the spinal cord and release substances such as endogenous opioids, serotonin, and norepinephrine that inhibit the transmission of nociceptive impulses. Tricyclic antidepressants may enhance normal modulation by interfering with the reuptake of serotonin and norepinephrine (Figure 7.1).

When a tricyclic antidepressant is coadministered with an opioid, some of the benefit may relate to a pharmacokinetic interaction that results in higher opioid concentrations. Such an interaction has been demonstrated when clomipramine or amitriptyline is added to a morphine regimen (Ventafridda, Bianchi, Ripamonti et al., 1990).

Adverse effects

Although serious adverse effects are uncommon at the doses usually administered for pain, less serious side effects are frequent (Baldessarini, 1990; Boyer, Blumhardt, 1992; Cooper, 1988). Even at low doses, patients with major organ dysfunction or those who use multiple other drugs may experience troublesome side effects. Moreover, some patients who receive low doses of the tricyclic antidepressants actually attain relatively high plasma drug concentrations (Preskorn, Irwin, 1982).

Orthostatic hypotension is a potentially serious side effect (Glassman, Bigger, 1981). Of the tricyclic compounds, nortriptyline is the least likely to cause this and should be considered in patients who develop orthostatic dizziness after treatment with another tricyclic or are otherwise predisposed to this symptom (Roose, Glassman, Giardina et al., 1986). Orthostatic hypotension appears to be much more likely in the elderly and, combined with the sedative effects of these drugs, probably accounts for an increased risk of hip fracture in this population (Ray, Griffin, Schaffner et al., 1987). Patients who are predisposed to orthostasis may be better candidates for one of the newer analgesic antidepressants, specifically an SSRI.

Sedation and mental clouding are common side effects of the tricyclic antidepressants. The likelihood of these effects is increased in the elderly. Within the class of tricyclic antidepressants, desipramine is perhaps the least likely to cause somnolence or confusion, and nortriptyline is less problematic than amitriptyline.

SSRIs are less likely to cause mental clouding, confusion, or somnolence (Boyer, Blumhardt, 1992; Cooper, 1988; Kerr, Fairweather, Mahendran et al., 1992). Although some patients experience somnolence, patients are more likely to report a sense of activation.

Anticholinergic side effects are also common during treatment with the tricyclic antidepressants. These effects are more likely during treatment with the tertiary amine drugs than the secondary amine drugs; they are not characteristic of the SSRIs. When relatively mild, anticholinergic side effects, such as dry mouth, blurred vision, or constipation, can usually be managed or tolerated. Occasionally, patients are distressed enough to warrant a trial of a less anticholinergic drug. In a small double-blind study of elderly patients receiving nortriptyline, side effects of dry mouth and blurred vision were safely reduced with bethanechol, 10 mg three times a day. The drug was well tolerated except for causing an increase in orthostatic hypotension (Rosen, Pollock, Altieri et al., 1993).

The decrease in salivation caused by the tricyclic antidepressants is especially troublesome for those patients

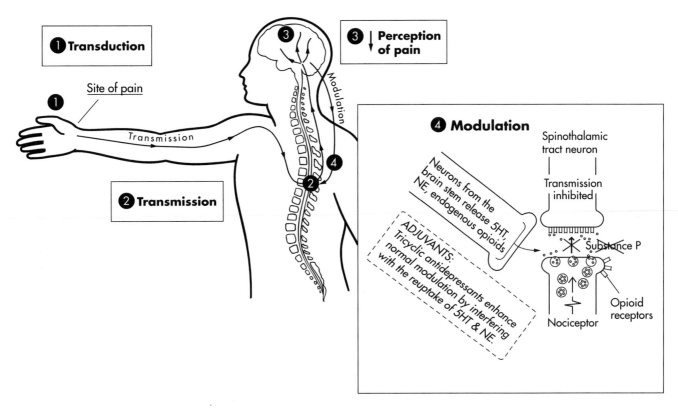

May be duplicated for use in clinical practice. As appears in McCaffery M, Pasero C: *Pain: Clinical manual,* p. 309, 1999, Mosby, Inc.

● ● ● ● ●

FIGURE 7.1 Analgesic action site for antidepressants. Adapted from Figure 4.2 *A* and *B*, pages 106-107, which the reader may return to for further details.

Key:

❶ **Transduction:** Conversion of one energy form to another. This process occurs in the periphery when a noxious stimulus causes tissue damage. Sensitizing substances are released by damaged cells and an action potential occurs.

❷ **Transmission:** The action potential continues from the site of damage to the spinal cord and ascends to higher centers. Transmission may be considered in three phases: injury site to spinal cord, spinal cord to brain stem and thalamus, and thalamus to cortex.

❸ **Perception of pain:** Conscious experience of pain.

❹ **Modulation:** Inhibition of nociceptive impulses. Neurons originating in the brain stem descend to the spinal cord and release substances, such as endogenous opioids, serotonin (5HT), and norepinephrine (NE), that inhibit the transmission of nociceptive impulses.

Antidepressants enhance normal modulation by interfering with the reuptake of serotonin (5HT) and norepinephrine (NE), which in turn decreases the perception of pain.

with dentures. Precautions should be taken, including regular dental examinations.

A troubling side effect for many patients taking tricyclic antidepressants or SSRIs is sexual dysfunction. A drug holiday is a potentially simple solution that may be helpful if the patient is taking an antidepressant with a short half-life, such as paroxetine (Paxil) or sertraline (Zoloft), as opposed to fluoxetine (Prozac) (Lipman, 1997). In a study of 30 depressed men and women who suffered sexual dysfunction as a result of SSRIs, a temporary discontinuance of the drug before the weekend (omission of doses after Thursday morning until Sunday noon) resulted in a marked increase in sexual satisfaction for those taking sertraline or paroxetine but not for those taking fluoxetine (Rothchild, 1995). These patients did not relapse into depression. Whether pain would return in patients taking these drugs for analgesia is unknown.

On the basis of anecdotal evidence, other suggestions for reducing sexual dysfunction associated with SSRIs include taking psychostimulants, such as 5 mg sublingually of dextroamphetamine or methylphenidate, 1 or more hours before intercourse (Bartlik, Kaplan, Kaplan, 1995). One literature review revealed numerous other anecdotal therapies for sexual dysfunction related to various antidepressants. These included cyproheptadine (2 to 16 mg/day), yohimbine (5.4 to 16.2 mg/day), dopamine antagonists (amantadine 100 to 200 mg/day), and buspirone (15 to 60 mg/day) (Gitlin, 1995). Unfortunately, research is lacking, and these suggestions must be viewed with caution.

The most serious adverse effect of the tricyclic antidepressants, cardiotoxicity, is very uncommon (Glassman, Bigger, 1981). Patients at risk are those who have significant heart disease, including conduction disorders, dysrhythmias, or failure. If these patients are treated with antidepressants, initial doses should be low, dose escalation should be gradual, and the electrocardiogram should be monitored as doses reach relatively high levels.

Tricyclic antidepressants and fluoxetine (Prozac) appear to be safe for the fetus. A study of infants of mothers who took antidepressants during pregnancy compared with those who did not found no differences in the infants regarding temperament, mood, activity levels, distractibility, or behavioral problems (Nulman, Rovet, Stewart et al., 1997).

Indications

As multipurpose analgesics, antidepressant drugs could potentially be considered for the treatment of any chronic pain syndrome. However, the available evidence does not support their use as analgesics for acute pain (Gordon, Heller, Gear et al., 1994; Kerrick, Fine, Lipman et al., 1993). In the palliative care setting, the strongest indication for the use of an antidepressant as an adjuvant analgesic is in the patient with neuropathic pain whose response to opioids has been inadequate.

Great variability exists in the range of symptoms presented by patients with neuropathic pains. Conceivably, specific symptoms may indicate the existence of mechanisms that respond differently to drugs with varying modes of action. Although little systematic investigation of this possibility has been done, the guidelines in the clinical literature reflect this perspective. For example, it is generally accepted that antidepressants are more useful for neuropathic pains characterized by continuous dysesthesias (e.g., burning pain or hypersensitivity to stimuli) than pains described as lancinating (stabbing). This impression continues despite controlled trials that have demonstrated the efficacy of amitriptyline and desipramine for continuous and lancinating dysesthesias in patients who are experiencing both (Kishore-Kuman, Max, Schafer et al., 1990; Max, Culnane, Schafer et al., 1987) and despite systematic literature review that fails to support this impression (McQuay, Tramer, Nye et al., 1996). In summation, the data suggest that an antidepressant may be appropriate for patients with lancinating neuropathic pains and continuous burning pain.

In terminally ill patients, early use of an adjuvant analgesic is also considered when pain is accompanied by other symptoms that may respond to a nonanalgesic effect of the drug. For example, antidepressants are commonly used when pain is complicated by depression, and the tricyclic antidepressants are especially useful when pain is accompanied by insomnia.

Drug selection

As mentioned earlier, a systematic review of the effectiveness and safety of antidepressants in neuropathic pain as revealed by controlled trials concluded that comparisons of tricyclic antidepressants do not reveal any significant differences among them (McQuay, Tramer, Nye et al., 1996). Given the extensive data from controlled clinical trials, amitriptyline might be considered first when an antidepressant is indicted. If treatment with amitriptyline has failed or is not indicated because of concerns about toxicity, numerous options remain.

If toxicity limits the trial of amitriptyline, a trial with an alternative tricyclic antidepressant is the most appropriate second-line approach. For example, desipramine might be considered because of its favorable side effect profile and evidence of analgesic efficacy (Kishore-Kumar, Max, Schafer et al., 1990; Max, Lynch, Muir et al., 1992). In fact, a comparison of fluoxetine, desipramine, and amitriptyline in postherpetic neuralgia revealed that all three have the potential to relieve pain but that desipramine was slightly more effective with fewer side effects, leading to the recommendation that this drug be the first choice unless contraindicated (Davies, Reisner-Keller, Rowbotham, 1996).

For patients who cannot tolerate any tricyclic compound one of the newer antidepressants may be tried. The SSRIs have the most favorable side effect profiles and might be considered in this circumstance. These drugs may vary in analgesic efficacy, and it is prudent to select one, such as paroxetine (Paxil) (Sindrup, Gram, Brosen et al., 1990), that has established analgesic effects.

Substantial variability exists in the analgesic response to the different antidepressants. Failure of one drug might reasonably be followed by a trial of an alternative drug. No guidelines exist for drug selection during these sequential trials, and the process usually proceeds by trial and error.

Dose selection

The starting dose of the tricyclic antidepressants, such as amitriptyline and desipramine, should be low, 10 mg in the elderly and 25 mg in younger patients. The usual dosing increases are the same size as the starting dose. Doses can be increased every few days. For example, an elderly patient may begin with 10 mg of desipramine. After 3 to 5 days, if the patient has no intolerable or unmanageable side effects, the dose may be increased to 20 mg. Again, after 3 to 5 days, the dose may be increased to 30 mg, then to 40 mg, continuing with 10 mg increases until pain relief is achieved or side effects become problematic.

The usual effective dose range for amitriptyline or desipramine is 50 to 150 mg. Some patients will benefit from doses less than or greater than this range. However, no evidence exists that analgesic doses need to be greater than or even as much as those recommended for depression.

If the patient does not benefit from the usual analgesic dose and has no side effects, the dose may be titrated upward until the antidepressant dose if reached. This course is clearly justified in patients with a coexistent depression but should be considered even in patients without depression. Also, monitoring plasma levels of the drug may reveal low levels, indicating rapid metabolism of the drug or the possibility that the patient is not taking all doses.

Most patients receive a single nighttime dose of the tricyclic drugs or a single daytime dose of the SSRIs. If pain relief is adequate throughout the day during treatment with a tricyclic antidepressant but the patient experiences "hangover" or double vision in the morning, the total daily dose may be divided into two doses given in the early and late evening. Similarly, if the patient has increased pain in the afternoon, the total daily dose may be divided into two doses given morning and evening.

Monitoring therapy

Changes in pain, mood, cognitive status, sleep pattern, and other effects must be carefully monitored during dose escalation. It is useful but not essential to monitor plasma drug concentration during therapy, if feasible.

A favorable analgesic effect is usually observed within a week after achieving an effective dosing level, and in some patients maximal effect appears to evolve over days or weeks thereafter. This delay, combined with the many days required to increase the dose to a therapeutic level, may result in a prolonged period during which patients experience unsatisfactory effects from the therapy, sometimes including uncomfortable side effects. Unless the patient is well informed about this potential, the patient is likely to discontinue the drug.

Corticosteroids

Research supports the classification of corticosteroids as multipurpose analgesics. The use of these drugs as analgesics has been suggested in reflex sympathetic dystrophy, a type of neuropathic pain (Kozin, Ryan, Carerra et al., 1981), and diverse types of cancer pain (e.g., Moertel et al., 1974; Schell, 1972), including bone pain, neuropathic pain from infiltration or compression of neural structures, headache caused by increased intracranial pressure, arthralgia, and pain caused by obstruction of hollow viscus (e.g., bowel or ureter). Analgesic effects have been described for a variety of corticosteroids and a broad range of doses. Specific examples are:

- A placebo-controlled trial in patients with far advanced cancer demonstrated that relatively low doses of methylprednisolone (16 mg twice daily) were analgesic, but that these effects waned over a 20-day evaluation period (Bruera, Roca, Cedaro et al., 1985).
- Low-dose prednisone (7.5 mg to 10 mg) produced substantial improvement in bone pain and quality of life in an uncontrolled survey of patients with metastatic prostate cancer (Tannock, Gospodarowicz, Meakin et al., 1989).

- A survey of patients administered high doses of dexamethasone (96 mg/day for 2 weeks) for malignant epidural spinal cord compression observed pain relief in 64% within hours of the initial dose (Greenberg, Kim, Posner, 1980).
- A recent randomized trial confirmed that dexamethasone was profoundly analgesic in spinal cord compression but could not identify any difference between a high (100 mg) and low (10 mg) initial dose (Vecht, Haaxma-Reiche, van Putten et al., 1989).
- Symptoms related to bowel obstruction have been shown to respond to dexamethasone, 8 to 60 mg/day (Fainsinger, Spanchynski, Hanson et al., 1994; Reid, 1988), and methylprednisolone, 30 to 50 mg/day (Farr, 1990).

This accumulated experience establishes the analgesic potential of corticosteroid drugs in a variety of chronic pain syndromes. Differences among drugs have not been discerned, and no data exist by which to judge dose-response relationships, relative potencies among drugs, and long-term efficacy.

Corticosteroid drugs have additional indications in the palliative care setting. Numerous studies have suggested that these drugs may improve appetite, nausea, malaise, and overall quality of life (Ettinger, Portenoy, 1988; Farr, 1990; Hanks, Trueman, Twycross, 1983; Wilcox, Corr, Shaw et al., 1984).

Mechanism of action

The mechanism of analgesia produced by corticosteroids is unknown. Any of several processes may be involved. Compression of pain-sensitive structures may be relieved by reduction of peritumoral edema (Yamada, Ushio, Hayakawa et al., 1983) or, in the case of steroid-responsive neoplasms, by shrinkage of tumor masses themselves (Posner, Howieson, Cvitkovic, 1977). Activation of nociceptors may be lessened by reduced tissue concentrations of some inflammatory mediators, specifically prostaglandins and leukotrienes. Aberrant electrical activity in damaged nerves may also be tempered by these agents (Devor, Govrin-Lippman, Raber, 1985).

Adverse effects

Well-recognized adverse effects are associated with short-term and long-term administration of corticosteroids and with the withdrawal of these drugs after chronic use (Haynes, 1990; Weissman, Dufer, Vogel et al., 1987). The risk of serious toxicity increases with the dose of the drug, the duration of therapy, and predisposing factors associated with the medical condition of the patient.

Short-Term Therapy

Although acute, transitory corticosteroid therapy is usually well tolerated, the potential toxicities include adverse neuropsychologic effects, hyperglycemia, fluid retention (which can lead to hypertension or volume overload in predisposed patients), and gastrointestinal disturbances ranging from dyspepsia to bowel perforation. A recent study of a high-dose dexamethasone regimen for epidural spinal cord compression (96 mg intravenously, followed by 96 mg orally for 3 days, then a taper for 10 days) noted three cases of serious toxicity among the 27 patients randomized to the steroid therapy (11%). One patient became hypomanic, one was in a confusional state, and one had a perforated gastric ulcer (Sorensen, Helweg-Larsen, Mouridsen et al., 1994).

The neuropsychologic toxicity associated with corticosteroid therapy ranges from delirium to relatively isolated changes in mood, cognitive functioning, or perception. Mood disturbances can themselves vary from euphoria to depression. In another study of patients who received a high-dose dexamethasone regimen for epidural spinal cord compression (100 mg, followed by 24 mg every 6 hours), the overall rate of psychiatric disorders was no greater than a comparison group, but a greater incidence of major depressive disorders and a trend toward a greater incidence of delirium in the steroid-treated group was noted. Those who received steroids also had more depressive and anxious symptoms (Breitbart, Stiefel, Kornblith et al., 1993).

Although neuropsychologic toxicity is usually observed early during treatment and when relatively high doses are administered, these adverse effects can complicate any steroid regimen at any time. No association with any specific drug has been proven, and the occurrence of acute toxicity during one course of therapy does not prefigure a similar response during subsequent courses.

Long-Term Therapy

Chronic administration of a corticosteroid can produce a cushingoid appearance (moon face, buffalo hump); skin diseases and changes in subcutaneous and connective tissues; weight gain; hypertension; severe osteoporosis; myopathy; increased risk of infection; hyperglycemia; gastrointestinal toxicity; and late neuropsychologic effects (Haynes, 1990; Weissman, Dufer, Vogel et al., 1987). In the palliative care setting, however, long-term treatment with relatively low doses is generally well tolerated. A study of advanced cancer patients chronically administered prednisolone or dexamethasone at varying doses noted oropharyngeal candidiasis in approximately one third of patients and edema or cushingoid appearance in less than one fifth; dyspepsia, weight gain, neuropsychologic changes and ecchymoses occurred in 5% to 10%, and the incidence of other adverse effects, such as hyperglycemia, myopathy, and osteoporosis, was even lower (Hanks, Trueman, Twycross, 1983).

Although chronic administration of a corticosteroid has been linked to an increased risk of peptic ulcer (Messer, Reitman, Sacks et al., 1983), the evidence of this association is weak, and concern about this risk in the absence of other predisposing factors should be minimal. For example, the risk of ulceration is clearly increased further by coadministration of a corticosteroid and a nonsteroidal antiinflammatory drug (Piper, Ray, Daugherty et al., 1991). This potentiation of gastrointestinal toxicity relatively contraindicates the combined use of a corticosteroid and a nonsteriodal antiinflammatory drug in the palliative care setting. Steroid use also increases the risk of gastrointestinal perforation, even during short-term therapy (Fadul, Lemann, Thaler et al., 1988; ReMine, McIlrath, 1980). An increased risk of perforation during treatment has been associated with constipation.

Steroid withdrawal after chronic therapy can produce a syndrome of muscle and joint pain known as steroid "pseudorheumatism" (Dixon, Christy, 1980). Withdrawal may also produce other symptoms, such as malaise, headache, and mood disturbance, or a flare of the symptoms for which steroid therapy had been initiated previously.

The symptoms associated with steroid withdrawal can occur with either dose reduction or discontinuation of therapy. In some cases symptoms appear after a relatively modest decline in a relatively high baseline dose. Escalation of the steroid dose can provide relief, and a slower, more gradual taper may avoid recurrence.

Indications

Corticosteroids are used routinely as part of the medical management of epidural spinal cord compression, raised intracranial pressure, and superior vena cava syndrome. Pain may accompany each of these syndromes, and symptomatic relief is one of the goals of therapy.

On the basis of anecdotal experience, corticosteroids are also administered for many other painful syndromes, including metastatic bone pain, neuropathic pain caused by compression or infiltration of peripheral nerves or nerve plexus, painful lymphedema, pain caused by obstruction of hollow viscus, and pain caused by organ capsule distention.

In patients with advanced illness, corticosteroids are usually added to an opioid regimen after the opioid dose has been increased to dose-limiting side effects. Patients with these pain syndromes commonly have other symptoms that could potentially be improved by steroid therapy, such as nausea or malaise, and corticosteroid therapy may be considered earlier if primarily indicated by these other symptoms.

Drug selection

The relative risks and benefits of the various corticosteroids are unknown. In the United States dexamethasone (Decadron) is usually selected, a choice that gains theoretical support from the relatively low mineralocorticoid effects (less fluid and electrolyte retention). Prednisone and methylprednisolone (Medrol) have also been used.

For convenience in prescribing, many clinicians consider these equivalencies: methylprednisolone 8 mg = prednisone 10 mg = dexamethasone 2 mg.

Dose selection

On the basis of clinical experience, corticosteroids are usually administered either in a high-dose regimen or a low-dose regimen.

High-Dose Regimen

A high-dose regimen (e.g., dexamethasone, 100 mg, followed initially by 96 mg/day in divided doses) has been used for patients who experience an acute episode of severe pain that cannot be promptly reduced with opioids, such as that associated with a rapidly worsening malignant plexopathy (Ettinger, Portenoy, 1988). This dosing regimen may also be appropriate when treating an oncologic emergency that may be steroid responsive, such as superior vena cava syndrome or epidural spinal cord compression. The dose can be tapered over weeks, concurrent with the initiation of other analgesic approaches, such as radiotherapy.

Low-Dose Regimen

A low-dose corticosteroid regimen (e.g., dexamethasone, 1 to 2 mg once or twice daily) has been used for patients with advanced medical illness who continue to have pain despite optimal dosing of opioid drugs. In most cases long-term therapy is planned. Although the risks associated with prolonged steroid use in this setting are more than balanced by the need for enhanced comfort, repeated assessments are required to ensure that benefits are sustained (Needham, Daley, Lennard, 1992). Ineffective regimens should be tapered and discontinued and, in all cases, the lowest dose that yields the desired results should be sought.

Alpha₂-Adrenergic Agonists

Classification of the alpha₂-adrenergic agonists as nonspecific, multipurpose analgesics is supported by both animal (Kayser, Desmeules, Guilbaud, 1995; Puke, Wiesenfeld-Hallin, 1993) and human studies. In humans analgesic effects in diverse pain syndromes have been established in controlled studies of systemic dexmedetomidine (Aho, Erkola, Scheinin et al., 1991) and both systemic and intraspinal clonidine (Byas-Smith, Max, Muir et al., 1995; Carroll, Jadad, King et al., 1993; Eisenach, Du Pen, Bubois et al., 1995; Max, Schafer, Culnane et al., 1988; Tan, Croese, 1986). The drug dexmedetomidine is currently being developed and is not available commercially. Another alpha₂-adrenergic agonist, tizanidine, is also analgesic and was recently approved in the United States as a treatment for spasticity.

Clonidine

Thus far, clonidine is the alpha₂-adrenergic agonist used most widely in the clinical setting for treatment of pain in humans. The above reports and others suggest that clonidine can be beneficial in pain syndromes that may be relatively less opioid responsive. These include:

- Chronic headache (Boisen, Deth, Hubbe et al., 1978; Shafar, Tallett, Knowlson, 1972)
- Nonmalignant neuropathic pains, such as sympathetically maintained reflex sympathetic dystrophy, chronic low back pain, pain from arachnoiditis, and deafferentation pain after spinal injury (Byas-Smith, Max, Muir et al., 1995; Glynn, Dawson, Sanders, 1988; Glynn, Teddy, Jamous et al., 1986; Max, Schafer, Culnane et al., 1988; Petros, Wright, 1987; Rauck, Eisenach, Jackson et al., 1993; Tan, Croese, 1986; Zeigler, Lynch, Muir et al., 1992)
- Some cancer pain syndromes (including neuropathic cancer related pain) (Coombs Saunders, Fratkin et al., 1986; Coombs, Saunders, Gaylor et al., 1984; Coombs, Saunders, La Chance et al., 1985; Eisenach, Du Pen, Dubois et al., 1995).

Two recent controlled trials have greatly illuminated the role of clonidine as an analgesic. In one study patients with painful diabetic polyneuropathy received transdermal clonidine (Byas-Smith, Max, Muir et al, 1995). This trial confirmed an earlier report (Shafar, Tallett, Knowlson, 1972) in demonstrating that less than one quarter of patients are potential responders, but that those who do respond can experience analgesia that is both substantial and sustained.

The second study compared a 14-day epidural infusion of clonidine (30 μg/h) with an epidural placebo infusion in patients with cancer pain who were also receiving titrated doses of epidural morphine PCA (Eisenach, Du Pen, Dubois et al., 1995). Overall, clonidine reduced pain but not opioid consumption. Increased pain relief occurred in 45% of those who received clonidine and 21% of those who received placebo. The greatest success was achieved in those patients with neuropathic pain. Epidural clonidine resulted in reduced pain in 56% of the patients with neuropathic pain.

Thus the data provide evidence that clonidine is a multipurpose analgesic that may be particularly useful in the management of neuropathic pain. Both systemic administration (by the oral or transdermal route) and epidural administration can yield favorable effects. Although a minority (less than one quarter during systemic administration) are likely to respond, those that do can experience clinically meaningful effects.

Mechanism of action

The mechanism of clonidine analgesia has not been established and is likely to be complex (Kayser, Desmeules,

Guilbaud, 1995). Noradrenergic receptors are clearly important in the modulation of nociceptive processing, and it is possible that interaction with alpha$_2$- receptors in the spinal cord (Puke, Wiesenfeld-Hallin, 1993; Yaksh, 1985) or brain stem (Sagan, Proudfit, 1985) activates endogenous systems that reduce nociceptive input to the central nervous system. Presumably, these systems may be relatively more or less involved in the processing of different types of noxious stimuli (Kayser, Desmeules, Guilbaud, 1995) or the development of different types of pain syndromes.

It is also possible that clonidine produces analgesia in some cases through interference with the mechanisms that perpetuate so-called sympathetically maintained pain, a subtype of neuropathic pain (more specifically, usually a subtype of reflex sympathetic dystrophy or causalgia) (Rauck, Eisenach, Jackson et al., 1993). Clonidine may reduce sympathetic tone and, in this way, ameliorate pains that are sustained, at least in part, by circulating catecholamines or efferent activity in the sympathetic nervous system.

Adverse effects

In placebo-controlled trials the most common adverse effects associated with systemic or epidural clonidine administration have been sedation, hypotension (usually orthostatic), and dry mouth (Byas-Smith, Max, Muir et al., 1995; Eisenach, Du Pen, Dubois et al., 1995). In patients without severe concurrent medical illness, the major toxicity produced by clonidine is usually sedation. The medical frailty of palliative care patients may increase this risk. The controlled trial of epidural clonidine in cancer pain demonstrated that the drug produced sustained hypotensive effects in almost one half of the patients, but was considered serious in only two patients (Eisenach, Du Pen, Dubois et al, 1995). However, for most patients hypotension was mild and the sedation transient.

Indications

Like other multipurpose analgesics, clonidine can be considered for a therapeutic trial in any chronic pain state. In patients with advanced illnesses, clonidine use is typically limited to patients with neuropathic pains that are not satisfactorily relieved with appropriate titration of opioids and also have not responded to other adjuvant analgesics, such as the antidepressants, oral local anesthetics, and anticonvulsants. Because of the potential for adverse effects, ideal candidates for treatment of neuropathic pain with clonidine are those patients who are hemodynamically stable, not predisposed to serious hypotension, and not markedly somnolent from other causes.

Routes

Although evidence is strong that intraspinal clonidine is an effective therapy for some patients with refractory pain, this route of administration is not readily available in all settings. Hence, treatment trials generally proceed using the oral or transdermal route. Currently, no evidence exists that one of these routes is better than the other for chronic pain, and the choice is usually made on the basis of patient preference.

Clinical experience with epidural clonidine for chronic pain is limited. Preliminary suggestions for patient selection, dosing, and monitoring are provided in Box 7.2.

Dose selection

To limit the risk of adverse effects, starting doses should be low (e.g., 0.1 mg orally per day). If doses lower than those commercially available are desirable, the transdermal system can be cut into pieces without change in its delivery properties.

Monitoring of both pain and adverse effects is necessary during gradual dose escalation. An analgesic ceiling dose has not been determined for systemic clonidine therapy. Consequently, gradual dose escalation should continue until significant side effects occur or blood pressure declines to a degree that is worrisome. Doses are typically increased by 0.1 mg/day at intervals of at least a few days. Anecdotally, some patients have benefited from relatively high doses (as high as 2 mg/day in rare cases), and it is reasonable to continue upward dose titration until dose-limiting toxicity is encountered.

Other Drugs With Nonspecific Analgesic Effects

Substantial evidence supports the analgesic effects of psychostimulant drugs in a variety of both acute and chronic pains. The psychostimulants include dextroamphetamine (Dexedrine), methylphenidate (Ritalin), and caffeine. With the exception of caffeine, which is a constituent of many proprietary analgesic products, these drugs are generally used only when pain is accompanied by another target symptom such as sedation.

Dextroamphetamine and Methylphenidate

Research has established the analgesia of dextroamphetamine in postoperative pain (Forrest, Brown, Brown et al., 1977) and methylphenidate in pain associated with Parkinson's disease (Cantello, Aguggia, Gillig et al., 1988) and cancer (Bruera, Chadwick, Brenneis et al., 1987). In addition to providing analgesia, controlled trials of methylphenidate in the cancer population have established that this drug can reduce opioid-induced sedation and cognitive impairment (Bruera, Chadwick, Brenneis et al., 1987; Bruera, Miller, Macmillan et al, 1992). Both dextroamphetamine and methylphenidate stimulate the medullary respiratory center and lessen the degree of central depression caused by various drugs, including opioids. They have been widely used to reverse opioid-induced somnolence.

BOX 7.2

GUIDELINES

EPIDURAL CLONIDINE FOR CHRONIC PAIN

Patient Screening
- Inadequate pain relief after conservative management has been optimized.
- Baseline orthostatic blood pressure is considered acceptable.

Initiating Therapy
- Consider initiating therapy in the inpatient setting if patient has severe pain, significant side effects or orthostasis.
- Obtain baseline orthostatic blood pressure before initiating therapy.
- Plan to hydrate patient with 1 to 2 L of IV fluids if blood pressure decreases >20% after initiation of therapy; consider hydration if blood pressure decreases 10% to 20%.
- Volume of epidural clonidine infusion is based on location of pathologic condition and tip of epidural catheter. Most common concentration is 10 μg/ml at 2 to 5 ml/h; however, very high concentrations at very low infusion rates also have been used (e.g., 100 μg/ml at 0.2 to 0.5 ml/h).
- Typical epidural clonidine starting dose is 20 μg/h by continuous infusion.
- Check orthostatic blood pressure and heart rate q4h × 2, then q8h × 24 h.

Continuing Care
- Monitor pain intensity regularly (e.g., q shift or q home visit).
- Monitor orthostatic blood pressure regularly (e.g., q shift or q home visit).
- Establish a system for addressing unrelieved pain, e.g., for pain rating of 4/10 to 6/10 with stable blood pressure, increase clonidine dose (continuous infusion rate) by 5% to 10%; for pain rating >6/10 with stable blood pressure, increase clonidine dose by 10% to 20%.
- Manage blood pressure changes, e.g., for significantly decreased blood pressure or >20% decrease in orthostatic blood pressure (when patient is raised from a flat position), maximize oral fluid intake; consider initiating fludrocortisone acetate (Florinef) 0.1 mg qd to tid.
- Manage unresolved symptomatic orthostasis or signs of excessive sedation or confusion, e.g., decrease clonidine dose by 50% and reevaluate within 24 h. Add epidural or systemic opioid to control pain.
- Never abruptly discontinue epidural clonidine because this can cause life-threatening rebound hypertension. To discontinue epidural clonidine, titrate dose downward in a stepwise fashion (e.g., 30% to 50% per 24-h period). Consider using transdermal clonidine during downward titration in patients with preexisting hypertension condition.

May be duplicated for use in clinical practice. As appears in McCaffery M, Pasero C: *Pain: Clinical manual*, p. 315, 1999, Mosby, Inc.

h, hour; *L*, liter; *tid*, three times daily; *q*, every; *qd*, daily.

Modified from DuPen S: Swedish Hospital Pain Management Service, Seattle, WA, 1997.

In the care of terminally ill patients the management of central nervous system side effects is an important issue. Accordingly, the practical use of psychostimulants in the palliative care setting has focused on this indication rather than the treatment of unrelieved pain.

Dextroamphetamine has been used to treat numerous conditions, including obesity, depression, narcolepsy, and attention-deficit hyperactivity disorder (Hoffman, Lefkowitz, 1996). When dextroamphetamine is considered for relieving pain or for counteracting opioid-induced sedation, the advantages and disadvantages of its other effects must also be evaluated. Other beneficial effects may include a decreased sense of fatigue, mood elevation (antidepressant effect), increased alertness and wakefulness, improved performance of simple mental tasks, and increased ability to concentrate. Problematic effects may include insomnia, anorexia, tremulousness, anxiety, agitation, and uncomfortable cognitive changes. The effects of methylphenidate are similar, but it is a milder CNS stimulant than dextroamphetamine.

Treatment with methylphenidate or dextroamphetamine is typically begun at 2.5 to 5 mg in the morning and again at midday, if necessary, to maintain effects throughout the day. The second dose is usually needed. Obviously, to avoid insomnia, doses later in the day are not advised. Doses are increased gradually until efficacy is established. Oral doses may be increased by 50% each day. Although few patients require more than 40 mg/day in divided doses, occasional patients benefit from higher doses. Some patients require dose escalation later in the course of therapy (Bruera, Miller, Macmillan et al., 1992).

The psychostimulants are usually well tolerated if they are titrated carefully. A survey of 50 patients treated with methylphenidate observed early toxicity in only two patients (hallucinations and a paranoid reaction, respectively) and no late toxicity (Bruera, Brenneis, Paterson et al., 1989).

There has been some anecdotal experience with a related compound, pemoline (Cylert). This drug has relatively minor sympathomimetic effects and is available in a chewable tablet, characteristics that may increase its usefulness. However, pemoline has recently been associated with a rare hepatopathy, which has been fatal in three cases (Berkovitch, Pope, Phillips et al., 1995), and this suggests that pemoline should be considered a second-line psychostimulant adjuvant in the medically ill.

Caffeine

Research has established the analgesia of caffeine in headache, sore throat, and oral surgery pain (Forbes, Beaver, Jones et al., 1991; Laska, Sunshine, Mueller et al., 1984; Sawynok, 1995; Schachtel, Fillingim, Lane et al., 1991; Ward, Whitney, Avery et al., 1991). Caffeine is widely available in both medications and food items, particularly coffee and tea. One well-controlled study of

53 patients with nonmigrainous headaches showed that caffeine has an analgesic effect that is independent of its ability to enhance nonopioid analgesia (Ward, Whitney, Avery et al., 1991). However, caffeine doses of either 65 or 130 mg orally provided only modest analgesia, less than that of acetaminophen, 648 mg. When a nonopioid is combined with caffeine, analgesia is enhanced. In six studies totaling 2400 patients with moderate to severe headache pain, caffeine-containing analgesics were significantly superior to placebo and to 1000 mg acetaminophen (Migliardi, Armenia, Freedman et al., 1994). A double-blind study comparing a combination of caffeine and ibuprofen with plain ibuprofen for relief of postoperative dental pain showed that ibuprofen, 100 mg or 200 mg, with 100 mg caffeine was more than twice as effective as ibuprofen alone (Forbes, Beaver, Jones et al., 1991).

Research has not confirmed the optimal dose of caffeine for increasing the analgesia of nonopioids, but the minimal effective dose appears to be 65 mg. A reasonable suggestion is 50 to 150 mg of caffeine per dose of nonopioid. This amount seems well tolerated by most adults (Beaver, 1984). Over-the-counter analgesic formulations containing caffeine and dietary sources of caffeine are discussed in detail in Chapter 5 on acetaminophen and NSAIDs.

Despite negative publicity about caffeine as a food additive, it is generally a safe drug (Laska, Sunshine, Mueller et al, 1984). Most research confirms that small doses of caffeine (e.g., 200 mg or less in normal subjects and in cardiac subjects) do not significantly affect heart rate, blood pressure, or cardiac rhythm (Schneider, 1987). However, allowance should be made for the possibility that caffeine users and nonusers react differently.

Cocaine

Studies of the analgesic effect of cocaine are limited, but historically it has been used for the relief of a variety of types of pain. In the early 1900s, cocaine was applied intranasally in a popular technique known as sphenopalatine ganglion nerve block, which was thought to be effective in a wide variety of painful disorders (Racz, Morton, Diede, 1996).

Several studies have suggested that intranasal cocaine produces analgesia (Marbach, Wallenstein, 1988; Yang, Clark, Dooley et al., 1982). In one study that used the intranasal route, the dose of cocaine was considerably higher, up to approximately 288 mg, than that used orally. At this dose, unequivocal relief of deafferentation neuralgia and myofascial facial pain occurred. Interestingly, a dose of "street" cocaine is estimated to be >1.5 mg/kg, 105 mg for a 70 kg adult (Van Dyke, Barash, Jatlow et al., 1976).

Although no adequate clinical trials have confirmed the efficacy of intranasal cocaine, this technique continues to be used today. It remains a controversial approach.

One method is to apply cocaine topically to the ganglion, which is located in the posterior nasal passage.

Cocaine was also common during the 1970s in the United States as an ingredient in Brompton's cocktail, a popular liquid analgesic mixture used for pain relief in the hospice setting. Brompton's cocktail included cocaine and an opioid such as heroin or morphine, along with varied ingredients such as an antiemetic. Some claimed that the cocaine enhanced analgesia, whereas others believed that its benefit was as a local anesthetic for the throat or as a stimulant to offset opioid-induced sedation. However, the doses of cocaine commonly used in Brompton's cocktail have not demonstrated analgesic effects. For example, in a study of postoperative patients and those with chronic cancer pain, 10 mg of oral cocaine did not produce pain relief (Kaiko, Kanner, Foley et al., 1987). A 10 mg dose of oral cocaine is considered a small dose, and it may be that higher oral doses are required for analgesia. The popularity of Brompton's cocktail faded as research revealed it to be devoid of any magic, and it has been replaced by single entity drugs such as plain oral morphine.

Indications

Psychostimulants are not widely used for their analgesic effect, probably because of their association with abuse and the likelihood that tolerance will develop rapidly. Current clinical use as analgesics is usually limited to situations when analgesia is secondary to usefulness in decreasing opioid-induced side effects, such as sedation.

Other possible multipurpose analgesics

Following are drugs discussed later in the text in relation to their use for specific pain problems. However, they are probably multipurpose adjuvant analgesics, although of limited usefulness currently.

- Systemic (oral or parenteral) local anesthetics: Many clinical series and controlled studies establish the analgesic potential of systemically administered local anesthetic drugs in patients with acute pain and various chronic pain syndromes (Backonja, 1994a,b; Glazer, Portenoy, 1991). Although the possibility of benefit in such diverse pains suggests that these drugs are multipurpose analgesics, both the controlled trials and a large clinical experience has focused on their use in the management of neuropathic pains.
- Neuroleptics: Except for methotrimeprazine (Levoprome), little evidence exists that neuroleptics are useful analgesics. However, studies of methotrimeprazine have shown that it is analgesic in patients with cancer pain, neuropathic pain, and acute pain (Beaver, Wallenstein, Houde et al., 1996; Bloomfield, Simard-Savoie, Bernier et al., 1964; Davidson, Lindenberg, Walsh, 1979; Lasagna,

DeKornfeld, 1961; Montilla, Frederick, Cass, 1963). The usefulness of this drug is limited because of its side effects, particularly sedation and hypotension.

- NMDA receptor blockers: At present, interest in *N*-methyl-D-aspartate (NMDA) receptor antagonists (specifically, dextromethorphan and ketamine) is focused on their use as new therapies for neuropathic pain. In addition, evidence shows that they may be multipurpose analgesics that could potentially ameliorate acute pain (Jahangir, Islam, Aziz, 1993) and diverse types of chronic pain (Cherry, Plummer, Gourlay et al., 1995; Mathisen, Skjelbred, Skoglund et al., 1995; Persson, Axelsson, Hallin et al., 1995; Stannard, Porter, 1993). New NMDA receptor antagonists are being developed and may ultimately prove useful for a variety of painful conditions.

ADJUVANT ANALGESICS FOR CHRONIC CONTINUOUS NEUROPATHIC PAIN

Continuous dysesthesias are often described by patients as continuous burning, electrical, or other abnormal sensations.

Antidepressants

Antidepressant analgesics are a first-line approach for this neuropathic pain syndrome. Antidepressants have already been discussed as multipurpose adjuvant analgesics. Systemic local anesthetics (oral or parenteral) are more appropriately considered second-line drugs for continuous neuropathic pain. Many other drugs may also be administered for continuous neuropathic pain (Table 7.4).

Oral and Parenteral (Systemic) Local Anesthetics

In pain management local anesthetics are used in three major ways:

1. For localized anesthesia by injection into tissues or near major nerves (nerve blocks), or intraspinal administration
2. For localized analgesia by absorption of a topical application (e.g., lidocaine patch or eutetic mixture of local anesthetics [EMLA]). EMLA produces analgesia or anesthesia, depending on the dose absorbed.
3. For generalized analgesia by systemic administration (oral or parenteral)

In this section the focus is on the systemic administration of local anesthetics for their general analgesic effects in the treatment of chronic pain.

Research and clinical experience have established the analgesic potential of systemic local anesthetic therapy. Diverse types of pain can potentially respond. Controlled trials have emphasized the value of this therapy in neuropathic pain, and this is the use that has been pursued in clinical practice.

However, information is limited about long-term safety and effectiveness of local anesthetics. Consequently, these drugs are considered second-line approaches for continuous neuropathic pain. Specifically, a trial with an oral local anesthetic is warranted in patients with continuous dysesthesias, such as burning pain, who do not respond adequately to antidepressants or who cannot tolerate them.

Surveys suggest that a brief intravenous infusion of lidocaine or procaine can be effective in a variety of chronic pains and that analgesia may continue for a prolonged period after the infusion. Types of pain that have responded favorably to brief intravenous infusions include neuropathic pains, arthritis, adiposis dolorosa, musculoskeletal pains, poststroke pain, and headache (Arner, Lindblom, Meyerson et al., 1990; Atkinson, 1982; Boas, Covino, Shahnarian, 1982; Edmondson, Simpson, Stubler et al., 1993; Edwards, Habib, Burney et al., 1985; Galer, Miller, Rowbotham, 1993; Graubard, Kovacs. Ritter, 1948; Iwane, Masanori, Matsuki et al., 1976; Juhlin, 1986; Marton, Spitzer, Steinbrocker, 1949; Petersen, Kastrup, 1987; Petersen, Kastrup, Zeeburg et al., 1986; Rosner, 1984). A single-blind, placebo-controlled trial suggested

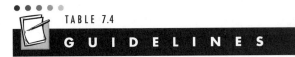

TABLE 7.4

G U I D E L I N E S

ADJUVANT ANALGESICS FOR CONTINUOUS NEUROPATHIC PAIN (CONTINUOUS DYSESTHESIAS)

Class	Examples
Usually Tried First	
Antidepressants	Amitriptyline, desipramine (See Table 7.3 for other examples)
Systemic local anesthetics	Mexiletine, tocainide, flecainide
Gabapentin	
For Refractory Cases	
Alpha$_2$-adrenergic agonists	Clonidine
Anticonvulsants	Carbamazepine, phenytoin, valproate, clonazepam
Topical agents	Capsaicin, local anesthetics
Neuroleptics	Prochlorperazine, haloperidol
NMDA receptor antagonists	Dextromethorphan, ketamine
Calcitonin	
Baclofen	

that intravenous lidocaine can relieve migraine but not tension headache (Maciewicz, Chung, Strassman et al., 1988), and another similarly designed trial suggested benefit from this therapy in central pain (Backonja, Gombar, 1992).

Other well-controlled studies yield conflicting results. Intravenous lidocaine has been effective in reducing the pain of postherpetic neuralgia (Rowbotham, Reisner-Kelelr, Fields, 1991) and painful diabetic neuropathy (Kastrup, Petersen, Dejgard et al., 1987). However, some research suggests IV lidocaine does not relieve neuropathic cancer pain (Elleman, Sjogren, Banning et al., 1989). Failure to achieve analgesia in this and another controlled study of patients with neuropathic cancer pain may have been due to low plasma lidocaine concentrations that were not measured (Bruera, Ripamonti, Brenneis et al., 1992; Tanelian, Victory, 1995). Anecdotally, long-term subcutaneous administration of lidocaine has been reported to yield sustained relief of refractory neuropathic pain in cancer patients (Brose, Cousins, 1991).

Oral formulations of local anesthetics (flecainide, tocainide, and mexilitine) have increased the availability of long-term systemic local anesthetic therapy. A survey of cancer patients suggested that flecainide can be effective in the treatment of pain caused by tumor infiltration of nerves (Dunlop, Davies, Hockley et al., 1989). In controlled trials tocainide was effective for trigeminal neuralgia (Lindstrom, Lindblom, 1987) and mexiletine lessened the pain of diabetic neuropathy (Dejgard, Petersen, Kastrup, 1988). Mexiletine has also been reported anecdotally to provide sustained pain relief for some patients with poststroke pain (Edmondson, Simpson, Stubler et al., 1993).

No systematic evaluation has been done of the safety or efficacy of the combination of an oral local anesthetic and other adjuvant drugs, such as a tricyclic antidepressant or anticonvulsant. On the basis of clinical experience, trials of such combinations, undertaken with close clinical monitoring, can be justified in patients with refractory neuropathic pain. If administration with one of these adjuvant analgesics yields meaningful partial analgesia, it should be continued as a trial with another drug initiated. If a risk of drug interaction or additive toxicities exists, dosing must be very cautious and monitoring must be intensified.

Mechanism of action

It is well known that local anesthetic drugs block sodium channels and thereby impose a nondepolarizing conduction block of the action potential, as shown in Figure 7.2 (Covino, 1993). A profound conduction block (localized anesthesia) can be produced in peripheral axons after the local instillation of these drugs. This type of peripheral effect, however, does not explain the analgesia produced by systemic administration

of these drugs. Nontoxic systemic doses of local anesthetics do not block the peripheral action potential, although amplitudes are decreased to a degree (deJong, Nace, 1968).

Studies of experimental models have revealed that systemic administration of local anesthetic drugs suppresses the activity of dorsal horn neurons that are activated by C fiber input (Woolf, Wiesenfeld-Halli, 1985) and the spontaneous firing of neuromas and dorsal root ganglion cells (Chabal, Russell, Burchiel, 1989; Devor, Wall, Catalan, 1992). Thus systemic local anesthetic drugs probably produce analgesic effects in neuropathic pain states through suppression of aberrant electrical activity or hypersensitivity in neural structures involved in causing the pain. These may include sensitized central neurons, neuroma associated with damaged peripheral axons, or both.

Adverse effects

The major dose-dependent toxicities associated with the local anesthetics affect the central nervous system and the cardiovascular system. The central nervous system effects generally occur at a lower concentration than cardiac changes. Dizziness, perioral numbness (numbness surrounding the mouth), other paresthesias (abnormal sensations), and tremor usually occur first. At higher plasma concentrations, progressive encephalopathy develops and seizures may occur (Covino, 1993). Toxic concentrations of local anesthetic drugs can also produce cardiac conduction disturbances and myocardial depression (Covino, 1993).

Thus all local anesthetics share a spectrum of serious, dose-dependent adverse effects, the existence of which mandates caution in dose selection and titration. Although variability across drugs in the propensity to produce these effects may be clinically relevant, comparative trials of systemically administered local anesthetic drugs have not been performed.

All local anesthetic drugs must be used cautiously in patients with preexisting heart disease. It is prudent to avoid this therapy in those patients with cardiac rhythm disturbances, those who are receiving antiarrhythmic drugs, and those who have cardiac insufficiency. Patients who have significant heart disease should undergo cardiologic evaluation before local anesthetic therapy is administered.

Long-term systemic treatment with a local anesthetic is usually accomplished with one of the oral formulations, mexiletine, tocainide, or flecainide. Mexiletine has been preferred in the United States.

Troublesome side effects occur commonly during therapy with mexiletine or tocainide (Kreeger, Hammill, 1987). A survey of patients administered tocainide for arrhythmia noted nausea in 34%, dizziness in 31%, light-headedness in 24%, tremors in 22%, palpitations in 17%, vomiting in 16%, and paresthesias in 16% (Horn,

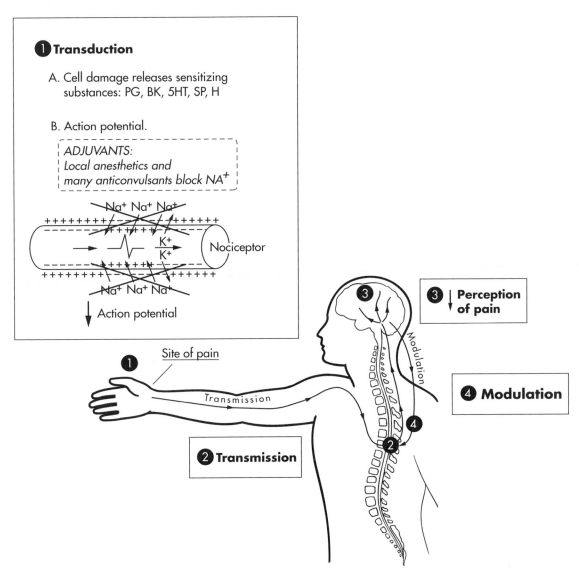

① Transduction

A. Cell damage releases sensitizing substances: PG, BK, 5HT, SP, H

B. Action potential.

ADJUVANTS:
Local anesthetics and many anticonvulsants block NA+

Na+ Na+ Na+

K^+
K^+

Nociceptor

Na+ Na+ Na+

↓ Action potential

① Site of pain

Transmission

② Transmission

③ Perception of pain

Modulation

④ Modulation

May be duplicated for use in clinical practice. As appears in McCaffery M, Pasero C: *Pain: Clinical manual,* p. 319, 1999, Mosby, Inc.

● ● ● ● ●
F I G U R E 7.2   Analgesic action site for local anesthetics and anticonvulsants. This figure is adapted from Figure 4.2 *A* and *B,* pages 106-107, which the reader may return to for further details.

Key:

❶ **Transduction:** Conversion of one energy form to another. This process occurs in the periphery when a noxious stimulus causes tissue damage. **A,** Sensitizing substances are released by damaged cells. **B,** An action potential results from release of the sensitizing substances (nociceptive pain) and a change in the charge along the neuronal membrane or abnormal processing of stimuli by the nervous system (neuropathic pain) and a change in the charge along the neuronal membrane.

The change in charge occurs when Na+ moves into the cell and other ion transfers occur.

Local anesthetics and many anticonvulsants reduce pain by blocking Na+, thereby decreasing the action potential. The mechanism underlying the analgesia of systemically administered (oral or parenteral) local anesthetics cannot, however, be explained by this mechanism.

❷ **Transmission:** The action potential continues from the site of damage to the spinal cord and ascends to higher centers. Transmission may be considered in three phases: injury site to spinal cord, spinal cord to brain stem and thalamus, and thalamus to cortex.

❸ **Perception of pain:** Conscious experience of pain.

❹ **Modulation:** Inhibition of nociceptive impulses. Neurons originating in the brain stem descend to the spinal cord and release substances such as endogenous opioids, serotonin (5HT), and norepinephrine (NE) that inhibit the transmission of nociceptive impulses.

Hadidian, Johnson et al., 1980). Serious but rare reactions include interstitial pneumonitis, severe encephalopathy, blood dyscrasia, hepatitis, and dermatologic reactions (Horn, Hadidina, Johnson et al., 1980; Kreeger, Hammill, 1987; Stein, Demarco, Gamsu et al., 1988; Vincent, Vincent, 1985).

Mexiletine often produces nausea and vomiting (diminished by ingesting the drug with food), tremor, dizziness, unsteadiness, and paresthesias, which may induce discontinuation of dosing in up to 40% (Campbell, 1987; Kreeger, Hammill, 1987). Serious side effects, including liver damage and blood dyscrasias, are very rare.

Indications

Data from controlled trials and clinical experience suggest that any one of a variety of chronic pains can be considered a potential indication for systemic local anesthetic therapy. A survey of patients treated with a brief lidocaine infusion found that neuropathic pains related to disorders of the peripheral nervous system are more likely to respond than pains related to central nervous system lesions, but some patients with central pain do attain at least partial relief (Galer, Miller, Rowbotham, 1993). Both continuous and lancinating dysesthesias can be ameliorated (Dejgard, Petersen Kastrup, 1988; Lindstrom, Lindblom, 1987).

In the palliative care setting the oral local anesthetic drugs are usually considered for the long-term management of opioid-refractory neuropathic pain. No comparative clinical trials have helped define the appropriate use of these drugs in relation to the many other adjuvant analgesics that may be used for this indication. On the basis of the limited data available concerning long-term safety and efficacy, it is appropriate to position the local anesthetics as second-line drugs for neuropathic pain. Specifically, a trial with an oral local anesthetic is warranted in patients with continuous dysesthesias who fail to respond adequately or who cannot tolerate other adjuvant analgesics, including the antidepressant analgesics and perhaps gabapentin, and in patients with lancinating pains who have been refractory to trials of anticonvulsant drugs or baclofen (see below).

The role of brief intravenous local anesthetic infusions is even less well defined. Some patients experience immediate analgesia with this technique, and in certain patients favorable effects may continue for some period of time after the infusion (Kastrup, Petersen, Dejgard et al., 1987). Furthermore, brief intravenous infusion may also be helpful in predicting response to oral local anesthetics. In a controlled study of nine patients with chronic neuropathic pain of peripheral origin, intravenous lidocaine infusions of 2 and 5 mg/kg over 45 minutes correlated with subsequent responses to a 4-week trial of oral mexiletine (Galer, Harle, Rowbotham, 1996). However, if the intravenous infusion fails to provide pain relief, a trial of oral therapy is still appropriate.

On the basis of clinical experience, a trial of a brief local anesthetic infusion is sometimes implemented in patients with severe neuropathic pain that has not responded promptly to an opioid and requires immediate relief. This technique, therefore, may be a useful approach to the uncommon circumstance of "crescendo" neuropathic pain (see pp. 335-340 for further discussion).

Drug selection

On theoretical grounds (less potency at the sodium channel) mexiletine may be the oral local anesthetic least likely to produce serious toxicity. Although intraindividual variability in the response to different drugs in this class has not been systematically assessed, such variability has been observed commonly with other drug classes and is likely to exist with the oral local anesthetics as well. Thus if mexiletine does not provide relief to a patient with severe neuropathic pain that has already proved refractory to opioids and other adjuvants, trials with tocainide or flecainide are justified.

With regard to brief intravenous infusions, no controlled comparisons of the analgesic effects of the various parenteral anesthetics have been made. The published experience is greatest with procaine and lidocaine, and it is reasonable to consider these drugs first.

Dose selection

Low initial doses followed with titration may reduce the likelihood of adverse effects. In the absence of contrary information, overall dosing levels should conform to those used in the treatment of cardiac arrhythmias. For example, mexiletine usually should be started at 150 mg once or twice per day. Doses are better tolerated when taken with food. If intolerable side effects do not occur, the dose can be increased by a like amount every few days until the usual maximum dose of 300 mg three times per day is reached. Plasma drug concentrations, if available, can provide information like that described previously for the tricyclic antidepressants.

Dosing guidelines for parenteral infusions of local anesthetics are derived from the large clinical experience with this approach and a limited number of trials in patients with neuropathic pain. Lidocaine infusions have been administered at varying doses, typically within a range of 2 to 5 mg/kg infused over 20 to 30 minutes. (Backonja, 1994a). In the medically frail patient it may be prudent to start even lower, for example, 0.5 mg/kg over 20 to 30 minutes. Central neuropathic pain may require larger doses of intravenous lidocaine than does peripheral neuropathic pain (Backonja, 1994a; Backonja, Gombar, 1992; Galer, Miller, Rowbotham, 1993). In all cases gradual dose escalation through repeated brief infusions should be considered if treatment initially fails (Ferrante, Paggioli, Cherukuri et al., 1996).

Other drugs are also tried for continuous neuropathic pain. Once a pain syndrome has been shown to be refractory to the drugs used conventionally for continuous neuropathic pain, it is common to undertake trials of drugs conventionally used first to treat lancinating pain, such as anticonvulsants. As an example, gabapentin has been used for numerous types of neuropathic pain.

ADJUVANT ANALGESICS FOR CHRONIC LANCINATING ("SHOOTING") NEUROPATHIC PAIN

Lancinating neuropathic pain is usually described by patients as sharp, shooting, stabbing, knifelike, and often sudden in onset. Anticonvulsants and baclofen, a γ-aminobutyric acid (GABA) agonist, are first-line analgesics for this type of pain. Anticonvulsants may be effective analgesics for other types of neuropathic pain, but baclofen is generally considered to be useful only in the treatment of lancinating or paroxysmal neuropathic pain. Other adjuvants are also useful for lancinating types of pain (Table 7.5).

Anticonvulsant Drugs

A systematic review of randomized controlled studies of anticonvulsants for pain management between 1966 and 1994 yielded 20 eligible publications (McQuay, Carroll, Jadad et al., 1995). Various anticonvulsants were effective for diabetic neuropathy and trigeminal neuralgia and for the prophylaxis of migraine. The superiority of one anticonvulsant over another was not evident because no study compared one anticonvulsant with another.

The clinical impression is that anticonvulsants are effective for neuropathic pain, especially pain that is lancinating, and there is good evidence for this (Swerdlow, 1984; Swerdlow, Cundill, 1981). Clinical experience also suggests that these agents may be useful in patients with other types of episodic neuropathic pains (particularly those that have paroxysmal onset) and in occasional patients with continuous neuropathic pain.

Overview of specific anticonvulsants

Following is a list of anticonvulsants along with types of pain for which they have been shown to be effective.

Carbamazepine (Tegretol)

The efficacy of carbamazepine in the treatment of neuropathic pain was suggested in numerous uncontrolled trials (Dunsker, Mayfield, 1976; Ekbom, 1972; Elliot, Little, Milbrandt, 1976; Espir, Millac, 1970; Gerson, Jones, Luscombe, 1977; Hatangdi, Boas, Richards, 1976; Martin, 1980; Mullan, 1973; Raskin, Levinson, Hoffman et al., 1974; Swerdlow, Cundill, 1981; Taylor, Brauer, Espir, 1980; Taylor, Gray, Bicknell et al., 1977; Tomson, Bertilsson, 1984).

Controlled studies have shown that carbamazepine is effective in the following varied neuropathic pains, suggesting that the drug has analgesic efficacy in lancinating neuropathic pain, regardless of the specific pathologic condition that induces it:

- Trigeminal neuralgia (Campbell, Graham, Zilkha, 1966; Killian, Fromm, 1968; Nicol, 1969; Rockliff, Davis, 1966)
- Postherpetic neuralgia (in which an effect against lancinating but not continuous pain was demonstrated) (Killian, Fromm, 1968)
- Painful diabetic neuropathy (Rull, Quibrera, Gonzalez-Millan et al., 1969)
- Glossopharyngeal neuralgia (Taylor, Gray, Bicknell et al., 1977)

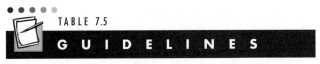

TABLE 7.5

GUIDELINES

ADJUVANT ANALGESICS TYPICALLY SELECTED FOR NEUROPATHIC PAIN WITH PREDOMINATING LANCINATING ("SHOOTING") OR PAROXYSMAL (SUDDEN ONSET) DYSESTHESIAS

Class	Examples
Usually Tried First	
Anticonvulsants	Carbamazepine, phenytoin, gabapentin, valproate, clonazepam
Baclofen	
For Refractory Cases	
Oral local anesthetics	Mexiletine, tocainide, flecainide
Tricyclic antidepressants	See Table 7.3
"Newer" antidepressants	See Table 7.3
Neuroleptics	Pimozide
Alpha$_2$-adrenergic agonists	Clonidine
Topical agents	Capsaicin, local anesthetics
NMDA receptor antagonists	Dextromethorphan, ketamine
Calcitonin	

May be duplicated for use in clinical practice. From McCaffery M, Pasero C: *Pain: Clinical manual*, p. 321. Copyright © 1999, Mosby, Inc.

- Tabetic lightning pains (Ekbom, 1972)
- Paroxysmal pain in multiple sclerosis (Espir, Millac, 1970)
- Postsympathectomy pain (Raskin, Levinson, Hoffman et al., 1974)
- So-called flashing dysesthesias in spinal cord injuries (Dunsker, Mayfield, 1976)
- Stabbing pains after laminectomy (Martin, 1980)
- Lancinating pains caused by cancer (Mullan, 1973)
- Phantom limb pain (Elliot, Little, Milbrandt, 1976)

Phenytoin (Dilantin)

In controlled trials phenytoin has been shown to be an effective analgesic for the following, all of which are characterized by a prominent lancinating component:
- Painful neuropathy in Fabry's disease (Lockman, Hunninghake, Drivit et al., 1973)
- Painful diabetic neuropathy (Chadda, Mathur, 1978).

Surveys and case reports also suggest that phenytoin is effective in:
- Trigeminal neuralgia (Braham, Saia, 1960; Ianmore, Baker, Morrell, 1958)
- Diabetic neuropathy (Ellenberg, 1968)
- Glossopharyngeal neuralgia (Taylor, Gray, Bicknell et al., 1977)
- Tabetic lightning pains (Green, 1961)

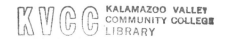

- Paroxysmal pain in postherpetic neuralgia (Hallag, Harris, 1968; Hatangdi, Boas, Richards, 1976)
- Central pain (Cantor, 1972)
- Postsympathectomy pain (Raskin, Levinson, Hoffman et al., 1974)
- Crescendo pelvic cancer–related pain with lancinating quality (Chang, 1997)

Gabapentin (Neurontin)

No double-blind placebo-controlled trials have been published regarding the effectiveness of gabapentin with neuropathic pain. However, case reports and patient surveys have suggested that gabapentin is effective in the following:
- Reflex sympathetic dystrophy (Mellick, Mellick, 1995)
- Deafferentation neuropathy of the face (Rosner, Rubin, Kestenbaum, 1996)
- HIV-related neuropathy (Rosner, Rubin, Kestenbaum, 1996)
- Mixed sympathetically maintained and sympathetically independent pain (Rosner, Rubin, Kestenbaum, 1996)
- Postherpetic neuralgia (Rosenberg, Harrell, Ristic et al., 1997; Rosner, Rubin, Kestenbaum, 1996; Segal, Rordorf, 1996)
- A variety of neuropathic pains (Benson, Parris, Cooper et al., 1996; Filadora, Sist, Patel et al., 1996; Saeger, 1996)

Clonazepam (Klonopin)

Clonazepam was reported to be effective for:
- Trigeminal neuralgia (Caccia, 1975)
- Paroxysmal postlaminectomy pain (Martin, 1981)
- Posttraumatic neuralgia (Swerdlow, Cundill, 1981).
- Lancinating phantom limb pain (Bartusch, Sanders, D'Alessio et al., 1996)

Valproic Acid (Depakene)

Valproate was beneficial for:
- Trigeminal neuralgia (Peiris, Perera, Devendra et al., 1980)
- Postherpetic neuralgia (Raftery, 1979)

Other Anticonvulsants

Lamotrigine was effective in reducing hyperalgesia in an animal model (Nakamura-Craig, Follenfant, 1994); it has yet to be described as an analgesic in humans. Felbamate has been used anecdotally to treat hemifacial spasm (Mellick, 1995), a painless syndrome characterized by paroxysmal contraction of facial muscles. Although this observation and anecdotal treatment of a small number of patients initially raised expectations, no follow-up studies of this drug have been done, and its recently recognized potential for lethal aplastic anemia has tempered enthusiasm.

Summary

Selected anticonvulsant drugs can relieve some types of dysesthesias in diverse neuropathic pain syndromes. The evidence of this effect is best for carbamazepine, but published reports and clinical experience suggest that phenytoin, clonazepam, and valproate may have similar effects. Newer anticonvulsants, particularly gabapentin, also have analgesic potential in neuropathic pain, but as yet experience is limited.

Mechanism of action

The efficacy of anticonvulsant drugs has been most clearly established for episodic lancinating pains, which are sudden in onset, peak very rapidly, and remit after a brief period. The benefits of these drugs for neuropathic pains that are nonlancinating but have a sudden onset is supported by extensive clinical experience. These observations suggest that pain phenomenology, such as the complaint of paroxysmal pain, associates with specific mechanisms and that these mechanism, in turn, have relatively selective responses to drugs with differing modes of action. Specifically, it may be hypothesized that mechanisms associated with recurrent pains of sudden onset respond relatively well to drugs that stabilize membranes, such as anticonvulsant drugs.

The specific mechanisms of the analgesia produced by the anticonvulsant drugs are not known but presumably relate to those actions underlying anticonvulsant effects. These include suppression of paroxysmal discharges and their spread from the site of origin and reduction of neuronal hyperexcitability (refer to Figure 7.2) (Weinberger, Nicklas, Berl, 1976). Aberrant electrical activity has been recorded from different levels of the neuraxis in experimental models of nerve injury (Albe-Fessard, Lombard, 1982; Chabal, Russell, Burchiel, 1989; Devor, 1994; Devor, Govrin-Lippman, Raber, 1985; Devor, Wall, Catalan, 1992; Guilbaud, Benoist, Levante et al, 1992) and in patients with chronic neuropathic pain (Lenz, Kwan, Dostrovsky et al., 1989; Loeser, Ward, White, 1968; Nystrom, Hagbarth, 1981). This is probably the pathophysiologic substrate for the experience of lancinating pains, and the analgesia from anticonvulsant drugs probably results from the suppression of these discharges (refer to Figure 7.2).

Adverse effects
Carbamazepine

Carbamazepine commonly causes sedation, dizziness, nausea, and unsteadiness. These effects can be minimized by low initial doses and gradual dose titration. The intensity diminishes in most patients maintained on the drug for several weeks. Of much greater concern, carbamazepine causes leukopenia or thrombocytopenia in approximately 2% of patients, and aplastic anemia is a rare complication (Hart, Easton, 1982). A complete blood count should be obtained before the start of therapy, after several weeks, then every 3 to 4 months thereafter. A leukocyte count less than 4000 is usually considered to be a contraindication to treatment, and a decline to less than 3000 (or an absolute neutrophil count of less than 1500) during therapy should lead to discontinuation of the drug. Other rare adverse effects of carbamazepine include hepatic damage, hyponatremia caused by inappropriate secretion of antidiuretic hormone, and congestive heart failure (Flegel, Cole, 1977; Terrence, Fromm, 1980). Baseline liver and renal function tests should also be obtained before therapy.

Phenytoin

Most of the common side effects of phenytoin are dose dependent and usually occur at plasma concentrations greater than the therapeutic range for seizure control. These include sedation or mental clouding, dizziness, unsteadiness, and diplopia (Ramsey, Wilder, Berger et al., 1983). Occasional patients experience toxicity at lower concentrations. Ataxia, progressive encephalopathy, and even seizures can occur at toxic levels (Troupin, Ojemann, 1975). Of the idiosyncratic effects, the most serious are hepatotoxicity and exfoliative dermatitis. The occurrence of a maculopapular rash, which can be the harbinger of the more severe cutaneous reactions, should lead to discontinuation of the drug. A rare permanent cerebellar degeneration has been reported in patients with chronic phenytoin intoxication (Ghatak, Santoso, McKinney, 1976).

Gabapentin

Gabapentin has a low side effect profile (McLean, 1995; Morris, 1995). In a survey of 122 patients taking gabapentin for chronic pain the most common side effect was sedation followed by dizziness and nausea or GI upset (Rosenberg, Harrell, Ristic et al., 1997). These usually decrease with continued use. Occasional patients report changes in mood, such as dysphoria, or cognitive impairment, which may be subtle. Movement disorders have been reported but appear to cease when the drug is discontinued (Buetefisch, Guiterrez, Gutmann et al., 1996; Reeves, So, Sharbrough et al., 1996). In children behavioral side effects have occurred, including aggression and hyperactivity (Hauck, Bhaumik, 1995; Lee, Steingard, Cesena et al., 1996; Tallian, Nahata, et al., 1996). However, most of the children had preexisting disorders (Berde, 1997). Because side effects are few, gabapentin may be particularly useful in elderly patients (Dichter, Brodie, 1996).

Gabapentin has few drug interactions. Unlike carbamazepine, gabapentin does not cause adverse hepatic effects (de Jong, 1996). The addition of tricyclic antidepressants in patients taking gabapentin for chronic pain did not change patient responses to gabapentin (Rosenberg, Harrell, Ristic et al., 1997).

Clonazepam

Drowsiness is the most common and troubling side effect of clonazepam. The sedation is usually additive to that produced by other drugs, including alcohol. Tolerance to the effect often develops within weeks after dosing is begun. Occasional patients develop ataxia, particularly at higher doses. Idiosyncratic reactions, including dermatitis, hepatotoxicity, and hematologic effects, appear to be very rare. Like other benzodiazepine drugs, a withdrawal syndrome may occur with abrupt discontinuation of relatively high doses.

Valproic Acid

At therapeutic doses, the side effects of valproate are usually mild, consisting of sedation, nausea, tremor, and sometimes increased appetite (Egger, Brett, 1981). An enteric-coated tablet minimizes GI disturbances, and dose-dependent side effects are reduced by the use of low initial doses and gradual upward dose titration. Hepatotoxicity, encephalopathy, dermatitis, alopecia, and a rare hyperammonemia syndrome are among the reported idiosyncratic reactions (Schmidt, 1984). The hyperammonemia syndrome can occur without abnormalities in other liver function tests. The development of confusion or any symptoms or signs compatible with hepatic dysfunction during valproate therapy should be evaluated with both liver function tests and serum ammonia level.

Other Anticonvulsants

The newer anticonvulsant drugs, including lamotrigine and felbamate, are generally associated with a favorable side effect profile (Fraught, Sacdeo, Remler et al., 1993; Goa, Sorkin, 1993; Matsuo, Bergen, Faught et al., 1993; Messenheimer, Ramsay, Willmore et al., 1994). Experience with these drugs is limited, however, and the recognized spectrum of toxicities is evolving. Felbamate has been associated with rare fatal aplastic anemia and liver failure, which has limited its use to patients with refractory epilepsy. This potential toxicity suggests that felbamate should not be administered for neuropathic pain unless other reasonable therapeutic options have been exhausted.

Indications

With the exception of gabapentin, which is now often given a trial in all types of neuropathic pain, lancinating and other episodic paroxysmal neuropathic pains are generally considered to be the primary indication for trials of anticonvulsant drugs. These drugs are often administered as a first-line approach for pains of this type. The treatment of lancinating or paroxysmal neuropathic pain may also be undertaken with other selected adjuvant analgesics such as baclofen (p. 324), local anesthetics, and antidepressants. As noted previously, data from controlled studies suggest that the tricyclic antidepressants can ameliorate pain of this type (Kishore-

Kumar, Max, Schafer et al., 1990; Max, Culnane, Schafer et al., 1987); nonetheless, conventional practice continues to view these drugs as a second-line approach in patients with lancinating pain.

For crescendo neuropathic pain, intravenous phenytoin may be an option for rapid pain control. One case report demonstrated relief of severe, rapidly escalating lancinating neuropathic pain within 1 hour after a 500 mg IV dose of phenytoin (Chang, 1997).

Drug selection

No studies have been done comparing the relative efficacy of the various anticonvulsant drugs in patients with neuropathic pain. The variability in the response to these drugs is great, and sequential trials in patients with refractory pain is amply justified by clinical experience.

Many practitioners begin with gabapentin because of its safety profile and favorable anecdotal experience or with carbamazepine because of the extraordinarily good response rate observed in trigeminal neuralgia. The use of carbamazepine is contraindicated, however, in patients with leukopenia, and the drug must be used cautiously in those with thrombocytopenia, those at risk for marrow failure (e.g., after chemotherapy), and those whose blood counts must be monitored to determine disease status. Patients with chronic pain associated with anxiety or insomnia might be considered for an early trial of clonazepam, which may also be effective for these symptoms.

Dose selection

Dosing guidelines used in the treatment of seizures are typically extrapolated for the management of pain. Low initial doses are appropriate for carbamazepine, valproate, and clonazepam, but the administration of phenytoin often begins with the presumed therapeutic dose (e.g., 300 mg/day) or a prudent oral loading regimen (e.g., 500 mg twice, separated by hours). Doses of gabapentin usually begin at 300 mg on day 1. Lower doses (e.g., 100 mg) can be started in the medically frail or elderly. Doses are then increased on a daily basis or more slowly, depending on response. The daily dose should be divided into three doses per day. The dose required for analgesia appears to vary widely. In a survey of 40 patients with a variety of neuropathic pains, 25 obtained good relief from gabapentin. Doses ranged from 300 to 1800 mg/day in three divided doses (Benson, Parris, Cooper et al., 1996). Some patients require 600 to 900 mg/day, divided into three doses, but others need as much as 3600/day, and rare patients have anecdotally benefited from even higher doses. Although an arbitrary upper limit of 2400 mg/day is set by some clinicians (de Jong, 1996), other clinicians will not stop dose titration in the absence of side effects until a total daily dose of 2700 to 3600 mg is reached.

When low initial doses of anticonvulsants are used, dose escalation should ensue until favorable effects occur, intolerable side effects supervene, or plasma drug concentration has reached some arbitrary level (customarily at the upper end of the therapeutic range for seizures).

Baclofen (GABA Agonist)

As noted previously, several nonanticonvulsant drugs have been used in the management of lancinating or paroxysmal neuropathic pains, including the neuroleptic pimozide (Lechin, van der Dijs, Lechin et al., 1989), systemically administered local anesthetics, and the tricyclic antidepressants (Kishore-Kumar, Max, Schafer et al., 1990; Max, Culnane, Schafer et al., 1987). Baclofen (Lioresal) is another alternative, a trial of which typically precedes other therapies listed in Table 7.5.

Baclofen, an agonist at the GABA type B receptor, has been conclusively demonstrated to have efficacy in trigeminal neuralgia (Fromm, Terrence, Chattha, 1984) and is widely considered to be a second-line pharmacologic approach in this condition, after carbamazepine (Fromm, 1994). Other neuropathic pains characterized by an episodic lancinating or paroxysmal phenomenology have also been reported to respond to this drug (Fromm, Graff-Radford, Terrence et al, 1990; Ringel, Roy, 1987; Terrence, Fromm, Tenicela, 1985). Although a few observations suggest a broader analgesic potential (Corli, Roma, Bacchini et al., 1984), baclofen is generally considered to have a relatively selective efficacy for lancinating or paroxysmal neuropathic pain.

Some evidence shows that baclofen enhances morphine analgesia for postoperative pain (Gordon, Gear, Heller et al., 1995). This may prove to be a role for baclofen in the management of acute pain.

The administration of baclofen for pain is undertaken in a manner similar to the use of the drug for its primary indication, spasticity. A starting dose of 5 mg two to three times per day is gradually escalated ot the range of 30 to 90 mg/day and sometimes higher if side effects do not occur. Occasional patients require more than 200 mg/day to benefit maximally. It is appropriate to continue dose escalation until pain is relieved or limiting side effects occur. The common side effects, dizziness, sedation, and gastrointestinal distress, are minimized by low starting doses and gradual dose escalation. The potential for a serious withdrawal syndrome including delirium and seizures, exists with abrupt discontinuation after prolonged use (Kofler, Leis, 1992); doses should always be tapered before discontinuation of the drug.

ADJUVANT ANALGESICS FOR CHRONIC BONE PAIN

Bone pain is a common problem in the palliative care setting. Radiation therapy is usually considered when bone pain is focal and poorly controlled with an opioid or is associated with a lesion that appears prone to fracture on radiographic examination. Anecdotally, multifocal bone pain has been observed to benefit from treatment with a nonsteroidal antiinflammatory drug or a corticosteroid (Payne, 1989). Other adjuvant analgesics that are potentially useful in this setting include calcitonin, bisphosphonate compounds, gallium nitrate, and selected radiopharmaceuticals (Table 7.6). No comparative trials of these adjuvant analgesics for bone pain have been done, and the selection of one over another is usually made on the basis of convenience, patient preference, and the clinical setting.

Calcitonin

Calcitonin has ameliorated bone pain in some (Hindley, Hill, Leyland et al., 1982; Roth, Kolariac, 1986), but not all (Blomquist, Elomaa, Porkka et al., 1988), controlled trials. Clinical experience with this drug suggests that it is relatively safe and can occasionally produce substantial pain relief.

The optimal dose and dosing frequency for calcitonin are unknown, and the durability of favorable effects, if they occur, has not been evaluated systematically. Calcitonin is now available as a nasal spray (Miacalcin Nasal Spray). The recommended dose is one puff in one nostril daily, providing 200 IU. Subcutaneous or IV therapy is usually initiated with a low dose, such as 25 IU daily. This may reduce the incidence of nausea, the major side effect. Skin testing with 1 IU before the start of therapy is sometimes recommended because of the small risk of serious hypersensitivity reactions. After therapy begins, gradual dose escalation may identify a minimal effective dose. The usual maximum dose, which is recommended solely on the basis of clinical experience, is in the range of 100 to 200 IU/day subcutaneously. The dosing frequency is usually daily at the start of therapy, then reduced, if possible, to the fewest weekly doses required to sustain effects.

Intrathecal calcitonin has also been suggested to produce analgesic effects (Fraioli, Fabbri, Gnessi et al., 1984), presumably independent of its putative mechanism of action in bone pain, but the long-term risks and benefits of this approach are not known, and this approach should be considered experimental at present.

Bisphosphonates

Bisphosphonates (previously known as diphosphonates) are analogs of inorganic pyrophosphate that inhibit osteoclast activity and, consequently, reduce bone resorption in a variety of illnesses. Many surveys and several controlled trials have established the analgesic efficacy of these compounds, particularly pamidronate (Aredia) and clodronate (Admi, Mian, 1989; Averbuch, 1993; Clarke, Holbrook, McClure et al., 1991; Coleman, Woll, Miles et al., 1988; Ernst, MacDonald, Paterson et al., 1992; Glover, Lipton, Keller et al., 1994; Kanis, McCloskey, Taube et al., 1991; Paterson, Powles, Kanis et al., 1993; Thiebaud, Leyvraz, von Fliedner et al., 1991; van Holten-

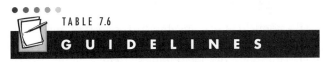

TABLE 7.6

GUIDELINES

ADJUVANT ANALGESICS USED FOR MALIGNANT BONE PAIN

Class	Comment
Calcitonin	Reduces bone pain; decreases rate of bone turnover; useful in osteoporosis; available IM, subcutaneous, and as nasal spray
Bisphosphonates (e.g., pamidronate, clodronate)	Reduces malignant bone pain and risk of skeletal morbidity
Radionuclides (e.g., strontium-89, samarium-153, rhenium-186, gallium nitrate)	Slow onset, used only if no further chemotherapy is planned
Corticosteroids	Anecdotal reports of effectness in bone pain
NSAIDs	Anecdotal reports of effectness in bone pain

May be duplicated for use in clinical practice. From McCaffery M, Pasero C: *Pain: Clinical manual*, p. 325. Copyright © 1999, Mosby, Inc.

Verzantvoort, Kroon, Bijvoet et al., 1993). For example, a recent controlled dose-ranging study of pamidronate (Glover, Lipton, Keller et al., 1994) noted that 60 mg every 2 to 4 weeks and 90 mg every 4 weeks produced at least partial pain relief in 50% of patients; almost one third of those who received the highest dose became pain-free. Although analgesic-effects from sodium etidronate have been suggested (Carey, Lippert, 1988), the benefits of this drug were not demonstrated in a controlled trial (Smith, 1989).

The bisphosphonates may also reduce other skeletal morbidity. For example, a placebo-controlled trial of oral clodronate in patients with metastatic breast cancer recorded a significant reduction in the number of hypercalcemic episodes, number of terminal hypercalcemic events, incidence of vertebral fractures, rate of vertebral deformity, and combined rate of all morbid skeletal events (Paterson, Powles, Kanis et al., 1993).

Optimal dosing regimens for the bisphosphonates have only begun to be clarified. The dose-ranging trial of pamidronate demonstrated efficacy and an acceptable safety profile for three different dosing regimens (60 mg every 2 weeks, 60 mg every 4 weeks, and 90 mg every 4 weeks) (Glover, Lipton, Keller et al., 1994). This study also suggested that analgesia begins after a period of weeks after treatment (as early as 2 weeks in some cases) and that several doses are needed to judge the full efficacy of the drug.

Radiopharmaceuticals

Radionuclides that are absorbed at areas of high bone turnover have been evaluated as potential therapies for metastatic bone disease (Holmes, 1993; Serafini, 1994). The first radionuclide introduced into clinical practice was phosphorus-32 orthophosphate. Numerous series suggest that this drug can relieve bone pain in as many as 80% of patients (Silberstein, 1993). Bone marrow suppression is the major toxicity, and the desire for a compound with a better therapeutic index has spurred the development of several new radionuclides.

Many newer radionuclides have been advocated as potential therapies for bone pain (Holmes, 1993; Serafini, 1994). Strontium chloride-89, samarium-153 ethylenediaminetetramethylenephosphonic acid, rhenium-186, and hydroxyethylenediphosphonic acid have been most promising thus far. Surveys of patients with bone metastases from a variety of tumor types have provided strong evidence that these compounds can reduce bone pain without undue risk to bone marrow or other vital structures.

Strontium-89, which is commercially available in the United States, has been most extensively evaluated as a treatment for bone pain. Favorable effects have been reported in numerous surveys (Laing, Achery, Bayly et al., 1991; Robinson, Spicer, Preston et al., 1987; Silberstein, Williams, 1985) and confirmed in placebo-controlled trials (Lewington, McEwan, Ackery et al., 1991; Porter, McEwan, Powe et al., 1993). The larger of these controlled trials evaluated strontium-89 as an adjunct to conventional radiotherapy in 126 patients with advanced prostate cancer; treatment reduced the need for both radiotherapy and analgesic drugs (Porter, McEwan, Powe et al., 1993). Strontium-89 has also been shown to compare favorably with hemibody irradiation in a randomized trial (Quilty, Kirk, Bolger et al., 1994).

Reviews of the extensive clinical experience with strontium-89 suggest that pain relief occurs in approximately 80% of patients, 10% of whom attain complete relief (Robinson, Preston, Baxter et al., 1993; Robinson, Preston, Schiefelbein et al., 1995). Initial clinical response occurs in 7 to 21 days and peak response may be delayed for a month or more. Approximately 5% to 10% of patients experience a transitory pain flare immediately after treatment. The usual duration of benefit is 3 to 6 months, after which retreatment may regain a favorable effect. After treatment, clinically significant leukopenia or thrombocytopenia occurs in approximately 10% and 33% of patients, respectively (Porter, McEwan, Powe et al., 1993). The nadir of bone marrow effects occurs 4 to 8 weeks after injection and usually undergoes at least partial return to baseline by 12 weeks.

In the absence of comparative trials, the profile of clinical effects produced by strontium-89 can help clarify its role in relation to the other strategies used for bone pain. Strontium-89 is only potentially effective in the treatment of pain caused by osteoblastic bone lesions or lesions with an osteoblastic component. An osteoblastic component should be considered by positive bone scintigraphy before treatment with this drug. Given the delayed onset and peak effects, treatment should not be administered unless patients have a life expectancy greater than 3 months. This delay also implies that this treatment should not be considered as the sole approach for patients with severe pain.

Because of the potential for bone marrow toxicity, treatment with strontium-89 should not be considered unless adequate bone marrow reserve has been documented. In the case of strontium-89 this is usually considered to be a platelet count greater than 60,000 and a white blood cell count greater than 2400 (Robinson, Preston, Schiefelbein et al., 1995). Patients who continue to be candidates for myelosuppressive chemotherapy should not be treated because the effects on bone marrow may worsen the toxicity of later cytotoxic therapy or limit the ability to rebound after therapy.

A second radiopharmaceutical, samarium-153, has been recently approved in the United States. Unlike strontium-89, this compound can be imaged and provides a scintigraphic picture of bone metastases at the same time treatment is given. No comparative studies of strontium-89 and samarium-153 have been done, and experience with the latter drug is yet very limited. For now, the indications and safety issues should be considered similar for both these radiopharmaceuticals.

Other Drugs for Bone Pain

Gallium nitrate is another osteoclast inhibitor that may be analgesic for multifocal malignant bone pain. Experience is currently limited to a series of cases (Warrell, Lovett, Dilmanian et al., 1993). Future studies are needed to clarify the value of this drug.

Anecdotal evidence strongly supports the usefulness of NSAIDs and corticosteroids in the relief of bone pain. Anecdotal reports also have suggested that L-dopa can ameliorate metastatic bone pain (Minton, 1974). More recent experience, however, has been disappointing and the approach cannot be recommended for routine trials.

ADJUVANT ANALGESICS FOR MALIGNANT BOWEL OBSTRUCTION

The management of symptoms associated with malignant bowel obstruction may be challenging (Ripamonti, 1994). If surgical decompression is not feasible, the need to control pain and other obstructive symptoms, including distention, nausea, and vomiting, becomes paramount. The use of opioids may be problematic because of dose-limiting toxicity (including gastrointestinal toxicity) or the intensity of breakthrough pain. Anecdotal reports suggest that anticholinergic drugs, the somatostatin analog octreotide, and corticosteroids may be useful adjuvant analgesics in this setting (Table 7.7). The use of these drugs may also ameliorate nonpainful symptoms and minimize the number of patients who must be considered for chronic drainage using nasogastric or percutaneous catheters.

Anticholinergic Drugs

Anticholinergic drugs could theoretically relieve the symptoms of bowel obstruction by reducing propulsive and nonpropulsive gut motility and decreasing intraluminal secretions. No controlled trials of this therapy have been done, and anecdotal experience is limited.

Some patients appear to benefit from the administration of scopolamine (De Conno, Caraceni, Zecca et al., 1991; Ventafridda, Ripamonti, Caraceni et al., 1990). This drug is available as a transdermal system, which simplifies treatment in patients with bowel obstruction. Problematic side effects include somnolence and confusion.

Octreotide

The somatostatin analog octreotide (Sandostatin) inhibits the secretion of gastric, pancreatic, and intestinal secretions and reduces GI motility. These effects probably underlie the analgesic effects that have been observed anecdotally in the symptomatic treatment of bowel obstruction (Mercadante, Maddaloni, 1992). Octreotide has also been used to manage severe diarrhea caused by enterocolic fistula, high output jejunostomies or ileostomies, or secretory tumors of the gastrointestinal tract (Ladefoged, Christensen, Hegnhoj et al., 1989; Mercadante, 1992; Mulvihill, Papas, Passaro et al., 1986).

Octreotide has a good safety profile but is expensive. The cost may be balanced by an excellent clinical result or the avoidance of the costs involved in the use of a GI drainage procedure.

Corticosteroids

Corticosteroid therapy may also be helpful with the symptoms associated with bowel obstruction. The mode of action is unclear, and the most effective drug, dose, and dosing regimen is unknown. A broad range of doses have been described anecdotally. For example, dexamethasone has been used for this indication in a dose range of 8 to 60 mg/day (Fainsinger, Spanchynski, Hanson et al., 1994; Reid, 1988), and methylprednisolone has been administered in a dose range of 30 to 50 mg/day (Farr, 1990). The potential for complications during long-term therapy, including an increased risk of bowel perforation, may limit this approach to patients with life expectancies that are likely to be short.

ADJUVANT ANALGESICS FOR CHRONIC MUSCULOSKELETAL PAIN

In the management of acute traumatic sprains or strains in the nonmedically ill, nonopioid and opioid analgesics are commonly supplemented by treatment with so-called muscle relaxant drugs or benzodiazepines (Table 7.8). Although pains that originate from injury to muscle or connective tissue are also prevalent in medically ill patients (Twycross, Fairfield, 1982), the role of these drugs remains ill defined.

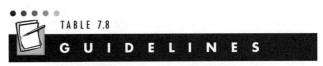

TABLE 7.8

G U I D E L I N E S

ADJUVANT ANALGESICS CUSTOMARILY USED FOR CHRONIC MUSCULOSKELETAL PAIN

Generic name	Brand name
*So-called Muscle Relaxants**	
Orphenadrine	Norflex
Cyclobenzaprine	Flexeril
Carisoprodol	Soma
Chlorzoxazone	Parafon Forte DSC
Methocarbamol	Robaxin
Benzodiazepines†	
Clonazepam	Klonopin
Diazepam	Valium

May be duplicated for use in clinical practice. From McCaffery M, Pasero C: *Pain: Clinical manual*, p. 327. Copyright © 1999, Mosby, Inc.

*No evidence that "muscle relaxants" relax muscle in humans; best viewed as alternatives to nonopioids and opioids.

†Evidence that benzodiazepines relax muscles is limited. Oral clonazepam may be more effective than oral diazepam.

TABLE 7.7

G U I D E L I N E S

ADJUVANT ANALGESICS FOR MALIGNANT BOWEL OBSTRUCTION

Class	Comment
Anticholinergic drugs (e.g. scopolamine)	Reduces peristalsis and secretions, anecdotal reports of analgesic effects
Octreotide (Sandostatin)	Reduces peristalsis and secretions, anecdotal reports of analgesic effects
Corticosteroids	Anecdotal reports of analgesic effects

May be duplicated for use in clinical practice. From McCaffery M, Pasero C: *Pain: Clinical manual*, p. 327. Copyright © 1999, Mosby, Inc.

Muscle Relaxants

The label "muscle relaxant" notwithstanding, no evidence exists that the drugs conventionally described in this way actually relax skeletal muscle in patients with muscle spasm or muscle tension. They do inhibit polysynaptic myogenic reflexes in animal models, but the relationship between this action and analgesia is not known. Although muscle relaxant drugs can relieve musculoskeletal pains, these effects may not be specific and do not depend on relaxation of skeletal muscle. They are administered primarily by the oral route.

The so-called muscle relaxants include drugs in a variety of classes, all of which are marketed for the treatment of acute musculoskeletal pain. This group includes drugs that are also administered as antihistamines such as orphenadrine (Norflex), tricyclic compounds structurally similar to the tricyclic antidepressants such as cyclobenzaprine (Flexeril), and other types of drugs such as carisoprodol (Soma), chlorzoxazone (Parafon Forte DSC), and methocarbamol (Robaxin).

The efficacy of the muscle relaxant drugs in common musculoskeletal pains has been established in placebo-controlled studies (Batterman, 1965; Bercel, 1977; Birkeland, Clawson, 1958; Gold, 1978). Some studies have demonstrated analgesic effects are superior to either aspirin or acetaminophen, and others have shown that the combination of a muscle relaxant and one of the latter drugs provides better analgesia than does aspirin or acetaminophen alone. There have been no controlled comparative trials or studies that have directly compared the efficacy and side effect profiles of these drugs with either nonsteroidal antiinflammatory drugs or opioids.

Thus the muscle relaxant drugs are best viewed as alternatives to the antiinflammatory drugs and opioids, which may be indicated in musculoskeletal pains because of the evidence of analgesic efficacy in these conditions. These drugs should not be administered in the mistaken belief that they relieve muscle spasm.

The muscle relaxant drugs are generally well tolerated but have sedative effects that may be additive to other centrally acting drugs, including the opioids. Anecdotally, some patients report differences among drugs in analgesic efficacy or sedative side effects, and it is reasonable to switch to an alternative drug if treatment is initially ineffective. Although the dose-response relationships of the muscle relaxant drugs have not been systematically explored, dose-dependent effects probably exist, and the use of a low initial dose followed by gradual dose escalation can be recommended as a means to identify the most salutary balance between analgesia and side effects. Experience with these drugs is too limited to pursue dose escalation beyond the usual recommended range.

Benzodiazepines

The evidence for use of benzodiazepines as muscle relaxants is limited. Diazepam is widely used for acute musculoskeletal pains, particularly those characterized by spasm. This use is based on a favorable clinical experience and evidence that this drug, unlike the so-called muscle relaxants, actually reduces myotonic activity (Tseng, Wang, 1971). However, other research has yielded inconsistent findings. Oral administration of diazepam, as opposed to parenteral, appears to be of little benefit (Baldessarini, 1996). On the other hand, clonazepam in nonsedating doses produces muscle relaxation (Hobbs, Rall, Verdoorn, 1996).

The usual oral dose of diazepam is 5 to 10 mg three to four times a day. The usual oral dose of clonazepam is 0.5 mg three times a day.

Because of their marked sedative effects, the use of benzodiazepines for muscle spasm should usually be limited to short courses. Other less sedating analgesics are more appropriate for patients in whom functional restoration is the goal.

ADJUVANT ANALGESICS FOR REFRACTORY CASES OF NEUROPATHIC PAIN

For either continuous or lancinating neuropathic pain, several other adjuvant analgesics are being investigated. Discussed below are some of the more promising drugs.

N-Methyl-D-Aspartate (NMDA) Receptor Blockers: Dextromethorphan and Ketamine

A variety of NMDA receptor antagonists are currently undergoing intensive investigation as potential analgesics. At present, two drugs are commercially available: the antitussive dextromethorphan (available orally in many nonprescription cough remedies, designated by DM) and the general anesthetic ketamine. Both have been shown to have analgesic effects in controlled studies of experimental pain (Park, Max, Robinovitz et al., 1994; Price, Mao, Frenk et al., 1994). Dextromethorphan may be useful for the prevention of morphine tolerance (Manning, Jianren, Frenk et al., 1996) or the enhancement of NSAID analgesia (Price, Mao, Lu et al., 1996).

Analgesia of ketamine for neuropathic pain, including phantom limb pain, has been demonstrated in both case reports (Edmonds, Davis, 1996; Persson, Axelsson, Hallin et al., 1995; Stannard, Porter, 1993) and controlled studies of short-term dosing (Backonja, Arndt, Gombar et al., 1994; Eide, Jorum, Stabhuag et al., 1994; Nikolajsen, Hansen, Nielsen et al., 1996). Sustained analgesia during long-term administration of ketamine has been observed anecdotally, and some of these reports describe patients with cancer pain (Mercadante, Lodi, Sapio et al., 1995; Oshima, Tei, Kayazawa et al., 1990; Persson, Axelsson, Hallin et al, 1995; Stannard, Porter, 1993).

In two controlled studies of patients with either diabetic neuropathy or postherpetic neuralgia, dextromethorphan was titrated in each patient to the highest level possible without disrupting normal activities (Nelson, Park, Robinovitz et al., 1997). Mean doses were 381 mg/day in patients with diabetic neuropathy and 439 mg/day for those with postherpetic neuralgia. Dextromethorphan reduced pain in diabetic neuropathy but not in postherpetic neuralgia. Side effects that caused five patients to drop out were ataxia and sedation.

New NMDA receptor antagonists are being developed and may ultimately prove useful for a variety of medical indications. Advances in this area have occurred rapidly, and it is likely that the role of these agents in the management of pain will be much better defined within a few years.

Mechanism of action

Excitatory amino acids, such as glutamate and aspartate, are released by primary afferent neurons in response to noxious stimuli and are important in the central processing of pain-related information. Interactions at the NMDA receptor are involved in the development of central nervous system changes that may underlie chronic pain and modulate opioid mechanisms, specifically tolerance (Mao, Price, Mayer, 1995). Preclinical studies have established that the NMDA receptor is involved in the sensitization of central neurons after injury and the development of the "wind-up" phenomenon, a change in the response of central neurons that has been associated with neuropathic pain (Dickenson, Sullivan, 1987; Woolf, Thompson, 1991). Antagonists at the NMDA receptor may offer a novel approach to the treatment of pain.

Indications

The most intense interest had focused on use of NMDA receptor antagonists as new therapies for neuropathic pain. In addition, evidence exists that such drugs may be multipurpose analgesics, which could potentially ameliorate acute pain (Jahangir, Islam, Aziz, 1993) and diverse types of chronic pain (Cherry, Plummer, Gourlay et al., 1995; Mathisen, Skjelbred, Skoglund et al., 1995; Persson, Axelsson, Hallin et al., 1995; Stannard, Porter, 1993).

Clinicians who are experienced in the use of parenteral ketamine may also consider this option in patients with refractory pain. In the palliative care setting this treatment may be useful, for example, in patients who have advanced disease and neuropathic pain that has not responded adequately to opioids. The side effect profile of ketamine, which includes delirium, severe night-

mares, hallucinosis, and dysphoria, can be daunting, particularly in the frail medically ill. However, the likelihood of serious toxicity is low at the relatively small, subanesthetic doses used to treat pain, and the risks may be justified when pain has been intractable to many routine approaches. At low doses, the most common side effect is sedation.

Ketamine has also been used for procedural pain (Shapiro, Warren, Egol et al., 1995) and is worth considering for brief episodes of increased pain in patients with chronic pain (see Chapter 8). For example, for patients with spinal metastases who experience severe pain on movement, transport from home to hospital has been accomplished comfortably with the use of ketamine, 100 mg IV bolus followed with 50 mg boluses as needed (Notcutt, 1994).

Although the role of NMDA receptor antagonists in the management of chronic pain is evolving, current data are sufficient to justify a trial of one of the commercially available drugs in patients with neuropathic pain that has been refractory to other measures.

Dose selection

Dextromethorphan has an extremely good safety profile and has been administered at doses higher than 1 g/day. At high doses, sedation or confusion can occur. On the basis of clinical experience, a trial of dextromethorphan may be initiated using a proprietary cough suppressant (ensuring that the product contains no alcohol or other active drugs). A prudent starting dose is 45 to 60 mg daily, which can be gradually escalated until favorable effects occur, side effects supervene, or a conventional maximum dose of 1 g is achieved. A commercially available source of dextromethorphan is cough syrup. At present, the most concentrated source is Delsym Extended Release suspension, which contains the equivalent of 30 mg dextromethorphan hydrobromide per 5 ml.

Typically, parenteral ketamine therapy for pain (subanesthetic doses) has been initiated at low doses, such as 0.1 to 1.5 mg/kg by brief infusion or the same dose administered hourly by continuous infusion. Onset of analgesia occurs within about 15 minutes of the full dose. A simple guide is an initial starting dose of 100 to 150 mg/day (Mercadante, 1996). The dose can be gradually escalated, with close monitoring of pain and side effects. Long-term therapy has been maintained with continuous subcutaneous infusion or repeated subcutaneous injections.

To prevent undue sedation, some suggest that the opioid dose be decreased to 50% when ketamine infusion is administered by continuous infusion throughout the 24-hour period. Further opioid reduction may be possible. If psychomimetic effects occur, haloperidol, 2 to 4 mg/day, may prevent them (Mercadante, 1996).

Ketamine may also be administered nasally, orally, and rectally. Both nasally and orally, ketamine produces a bitter taste and burning of the throat. Case reports of patients with neuropathic pain, such as postherpetic neuralgia and peripheral neuropathy, suggest that successful parenteral therapy may be maintained by the oral route (Broadley, Kurowska, Tookman, 1996; Hoffmann, Coppejans, Vercauteren et al., 1994). Calculation of the oral dose is made on the basis of clinical observations that when the same dose given parenterally is administered orally, analgesia is approximately equal and, in fact, may be greater by the oral route (Broadley, Kurowska, Tookman, 1996; Grant, Nimmo, Clements, 1981). Transition from parenteral to oral may be initiated by decreasing the parenteral dose by 50% and starting an oral dose. Both dose and interval must be adjusted on the basis of the effects experienced by the patient. When the injectable formulation is used orally, the bitter taste may be masked with orange juice or cola drinks.

Calcitonin

The use of calcitonin in the treatment of bone pain has been discussed previously in this chapter. Evidence also exists that calcitonin is effective in various neuropathic pains such as reflex symapthetic dystrophy (Gobelet, Waldburger, Meier, 1992) and phantom limb pain (Jaeger, Maier, 1992).

In a controlled study of 10 patients with painful diabetic neuropathy of the legs who had not benefited from other analgesics, 100 IU of intranasal calcitonin daily for 2 weeks resulted in pain relief for four patients (Quatraro, Minei, 1992). Three obtained complete relief and the fourth experienced a 50% improvement. Analgesic effects tended not to be apparent until after 2 weeks of therapy. The drug proved to be safe for these patients and did not negatively affect carbohydrate metabolism.

Although the mechanisms that may be responsible for these analgesic effects are unknown, these observations justify an empirical trial of calcitonin in refractory neuropathic pain of diverse types.

The optimal dose and dosing frequency for calcitonin are unknown. Dosing recommendations discussed previously in relation to bone pain may be used for neuropathic pain (p. 325). Calcitonin is now available as a nasal spray (Miacalcin Nasal Spray), and the recommended dose is one puff in one nostril daily, providing 200 IU. Parenteral therapy is started at a lose dose, such as 25 IU subcutaneously daily, followed by gradual dose escalation to identify a minimal effective dose. The usual maximum dose is in the range of 100 to 200 IU/day. The dosing frequency is usually daily at the start of therapy, then reduced, if possible, to the fewest weekly doses required to sustain effects.

Other Drugs for Sympathetically Maintained Pain

Sympathetically maintained pain is a form of neuropathic pain in which dysesthesias, such as burning and tingling, are believed to be sustained through efferent activity in the sympathetic nervous system (Backonja, 1994b). This type of pain is believed to occur most often in patients with a clinical syndrome consistent with reflex sympathetic dystrophy or causalgia (recently termed complex regional pain syndrome Type I and Type II). The latter syndromes are characterized by the occurrence of focal autonomic dysregulation (e.g., swelling, vasomotor disturbances, and sweating abnormalities), focal motor disturbances (e.g., tremor or dystonia), or trophic changes (e.g., focal osteoporosis, atrophy of skin or subcutaneous tissues, and changes in nail or hair growth) in the region of the pain. Sympathetic nerve blocks are an important diagnostic test and, if positive, a first-line of treatment. Drug therapy is usually considered if nerve blocks are contraindicated or fail.

Drug treatments for pain that is presumed to be sympathetically maintained may involve the nonspecific use of any of the aforementioned classes of adjuvant analgesics, either multipurpose drugs or drugs used specifically for neuropathic pain. Alternately, therapy may focus on trials of drugs that either influence sympathetic function or have been specifically studied in this condition.

As noted previously, calcitonin has been evaluated as a treatment for reflex sympathetic dystrophy in a controlled trial (Gobelet, Waldburger, Meier, 1992). The findings from this study suggest that this drug may be useful when combined with physical therapy. A trial for neuropathic pains that may be sympathetically maintained is warranted.

Drugs that modulate sympathetic nervous system function have been explored in single cases or small series of patients. The analgesic effects that have been associated with phentolamine infusion, which has been developed as a diagnostic tool for sympathetically maintained pain (Raja, Treede, Davis et al., 1991), indicate the potential viability of this therapeutic strategy. In separate surveys phenoxybenzamine, prazosin, and guanethidine were reported to be effective for patients with causalgia (Abram, Lightfoot, 1981; Ghostine, Comair, Turner et al., 1984; Tabira, Shibasaki, Kuroiwa, 1983). Although propranolol has been recommended on the basis of uncontrolled observations (Meyers, Meyers, 1992; Simson, 1974), another survey yielded disappointing results (Scadding, 1982). The risk of orthostatic hypotension limits trials of all these treatments to younger patients with intact cardiovascular reflexes.

Nifedipine, a calcium channel blocker, has also been reported to have favorable effects in a small survey of patients with reflex sympathetic dystrophy (Prough, McLoskey, Borshy et al., 1985).

Topical Analgesics

Topical therapies for neuropathic pain have been used for those syndromes characterized by both a predominating peripheral mechanism and continuous dysesthesia. Available topical therapies include capsaicin preparations, formulations containing aspirin or a nonsteroidal antiinflammatory drug, and local anesthetic preparations (Rowbotham, 1994). These are summarized in Table 7.9.

Topical capsaicin

The potential value of topical capsaicin (Zostrix) in painful neuropathies has been suggested from surveys of patients with postherpetic neuralgia or postmastectomy pain (Berstein, Bickers, Dahl et al., 1987; Watson, Evans, Watt, 1988, 1989) and controlled trials in populations with postherpetic neuralgia (Watson, Tyler, Bickers et al., 1993), painful diabetic neuropathy (Capsaicin Study Group, 1991; Tandan, Lewis, Krusinski et al., 1992) and postmastectomy pain (Watson, Evans, 1992). In an open-label series of 12 patients with trigeminal neuralgia, topical capsaicin provided sustained relief in 10 (six complete and four partial) (Fusco, Alessandri, 1992). Other controlled trials, which demonstrate that topical capsaicin may relieve the pain associated with osteoarthritis of the finger joints (McCarthy, McCarty, 1992), also suggest that some painful somatic disorders may be amenable to this therapy. The benefit of topical capsaicin in painful diabetic neuropathy, osteoarthritis, and one nonpainful condition, psoriasis, was confirmed in a metaanalysis of available controlled trials (Zhang, Li Wan Po, 1994).

Presumably, topical capsaicin lessens pain by reducing the concentration of small peptides in primary afferent neurons. These peptides, which include substance P, may activate nociceptive systems in the dorsal horn of the spinal cord. Their depletion may reduce the central transmission of information about noxious stimuli or reduce peripheral input to sensitized central neurons (Dubner, 1991).

Topical antiinflammatory drugs

The effectiveness of topical antiinflammatory drugs for neuropathic pain remains unproved. Numerous antiinflammatory drugs have been investigated for topical use in populations with neuropathic pain, particularly postherpetic neuralgia, and results have been mixed. Survey data have been conflicting (Rowbotham, 1994), and one controlled trial found no efficacy whatsoever for topical treatment with a benzydamine cream in a patient with acute herpes and postherpetic neuralgia (McQuay, Carroll, Moxon, 1990).

However, double-blind comparison of topical aspirin, indomethacin, and diclofenac in patients with acute herpetic neuralgia and postherpetic neuralgia revealed that aspirin, but not indomethacin or diclofenac, was superior

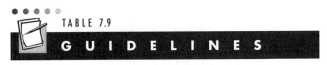

TABLE 7.9

GUIDELINES

TOPICAL ANALGESICS

Type	Example
Topical capsaicin	Zostrix
Topical antiinflammatory drugs	Aspirin in chloroform
Topical local anesthetics	EMLA, patches of 5% lidocaine

May be duplicated for use in clinical practice. From McCaffery M, Pasero C: *Pain: Clinical manual*, p. 331. Copyright © 1999, Mosby, Inc.

to placebo, confirming earlier suspicions made on the basis of an open-label study (De Beneditis, Lorenzetti, 1996; De Beneditis, Besana, Lorenzettit, 1992). Also, a double-blind study of patients with *acute* herpes zoster found topical aspirin applied twice daily resulted in substantial pain relief (Steen, Reeh, Kreysel et al., 1996). Another uncontrolled study of 15 patients with severe neuropathic pain reported that 11 patients (74%) experienced good pain relief (pain rating of 25/100) from topical aspirin in chloroform (Tharion, Bhattacharji, 1997). Pain relief tended to occur within 20 minutes of application, reached maximum effect in 30 minutes, and lasted up to 4 hours. The authors pointed out that this is an inexpensive and easy method.

Topical local anesthetics

A commercially available mixture of local anesthetics, which contains a 1:1 mixture of prilocaine and lidocaine, is capable of penetrating the skin and producing a dense local cutaneous anesthesia. This product, known as eutectic mixture of local anesthetics (EMLA), is widely used to prevent the pain of needle puncture or incision. A limited study in patients with postherpetic neuralgia suggests its use in the management of some chronic neuropathic pains (Stow, Glynn, Minor, 1989).

Surveys of relatively high concentrations of topical lidocaine (Rowbotham, 1994, Rowbotham, Fields, 1989) and a controlled trial of 5% lidocaine gel (Rowbotham, Davies, Fields, 1995) have also been positive in patients with postherpetic neuralgia. Further study of 150 patients comparing lidocaine 5% and vehicle (placebo) patches confirmed that lidocaine patches produce significant decreases in pain and allodynia (pain cause by nonpainful stimuli such as touch) and are well tolerated with few side effects (Davies, Galer, 1996). Maximum analgesia occurred after approximately 8 days and was maintained over the 4-week period of the study. This lidocaine preparation produces localized analgesia as opposed to local anesthesia. Vehicle patches also provided some pain relief probably because they protected the area from stimuli that cause pain, such as air currents and clothing.

Recently lidocaine patches have become commercially available without a prescription. For example, MediPad-L Plus, manufactured by Henley ([800] 634-1887), is a 3 inch by 5 inch pad containing 4% lidocaine with 0.2% menthol.

Anecdotal experience with commercially available, relatively low concentrations of local anesthetic topical ointments (e.g., Foille Plus Medicated First Aid with benzocaine 5%) and sprays (e.g., Medi-Quick First Aid with lidocaine 2%) has not been favorable, however, unless the painful area involves mucosal surfaces. Hemorrhoidal products often contain an anesthetic (Medicone ointment with 20% benzocaine).

Indications

On the basis of these data, a trial of a topical drug may be considered for neuropathic pains presumed to be sustained, at least in part, by peripheral input. With the exception of topical capsaicin in the treatment of pain caused by disease of small joints, the usefulness of the topical analgesics for nociceptive pains caused by injury of the skin, subcutaneous tissues, muscles or joints, has not been clarified. Nonetheless, a trial in one of the latter pain syndromes is often warranted by the potential advantages of topical therapy, especially in medically ill patients, who are often predisposed to side effects from systemically administered drugs.

Adverse Effects

The adverse effects associated with topical analgesic therapy have been minimal. Capsaicin can cause local burning, which is sometimes intense. Although this symptom is not related to tissue damage and poses no risk to the patient, it can create significant discomfort and lead to discontinuation of the treatment. For those who are able to tolerate the burning initially, it may disappear with repeated administrations over days to weeks. Some patients are able to tolerate the drug if administration is preceded by application of a local anesthetic or ingestion of an analgesic.

A remote risk of toxicity exists from systemic absorption of a topical local anesthetic (Rowbotham, Davies, Fields, 1995; Stow, Glynn, Minor, 1989). When EMLA is used, a small risk of methemoglobinemia from prilocaine also occurs in predisposed patients. This rare event suggests that the drug should be used cautiously in infants, patients with histories of prior methemoglobinemia, and those who are coadministered drugs that may also cause this complication, such as sulfonamides (Frayling, Addison, Chattergee et al., 1990). (See Chapter 14 for details on the use of EMLA with infants.)

Dosing guidelines for various topical therapies

No comparative trials have been done of the various topical therapies. Most clinicians begin with a trial of capsaicin, a local anesthetic, or both applied concurrently. In the United States capsaicin is available in 0.025% and 0.075% concentrations. The latter concentration has been tested most often in controlled trials (Zhang, Li Wan Po, 1994), and it is reasonable to use this compound in most circumstances. On the basis of clinical observations, an adequate trial is usually considered to be three to four applications per day for a minimum of 4 weeks. The patient or whoever applies the capsaicin should be taught to take precautions against the spread of the capsaicin to other parts of the body of both patient and caregivers. Suggestions include wearing gloves or using applicators such as cotton tip and covering the area with cloth.

Guidelines for a trial of topical local anesthetic are ill defined. To create an area of dense sensory loss using EMLA, a relatively thick application must remain in contact with the skin under an occlusive dressing for at least 1 hour. This mode of administration may be difficult if the painful area is large or adjacent to the face or a mobile region of the body. No evidence exists that cutaneous anesthesia is necessary to gain benefit from a topical local anesthetic and, anecdotally, some patients seem to respond favorably to a thin application applied without a dressing. In the absence of any systematic evaluation of dosing techniques, the patient should be encouraged to try various modes of administration in an effort to identify a salutary approach. If possible, one of these trials should include an occlusive dressing of some type (ordinary plastic wrap can be used for large areas) and a duration of application under this dressing of at least 1 hour.

A trial of a topical antiinflammatory drug may consist of applying to the painful area a solution in which aspirin (or other antiinflammatory drug such as diclofenac) is dissolved in ether or chloroform. The solvent evaporates, leaving the drug in contact with the skin. One way to make the mixture is to crush one or two tablets into a fine powder, stir into approximately 15 mg of chloroform to make a suspension, and apply to the skin with a cotton ball (King, 1993).

ADJUVANT ANALGESICS OF LIMITED USEFULNESS
Neuroleptics

Certain neuroleptics may be considered nonspecific multipurpose analgesics. For some neuroleptics, analgesia has been demonstrated in animal models (Yjritsy-Roy, Standish, Terry, 1989) and several controlled clinical trials in diverse pain syndromes (Beaver, 1996; Bloomfield, Simard-Savoie, Bernier et al., 1964; Hakkarainen, 1977; Lasagna, DeKornfeld, 1961; Lechin, van der Dijs, Lechin et al., 1989). Nonetheless, relatively little evidence of analgesic activity exists for most neuroleptic compounds, and their role as adjuvant analgesics is limited by this lack of research and the potential for adverse effects (Patt, Proper, Reddy, 1994). Neuroleptics that may have some clinical value as analgesics include methotrimeprazine (Levoprome), pimozide (Orap), and fluphenazine (Prolixin).

The strongest evidence of analgesic efficacy has been acquired in studies of the phenothiazine, methotrimeprazine (Levoprome). Favorable studies of this drug have been conducted in patients with cancer pain, other chronic pain states (including some with neuropathic pain), and acute pain after surgery or myocardial infarction (Beaver, Wallenstein, Houde et al., 1966; Bloomfield, Simard-Savoie, Bernier et al., 1964; Davidson, Lindenberg, Walsh, 1979; Lasagna, DeKornfeld, 1961; Montilla, Frederick, Cass, 1963). In these studies the analgesic potency of parenteral methotrimeprazine, 10 to 20 mg, approximated morphine, 10 mg IM.

A controlled comparison of pimozide (Orap) 4 to 12 mg orally per day and carbamazepine in patients with trigeminal neuralgia demonstrated that pimozide has analgesic efficacy in this lancinating neuropathic pain syndrome (Lechin, van der Dijs, Lechin et al., 1989). Unfortunately, a very high incidence of disturbing side effects, including physical and mental slowing, tremor, and parkinsonian symptoms, limited the value of this therapy. The analgesic efficacy of fluphenazine (Prolixin) in headache was similarly suggested in a controlled, multiple-dose (1 mg/day) study of 50 patients with chronic tension headache (Hakkarainen, 1977).

The analgesic efficacy of neuroleptic drugs was *not* confirmed in other controlled single-dose studies. These evaluated chlorpromazine (Thorazine) (Houde, Wallenstein, 1966), promethazine (Phenergan) (Keats, Telford, Kurosu, 1961), and haloperidol (Haldol) (Judkins, Harmer, 1982) in varied pain models.

The possibility of neuroleptic-mediated analgesic effects has also been suggested in numerous anecdotal reports. Trifluoperazine, chlorprothixine, haloperidol, and fluphenazine have been administered for a variety of pain syndromes, including chronic headache and neuropathic pain (Cavenar, Maltbie, 1976; Daw, Cohen-Cole, 1981; Kocher, 1976; Merskey, Hester, 1976; Nathan, 1978), and various neuroleptics have been reported to be coanalgesic when added to another psychotropic or an opioid (Breivik, Rennemo, 1982; Cavenar, Maltbie, 1976; Gomez-Perez, Riell, Dies et al., 1985; Taub, 1973; Weiss Sriwatanakul, Weintraub, 1982). An opioid-sparing effect has been described in several (Breivik, Rennemo, 1982; Cavenar, Maltbie, 1976), but not all (Hanks, Thomas, Trueman et al., 1983), surveys of patients with cancer pain.

Thus the available data establish the analgesic potential of one neuroleptic, methotrimeprazine, and suggests that others may be similarly characterized. The evidence is limited, however, and some well-controlled studies have failed to confirm this effect.

Mechanism of action

The mechanism of neuroleptic analgesia is unknown, but may involve the effect of dopaminergic blockade on endogenous pain-modulating systems. Dopamine receptors, specifically the D2 subtype, are represented among the numerous pathways that subserve pain modulation (Yaksh, Malmberg, 1994). Studies in animals have suggested that selective dopamine antagonists can potentiate morphine analgesia (Bodnar, Nicotera, 1982; Yjritsy-Roy, Standish, Terry, 1989) and controlled clinical trials have demonstrated that metoclopramide, a relatively selective blocker of the D2 receptor, is analgesic in humans (Kandler, Lisander, 1993; Rosenblatt, Cioffi, Sinatra et al, 1991). This evidence, however, does not confirm that a dopaminergic mechanism underlies the analgesic effects of neuroleptic drugs because all these drugs interact with other receptors that could potentially mediate analgesic effects. Even metoclopramide has effects on another central nervous system receptor, specifically the serotonin (5-HT) receptor, that could mediate analgesia (Moss, Sanger, 1990).

Adverse effects

Common side effects of neuroleptic drugs include sedation, orthostatic dizziness, and anticholinergic effects. Some patients experience mental clouding or confusion. Phenothiazines, such as chlorpromazine and fluphenazine, are more likely to produce these effects than other subclasses, such as the butyrophenones (e.g., haloperidol). The sedation produced by the neuroleptics can be additive to other central nervous system depressants.

The possibility of extrapyramidal side effects is perhaps the greatest concern in the clinical use of neuroleptic drugs. The incidence of these disorders varies with the drug, duration of therapy, and dose (Baldessarini, 1990). Compared with other neuroleptics, both fluphenazine and haloperidol are relatively more likely to produce these effects.

The most serious extrapyramidal reaction is the neuroleptic malignant syndrome that is characterized by rigidity, autonomic instability, and encephalopathy. Successful management requires prompt diagnosis, discontinuation of the neuroleptic, and intensive supportive measures. The use of dantrolene and bromocriptine has been suggested in severe cases (Kocher, 1976).

Other extrapyramidal effects can be distressing or seriously impair function. These include acute dystonic reactions (muscle contraction and jerking movements), akithisia (restlessness), parkinsonism, and tardive dyskinesia. The management of these complications usually involves discontinuation of the neuroleptic, with or without the administration of an anticholinergic drug, such as benztropine.

Indications

Ordinarily neuroleptics are not suitable for the ambulatory patient. Their specific use as analgesics has been limited by concerns about side effects. Nonetheless, some indications have evolved on the basis of anecdotal experience.

Methotrimeprazine may be useful in bedridden patients with advanced illnesses such as cancer, who experience pain associated with anxiety, restlessness, or nausea. Consistent with the view of neuroleptics as possible nonspecific multipurpose analgesics, any type of pain may be responsive. For patients with advanced disease, the sedative, anxiolytic, and antiemetic effects of this drug can be highly favorable, and side effects, such as orthostatic hypotension, are less an issue. In the palliative care setting, neuroleptics are also commonly used in the management of delirium.

The efficacy of pimozide in patients with trigeminal neuralgia (Lechin, van der Dijs, Lechin et al., 1989) has suggested a role for this drug in the treatment of patients with refractory neuropathic pains characterized by a predominating lancinating or paroxysmal component. Given its side effect liability, this drug is used after failed trials of other adjuvant analgesics that are indicated for this type of pain. Other neuroleptics, such as haloperidol and fluphenazine, are sometimes considered for patients with various neuropathic pains that have not responded to opioids or preferred adjuvant analgesics, such as antidepressants, local anesthetics, or anticonvulsants.

Dose selection

The neuroleptics are started at low doses and increased to whatever dose the literature suggests is usually analgesic and then discontinued if no analgesia ensues. For example, low initial doses of fluphenazine can be escalated to 1 to 2 mg three times daily, and the dose of haloperidol can be slowly increased to 2 to 5 mg two to three times a day.

In the United States methotrimeprazine is approved only for repetitive intramuscular administration, but extensive experience has affirmed that it may also be given by continuous or bolus subcutaneous or intravenous administration (Storey, Hill, St. Louis et al., 1990). Bolus doses should be administered over 20 to 30 minutes. A useful dosing schedule begins with 5 mg every 6 hours or a comparable dose delivered by infusion, which is gradually increased as needed. Most patients will not require more than 20 mg every 6 hours to gain desired effects.

Antihistamines

Favorable effects from antihistamine-containing proprietary pain relievers has been observed (Gilbert, 1976; Lipman, 1996), and some data suggest that antihistaminic drugs may be nonspecific analgesics. Controlled single-dose studies have established that the following can have some analgesic effects (Batterman, 1965; Beaver, Feise, 1976; Birkeland, Clawson, 1958; Campos, Solis, 1980; Hupert, Yacoub, Turgeon, 1980; McColl, Durkin, 1982; Stambaugh, Lance, 1983; Sunshine, Zighelboim, De Castro et al., 1989):

- Diphenhydramine (Benadryl)
- Hydroxyzine (Vistaril parenterally)
- Orphenadrine (one ingredient in Norgesic)
- Phenyltoloxamine (Phenylgesic, a nonprescription cold remedy)
- Pyrilamine (an ingredient in several cold remedies [e.g., Codimal PH syrup, ND-Gesic tablets])

Despite research evidence of their analgesic effects, clinical experience has been disappointing. The failure to observe substantial analgesia from the addition of an antihistamine suggests that treatment should be considered only for patients who have other indications other than pain. Hydroxyzine, for example, is sometimes administered to patients with pain complicated by anxiety, nausea, or itch in the hope that analgesia will be augmented while these other symptoms are relieved. The use of these agents must also be tempered by the potential for side effects (e.g., sedation) that add to those produced by other centrally acting drugs, including the opioids.

Cannabinoids

The synthesized form of one of marijuana's active ingredients is delta-9-tetrahydrocannabinol (THC), which has been marketed as dronabinol (Marinol) and is available in 2.5, 5, and 10 mg capsules. In a single-dose study of patients with cancer pain, THC, 10 mg orally, was well tolerated and produced analgesic effects similar to 60 mg codeine, but a higher dose yielded severe side effects in many patients (Noyes, Brunk, Avery et al., 1976). Thus the therapeutic window for this drug appears narrow, and maximal efficacy at tolerable doses is limited. For these reasons, cannabinoids have not become accepted as adjuvant analgesics.

Alcohol (Ethanol)

For centuries, alcohol has served as an analgesic in the absence of other more effective alternatives. This practice continues today as a socially, although not medically, accepted remedy for dealing with pain. For example, according to Kotarba's (1983) observations of social drinking in neighborhood cocktail lounges, many pain-afflicted working class bar drinkers use alcohol as an analgesic. Some drinkers consciously take advantage of the relationship between drinking alcohol and "feeling no pain."

Years ago IV alcohol in 5% to 10% solution was used to relieve mild to moderate pain (Cutter, O'Farrell, Whitehouse et al., 1986). The effects of IV administration appear to be the same as those that occur with oral administration.

Research based on experimentally induced pain suggests that the analgesia of alcohol is related to increased pain tolerance rather than decreased pain perception (Woodrow, Eltherington, 1988). The alcohol equivalent of two cocktails induced analgesia (in the form of pain tolerance) that was comparable to that of 11.6 mg of subcutaneous morphine. This occurred at a blood concentration of approximately 70 mg/100 ml.

The therapeutic value of alcohol is extremely limited because of the intoxicating effects that accompany acute consumption and the medical problems associated with chronic use. Furthermore, alcohol used in conjunction with opioids increases sedation and may decrease respirations (Hobbs, Rall, Verdoorn, 1996). Chronic use of alcohol in conjunction with acetaminophen increases the risk of hepatic damage. Use with NSAIDs increases the risk of gastric injury. Thus alcohol is not recommended as an adjuvant analgesic. However, clinicians should be aware of why patients with pain may consume alcohol and attempt to replace the perceived benefits of alcohol with other pain relief methods.

Benzodiazepines

The benzodiazepines clonazepam (Caccia, 1975; Martin, 1981; Swerdlow, Cundill, 1981) and alprazolam (Fernandez, Adams, Holmes, 1987) have been used in the management of lancinating and cancer-related neuropathic pain, respectively. Although these data suggest a broad role for the benzodiazepines as adjuvant analgesics for neuropathic pain, the critical reviews of the current information about these drugs do not support this position (Dellemijn, Fields, 1994; Reddy, Patt, 1994). Negative findings have been reported in a controlled trial of lorazepam for postherpetic neuralgia (Max, Schafer, Culnane et al., 1988) and a small controlled repeated-dose study of oral chlordiazepoxide for chronic pain (Yosselson-Superstine, Lipman, Saunders, 1985).

The evidence for benzodiazepine-induced analgesia in acute pain is mixed. One study of 105 patients receiving intramuscular morphine (10 mg), diazepam (10 mg), and a combination of both (morphine, 5 mg, and diazepam, 5 mg) revealed that all three treatments produced pain relief, with diazepam alone being the least effective and the combination being the most effective (Singh, Sharma, Gupta et al., 1981). However, in another controlled study of IV midazolam and morphine for postoperative pain, the addition of midazolam decreased anxiety but did not influence pain scores or amount of morphine required (Egan, Ready, Nessly et al., 1992). In a human experimental pain paradigm, the addition of alprazolam to a morphine infusion did not potentiate analgesia (Reddy, Patt, 1994). In a controlled study of postoperative pain the addition of midazolam to meperidine did not enhance analgesia but did produce significantly more sedation than meperidine alone (Miller, Eisenkraft, Cohen et al.,

1986). In a controlled study of postoperative dental pain the administration of diazepam preoperatively was shown to have an ongoing antianalgesic effect on morphine analgesia (Gear, Miaskowski, Heller et al., 1997).

Another study of diazepam in a model of laboratory-induced pain suggested that the analgesic effects produced by diazepam were attributable to a change in response bias, the psychologic inclination to describe a nociceptive stimulus as painful rather than a change in the sensorineural processing of the stimulus (Yang, Clark, Ngai et al., 1979). Interestingly, in one study of morphine and midazolam for postoperative pain, nursing assessments of pain were lower than those of the patients, suggesting that observers have response biases toward inferring less pain when patients are less anxious (Fragen, Tobin, 1984).

Thus the evidence for benzodiazepine analgesia is limited and conflicting. Regarding acute pain, the American Pain Society (1992) concludes that benzodiazepines are not effective analgesics except for muscle spasm, and opioid titration should precede treatment with benzodiazepines. Although a trial of clonazepam or alprazolam can be justified in refractory neuropathic pain on the basis of anecdotal experience, the relative safety of these drugs, and the common coexistence of pain and anxiety, wider use of benzodiazepines as adjuvant analgesics is not warranted. Clinical experience with clonazepam has generally been favorable in those patients with lancinating or paroxysmal pain.

As discussed previously, the evidence for use of benzodiazepines as muscle relaxants is also limited. Diazepam and other benzodiazepines are widely used for this purpose, but benefits are limited, especially when given orally (Baldessarini, 1996).

ROLE OF ADJUVANT ANALGESICS IN ACUTE PAIN AND CRESCENDO PAIN

Certain adjuvant analgesics used in the treatment of chronic pain may also be useful in the relief of acute pain, including acute exacerbations of chronic pain, sometimes referred to as crescendo pain. Others have been shown to be ineffective. For example, in a controlled study of relief of experimentally induced acute pain in volunteers, parenteral administration of amitriptyline alone and with alfentanil failed to demonstrate that amitriptyline relieves pain or potentiates opioid analgesia for acute pain (Eisenach, Hood, Curry et al., 1997). Postoperative pain was not responsive to sodium valproate (Martin, Martin, Rud et al., 1988), and postherpetic neuralgia was not relieved by carbamazepine (Keczkes, Basheer, 1980).

However, some of the previously discussed adjuvant analgesics may be useful in acute pain. Following is a discussion of the potential role of certain adjuvant analgesics that may be used in addition to or instead of the more traditional approaches to episodes of acute pain.

Clonidine

The benefits of epidural clonidine (now available as Duraclon) for chronic neuropathic pain in patients with cancer were demonstrated and discussed earlier in this chapter. Clonidine is also useful for acute pain. A clinical review of publications from 1984 through 1995 on clonidine administered spinally and peripherally for anesthesia and analgesia reveals that clonidine added to local anesthetics prolongs and intensifies anesthesia for surgery and that clonidine combined with epidural opioids postoperatively reduces the dose of opioid required with correspondingly fewer side effects. Epidural clonidine has demonstrated opioid dose-sparing effects postoperatively in combination with fentanyl, sufentanil, butorphanol, and morphine (Eisenach, De Kock, Klimscha, 1996). Research also confirms that clonidine alone provides analgesia for postoperative pain, but these doses tend to be much higher than those required for potentiation of opioid analgesia (De Kock, Wiederkher, Laghmiche et al., 1997). Further, epidural clonidine alone was not sufficient analgesia for most patients.

Because clonidine is lipophilic, it is rapidly absorbed into the systemic circulation after epidural administration. However, clonidine is approximately twice as effective given epidurally as intravenously. This fact indicates a spinal site of action for analgesia (Eisenach, De Kock, Klimscha, 1996). The superiority of the epidural route over intravenous administration of clonidine is further confirmed in a controlled trial of intravenous versus epidural clonidine after major orthopedic surgery. These data revealed that intravenous clonidine causes more sedation (Bernard, Kick, Bonnet, 1995).

Side effects of clonidine are mainly hypotension, bradycardia, and sedation. However, experience with more than 2000 patients, mostly in the perioperative period, suggests that epidural clonidine is safe. Unlike opioids, clonidine does not produce severe respiratory depression (even after massive overdose) nor does it potentiate opioid-induced respiratory depression (Eisenach, De Kock, Klimscha, 1996).

Hemodynamic effects of spinal or systemic clonidine begin within 30 minutes of administration, reach a peak at 1 to 2 hours, and last approximately 6 to 8 hours after injection. Delayed onset of hypotension has not been observed. Epidural clonidine administered at low thoracic or lumbar levels is much less likely to produce hypotension than with higher thoracic epidural injection. In studies of epidural clonidine by continuous infusion for postoperative analgesia, no cases of serious hypotension or respiratory depression have been found. However, blood pressure and heart rate should be monitored for at least 2 hours after a bolus injection, and intravenous access should be maintained (Eisenach, De Kock, Klimscha, 1996).

Sedation occurs within 20 minutes of administration. It increases with increasing doses and reflects systemic absorption that affects higher centers in the CNS. After a large epidural bolus, such as 700 μg, sedation is intense for 4 to 6 hours. Delayed onset of sedation has not been observed. With epidural continuous infusion, doses of 30 and 40 μg/h epidurally for cancer pain and postoperative pain, respectively, produce no more sedation than placebo (Eisenach, De Kock, Klimscha, 1996).

Onset of analgesia after epidural injection of clonidine is usually within 1 hour (30 to 60 minutes). In postoperative patients analgesia after an epidural bolus of clonidine lasts approximately 2 to 6 hours. Duration of analgesia increases with increasing doses up to a 400 μg epidural bolus. A continuous infusion is required for sustained analgesia. Infusion rates of about 25 μg/h reduce morphine requirements, and infusion rates of 120 to 150 μg/h may provide complete analgesia (Eisenach, De Kock, Klimscha, 1996).

For women in labor, studies suggest that 75 μg may be the appropriate dose to combine with bupivacaine as a single epidural bolus to prolong analgesia. Sedation is not evident at this dose and labor is not prolonged. Most studies demonstrate no adverse effects on the infant (Eisenach, De Kock, Klimscha, 1996).

After cesarean section, studies suggest that the appropriate loading dose is 400 μg. Continuous infusion (20 to 40 μg) is necessary for sustained analgesia. Clonidine has also been combined with an epidural opioid for analgesia after cesarean section. Side effects are similar to those following other types of surgery (Eisenach, De Kock, Klimscha, 1996).

In children clonidine has been combined with bupivacaine for caudal and lumbar epidural analgesia. This has successfully increased the duration of analgesia postoperatively (Eisenach, De Kock, Klimscha, 1996; De Negri, Visconte, De Vivo et al., 1997).

Thus epidural clonidine shows promise in the treatment of acute pain of nociceptive origin and chronic pain of neuropathic origin. Table 7.10 summarizes this clinical experience.

A recent study investigated the effect of oral clonidine premedication on postoperative analgesia. Data suggest that oral clonidine (5 μg/kg) increases the duration of analgesia of intrathecal morphine plus tetracaine without increasing the intensity of opioid side effects (Goyagi, Nishikawa, 1996). Another study suggests that premedication of oral clonidine, 4 μg/kg, alone may provide analgesia postoperatively in children (Mikawa, Nishina, Maekawa et al., 1996).

Ketamine

Although interest in the use of ketamine (an NMDA receptor antagonist) for analgesia has focused mostly on

TABLE 7.10

SUMMARY OF CLINICAL EXPERIENCE WITH CLONIDINE FOR REGIONAL ANESTHESIA AND ANALGESIA				
PATIENT GROUP	USE	DOSE	EFFECT	SIDE EFFECTS
Epidural Administration				
Cancer pain	+ Morphine	30 μg/h	Improved pain, reduced morphine especially neuropathic pain	Transient sedation, ↓ blood pressure
Chronic pain	Alone	30 μg/h	Pain relief, especially in sympathetically maintained pain, deafferentation	Transient sedation, ↓ blood pressure
Intraoperative	Alone	300-500 μg	↓ Anesthetic use by 50%-75%	↓ Blood pressure
	+ Local anesthetic	150 μg	Prolongs anesthesia by 50%-100%	Sedation, blood pressure similar to local anesthetic alone
Postoperative	Alone	400 μg	Analgesia for 5 h	Intense sedation, ↓ blood pressure
	+ Opioid	75-150 μg	Prolongs analgesia by 100%	Minimal
		20 μg/h	Reduces opioid use by 50%, improves pain relief	Less hypoxemia than opioid alone
Obstetrics (labor)	+ Bupivacaine	75 μg	Prolongs analgesia by 100%	Minimal
Pediatrics (caudal)	+ Bupivacaine	1-3 μg/kg	Prolongs anesthesia/analgesia by 100%	Minimal
Spinal Administration				
Intraoperative	+ Bupivacaine	75-150 μg	Prolongs anesthesia/analgesia by 30%, reduces tourniquet pain	Minimal
Postoperative	Alone	150-300 μg	7-10 h of complete analgesia	Sedation, ↓ blood pressure
Peripheral Nerve Block				
Intraoperative	+ Mepivacaine	10-100 μg	Prolongs anesthesia/analgesia 50%-100%	Minimal

Minimal, no difference from control (opioid or local anesthetic alone).
From Eisenach JC, De Kock M, Klimscha W: α2-Adrenergic agonists for regional anesthesia: A clinical review of clonidine (1984-1995), *Anesthesiology* 85:655-674, 1996.

treatment of chronic neuropathic pain, evidence also suggests that ketamine may be a multipurpose analgesic for acute pain (Dich-Hielsen, Svendsen, Berthelsen, 1992; Jahangir, Islam, Aziz, 1993). At subanesthetic doses ketamine has several advantages over opioids. It does not suppress cardiovascular function, it does not depress the laryngeal protective reflexes, and it causes less respiratory depression than opioids. However, tolerance can occur and adverse effects include dizziness, frightening dreams, and possibly hallucinations (Javery, Ussery, Steger et al., 1996).

Parenteral

IV PCA administration of ketamine (1 mg/ml) plus morphine (1 mg/ml) compared with morphine (1 mg/ml) alone for postoperative pain revealed that morphine with ketamine provided superior analgesia with almost half as much morphine. Patients receiving morphine with ketamine also had fewer side effects. Because keta-

mine is known to cause adverse psychomimetic effects, it is noteworthy that only one patient in the morphine/ketamine group reported dysphoria (Javery, Ussery, Steger et al., 1996).

These findings are in contrast with those of a comparable study of elderly patients postoperatively in which variable doses of ketamine (5, 10, or 15 mg/h) were added to morphine (1 mg/h) IV continuous infusion and compared with morphine alone (Edwards, Fletcher, Cole et al., 1993). Additional morphine was available by IV PCA. No difference was found between the groups with respect to analgesia, morphine consumption, or pulmonary function. Patients on the higher doses of ketamine were more likely to report dreams. Still another study comparing intramuscular ketamine with IM meperidine found that the two were comparable in providing analgesia with few side effects (Dich-Hielsen, Svendsen, Berthelsen, 1992).

A controlled study of postoperative pain found that ketamine (0.5 mg/kg followed by IV infusion of 10 μg/kg/min) given preemptively (before surgery) reduced postoperative opioid requirements (Fu, Miguel, Scharf, 1997). However, the value of using ketamine for preemptive analgesia remains unclear, and it is certainly far less effective than spinally administered bupivacaine (Hirota, Lambert, 1996; Tverskoy, Oz, Isakson et al., 1994).

Because opioids may release histamine and cause bronchospasm in asthmatic patients, the role of ketamine for postoperative analgesia for patients with asthma has been explored (Jahangir, Islam, Aziz, 1993). Preliminary observations suggest that a ketamine and midazolam infusion is worthy of consideration in these patients. Benzodiazepines are often used with ketamine to prevent psychomimetic effects (Beltrutti, Coletta, Di Santo et al., 1997).

Ketamine has also been used for procedural pain such as burn wound care and peribulbar block (Martinez, Achauer, de Rios, 1985; Rosenberg, Raymond, Bridge, 1995). Doses IV begin at 0.5 to 1 mg/kg. The use of ketamine for procedural pain is discussed further in Chapter 8. For patients with spinal metastases who experience severe pain on movement, transport from home to hospital has been accomplished comfortably with the use of ketamine 100 mg IV with 50 mg boluses as needed (Notcutt, 1994).

The role of IV ketamine in relief of crescendo neuropathic pain remains to be clarified. A controlled study of six patients with chronic neuropathic pain demonstrated that IV ketamine produces prompt but partial analgesia in some patients, but it lasts only 2 to 3 hours (Backonja, Arndt, Gombar et al., 1994). Each patient was premedicated with a benzodiazepine and received 250 μg/kg by slow push over 5 minutes. Side effects after a single dose were mild, most commonly sedation. Continuous infusion resulted in much more pronounced side effects.

Epidural

Epidural ketamine alone has also been evaluated as a postoperative analgesic, but most studies indicate inadequate analgesia. The mechanism of action for epidural ketamine analgesia may be the result of local anesthetic or opioid agonist activity (Littrell, 1991). In one uncontrolled study of 50 patients after relatively minor surgical procedures, ketamine (4 mg epidurally) was found to be a safe and effective analgesic (Islas, Astorga, Laredo, 1985).

A controlled study of epidural ketamine for surgical pain demonstrated that 30 mg was safe and effective (Naguib, Adu-Gyamfi, Absood et al., 1986). Other double-blind studies, however, do not confirm the usefulness of epidural ketamine (7 mg bolus followed by continuous infusion of 10 mg/h) and suggest that morphine and/or bupivacaine epidurally are superior (Cullen, Starren, El-Ganzouri et al., 1985; Ivankovich, McCarthy, 1986; Logas, Faber, El-Ganzouri et al., 1984).

A review of these and other studies of epidural ketamine for postoperative analgesia points to two levels of dosing, one in the range of 30 to 50 mg and the other at lower doses of 4 to 12 mg. Results do not establish that higher doses are better than the lower doses. One of the problems is the lack of controlled studies. Ketamine alone epidurally does not appear to be a good choice for postoperative pain management (Beltrutti, Coletta, Di Santo et al., 1997).

However, ketamine may have a role in combination with opioids epidurally. In a controlled study of surgical patients undergoing major joint replacement, the results indicated that ketamine, 30 mg, epidurally alone produced no significant pain relief, but coadministration of ketamine, 10 mg, and morphine, 0.5 mg, epidurally produced a strong analgesic effect with fewer adverse effects than morphine alone (Wong, Liaw, Tung et al., 1996). Another study shows that ketamine combined with bupivacaine increases the duration of analgesia (Cook, Grubb, Aldridge et al., 1995).

Further studies are needed before encouraging the use of epidural ketamine. The extent of the neurotoxic effects needs to be identified, and clarification is needed regarding the use of ketamine spinally as a single drug or in support of local anesthetics or opioids (Beltrutti, Coletta, Di Santo et al., 1997).

Parenteral Lidocaine

Systemic (oral or parenteral) local anesthetics are effective analgesics in a variety of acute and chronic pain syndromes, suggesting that they are multipurpose analgesics. Most of the focus of controlled trials and clinical experience has been on the management of chronic neuropathic pain, discussed previously in this chapter.

The role of parenteral local anesthetics in acute pain is promising but less well established. Because of its rapid onset of analgesia, parenteral infusion of lidocaine is a reasonable consideration in patients with crescendo neuropathic pain that is unresponsive to more traditional approaches. Furthermore, parenteral lidocaine may be beneficial for some patients who have not responded to oral local anesthetics (Brose, Cousins, 1991).

Intravenous lidocaine may provide immediate relief for some patients with chronic neuropathic pain. In a study of 13 patients with neuropathic pain, lidocaine, 500 mg IV, administered over 60 minutes resulted in complete pain relief for 10 patients. Analgesia occurred rapidly, within 15 minutes, and peaked within 1 hour of administration. Six patients experienced light-headedness, two felt "drunk," and another two were slightly sedated but it was not necessary to adjust the infusion. An important finding was that pain scores increased and decreased abruptly with small changes in dose (Ferrante, Paggioli, Cherukuri et al., 1996).

In another study of three patients with neuropathic pain unresponsive to a variety of other more traditional analgesic regiments, intravenous lidocaine (4 mg/kg over 30 minutes) was effective and led to initiation of continuous infusion of subcutaneous lidocaine. Subcutaneous doses ranging from 100 to 160 mg/hour continued to provide pain relief for all three patients, and therapy was continued for up to 6 months (Brose, Cousins, 1991).

Brief intravenous infusions of lidocaine or procaine can relieve acute postoperative pain and pain caused by burns as demonstrated in numerous surveys (Gilbert, Hanson, Brown et al., 1951; Gordon, 1943, 1948; McLachlin, 1945) and several controlled trials (Bartlett, Hutaserani, 1961; Birch, Jorgensen, Chraemer-Jorgensen et al., 1987; Cassuto, Wallin, Hogstrom et al., 1985; Keats, D'Allessandro 1951). For example, a survey of seven patients with second-degree burns illustrates how IV lidocaine may be used (Jonsson, Cassuto, Hanson, 1991). For these patients, IV lidocaine was begun within 6 hours of injury and continued up to 3 days. Using a pain rating scale of 0 to 100 (0 = no pain; 100 = unbearable pain), pain scores fell from the 80s and 90s to an average of 17 two hours after the infusion was started. Starting dose was a bolus of 1 mg/kg, followed by a continuous infusion of 40 μg/kg per minute. A bolus dose of 50 mg was given either before dressing changes or as needed. Additional opioid analgesia was available, but no patient requested it. Side effects included euphoria and light-headedness, but no cardiovascular or other side effects were noted.

Brief intravenous infusion of lidocaine is also effective in relieving some types of headache. A controlled study confirmed the effectiveness of lidocaine, 100 mg IV slow push, in migraine headaches but not tension headaches (Maciewicz, Chung, Strassman et al., 1988).

A controlled study of postoperative PCA analgesia with lidocaine plus morphine compared with morphine alone yielded disappointing results (Cepeda, Delgado, Ponce et al., 1996). The addition of lidocaine, 10 or 20 mg/ml, to morphine, 1 mg/ml, resulted in no difference in opioid use, pain levels, or side effects. However, the dose may have been too low or the infusion technique (PCA as opposed to continuous infusion) may be responsible. Analgesia may occur only within a narrow dose range (Ferrante, Paggioli, Cherukuri et al., 1996).

The narrow therapeutic range for analgesia requires monitoring of lidocaine concentration in the blood. In one anecdotal report analgesia occurred with plasma concentrations in the range of 2 to 5 μg/ml (Brose, Cousins, 1991).

Lidocaine infusions have been administered at varying doses, typically within a range of 2 to 5 mg/kg infused intravenously over 20 to 30 minutes (Backonja, 1994a; Portenoy, Kanner, 1996). These are the dose ranges currently chosen by most clinicians. In the medically frail patient it is prudent to start at the lower end of this range.

Adverse effects with parenteral administration of lidocaine have been minimal. They occur with increasing serum concentrations and include light-headedness, numbness around the mouth, dizziness, tinnitus, and visual changes. The dose must be adjusted downward to prevent progression to muscle spasm and convulsions (Brose, Cousins, 1991).

Adenosine

Adenosine (Adenocard, Adenoscan) is an antiarrhythmic commercially available for intravenous administration. A recent study of adenosine in the postoperative setting suggests that this compound may have analgesic effects (Segerdahl, Ekblom, Sandelin et al., 1995). In addition, in two patients with peripheral neuropathic pain, an intravenous infusion of 50 to 70 μg/kg per minute produced pain relief within 30 minutes that lasted for hours after the infusion (Sollevi, Belfrage, Lundeberg et al., 1995). A clinical role for adenosine is yet to be clarified.

IV Phenytoin

For crescendo neuropathic pain, phenytoin IV may be an option for rapid pain control. One case report demonstrated relief of severe, rapidly escalating lancinating neuropathic pain within 1 hour after a 500 mg IV dose of phenytoin (Chang, 1997).

Dextroamphetamine

Efficacy of dextroamphetamine in postoperative pain management was clearly illustrated in a study of 450 patients who received combinations of morphine and dextroamphetamine. Intramuscular doses of dextroamphetamine, 5 or 10 mg, added to morphine resulted in 50% to 100% increases in analgesia without accompanying sedation or respiratory depression (Forrest, Brown, Brown et al., 1977). The use of this drug or other psychostimulants combined with opioids for acute pain may be worthy of consideration and further investigation.

Corticosteroids

As discussed previously, the role of corticosteroids in the management of spinal cord compression, superior vena cava syndrome, and raised intracranial pressure is well recognized. Short-term, high-dose therapy is appropriate for crescendo cancer pain.

A survey of patients administered high doses of dexamethasone (96 mg per day for 2 weeks) for malignant epidural spinal cord compression observed pain relief in 64% within hours of the initial dose (Greenberg, Kim,

Posner, 1980). A recent randomized trial confirmed that dexamethasone was profoundly analgesic in spinal cord compression but could not identify any difference between a high (100 mg) and low (10 mg) initial dose (Vecht, Haaxma-Reiche, van Putten et al., 1989). Clinically, a high-dose regimen is often used for severe, acute pain (Ettinger, Portenoy, 1988). This is tapered over weeks as other analgesic approaches are initiated and become effective.

USE OF ADJUVANT ANALGESICS IN CHILDREN

A number of conditions that occur in adults and are treated with adjuvant analgesics also occur in children. For example, reflex sympathetic dystrophy, phantom pain, neuropathic pain resulting from chemotherapy, and neuropathy associated with HIV are a few of many painful problems that occur in both adults and children and may be responsive to the same treatment, such as adjuvant analgesics.

Little research is available, however, regarding how the use of adjuvant analgesics in children might differ from their use in adults. Meanwhile, the same guidelines are used for both children and adults, except for dosing. Table 7.11 provides pediatric dosing guidelines for selected adjuvant analgesics. Most of the dosing is based on recommendations given when the drugs are used for their original indications; dosing for anticonvulsants are essentially the same whether they are used for seizure disorder or for pain relief.

CONCLUSIONS

Although the use of adjuvant analgesics in chronic and acute pain remains largely guided by anecdotal experience, controlled clinical trials have begun to provide a scientific rationale for many therapies. Future investigations of nociceptive processes and pain pathophysiology will undoubtedly lead to the development of novel drugs. For example, the adjuvant analgesics may one day include drugs that modulate peripheral nociceptive processes, such as substance P or bradykinin antagonists, or drugs that alter central processing by interacting with gangliosides or second messenger systems activated by excitatory amino acids.

For many patients with pain, particularly those in the palliative care and acute care settings, opioid drugs continue to be the mainstay of analgesia. However, adjuvant analgesics offer opportunities for improved outcomes in those patients who cannot attain an acceptable balance between pain relief and opioid or NSAID-induced side effects. For many patients with chronic nonmalignant pain, adjuvants are an alternative to opioids or more invasive therapies. Table 7.12 provides guidelines for adults for the more commonly used adjuvant analgesics discussed in this chapter.

PATIENT INFORMATION

As mentioned at the beginning of this chapter, use of adjuvant analgesics is "labor intensive," requiring frequent assessment and dose titration. Enlisting the patient's cooperation is essential for success. Form 7.1 (p. 345) presents a format for teaching the patient and family about adjuvant analgesics in general along with blanks for information about the specific one the patient is taking.

Another approach to teaching patients about their medications is to develop an information sheet about the most commonly prescribed drugs in that particular clinical setting. Examples are provided for desipramine (Box 7.3), nortriptyline (Box 7.4), gabapentin (Box 7.5), and mexiletine (Box 7.6) (pp. 346–353). The information covers physical description of the medication, why it is prescribed, dosage, frequency, and possible side effects. To ensure safety the patient needs to know which adverse effects may occur. Research has shown that informing patients about adverse effects of therapy does not itself have any detectable adverse effects (Howland, Baker, Poe, 1990). In other words, educating the patient about potential side effects does not increase the likelihood that these side effects will occur.

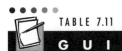

TABLE 7.11

GUIDELINES

PEDIATRIC DOSING GUIDELINES FOR SELECTED ADJUVANT ANALGESICS

Drug class: generic (brand)	Dosing (oral)
Anticonvulsants	

Carbamazepine (Tegretol)	< 6 years:
	    Initial: 5-10 mg/kg/24 h PO ÷ bid
	    Increment: up to 20 mg/kg/24 h q week
	6-12 years:
	    Initial: 10 mg/kg/24 h PO ÷ bid
	    Maximum dose: 100 mg/dose bid
	    Increment: 10 mg/kg/24 h ÷ bid q week
	> 12 years:
	    Initial: 200 mg PO bid
	    Increment: 200 mg/24 hr ÷ bid q week
	    Maximum dose: 1.6-2.4 g/24 h

Gabapentin (Neurontin)	Initial: 5 mg/kg or 300 mg PO qhs Day 2: increase to bid Day 3: increase to tid
Phenytoin (Dilantin)	Initial: 2-3 mg/kg or 100-150 mg PO, bid, qid Titrate: increase 0.5 mg/kg or 25-50 mg q 3-4 wk Maximum dose: 5 mg/kg/day or 1000 mg/day
Valproic acid (Depakene)	Initial: 5-15 mg/kg or 250-2000 mg PO qhs or tid Titrate: increase 5-10 mg/kg or 25-50 mg q 5-7 days Maintenance: 0.5-4.0 mg/kg or 25-200 mg PO Maximum dose: 60 mg/kg/day
Antidepressants	
Amitriptyline (Elavil)	Initial: 0.2-0.5 mg/kg or 10-25 mg PO qhs Titrate: increase by 0.25 mg/kg or 10-25 mg q 5-7 days Maintenance: 0.2-3 mg/kg or 10-150 mg
Desipramine (Norpramin)	Initial: 1-2 mg/kg or 50-100 mg PO qhs Titrate: increase by 0.5 mg/kg (25-50 mg) q 5-7 days Maintenance: 1-4 mg/kg or 50-200 mg
Imipramine (Tofranil)	Initial: 0.5-2.0 mg/kg or 25-100 mg PO qhs Titrate: increase by 0.5 mg/kg or 25-50 mg PO q 5-7 days Maintenance: 0.5-4.0 mg/kg or 25-200 mg Maximum dose: 5 mg/kg/day
Nortriptyline (Aventyl, Pamelor)	Initial: 0.2-1.0 mg/kg or 10-50 mg PO q AM Titrate: increase 0.25 mg/kg or 10-25 mg PO q 5-7 day Maintenance: 0.2-3 mg/kg or 10-150 PO mg q AM
Oral Local Anesthetic	
Mexiletine (Mexitil)	Initial: 2-3 mg/kg or 150-200 mg PO qd-tid Titrate: increase 0.5 mg/kg or 25-50 mg q 2-3 wk Maintenance: 2-8 mg/kg or 150-400 mg PO qd tid Maximum dose: 1800 mg qd
Psychostimulants	
Dextroamphetamine (Dexedrine)	Initial: 2.5 mg dose after breakfast and lunch Titrate: 2.5 mg/dose Maintenance: 2.5-10 mg/dose
Methylphenidate (Ritalin)	Initial: 2.5 mg dose after breakfast and lunch Titrate: 2.5 mg/dose Maintenance: 5-20 mg/dose

May be duplicated for use in clinical practice. From McCaffery M, Pasero C: *Pain: Clinical manual*, p. 341. Copyright © 1999, Mosby, Inc.

Information from Heiligenstein D, Gerrity S: Psychotropics as adjuvant analgesics. In Schechter NL, Berde CB, Yaster M, editors: *Pain in infants, children, and adolescents*, pp 173-177, Baltimore, 1993, Williams & Wilkins; Yaster M, Krane EJ, Kaplan RF et al., editors: *Pediatric pain management and sedation handbook*, St. Louis, 1997, Mosby.

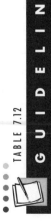

TABLE 7.12

COMMONLY USED ADJUVANT ANALGESICS

Drug Class	Indications	Preferred Drugs/Routes	Usual Starting Dose (mg/day)	Usual Effective Dose Range (mg/day)	Dosing Schedule	Comments
Alpha₂-adrenergic agonist	Multipurpose for chronic pain	Clonidine Transdermal (Catapres)	0.1	?	qd	Doses may be increased by 0.1 mg/day q3-5 days.
		PO	0.1	?	qd	
	Acute nociceptive pain or chronic neuropathic pain	Epidural	25 μg/h	Same	q1h	Added to local anesthetics, clonidine prolongs anesthesia for surgery; combined with epidural opioids, it reduces the opioid dose required. Onset of side effects and analgesia within 30-60 min. Epidural superior to IV.
	Multipurpose for chronic pain	Tizanidine PO (Zanaflex)	6	bid		
Anticonvulsants	First line for paroxysmal (sudden onset) or "shooting" neuropathic pain; second line for nonparoxysmal	Carbamazepine (Tegretol) PO	200	600-1200	q6-8h	
		Clonazepam (Klonopin) PO	0.5	0.5-3	q8h	
		Divalproex sodium (Depakote) PO	500	1500-3000	q8h	
		Phenytoin (Dilantin) PO	300	300	hs	Loading doses may be used (e.g., 500 mg × 2).
		IV	500-1000	?	?	IV dose used for rapidly escalating neuropathic pain.
		Valproate sodium (Depacon) IV	max 20 mg/kg over 5 min	?	?	IV dose used for rapidly escalating neuropathic pain; followed by PO doses.
	Multipurpose for all types of neuropathic pain	Gabapentin (Neurontin) PO	100-300	300-3600	q8h	May increase dose daily.

Continued.

May be duplicated for use in clinical practice. From McCaffery M, Pasero C: *Pain: Clinical manual,* pp. 342-344. Copyright © 1999, Mosby, Inc.

?, unknown, unclear; *h,* hour; *hs,* bedtime; *IU,* international units; *q,* every; *qd,* every day.

Table based on clinical experience of the authors and a variety of published sources, including Coyle N, Cherny NI, Portenoy RK: Pharmacologic management of cancer pain. In McGuire DB, Yarbro CH, Ferrell BR, editors: *Cancer pain management,* ed 2, pp 118-119, Boston, 1995, Jones & Bartlett Publishers.

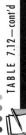

TABLE 7.12—cont'd

GUIDELINES

GUIDELINES FOR COMMONLY USED ADJUVANT ANALGESICS—cont'd

Drug Class	Indications	Preferred Drugs/Routes	Usual Starting Dose (mg/day)	Usual Effective Dose Range (mg/day)	Dosing Schedule	Comments
Antidepressants						
Tricyclics	Multipurpose for chronic pain; effective for both continuous and "shooting" neuropathic pain, but generally used as second-line agents for paroxysmal (sudden onset) pain	Amitriptyline (Elavil) PO	10–25	50–150	hs	Traditionally amitriptyline was first line. Because of side effects and recent evidence of comparable analgesia, desipramine is preferred for many patients, especially elderly. Less hypotension with nortriptyline. Evaluate and titrate upward q3-5 days. Some patients may prefer divided doses (e.g., q8h).
		Clomipramine (Anafranil) PO	10–25	50–150	hs	
		Desipramine (Norpramin) PO	10–25	50–150	hs	
		Doxepin (Sinequan) PO	10–25	50–150	hs	
		Imipramine (Tofranil) PO	10–25	50–150	hs	
		Nortriptyline (Aventyl, Pamelor) PO	10–25	50–150	hs	
"Newer"	Same as above	Fluoxetine (Prozac) PO	10–20	20–40	qd	Fewer side effects than tricyclics; less evidence of effectiveness.
		Paroxetine (Paxil) PO	20	20–40	qd	
		Sertraline (Zoloft) PO	50	150–200	qd	
Corticosteroids	Multipurpose analgesics	Dexamethasone (Decadron) PO	Low-dose regimen: 1-2 mg	Same	qd or bid	May also improve appetite, nausea, and malaise. In patients with advanced medical illness, long-term treatment with low doses is generally well tolerated; used when pain persists after optimal opioid dosing.
			High-dose regimen: 100 mg then 96 mg in 4 divided doses	Same	qid	High doses used for acute episode of severe pain unresponsive to opioids. Risk of serious toxicity increases with dose, duration of therapy, and coadministration of a NSAID.
GABAergic	"Shooting" neuropathic pain	Baclofen (Lioresal) PO	15	30–200	q8h	

May be duplicated for use in clinical practice. From McCaffery M, Pasero C: *Pain: Clinical manual*, pp. 342-344. Copyright © 1999, Mosby, Inc.

Continued.

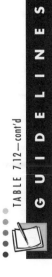

TABLE 7.12—cont'd

GUIDELINES FOR COMMONLY USED ADJUVANT ANALGESICS—cont'd

Drug Class	Indications	Preferred Drugs/Routes	Usual Starting Dose (mg/day)	Usual Effective Dose Range (mg/day)	Dosing Schedule	Comments
Local anesthetics	Neuropathic pain of any type	Mexiletine (Mexitil) PO	150	900–1200	q8h	Mexiletine is safer than tocainide and should be tried first. Plasma concentrations should be followed to reduce risk of toxicity.
		Tocainide (Tonocard) PO	400	1200–1600	q8h	
		Lidocaine IV	Brief infusion: 2–5 mg/kg over 20–30 min.	—	—	Analgesia occurs within 15–30 min. May be appropriate for procedural pain or rapidly escalating neuropathic pain.
		SC, IV	Continuous infusion 2.5 mg/kg/h	Same	—	
Psychostimulants, oral	Multipurpose for acute or chronic pain; neuropathic or nociceptive; conventionally used to reverse somnolence caused by opioids	Caffeine PO	50–150/dose of opioid or NSAID	?	?	Used in combination products for headache.
		Dextroamphetamine (Dexedrine) PO	2.5 after breakfast	10–30	2/day	Administer after breakfast and/or lunch. Avoid evening doses.
		Methylphenidate (Ritalin) PO	2.5 after breakfast	10–30	2/day	Administer after breakfast and/or lunch. Avoid evening doses.
Miscellaneous	Various neuropathic pains; bone pain; osteoarthritis?	Calcitonin Subcutaneous, IV	25 IU	100–200 IU	qd	
		Nasal spray (Miacalcin)	200 IU	200–400 IU	qd	
Neuroleptics	Pain associated with anxiety, restlessness, or nausea; multipurpose analgesic.	Methotrimeprazine (Levoprome) IV, SC	20	80	q6h	Side effects usually limit use to bedridden patients with advanced cancer. 10–20 mg approximately equal to 10 mg morphine. May administer by continuous infusion.
	Trigeminal neuralgia; refractory; paroxysmal (sudden onset) or "shooting" neuropathic pain	Pimozide (Orap) PO	2	4–12	q8h	Neuroleptic drug with side effects typical of this class (e.g., sedation).

● ● ● ● ●

FORM 7.1 **Patient/Family Information: "New" Group of Pain Relievers**

To: _____ Date: _____

You are taking _____, a pain reliever from a new group called "adjuvant analgesics."

Pain relievers are divided into three main groups:
1. Nonnarcotics or nonopioids, such as aspirin or ibuprofen.
2. Narcotics or opioids, such as morphine or codeine.
3. Adjuvants: This group includes many different medicines that are used to treat problems other than pain. Now we know that adjuvant analgesics also relieve pain. These medicines include some medicines used for high blood pressure, depression, convulsions, and heart problems.

The medicine you are taking for pain relief is:

Brand name: _____

Generic name: _____

You are taking _____ for pain relief.

_____ is also used for _____.

Take as follows:

How much? _____

How often? _____

When will I feel pain relief? If may take a few days or several weeks to find the dose that works for you. The medicine is started at a low dose and gradually increased until we know what works for you. If this medicine doesn't work, we will try another one.

With this group of pain relievers, it takes time to find the best one and the right dose. Keep taking the medicine even if it doesn't work. If you have side effects that bother you, call your nurse or doctor. You may need to put up with the side effects for a few days until your system adjusts and the side effects stop, or you may need to stop taking the medicine.

Next visit (or phone call) to adjust your medicine: (We will want to know whether you have had any pain relief or side effects.)

Date: _____ Time: _____

If you have any questions or problems, contact:

_____ (RN or MD)

Phone number: _____

Best days/times to call are: _____

BOX 7.3

PATIENT MEDICATION INFORMATION

Desipramine (generic name)

BRAND NAME: Norpramin

DESCRIPTION:
Norpramin Tablets come in six strengths:
   10 mg: blue
   25 mg: yellow
   50 mg: green
   75 mg: orange
   100 mg: peach
   150 mg: white
Generics may look different.

TYPE OF MEDICINE: Antidepressant

USES:
Relieves pain caused by nerve damage.
Relieves depression.

DOSAGE AND ADMINISTRATION:
- Take only as directed.
- These directions may change. Norpramin is usually started at a low dose and then increased slowly every 3 to 4 days to find the best dose.
- Starting dose is usually 10 mg or 25 mg.
- May be taken with or without food.
- Pain relief usually takes 2 to 4 weeks after starting medication. It may take this much time to get to the right dose for you and to allow the medicine to build up in your body.

POSSIBLE SIDE EFFECTS:
- Dry mouth: May be relieved by chewing sugarless gum, sucking sugarless or sour hard candy, or drinking fluids frequently.
- Drowsiness: May occur as your dose is increased. If this happens, your dose may need to be lowered.
- Constipation: Constipation can be controlled with daily laxatives.
- Dizziness: May occur when moving from lying to sitting or sitting to standing. Change position slowly. If this does not help, call your doctor or nurse.
- Difficulty starting your urine: If this happens, call your doctor or nurse.

PRECAUTIONS:
- Be careful when driving or using machinery such as lawn mowers, power tools, or saws.
- Be careful when drinking alcohol. Alcohol could increase drowsiness and dizziness.

Continued.

PATIENT MEDICATION INFORMATION—cont'd

Desipramine (generic name)

BRAND NAME: Norpramin

STOPPING MEDICATIONS: Do not suddenly stop taking your medicine. The Norpramin dose should be lowered gradually. Call your doctor or nurse for directions.

REMEMBER!
- Don't run out of medicine.
- Keep count of your pills.
- Get your prescription refilled by or phoned into your pharmacy or drug store a few days before you run out of medicine.

COMMENTS:

WARNING: Keep this and all medicines out of the reach of children.

May be duplicated for use in clinical practice. As appears in McCaffery M, Pasero C: *Pain: Clinical manual,* pp. 346-347, 1999, Mosby, Inc.
Courtesy Fox Chase Cancer Center/Pain Management, Philadelphia, Pa, 1997.

BOX 7.4

PATIENT MEDICATION INFORMATION

Nortriptyline (generic name)

BRAND NAME: Pamelor

DESCRIPTION:
Pamelor capsules come in four strengths:
  10 mg, 25 mg: half orange, half white
  50 mg: solid white
  75 mg: solid orange
Pamelor solution: 10 mg/teaspoon (5 ml)
Generics may look different.

TYPE OF MEDICINE: Antidepressant

USES:
Relieves pain caused by nerve damage.
Relieves depression.
Improves sleep.

DOSAGE AND ADMINISTRATION:
- Take only as directed.
- These directions may change. Pamelor is usually started at a low dose and then increased slowly every 3 to 4 days to find the best dose.
- Starting dose is usually 10 mg or 25 mg.
- Usually taken at bedtime.
- May be taken with or without food.
- Pain relief usually takes 2 to 4 weeks after starting medication. It may take this much time to get to the right dose for you and to allow the medicine to build up in your body.

POSSIBLE SIDE EFFECTS:
- Dry mouth: May be relieved by chewing sugarless gum, sucking sugarless or sour hard candy, or drinking fluids frequently.
- Drowsiness: May occur as your dose is increased. If this happens, your dose may need to be lowered.
- Constipation: Constipation can be controlled with daily laxatives.
- Dizziness: May occur when moving from lying to sitting or sitting to standing. Change position slowly. If this does not help, call your doctor or nurse.
- Difficulty starting your urine: If this happens, call your doctor or nurse.

PRECAUTIONS:
- Be careful when driving or using machinery such as lawn mowers, power tools, or saws.
- Be careful when drinking alcohol. Alcohol could increase drowsiness and dizziness.

Continued.

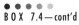
BOX 7.4—cont'd

PATIENT MEDICATION INFORMATION—cont'd

Nortriptyline (generic name)

BRAND NAME: Pamelor

STOPPING MEDICATIONS: Do not suddenly stop taking your medicine. The Pamelor dose should be lowered gradually. Call your doctor or nurse for directions.

REMEMBER!
- Don't run out of medicine.
- Keep count of your pills.
- Get your prescription refilled by or phoned into your pharmacy or drug store a few days before you run out of medicine.

COMMENTS:

WARNING: Keep this and all medicines out of the reach of children.

May be duplicated for use in clinical practice. As appears in McCaffery M, Pasero C: *Pain: Clinical manual,* pp. 348-349, 1999, Mosby, Inc. Courtesy Fox Chase Cancer Center/Pain Management, Philadelphia, Pa, 1997.

BOX 7.5

PATIENT MEDICATION INFORMATION

Gabapentin (generic name)

BRAND NAME: Neurontin

DESCRIPTION:
Neurontin capsules come in three strengths:
    100 mg: white
    300 mg: yellow
    400 mg: orange

TYPE OF MEDICINE: Antiseizure, anticonvulsant

USES:
Relieves pain caused by nerve damage.
Controls seizures.

DOSAGE AND ADMINISTRATION:
- Take only as directed.
- These directions may change. Neurontin is usually started at a low dose and then increased slowly to find the best dose.
- It may take a few days or longer before you feel pain relief. It may take this much time to get to the right dose for you and to allow the medicine to build up in your body.
- May be taken with or without food.

POSSIBLE SIDE EFFECTS: If these occur, call your doctor or nurse:
- Sleepiness
- Dizziness
- Unsteady hands
- Unsteady walking
- Increased fatigue

PRECAUTIONS:
- Do not take with antacids.
- Tell your nurse or doctor if you are taking Maalox.

STOPPING MEDICATIONS: Do not suddenly stop taking your medicine. The Neurontin dose should be lowered gradually. Call your doctor or nurse for directions.

REMEMBER!
- Don't run out of medicine.
- Keep count of your pills.
- Get your prescription refilled by or phoned into your pharmacy or drug store a few days before you run out of medicine.

May be duplicated for use in clinical practice. As appears in McCaffery M, Pasero C: *Pain: Clinical manual*, pp. 350-351, 1999, Mosby, Inc.   *Continued.*

● ● ● ● ●
B O X 7.5—cont'd

PATIENT MEDICATION INFORMATION—cont'd

Gabapentin (generic name)

BRAND NAME: Neurontin

COMMENTS:

WARNING: Keep this and all medicines out of the reach of children.

May be duplicated for use in clinical practice. As appears in McCaffery M, Pasero C: *Pain: Clinical manual*, pp. 350-351, 1999, Mosby, Inc. Courtesy Fox Chase Cancer Center/Pain Management, Philadelphia, Pa, 1997.

PATIENT MEDICATION INFORMATION

Mexiletine (generic name)

BRAND NAME: Mexitil

DESCRIPTION:
Mexitil capsules come in three strengths:
  150 mg: red and caramel
  200 mg: red
  250 mg: red and aqua green
Generics may look different.

TYPE OF MEDICINE: Antiarrhythmic (heart medicine)

USES:
Relieves pain caused by nerve damage.
Controls irregular heartbeats.

DOSAGE AND ADMINISTRATION:
- Take only as directed.
- Mexitil is usually started at a low dose and then increased slowly to find the best dose.
- Pain relief may take 2 to 4 weeks. It may take this much time to get to the right dose for you and to allow the medicine to build up in your body.
- Take with food or antacid.

POSSIBLE SIDE EFFECTS: If these occur, call your nurse or doctor:
- Stomach irritation or heartburn: Can be controlled by taking medicine with food or antacid.
- Nausea and vomiting: Can be controlled with other medication.

LESS COMMON SIDE EFFECTS:
- Dizziness or light-headedness. May occur when moving from lying to sitting or sitting to standing. Change position slowly.
- Unsteady hands
- Nervousness
- Headache
- Blurred vision
- Chest pain or pounding in chest

PRECAUTIONS:
- Tell your nurse or doctor if you are taking any of these medications:
  Metoclopramide (Reglan)
  Theophylline (Theo-Dur, Uniphyl)

May be duplicated for use in clinical practice. As appears in McCaffery M, Pasero C: *Pain: Clinical manual*, pp. 352-353, 1999, Mosby, Inc.   *Continued.*

BOX 7.6—cont'd

PATIENT MEDICATION INFORMATION—cont'd

Mexiletine (generic name)

BRAND NAME: Mexitil

STOPPING MEDICATIONS: Do not suddenly stop taking your medicine. The Mexitil dose should be lowered gradually. Call your doctor or nurse for directions.

REMEMBER!
- Don't run out of medicine.
- Keep count of your pills.
- Get your prescription refilled by or phoned into your pharmacy or drug store a few days before you run out of medicine.

COMMENTS:

WARNING: Keep this and all medicines out of the reach of children.

May be duplicated for use in clinical practice. As appears in McCaffery M, Pasero C: *Pain: Clinical manual,* pp. 352-353, 1999, Mosby, Inc. Courtesy Fox Chase Cancer Center/Pain Management, Philadelphia, Pa, 1997.

References

Abram SE, Lightfoot RW: Treatment of longstanding causalgia with prazosin, *Reg Anesth* 6:79-81, 1981.

Admi S, Mian M: Clodronate therapy of metastatic bone disease in patients with prostatic carcinoma, *Cancer Res* 116:67-72, 1989.

Aho MS, Erkola OA, Scheinin H et al.: Effect of intravenously administered dexmedetomidine on pain after laparoscopic tubal ligation, *Anesth Analg* 73:112-118, 1991.

Albe-Fessard D, Lombard MC: Use of an animal model to evaluate the origin of deafferentation pain and protection against it. In Bonica JJ, Lindblom U, Iggo A, editors: *Adv Pain Res Ther*, 5:691-700, 1982.

Alcoff J, Jones E, Rust P et al.: Controlled trial of imipramine for chronic low back pain, *J Fam Pract* 14:841-846, 1982.

American Pain Society: *Principles of analgesic use in the treatment of acute and cancer pain*, Skokie, Ill, 1992, The Society.

Arner S, Lindblom U, Meyerson BA et al.: Prolonged relief of neuralgia after regional anesthetic blocks: a call for further experimental and systemic clinical studies, *Pain* 43:287-297, 1990.

Atkinson RL: Intravenous lidocaine for the treatment of intractable pain of adiposis dolorosa, *Int J Obstet* 6:351-357, 1982.

Averbuch SD: New bisphosphonates in the treatment of bone metastases, *Cancer* 72:3443-3452, 1993.

Backonja M: Local anesthetics as adjuvant analgesics, *J Pain Symptom Manage* 9:491-499, 1994a.

Backonja M: Reflex sympathetic dystrophy/sympathetically-maintained pain/ causalgia: the syndrome of neuropathic pain with dysautonomia, *Semin Neurol* 14:263-271, 1994b.

Backonja M, Arndt G, Gombar KA et al.: Response of chronic neuropathic pain syndromes to ketamine: a preliminary study, *Pain* 56:51-57, 1994.

Backonja M, Gombar K: Response of central pain syndromes to intravenous lidocaine, *J Pain Symptom Manage* 7:172-178, 1992.

Baldessarini RJ: Drugs and the treatment of psychiatric disorders. In Gilman AG, Rall TW, Nies AS, Taylor P, editors: *The pharmacological basis of therapeutics*, ed 8 pp. 383-435, New York; 1990, Pergamon Press.

Baldessarini RJ: Drugs and the treatment of psychiatric disorders. In Hardman JL, Limbird LE: *Goodman and Gilman's the pharmacological basis of therapeutics*, ed 9, pp. 399-430, New York, 1996, McGraw-Hill.

Bartlett E, Hataserani O: Xylocaine for the relief of postoperative pain, *Anesth Analg* 40:296-304, 1961.

Bartlik BD, Kaplan P, Kaplan HS: Psychostimulants apparently reverse sexual dysfunction secondary to selective serotonin re-uptake inhibitors, *J Sex Marital Ther* 21:264-271, 1995.

Bartusch SL, Sanders BF, D'Alessio JG et al.: Clonazepam for the treatment of lancinating phantom limb pain, *Clin J Pain* 12:59-62, 1996.

Basbaum AI, Fields HL: Endogenous pain control systems: brainstem spinal pathways and endorphin circuitry, *Annu Rev Neurosci* 7:309-338, 1984.

Batterman RC. Methodology of analgesic evaluation: experience with orphena-drine citrate compound, *Curr Ther Res* 7:639-647, 1965.

Beaver W: Caffeine revisited, *JAMA* 251:1732-1733, 1984.

Beaver WT, Feise G: Comparison of the analgesic effect of morphine, hydroxyzine and their combination in patients with postoperative pain. In Bonica JJ, editor: *Adv Pain Res Ther* 1:553-557, 1976.

Beaver WT, Wallenstein S, Houde RW et al.: A comparison of the analgesic effects of methotrimeprazine and morphine in patients with cancer, *Clin Pharmacol Ther* 7:436-446, 1966.

Beltrutti DPC, Colleta P, Di Santo S et al.: The spinal administration of ketamine: lights and shadows, *Pain Digest* 7:127-135, 1997.

Benson RF, Parris WCV, Cooper J et al.: Efficacy of gabapentin in neuropathic pain. In *Abstracts of the 8th world congress on pain*, p 373, Seattle, 1996, IASP Press.

Bercel NA: Cyclobenzaprine in the treatment of skeletal muscle spasm in osteo-arthritis of the cervical and lumbar spine, *Curr Ther Res* 22:462-468, 1977.

Berde CB: New and old anticonvulsants for management of pain, *IASP Newsletter* 3-5, January/February 1997.

Berkovitch M, Pope E, Phillips J et al.: Pemoline-associated fulminant liver failure: testing the evidence for causation, *Clin Pharmacol Ther* 57:696-698, 1995.

Bernard JM, Kick O, Bonnet F: Comparison of intravenous and epidural clonidine for postoperative patient-controlled analgesia, *Anesth Analg* 81:706-712, 1995.

Bernstein JE, Bickers RR, Dahl MV et al.: Treatment of chronic postherpetic neuralgia with topical capsaicin: a preliminary study, *J Am Acad Dermatol* 17:93-96, 1987.

Besson JM, Chaouch A: Peripheral and spinal mechanisms of nociception, *Physiol Rev* 67:67-186, 1987.

Birch K, Jorgensen B, Chraemer-Jorgensen B et al.: Effect of i.v. lignocaine on pain and the endocrine metabolic responses after surgery, *Br J Anaesth* (59)721-724, 1987.

Birkeland IW, Clawson DK: Drug combinations with orphenadrine for pain relief associated with muscle spasm, *Clin Pharmacol Ther* 9:639-46, 1958.

Blomquist C, Elomaa I, Porkka L et al.: Evaluation of salmon calcitonin treatment in bone metastases from breast cancer: a controlled trial, *Bone* 9:45-51, 1988.

Bloomfield S, Simard-Savoie S, Bernier J et al.: Comparative analgesic activity of levomepromazine and morphine in patients with chronic pain, *Can Med Assoc J* 90:1156-1159, 1964.

Boas RA, Covino BG, Shahnarian A: Analgesic responses to IV lignocaine, *Br J Anaesth* 54:501-505, 1982.

Bodnar RJ, Nicotera N: Neuroleptic and analgesic interactions upon pain and activity measures, *Pharmacol Biochem Behav* 16:411-416, 1982.

Boisen E, Deth S, Hubbe P et al.: Clonidine in the prophylaxis of migraine, *Acta Neurol Scand* 58:288-295, 1978.

Boyer WF, Blumhardt CL: The safety profile of paroxetine, *J Clin Psychiatry* 53(suppl 2):61-66, 1992.

Braham J, Saia A: Phenytoin in the treatment of trigeminal and other neuralgias, *Lancet* 2:892-893, 1960.

Breitbart W, Stiefel F, Kornblith AB et al.: Neuropsychiatric disturbance in cancer patients with epidural spinal cord compression receiving high dose corticosteroids: a prospective comparison study, *Psycho-oncology* 2:233-245, 1993.

Breivik H, Rennemo F: Clinical evaluation of combined treatment with meth-adone and psychotropic drugs in cancer patients, *Acta Anaesth Scand* 74:135-40, 1982.

Broadley KE, Kurowska A, Tookman A: Ketamine injection used orally, *Palliat Med* 10:247-250, 1996.

Brose WG, Cousins MJ: Subcutaneous lidocaine for treatment of neuropathic cancer pain, *Pain* 45:145-148, 1991.

Bruera E, Brenneis C, Paterson AH et al.: Use of methylphenidate as an adjuvant to narcotic analgesics in patients with advanced cancer, *J Pain Symptom Manage* 4:306, 1989.

Bruera E, Chadwich S, Brenneis C et al.: Methylphenidate associated with narcotics for the treatment of cancer pain, *Cancer Treatment Rep* 71:67-70, 1987.

Bruera E, Miller MJ, Macmillan K et al.: Neuropsychological effects of methylphenidate in patients receiving a continuous infusion of narcotics for cancer pain, *Pain* 48:163-166, 1992.

Bruera E, Ripamonti C, Brenneis C et al.: A randomized double-blind crossover trial of intravenous lidocaine in the treatment of neuropathic cancer pain, *J Pain Symptom Manage* 7:138-140, 1992.

Bruera E, Roca E, Cedaro L et al.: Action of oral methylprednisolone in terminal cancer patients: a prospective randomized double-blind study, *Cancer Treat Rep* 69:751-754, 1985.

Buetefisch CM, Gutierrez MA, Gutmann L: Choreoathetotic movements: a possible side effect of gabapentin, *Neurology* 46:851-852, 1996.

Byas-Smith MG, Max MB, Muir H et al.: Transdermal clonidine compared to placebo in painful diabetic neuropathy using two-staged "enriched enrollment" design, *Pain* 60:267-274, 1995.

Caccia MR: Clonazepam in facial neuralgia and cluster headache: clinical and electrophysiological study, *Eur Neurol* 13:560-563, 1975.

Campbell FG, Graham JC, Zilkha KJ: Clinical trial of carbamazepine (Tegretol) in trigeminal neuralgia, *J Neurol Neurosurg Psychiatry* 29:265-267, 1966.

Campbell RWF: Mexiletine, *N Engl J Med* 316:29-34, 1987.

Campos VM, Solis EL: The analgesic and hypothermic effects of nefopam, morphine, aspirin, diphenhydramine and placebo, *J Clin Pharmacol* 20:42-49, 1980.

Cannon RO, Quyyumi AS, Mincemoyer R et al.: Imipramine in patients with chest pain despite normal coronary angiograms, *N Engl J Med* 330:1411-1417, 1994.

Cantello R, Aguggia M, Gillig M et al.: Analgesic action of methylphenidate on parkinsonian sensory symptoms: mechanisms and pathophysiological implications, *Arch Neurol* 45:973-976, 1988.

Cantor FK: Phenytoin treatment of thalamic pain, *BMJ* 2:590, 1972.

Capsaicin Study Group: Treatment of painful diabetic neuropathy with topical capsaicin: a multicenter, double-blind, vehicle-controlled study, *Arch Intern Med* 151(11):2225-2229, 1991.

Carey PO, Lippert MC: Treatment of painful prostatic bone metastases with oral etidronate disodium, *Urology* 32:403-407, 1988.

Carrette S, McCain GA, Bell DA et al.: Evaluation of amitriptyline in primary fibrositis, *Arthritis Rheum* 29:655-659, 1986.

Carroll D, Jadad A, King L et al.: Single-dose, randomized, double-blind, double- dummy, cross-over comparison of extradural and i.v. clonidine in chronic pain, *Br J Anaesth* 7:665-669, 1993.

Cassuto J, Wallin G, Hogstrom S et al.: Inhibition of postoperative pain by continuous low-dose infusion of lidocaine, *Anesth Analg* 64:971-974, 1985.

Cavernar JO, Maltbie AA: Another indication for haloperidol, *Psychosomatics* 17:128-130, 1976.

Cepeda ML, Delgado M, Ponce M et al.: Equivalent outcomes during postoperative patient-controlled intravenous analgesia with lidocaine plus morphine versus morphine alone, *Anesth Analg* 83:102-106, 1996.

Chabal C, Russell LC, Burchiel KJ: The effect of intravenous lidocaine, tocainide and mexiletine on spontaneously active fibers originating in rat sciatic neuromas, *Pain* 38:333-338, 1989.

Chadda VS, Mathur MS: Double-blind study of the effects of diphenylhydantoin sodium in diabetic neuropathy, *J Assoc Physicians India* 26:403-406, 1978.

Chang VT: Intravenous phenytoin in the management of crescendo pelvic cancer- related pain, *J Pain Symptom Manage* 13:238-240, 1997.

Cherry DA, Plummer JL, Gourlay GK et al.: Ketamine as an adjunct to morphine in the treatment of pain, *Pain* 62:119-121, 1995.

Clarke NW, Holbrook IB, McClure J et al.: Osteoclast inhibition by pamidronate in metastatic prostate cancer: a preliminary report, *Br J Cancer* 63:420-423, 1991.

Coleman RE, Woll PF, Miles M et al.: Treatment of bone metastases from breast cancer with (3 amino-1-hydroxypropylidene)-1, 1-bisphosphonate (APD), *Br J Cancer* 58:621-625, 1988.

Cook B, Grubb DJ, Aldridge LA et al.: Comparison of the effects of adrenaline, clonidine, and ketamine on the duration of caudal analgesia produced by bupivacaine in children, *Br J Anaesth* 75:698-701, 1995.

Coombs DW, Saunders RL, Fratkin JD et al.: Continuous intrathecal hydromorphone and clonidine for intractable cancer pain, *J Neurosurg* 64:890-894, 1986.

Coombs DW, Saunders R, Gaylor M et al.: Clinical trial of intrathecal clonidine for cancer pain, *Reg Anesth* 9:34-35, 1984.

Coombs DW, Saunders RL, LaChance D et al.: Intrathecal morphine tolerance: use of intrathecal clonidine, DADLE and intraventricular morphine, *Anesthesiology* 62:357-363, 1985.

Cooper GL: The safety of fluoxetine: an update, *Br J Psychiatry* 153(suppl 3):77-86, 1988.

Corli O, Roma G, Bacchini M et al.: Double-blind placebo-controlled trial of baclofen, alone and in combination, in patients undergoing voluntary abortion, *Clin Ther* 6:800-807, 1984.

Couch JR, Ziegler DK, Hassanein R: Amitriptyline in the prophylaxis of migraine: effectiveness and relationship of antimigraine antidepressant effects, *Neurology* (Minneap), 26:121-127, 1976.

Covino BG: Local anesthetics. In Ferrante FM, VadeBoncouer TR, editors: *Postoperative pain management*, pp 211-253, New York, 1993, Churchill Livingstone.

Cullen ML, Starren Ed, El-Ganzouri A et al.: Continuous epidural infusion for analgesia after major abdominal operations: a randomized prospective, double-blind study, *Surgery* 98:718-728, 1985.

Cutter HSG, O'Farrell TJ, Whitehouse J et al.: Pain changes among men from before to after drinking: effects of expectancy set and dose manipulations with alcohol and tonic as mediated by prior experience with alcohol, *Int J Addict* 21:937-945, 1986.

Davidoff G, Guarracini- M, Roth E et al.: Trazodone hydrochloride in the treatment of dysesthetic pain in traumatic myelopathy: a randomized, double-blind, placebo-controlled study, *Pain* 29:151-61, 1987.

Davidson O, Lindenberg O, Walsh M: Analgesic treatment with levomedromazine in acute myocardial infarction, *Acta Med Scand* 205:191-194, 1979.

Davies PS, Galer BS: Multicenter, double-blind vehicle-controlled trial of longer term use of lidocaine patches for postherpetic neuralgia [abstract], p 274. In *Abstracts: 8th world congress on pain*, Seattle, 1996, IASP Press.

Davies PS, Reisner-Keller L, Rowbotham MC: Randomized, double-blind comparison of fluoxetine, desipramine and amitriptyline in postherpetic neuralgia [abstract] p 276. In *Abstracts: 8th world congress on pain*, Seattle, 1996, IASP Press.

Daw JL, Cohen-Cole SA: Haloperidol analgesia, *South Med J* 74:364-365, 1981.

De Benedittis G, Besana F, Lorenzettit A: A new topical treatment for acute herpetic neuralgia and postherpetic neuralgia: the aspirin/diethyl ether mixture: an open-label study plus a double-blind controlled clinical trial, *Pain* 48:383-390, 1992.

De Benedittis G, Lorenzetti A: Topical aspirin/diethyl ether mixture versus indomethacin and diclofenac/diethyl ether mixtures for acute herpetic neuralgia and postherpetic neuralgia: a double-blind crossover placebo-controlled study, *Pain* 65:45-51, 1996.

De Conno F, Caraceni A, Zecca E et al.: Continuous subcutaneous infusion of hyoscine butylbromide reduces secretions in patients with gastrointestinal obstruction, *J Pain Symptom Manage* 6:484-486, 1991.

Dejgard A, Petersen P, Kastrup J: Mexiletine for treatment of chronic painful diabetic neuropathy, *Lancet* 1:9-11, 1988.

de Jong RH: Neurontin: pie in the sky or pie on the plate? *Pain Digest* 6:143-14, 1996.

deJong RH, Nace R: Nerve impulse conduction during intravenous lidocaine injection, *Anesthesiology* 29:22-28, 1968.

De Kock M, Wiederkher P, Laghmiche JA et al.: Epidural clonidine used as the sole analgesic agent, *Anesthesiology* 86:285-292, 1997.

Dellemijn PLI, Fields HL: Do benzodiazepines have a role in chronic pain management? *Pain* 57:137-152, 1994.

De Negri P, Visconte JC, De Vivo P et al.: Continuous epidural postoperative analgesia with bupivacaine-clonidine mixture in children, *Regional Anesth* 22(2S)32, 1997.

Devor M: The pathophysiology of damaged peripheral nerves. In Wall PD, Melzack R, editors: *Textbook of pain*, pp 79-100, Edinburgh, 1994, Churchill Livingstone.

Devor M, Govrin-Lippman R, Raber P: Corticosteroids reduce neurona hyperexcitability. In Fields HL, Dubner R, Cervero F, editors: *Adv Pain Res Ther* 9:451-455, 1985.

Devor M, Wall PD, Catalan N: Systemic lidocaine silences ectopic neuroma and DRG discharge without blocking nerve conduction, *Pain* 48:261-268, 1992.

Diamond S, Baltes BJ: Chronic tension headache: treatment with amitriptyline—a double-blind study, *Headache* 11:110-116, 1971.

Diamond S, Frietag FG: The use of fluoxetine in the treatment of headache, *Clin J Pain* 5:200-201, 1989.

Dich-Hielsen JO, Svendsen LB, Berthelsen P: Intramuscular low-dose ketamine versus pethidine for postoperative pain treatment after thoracic surgery, *Acta Anaesthesiol Scand* 36:583-587, 1992.

Dichter MA, Brodie MJ: New antiepileptic drugs, *N Engl J Med* 334:1583-1590, 1996.

Dickenson AH, Sullivan AF: Evidence for a role of the NMDA receptor in the frequency dependent potentiation of deep dorsal horn nociceptive neurons following C fibre stimulation, *Neuropharmacology* 26:1235-1238, 1987.

Dinerman H, Felsen D, Goldenberg D: A randomized clinical trial of naproxen and amitriptyline in primary fibromyalgia, *Arthritis Rheum* 159(S):28-33, 1985.

Dixon RA, Christy NP: On the various forms of corticosteroid withdrawal syndrome, *Am J Med* 68:224-230, 1980.

Dubner R: Topical capsaicin therapy for neuropathic pain, *Pain* 47:247-248, 1991.

Dunlop R, Davies RJ, Hockley J et al.: Letter to the editor, *Lancet* 1:420-421, 1989.

Dunsker SB, Mayfield FH: Carbamazepine in the treatment of flashing pain syndrome, *J Neurosug* 45:49-51, 1976.

Eberhard G, von Knorring L, Nilsson ML et al.: A double-blind randomized study of clomipramine versus maprotiline in patients with idiopathic pain syndromes, *Neuropsychobiology* 19:25-34, 1988.

Edmonds P, Davis C: Experience of the use of subcutaneous ketamine in patients with cancer-related neuropathic pain, *Palliat Med* 10:76-77, 1996.

Edmondson EA, Simpson RK, Stubler DK et al.: Systemic lidocaine therapy for poststroke pain, *South Med J* 86:1093-1096, 1993.

Edwards ND, Fletcher A, Cole JR et al.: Combined infusions of morphine and ketamine for postoperative pain in elderly patients, *Anaesthesia* 48:124-127, 1993.

Edwards WT, Habib F, Burney RG et al.: Intravenous lidocaine in the management of various chronic pain states, *Reg Anesth* 10:1-6, 1985.

Egan KJ, Ready LB, Nessly M et al.: Self-administration of midazolam for postoperative anxiety: a double blinded study, *Pain* 49:3-8, 1992.

Egbunike IG, Chaffee BJ: Antidepressants in the management of chronic pain syndromes, *Pharmacotherapy* 10:262-270, 1990.

Egger J, Brett EM: Effects of sodium valproate in 100 children with special reference to weight, *BMJ* 283:577-581, 1981.

Eide PK, Jorum E, Stubhaug A et al.: Relief of post-herpetic neuralgia with the N-methyl-D-aspartic receptor antagonist ketamine: a double-blind, cross-over comparison with morphine and placebo, *Pain* 58:347-354, 1994.

Eisenach JC, De Kock M, Kimscha W: α-adrenergic agonists for regional anesthesia, *Anesthesiology* 85:655-674, 1996.

Eisenach JC, Du Pen S, Dubois M et al.: Epidural clonidine analgesia for intractable cancer pain, *Pain* 61:391-400, 1995.

Eisenach JC, Hood DD, Curry R et al.: Alfentanil, but not amitriptyline, reduces pain, hyperalgesia, and allodynia from intradermal injection of capsaicin in humans, *Anesthesiology* 86:1279-1287, 1997.

Ekbom K: Carbamazepine in the treatment of tabetic lightning pains, *Arch Neurol* 26:374-378, 1972.

Elleman K, Sjogren P, Banning A et al.: Trial of intravenous lidocaine on painful neuropathy in cancer patients, *Clin J Pain* 5:291-294, 1989.

Ellenberg M: Treatment of diabetic neuropathy with diphenylhydantoin, *NY State J Med* 68:2633-55, 1968.

Elliot F, Little A, Milbrandt W: Carbamazepine with phantom limb phenomena, *N Engl J Med* 295:678, 1976.

Ernst DS, MacDonald RN, Paterson AHG et al.: A double blind, cross-over trial of IV clodronate in metastatic bone pain, *J Pain Symptom Manage* 7:4-11, 1992.

Espir MLE, Millac P. Treatment of paroxysmal disorders in multiple sclerosis with carbamazepine (Tegretol), *J Neurol Neurosurg Psychiatry* 33:528-31, 1970.

Ettinger AB, Portenoy RK: The use of corticosteroids in the treatment of symptoms associated with cancer, *J Pain Symptom Manage* 3:99-103, 1988.

Evans W, Gensler F, Blackwell B et al.: The effects of antidepressant drugs on pain relief and mood in the chronically ill, *Psychosomatics* 14:214-219, 1973.

Fadul CE, Lemann W, Thaler HT et al.: Perforation of the gastrointestinal tract in patients receiving steroids for neurologic disease, *Neurology* 38:348-352, 1988.

Fainsinger RL, Spanchynski K, Hanson J et al.: Symptom control in terminally ill patients with malignant bowel obstruction, *J Pain Symptom Manage* 9:12-18, 1994.

Farr WC: The use of corticosteroids for symptom management in terminally ill patients, *Am J Hospice Care* 7:41-46, 1990.

Fernandez F, Adams F, Holmes VF: Analgesic effect of alprazolam in patients with chronic, organic pain of malignant origin, *J Clin Psychopharmacol* 3:167-169, 1987.

Ferrante FM, Paggioli J, Cherukuri S et al.: The analgesic response to intravenous lidocaine in the treatment of neuropathic pain, *Anesth Analg* 82:91-97, 1996.

Filadora V, Sist T, Patel N et al.: Gabapentin treatment of neuropathic pain: report of 12 cases [abstract]. In *American Pain Society 15th Annual Scientific Meeting*, p A-56, 1996.

Flegel KM, Cole GH: Inappropriate antidiuresis during carbamazepine treatment, *Ann Intern Med* 87:722-723, 1977.

Forbes JA, Beaver WT, Jones KF et al.: Effect of caffeine on ibuprofen analgesia in postoperative oral surgery pain, *Clin Pharmacol Ther* 49:674-684, 1991.

Forrest WH, Brown BW, Brown CR et al.: Dextroamphetamine with morphine for the treatment of postoperative pain, *N Engl J Med* 296:712-715, 1977.

Fragen RJ, Tobin M: Does midazolam augment morphine analgesia for postoperative pain? *Anesthesiology* 61(3A):A192, 1984.

Fraioli F, Fabbri A, Gnessi L et al.: Calcitonin and analgesia. In Benedetti JC, Chapman CR, Moricca G, editors: *Adv Pain Res Ther* 7:237-250, 1984.

Frank RG, Kashini JH, Parker JC et al.: Antidepressant analgesia in rheumatoid arthritis, *J Rheumatol* 15:1632-1638, 1988.

Fraught E, Sacdeo RC, Remler MP et al.: Felbamate monotherapy of partial-onset seizures: an active control trial, *Neurology* 43:688-692, 1993.

Frayling IM, Addison GM, Chattergee K et al.: Methaemoglobinaemia in children treated with prilocaine-lignocaine cream, *BMJ* 301:153-154, 1990.

Fromm GH: Baclofen as an adjuvant analgesic, *J Pain Symptom Manage* 9:500-509, 1994.

Fromm GH, Graff-Radford SB, Terrence CF et al.: Pretrigeminal neuralgia, *Neurology* 40:1493-1495, 1990.

Fromm GH, Terrence CF, Chattha AS: Baclofen in the treatment of trigeminal neuralgia: double-blind study and long-term follow-up, *Ann Neurol* 15:240-244, 1984.

Fu ES, Miguel R, Scharf JE: Preemptive ketamine decreases postoperative narcotic requirements in patients undergoing abdominal surgery, *Anesth Analg* 84:1086-1090, 1997.

Fusco BM, Alessandri M: Analgesic effect of capsaicin in idiopathic trigeminal neuralgia, *Anesth Analg* 74:375-377, 1992.

Galer BS, Harle J, Rowbotham MD: Response to intravenous lidocaine infusion predicts subsequent response to oral mexiletine: a prospective study, *J Pain Symptom Manage* 12:161-167, 1996.

Galer BS, Miller KV, Rowbotham MC: Response to intravenous lidocaine infusion differs based on clinical diagnosis and site of nervous system injury, *Neurology* 43:1233-1235, 1993.

Gear RW, Miaskowski C, Heller PH et al.: Benzodiazepine mediated antagonism of opioid analgesia, *Pain* 71:25-29, 1997.

Geller SA: Treatment of fibrositis with fluoxetine hydrochloride (Prozac), *Am J Med* 87:594-595, 1989.

Gerson GR, Jones RB, Luscombe DK: Studies on the concomitant use of carbamazepine and clomipramine for the relief of postherpetic neuralgia, *Postgrad Med J* 53:104-109, 1977.

Getto CJ, Sorkness CA, Howell T: Antidepressants and chronic non-malignant pain: a review, *J Pain Symptom Manage* 2:9-18, 1987.

Ghatak NR, Santoso RA, McKinney WM: Cerebellar degeneration following long-term phenytoin therapy, *Neurology* 26:818-824, 1976.

Ghostine SY, Comair YG, Turner DM et al.: Phenoxybenzamine in the treatment of causalgia, *J Neurosurg* 60:1263-1268, 1984.

Gilbert CRA, Hanson IR, Brown AB et al.: Intravenous use of xylocaine, *Curr Res Anesth Analg* 30:301-313, 1951.

Gilbert MM: The efficacy of Percogesic in relief of musculoskeletal pain associated with anxiety, *Psychosomatics* 17:190-193. 1976.

Gitlin MJ: Effects of depression and antidepressants on sexual functioning, *Bull Menninger Clin* 59:232-248, 1995.

Glassman AH, Bigger JT: Cardiovascular effects of therapeutic doses of tricyclic antidepressants, *Arch General Psychiatry* 38:815-820, 1981.

Glazer S, Portenoy RK: Systemic local anesthetics in pain control, *J Pain Symptom Manage* 6:30-39, 1991.

Glick EN, Fowler PD: Imipramine in chronic arthritis, *Pharmacol Med* 1:94-96, 1979.

Glover D, Lipton A, Keller A et al.: Intravenous pamidronate disodium treatment of bone metastases in patients with breast cancer, *Cancer* 74:2949-2955, 1994.

Glynn C, Dawson D, Sanders R: A double-blind comparison between epidural morphine and epidural clonidine in patients with chronic non-cancer pain, *Pain* 34:123-128, 1988.

Glynn CJ, Teddy PJ, Jamous MA et al.: Role of spinal noradrenergic system in transmission of pain in patients with spinal cord injury, *Lancet* 2:1249-1250, 1986.

Goa KL, Sorkin EM: Gabapentin: a review of its pharmacological properties and clinical potential in epilepsy, *Drugs* 46:409-427, 1993.

Gobel H, Hamouz V, Hansen C et al.: Chronic tension-type headache: amitriptyline reduces clinical headache duration and experimental pain sensitivity but does not alter pericranial muscle activity readings, *Pain* 59:241-250, 1994.

Gobelet C, Waldburger M, Meier JL: The effect of adding calcitonin to physical treatment on reflex sympathetic dystrophy, *Pain* 48:171-175, 1992.

Gold RH: Treatment of low back pain syndrome with oral orphenadrine citrate, *Curr Ther Res* 23:271-276, 1978.

Gomersall JD, Stuart A: Amitriptyline in migraine prophylaxis, *J Neurol Neurosurg Psychiatry* 3C:684-690, 1973.

Gomez-Perez FJ, Riell JA, Dies H et al.: Nortriptyline and fluphenazine in the symptomatic treatment of diabetic neuropathy. A double-blind crossover study, *Pain* 23:395-400, 1985.

Gordon RA: Intravenous novocaine for analgesia in burns, *Can Med Assoc J* 49:478-481, 1943.

Gordon RA: Intravenous procaine: clinical applications, *Can Med Assoc J* 59:534-535, 1948.

Gordon NC, Gear RW, Heller PH et al.: Enhancement of morphine analgesia by the GABA-B agonist baclofen, *Neuroscience* 69:345-349, 1995.

Gordon NC, Heller PH, Gear RW et al.: Interactions between fluoxetine and opiate analgesia for postoperative dental pain, *Pain* 58:85-88, 1994.

Gordon RA: Intravenous novocaine for analgesia in burns, *Can Med Assoc J* 49:478-481, 1943.

Goyagi T, Nishikawa T: Oral clonidine premedication enhances the quality of postoperative analgesia by intrathecal morphine, *Anesth Analg* 82:1192-1196, 1996.

Grant IS, Nimmo WS, Clements JA: Pharmacokinetics and analgesic effects of IM and oral ketamine, *Br J Anaeth* 53:805-809, 1981.

Graubard DJ, Kovacs J, Ritter HH: The management of destructive arthritis of the hip by means of intravenous procaine, *Ann Intern Med* 28:1106-1116, 1948.

Green JB: Dilantin in the treatment of lightning pains, *Neurology* (Minneap) 11:257-258, 1961.

Greenberg HS, Kim J, Posner JB: Epidural spinal cord compression from metastatic tumor: results with a new treatment protocol, *Ann Neurol* 8:361-366, 1980.

Gringas M: A clinical trial of tofranil in rheumatic pain in general practice, *J Int Med Res* 4:41-49, 1976.

Guilbaud G, Benoist JM, Levante A et al.: Primary somatosensory cortex in rats with pain-related behaviors due to a peripheral mononeuropathy after moderate ligation of one sciatic nerve: neuronal responsivity to somatic stimulation, *Exp Brain Res* 92:227-245, 1992.

Hakkarainen H: Fluphenazine for tension headache: double-blind study, *Headache* 17:216-218, 1977.

Hallaq IY, Harris JD: The syndrome of postherpetic neuralgia: complications and an approach to therapy, *J Am Osteopathic Assoc* 681:1265-1268, 1968.

Hameroff SR, Cork RC, Scherer K et al.: Doxepin effects on chronic pain, depression and plasma opioids, *J Clin Psychiatry* 43:22-27, 1982.

Hanks GW, Thomas PJ, Trueman T et al.: The myth of haloperidol potentiation, *Lancet* 2:523-524, 1983.

Hanks GW, Trueman T, Twycross RG: Corticosteroids in terminal cancer, Postgd D, editors: *Adv Pain Res Ther* 1:583-587, 1976.

Hauck A, Bhaumik S: Hypomania induced by ga*bapentin, Br J Psychiatry* 167:549, 1995 (letter).

Haynes RC: Adrenocorticotrophic hormone: adrenocortical steroids and their synthetic analogs: inhibitors of the syd D, editors: *Adv Pain Res Ther* 1:583-587, 1976.

Hauck A, Bhaumik S: Hypomania induced by gabapentin, *Br J Psychiatry* 167:549, 1995 (letter).

Haynes RC: Adrenocorticotrophic hormone: adrenocortical steroids and their synthetic analogs: inhibitors of the synthesis and actions of adrenocortical hormones, pp 1431-1462, In Gilman AG, Rall TW, Nies et al., editors: *The pharmacological basis of therapeutics,* ed 8, New York, 1990, Pergamon Press.

Hindley AC, Hill AB, Leyland MI et al.: A double-blind controlled trial of salmon calcitonin in pain due to malignancy, *Cancer Chemother Pharmacol* 9:71-74, 1982.

Hirota K, Lambert DG: Ketamine: its mechanism(s) of action and unusual clinical uses, *Br J Anaesthesia* 77:441-444, 1996.

Hobbs WR, Rall TW, Verdoorn TA: Hypnotics and sedatives: ethanol. In Hardman JG, Limbird LE, editors: *Goodman & Gilman's the pharmacological basis of therapeutics,* ed 9, pp. 361-396, New York, 1996, McGraw-Hill.

Hoffman BB, Lefkowitz RJ: Catecholamines, sympathomimetic drugs, and adrenergic receptor antagonists. In Hartman JL, Limbird LE, editors: *Goodman & Gilman's the pharmacological basis of therapeutics,* ed 9, pp. 199-248, New York, 1996, McGraw-Hill.

Hoffmann V, Coppejans H, Vercauteren M et al.: Successful treatment of postherpetic neuralgia with oral ketamine, *Clin J Pain* 10:240-242, 1994.

Holmes RA: Radiopharmaceuticals in clinical trials, *Semin Oncol* 20:22-26, 1993.

Horn HR, Hadidian Z, Johnson JL et al.: Safety evaluation of tocainide in an American emergency use program, *Am Heart J* 100:1037-1040, 1980.

Houde RW, Wallenstein SL: Analgesic power of chlorpromazine alone and in combination with morphine, *Fed Proc* 14:353, 1966 (abstract).

Howland JS, Baker MG, Poe T: Does patient education cause side effects? *J Fam Pract* 31:62-64, 1990.

Hupert C, Yacoub M, Turgeon LR: Effect of hydroxyzine on morphine analgesia for the treatment of postoperative pain, *Anesth Analg* 59:690-696, 1980.

Ianmore A, Baker AR, Morrell F: Dilantin in the treatment of trigeminal neuralgia, *Neurology* 8:12, 1958.

Indaco A, Carrieri PB: Amitriptyline in the treatment of headache in patients with Parkinson's disease: a double-blind placebo-controlled study, *Neurology* 38:1720-1722, 1988.

Islas JA, Astorga J, Laredo M: Epidural ketamine for control of postoperative pain, *Anesth Analg* 64:1161-1162, 1985.

Ivankovich AD, McCarthy RJ: Epidural ketamine for control of postoperative pain: two comments, *Anesth Analg* 65:989-990, 1986.

Iwane T, Masanori M, Matsuki M et al.: Management of intractable pain in adiposis dolorosa with intravenous administration of lidocaine, *Anesth Analg* 55:257-259, 1976.

Jaeger H, Maier C: Calcitonin in phantom limb pain: a double blind study, *Pain* 48:21-27, 1992.

Jahangir SM, Islam F, Aziz L: Ketamine infusion for postoperative analgesia in asthmatics: a comparison with intermittent meperidine, *Anesth Analg* 76:45-49, 1993.

Jain AK, Ryan JR, McMahon FG et al.: Evaluation of intramuscular levonan-tradol and placebo in acute postoperative pain, *J Clin Pharmacol* 21:320S-326S, 1981.

Javery KB, Ussery TW, Steger HG et al.: Comparison of morphine and morphine with ketamine for postoperative analgesia, *Can J Anaesth* 43:212-215, 1996.

Jonsson A, Cassuto J, Hanson B: Inhibition of burn pain by intravenous lignocaine infusion, *Lancet* 338:151-152, 1991.

Judkins KC, Harmer M: Haloperidol as an adjuvant analgesic in the management of postoperative pain, *Anaesthesia* 37:1118-1120, 1982.

Juhlin L: Long-standing pain relief of adiposa dolorosa (Dercum's disease) after intravenous infusion of lidocaine, *J Am Acad Dermatol* 15:383-384, 1986.

Kaiko RF, Kanner R, Foley KM et al.: Cocaine and morphine interaction in acute and chronic cancer pain, *Pain* 31:35-45, 1987.

Kandler D, Lisander B: Analgesic action of metoclopramide in prosthetic hip surgery, *Acta Anaesthesiol Scand* 37:49-53, 1993.

Kanis JA, McCloskey EV, Taube T et al.: Rationale for the use of bisphosphonates in bone metastases, *Bone* 12:8-13, 1991.

Kastrup J, Petersen P, Dejgard A et al.: Intravenous lidocaine infusion: a new treatment for chronic painful diabetic neuropathy, *Pain* 28:69-75, 1987.

Kayser V, Desmeules J, Guilbaud G: Systemic clonidine differentially modulates the abnormal reactions to mechanical and thermal stimuli in rats with peripheral mononeuropathy, *Pain* 60:275-285, 1995.

Keats AS, D'Allessandro GL: A controlled study of pain relief by intravenous procaine, *JAMA* 147:1761-1763, 1951.

Keats AS, Telford J, Kurosu Y: Potentiation of meperidine by promethazine, *Anesthesiology* 22:31-41, 1961.

Keczkes K, Basheer AM: Do corticosteroids prevent post-herpetic neuralgia? *Br J Dermatol* 102:551-555, 1980.

Kerr JS, Fairweather DB, Mahendran R et al.: The effects of paroxetine, alone and in combination with alcohol on psychomotor performance and cognitive function in the elderly, *Int Clin Psychopharmacol* 7:101-108, 1992.

Kerrick JM, Fine PG, Lipman AG et al.: Low-dose amitriptyline as an adjunct to opioids for postoperative orthopedic pain: a placebo-controlled trial, *Pain* 52:325-330, 1993.

Killian JM, Fromm GH: Carbamazepine in the treatment of neuralgia: use and side effects, *Arch Neurol* 19:129-136, 1968.

King RB: Topical aspirin and chloroform and the relief of pain due to herpes zoster and post-herpetic neuralgia, *Arch Neurol* 50:1046-1053, 1993.

Kishore-Kumar R, Max MB, Schafer SC et al.: Desipramine relieves postherpetic neuralgia, *Clin Pharmacol Ther* 47:305-312, 1990.

Kocher R: Use of psychotropic drugs for the treatment of chronic severe pain. In Bonica JJ, Albe-Fessard D, editors. *Adv Pain Res Ther* 1:579-582, 1976.

Kofler M, Leis AA: Prolonged seizure activity after baclofen withdrawal, *Neurology* 42:697, 1992.

Kotarba JA: *Chronic pain: its social dimensions,* Beverly Hills, 1983, Sage Publications.

Kozin F, Ryan LM, Carerra GF et al.: The reflex sympathetic dystrophy syndrome (RSDS). III. Scintigraphic studies, further evidence for the therapeutic efficacy of systemic corticosteroids, and proposed diagnostic criteria, *Am J Med* 70:23-29, 1981.

Kreeger W, Hammill SC: New antiarrhythmic drugs: tocainide, mexiletine, flecainide, encainide and amiodarone, *Mayo Clin Proc* 62:1033-1050, 1987.

Kvinesdal B, Molin J, Froland A et al.: Imipramine treatment of painful diabetic neuropathy, *JAMA* 251:1727-1730, 1984.

Ladefoged K, Christensen KC, Hegnhoj J et al.: Effect of a long acting somatostatin analogue SMS 201-995 on jejunostomy effluents in patients with severe short bowel syndrome, *Gut* 30:943-949, 1989.

Laing AH, Achery DM, Bayly RJ et al.: Strontium-89 chloride for pain palliation in prostatic skeletal malignancy, *Br J Radiol* 64:816-822, 1991.

Lance JW, Curran DA: Treatment of chronic tension headache, *Lancet* 1:1236-1239, 1964.

Langohr HD, Stohr M, Petruch F: An open and double-blind crossover study on the efficacy of clomipramine (Anafranil) in patients with painful mono- and polyneuropathies, *Eur Neurol* 21:309-317, 1982.

Lasagna L, DeKornfeld TJ: Methotrimeprazine, a new phenothiazine derivative with analgesic properties: *JAMA* 178:887-890, 1961.

Laska EM, Sunshine A, Mueller F et al.: Caffeine as an analgesic adjuvant, *JAMA* 251:1711-1718, 1984.

Lechin F, van der Dijs B, Lechin ME et al.: Pimozide therapy for trigeminal neuralgia, *Arch Neurol* 9:960-962, 1989.

Lee DO, Steingard RJ, Cesena M et al.: Behavioral side effects of gabapentin in children, *Epilepsia* 37:87-90, 1996.

Leijon G, Boivie J: Central post-stroke pain: a controlled trial of amitriptyline and carbamazepine, *Pain* 36:27-36, 1989.

Lenz FA, Kwan HC, Dostrovsky JO et al.: Characteristics of bursting pattern of action potentials that occurs in the thalamus of patients with central pain, *Brain Res* 496:357-360, 1989.

Lewington VJ, McEwan AJB, Ackery DM et al.: A prospective, randomized double- blind cross-over study to examine the efficacy of strontium-89 in pain palliation in patients with advanced prostate cancer metastatic to bone, *Eur J Cancer* 27:954-958, 1991.

Lindstrom P, Lindblom U: The analgesic effect of tocainide in trigeminal neuralgia, *Pain* 28:45-50, 1987.

Lipman AG: Internal analgesic and antipyretic products. In *Handbook of nonprescription drugs,* pp 45-74, Washington DC, 1996, American Pharmaceutical Association.

Lipman AG: Letter to the editor, *Topics Pain Manage* 12(8):32, 1997.

Littrell RA: Epidural analgesia, *Am J Hosp Pharm* 48:2460-2474, 1991.

Lockman LA, Hunninghake DB, Drivit W et al.: Relief of pain of Fabry's disease by diphenylhydantoin, *Neurology* (Minneap) 23:871-875, 1973.

Loeser JD, Ward AA, White LE: Chronic deafferentation of human spinal cord neurons, *J Neurosurg* 29:48-50, 1968.

Logas WG, Faber LP, El-Ganzouri A et al.: A prospective don, *J Pain* 4:11-16, 1988.

Magni G: The use of antidepressants in the treatment of chronic pain: a review of the current evidence, *Drugs* 42:130-748, 1991.

Magni G, Arsie D, DeLeo D: Antidepressants in the treatment of cancer pain: a survey in Italy, *Pain* 29:347-n *J Pain* 4:11-16, 1988.

Magni G: The use of antidepressants in the treatment of chronic pain: a review of the current evidence, *Drugs* 42:130-748, 1991.

Magni G, Arsie D, DeLeo D: Antidepressants in the treatment of cancer pain: a survey in Italy, *Pain* 29:347-353, 1987.

Manning BH, Jianren M, Frenk H et al.: Continuous co-administration of dextromethorphan or MK-801 with morphine: attenuation of morphine dependence and naloxone-reversible attenuation of morphine tolerance, *Pain* 67:79-88, 1996.

Mao J, Price DD, Mayer DJ: Experimental mononeuropathy reduces antinociceptive effects of morphine: implications for common intracellular mechanisms involved in morphine tolerance and neuropathic pain, *Pain* 61:353-364, 1995.

Marbach JJ, Wallenstein SL: Analgesia, mood and hemodynamic effects of intranasal cocaine and lidocaine in chronic facial pain of deafferentation and myofascial origin, *J Pain Symptom Manage* 3:73-79, 1988.

Martin G: Recurrent pain of a pseudotabetic variety after laminectomy for a lumbar disc lesion, *J Neurol Neurosurg Psychiatry* 43:283-284, 1980.

Martin G: The management of pain following laminectomy for lumbar disc lesions, *Ann R Coll Surg Engl* 63:244-252, 1981.

Martin C, Martin A, Rud C et al.: Comparative study of sodium valproate and ketoprofen in the treatment of postoperative pain, *Am Fr Anesth Reanim* 7:387-392, 1988.

Martinez S, Achauer B, de Rios MD: Ketamine use in a burn center: hallucinogen or debridement facilitator? *J Psychoactive Drugs* 17(1):45-49, 1985.

Marton R, Spitzer N, Steinbrocker O: Intravenous procaine as an analgesic and therapeutic procedure in painful, chronic neuromusculoskeletal disorders, *Ann Intern Med* 10:629-633, 1949.

Mathisen LC, Skjelbred P, Skoglund LA et al.: Effect of ketamine an NMDA receptor inhibitor, in acute and chronic orofacial pain, *Pain* 61:215-220, 1995.

Matsuo F, Bergen D, Faught E et al.: Placebo-controlled study of the efficacy and safety of lamotrigine in patients with partial seizures, *Neurology* 43:2284-2291, 1993.

Max MB, Culnane M, Schafer SC et al.: Amitriptyline relieves diabetic neuropathy pain in patients with normal or depressed mood, *Neurology* 37:589-596, 1987.

Max MB, Lynch SA, Muir J et al.: Effects of desipramine, amitriptyline, and fluoxetine on pain in diabetic neuropathy, *N Engl J Med* 326:1250-1256, 1992.

Max MB, Schafer SC, Culnane M et al.: Association of pain relief with drug side effects in postherpetic neuralgia: a single dose study of clonidine, codeine, ibuprofen and placebo, *Clin Pharmacol Ther* 43:363-371, 1988.

McCarthy GM, McCarty DJ: Effect of topical capsaicin in the therapy of painful osteoarthritis of the hands, *J Rheumatol* 19:604-607, 1992.

McColl JD, Durkin W: The effect of pyrilamine on relief of symptoms of the premenstrual syndrome (PMS) and primary dysmenorrhea, *Fed Proc* 41:5572, 1982.

McDonald-Scott WA: The relief of pain with an antidepressant in arthritis, *Practitioner* 202:802-807, 1969.

McLachlin JA: The intravenous use of novocaine as a substitute for morphine in postoperative care, *Can Med Assoc J* 52:383-386, 1945.

McLean MJ: Gabapentin, *Epilepsia* 36(suppl 2):S73-S86, 1995.

McQuay H, Carroll D, Jadad AR et al.: Anticonvulsant drugs for management of pain: a systematic review, *BMJ* 311:1047-1052, 1995.

McQuay HJ, Carroll D, Moxon A: Benzydamine cream for the treatment of postherpetic neuralgia: minimum duration of treatment periods in a cross-over trial, *Pain* 40:131-135, 1990.

McQuay HJ, Tramer M, Nye BA et al.: A systematic review of antidepressants in neuropathic pain, *Pain* 68:217-227, 1996.

Mellick GA: Hemifacial spasm: successful treatment with felbamate, *J Pain Symptom Manage* 10:392-395, 1995.

Mellick GA, Mellick LB: Gabapentin in the management of reflex sympathetic dystrophy, *J Pain Symptom Manage* 10:265-266, 1995 (letter).

Mercadante S: Ketamine in cancer pain: an update, *Palliat Med* 10:225-230, 1996.

Mercadante S: Treatment of diarrhea due to enterocolic fistula with octreotide in a terminal cancer patient, *Palliat Med* 6:257-259, 1992.

Mercadante S, Lodi F, Sapio M et al.: Long-term ketamine subcutaneous continuous infur RA: The treatment of chronic pain with psychotropic drugs, *Postgrad Med J* 48:594-598, 1976.

Mercadante S, Maddaloni S: Octreotide in the management of inoperable gastrointestinal obstruction in terminal cancer patients, *J Pain Symptom Manage* 7:496-498, 1992.

Merskey H, Hester RA: The treatment of chronic pain with psychotropic drugs, *Postgrad Med J* 48:594-598, 1976.

Messenheimer J, Ramsay RE, Willmore LJ et al.: Lamotrigine therapy for partial seizures: a multicenter, placebo-controlled, double-blind, cross-over trial, *Epilepsia* 35:113-121, 1994.

Messer J, Reitman D, Sacks HS et al.: Association of adrenocorticosteroid therapy and peptic ulcer disease, *N Engl J Med* 309:21-24, 1983.

Meyers FH, Meyers FJ: Patients with neuropathic pain regularly benefit from treatment with propranolol, *Am J Pain Manage* 2:89-92, 1992.

Migliardi JR, Armenia DU, Freedman M et al.: Caffeine as an analgesic adjuvant in tension headache, *Clin Pharmacol Ther* 56(5):576-586, 1994.

Mikawa K, Nishina K, Maekawa N et al.: Oral clonidine premedication reduces postoperative pain in children, *Anesth Analg* 82:225-230, 1996.

Miller R, Eisenkraft JB, Cohen M et al.: Midazolam as an adjunct to meperidine analgesia for postoperative pain, *Clin J Pain* 2:37-43, 1986.

Minton JP: The response of breast cancer patient with bone pain to L-dopa, *Cancer* 33:358-63, 1974.

Moertel CG et al.: Corticosteroid therapy of preterminal gastrointestinal cancer, *Cancer* 33:1607-1609, 1974.

Monks R: Psychotropic drugs. In Wall PD, Melzack R, editors: *Textbook of pain*, ed 3, pp 963-990, New York, 1994, Churchill Livingstone.

Montilla E, Frederick WS, Cass LJ: Analgesic effects of methotrimeprazine and morphine, *Arch Intern Med* 111:725-728, 1963.

Morland TJ, Storli OV, Mogstad TE: Doxepin in the treatment of mixed vascular and tension headaches, *Headache* 1979;19:382-383, 1979.

Morris GL: Efficacy and tolerability of gabapentin in clinical practice, *Clin Ther* 17:891-900, 1995.

Moss HE, Sanger GJ: The effects of granisetron, ICS 205-930 and ondansetron on the visceral pain reflex induced by duodenal cistension, *Br J Pharmacol* 100:497-501, 1990.

Mullan S: Surgical management of pain in cancer of the head and neck, *Surg Clinic North Am* 53:203-210, 1973.

Mulvihill S, Pappas TN, Passaro E et al.: The use of somatostatin and its analogues, *Surgery* 100:467-476, 1986.

Naguib M, Adu-Gyamfi Y, Absood GH et al.: Epidural ketamine for postoperative analgesia, *Can Anaesth Soc J* 33(1)16-21, 1986.

Nakamura-Craig M, Follenfant RL: Lamotrigine and analogs: a new treatment for chronic pain? In Gebhardt GF, Hammond DL, Jensen TS, editors: *Progress in pain research and management*, Vol 2, pp 725-730, Seattle, 1994, IASP Press.

Nathan PW: Chlorprothixene (Taractan) in postherpetic neuralgia and other severe pains, *Pain* 5:367-371, 1978.

Needham PR, Daley AG, Lennard RF: Steroids in advanced cancer: survey of current practice, *BMJ* 305:999, 1992.

Nelson KA, Park KM, Robinovitz E et al.: High-dose oral dextromethorphan versus placebo in painful diabetic neuropathy and postherpetic neuralgia, *Neurology* 48:1212-1218, 1997.

Nicol CF: A four year double-blind study of carbamazepine in facial pain, *Headache* 9:54-57, 1969.

Nikolajsen L, Hansen CL, Nielsen J et al.: The effect of ketamine on phantom pain: a central neuropathic disorder maintained by peripheral input, *Pain* 67:69-77, 1996.

Notcutt WG: Transporting patients with overwhelming pain, *Anaesthesia* 49:145-147, 1994.

Noyes R, Brunk SF, Avery DH et al.: The analgesic properties of delta-9-tetrahydrocannabinol and codeine, *Clin Pharmacol Ther* 18:84-89, 1976.

Nulman I, Rovet J, Stewart DE et al.: Neurodevelopment of children exposed in utero to antidepressant drugs, *N Engl J Med* 336:258-262, 1997.

Nystrom B, Hagbarth KE: Microelectrode recordings from transected nerves in amputees in phantom limb pain, *Neurosci Lett* 27:211-216, 1981.

Okasha A, Ghaleb AA, Sadek A: A double-blind trial for the clinical management of psychogenic headache, *Br J Psychiatry* 122:181-183, 1973.

Onghena P, Van houdenhove B: Antidepressant-induced analgesia in chronic nonmalignant pain: a meta-analysis of 39 placebo-controlled studies, *Pain* 49:205-219, 1992.

Oshima E, Tei K, Kayazawa H et al.: Continuous subcutaneous injection of ketamine for cancer pain, *Can J Anaesth* 37:385-392, 1990.

Panerai AE, Monza G, Movillia P et al.: A randomized, within-patient crossover, placebo-controlled trial on the efficacy and tolerability of the tricyclic antidepressants clomipramine and nortriptyline in central pain, *Acta Neurol Scand* 82:34-38, 1990.

Park KM, Max MB, Robinovitz E et al.: Effects of intravenous ketamine and alfentanil on hyperalgesia induced by intradermal capsaicin. In Gebhardt GF, Hammond DL, Jensen TS, editors: *Proceedings of the 7th World Congress on Pain*, pp 647-655, Seattle, IASP Press.

Paterson AHG, Powles TJ, Kanis JA et al.: Double-blind controlled trial of 1994, oral clodronate in patients with bone metastases from breast cancer, *J Clin Oncol* 11:59-65, 1993.

Patt RB, Proper G, Reddy S: The neuroleptics as adjuvant analgesics, *J Pain Symptom Manage* 9:446-453, 1994.

Payne R: Pharmacologic management of bone pain in the cancer patient, *Clin J Pain* 5:S43-S50, 1989.

Peiris JB, Perera GLS, Devendra SV et al.: Sodium valproate in trigeminal neuralgia, *Med J Aust* 2:278, 1980.

Persson J, Axelsson G, Hallin RG et al.: Beneficial effects of ketamine in a chronic pain state with allodynia, possibly due to central sensitization, *Pain* 60:217-222, 1995.

Petersen P, Kastrup J: Dercum's disease (adiposa dolorosa): treatment of severe pain with intravenous lidocaine, *Pain* 28:77-80, 1987.

Petersen P, Kastrup J, Zeeburg I et al.: Chronic pain treatment with intravenous lidocaine, *Neurol Res* 8:189-190, 1986.

Petros AJ, Wright RMB: Epidural and oral clonidine in domiciliary control of deafferentation pain, *Lancet* 1:1034, 1987.

Pilowsky I, Hallett EC, Bassett DL et al.: A controlled study of amitriptyline in the treatment of chronic pain, *Pain* 14:169-179, 1982.

Piper JM, Ray WA, Daugherty JR et al.: Corticosteroid use and peptic ulcer disease: role of nonsteroidal anti-inflammatory drugs, *Ann Intern Med* 114:735-740, 1991.

Portenoy RK: Cancer pain: epidemiology and syndromes, *Cancer* 63:2298-2307, 1989.

Portenoy RK, Kanner RM: Nonopioid and adjuvant analgesics. In Portenoy RK, Kanner RM, editors: *Pain management: theory and practice*, pp 219-247, Philadelphia, 1996, FA Davis.

Porter AT, McEwan AJ, Powe JE et al.: Results of a randomized phase-III trial to evaluate the efficacy of strontium-89 adjuvant to local field external beam irradiation in the management of endocrine resistant metastatic prostate cancer, *Int J Radiat Oncol Biol Phys* 25:805-813, 1993.

Posner JB, Howieson J, Cvitkovic E: "Disappearing" spinal cord compression: oncolytic effects of glucocorticoids (and other chemotherapeutic agents) on epidural metastases, *Ann Neurol* 2:409-413, 1977.

Preskorn SH, Irwin HA: Toxicity of tricyclic antidepressants: kinetics, mechanism, intervention: a review, *J Clin Psychiatry* 43:151-156, 1982.

Price DD, Mao J, Frenk H et al.: The N-methyl-D-aspartate antagonist dextromethorphan selectively reduces temporal summation of second pain in man, *Pain* 59:165-174, 1994.

Price DD, Mao J, Lu J et al.: Effects of the combined oral administration of NSAIDs and dextromethorphan on behavioral symptoms indicative of arthritic pain in rats, *Pain* 68:119-127, 1996.

Prough DS, McLeskey CH, Borshy GG et al.: Efficacy of oral nifedipine treatment of reflex sympathetic dystrophy, *Anesthesiology* 62:796-799, 1985.

Puke MJC, Wiesenfeld-Hallin Z: The differential effects of morphine and the alpha 2 adrenoceptor agonists clonidine and dexmedetomidine on the prevention and treatment of experimental neuropathic pain, *Anesth Analg* 77:104-109, 1993.

Quatraro A, Minei A: Calcitonin in painful diabetic neuropathy, *Lancet* 339:746-747, 1992.

Quilty PM, Kirk D, Bolger JJ et al.: A comparison of the palliative effects of strontium-89 and external beam radiotherapy in metastatic prostate cancer, *Radiother Oncol* 31:33-40, 1994.

Racz GB, Morton AB, Diede JH: Sphenopalatine ganglion block. In Waldman SD, Winnie AP, editors. *Interventional pain management*, pp 223-225, Philadelphia, 1996, WB Saunders.

Raftery H: The management of postherpetic pain using sodium valproate and amitriptyline, *J Irish Med Assoc* 72:399-401, 1979.

Raja SN, Treede RD, Davis KD et al.: Systemic alpha-adrenergic blockade with phentolamine: a diagnostic test for sympathetically-maintained pain, *Anesthesiology* 74:691-698, 1991.

Ramsey RE, Wilder BJ, Berger JR et al.: A double-blind study comparing carbM et al.: Postsympathectomy neuralgia: amelioration with diphenylhydantoin and carbamazepine, *Am J Surg* 1974.

Rani PU, Naidu MUR, Prasad VBN et al.: An evaluation of antidepressants in rheumatic pain conditions, *Anesth Analg* 83:371-375, 1996.

Raskin NH, Levinson SA, Hoffman PM et al.: Postsympathectomy neuralgia: amelioration with diphenylhydantoin and carbamazepine, *Am J Surg* 1974.

Rauck RL, Eisenach JC, Jackson K et al.: Epidural clonidine treatment for refractory reflex sympathetic dystrophy, *Anesthesiology* 79:1163-1169, 1993.

Ray WA, Griffin MR, Schaffner W et al.: Psychotropic drug use and the risk of hip fracture, *N Engl J Med* 316:363-369, 1987.

Reddy S, Patt RB. The benzodiazepines as adjuvant analgesics, *J Pain Symptom Manage* 9:510-514, 1994.

Reeves AL, So EL, Sharbrough FW et al.: Movement disorders associated with the use of gabapentin, *Epilepsia* 37:988-990, 1996.

Reid DB: Palliative management of bowel obstruction, *Med J Aust* 148:54, 1988.

ReMine Sg, McIlrath D: Bowel performation in steroid-treated patients. *Ann Surg* 192:581-586, 1980.

Ringel RA, Roy EP: Glossopharyngeal neuralgia: successful treatment with baclofen, *Ann Neurol* 21:514-515, 1987.

Ripamonti C: Management of bowel obstruction in advanced cancer patients, *J Pain Symptom Manage* 9:193-200, 1994.

Robinson RG, Preston DF, Baxter KG et al.: Clinical experience with strontium-89 in prostatic and breast cancer patients, *Semin Oncol* 20:44-48, 1993.

Robinson RG, Preston DF, Schiefelbein M et al.: Strontium-89 therapy for the palliation of pain due to osseous metastases, *JAMA* 274:420-424, 1995.

Robinson RG, Spicer JA, Preston DF et al.: Treatment of metastatic bone pain with strontium-89, *Nucl Med Biol* 14:219-222, 1987.

Rockliff BW, Davis EH: Controlled sequential trials of carbamazepine in trigeminal neuralgia, *Arch Neurol* 15:129-136, 1966.

Roose SP, Glassman AH, Giardina EG et al.: Nortriptyline in depressed patients with left ventricular impairment, *JAMA* 256:3253-3257, 1986.

Rosen J, Pollock BG, Altieri L et al.: Treatment of nortriptyline's side effects in elderly patients: a double-blind study of bethanechol, *Am J Psychiatry* 150:1249-1251, 1993.

Rosenberg JM, Harrell C, Ristic H et al.: The effect of gabapentin on neuropathic pain, *Clin J Pain* 13:251-255, 1997.

Rosenberg MK, Raymond C, Bridge PD: Comparison of midazolam/ketamine with methohexital for sedation during peribulbar block, *Anesth Analg* 81:173-174, 1995.

Rosenblatt WH, Cioffi AM, Sinatra R et al.: Metoclopramide: an analgesic adjunct to patient-controlled analgesics, *Anesth Analg* 73:553-555, 1991.

Rosner H, Rubin L, Kestenbaum A: Gabapentin adjunctive therapy in neuropathic pain states, *Clin J Pain* 12:56-58, 1996.

Rosner S: A simple method of treatment for acute headache, *Headache* 24:50, 1984.

Roth A, Kolaric K: Analgesic activity of calcitonin in patients with painful osteolytic metastases of breast cancer: results of a controlled randomized study, *Oncology* 43:283-287, 1986.

Rothchild AJ: Selective serotonin reuptake inhibitor-induced sexual dysfunction: efficacy of a drug holiday, *Am J Psychiatry* 152:1514-1516, 1995.

Rowbotham MC: Topical analgesic agents. In: Fields HL, Liebeskind JC, editors: *Pharmacological approaches to the treatment of chronic pain: new concepts and critical issues*, pp 211-229, Seattle, 1994, IASP Press.

Rowbotham MC, Davies PS, Fields HL: Topical lidocaine gel relieves postherpetic neuralgia, *Ann Neurol* 37:246-253, 1995.

Rowbotham MC, Fields H: Topical lidocaine reduces pain in postherpetic neuralgia, *Pain* 38:297-302, 1989.

Rowbotham MC, Reisner-Keller LA, Fields HL: Both intravenous lidocaine and morphine reduce the pain of postherpetic neuralgia, *Neurology* 41:1024-1028, 1991.

Rull JA, Quibrera R, Gonzalez-Millan H et al.: Symptomatic treatment of peripheral diabetic neuropathy with carbamazepine (Tegretol): double-blind cross-over trial, *Diabetologia* 5:215-218, 1969.

Saeger LC: Clinical use of gabapentin for neuropathic and chronic pain: efficacy, side-effects and dose ranges in a community based pain medicine practice. In *American Pain Society 15th Annual Scientific Meeting* p A-109, 1996 (abstract).

Sagen J, Proudfit H: Evidence for pain modulation by pre- and postsynaptic noradrenergic receptors in the medulla oblongota, *Brain Res* 331:285-293, 1985.

Sawynok J: Pharmacological rationale for the clinical use of caffeine, *Drugs* 49:37-50, 1995.

Scadding JW: Clinical trial of propranolol in post-traumatic neuralgia, *Pain* 14:283-92, 1982.

Schachtel BP, Fillingim JM, Lane AC et al.: Caffeine as an analgesic adjuvant: a double-blind study comparing aspirin with caffeine to aspirin and placebo in patients with severe sore throat, *Arch Intern Med* 151:733-737, 1991.

Schell HW: Adrenal corticosteroid therapy in far advanced cancer, *Geriatrics* 27:131-141, 1972.

Schmidt D: Adverse effects of valproate, *Epilepsia* 25:44S-49S, 1984.

Schneider JR: Effects of caffeine ingestion on heart rate, blood pressure, myo-cardial oxygen consumption, and cardiac rhythm in acute myocardial infarction patients, *Heart Lung* 16(2)167-174, 1987.

Schug SA, Zech D, Dorr U: Cancer pain management according to WHO analgesic guidelines, *J Pain Symptom Manage* 5:27-32, 1990.

Schug SA, Zech D, Grond S et al.: A long-term survey of morphine in cancer pain patients, *J Pain Symptom Manage* 7:259-266, 1992.

Segal AZ, Rordorf G: Gabapentin as a novel treatment for postherpetic neuralgia, *Am Academy Neurol* 1173-1174, 1996.

Segerdahl M, Ekblom A, Sandelin K et al.: Perioperative adenosine infusion reduces the requirements for isoflurane and postoperative analgesics, *Anesth Analg* 80:1145-1149, 1995.

Serafini AN: Current status of systemic intravenous radiopharmaceuticals for the treatment of painful metastatic bone disease, *Int J Radiat Oncol Biol Phys* 30:1187-1194, 1994.

Shafar J, Tallett ER, Knowlson PA: Evaluation of clonidine in prophylaxis of migraine, *Lancet* 1:403-407, 1972.

Shapiro BA, Warren J, Egol AB et al.: Practice parameters for intravenous analgesia and sedation for adult patients in the intensive care unit: an executive summary, *Critical Care Med* 23:1596-1600, 1995.

Sharav Y, Singer E, Schmidt E et al.: The analgesic effect of amitriptyline on chronic facial pain, *Pain* 31:199-209, 1987.

Silberstein EB: The treatment of painful osseous metastases with phosphorus-32-labeled phosphates, *Semin Oncol* 20:10-21, 1993.

Silberstein EB, Williams C: Strontium-89 therapy for the pain of osseous metastases, *J Nucl Med* 26:345-348, 1985.

Simson G: Propranolol for causalgia and Sudek's atrophy, *JAMA* 227:327-332, 1974.

Sindrup SH, Ejlertsen B, Froland A et al.: Imipramine treatment in diabetic neuropathy: relief of subjective symptoms without changes in peripheral and autonomic nerve function, *Eur J Clin Pharmacol* 151-153, 1989.

Sindrup SH, Gram LF, Brosen K et al.: The selective serotonin reuptake inhibitor paroxetine is effective in the treatment of diabetic neuropathy symptoms, *Pain* 42:135-144, 1990.

Sindrup SH, Gram LF, Skjold T et al.: Concentration-response relationship in imipramine treatment of diabetic neuropathy symptoms, *Clin Pharmacol Ther* 47:509-515, 1990.

Sindrup SH, Gram LF, Skjold T et al.: Clomipramine vs. desipramine vs. placebo in the treatment of diabetic neuropathy symptoms: a double-blind crossover study, *Br J Clin Pharmacol* 30:683-691, 1990.

Singh PH, Sharma P, Gupta PK et al.: Clinical evaluation of diazepam for relief of postoperative pain, *Br J Anaesth* 53:831-836, 1981.

Smith JA: Palliation of painful bone metastases from prostate cancer using sodium etidronate: results of a randomized, prospective, double-blind, placebo-controlled study, *J Urol* 141:85-87, 1989.

Sollevi A, Belfrage M, Lundeberg T et al.: Systemic adenosine infusion: a new treatment modality to alleviate neuropathic pain, *Pain* 671:155-158, 1995.

Sorensen PS, Helweg-Larsen S, Mouridsen H et al.: Effect of high-dose dexamethasone in carcinomatous metastatic spinal cord compression treated by radiotherapy: a randomized trial, *Eur J Cancer* 30A:22-27, 1994.

Spiegel K, Kalb R, Pasternak GW: Analgesic activity of tricyclic antidepressants, *Ann Neurol* 13:462-465, 1983.

Stambaugh JE, Lance C: Analgesic efficacy and pharmacokinetic evaluation of meperidine and hydroxyzine, alone and in combination, *Cancer Invest* 1:111-117, 1983.

Stannard CF, Porter GE: Ketamine hydrochloride in the treatment of phantom limb pain, *Pain* 54:227-230, 1993.

Steen AE, Reeh PW, Kreysel HW et al.: Topical acetylsalicylic acid applied to the skin of herpes zoster patients strongly reduces their acute neuralgia (abstract) p 276. In *Abstracts: 8th world congress on pain*, Seattle, 1966, IASP Press.

Stein MG, Demarco T, Gamsu G et al.: Computed tomography: pathologic correlates in lung disease due to tocainide, *Am Rev Respir Diseases* 137:458-460, 1988.

Storey P, Hill HH, St. Louis R et al.: Subcutaneous infusions for control of cancer symptoms, *J Pain Symptom Manage* 5:33-41, 1990.

Stow PJ, Glynn CJ, Minor B: EMLA cream in the treatment of postherpetic neuralgia: efficacy and pharmacokinetic profile, *Pain* 39:301-305, 1989.

Sunshine A, Zighelboim I, De Castro A et al.: Augmentation of acetaminophen analgesia by antihistamine phenyltoloxamine, *J Clin Pharmacol* 29:660-664, 1989.

Swerdlow M: Anticonvulsant drugs and chronic pain, *Clin Neuropharmacol* 7:51-82, 1984.

Swerdlow M, Cundill JG: Anticonvulsant drugs used in the treatment of lancinating pains: a comparison, *Anesthesia* 36:1129-1132, 1981.

Tabira T, Shibasaki H, Kuroiwa Y: Reflex sympathetic dystrophy (causalgia) treatment with guanethidine, *Arch Neurol* 40:430-432, 1983.

Tallian KB, Nahata MC et al.: Gabapentin associated with aggressive behavior in pediatric patients with seizures, *Epilepsia* 37:501-502, 1996.

Tan Y-M, Croese J: Clonidine and diabetic patients with leg pains, *Ann Intern Med* 105:633, 1986.

Tandan R, Lewis GA, Krusinski PB et al.: Topical capsaicin in painful diabetic neuropathy: controlled study long-term followup, *Diabetes Care* 15(1):8-14, 1992.

Tanelian DL, Victory RA: Sodium channel-blocking agents: their use in neuropathic pain conditions, *Pain Forum* 4(2):75-80, 1995.

Tannock I, Gospodarowicz M, Meakin W et al.: Treatment of metastatic prostatic cancer with low-dose prednisone: evaluation of pain and quality of life pragmatic indices of response, *J Clin Oncol* 7:590-597, 1989.

Taub A: Relief of postherpetic neuralgia with psychotropic drugs, *J Neurosurgy* 39:235-239, 1973.

Taylor JC, Brauer S, Espir MLE: Long-term treatment of trigeminal neuralgia with carbamazepine, *Postgrad Med J* 57:16-18, 1980.

Taylor PH, Gray K, Bicknell RG et al.: Glossopharyngeal neuralgia with syncope, *J Laryngol Otol* 91:859-368, 1977.

Terrence CF, Fromm GH: Congestive heart failure during carbamazepine therapy, *Ann Neurol* 8:200-201, 1980.

Terrence CF, Fromm GH, Tenicela R: Baclofen as an analgesic in chronic peripheral nerve disease, *Eur Neurol* 24:380-385, 1985.

Tharion G, Bhattacharji S: Aspirin in chloroform as an effective adjuvant in the management of chronic neurogenic pain, *Arch Phys Med Rehabil* 78:437-439, 1997.

Thiebaud D, Leyvraz S, von Fliedner V et al.: Treatment of bone metastases from breast cancer and myeloma with pamidronate, *Eur J Cancer* 27:37-41, 1991.

Tomson T, Bertilsson L: Potent therapeutic effects of carbamazepine-10, 11-epoxide in trigeminal neuralgia, *Arch Neurol* 41:598-601, 1984.

Troupin A, Ojemann LM: Paradoxical intoxication: a complication of anticonvulsant administration, *Epilepsia* 16:753-758, 1975.

Tseng TC, Wang SC: Locus of action of centrally-acting muscle relaxants, diazepam and tybamate, *J Pharmacol Exp Ther* 178:350-360, 1971.

Turkington RW: Depression masquerading as diabetic neuropathy, *JAMA* 243:1147-1150, 1980.

Tverskoy M, Oz Y, Isakson A et al.: Preemptive effect of fentanyl and ketamine on postoperative pain and wound hyperalgesia, *Anesth Analg* 78:205-209, 1994.

Twycross RG, Fairfield: Pain in far-advanced cancer, *Pain* 14:303-310, 1982.

Van Dyke D, Barash PG, Jatlow P et al.: Cocaine: plasma concentrations after intranasal application in man, *Science* 191d:859-861, 1976.

van Holten-Verzantvoort AT, Kroon HM, Bijvoet OK et al.: Palliative pamidronate treatment in patients with bone metastases from breast cancer, *J Clin Oncol* 11:491-498, 1993.

Vecht Ch J, Haaxma-Reiche H, van Putten WLJ et al.: Initial bolus of conventional versus high-dose dexamethasone in metastatic spinal cord compression, *Neurology* 39:1255-1257, 1989.

Ventafridda V, Bianchi M, Ripamonti C et al.: Studies on the effects of antidepressant drugs on the antinociceptive action of morphine and on plasma morphine in rat and man, *Pain* 43:155-162, 1990.

Ventafridda V, Bonezzi C, Caraceni A et al.: Antidepressants for cancer pain and other painful syndromes with deafferentation component: comparison of amitriptyline and trazadone, *Ital J Neurol Sci* 8:579-587, 1987.

Ventafridda V, Ripamonti C, Caraceni A et al.: The management of inoperable gastrointestinal obstruction in terminal cancer patients, *Tumori* 76:389-393, 1990.

Ventafridda V, Tamburini M, Caraceni A et al.: A validation study of the WHO method for cancer pain relief, *Cancer* 59:850-856, 1990.

Vincent FM, Vincent T: Tocainide encephalopathy, *Neurology* 35:1804-1805, 1985.

Walsh TD. Controlled study of imipramine and morphine in chronic pain due to advanced cancer, *Proc Am Soc Clin Oncol* 5:237, 1986 (abstract).

Ward NG: Tricyclic antidepressants for chronic low back pain: mechanism of action and predictors of response, *Spine* 11:661-665, 1986.

Ward NG, Bloom VL, Friedel RP: The effectiveness of tricyclic antidepressants in the treatment of coexisting pain and depression, *Pain* 7:331-341, 1979.

Ward N, Whitney C, Avery D et al.: The analgesic effects of caffeine in headache, *Pain* 44:151-155, 1991.

Warrell RP, Lovett D, Dilmanian FA et al.: Low-dose gallium nitrate for prevention of osteolysis in myeloma: results of a pilot randomized study, *J Clin Oncol* 11:2443-2450, 1993.

Watson CPN, Chipman M, Reed K et al.: Amitriptyline versus maprotiline in postherpetic neuralgia: a randomized double-blind, crossover trial, *Pain* 48:29-36, 1992.

Watson CPN, Evans RJ: The postmastectomy pain syndrome and topical capsaicin: a randomized trial, *Pain* 51:375-379, 1992.

Watson CPN, Evans RJ, Reed K et al.: Amitriptyline versus placebo in postherpetic neuralgia, *Neurology* (NY) 32:671-673, 1982.

Watson CPN, Evans RJ, Watt VR: Postherpetic neuralgia and topical capsaicin, *Pain* 33:333-340, 1988.

Watson CPN, Evans RJ, Watt VR: The post-mastectomy pain syndrome and the effect of topical capsaicin, *Pain* 33:177-186, 1989.

Watson CPN, Tyler KL, Bickers DR et al.: A randomized vehicle-controlled trial of topical capsaicin in the treatment of postherpetic neuralgia, *Clin Ther* 15:510-526, 1993.

Weinberger J, Nicklas WJ, Berl S: Mechanism of action of anticonvulsants, *Neurology* (Minneap) 26:162-173, 1976.

Weis O, Sriwatanakul K, Weintraub M: Treatment of postherpetic neuralgia and acute herpetic pain with amitriptyline and perphenazine, *South Afr Med J* 62:274-275, 1982.

Weissman DE, Dufer D, Vogel V et al.: Corticosteroid toxicity in neuro-oncology patients, *J Neurooncol* 5:125-128, 1987.

Wilcox JC, Corr J, Shaw J et al.: Prednisolone as an appetite stimulant in patients with cancer, *BMJ* 288:27, 1984.

Wong CS, Liaw WJ, Tung CS et al.: Ketamine potentiates analgesic effect of morphine in postoperative epidural pain control, *Reg Anesth* 21:534-541, 1996.

Woodrow KM, Eltherington LG: Feeling no pain, alcohol as an analgesic, *Pain* 32:159-163, 1988.

Woolf CJ, Thompson SWN: The induction and maintenance of central sensitization is dependent on N-methyl-D-aspartic acid receptor activation: implications for the treatment of post-injury pain hypersensitivity states, *Pain* 44:293-299, 1991.

Woolf CJ, Wiesenfeld-Halli Z: The systemic administration of local anesthetic produces a selective depression of C-afferent evoked activity in the spinal cord, *Pain* 23:361-374, 1985.

World Health Organization: *Cancer pain relief and palliative care*, Geneva, 1990, The Organization.

Yaksh TL: Direct evidence that spinal serotonin and noradrenaline terminals mediate the spinal antinociceptive effects of morphine in the periaqueductal gray, *Brain Res* 160:180-185, 1979.

Yaksh TL: Pharmacology of spinal adrenergic systems which modulate spinal nociceptive processing, *Pharmacol Biochem Behav* 22:845-858, 1985.

Yaksh TL, Malmberg AB: Central pharmacology of nociceptive transmission. In Wall PD, Melzack R, editors: *Textbook of pain*, ed 3, pp 165-200, Edinburgh, 1994, Churchill Livingstone.

Yamada K, Ushio Y, Hayakawa T et al.: Effects of methylprednisolone on peritumoral brain edema, *J Neurosurg* 59:612-619, 1983.

Yang JC, Clark WC, Dooley JC et al.: Effect of intranasal cocaine on experimental pain in man, *Anesth Analg* 61:358-361, 1982.

Yang JC, Clark WC, Ngai SH et al.: Analgesic action and pharmacokinetics of morphine and diazepam in man: an evaluation by sensory decision theory, *Anesthesiology* 51:495-502, 1979.

Yjritsy-Roy JA, Standish SM, Terry LC: Dopamine D-1 and D-2 receptor antagonists potentiate analgesic and motor effects of morphine, *Pharmacol Biochem Behav* 32:717-721, 1989.

Yosselson-Superstine S, Lipman AG, Saunders SH: Adjunctive antianxiety agents in the management of chronic pain, *Israel J Med Sci* 21:113-117, 1985.

Zeigler D, Lynch SA, Muir J et al.: Transdermal clonidine versus placebo in painful diabetic neuropathy, *Pain* 48:403-408, 1992.

Zhang WY, Li Wan Po A: The effectiveness of topically applied capsaicin: a meta-analysis, *Eur J Clin Pharmacol* 46:517-522, 1994.

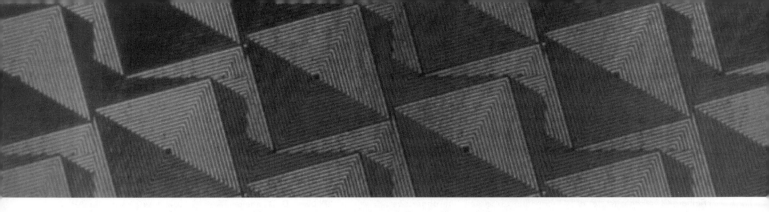

chapter eight
PROCEDURAL PAIN MANAGEMENT

Chris Pasero and Margo McCaffery
Reviewer: Donna Wong

CHAPTER OUTLINE

TERMINOLOGY

Analgesic ceiling: A dose beyond which further increases in dose do not provide additional analgesia.

Dermatome: An area of skin that is primarily innervated by a single spinal cord segment.

Mu agonist: A type of opioid; includes morphine and other opioids that relieve pain by binding to the mu receptor sites in the nervous system. Used interchangeably with the terms full agonist, pure agonist, and morphine-like drug.

Opioid: Preferred to "narcotic." Refers to natural, semisynthetic, and synthetic drugs that relieve pain by binding to multiple types of opioid receptors in the nervous system.

Opioid agonist-antagonist: A type of opioid (e.g., nalbuphine and butorphanol) that binds to the kappa opioid receptor sites acting as an agonist (capable of producing analgesia) and simultaneously to the mu opioid receptor sites acting as an antagonist (reversing agonist effects).

Opioid antagonist: Competes with agonists for opioid receptor binding sites; can displace agonists, thereby inhibiting their action. Examples include naloxone and naltrexone.

Preemptive analgesia: Preinjury pain treatments, (e.g., preprocedure analgesics or preincision local anesthetic infiltration) to prevent the establishment of peripheral and central sensitization of pain.

 Advances in diagnostic and therapeutic modalities have resulted in patients being subjected to an increasing number of relatively brief, but sometimes very painful, procedures. These procedures occur in many settings, such as the hospital, home, and outpatient clinic, and they are performed by a variety of individuals, including nurses, physicians, and family members. Often they are performed without appropriate analgesics or anesthetics. Although the frequency of undertreated procedural pain is unknown, most health care professionals would have little difficulty listing a number of painful procedures they know are performed routinely without pain control.

Procedural pain serves no useful purpose and has many damaging consequences. Without adequate analgesic treatment, patients who are subjected to repetitive painful procedures become fearful and anxious in anticipation of procedural pain (Barr, 1994). Patients often describe feeling victimized, violated, and even attacked when forced to endure painful procedures without pain control. Many are reluctant to return for further treatment or diagnostic procedures. Some seek other health care professionals who are attentive to their analgesic needs.

Consideration also must be given to the adverse physiologic effects of unrelieved pain, even if the pain is temporary (see Chapter 2). For patients who already are stressed and compromised, such as the critically ill and individuals immediately following a traumatic injury, painful procedures are another physical insult.

Although all patients are at risk for undertreated procedural pain, specific populations of patients who are at particularly high risk include premature and full-term infants, children, and the elderly. Other vulnerable patients are those who are paraplegic or quadriplegic, chronically ill, cognitively impaired, comatose or unconscious, and patients who are chemically paralyzed by neuromuscular blocking agents.

This chapter identifies procedures that require pain management and presents strategies for reducing the anxiety and pain that accompany many procedures. These strategies focus on patient teaching, medication use, and nondrug methods for pain and anxiety reduction. In addition, common barriers to effective pain control during procedures are listed and suggestions are provided throughout the chapter for overcoming these obstacles. Included is a protocol on conscious sedation and analgesia and recommendations for developing standardized pain management plans that can be implemented to ensure that pain is systematically assessed and managed during known or suspected painful procedures. Central to all the information provided in this chapter is the health care professional's accountability for pain assessment and management during procedures. Selected terms and definitions (terminology) are listed at the beginning of this chapter to facilitate an understanding of the chapter content.

BARRIERS TO EFFECTIVE PROCEDURAL PAIN MANAGEMENT

Despite efforts to improve pain control in institutions across the country, many barriers remain. Some of the most bothersome are those that result in the undertreatment of pain during procedures. Traditional clinical practice has largely ignored the pain related to procedures, and clinicians have continued to rationalize this on the basis of outdated information about methods of pain control. Patients themselves fail to demand pain relief because of their own misconceptions and faulty assumptions. Table 8.1 lists some of the misconceptions that present barriers to effective procedural pain management.

DETERMINING THE NEED FOR PROCEDURAL PAIN MANAGEMENT

Not all procedures are painful. Some produce anxiety and no pain. For example, magnetic resonance imaging (MRI) and computed tomography (CT) usually are not

TABLE 8.1 ● ● ● ● ●

Misconceptions Procedural Pain

MISCONCEPTION	CORRECTION
1. Giving local anesthetics and analgesics for procedures is complex. They require special administration techniques and have unmanageable side effects and risks, especially for premature infants, neonates, infants, children, and the elderly.	When administered correctly, local anesthetics and analgesics used for procedural pain are safe and effective in almost all populations of patients with minimal side effects that are easy to detect and manage. The techniques used to administer the local anesthetics and analgesics for many procedures are simple to master with proper training.
2. Giving the analgesic/anesthetic hurts as much as the procedure.	A number of easy-to-apply techniques can be used to reduce the discomfort associated with drugs that are painful when administered (e.g., buffering and warming lidocaine and adding lidocaine to propofol).
3. There is not enough time available to provide anesthesia and analgesia before procedures, and most procedures are brief and over before the anesthetic or analgesic takes effect.	Poor planning is not justification for failing to provide adequate procedural pain control. Most anesthetics and analgesics recommended for procedural pain have a rapid onset of action and can be titrated or redosed if necessary during the procedure to maintain adequate pain control. Institutional protocols and standardized pain management plans can be developed for the routine management of most procedural pain, making preplanning easier.
4. If the procedure is brief, the pain will be brief and tolerable.	Procedural pain serves no useful purpose and has many damaging consequences. Research shows that a number of adverse physiologic, psychologic, and emotional effects of unrelieved pain exist, even if the pain is brief and temporary.
5. If given enough sedation, patients will not feel or remember the pain.	Benzodiazepines do not have any analgesic properties except for muscle spasm. Sedation does not reduce pain and it does not eliminate the memory of it.
6. Caregivers know that the procedure is painful and will do all they can to relieve pain during the procedure.	For years patients have tolerated without analgesia or anesthesia procedures such as venipuncture, immunization, circumcision, and tubing and line placement, believing that their caregivers are doing all they can to relieve their pain. Subjecting patients to this practice is no longer justified in light of the many drugs and methods available to control pain. Patients have a right to aggressive pain management, including the control of procedural pain.

May be duplicated for use in clinical practice. From McCaffery M, Pasero C: *Pain: Clinical manual*, p. 364. Copyright © 1999, Mosby, Inc. See text for references.

painful procedures but require the patient to be as motionless as possible. Some patients find these procedures frightening or claustrophobic. Others have difficulty remaining motionless. In these cases providing sedation during the procedure may decrease anxiety and enhance cooperation.

However, most therapeutic and diagnostic procedures performed today are painful. The decision to provide analgesia during a procedure must be made on the basis of knowledge of the likelihood that the procedure produces pain. If any question exists about whether pain is associated with the procedure, the health care team must assume that pain is present. To ensure clear communication, standardized pain management plans and protocols

can be established. Before beginning the procedure, the health care team can address whether analgesic agents will be administered. If no analgesics are administered, they must be added if it becomes apparent that a procedure thought not to be associated with pain is causing pain.

Table 8.2 lists several common procedures and attempts to delineate which ones are likely to require sedation alone or which probably necessitate both sedation and analgesia. The decision to add sedation may vary from what is suggested in the table, depending on the patient's age, condition, and anxiety level. For example, chest tube removal and lumbar puncture may require sedation in addition to analgesia for some patients. Previous experience with the painful procedure may con-

• • • • •

TABLE 8.2 **Procedures That May Require Analgesia and/or Sedation**

PROCEDURE	ANALGESIA/ ANESTHESIA	SEDATION
Bone marrow aspiration or biopsy	X	X
Burn debridement	X	X
Cardioversion	X	X
Chest tube placement	X	X
Chest tube removal	X	X*
Circumcision	X	
Dressing changes	X	X*
Endoscopy	X	X
Incision and drainage of abscess	X	X*
Immunization	X	
Lumbar puncture	X	X*
Minor dental, podiatric, plastic, urologic, and ophthalmic surgical procedures	X	X*
Paracentesis	X	X
Placement or removal of implanted devices	X	X
Placement of catheters, lines, and tubings	X	X*
Radiologic procedures (CT, MRI)		X*
Reduction and immobilization of fractures	X	X
Suturing of lacerations	X	X*
Thoracentesis	X	X
Tissue biopsies	X	X*
Venipuncture	X	
Mechanical ventilation	X†	X*

May be duplicated for use in clinical practice. From McCaffery M, Pasero C: *Pain: Clinical manual*, p. 365. Copyright © 1999, Mosby, Inc.

Table 8.2 lists a number of procedures that may require the use of analgesics, sedatives, or both.

*The decision to add sedation may vary from what is suggested in the table depending on the patient's age, condition, and anxiety level. Opioid analgesics alone may provide adequate sedation in some instances. If the patient has high anxiety or previous experience with uncontrolled pain, additional sedation may be needed.

†Discontinuation of analgesics before weaning from mechanical ventilation is not recommended.

Information from Carroll KC, Magruder CC: The role of analgesics and sedatives in the management of pain and agitation during weaning from mechanical ventilation, *Crit Care Nurs Q* 15(4):68-77, 1993.

tribute to high or low levels of anxiety about the procedure. For example, a previous painful and frightening experience with lumbar puncture may indicate the need for sedation, whereas a previous experience with minimal discomfort during a lumbar puncture may negate the need for sedation.

GOALS OF PROCEDURAL PAIN MANAGEMENT

Identifying the goals of effective procedural pain management is one of the first steps in establishing standardized pain management plans and protocols. The primary goal is for the patient to experience adequate pain relief during the procedure. Other goals include minimal or no anxiety and fear related to the procedure, ability to cooperate during the procedure, and a prompt, safe recovery from the effects of the procedure. To accomplish these goals caregivers must ensure that the patient understands the procedure and the pain management plan and also experiences safe and effective anxiety and pain control during the procedure and recovery period.

INFORMED CONSENT AND PATIENT TEACHING

Obtaining informed consent is an important function of health care professionals who perform and assist with procedures. Informed consent indicates that the patient understands the nature of the procedure, including its benefits, risks, and potential complications. The process of obtaining informed consent forces patients to recognize that their control and the health care professional's control over the outcome of the procedure is limited (Syrjala, 1993). This, plus the abundance of unfamiliar and often confusing information patients must comprehend, magnifies their feelings of helplessness when exposed to the health care system. However, the need to obtain informed consent can be viewed as the ideal opportunity for the health care professional to use teaching methods that can help patients view their situation from a less threatening perspective.

Procedures and the pain they produce are predictable, at least in terms of the timing of their occurrence. This characteristic lends itself particularly well to the use of teaching methods that can reduce patients' fears and anxiety. Providing three types of information for patients is recommended: procedural, temporal, and sensory. These types of information help patients "reframe" their thinking and label their experiences and sensations with familiar and less threatening terms than what are evoked through traditional methods of obtaining informed consent (Syrjala, 1993).

Ideally, caregivers provide all three types of information to patients both before and during a procedure. For most patients, preparation for the procedure begins with procedural information (what will happen) and then the focus turns to temporal (timing of events) and sensory information (characteristics of the sensations the patient is likely to feel). During the procedure, caregivers tend to provide primarily temporal information, such as how much longer various segments of the procedure will take (Syrjala, 1993).

Procedural Information

Providing procedural information consists of telling the patient exactly what will happen or is happening. Information about what the clinicians will do and are doing helps the patient feel that the situation is under control. Generally, health care professionals provide this type of information more often than temporal or sensory information. However, temporary and sensory information are more helpful in reducing feelings of threat and helplessness (Syrjala, 1993).

Some patients may prefer not to know specific details of a procedure. They can become anxious if each step of a procedure is discussed, especially when the steps are discussed during the procedure. For these patients, outlining what will happen or is happening is counterproductive. Distraction strategies may be helpful for patients who do not want procedural information (see Nondrug Approaches, Chapter 9).

Other patients benefit more from ongoing details of the procedure during the procedure and are made more anxious by attempts to distract them from it. Therefore it is wise to ask all patients if they would like to know details about their procedure and if they think repeating information during the procedure will be helpful (Syrjala, 1993).

Temporal Information

The most important information to provide is temporal information. Most individuals find an unpleasant situation, such as a painful procedure, considerably easier to tolerate if they know when it will begin and end.

Temporal information includes telling patients when something is going to happen and approximately how long it will last. The explanation of a procedure can also be broken down into small time frames or steps, which patients may find easier to understand and more tolerable (Syrjala, 1993). For example, the patient may be told that positioning and draping for a procedure takes about 2 minutes, whereas inserting the needle and numbing the site takes about 30 seconds.

Sensory Information

Providing sensory information includes telling patients how they will feel and providing descriptors other than "pain" to label what they will feel. Using descriptors that are familiar terms, such as "stinging" or

"aching," may be less threatening than the word "pain" (Syrjala, 1993).

Making sure patients understand exactly what will happen and is happening and how long it will last can give them a stronger sense of control. However, a small number of patients may be so afraid of being in a situation they cannot control that they are phobic and refuse care. It may be impossible to reduce their fears and anxiety related to the procedure by providing information alone. In these cases the use of systematic desensitization and/or anxiolytics may be helpful (Syrjala, 1993).

Patient Example

Mr. R. wants to know everything about the epidural catheter placement procedure he is going to have later today. His nurse decides to provide a thorough explanation of the procedure using procedural, temporal, and sensory information.

"You'll be in a sitting position or lying on your side for the procedure. The doctor will be behind you facing your back. First he'll wash a small area on your back with a sponge. This may feel cool. Then he'll put paper drapes on your back to keep the area as clean as possible. You'll need to roll your shoulders inward and push your back out slightly like this (nurse demonstrates). The doctor will use a local anesthetic to numb the place where the small tubing, called the catheter, will go. Sometimes injecting the local anesthetic causes a burning, stinging sensation that lasts less than a minute. It usually takes the doctor about 2 or 3 minutes to insert the epidural needle into the numb area. This will feel like dull pressure against your back. Next the doctor inserts the catheter through the needle into the epidural space, which takes less than a minute. As he inserts the catheter you may feel some sparklike sensations in your legs and feet. These will go away very quickly. The doctor will remove the epidural needle and tape the catheter in place up your back to your shoulder. After the catheter is taped in place you'll be able to move and turn and lay on your back like you did before the procedure. The whole procedure usually takes less than 30 minutes. You may feel a very slight irritation for an hour or two after the procedure just at the site where the catheter goes into your back. If you feel any more discomfort in your back than that at any time while the catheter is in place, you'll need to let us know. Can I answer any questions?"

ASSESSMENT OF PROCEDURAL PAIN

The process that will be used to assess procedural pain is discussed with patients before the procedure. A baseline pain assessment, including the existence of preexisting pain and the patient's current use of analgesics, sedatives, and nondrug methods, provides important information that can be used to manage pain during and after the procedure. Before the procedure, patients are introduced to the pain rating scale (see Chapter 3). As in any other situation, during a procedure the patient's report is the most reliable indicator of the existence and intensity of pain (AHCPR, 1992).

If patients are unable to talk during the procedure, they may be afraid that they will not be able to report pain. In these cases establishing an alternative method for alerting the health care team of their pain is helpful. For example, give the patient a squeak toy to hold during the procedure. The patient can squeeze it to signal to the health care team that pain control is inadequate. Or the patient may prefer signaling by raising a hand or lifting a finger.

Overt physical signs, such as muscle rigidity, tearing of eyes, facial grimacing, groaning, agitation, and changes in vital signs can be signs of pain and may be included in procedural pain assessment. However, the absence of overt physical signs must not be interpreted as an absence of pain.

PHARMACOLOGIC APPROACHES TO PROCEDURAL PAIN

Local anesthetics and opioids are the mainstay pharmacologic agents for managing pain during procedures. Benzodiazepines are added if necessary to provide sedation and reduce anxiety. Local anesthetics, opioids, and NSAIDs can be used to provide preemptive analgesia (treatment of pain before tissue damage occurs) (Anderson, Zeltzer, Fanurik, 1993) (see Chapter 4). Other agents used for procedural pain include general anesthetics, such as ketamine, propofol, and nitrous oxide. The choice of pharmacologic agent, route of administration, and dose depends on the nature of the procedure, the setting in which it is performed, and the patient's age and condition.

Institutional commitment to aggressive pain control and the use of potent analgesic and anesthetic agents to meet this commitment has resulted in role expansion for registered nurses. Before delineating the role of nursing in administering and monitoring these agents in your institution, it is recommended that a representative from your institution contact your state's board of nursing to determine the scope of practice for the nursing staff. Scope of nursing practice can vary from state to state (Pasero, 1994).

In addition, the Agency for Health Care Policy and Research (AHCPR) acute pain management guideline (1992) emphasizes that "no anesthetic or analgesic agent should be used unless the clinician understands the proper technique of administration, dosage, contraindications, side effects, and treatment of overdose" (p. 68). Mechanisms for ensuring medical and nursing staff are competent to administer anesthetic and analgesic agents must be established. When large doses of general anesthetics, seda-

tives, or opioids are required for procedural sedation and pain management, it is wise to implement a conscious sedation/analgesia protocol (see example, pp. 382-384).

Local Anesthetics

Local anesthetics are used to control the pain of procedures ranging from minor ones, such as venipuncture, injection, and suturing, to major ones, such as bone marrow aspiration, thoracentesis, and minor surgeries. Local anesthetics are inexpensive, simple to use, and relatively safe for a wide variety of patients (Illingworth, Simpson, 1994). Hypersensitivity (allergy) to local anesthetics is rare and is manifested usually as allergic dermatitis or a typical asthma attack (Catterall, Mackie, 1996). (See Box 8.1 for practical information on the use of local anesthetics.)

Local anesthetics work by blocking nerve conduction and thus have the capability of stopping the transmission of pain completely (see Chapter 2). Most often they are injected intradermally or subcutaneously at the site of sensory nerve endings before a procedure to anesthetize

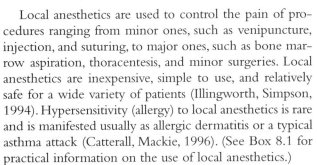

BOX 8.1

GUIDELINES

USE OF LOCAL ANESTHETICS

- Review medical history and allergies to determine correct local anesthetic agent to use.
- Check container of local anesthetic for presence of epinephrine and do not give if contraindicated, such as for IV regional anesthesia or on tissues with end arteriole blood supply, such as fingers, toes, penis, nose, or ears.
- Do not inject directly into an infected area.
- Before injecting or applying, check maximum dose of local anesthetic and epinephrine and be especially careful not to exceed it in children. Children are not more resistant to local anesthetics than are adults.
- Inject local anesthetics slowly.
- Stop injection immediately if patient reports significant pain from the injection or signs of toxicity, such as tinnitus or tingling around the mouth.
- Document the use of even small amounts of local anesthetic in the medical record.

May be duplicated for use in clinical practice. From McCaffery M, Pasero C: Pain: Clinical manual, p. 367. Copyright © 1999, Mosby, Inc.

IV, intravenous.

Information from Franck LS, Gregory GA: Clinical evaluation and treatment of infant pain in the neonatal intensive care unit. In Schechter N, Berde CB, Yaster M, editors: *Pain in infants, children, and adolescents,* pp 519-535, Baltimore, 1993, Williams & Wilkins; Catterall W, Mackie K: Local anesthetics. In Hardman JG, Limbird LE, editors: *Goodman and Gilman's the pharmacological basis of therapeutics,* ed 9, pp 331-347, New York, 1996, McGraw-Hill; Illingworth KA, Simpson KH: *Anaesthesia and analgesia in emergency medicine,* New York, 1994, Oxford University Press; Rice LJ: Regional anesthesia and analgesia. In Motoyama EK, Davis PJ, editors: *Smith's anesthesia for infants and children,* pp 403-442, St. Louis, 1996, Mosby.

a small area, such as for venipuncture or suturing. For more complex procedures, they are used to block selected nerves or to produce a regional block that covers a large area in a dermatomal pattern (see Chapter 6, p. 221). Local anesthetics also can be administered topically, in solution, cream, gel, and spray form, and by dermal iontophoresis. Local anesthetics should not be injected into an infected area (Illingworth, Simpson, 1994). Table 8.3 lists the characteristics of local anesthetics commonly used for procedural analgesia.

Local anesthetic toxicity

Because local anesthetics, by any route, are absorbed rapidly into the circulation, they can produce systemic toxic reactions. Early signs of local anesthetic toxicity include circumoral numbness, metallic taste, dizziness, blurred vision, tinnitus, and decreased hearing. The presence of any of these signs warrants immediate discontinuation of the local anesthetic. Increasing plasma concentrations can eventually result in restlessness and tremors, which can progress to seizures and decreases in cardiac electrical excitability, conduction rate, and force of contraction (Catterall, Mackie, 1996). The presence of any of these manifestations also requires immediate discontinuation of the local anesthetic and may warrant emergency management. It is, therefore, important to have emergency equipment and drugs readily available in areas where local anesthetics are used.

Pediatric patients should be watched closely for local anesthetic toxicity. It is a misconception that children are more resistant to local anesthetic toxicity than are adults. Plasma proteins, which are responsible for binding of local anesthetics, are low in the neonate. Plasma protein binding does not approach adult levels until after the first year of life. This lower level of protein binding allows more of the drug to remain active. It is important to remember that although children eliminate drugs faster than newborns and infants, they eliminate drugs slower than adults (Rice, 1996).

The risk of toxicity when large amounts of the local anesthetic are required, such as might be necessary for a long procedure, can be reduced by using low concentrations (e.g., lidocaine is available for local infiltration in 0.5% to 2.0% concentration) and by adding epinephrine (Illingworth, Simpson, 1994). Epinephrine is a vasoconstrictor and prevents the local anesthetic from being perfused away from the anesthetized site. Adding epinephrine also minimizes bleeding and lengthens the duration of action of local anesthetics, such as lidocaine, by 50% (Anderson, Zeltzer, Fanurik, 1993).

Care must be taken not to use local anesthetics with vasoconstrictors for IV regional anesthesia or on tissues with end arteriole blood supply, such as fingers, toes, the penis, the nose, or ears (Anderson, Zeltzer, Fanurik, 1993; Illingworth, Simpson, 1994; Wong, 1996a). Local anes-

thetic solutions containing epinephrine or norepinephrine should be used with extreme caution in patients receiving monoamine oxidase (MAO) inhibitors or tricyclic antidepressants because severe prolonged hypertension can occur (Catterall, Mackie, 1996).

Injectable lidocaine and other local anesthetics

Lidocaine (0.5% to 2.0%) is the local anesthetic used most often for procedural pain because it has a fast onset of action and can be prescribed in a wide range of doses without producing toxicity (Anderson, Zeltzer, Fanurik, 1993). Onset of action usually is within 2 minutes of subcutaneous (SC) infiltration, and anesthesia can last up to 30 minutes (Illingworth, Simpson, 1994). It is used frequently and safely in both children and adults (Rice, 1996). The maximum safe dose for SC administration of lidocaine in children is 7 mg/kg (Zeltzer, Jay, Fisher, 1989).

When a longer duration of anesthesia is needed than can be produced by lidocaine, bupivacaine (Marcaine, Sensorcaine) may be used. Bupivacaine is commonly used for children. Doses of 0.25% bupivacaine should not exceed 2.5 mg/kg (Berde, Kain, 1996). Penile blocks that use bupivacaine without epinephrine are used for repair of hypospadias (Anderson, Zeltzer, Fanurik, 1993; Serour, Mori, Barr, 1994). Both lidocaine and bupivacaine are safe for infiltration and retrobulbar block anesthesia for ophthalmic surgical procedures (Moroi, Lichter, 1996).

Local anesthetics often are combined so that the properties of one (e.g., onset and duration of action) can be compensated for by another (Covino, Wildsmith, 1998). For example, bupivacaine has a slower onset of action (up to 10 minutes) than lidocaine (2 minutes), so some practitioners administer lidocaine at the beginning of a procedure and bupivacaine during or at the end of the procedure to prolong the block and provide continued pain relief after the procedure. However, the use of a lidocaine-bupivacaine combination approach for digital nerve block may provide no advantage. In one study of this procedure, bupivacaine, 0.25%, induced anesthesia in the same period of time and with equivalent pain on injection as a 1:1 lidocaine and bupivacaine, 0.25%, combination (Valvano, Leffler, 1996).

A relatively new local anesthetic, ropivacaine (Naropin), is gaining popularity. It is closely related in structure to bupivacaine, but it is less cardiotoxic and slightly less potent in producing anesthesia, with reports of less motor blockade than bupivacaine (Covino, Wildsmith, 1998). Its duration of action (2 to 6 hours) is similar to bupivacaine (Catterall, Mackie, 1996) (see Chapter 6 on p. 227). Its use for retrobulbar block has not been studied (ASTRA, 1996).

TABLE 8.3

GUIDELINES

USE OF LOCAL ANESTHETICS FOR PROCEDURAL ANALGESIA

Local Anesthetic*	Route	Onset (min)	Peak (min)	Duration (h)	Dose†	Dosing
Lidocaine, 0.25%–1%	Local infiltration	Rapid	2-5	0.5-2	Adult: With epinephrine: 7 mg/kg, not to exceed 500 mg; without epinephrine: 4.5 mg/kg, not to exceed 300 mg Child: 3-5 mg/kg	Duration of action and sometimes dose is increased with addition of epinephrine.
Bupivacaine 0.05%–0.25%	Local infiltration	2-10		3-7	Adult and child: 2 mg/kg	Duration of action and sometimes dose is increased with addition of epinephrine.
Ropivacaine (Naropin) 0.2%–0.5%	Local infiltration	1-15		0.5-6	Adult: 2-200 mg (0.2%); 5-200 mg (0.5%)	Less cardiotoxic and less motor block than bupivacaine. Although used, safety is not fully established in neonates and children.
Lidocaine 4%	Topical spray	2-5		2-3	Adult and child: 2 mg/kg	Absorption is particularly rapid when instilled in the tracheobronchial tree; concentrations in the blood approximate those that follow IV injection.
Benzocaine 20%	Topical lubricant	Slow	UK	0.5-1	Apply evenly to exterior of tube or instrument before use.	May cause methemoglobinemia; not recommended for use in infants < 12 mo old.
EMLA cream (lidocaine 2.5%, prilocaine 2.5%)	Topical cream	60	120-180	1-2 after removal of cream	Adult and child: 2.5 g over 20-25 cm² skin surface (minor); 2 g per 10 cm² skin surface (major) (See Box 8.5, p. 375.)	Application time: 1 h (minor procedures); 2 h (major). Maximum application area for weight to 10 kg = up to 100 cm²; for weight 10-20 kg = up to 600 cm²; for weight > 20 kg = up to 2000 cm². Do not use on mucous membranes or abraded skin. Not recommended in infants < 1 mo old or < 12 mo old and receiving methemoglobin-inducing agents (see p. 376).

TABLE 8.3—cont'd

GUIDELINES

Table 8.3 presents information on the pharmacokinetics, pharmacodynamics, and use of common local anesthetics for procedural pain.

*Do not use solutions with vasoconstrictors on tissues with end arteriole blood supply, such as fingers, toes, penis, nose, or ears.

†These doses are only approximate and should be calculated individually. (NOTE: This footnote does not apply to cm².)

cm², square centimeter; *kg*, kilogram; *mg*, milligram; *ml*, milliliter; *UK*, unknown.

Information from ASTRA USA, Inc: EMLA cream package insert, *Dollops* 4(1), 1997; ASTRA USA, Inc: *Naropin* (ropivacaine) package insert, Westborough, Mass, ASTRA 1996; Bonica JJ, Butler SH: Local anesthesia and regional blocks. In Wall PD, Melzack R, editors: *Textbook of pain,* ed 3, pp 997-1023, New York, 1994, Churchill Livingstone; Catterall W, Mackie K: Local anesthetics. In Hardman JG, Limbird LE, editors: *Goodman and Gilman's the pharmacological basis of therapeutics,* ed 9, pp 331-347, 1996, New York, McGraw-Hill, Inc; Covino BG, Wildsmith JA: Clinical pharmacology of local anesthetic agents. In Cousins MJ, Bridenbaugh PO, editors: *Neural blockade in clinical anesthesia and management of pain,* ed 3, pp. 97-128, Philadelphia, 1998, Lippincott-Raven Publishers; Deglin JH, Vallerand AH: *Davis's drug guide for nurses,* ed 5, Philadelphia, 1995, FA Davis; Illingworth KA, Simpson KH: *Anaesthesia and analgesia in emergency medicine,* New York, 1994, Oxford University Press; Rice LJ: Regional anesthesia and analgesia. In Montoyama EK, Davis PJ, editors: *Smith's anesthesia for infants and children,* pp 403-442, St. Louis, 1996, Mosby.

Reducing the Discomfort of Lidocaine Injection

Many patients report a burning and stinging sensation when lidocaine is injected intradermally or subcutaneously. It is believed that the pain is a consequence, in part, of the acidity of lidocaine (Richtsmeier, Hatcher, 1995). This explains why buffering lidocaine with sodium bicarbonate before infiltration can reduce the pain associated with its infiltration (Wong, 1996a) (see Box 8.2 for directions on how to buffer lidocaine).

Several researchers point out the importance of using correct technique when infiltrating lidocaine. To minimize the pain, injecting the lidocaine very slowly (4 seconds or longer/ml) is recommended (McGlone, Bodenham, 1990; Richtsmeier, Hatcher, 1995).

Lidocaine also can be warmed to further reduce the stinging associated with its infiltration. Four solutions of 1% lidocaine were compared for pain at infiltration: (1) room temperature unbuffered, (2) warmed only, (3) buffered only, and (4) warmed and buffered (Mader, Playe, Garb, 1994; Waldbilling, Quinn, Stiell et al., 1995). Warmed and buffered lidocaine was found to be significantly less painful than the others, suggesting that warming and buffering have a synergistic effect. It is recommended that buffered lidocaine be warmed to 40° to 42° C in a warm water bath, blanket warmer, or an IV solution warmer before use. Microwaves should not be used to warm lidocaine. Many caregivers simply roll the syringe of lidocaine back and forth between the palms of their hands several times to warm it before injection.

Patient Example

Mrs. J. is admitted in labor with her second child. The physician has prescribed an IV. Mrs. J. tells the nurse who admits her that she is terrified to have an IV started because it was so painful when she had one started with her last baby. The nurse who will start the IV explains to Mrs. J. that she routinely uses the local anesthetic, lidocaine, to numb the site where the IV will be started. The

nurse tells Mrs. J. that she will buffer it before infiltration to reduce the burning and stinging lidocaine sometimes can cause. To buffer the lidocaine, the nurse adds 0.1 ml of sodium bicarbonate as a buffering agent to 1 ml lidocaine in a TB syringe. She replaces the needle that was used to draw up the solutions with a 30-gauge needle for the intradermal injection. To warm the buffered lidocaine the nurse rolls the syringe back and forth between her palms several times. Before the venipuncture, she slowly (2 to 3 seconds) injects about 0.1 to 0.2 ml of the buffered lidocaine intradermally directly over the intended puncture site. The nurse was able to insert an 18-gauge angiocatheter painlessly in the patient.

Bacteriostatic saline has been used as an alternative to lidocaine to start an IV painlessly (Welch, 1996). The preservative in bacteriostatic saline, 0.9% benzyl alcohol, eliminates the pain, so preservative-free water or saline will not produce the same results. A wheal of bacteriostatic saline 1 cm in diameter is injected intradermally with a 30-gauge needle over or just distal to the vein. This allows painless searching for a vein at that site. Advantages of this method over lidocaine are that it does not burn on injection, does not require a physician's order, no one is allergic to it, and it is inexpensive. Researchers found that when bacteriostatic saline is mixed with 1% lidocaine, it provides effective anesthesia and less pain on infiltration than 1% lidocaine buffered with sodium bicarbonate for superficial surgical procedures, such as shave and scissors excision and superficial laser vaporization (Lugo-Janer, Padial, Sanchez, 1993).

Drugs That Are Painful on Injection

Many patients report the IV infusion of potassium chloride as an extremely painful experience (Puntillo, 1990). Adding lidocaine to the infusion can help reduce this intense pain. The recommended dose is 10 mg of lidocaine hydrochloride in a mixture of 50 ml of 5%

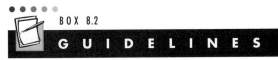

PREPARATION AND USE OF BUFFERED LIDOCAINE (BL)

Supplies
- 8.4% sodium bicarbonate (1 mEq/ml)
- 1% lidocaine
- TB syringe with removable needle (use larger syringe for larger doses), 30-gauge needle

Instructions
- Use 1 part sodium bicarbonate to 10 parts lidocaine (e.g., draw up 1 ml of lidocaine and 0.1 ml of sodium bicarbonate).
- Change needle used to withdraw BL to 30-gauge needle for intradermal injection.
- For venipuncture or port access, inject 0.1 ml or less (child) or 0.5 ml or less (adult) BL intradermally directly over intended puncture site; anesthesia occurs almost immediately.
- Suggested maximum dose of lidocaine for local anesthesia is 4.5 mg/kg.
- If buffering lidocaine vial (e.g., 20 ml lidocaine with 2 ml sodium bicarbonate), use solution for 7 days or less and preferably when freshly prepared.

May be duplicated for use in clinical practice. As appears in McCaffery M, Pasero C: *Pain: Clinical manual*, p. 371, 1999, Mosby, Inc.

kg, kilogram; *mEq*, milliequivalent; *mg*, milligram; *ml*, milliliter; *TB*, tuberculin.
Modified from Wong DL: *Whaley and Wong's essentials of pediatric nursing*, ed 5, St. Louis, 1997, Mosby.

dextrose in water and 10 mEq of potassium chloride (Morrill, Katz, 1988).

Lidocaine also can reduce the pain associated with ceftriaxone (Rocephin) IM injection. In one study subjects received ceftriaxone diluted either with sterile water or with 1% lidocaine (Schichor, Bernstein, Weinerman et al., 1994). Subjects who received ceftriaxone diluted with lidocaine reported significantly less pain at the time of injection and at 10 and 20 minute and 6 hour intervals than those who received it diluted with sterile water. In another study, sterile water, 1% lidocaine, and buffered 1% lidocaine were compared as diluents for ceftriaxone (Hayward, Nafziger, Kohlhepp et al., 1996). Injections with water diluent were significantly more painful than with the other two diluents, but no difference in injection pain was noted between lidocaine and buffered lidocaine.

Newborn Circumcision

One of the most painful procedures physicians perform is circumcision, yet when performed on newborns, many physicians do not provide any anesthesia or analgesia whatsoever. A number of unsupported explanations are offered for this lack of attentive analgesic care, including myths that babies do not feel pain or remember pain and will not be able to urinate if the penis is anesthetized. This flagrant disregard for this vulnerable group of patients is no longer acceptable in light of the number of studies that have shown that the use of local anesthetics for this procedure in newborns is safe, effective, and relatively easy to administer (Lander, Brady-Fryer, Metcalfe et al., 1997; Maxwell, Yaster, Wetzel et al., 1987; Rice, 1996; Spencer, Miller, O'Quin et al., 1992; Taddio, Stevens, Craig et al., 1997; Williamson, Williamson, 1983; Williamson, 1997) (see Chapter 2 for more on the harmful effects of unrelieved circumcision pain and Chapter 14 for more on pain and circumcision in neonates).

Topical local anesthetics

Topical local anesthetics are ideal for reducing the pain associated with many procedures. When topical anesthetics are applied, they must diffuse through the mucous membrane or skin to produce anesthesia. The onset of action of topical anesthetics varies from rapid (tracheobronchial tree application) to slow (eutectic mixtures). The duration of the topical anesthetics also varies widely from seconds (refrigerated spray) to hours (lidocaine gel), depending on how quickly it is eliminated (Illingworth, Simpson, 1994). It is important to remember that, even when administered topically, local anesthetics can be absorbed into circulation and may produce systemic toxic reactions (Catterall, Mackie, 1996) (see Local Anesthetic Toxicity, p. 368). In choosing topical anesthetic agents, the same considerations apply to both adults and children (Rice, 1996).

Lubricants with 20% benzocaine (Americaine, Hurricane) can be used to facilitate passage of fiberoptic gastroscopes, laryngoscopes, bronchoscopes, airways, proctoscopes, and sigmoidoscopes. They are helpful in suppressing the pharyngeal and tracheal gag reflex during placement of nasogastric tubes. They are effective also for controlling the discomfort of a number of gynecologic procedures, including intrauterine device insertion and vaginal speculum placement.

Hurricane is available in liquid and spray form, on swabsticks, and in a number of flavors. For example, before infiltration of lidocaine for a nerve block, many dentists swab cherry-flavored Hurricane to reduce the discomfort of the needle stick and the infiltration of lidocaine used for the nerve block.

A spray containing benzocaine (14%) and tetracaine (2.0%) (Cetacaine) is used for anesthesia of accessible mucous membranes, such as in the throat to control the gagging reflex. It is not recommended for anesthesia of large areas. Cetacaine is applied directly to the mucous membrane for 1 second (200 mg) or less to produce normal anesthesia. Spray in excess of two seconds is contraindicated. This combination is also available in liquid and ointment and can be applied with a cotton pledget or directly to tissue. To prevent local reaction, the pledget should not be held in position for an extended period of time.

Because benzocaine is poorly soluble in water, it is thought to be too slowly absorbed to be toxic. However, local reactions can occur and are related to the length of application time. It is not known whether benzocaine preparations cause fetal harm, so they should be administered with caution during pregnancy. Because benzocaine can cause methemoglobinemia, careful dosing is recommended (Catterall, Mackie, 1996) (see p. 376 for more on methemoglobinemia).

Lidocaine can be used as a gel (5%) or can be sprayed (4%), swabbed, or squirted into the nose, nasopharynx, pharynx, larynx, and tracheal area to produce local anesthesia. Absorption is particularly rapid when local anesthetics are instilled in the tracheobronchial tree; concentrations in the blood are nearly the same as those that follow IV injection (Catterall, Mackie, 1996). Onset of action is 2 to 5 minutes and duration is 2 to 3 hours (Illingworth, Simpson, 1994).

In children, an appropriate dose of 4% lidocaine by topical spray is 2 mg/kg. Because the delivery of atomizers can vary greatly with the position in which the atomizer is held, it is important to pretest spraying while holding the atomizer at the angle at which it will be used (Rice, 1996). Lidocaine by a 5% sprayer produced safe and effective laryngeal anesthesia in children age 3 to 24 months before laryngoscopy or bronchoscopy (Sitbon, Laffron, Lesage et al., 1996). Doses of lidocaine ranged between 0.9 mg and 2.6 mg/kg, and maximum plasma lidocaine concentration was acceptable at 1.05 μg/ml.

Uretheral catheterization can be anxiety provoking and painful for patients of all ages. Lidocaine 2% in gel form injected through a nozzlelike adapter into the urethra before urethral catheterization or cystoscopic procedures can make this procedure significantly less painful (Box 8.3). Aqueous preparations may be used, but the gel form has the advantage of providing lubrication for instrumentation. The lidocaine is absorbed into the mucous membranes, and toxicity may occur if mucosal damage is present. Care must be taken if bleeding from the meatus occurs, and instillation under high pressure may cause injection into the bloodstream. The recommended dose must be reduced for premature infants and infants with hyperbilirubinemia because the drug can accumulate (Anderson, Zeltzer, Fanurik, 1993; Illingworth, Simpson, 1994).

Dyclonine hydrochloride (Dyclone) has a rapid onset and short duration of action. A solution of 0.5% to 1.0% is used as a topical anesthetic for anogenital procedures and endoscopy. It is absorbed through the skin and mucous membranes (Catterall, Mackie, 1996).

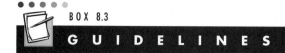

BOX 8.3

GUIDELINES

ATRAUMATIC URETHRAL CATHETERIZATION

Supplies

- 2% Xylocaine lubricant gel (available from Astra USA, Inc. and International Medication Systems, Limited [IMS])
- Appropriate type and size catheter
  - Use lubricious-coated or silicone catheters for indwelling catheterization because these produce less irritation of the urethral mucosa than plastic, latex catheters.
  - For obtaining a urine sample in children: Use a soft 5-8 F feeding tube or 6-8 F rubber or polyvinylchloride catheter for girls and prepubescent boys; a coudé-tipped catheter can be used for adolescent boys and children and adults with history of urethral surgery.

Procedure

1. Check label on 2% Xylocaine container for sterilizing instructions.
2. Tell patient that introduction of the catheter will produce pressure and a desire to urinate but should not be painful.
3. Use strict aseptic technique.
4. Assemble 2% Xylocaine lubricant with applicator according to manufacturer directions.
5. Cleanse area with appropriate cleansing agent.
6. Wipe dry with sterile towel or cotton balls.
7. Place several drops of the Xylocaine lubricant on meatus.
   - In males, gently introduce the tip of the xylocaine applicator into the urethra 1 to 2 cm and slowly insert 15 ml (5 to 10 ml for prepuberal males) of lubricant. The lubricant is held in place by gently squeezing the distal penis for 3 to 5 minutes. This will allow the mucosa to absorb the active Xylocaine.
   - For females, 3 to 5 ml of the Xylocaine lubricant is placed on the periurethral mucosa and 3 to 5 ml (1 to 2 ml for prepuberal females) is inserted into the uretheral meatus. Delay catheterization for 2 to 3 minutes for maximum absorption.
8. Place additional lubricant without local anesthetic on the catheter to promote opening of the sphincter mechanism.
9. Gently insert catheter until urine flows. Be patient; urine flow usually takes longer than when minimal lubricant is used.

May be duplicated for use in clinical practice. From McCaffery M, Pasero C: *Pain: Clinical manual,* p 372. Copyright © 1999, Mosby, Inc.

cm, centimeter; F, French; ml, milliliter.

Information from Gray ML: Atraumatic uretheral catheterization of children, *Pediatr Nurs* 22(4):306-310, 1996; Wong D: *Wong and Whaley's essentials of pediatric nursing,* ed 5, St. Louis, 1997, Mosby.

Topical anesthesia is invaluable for the management of pain associated with ophthalmic procedures, such as the measurement of intraocular tension (tonometry), removal of a foreign body from the cornea or conjunctiva, and manipulation of the nasolacrimal canalicular system. For these procedures, ophthalmologists instill proparacaine or tetracaine a single drop at a time onto the eye to produce local anesthesia. Initial ophthalmic instillation may cause a stinging sensation, which disappears after 30 seconds. The onset of anesthesia is approximately 30 seconds and duration depends on the vascularity of the tissue; it is longest in normal cornea and shortest in inflamed cornea. Topical anesthesia also is combined with cocaine for anesthesia during nasolacrimal system cannulation (Catterall, Mackie, 1996; Illingworth, Simpson, 1994).

Long-term use of ophthalmic local anesthetics can retard healing and cause pitting and sloughing of the corneal epithelium. Thus they should not be prescribed for self-administration (Catterall, Mackie, 1996).

TLC, TAC, and LET

A mixture of tetracaine (2%), lidocaine (2% to 10%), and cocaine (1% to 4%) (TLC) can be applied topically in solution or gel form to produce skin anesthesia in adults. The maximum safe total dosages for a healthy 70 kg adult are 50 mg of tetracaine, 500 mg of lidocaine, 200 mg of cocaine (Catterall, Mackie, 1996). For children, tetracaine, 0.5%, can be combined with epinephrine (adrenaline), 0.05%, and cocaine, 11.8% (TAC) or with lidocaine, 4%, and epinephrine, 0.05% (LET) for topical anesthesia (Ochsenreither, 1996).

These combinations are used most often before wound cleaning and repairing uncomplicated facial and scalp lacerations. They are prepared by the hospital's pharmacy in gel or liquid form. The gel form is preferred because it is easier to control the application (see Box 8.4 for guidelines for the preparation and use of LET). It is recommended that the gel or solution be painted into and around the wound with cotton-tipped applicators. The anesthetic is left for a minimum of 10 minutes and a maximum of 30 minutes. Peak anesthetic effect after topical application of mixtures that contain cocaine or lidocaine is 2 to 5 minutes and 3 to 8 minutes for tetracaine combinations. Anesthesia is superficial and does not extend to the submucosal structures (Catterall, Mackie, 1996).

TAC and LET have been found to be 90% effective in producing anesthesia of the area of application (Schilling, Bank, Borchert et al., 1995; Ochsenreither, 1996) lasting for approximately 15 minutes (Wong, 1996a). LAT gel compared favorably with injected buffered lidocaine for local anesthesia effectiveness and was significantly less painful to apply before suturing lacerations (Houry, 1997).

When using TAC and LET, care must be taken to avoid the eyes because of the risk of corneal abrasions and the mucous membranes because of the risk of systemic absorption and toxicity (Ernst, Marvez, Nick et al.,

1995; Schilling, Bank, Borchert et al., 1995; Wong, 1996a). Because these combinations contain epinephrine, they should not be used on tissues with end arteriole blood supply, such as fingers, toes, penis, nose, or ears (Anderson, Zeltzer, Fanurik, 1994; Wong, 1996a). Also, caregivers must be sure to wear gloves when in contact with the solutions because vasoconstriction can occur in intact skin.

Adverse effects are associated with the use of TAC. These include seizures, hyperexcitability, euphoria, tachycardia, hypertension, and even death. TAC is also expensive to produce, and tracking is required for substance control because cocaine is an ingredient. Fewer adverse effects are associated with LET. Also LET is less expensive to produce and does not contain a controlled substance (Ernst, Marvez, Nick et al., 1995; Ochsenreither, 1996; Schilling, Bank, Borchert et al., 1995).

Several alternatives to TAC and LET exist. Three that do not contain cocaine have been studied (Smith, Strausbaugh, Harbeck-Weber et al., 1997). They are prilocaine-phenylephrine (Prilophen), tetracaine-phenylephrine (Tetraphen), and tetracaine-lidocaine-phenylephrine (Tetralidophen). No statistical differences between TAC and Tetraphen could be found in this study.

Another alternative is a topical anesthetic solution of 0.48% bupivacaine and 1:26,000 norepinephrine (Bupivanor). Bupivanor was compared with TAC and 1% lidocaine infiltration for wound laceration repair in children. It was found to be an effective alternative to both TAC and lidocaine, especially for repair of face and scalp lacerations. The researchers point out that the effectiveness of Bupivanor on the face is important because it is here that TAC can come into contact with mucous membranes and cause systemic toxicity (Smith, Strausbaugh, Harbeck-Weber et al., 1996). Bupivanor is not available commercially, and little information exists about its use clinically, but it merits further investigation.

EMLA Cream

Eutectic mixture of local anesthetics (EMLA) combines lidocaine, 2.5%, and prilocaine, 2.5%, in a cream for topical application. A eutectic mixture, which has a melting point lower than that of the two anesthetics alone, permits the drug to penetrate intact skin. EMLA has increased efficacy with enhanced safety because the dose of the drugs in EMLA is small and plasma concentrations are less than toxic levels (Covino, Wildsmith, 1998).

EMLA can be used to reduce the pain of many procedures in children and adults. These include venous, arterial, lumbar, finger, and heel punctures (see following discussion); implanted port access; peripheral insertion of central catheters (PICC lines); removal of sutures, staples, cardiac catheterization lines, and epicardial wires; superficial biopsies; skin grafts; insertion and removal of Norplant contraception; and IM and SC injections

BOX 8.4

G U I D E L I N E S

PREPARATION AND USE OF LIDOCAINE, EPINEPHRINE, TETRACAINE (LET) TOPICAL GEL

Preparation A

Concentrations
- 4% lidocaine
- 0.05% epinephrine
- 0.5% tetracaine

Ingredients
- 0.90 g of lidocaine powder
- 0.15 g of tetracaine powder
- 15.0 ml of epinephrine 1:1000 multidose injections
- qs ad 30.0 ml of 2% Xylocaine jelly (in hydroxypropyl-methylcellulose)

Procedure
- Weigh 0.9 g lidocaine powder and 0.15 g tetracaine powder.
- Combine weighed powders in a graduate or calibrated amber bottle.
- With a syringe, draw up 15 ml epinephrine 1:1000 injection from multidose vial.
- Add to graduate or calibrated bottle and stir until dissolved.
- Draw this solution through a 5 μm filter and place in a calibrated amber bottle.
- Slowly add 2% Xylocaine jelly to a volume of 30 ml and mix thoroughly.
- Dispense in an airtight amber bottle and refrigerate.
- Store up to 30 days.

Preparation B

Concentrations
- 4% lidocaine
- 0.1% epinephrine
- 0.5% tetracaine

Ingredients
- 40 ml of 20% lidocaine
- 15 ml of 2.25% racemic epinephrine
- 1.72 g of tetracaine added to 0.26 g of sodium bisulfate

Procedure
- To make a gelatinous form, use 300 ml of 2% lidocaine jelly.
- This preparation yields 114 doses of LET (3 ml/dose).
- Refrigerate and protect from light.

Directions for Applying LET

1. Review LET order for correct dose, time, and route.
2. Inspect LET for discoloration or broken seal.
3. Gather supplies needed for application: nonsterile gloves, sterile cotton-tipped applicator, LET gel/solution in 3 ml syringe, and bacteriostatic normal saline for irrigation.
4. Inform patient/family members of the application procedure for LET and why it is needed.
5. Wash hands and put on nonsterile gloves.
6. Apply LET with sterile cotton-tipped applicator into the wound bed and around its edges (1.5 to 3 ml depending on size of laceration) or squirt LET into and around laceration with syringe tip.
7. Avoid contact with or application near mucous membranes because these membranes may more readily absorb LET than a wound bed.
8. Allow LET to remain on wound for at least 10 minutes but no more than 30 minutes (It may be covered with gauze secured in place.)
9. Practitioner may choose to check laceration after 10 minutes to assess degree of anesthesia. Skin may blanch because of vasoconstriction as LET takes effect.
10. If a wound is still sensitive after 20 minutes, more LET may be applied and left on for an additional 10 min.
11. Once anesthesia is achieved, irrigate wound to remove LET and any remaining dirt or foreign bodies. Laceration is then sutured.
12. Wash hands and discard supplies.

May be duplicated for use in clinical practice. From McCaffery M, Pasero C: *Pain: Clinical manual*, p. 374. Copyright © 1999, Mosby, Inc.

Box 8.4 provides guidelines for compounding and applying two preparations for lidocaine, epinephrine, tetracaine (LET) topical gel.

ad, increase; *ml*, milliliter; *qs*, quantity sufficient.

Information from United Healthcare System, Department of Pharmacy, Newark, NJ, 1996 (Preparation A); Jacqueline Ochsenreither, RN, Rita Jew, Pharm D, Children's Hospital of Philadelphia, Philadelphia, PA, personal communication, October 1996 (Preparation B); Ochsenreither JM: Better topical anesthetic, *Am J Nurs* 96(5):21-22, May 1996 (Directions for applying LET).

(Wong, 1995a; Wong, 1996a). Only partial pain control is provided when EMLA is used for bone marrow aspiration and chest tube removal.

Studies conflict on the effectiveness of EMLA in reducing pain from heel punctures. A review of 11 studies led researchers to recommend EMLA for circumcision but not for heel puncture (Taddio, Ohlsson, Einarson, 1998). However, a study of premature infants showed that newborns are capable of a chronic pain response to local injury from heel puncture and that EMLA reduced this response (Fitzgerald, Millard, McIntosh, 1989). Further research on the use of EMLA for reducing the pain of heel puncture is warranted.

EMLA should be used on intact skin only and not on mucous membranes. Abraded skin surfaces and mucous membranes allow rapid absorption, which can result in systemic toxicity (Catterall, Mackie, 1996), although EMLA has been used safely to numb the gums before lo-

BOX 8.5

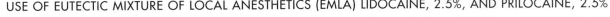

G U I D E L I N E S

USE OF EUTECTIC MIXTURE OF LOCAL ANESTHETICS (EMLA) LIDOCAINE, 2.5%, AND PRILOCAINE, 2.5%

Explain to child that EMLA is like a "Magic cream that takes hurt away." Tap or lightly scratch site of procedure to show child that "skin is now awake."

Apply thick layer (dollop) of EMLA over normal intact skin to anesthetize site (about ½ of 5-g tube; can use ⅓ of tube if puncture site is localized and superficial, e.g., intradermal injection or heel/finger puncture).

For venous access, apply to two sites; place enough cream on antecubital fossa to cover medial and lateral veins. Do not rub.

Place transparent adhesive dressing (e.g., Tegaderm) over EMLA. Make sure cream remains dollop. A piece of plastic film (e.g., Saran Wrap) with tape to seal the edges can be used. Use only as much adhesive as needed to prevent leakage.

To make the dressing less accessible, cover it with a self-adhering Ace-type bandage, such as *Coban,* or an IV protector, such as *IV House.** Label the dressing with "EMLA applied," the date, and the time to distinguish it from other types of dressings. Instruct older children not to disturb the dressing. (Covering the dressing with an opaque material may reduce the attraction and discourage "fingering.") Supervise younger or cognitively compromised children throughout the application time.

Leave EMLA on skin for at least 60 minutes for superficial puncture and 120 min for deep penetration (e.g., IM injection, biopsy). EMLA may be applied at home and may need to be kept on longer in persons with dark and/or thicker skin. Anesthesia may last up to 3 h after EMLA is removed.

Remove dressing before procedure and wipe cream from skin. With transparent adhesive, grasp opposite sides, and while holding dressing *parallel* to skin, pull sides away from each other to stretch and loosen dressing. An adhesive remover may be used.

Observe skin reaction, either blanched or reddened. If no obvious skin reaction occurs, EMLA may not have penetrated adequately; test skin sensitivity and if needed, reapply.

Repeat tapping or lightly scratching skin to show child that "skin is asleep" so that "it cannot feel a needle either."

After procedure, assess behavioral response. If chid was upset, use pain scale (e.g., FACES, to help child distinguish between pain and fear).

EMLA should not be used in those rare patients with congenital or idiopathic *methemoglobinemia* and in infants under the age of 12 months who are receiving treatment with methemoglobin-inducing agents (e.g., sulfonamides, phenytoin [Dilantin], phenobarbital, and acetaminophen [Tylenol]). *Methemoglobin,* a dysfunctional form of hemoglobin, reduces the blood's oxygen-carrying capacity, causing cyanosis and hypoxemia. The use of intravenous methylene blue promptly eliminates the methemoglobinemia.

NOTE: EMLA is contraindicated in anyone with a known history of sensitivity or allergy to amide-type local anesthetics (lidocaine, prilocaine, mepivacaine, bupivacaine, etidocaine) or to any other component of the product.

AGE AND BODY WEIGHT REQUIREMENTS	MAXIMUM TOTAL DOSE OF EMLA	MAXIMUM APPLICATION AREA	MAXIMUM APPLICATION TIME
0 up to 3 months or <5 kg	1 g	10 cm²	1 hour
3 up to 12 months and >5 kg	2 g	20 cm²	4 hours
1 to 6 years and >10 kg	10 g	100 cm²	4 hours
7 to 12 years and >20 kg	20 g	200 cm²	4 hours

Please note: If a patient greater than 3 months old does not meet the minimum weight requirement, the maximum total dose of EMLA should be restricted to that which corresponds to the patient's weight. In neonates (minimum gestation: 37 weeks) and children weighing less than 20 kg, the area and duration of application should be limited.

These are broad guidelines for avoiding systemic toxicity in applying EMLA to patients with normal, intact skin and with normal renal function and hepatic function.

For more individualized calculation of how much lidocaine and prilocaine may be absorbed, practitioners can use the following estimates of lidocaine and prilocaine absorption for children and adults:

The estimated mean (± SD) absorption of lidocaine is 0.045 (±0.016) mg/cm²/h.

The estimated mean (± SD) absorption of prilocaine is 0.077 (±0.036) mg/cm²/h.

May be duplicated for use in clinical practice. As appears in McCaffery M, Pasero C: *Pain: Clinical manual,* p. 375, 1999, Mosby, Inc.

*For more information, contact I.V. House, 7400 Foxmont Dr., Hazelwood, MO 63042-2198: 800-530-0400: Fax 314-831-3683.

†In Canada, EMLA is not approved for use in infants less than 6 months of age. See p. 376 for exceptions and discussion.

Modified from Wong DL: Overcoming 'needle phobia' with EMLA, *Am J Nurs* 65(2):24, 1995.

From Wong D: *Wong and Whaley's clinical manual of pediatric nursing,* ed 4, p 327, St. Louis, 1996, Mosby.

cal anesthetic blocks for dentistry (Covino, Wildsmith, 1998).

EMLA's duration of analgesia can be up to 4 hours (Wong, 1995a). It is recommended that 2.5 g (1/2 of a 5 g tube) of EMLA be applied per 20 to 25 cm² (2 inch by 2 inch) area, then covered with an occlusive dressing for 1 hour. If deeper penetration is needed, such as for taking split-thickness grafts or IM injections, the application time should be increased to 2 to 3 hours (ASTRA, 1997). See Box 8.5 for guidelines on the use of EMLA.

EMLA is available over-the-counter in patch form in Canada. Patients or parents are instructed to apply the patch over the site before a painful procedure or neural blockade (Covino, Wildsmith, 1998).

Sometimes EMLA provides incomplete anesthesia and additional analgesics or anesthetics are necessary. It is, therefore, wise to explain EMLA to patients as a pain reliever (analgesic), rather than as a numbing agent (anesthetic) (Wong, 1996b). A study that used EMLA for anesthesia during circumcision of adult males was terminated when marked differences in pain relief were found (Siddique, D'Alessio, Dmochowski, 1997). Patients who received a total of 10 ml of EMLA 1 hour before circumcision experienced excruciating pain (rating 10 on a 10 cm VAS) when the foreskin was clamped compared with no pain (rating 1 on a 10 cm VAS) in patients who received a dorsal penile block. It was interesting to note that although circumcision is routinely performed on newborn males without anesthesia, this study of adult males was terminated because of the marked differences in the pain control experienced by the control and experimental groups.

EMLA was compared with a preparation of 4% amethocaine (a local anesthetic available in the United Kingdom) (McCafferty, Woolfson, Boston, 1989). EMLA produced anesthesia in 95% of the patients studied, and the amethocaine preparation produced anesthesia in 100%. Most appealing was the finding that amethocaine had a faster onset and longer duration than EMLA and an application time 50% (30 minutes) that of EMLA (60 minutes). At 30 minutes after application, EMLA produced transient anesthesia lasting only 6 minutes, whereas the amethocaine preparation had a 3.8 hour mean duration of anesthesia. When the application time was increased from 30 to 60 minutes for both preparations, the amethocaine preparation had a significantly longer mean duration of action (4.5 hours) compared with EMLA (1 hour). The researchers attribute these findings to the differences between EMLA and amethocaine in solubility. Because amethocaine is more readily dissolved in fatty tissue (lipophilic), it diffuses more rapidly across membranes (shorter application time) and remains sequestered in fatty tissues for slow release (longer duration).

In a more recent study placebo, 4% amethocaine gel, and EMLA were compared for pain relief in patients after laser treatment of port-wine stains. Researchers found that both the amethocaine gel and the EMLA cream were superior to the placebo; however, the amethocaine provided significantly better pain relief than EMLA (McCafferty, Woolfson, Handley et al., 1997).

The manufacturers of EMLA warn against its use in infants less than 1 month old and in infants less than 12 months old who are receiving treatment with methemoglobin-inducing agents, such as acetaminophen and sulfonamides (ASTRA, 1997). Methemoglobinemia is a condition in which more than 1% of the blood's hemo-globin has been oxidized to the ferric form, which is incapable of binding molecular oxygen for transfer to cells (Wong, 1997). Very young patients and those with glucose-6-phosphate deficiency are more susceptible to methemoglobinemia than others. The signs of methemoglobinemia include cyanosis and hypoxemia; the blood has a chocolate hue. It is reversible when treated promptly with IV methylene blue (Wong, 1995b).

Methemoglobinemia is relatively rare in infants. One reported case was a 3-month-old prematurely born male (5.3 kg) who had 5 g of EMLA applied to the back of his hands and cubital region for 5 hours. The infant was receiving sulfonamides concomitantly. In another situation a 2-month-old infant who had EMLA for removal of a port-wine stain was given acetaminophen postoperatively. Both these infants had methemoglobinemia develop and responded satisfactorily to treatment (ASTRA, 1997; Wong, 1995b).

These cases have led many practitioners to avoid the use of EMLA for painful procedures in infants less than 12 months old. However, researchers have found EMLA to be safe and efficacious for this age group. In one study EMLA was used for pain control during neonatal circumcision. Blood methemoglobin concentrations were similar in the neonates treated with EMLA and those treated with placebo cream in this study (Taddio, Stevens, Craig et al., 1997). (See Chapter 14 for more on anesthesia for circumcision.)

In another study EMLA was compared with a placebo for pain associated with vaccination. The mean age of infants receiving EMLA was 9.2 months; 8.8 months for those receiving placebo. Parents and nurses evaluated the infants' responses, and both rated the amount of pain and crying as significantly less in infants receiving EMLA. After discharge, the parents of the EMLA infants also reported less site tenderness. No significant side effects were noted in either group (Uhari, 1993).

Patient Example

The staff in a newborn nursery in a local hospital has taken a creative approach to help reduce the pain newborn babies experience from heelsticks. One of the first procedures the day shift nurses perform is drawing blood by heelstick for the phenylketonuria (PKU) test. The night shift nurses apply EMLA cream to the babies' heels and cover them with an occlusive dressing 1 hour before the heelsticks. In addition to using EMLA, the nurses try to minimize the number of heelsticks the babies must have by correlating, whenever possible, other necessary tests that require blood drawing, such as glucose and hematocrit, with the PKU blood draw. The nurses explain to the babies' parents what tests the babies will be having, how the heelstick is performed, and the purpose of the EMLA. While holding and caring for their babies

during the time before the heelstick, parents are asked to help keep the dressing in place over the EMLA cream on the heel. Parents also are invited to hold their babies during the procedure to comfort and soothe them.

Clinicians occasionally voice concerns about the local circulatory effects of EMLA, such as vasoconstriction and vasospasm at the site of application (Bahruth, 1996). Mild pallor at the site has been reported (Taddio, Stevens, Craig et al., 1997); however, no evidence suggests that these circulatory changes produce adverse effects.

Refrigerant Sprays

As discussed, a limitation of EMLA is that it must be applied at least 60 minutes before a procedure. For superficial procedures, the use of refrigerant topical anesthetic sprays should be considered when time is insufficient for EMLA to take effect. When a refrigerant anesthetic is sprayed on the skin, it vaporizes and causes the area to be rapidly cooled (<10°C). This produces superficial anesthesia or analgesia within 10 to 15 seconds. Refrigerant topical anesthetic sprays do not provide deep anesthesia, and their use should be limited to short-term painful procedures when "pinpoint" analgesia is desired, such as for needle insertion (Illingworth, Simpson, 1994).

Several types of refrigerant topical anesthetic sprays are available, such as ethylchloride, fluroethyl, and Frigiderm. This form of local anesthetic has been used safely in both adults and children (Abbott, Fowler-Kerry, 1995; Illingworth, Simpson, 1994). Two disadvantages of refrigerant sprays are that incorrect application can produce frostbite and children may object to the extreme cold refrigerant sprays can produce (Wong, 1996b).

The fact that both placebo spray (compressed air with freon) and refrigerant anesthetic spray reduce pain (Abbott, Fowler-Kerry, 1995) may be because both sprays cool the skin. The cooling, rather than the anesthetic, may be all that is necessary to reduce pain before injection (Broadley, Ling, 1996).

Patient Example

The staff at a children's health clinic gives preschool children their diphtheria-pertussis-tetanus (DPT) immunizations. Several staff members were concerned about the pain the children experience from the injection and decided to implement pain control measures. First they tried to teach parents to apply EMLA cream to the injection site 60 minutes before bringing the children in for immunization. This proved unsuccessful for a variety of reasons, including parents forgetting to apply the cream, applying the cream to the wrong site, and applying the cream too early or too late. Next the staff tried to use an ethylchlo-

ride refrigerant spray 15 seconds before injecting. They found the spray provided excellent "pinpoint" anesthesia just at the site of needle penetration. To monitor effectiveness, the staff taught children to use the Wong-Baker FACES Pain Rating Scale. The children's pain rating scores immediately after immunization consistently range between no hurt (0) to hurts a little bit (1) (see Chapter 3 for more on the Wong-Baker FACES Pain Rating Scale).

Dermal anesthesia by iontophoresis

Iontophoresis is a method of transdural drug administration in which ionizable drug molecules are rapidly transported into the skin by external mild, low-level electric currents. Drugs that have been administered by iontophoresis include steroids, opioids, and local anesthetics. (Ashburn, Gauthier, Love et al., 1997).

An anesthetic product called Numby Stuff (IOMED, 1996) delivers lidocaine HCl, 2%, and epinephrine, 1:100,000 (Iontocaine), by iontophoresis safely to children and adults. To use Numby Stuff, a disposable single-use electrode is applied to the area of skin to be anesthetized. A small reusable battery-powered electronic unit produces the electric currents to transport the drug painlessly into the skin (Ashburn, Gauthier, Love et al., 1997; IOMED, 1996; Rust, 1997).

Before beginning iontophoresis, patients should be told to expect to feel a slight current under the skin as the drug is delivered. Young children may be frightened by the delivery system and the sensation of the current. Ample time should be spent explaining and letting children see and become familiar with the delivery equipment.

The amount of drug delivered by iontophoresis is directly proportional to the total charge applied (current multiplied by time) and is expressed in milliampere-minutes (mAmin). The typical iontophoresis treatment delivers a 4.0 mA current over a 10-minute period for a total current dose of 40 mAmin. Children can be given the same 40 mAmin treatment that is given to adults. If a patient reports discomfort from the current, the current level can be lowered (2.0 mA) and the treatment time lengthened (20 minutes) so a total dose of 40 mAmin is given (IOMED, 1996).

Numby Stuff produces local dermal anesthesia to a depth of 10 mm lasting up to 100 minutes. It can be used for IV catheter insertions, injections, implantable port needle insertion, shave biopsies, pulsed dye laser therapy, and blood drawing, but should not be used for placement of portacatheters containing metal (IOMED, 1996).

Side effects of Numby Stuff are mild and resolve within 48 hours. These include mild urticaria, transient erythema, blanching, or redness at the site of drug delivery electrode. Doses of lidocaine delivered by iontophoresis do not result in lidocaine blood levels high enough to cause any hemodynamic adverse effects. In fact, plasma concentrations of lidocaine are not even detectable after short delivery periods (40 mAmin) (Ashburn, Gauthier, Love et al., 1997; Rust, 1997).

Opioid Analgesics

Opioid analgesics are used alone for procedural pain management or in combination with any of the other analgesics and sedatives discussed in this section on pharmacologic approaches. Opioids act by binding to opioid receptor sites in the brain and spinal cord to block the production of neurotransmitters and thereby inhibit the transmission of pain (see Chapters 2 and 6).

The mu agonist opioid analgesics, such as morphine, fentanyl, hydromorphone (Dilaudid), and meperidine (Demerol), are the most common opioids used for procedural pain management because they produce the most reliable pain control. No analgesic ceiling (dose beyond which further dose increases do not provide additional analgesia) exists with the mu agonist opioid analgesics so doses can be adjusted to meet patients' individual requirements. Agonist-antagonists, such as nalbuphine (Nubain) and butorphanol (Stadol), are occasionally used, but because they have an analgesic ceiling, they are less suitable for procedural pain than the mu agonists (AHCPR, 1992; APS, 1992, Jacox, Carr, Payne et al., 1994) (see Chapter 6). Table 8.4 summarizes the characteristics of opioid analgesics used for procedural pain control.

Fentanyl is preferred most often for pain management during short procedures because of its particularly rapid onset of action (1 to 2 minutes) and peak effect (3 to 5 minutes) and short duration of action (3.6 hours). It should be diluted and administered slowly (over 2 to 5 minutes) to prevent respiratory muscle rigidity ("rigid chest"). This adverse effect is treated with muscle relaxants and mechanical ventilation. Morphine, with its longer duration of action, may be more suitable for longer procedures and when pain is expected to continue after the procedure (Anderson, Zeltzer, Fanurik, 1993).

Before administering opioids, it is important to determine the patient's history of drug use. Chemically dependent patients usually require higher than recommended doses of opioids during procedures. Agonist-antagonist opioids should not be used in patients who have been receiving mu agonist opioids before a procedure because of their potential to reverse analgesia and precipitate a withdrawal syndrome (AHCPR, 1992; APS, 1992; Jacox, Carr, Payne et al., 1994) (see Chapter 6).

Routes of administration

The IV route is preferred for administering opioids for procedural pain control. It has a fast onset of action, and absorption is more predictable than it is by the IM,

SC, oral, and rectal routes (AHCPR, 1992). It is also easier to titrate doses given by the IV route (Weinreb, 1996).

The oral route is used for anesthetic premedication in the operating room and before conscious sedation for therapeutic or diagnostic procedures. Occasionally, intranasal sufentanil is administered cautiously to children (0.2 to 0.4 μg/kg) when IV access is not possible (Berde, Kain, 1996) (see Chapter 6).

The oral transmucosal route is also used to administer analgesia and sedation for procedures (see Chapter 6). Oral transmucosal fentanyl citrate (OTFC) has been incorporated within a sweetened matrix and placed on a stick (Oralet) for this purpose. To administer OTFC, patients are instructed to suck on the matrix and, holding onto the stick, move it around the inside of the mouth and gums and above and below the tongue so that it dissolves in the salvia. A portion of the fentanyl diffuses across the oral mucosa (25%) and the rest is swallowed and partially absorbed through the stomach and the intestine (75%) (Berryman, 1997; Streisand, Varvel, Stanski, 1991).

Because OTFC has a rapid onset (5 minutes) and peak effect (within 15 minutes) and a short duration of action (2.5 to 5 hours) with single dosing (Berryman, 1997), it is ideal for providing conscious sedation and as a premedication for surgery and procedures. OTFC is approved by the Food and Drug Administration for these purposes in adults and children weighing more than 15 kg (33 lb). It has the benefits of providing analgesia, sedation, and anxiolysis rapidly, noninvasively, and painlessly (Streisand, Varvel, Stanski, 1991), so it is especially appealing for use with children. Because these patients usually are opioid naive, the manufacturer recommends that OTFC be administered only by trained personnel in an anesthesia-monitored setting. It is also used in areas such as the emergency department (ED).

Adverse effects

Concern over the adverse effects of opioids is a persistent barrier to effective procedural pain management. Probably the most feared of all adverse effects is respiratory depression. At equianalgesic doses all opioids, including the agonist-antagonist opioids, have a similar dose-dependent respiratory depressant effect (APS, 1992; Anderson, Zeltzer, Fanurik, 1993). Using the correct technique to administer opioids during procedures can help to prevent adverse events from occurring. Both analgesia and adverse effects of opioids vary considerably from one individual to another; therefore opioids must be titrated according to the patient's response. The adage "start low and go slow" is applicable. Large bolus doses are avoided, and when adequate pain control is achieved, boluses are administered steadily to maintain control.

Monitoring sedation and respiratory status during procedures is crucial to preventing excessive opioid-

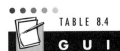

TABLE 8.4

GUIDELINES

USE OF OPIOID ANALGESICS FOR PROCEDURAL ANALGESIA

Opioid	Route	Onset (min)	Peak (min)	Half-life (h)	Dosing
Mu Agonist					
Morphine	IV	5-10	20	2-4	Dilute 1 mg/ml; 1-2 mg increments over 30 sec periods q5-10 min. Pediatric dosing: 0.05-0.1 mg/kg IV over 2 min period. Ideal for long procedures and when pain is expected after the procedure.
Fentanyl (Sublimaze)	IV	1-2	3-5	3.6	0.5-2 μg/kg; dilute 10 μg/ml; administer doses very slowly over 2-5 min; 25-100 μg increments q10-15 min. Pediatric dosing: 0.5-1 μg/kg increments over 3 min to maximum of 3 doses. Rapid IV injection may cause "rigid chest," which can be treated with muscle relaxant and mechanical ventilation. Ideal for short procedures.
Oral transmucosal fentanyl citrate (OTFC)	Oral mucosal	5-15	20-30	6.6	Dosed by sucking on sweetened matrix and, holding onto stick, moving it around the inside of mouth and gums and above and below tongue so it dissolves in the saliva; 100-, 200-, 300-, and 400 μg dose strengths. Pediatric dosing: 10-15 μg/kg/h. Use in monitored hospital setting for conscious sedation or premedication.
Hydromorphone (Dilaudid)	IV	5	10-20	2-3	Dilute 0.1-0.2 mg/ml; 0.1-0.5 mg increments over 30 sec periods q5-10 min. Pediatric dosing: 0.015-0.02 mg/kg.
Meperidine (Demerol)	IV	5-10	10-15	2-3	Dilute 10 mg/ml saline, administer in 10 mg increments q5-10 min. Pediatric dosing: 0.5-1.0 mg/kg IV over 2 min. Painful on injection, so inject slowly.
Antagonist Naloxone (Narcan)	IV	1-2	UK	Adult: 1.1; Neonate: 3.1	Dilute 0.4 mg in 10 ml saline; administer by titration-to-effect technique (i.e., no more than 0.5 ml over 2 min up to 0.8 mg). Pediatric dosing: weight < 40 kg: dilute 0.1 mg in 10 ml saline (10 μg/ml). Administer 0.5 μg/kg q2 min until desired effect is achieved. May be given SC, IM.
Nalmefene (Revex)	IV	1-2	UK	10.8	As with naloxone, dilute and titrate-to-effect technique applies. Parenteral nalmefene, 0.5 μg/kg, is comparable in safety and efficacy to 1.0 μg/kg of parenteral naloxone. A cumulative dose > 1.0 mg/70 kg is unlikely to yield additional therapeutic effect. May be given SC, IM. Long duration complicates pain control because it is much longer than that of opioids. Safety not established in neonates and children.

May be duplicated for use in clinical practice. From McCaffery M, Pasero C: *Pain: Clinical manual,* p. 379. Copyright © 1999, Mosby, Inc.

Table 8.4 presents information on the pharmacokinetics, pharmacodynamics, and use of common opioid analgesics for procedural pain. Included also is information on opioid antagonist drugs.

h, hour; *IM,* intramuscular; *IV,* intravenous; *kg,* kilogram; *min,* minutes; *μg,* microgram; *ml,* milliliter; *mg,* milligram; *q,* every; *SC,* subcutaneous; *sec,* seconds; *UK,* unknown.

Information from Abbott Laboratories: Fentanyl oralet package insert, Abbott Park, IL, 1995, Abbott Laboratories; Berde CB, Kain ZN: Pain management in infants and children. In Motoyama EK, Davis PJ, editors: *Smith's anesthesia for infants and children,* pp 385-402, St. Louis, 1996, Mosby; Deglin JH, Vallerand AH: *Davis's drug guide for nurses,* ed 5, Philadelphia, 1995, FA Davis; Ohmeda Pharmaceutical Products Division, Inc: Revex (nalmefene HCL injection) package insert, Liberty Corner, NJ, 1995, Ohmeda Pharmaceuticals; Reisine T, Pasternak G: Opioid analgesics and antagonists. In Hardman JG, Limbird LE, editors: *Goodman and Gilman's the pharmacological basis of therapeutics,* ed 9, pp 521-555, New York, 1996, McGraw-Hill, Inc; Wong D: *Wong and Whaley's clinical manual of pediatric nursing,* ed 4, St. Louis, 1996, Mosby; Yaster M, Krane EJ, Kaplan RF, et al., editors: *Pediatric pain management and sedation handbook,* St. Louis, 1997, Mosby.

induced sedation and clinically significant respiratory depression. Sedation precedes respiratory depression because more opioid is required to produce respiratory depression than is required to produce sedation. Signs that a patient is becoming excessively sedated are severely slurred speech and inability to complete a sentence without falling asleep.

Combining drugs, such as benzodiazepines and opioids, may potentiate adverse effects, such as sedation and respiratory depression (Anderson, Zeltzer, Fanurik, 1993; Somerson, Husted, Sicilia, 1995); therefore when they are combined, initial doses of both should be reduced (Somerson, Husted, Sicilia, 1995). When a benzodiazepine and an opioid are combined and excessive sedation occurs during a procedure, it is best to try decreasing the dose of the benzodiazepine before decreasing the dose of the opioid. Because benzodiazepines have no analgesic properties, decreasing the dose will not affect pain control. However, if the opioid dose is decreased first, pain control could be lost. Because opioids provide sedation and analgesia, many times a desirable level of sedation and pain control is achieved in this type of situation by simply decreasing the benzodiazepine dose while maintaining the opioid dose. When excessive sedation is detected during a procedure and an opioid is the only agent being administered, the opioid dose must be decreased (Pasero, McCaffery, 1994).

If opioid-induced clinically significant respiratory depression occurs, it can be reversed with the opioid antagonist, naloxone (Narcan). (If it is necessary to reverse the sedative effects of benzodiazepines, the benzodiazepine antagonist flumazenil [Romazicon] can be given IV. See p. 381.) To prevent giving too much naloxone too quickly and reversing analgesia, it must be carefully titrated to effect. Naloxone must be used with extreme caution in patients who are receiving opioids on a long-term basis because of its potential to precipitate a withdrawal syndrome (APS, 1992; Jacox, Carr, Payne et al., 1994) (see pp. 269-270 and Box 6.29 for recommended guidelines for administering naloxone).

Nalmefene (Revex) is a relatively new opioid antagonist. Parenteral nalmefene, 0.5 μg/kg, is comparable in safety and efficacy to 1.0 μg/kg of parenteral naloxone. A 1 mg parenteral dose of nalmefene is capable of blocking 80% of the opioid receptors within 5 minutes of administration (Ohmeda, 1995). The recommendations and precautions for naloxone apply to nalmefene, particularly careful titration to effect.

The half-life of nalmefene (approximately 10 hours) is much longer than that of naloxone (approximately 1 hour) so reversal effects will last much longer with nalmefene than naloxone. Whereas repeated doses of naloxone sometimes are necessary to maintain reversal of most opioids, a single dose of nalmefene with its long duration usually is sufficient. However, maintaining pain control may be particularly difficult after nalmefene administration because its duration is much longer than most opioids. More research is needed to address these issues.

Demerol, phenergan, and thorazine (DPT)

DPT, the meperidine (Demerol), promethazine (Phenergan), and chlorpromazine (Thorazine) combination, sometimes called the lytic cocktail or pedi-cocktail, has been prescribed for years to sedate pediatric patients for painful procedures. Although this is a persistent practice, it no longer is recommended. The American Academy of Pediatrics (AAP) (1995) warns that DPT is associated with a high rate of therapeutic failure and serious adverse reactions. The AAP (195) states, ". . . the dose (of DPT) cannot be titrated easily and individually, the onset of action is significantly delayed (20-30 minutes), the duration of sedation is protracted (5-20 hours), the duration of analgesia is much shorter (1-3 hours), and no anxiolytic or amnestic properties exist" (p. 601).

Excessive and prolonged CNS depression after DPT administration can be especially dangerous when pediatric patients are discharged shortly after a procedure and family members must observe them during their recovery (Wong, 1996c). The AHCPR acute pain management clinical practice guideline (1992) states a warning about DPT, "Exercise caution when using the mixture . . . DPT—given intramuscularly. . . . The efficacy of this mixture is poor when compared with alternative approaches and it has been associated with a high frequency of adverse effects . . . It is not recommended for general use and should only be used in exceptional circumstances" (p. 45). *The Harriet Lane Handbook* no longer lists DPT among the drugs suggested for procedural pain management (Johnson, 1993).

Nonsteroidal Antiinflammatory Drugs (NSAIDs)

NSAIDs inhibit the release of substances that facilitate the movement of pain impulses from the periphery to the spinal cord. These substances are released at the periphery as a result of tissue damage or potential damage (see Chapter 2). NSAIDs may have limited use for treatment of the immediate pain associated with procedures because of the latency of their action. However, they may be used to provide preemptive analgesia for procedural pain and for the relief of pain after procedures (see Chapter 5).

Although the manufacturer does not recommend the use of ketorolac preoperatively, it has been used safely and effectively as a preemptive analgesic (Varrassi, Panella, Piroli et al., 1994) and as an adjuvant to opioids for moderate to severe pain (Grass, Sakima, Valley et al., 1993). Ketorolac has been shown to improve pain relief also when given before painful procedures in the ICU (Puntillo, 1996). Protocol in many outpatient surgery centers includes administering a dose of IV ketorolac at the end of a procedure and sending patients home with instructions to take ibuprofen ATC for mild pain or in combination with an opioid for moderate pain.

Ketorolac is also safe for use in children. A dose of 0.5 mg/kg gives plasma concentrations comparable to those with maximal analgesic effects in adults (Berde, Kain, 1996).

Benzodiazepines

Benzodiazepines can diminish skeletal muscle spasm, reduce anxiety, and at high doses produce amnesia for the procedure, but they lack analgesic properties for acute tissue injury. For painless procedures it may be appropriate to use benzodiazepines alone to provide sedation and reduce anxiety if necessary. However, if a procedure is expected to produce pain, an analgesic must be added (AHCPR, 1992). (See Guidelines for conscious sedation and analgesia Box 8.6 on pp. 382-384.)

The importance of adding opioids to sedative drugs when procedures are expected to be painful cannot be overemphasized, especially for patients who must endure repetitive procedures. Managing pain adequately during the first procedure the patient experiences usually helps to reduce the anxiety associated with future procedures. This can help to prevent the continual use of benzodiazepines for controlling anticipatory anxiety in these patients (Choiniere, 1994).

The two benzodiazepines used most often for procedural sedation are diazepam (Valium) and midazolam (Versed). Lorazepam (Ativan) is occasionally used for procedural sedation, but it can produce prolonged sedation (Marshall, Longnecker, 1996).

Midazolam is recommended as a replacement for diazepam as the drug of choice for conscious sedation (Lee, Hanna, Harding, 1989; Somerson, Husted, Sicilia, 1995) and induction and maintenance of anesthesia (Marshall, Longnecker, 1996). Diazepam is associated with greater variation in effect, prolonged action with a second peak effect at 6 to 8 hours, pain on injection, and thrombophlebitis at the site of injection (Marshall, Longnecker, 1996; Lee, Hanna, Harding, 1989). Midazolam has a rapid onset of action (1 to 5 min), short half-life (1 to 12 h), and is not associated with pain at the site of injection. However, it should be administered very slowly, and time must be taken to assess the effect of each dose before administering more (*Drug facts and comparisons,* 1996). Table 8.5 on pp. 385-386 summarizes the characteristics of the benzodiazepines used for procedural pain.

Routes of administration

Although the IV route is the most common route for administering midazolam, it may be given IM, orally, rec-

tally, and intranasally. The intranasal route has been used for pediatric conscious sedation because it is noninvasive and has been shown to be effective and safe with minimal respiratory depression and no effect on blood pressure. By the intranasal route, midazolam produces sedation within 5 minutes and has a recovery time of 60 minutes (Adrian, 1994). However, the use of midazolam by the intranasal route is controversial and may be traumatic and frightening for children (Wong, 1996a). It is reported to cause intense burning, irritation, and lacrimation on instillation into the nares (Lugo, Fishbein, Nahata et al., 1993). For these reasons, the oral or IV route for administration of midazolam is preferable. By the oral route, midazolam should be administered 30 to 45 minutes before the procedure (Mitchell, Grange, Black et al., 1997; Wong, 1996a); by the IV route, 3 minutes before (Wong, 1996a).

Adverse effects

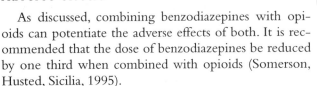

As discussed, combining benzodiazepines with opioids can potentiate the adverse effects of both. It is recommended that the dose of benzodiazepines be reduced by one third when combined with opioids (Somerson, Husted, Sicilia, 1995).

If it is necessary to reverse the sedative effects of benzodiazepines, the benzodiazepine antagonist flumazenil (Romazicon) can be given IV. Just as with naloxone, the titration-to-effect technique is used to administer flumazenil. Partial reversal of sedation is produced by giving 0.1 to 0.2 mg doses over a period of 1 to 3 min/dose; complete reversal is possible with 1 mg. If a patient does not respond to a cumulative dose of 1 to 5 mg over 2 to 10 minutes, causes other than benzodiazepine overdose should be considered. Flumazenil may precipitate seizures and other withdrawal symptoms in patients who have been taking benzodiazepines on a long-term basis. It should not be given in an effort to reverse the sedative effects of barbiturates or tricyclic antidepressants. This can precipitate life-threatening seizures (Hobbs, Rall, Verdoorn, 1996).

Barbiturates

Barbiturates are used less frequently than benzodiazepines to produce sedation during procedures, probably because their potential for adverse effects and their anxiolytic properties are greater than benzodiazepines, especially with respect to the degree of sedation that is produced (Hobbs, Rall, Verdoorn, 1996). Barbiturates can produce all degrees of CNS depression, ranging from mild sedation to general anesthesia. They do not possess analgesic properties and, in fact, increase the reaction to painful stimuli. Barbiturates must be used with caution because of their potential to cause seizures and life-threatening respiratory and cardiovascular effects (Anderson, Zeltzer, Fanurik, 1993).

Text continued on p. 386.

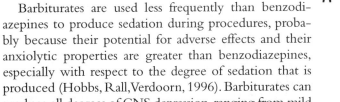

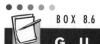

BOX 8.6

GUIDELINES

CONSCIOUS SEDATION AND ANALGESIA
(ADULTS AND CHILDREN)

Purpose
To provide safe and effective conscious sedation and analgesia for adults and children during diagnostic and therapeutic procedures.

Definition
1. Conscious sedation/analgesia is defined as combinations of pharmacologic agents administered by one or more routes to produce a minimally depressed level of consciousness and satisfactory analgesia while retaining the patient's ability to independently and continuously maintain an airway and to respond to physical stimulation and verbal commands.
2. Optimal conscious sedation/analgesia is achieved when the patient:
   - Maintains consciousness
   - Independently maintains his or her airway
   - Retains protective reflexes (swallow and gag)
   - Responds to physical and verbal commands
   - Is not anxious or afraid
   - Experiences acceptable pain relief
   - Has minimal changes in vital signs
   - Is cooperative during the procedure
   - Has mild amnesia for the procedure
   - Recovers to baseline (preprocedure) status safely and promptly

Designated Team Members
1. Physician who has met competency requirements
2. Registered nurse (RN) who has met competency requirements

Competency Requirements
1. Physician
   - Validated current Advanced Cardiac Life Support (ACLS) training for adults; Pediatric Advanced Life Support (PALS) for children
   - Validated current competency in prescribing and administering conscious sedation/analgesia
2. Registered nurse
   - Validated current ACLS or PALS training
   - Validated current competency in administering and monitoring conscious sedation/analgesia

Roles and Responsibilities
1. Physician
   - Determines the need for conscious sedation/analgesia
   - Performs preprocedure health evaluation (risk assessment, health history, review of systems, statement as to airway patency, vital signs, and physical examination)
   - Provides patient and family with information to obtain informed consent
   - Prescribes drugs for conscious sedation/analgesia, side effects, and complications
   - Administers drugs for conscious sedation/analgesia when indicated
   - Administers drugs for treatment of side effects and complications of conscious sedation/analgesia when indicated
   - Manages emergency situations
   - Documents preprocedure health evaluation, vital statistics (weight and age), rationale for sedation/analgesia, information to patient/family, dietary precautions, procedure, pharmacologic agents used, and patient response
2. Registered Nurse
   - Reviews and ensures documentation of preprocedure health evaluation
   - Ensures appropriate preprocedure dietary precautions have been taken (e.g., fasting or clear liquids up to 2 hours before procedure)
   - Provides patient and family with information regarding procedure and aftercare
   - Administers drugs for conscious sedation/analgesia under direct supervision of responsible physician
   - Monitors and assesses patient response
   - Administers drugs for treatment of side effects and complications of conscious sedation/analgesia
   - Manages emergency situations
   - Documents preprocedure health evaluation (see above), procedure, pharmacologic agents used, and patient response

Policy
1. Before the procedure, team members will discuss what drugs will be used and whether analgesia will be needed for the procedure.
   ⇒ The decision to provide analgesia for a procedure will be made on the basis of knowledge of the likelihood that the procedure is painful. If any question exists as to whether pain is associated with the procedure, the health care team will assume that it is.
   ⇒ Analgesic agents will be added if it becomes apparent that a procedure thought not to be associated with pain is causing pain.
2. If the amount of sedation required is likely to produce deep sedation, rendering the patient unable to respond to physical or verbal stimulation and independently maintain an airway, it will be administered and monitored by a trained anesthesia provider.
3. Consideration will be given to consulting a trained anesthesia provider before administering conscious sedation/analgesia to patients with:
   - Liver or kidney disease
   - Respiratory compromise

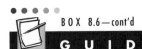

BOX 8.6—cont'd

GUIDELINES

CONSCIOUS SEDATION AND ANALGESIA
(ADULTS AND CHILDREN)—cont'd

- Acute narrow angle glaucoma
- Unstable dysrhythmias
- Young children, infants, neonates, premature infants
- Frail, debilitated elderly
- Possible or confirmed pregnancy, nursing mothers

⇒ In some of these cases it may be wise to ask a trained anesthesia provider to administer the conscious sedation/analgesia or to administer it in a location where anesthesia providers are immediately accessible.

4. Informed consent will be obtained before administering conscious sedation/analgesia.

5. Chemical dependency or substance abuse is not a contraindication to the use of conscious sedation/analgesia.

6. The responsible physician will be present when conscious sedation/analgesia is initiated and throughout its administration.

7. Long-term conscious sedation will be administered only in the intensive care units where a physician is immediately accessible.

8. A one-to-one RN/patient ratio will be maintained during the administration of conscious sedation/analgesia (i.e., the RN will have no other responsibilities during the procedure and will not leave the patient unattended or engage in tasks that will compromise continuous monitoring).

9. All equipment and supplies will be age appropriate, failsafe, and calibrated according to the manufacturers' recommended highest standards at least annually.

Equipment and Supplies

- Fully equipped crash cart, including emergency and resuscitative drugs, airway and ventilatory equipment, and defibrillator, immediately available in all locations where conscious sedation/analgesia is administered
- 100% oxygen source and administration supplies in room capable of providing > 90% oxygen for > 60 min
- Airways and positive-pressure breathing device in room capable of providing appropriate flow rate for age
- Suction source and supplies in room
- Electrocardiogram (ECG) monitor with display
- Noninvasive blood pressure (BP) monitor
- Means to monitor oxygen saturation and carbon dioxide (CO_2) level
- Means to monitor body temperature
- Stethoscope
- IV supplies
- Sedative, analgesic, and reversal agents

Procedure: Preparation Phase

- Ensure all supplies and equipment are fully stocked, age-appropriate, and functional.
- Review patient's history and physical information to determine current condition, chief complaint, reason for conscious sedation/analgesia, and identify risk factors or contraindications to receiving conscious sedation/analgesia.

- Determine current medications and substances patient is taking; existence of allergies; history of drug use or abuse, including tobacco and alcohol; adverse experience with anesthesia, analgesics, or sedatives; and last oral intake.

- Outpatient setting: Ensure responsible person is available to drive patient home after recovery and that a responsible person will remain with patient the length of two half-lives of the drugs administered for conscious sedation/analgesia.

- Reinforce to patient and family the physician's explanations of procedure and conscious sedation/analgesia including:
  - Purpose and goal of conscious sedation/analgesia
  - Procedure for administering conscious sedation/analgesia, including roles
  - Approximate length of procedure
  - Sensations patient may experience
  - Monitoring and assessment
  - Use of pain rating scale and/or signaling system
  - Drugs to be administered
  - Side effects and complications and their treatment
  - Nondrug interventions
  - Postrecovery expectations

- Ensure written consent is obtained.

- Attach monitoring equipment to patient (e.g., ECG, BP, temperature, oximetry).

- Obtain and document baseline data: temperature, heart rate and rhythm, respiratory status, blood pressure, skin condition, level of sedation (LOS) and mental status, ability to ambulate, weakness or sensory loss in extremities (if pertinent), and description and intensity of current painful condition.

- Insert IV (no exceptions) and regulate continuous infusion at a keep-open rate.

- Prepare all drugs to be administered; ready reversal agents.

Procedure: Administration Phase

- Administer drugs for conscious sedation/analgesia when responsible physician is present and able to directly supervise.

- Continuously observe and document patient responses to conscious sedation/analgesia.

⇒ Monitoring all the parameters as frequently as outlined in the following may not be possible during some procedures. If this is the case, close observation and monitoring of other parameters is invaluable.

- ECG, BP, temperature, oxygen saturation or CO_2 level every 5 min.

- Auscultate breath sounds, observe respiratory depth and rate every 5 min.

Continued.

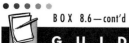

BOX 8.6—cont'd

GUIDELINES

CONSCIOUS SEDATION AND ANALGESIA
(ADULTS AND CHILDREN)—cont'd

- LOS, mental status every 5 min
  N = Normal sleep
  1 = Anxious, agitated, or restless
  2 = Calm, cooperative to tranquil (patient's baseline without sedation)
  3 = Quiet, drowsy, responds to verbal commands
  4 = Asleep, brisk response to forehead tap or loud verbal stimuli
  5 = Asleep, sluggish response to increasingly vigorous stimuli
  6 = Unresponsive to painful stimuli
- Skin color and condition every 10 min
- Pain assessment every 10 minutes
  - Self report (e.g., 0 to 10, Wong-Baker FACES Pain Rating Scale); use of signaling system for patients unable or afraid they will not be able to report
  - Overt physical signs (e.g., muscle rigidity, tearing of eyes, facial changes, groaning, agitation, changes in vital signs)
⇒ Absence of overt physical signs will not be interpreted as absence of pain.
- Provide reassurance and emotional support; encourage use of nondrug interventions if appropriate.
- Inform physician immediately of adverse responses or significant changes in baseline parameters.
- Maintain continuous IV access.
- Manage emergency situations.

Procedure: Recovery Phase
- Continue mechanical monitoring: ECG, BP, temperature, oximetry.
- Assess and document vital signs, skin condition, LOS, mental status, and pain every 15 min for at least 60 min after last sedative or analgesic drug dose is given and until discharge criteria are met.
- Inform physician immediately of adverse responses or significant changes in baseline parameters.
- Maintain IV access for at least 60 min after last sedative/analgesic drug dose is given and until discharge criteria are met.
- Discharge 60 min after last dose of sedative or analgesic drug is administered if *all* of the following discharge criteria are met (variations must be approved by responsible physician):
  - Alert and oriented as baseline
  - Protective reflexes (swallow and gag) present
  - Vital signs stable and consistent with baseline for 30 min after last drug dose

- Oxygen saturation on room air at least 95% or at baseline for 30 min after last drug dose
- Cardiac rhythm consistent with baseline
- BP and heart rate within normal limits or within 20 points of baseline
- Temperature ≤ 101°F
- Pain rating is at baseline or less
- When applicable, no visible site drainage or excessive swelling
- Ambulation consistent with baseline
- Responsible adult present to drive patient home and remain with patient the length of two half-lives of the drugs administered for conscious sedation/analgesia
- If reversal agent was administered, enough time has elapsed to ensure adverse reaction will not recur
- Review discharge instructions:
  - When to resume taking medications taken before procedure
  - New prescriptions
  - Wound care
  - Diet and activity restrictions, including no driving or operating dangerous machinery for at least 24 h.
  - Follow-up care, telephone contact numbers
  - Written materials

Suggested Teaching Content for Competency Validation
- Definitions, differences between analgesia, conscious sedation, deep sedation, and anesthesia, including the implications for scope of practice
- Goal and purpose of conscious sedation/analgesia
- Review of institutional protocol for administering and monitoring conscious sedation/analgesia
- Procedures for which conscious sedation/analgesia is commonly administered
- Patient selection criteria
- Guidelines and indications for adding analgesia to sedation
- Patient advocacy
- Informed consent
- Patient teaching and discharge planning
- Pharmacology of drugs administered for conscious sedation/analgesia, routes of administration, recommended doses, adverse effects, and complications
- Assessment, monitoring, and documentation during all phases of care
- Equipment operation
- Emergency management

This is an example of an institutional protocol for the administration of conscious sedation and analgesia.

Information from Acute Pain Management Guideline Panel: *Acute pain management: Operative or medical procedures and trauma: Clinical practice guideline*, AHCPR Pub. No. 92-0032, Rockville, Md, Agency for Health Care Policy and Research, Public Health Service, US Department of Health and Human Services, February 1992; Committee on Drugs, American Academy of Pediatrics (AAP): Guidelines for monitoring and management of pediatric patients during and after sedation for diagnostic therapeutic procedures, *Pediatrics* 89:1110-1115, 1992; Pasero C, Bennett P: Combining analgesia with sedation on the unit, *Am J Nurs* 96(11):17, 19, 1996; Somerson SJ, Husted CW, Sicilia MR: Insights into conscious sedation, *Am J Nurs* 95(6):26-33, 1995; University of Wisconsin Hospital and Clinics: Guidelines for continuous opioid intravenous infusions (for inpatients), 1997.

TABLE 8.5

GUIDELINES

USE OF BENZODIAZEPINES FOR PROCEDURAL SEDATION

Drug	Route	Onset (min)	Peak (min)	Duration (h)	Half-life (h)	Dosing
Midazolam (Versed)	IV	1-5	Rapid	2-6	1-12	Reduce dose by one third initially when combining with opioid; dilute 1 mg/ml saline; 0.5-1 mg increments; no more than 2.5 mg should be administered over 3 min period; allow at least 3 min between doses to assess full effect. Once sedation is achieved, additional doses should be 25% of dose required to produce sedative endpoint. A total dose of >5 mg is usually not necessary. Maintenance dose: 0.25-1 mg. Pediatric dosing: 0.03-0.1 mg/kg increments to maximum of 3 doses IV; oral dose 0.5-0.75 mg/kg. Because of rapid onset of action, short half-life, and no pain at site of injection, midazolam is recommended as first choice for conscious sedation.
Diazepam (Valium)	IV	1-5	15-30	15-60	20-70	Reduce dose by one third initially when combining with opioid; 1-5 mg increments; 20 mg maximum dose in 1 h. Pediatric dosing: 0.1-0.3 mg/kg before procedures such as a regional block. Associated with great variation in response, prolonged action with a second peak effect at 6-8 h, pain on injection, and thrombophlebitis at the site of injection. Midazolam is recommended as a replacement for diazepam as drug of choice for conscious sedation.
Lorazepam (Ativan)	IV	5-15	UK	Up to 48	10-20	Reduce dose by one third initially when combining with opioid; dilute 1:1 in compatible solution immediately before administering; 0.05 mg/kg to 4 mg maximum total dose. Pediatric dosing: 0.02-0.1 mg/kg. Long half-life of lorazepam makes midazolam a preferable choice.
Antagonist Flumazenil (Romazicon)	IV	1-3	6-10	Depends on dose and plasma concentration of benzodiazepine	Initial = 7-10; terminal = 41-79	Administer by titration-to-effect technique: 0.1-0.2 mg over 1 to 3 min. After waiting 45 sec, an additional 0.2 mg can be repeated at 60 sec intervals up to 1 mg. Pediatric dosing: 0.01 mg/kg loading dose followed by 0.005 mg/kg per minute until awake or to maximum dose of 1 mg. Can cause life-threatening seizures in patients receiving benzodiazepines on long-term basis and in patients who have overdosed on barbiturates or tricyclic antidepressants.

TABLE 8.5—cont'd

GUIDELINES

May be duplicated for use in clinical practice. From McCaffery M, Pasero C: *Pain: Clinical manual*, pp. 385-386. Copyright © 1999, Mosby.

Table 8.5 presents information on the pharmacokinetics, pharmacodynamics, and use of common benzodiazepines for procedural sedation. Included also is information on the benzodiazepine antagonist drug.

h, hour; *IV,* intravenous; *kg,* kilogram; *min,* minutes; *ml,* milliliter; *mg,* milligram; *q,* every; *sec,* seconds; *UK,* unknown.

Information from Berde CB, Kain ZN: Pain management in infants and children. In Motoyama EK, Davis PJ, editors: *Smith's anesthesia for infants and children,* pp 385-402, St. Louis, 1996, Mosby; Deglin JH, Vallerand AH: *Davis's drug guide for nurses,* ed 5, Philadelphia, 1995, FA Davis; Lee MG, Hanna W, Harding H: Sedation for upper gastrointestinal endoscopy: A comparative study of midazolam and diazepam, *Gastrointest Endosc* 35(2):82-84, 1989; Marshall BE, Longnecker DE: General anesthetics. In Hardman JG, Limbird LE, editors: *Goodman and Gilman's the pharmacological basis of therapeutics,* ed 9, pp 307-330, New York, 1996, McGraw-Hill, Inc; Rice LJ: Regional anesthesia and analgesia. In Motoyama EK, Davis PJ, editors: *Smith's anesthesia for infants and children,* pp 403-442, St. Louis, 1996, Mosby. Wong D: *Wong and Whaley's clinical manual of pediatric nursing,* ed 4, St. Louis, 1996, Mosby; Yaster M, Krane EJ, Kaplan RF, et al., editors: *Pediatric pain management and sedation handbook,* St. Louis, 1997, Mosby.

Continuous IV infusion of the ultrashort–acting barbiturate, methohexital (Brevital), sometimes is used to produce sedation for brief painless procedures (Gronert, Motoyama, 1996). IV methohexital has an onset of action within 60 seconds and its duration is just 5 to 7 minutes (Anderson, Zeltzer, Fanurik, 1993).

Although rectal methohexital is not recommended as a premedication (Gronert, Motoyama, 1996), sometimes it is given to children before minor painless procedures or to ease separating them from their parents before surgery. When given rectally, it can induce sedation within 6 to 10 minutes (Anderson, Zeltzer, Fanurik, 1993). Pentobarbital (Nembutal) was used extensively in the past as a premedication. Today it is given only occasionally to children as a premedication for conscious sedation. It is given IV, orally (3 mg/kg), and rectally (4 mg/kg) (Krane, Davis, Smith, 1996; Wong, 1996a).

Chloral Hydrate

Chloral hydrate is a sedative/hypnotic with minimal analgesic properties. It has been used as a sedative for many years. Although it is used occasionally for procedural sedation, it is not recommended. Chloral hydrate is irritating to skin and mucous membranes and has an extremely unpleasant taste. It can cause epigastric distress, GI hemorrhage, esophageal stricture, nausea, vomiting, hypotension, malaise, ataxia, delirium, and nightmares. Recovery from chloral hydrate is accompanied by a "hangover" (Anderson, Zeltzer, Fanurik, 1993; Deglin, Vallerand, 1995; Hobbs, Rall, Verdoorn, 1996).

General Anesthetics Used for Analgesia and Sedation

General anesthetics, given at subanesthetic doses, to manage the pain and anxiety of procedures is becoming increasingly common. The use of general anesthetics should be guided by policies and procedures that establish safe administration. It is recommended that they be administered only by personnel experienced in their effects

and comfortable with maintaining an airway (AHCPR, 1992). Table 8.6 summarizes some of the general anesthetics used for procedural pain and sedation.

Ketamine

Ketamine is a dissociative (see following discussion) anesthetic agent capable of producing amnesia, marked analgesia, and all degrees of sedation, including general anesthesia. It can also produce local anesthetic effects, causing sensory and motor blockade. Subanesthetic doses of ketamine have been shown to produce safe and effective pain control during a wide variety of procedures ranging from debridement and grafting of burn wounds (Choiniere, 1994) to transporting patients with overwhelming pain (Notcutt, 1994). Advantages of ketamine include availability by many routes (IV, IM, oral, rectal, and intranasal), rapid onset (30 seconds), and less respiratory depression at subanesthetic doses than opioids (Anderson, Zeltzer, Fanurik, 1993; Choiniere, 1994; Notcutt, 1994).

The dissociative state produced by ketamine must be understood by the staff and explained to the patient. The term dissociative anesthesia refers to the feelings of separateness from the environment, loss of control, hallucinations, and vivid dreams that patients report while recovering from ketamine administration (Anderson, Zeltzer, Fanurik, 1993; Marshall, Longnecker, 1996). Providing patients with a thorough explanation of the dissociative state before ketamine administration may help them adjust better to the drug (Martinez, Achauer, Dobkin de Rios, 1985). Benzodiazepines can reduce the incidence of the unpleasant experiences of dissociation. Preprocedural or postprocedural administration of midazolam rather than diazepam is recommended. Concurrent administration of diazepam inhibits the metabolic breakdown of ketamine, which would prolong its half-life (Anderson, Zeltzer, Fanurik, 1993).

Other adverse effects of ketamine include increases in heart rate, cardiac output, blood pressure, cardiac work, systemic vascular resistance, and stroke volume. Although

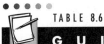

TABLE 8.6

GUIDELINES

USE OF GENERAL ANESTHETICS FOR PROCEDURAL ANALGESIA AND SEDATION

Drug	Route	Onset	Peak	Duration	Half-life	Dosing
Ketamine	IV	30 sec	UK	5-10 min	2.3 h	Subanesthetic dose: 0.5 mg/kg; anesthetic dose: ≥ 1.0 mg/kg. Analgesic and sedative.
Ketamine	IM	3-4 min	UK	12-25 min	2.5 h	Pediatric dosing for anesthesia induction premedication: 2-3 mg/kg.
Propofol (Diprivan)	IV	40 sec	UK	3-5 min	3-12 h	5-200 mg/h for sedation; time to recovery is 8 min; 19 min if opioids have also been used. Pediatric dosing for light sedation: 0.5-1 mg/kg. Not analgesic at subanesthetic doses.
Nitrous oxide	Inhalation	20 sec	1-3 min	As long as treatment is in progress	UK	For analgesia, use self-administration of 50% nitrous oxide/50% oxygen mixture. Must be stored in pressurized tanks. Use scavenger system to prevent environmental contamination.
Reversal of effects						To reverse most general anesthetics, discontinue administration immediately and wait for effects to dissipate.

May be duplicated for use in clinical practice. From McCaffery M, Pasero C: *Pain: Clinical manual,* p. 387. Copyright © 1999, Mosby, Inc.

Table 8.6 presents information on the pharmacokinetics, pharmacodynamics, and use of various general anesthetic agents for procedural pain and sedation.

h, hour; *IM,* intramuscular; *IV,* intravenous; *kg,* kilogram; *min,* minutes; *mg,* milligram; *q,* every; *sec,* seconds; *UK,* unknown.

Information from Acute Pain Management Guideline Panel: *Acute pain management: Operative or medical procedures and trauma: Clinical practice guideline,* AHCPR Pub. No. 92-0032, Rockville, Md, Agency for Health Care Policy and Research, Public Health service, US Department of Health and Human Services, February 1992; Anderson CTM, Zeltzer LK, Fanurik D: Procedural pain. In Schechter N, Berde CB, Yaster M, editors: *Pain in infants, children, and adolescents,* pp 435-458, Baltimore, 1993, Williams & Wilkins; Berde CB, Kain ZN: Pain management in infants and children. In Motoyama EK, Davis PJ, editors: *Smith's anesthesia for infants and children,* pp 385-402, St. Louis, 1996, Mosby; Boyd MJ: Nitrous oxide/oxygen: An additional method of pain control, *Oncol Nurs Forum* Suppl 11(2):119, 1984; Deglin JH, Vallerand AH: *Davis's drug guide for nurses,* ed 5, Philadelphia, 1995, FA Davis; Illingworth KA, Simpson KH: *Anesthesia and analgesia in emergency medicine,* New York, 1994, Oxford, University Press; Rice LJ: Regional anesthesia and analgesia, In Motoyama EK, Davis PJ, editors: *Smith's anesthesia for infants and children,* pp 403-442, St. Louis, 1996, Mosby; Lee MG, Hanna W, Harding H: Sedation for upper gastrointestinal endoscopy: A comparative study of midazolam and diazepam, *Gastrointest Endosc* 35(2):82-84, 1989; Marshall BE, Longnecker DE: General anesthetics. In Hardman JG, Limbird LE, editors: *Goodman and Gilman's the pharmacological basis of therapeutics,* ed 9, pp 307-330, New York, 1996, McGraw-Hill, Inc; Rice LJ: Regional anesthesia and analgesia. In Motoyama EK, Davis PJ, editors: *Smith's anesthesia for infants and children,* pp 403-442, St. Louis, 1996, Mosby.

tracheal aspiration and apnea have also been reported, airway reflexes typically are preserved at subanesthetic doses (Anderson, Zeltzer, Fanurik, 1993). Ketamine should not be used for pain control during tonometry because it is contraindicated in patients with elevated intraocular pressure (Marshall, Longnecker, 1996).

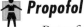

Propofol

Propofol (Diprivan) is a hypnotic general anesthetic that, when administered in subanesthetic doses, has no significant analgesic effect but is capable of producing excellent sedation for a wide variety of procedures (Choiniere, 1994; Klafta, Klock, Young et al., 1995). It must be given by the IV route only. A continuous IV infusion of propofol often is administered to provide sedation for children and adults receiving regional anesthesia, intensive care, or palliative care (Marshall, Longnecker, 1996; Moyle, 1995; Shapiro, Warren, Egol et al., 1995). Recently it has gained popularity as a sedative for burn patients undergoing painful procedures (Choiniere, 1994).

Propofol is effective as an adjuvant to opioids and benzodiazepines, allowing clinicians to significantly decrease the doses of each (Graves, Moran, Porter et al., 1996). However, subanesthetic propofol provides only minimal analgesia. The analgesic effect of subanesthetic propofol has been shown to be weak compared with fentanyl (Klafta, Klock, Young et al., 1995). Therefore when propofol is administered at subanesthetic doses for sedation during painful procedures or for painful conditions, an opioid must be added for pain control (Choiniere, 1994; Deglin, Vallerand, 1995; Klafta, Klock, Young et al., 1995; Shapiro, Warren, Egol et al., 1995). When used for continuous sedation in the terminally ill with intractable pain, recommended dosing is 0.6 mg/kg per hour to 6.0 mg/kg per hour (Smith, 1995).

Advantages of propofol are that its dosage can be titrated accurately minute to minute and, whether administered by single bolus or infusion, recovery is extremely rapid and free from the "hangover" effects associated with other anesthetics. Unlike ketamine, no hallucinogenic reactions are associated with propofol. At subanesthetic doses, patients remain in full communication with staff and relatives (Choiniere, 1994; Moyle, 1995).

Adverse effects of propofol include bradycardia, hypotension, and apnea (Deglin, Vallerand, 1995). Clearance and elimination of the drug may cause the urine to be green (Moyle, 1995). Patients report burning and stinging at the IV site, which is rarely followed by phlebitis or thrombosis (Deglin, Vallerand, 1995; Marshall, Longnecker, 1996). Injecting lidocaine (0.2 mg/kg) into a large vein before the propofol and slowing the rate of administration are helpful in reducing this discomfort (Morton, 1990; Welborn, 1996). Another recommendation is to mix one part of 1% lidocaine with 10 parts of 1% propofol to reduce the pain at the injection site and at more proximal sites as well (Eriksson, Englesson, Niklasson et al., 1997).

Patient-Controlled Analgesia and Sedation

IV patient-controlled analgesia (PCA) is used extensively for acute and chronic pain of a continuous nature (see Chapter 6, p. 248). The concept of PCA also has been used safely and effectively to administer analgesia and sedation for elective surgery in a monitored care setting (Irwin, Thompson, Kenny, 1997; Thorpe, Balakrishman, Cook, 1997; Wallace, 1997). A number of short-acting opioids, such as alfentanil and fentanyl, and hypnotic drugs, such as propofol, have been administered with a standard PCA pump and patients controlling the amount of analgesia and sedation they receive (Wallace, 1997). To administer PCA sedation, the pump is modified to a zero (Thorpe, Balakrishman, Cook, 1997) to 2-minute (Irwin, Thompson, Keeny, 1997) delay (lockout) interval.

The most common drug administered by PCA seems to be propofol. It is ideal for this method of administra-

tion because of its extremely rapid onset and short duration. One study started patients on IV propofol at a target plasma level of 1 μg/ml. Patients could self-administer propofol doses in 0.2 μg/ml increments as often as every 2 minutes to a maximum concentration of 3 μg/ml (Irwin, Thompson, Kenny, 1997). Considerable interindividual variability in propofol consumption, ranging from 3 to 131 μg/kg per minute and no oversedation or cardiovascular instability were noted. Optimal sedation was provided at median concentrations of 0.8 to 0.9 μg/ml. Patient satisfaction was high.

Nitrous oxide

The short-acting inhalational anesthetic, nitrous oxide, is gaining popularity for use in procedural pain management. It has been used safely for dressing changes in both pediatric and adult burn patients (Choiniere, 1994), fracture reductions in children (Wattenmaker, Kasser, McGravey, 1990), patients during labor and delivery, a number of diagnostic and therapeutic procedures for both adults and children, and in the oncology and ED settings (AHCPR, 1992; Boyd, 1984; Driscoll, Gwinnutt, Nancarrow et al., 1995; Ducharme, 1994; Jacox, Carr, Payne et al., 1994).

Nitrous oxide provides rapid (within 20 seconds) and potent analgesia with minimal depression of the respiratory, cardiovascular, and central nervous systems (Boyd, 1984; Scott, 1981). In addition to providing analgesia, nitrous oxide is mildly anxiolytic and sedating. The exact mechanism by which nitrous oxide produces analgesia is not known; however, it is partially reversible by administration of naloxone. The analgesic effect of nitrous oxide diminishes rapidly when administration is discontinued (Boyd, 1984).

For analgesia, nitrous oxide is given as a mixture in oxygen. Varying concentrations of nitrous oxide in oxygen ranging from 20% to 65% have been used in the clinical setting for pain control. Analgesia equivalent to morphine is possible with inhalation of 20% nitrous oxide (Driscoll, Gwinnutt, Nancarrow et al., 1995). Commercial mixtures of 50% nitrous oxide and 50% oxygen (Etonox, Nitronox. Scavenger) are used most often (Boyd, 1984; Driscoll, Gwinnutt, Nancarrow et al., 1995; Wattenmaker, Kasser, McGravey, 1990).

Perhaps the safest method of providing nitrous oxide is self-administration, a form of PCA. The patient holds a mouthpiece or face mask and breathes the mixture of nitrous oxide and oxygen. If excessive sedation occurs, the patient will drop the mouthpiece or mask, preventing further delivery (AHCPR, 1992). The patient must be instructed to maintain an airtight seal between the face and mask or not to nose-breathe if a mouthpiece is used (Driscoll, Gwinnutt, Nancarrow et al., 1995). The self-administration technique has been used successfully by both adults and children (Driscoll, Gwinnutt,

Nancarrow et al., 1995; Scott, 1981; Wattenmaker, Kasser, McGravey, 1990).

Caution is recommended when using nitrous oxide because of the possibility of toxicity, especially in patients who are exposed to it repeatedly over a prolonged period of time (Choiniere, 1994). It is contraindicated in patients with altered sensorium, pulmonary disorders (pneumothorax, pulmonary blebs), bowel obstruction, air embolism, chronic pulmonary disease, or suspected decompression sickness (AHCPR, 1992; Choiniere, 1994).

Appropriate precautions should be taken to prevent environmental contamination with nitrous oxide and possible inhalation of pure nitrous oxide. This can be accomplished by using a commercially available scavenger system as described earlier (AHCPR, 1992; Jacox, Carr, Payne et al., 1994; Wattenmaker, Kasser, McGravey et al., 1990).

NONDRUG APPROACHES TO PROCEDURAL PAIN

Although local anesthetics, opioids, and benzodiazepines are the mainstay of procedural pain and sedation management, nondrug pain relief methods may be beneficial as supplements. In fact, the AHCPR acute and cancer pain management clinical practice guidelines recommend the use of nondrug interventions to complement pharmacologic pain management plans (AHCPR, 1992; Jacox, Carr, Payne et al., 1994).

Before using nondrug interventions, patients need clarification of the relationship between nondrug pain relief measures and the use of analgesics to control pain. It is important that patients, families, and caregivers understand that nondrug methods are used most often when pain is reasonably well controlled with analgesics. They are not used as a substitute for analgesics when analgesics are indicated. Although helpful in reducing anxiety and promoting relaxation, nondrug methods have been shown to actually relieve pain in only a few well-controlled studies.

Patients should be asked before their procedure if they are interested in the use of nondrug interventions. Describing a few will help patients understand better what is meant. They can then be asked what methods they have found effective in the past in dealing with painful or stressful situations. If they are familiar with a technique, they can describe what happened when they used it. If they had good results with the technique, they should be encouraged to use it before and during the procedure. For example, if a patient is a woman and has children, she may have used relaxation and distraction techniques to help control her labor pain. Many women find these same nondrug methods effective for the stressful time before and during a procedure.

Caregivers can suggest a few methods to patients who are unfamiliar with nondrug interventions and want to learn. Not everyone will benefit from the same nondrug method. The type of procedure and whether the patient will need to participate must be considered. It is important to assess a patient's capabilities, such as attention span, concentration, and energy, if the nondrug method requires patient participation. Patients who are sedated, confused, exhausted, frustrated, or in pain will have a difficult time learning. In these cases or until patients are able to learn, physical methods, such as cold and massage, can be used (Syrjala, 1993).

It is important to consider the time it takes to teach patients how to use a nondrug method. The short notice and brevity of many procedures will prohibit teaching some of the methods, such as guided imagery and meditation, if these are completely unfamiliar concepts to the patient. However, when patients are faced with the prospect of repetitive procedures, no matter how brief, caregivers should take time to help them perfect methods that can be used with each procedure.

Patients should be encouraged to practice their nondrug technique before their procedure. During the procedure they may be embarrassed or not remember to use the techniques, so it may be necessary to remind them.

In addition to nondrug interventions, caregivers can implement a number of very simple approaches to help reduce the anxiety, distress, and discomfort patients experience with procedures and hospitalization in general. Box 8.7 lists approaches that can be used for patients of various ages and in a variety of health care settings. Also see Chapter 9 for more on nondrug pain relief methods.

Cognitive-Behavioral Methods

The basis for use of cognitive-behavioral methods is that thoughts influence feelings, and if thoughts (and behaviors) can be changed, so can feelings and even sensations, such as pain (Syrjala, 1993). Cognitive-behavioral methods require the patient's active participation. They include distraction, imagery, and relaxation (AHCPR, 1992).

Distraction has been found to be an effective technique, preferred by patients over other techniques, for coping with pain (McCaul, Malott, 1984). A wide variety of distraction techniques can be used by patients during procedures. Some, such as imagining a pleasant place, praying, reading, and looking at a kaleidoscope, involve focusing on mental activity. Self-statements, such as "I will feel better" or "Relaxing will help me feel better," also involve mental activity (Wong, 1996a; Syrjala, 1993).

Other distraction activities focus on active behaviors. These include rhythmic breathing and progressive relaxation. Talking with a family member or friend, which is also an active behavior, is a highly effective distracter (Syrjala, 1993).

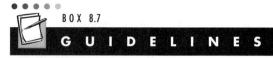

BOX 8.7

GUIDELINES

REDUCING ANXIETY, DISTRESS, AND DISCOMFORT

- Reduce environmental stimuli: Reduce noise, speak softly, set telephone and intercom volumes as low as possible, pad trash receptacles, close doors softly, limit traffic, and after procedures, lower lights if possible.
- Slow down; allow patients "time out" to "catch up" with the pain; allow recovery between procedures and interventions.
- Handle tubes, catheters, and drains gently.
- Remove tape and dressings slowly and gently.
- Ask patients if they would like to perform their own dressing changes and apply topical medications.
- Use moisture-retentive dressings that will not adhere to the wound bed; use adhesive dissolvents if not contraindicated.
- Ask patients how best to turn and position them; do this slowly and gently.
- Allow uninterrupted sleep; cluster care activities so that patients are rested.
- Establish central line instead of repeated venous and arterial punctures when appropriate; in premature infants and neonates, use umbilical catheter, if in place, instead of repeated venous and arterial punctures.
- Allow parent or guardian to stay with infants and children during procedures (e.g., venipuncture, heelstick, immunization, circumcision); for adult patients, ask if they wish to have a family member or friend stay.
- Swaddle infants; use cutaneous stimulation techniques (e.g., for term neonates, rub the opposite extremity during heel puncture); provide neonates and premature infants with objects for sucking and grasping.

May be duplicated for use in clinical practice. From McCaffery M, Pasero C: *Pain: Clinical manual*, p. 390. Copyright © 1999, Mosby, Inc.

Box 8.7 provides guidelines that can be used to reduce the anxiety, distress, and discomfort of procedures and hospitalization in general.

Information from Franck LS, Gregory GA: Clinical evaluation and treatment of infant pain in the neonatal intensive care unit. In Schechter N, Berde CB, Yaster M, editors: *Pain in infants, children, and adolescents*, pp 519-535, Baltimore, 1993, Williams & Wilkins; Kain ZN, Mayes LC, Caramico MD et al.: Parental presence during induction of anesthesia, *Anesthesiology* 84:1060-1067, 1996; Krasner D: Managing pain from pressure ulcers, *Am J Nurs* 95(6):22, 24, June 1995.

Patients can learn to use music for both distraction and relaxation. Providing background music or providing patients with the materials and equipment for listening to music is a method that is used effectively for relaxation in many settings, including chronic and cancer pain care centers, cancer treatment centers, preoperative holding areas, outpatient surgery, pediatric units, and postanesthesia care units (PACUs) (Smith, Pasero, McCaffery, 1997).

Researchers who study music have found that patients who listen to music may have more satisfying experiences in the hospital. For example, in a 1992 study, patients who listened to music in the PACU reported their PACU experience as significantly more pleasant than those who did not listen to music (Heitz, Symreng, Scamman, 1992).

The use of music for relaxation in the hospital setting has some drawbacks. One potential obstacle is that equipment is needed to play the music. Quite often hospital volunteers enjoy raising money for projects like the purchase of compact disc (CD) or cassette players, CDs, cassettes, portable tape recorders, and headphones. Until equipment can be purchased, interested patients can be encouraged to bring their own portable equipment from home. Another consideration is that hospital equipment will be shared by many patients. If headphones are reused, they will need to be made of a material that can be cleaned repeatedly (Smith, Pasero, McCaffery, 1997).

Another potential drawback is that listening to music can be an unpleasant experience if patients are not allowed to choose the type of music they want to hear. This makes it necessary to maintain a wide variety of music selections to accommodate different patient preferences (Smith, Pasero, McCaffery, 1997). Box 8.8 lists tips on using music for distraction and relaxation.

Cutaneous Stimulation

Cold can be very effective in reducing the pain of many procedures, especially when pain is expected to be localized or caused by inflammation. Well-wrapped cold packs can be applied to the site before a procedure and applied again afterwards for continued pain relief. Although patients tend to be reluctant to try cold, some research has shown that it relieves pain more effectively than heat. Compared with heat, cold tends to relieve pain faster and longer. Cold also has the beneficial therapeutic effect of vasoconstriction to reduce bleeding and edema. Patients can be shown a lightweight, well-wrapped cold pack and asked to evaluate whether it is too cool or too heavy. Modifications can be made on the basis of their comments.

Counterirritation techniques that involve applying peripheral, nonpainful stimulation to block pain sensations include simple massage, pressure, or scratching. For example, massaging the opposite leg of a full-term infant during a heelstick may reduce the pain of the procedure (Franck, Gregory, 1993). The simple act of scratching the skin before and during local anesthetic infiltration has been found to reduce the number of patients who report feeling the needle stick and infiltration (Bourke, 1985).

COMMENTS ON SELECTED PROCEDURES

Ensuring correct body alignment and positioning patients for comfort during procedures is important to re-

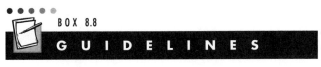

BOX 8.8

GUIDELINES

USING MUSIC FOR DISTRACTION AND RELAXATION

1. Use small, portable tape players with headsets. Headsets block out environmental noises, allow for a variety of music to be played by several patients in the same care area, and patients can fast-forward and reverse their music selection as desired.
2. Build a library of tapes with a variety of musical styles and artists. Become familiar with the tapes in the library so that recommendations can be made to patients.
3. Ask patients before their procedures and before surgery if they enjoy listening to music. Explain the purposes and benefits of listening to music to relax. Tell them that the use of music is not intended to reduce pain and that analgesics will be given for pain control and sedation for anxiety. If they want to listen to music, ask them what kind of music makes them feel happy and relaxed. Make suggestions on the basis of their responses. Music can be offered postoperatively when it is not possible to talk to patients before surgery. Be sure their pain is under control and that they are lucid enough to understand instructions.
4. Allow patients to select their own music.
5. Teach patients how to use the tape player and headsets. Be sure the headset fits and that the patient is satisfied with the volume.
6. At regular intervals, assess the patient's ability to use the tape player and offer other music selections.

May be duplicated for use in clinical practice. From McCaffery M, Pasero C: *Pain: Clinical manual,* p. 391. Copyright © 1999, Mosby, Inc.

Box 8.8 provides tips on the effective use of music to help patients relax during procedures and hospitalization.

Information from Smith NK, Pasero C, McCaffery M: Using nondrug methods during procedures, *Am J Nurs* 97(8):18-20, August 1997.

duce the pain of long procedures and to prevent later pain. For example, taking care to correctly position patients in stirrups for obstetric and gynecologic procedures can help prevent postprocedure neuropathies. In addition, when positioned comfortably with pain adequately controlled, patients are better able to remain still so that the procedure can be completed expeditiously.

Reducing Back Pain After Angiography

Traditional practice after femoral access for cardiac angiography is bedrest and immobilization for 4 to 24 hours after the procedure to prevent delayed bleeding (bleeding after 24 hours of initial hemostasis of the ves-

sel). Patients who receive heparin and undergo this procedure are at higher risk for delayed bleeding than those who do not receive heparin (Pooler-Lunse, Barkman, Bock et al., 1996).

Traditional practice and modified positioning and mobilization were compared for their effect on back pain and delayed bleeding in patients who had received heparin and undergone angiography (Pooler-Lunse, Barkman, Bock et al., 1996). Patients in group one were treated according to traditional protocol with 6 hours of bedrest and immobilization of the affected limb. Patients in group two were treated according to a modified routine that included raising the head of the bed 45 degrees for a minimum of 15 minutes, after which time patients could choose the head of bed height from flat to 45 degrees. Patients in group two also stood at the bedside for a minimum of 2 minutes at 4 hours after angiography, and they were given the opportunity to sit on a commode or stand to void. Patients in both groups received analgesics, backrubs, and a flat pillow for the lumbar area of the back. The researchers found no differences between the two groups in incidence or severity of delayed bleeding (one patient in each group), and the patients in group two experienced significantly less pain intensity, less pain at each assessment interval, and less pain overall.

Reducing the Discomfort of IM Injections

Because of unreliable absorption, the IM route is no longer recommended for the administration of opioid analgesics. The IM route should also be avoided with all other drugs whenever possible, especially in children and the elderly. Children find IM injections especially painful and frightening, and the elderly suffer from muscle wasting (AHCPR, 1992). Nevertheless, IM injections continue to be a frequent occurrence, sometimes because equipment, such as PCA pumps, for using another route, is not available. Clinicians may lack the skill and knowledge required for delivering analgesics by other routes, such as the epidural route, or the drug may be available only in the IM form, such as with immunizations. However, when the IM route cannot be avoided, pain and tissue trauma of injections may be reduced by improving the technique used to administer them (Box 8.9).

The Z-track method for administering IM injections has been found to be less painful than the traditional injection technique. The traditional IM technique allows leakage of the solution from the site, which can cause significant pain and irritation. The Z-track method involves pulling the skin down or to one side before the injection, then injecting slowly, removing the needle smoothly, and then allowing the skin to return to its original position. This prevents painful leakage by sealing

Text continued on p. 394.

GUIDELINES

REDUCING THE DISCOMFORT OF IM INJECTIONS

1. Match syringe size as closely as possible to volume injected.
2. Use a filter needle to draw up medication from vial or ampule.
3. If a prefilled syringe is used to draw up more medication, instill the complete dose into another syringe.
4. Change to a new dry, sterile needle before injecting.
5. If medication has dripped from the needle of a prefilled unit-dose syringe, wipe it clean with a dry, sterile pad before injecting.
6. Assess the amount of subcutaneous tissue at the site to determine needle length required to penetrate the muscle. Generally, use a 1.5 inch needle for adults, a 1 inch needle for children and infants as young as 4 months old and possibly as young as 2 months old.
7. Use the ventrogluteal site (Figure 8.1) as the primary site of injection for patients of any age. As an alternative, the vastus lateralis site (Figure 8.2) is preferred over the dorsogluteal site (Figure 8.3) because it contains no major nerves or vessels. The deltoid site (Figure 8.4) is associated with less site pain and fewer local side effects from vaccines compared with the vastus lateralis site.

8. Position patient correctly:
   - Side-lying: Flex knee of the side on which injection will be given, then pivot leg forward from the hip 20 degrees.
   - Supine: Flex knee of the side on which injection will be given.
   - Prone: Point toes in to internally rotate the femur.
   - Standing and using dorsogluteal site: Lean against a counter, put weight on side opposite injection site, point toes on injection side toward opposite foot.
   - Prone or on side and using dorsogluteal site: Point toes inward to internally rotate femur and relax muscle.
9. Allow skin antiseptic to dry completely.
10. Use the Z-track method (Figure 8.5): Pull skin down or to one side, insert needle quickly and smoothly at a 90-degree angle, inject slowly (10 sec/ml), wait 10 sec before smoothly withdrawing the needle, apply pressure at the site.
11. Limit volume of injection; if the muscle is large and healthy, up to 4 ml may be injected. If injections are to be given on an ongoing basis, consider concentrating the medication to reduce the volume.
12. Do not massage the site after injection.
13. Avoid using the same site twice in a row.

Box 8.9 provides suggestions for reducing the discomfort of IM injections.

ml, milliliter; *sec,* second.

Information from Barnhill BJ, Holbert MD, Jackson NM et al.: Using pressure to decrease the pain of intramuscular injections, *J Pain Symptom Manage* 12(1):52-58, 1996; Beecroft PC, Kongelbeck SR: How safe are intramuscular injections? *AACN Clin Issues* 5(2):207-215, 1994; Beyea SC, Nicoll LH: Back to basics: Administering IM injections the right way, *Am J Nurs* 96(1):34-35, January 1996; Feldman HR: Practice may make perfect but research makes a difference, *Nursing* 87(7): 82, 1987; Meissner JE: Using the vastus lateralis for injections, *Nursing* 87(7):82, 1987; Rettig FM, Southby J: Using different body positions to reduce discomfort from dorsogluteal injection, *Nurs Res* 31:219, July/August 1982; Wong D: *Wong and Whaley's clinical manual of pediatric nursing,* ed 4, St. Louis, 1996, Mosby; Wong D: *Wong and Whaley's essentials of pediatric nursing,* ed 5, St. Louis, 1997, Mosby.

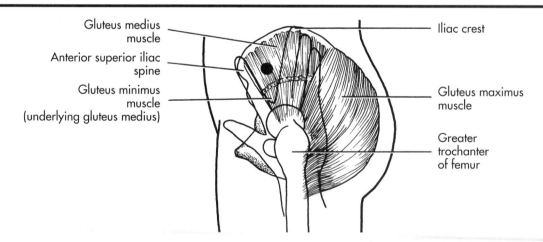

Gluteus medius muscle
Anterior superior iliac spine
Gluteus minimus muscle (underlying gluteus medius)
Iliac crest
Gluteus maximus muscle
Greater trochanter of femur

● ● ● ● ●
FIGURE 8.1   Ventrogluteal site for IM injections. To locate the ventrogluteal site, palpate the greater trochanter of the femur with the heel of the hand. The index and middle fingers are spread to form a V from the anterior superior iliac spine to just below the iliac crest. The triangle formed between the index finger, the middle finger, and the crest of the ilium is the injection site.

From Pagliaro AM, Pagliaro LA: *Pharmacologic aspects of nursing,* St. Louis, 1986, Mosby.

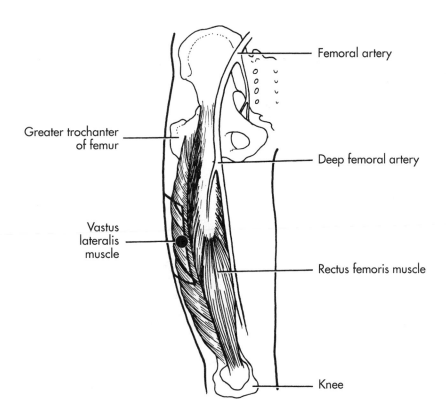

Femoral artery

Greater trochanter of femur

Deep femoral artery

Vastus lateralis muscle

Rectus femoris muscle

Knee

May be duplicated for use in clinical practice. As appears in McCaffery M, Pasero C: *Pain: Clinical manual,* p. 393, 1999, Mosby, Inc.

FIGURE 8.2   **Vastus lateralis site for IM injections.** The vastus lateralis site is the preferred site in patients of all ages. The site is located on the medial outer aspect in the center third portion of the thigh in children. The belly of the muscle is one third the distance between the greater trochanter and the knee. In adults, the site for injection is from one hand's breadth below the greater trochanter to a hand's breadth above the knee.

From Pagliaro AM, Pagliaro LA: *Pharmacologic aspects of nursing,* St. Louis, 1986, Mosby.

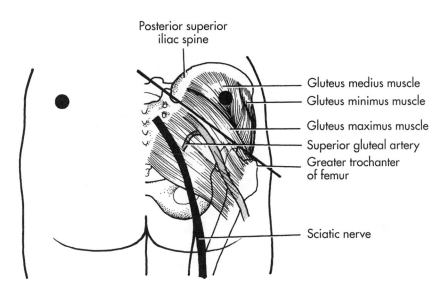

Posterior superior iliac spine

Gluteus medius muscle
Gluteus minimus muscle

Gluteus maximus muscle
Superior gluteal artery
Greater trochanter of femur

Sciatic nerve

May be duplicated for use in clinical practice. As appears in McCaffery M, Pasero C: *Pain: Clinical manual,* p. 393, 1999, Mosby, Inc.

FIGURE 8.3   **Dorsogluteal site for IM injections.** To locate the dorsogluteal site for injection, draw an imaginary line from the posterior superior iliac spine to the greater trochanter of the femur. Because this line is lateral and parallel to the sciatic nerve, a site selected laterally and superiorly will be away from the nerve and the superior gluteal artery.

From Pagliaro AM, Pagliaro LA: *Pharmacologic aspects of nursing,* St. Louis, 1986, Mosby.

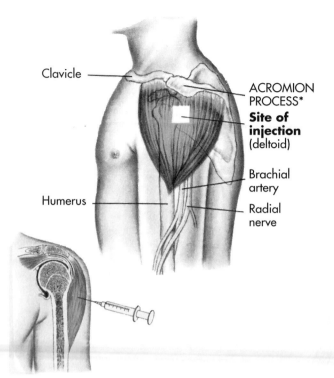

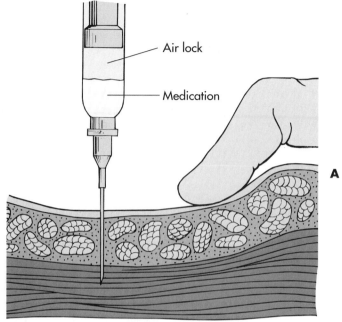

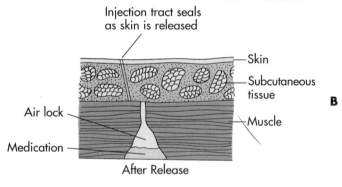

May be duplicated for use in clinical practice. As appears in McCaffery M, Pasero C: *Pain: Clinical manual*, p. 394, 1999, Mosby, Inc.

 FIGURE 8.4 **Deltoid site for IM injections.** To locate the densest area of the deltoid muscle and to avoid the radial nerve and deep brachial artery, locate the site 1 to 2 inches below the lower edge of the acromion process.

From Wong DL: *Whaley and Wong's essentials of pediatric nursing*, ed 5, St. Louis, 1997, Mosby.

May be duplicated for use in clinical practice. As appears in McCaffery M, Pasero C: *Pain: Clinical manual*, p. 394, 1999, Mosby, Inc.

 FIGURE 8.5 **Z-track method for administering IM injections. A,** Z-track method involves pulling the skin down or to one side, inserting the needle quickly and smoothly at a 90-degree angle, injecting slowly (10 sec/ml), and waiting 10 seconds before smoothly withdrawing the needle and applying pressure at the site. **B,** The Z-track left after injection prevents the deposit of medication through sensitive tissue.

From Potter PA, Perry AG: *Fundamentals of nursing*, ed 4, St. Louis, 1997, Mosby.

the injected solution into the musculature (Beyea, Nicoll, 1996; Keen, 1986) (See Box 8.9 and Figure 8.5).

A pinch-grasp technique has been shown to reduce the discomfort of IM injections into the deltoid muscle. This technique involves grasping the muscle, pulling it about 1/2 to 1 inch toward the person administering the injection, and applying a pinching pressure hard enough to cause mild discomfort. Resting the wrist about 3 inches from the site of injection, the injection is given at a 90 degree angle (Locsin, 1985) (Figure 8.6). Before pinching the skin, warn the patient and explain the purpose.

Manual pressure over the injection site may help reduce the pain associated with dorsogluteal IM injections of immune globulin in adults. In one study investigators applied pressure over the injection site with the noninjecting thumb until resistance was felt, then maintained that pressure for 10 seconds in patients in group 1 (Barnhill, Holbert, Jackson et al., 1996). They applied no manual pressure over the injections sites of patients in group 2. For both groups, the skin at the injection site was held taut between the noninjecting thumb and index finger, and the immune globulin was injected over a period of 5 to 10 seconds. Patients in group 1 reported signifi-

cantly less injection pain on injection compared with patients in group 2.

The use of cold in addition to manual pressure to reduce the pain of IM injection also has been studied (Hillman, Jarman, 1986). Ice and "slight" pressure applied to the IM injection site for 15 to 20 seconds before injection was found to reduce pain at deeper penetrations than without ice and pressure.

Application of cold alone can be an effective pain reliever in some patients. A 5-minute ice massage to the site contralateral to that used for a bone marrow aspira-

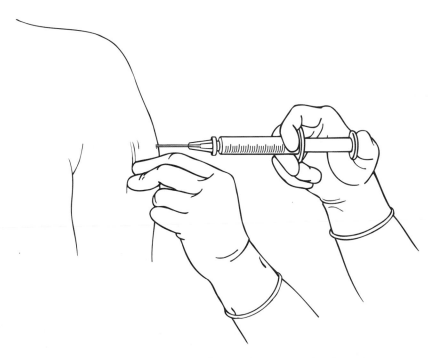

May be duplicated for use in clinical practice. From McCaffery M, Pasero C: *Pain: Clinical manual,* p. 395. Copyright © 1999, Mosby, Inc.

● ● ● ● ●
F I G U R E 8.6   **Pinch-grasp technique for administering IM injections.** A pinch-grasp technique has been shown to reduce the discomfort of IM injections into the deltoid muscle. This technique involves grasping the muscle, pulling it about 1/2 to 1 inch toward the person administering the injection, and applying a pinching pressure hard enough to cause mild discomfort. The injection is given at a 90-degree angle.

tion reduced pain during the aspiration procedure (Hudziak, 1983). It seems likely that ice massage would be effective in reducing the pain of injection as well. However, in preschool children, the use of ice failed to reduce the children's pain-distress associated with injections (Gedaly-Duff, Burns, 1992).

Refrigerant topical anesthetic sprays, such as ethyl chloride, provide ideal "pinpoint" analgesia for IM injections (see p. 377). Even gentle slapping of the area before an IM injection can reduce its discomfort (Goodfriend, 1987). Obviously, before the slap, the patient should be warned and the reason explained.

Atraumatic Suturing of Lacerations

Noninvasive tissue adhesive (Histoacryl blue) may be a less painful method for closing laceration wounds than traditional suturing (Osmond, Klassen, Quinn, 1995). It is recommended that, after cleansing the laceration and approximating the wound edges, a few drops of the tissue adhesive be applied to the opposed edges. Manual approximation of the wound should be maintained for 30 seconds while adhesion takes place.

Compared with invasive suturing, the noninvasive tissue adhesive method for closing lacerations was found to be similar in terms of efficacy, complication rate, cosmetic outcome, rate of dehiscence, and infection (Osmond, Klassen, Quinn, 1995). The noninvasive tissue adhesive took less time to apply and required less additional supply cost and fewer follow-up appointments. Although the noninvasive tissue adhesive is relatively expensive compared with suture materials, a cost analysis found that the undissolvable suture method had the highest total cost and the noninvasive tissue adhesive method the lowest.

References

Abbott K, Fowler-Kerry S: The use of a topical refrigerant anesthetic to reduce injection pain in children, *J Pain Symptom Manage* 10(8):584-590, 1995.
Abbott Laboratories: Fentanyl oralet® package insert, Abbott Park, Ill, 1995, Abbott Laboratories.
Adrian ER: Intranasal Versed: the future of pediatric conscious sedation, *Pediatr Nurs* 20(3):287-292, 1994.
Agency for Health Care Policy and Research (AHCPR): *Acute pain management: operative or medical procedures and trauma: clinical practice guideline,* AHCPR Pub. No. 92-0032, Rockville, Md, Agency for Health Care Policy and Research, Public Health Service, US Department of Health and Human Services, February 1992.
American Academy of Pediatrics (AAP) Committee on drugs: Reappraisal of lytic cocktail/demerol, phenergan, and thorazine (DPT) for the sedation of children, *Pediatrics* 95(4):598-602, 1995.
American Pain Society (APS): *Principles of analgesic use in the treatment of acute pain and cancer pain,* ed 3, Glenview, Ill, 1992, APS.
Anderson CTM, Zeltzer LK, Fanurik D: Procedural pain. In Schechter N, Berde CB, Yaster M, editors: *Pain in infants, children, and adolescents,* pp 435-458, Baltimore, 1993, Williams & Wilkins.

Ashburn MA, Guathier M, Love G et al.: Iontophoretic administration of 2% lidocaine HCl and 1:100,000 epinephrine in humans, *Clin J Pain* 13(1):22-26, 1997.

ASTRA USA, Inc: *Naropin (ropivacaine) package insert*, Westborough, Mass, 1996, ASTRA.

ASTRA USA, Inc: EMLA cream package insert, *Dollops* 4(1), 1997.

Bahruth AJ: Peripherally inserted central catheter insertion problems associated with topical anesthesia, *J Intravenous Nurs* 19(1):32-34, 1996.

Barnhill BJ, Holbert MD, Jackson NM et al.: Using pressure to decrease the pain of intramuscular injections, *J Pain Symptom Manage* 12(1): 52-58, 1996.

Barr RG: Pain experiences in children: developmental and clinical characteristics. In Wall PD, Melzack R, editors: *Textbook of pain*, New York, 1994, Churchill Livingstone.

Berde CB, Kain ZN: Pain management in infants and children. In Motoyama EK, Davis PJ, editors: *Smith's anesthesia for infants and children*, pp 385-402, St. Louis, 1996, Mosby.

Berryman D, Marketing Manager, Anesta Corp., Salt Lake City, UT: personal communication by telephone with Chris Pasero, August 21, 1997.

Beyea SC, Nicoll LH: Back to basics: administering IM injections the right way, *Am J Nurs* 96(1):34-35, January 1996.

Bonica JJ, Butler SH: Local anesthesia and regional blocks. In Wall PD, Melzack R, editors: *Textbook of pain*, ed 3, pp 997-1023, New York, 1994, Churchill Livingstone.

Bourke DL: Counter-irritation reduces pain during cutaneous needle insertion, *Anesth Analg* 6:266, 1985 (letter).

Boyd MJ: Nitrous oxide/oxygen: an additional method of pain control, *Oncol Nurs Forum* Suppl 11(2):119, 1984.

Broadley K, Ling J: The use of topical refrigerant anesthetic to reduce injection pain in children, *J Pain Symptom Manage* 12(4):208, 1996 (letter).

Carroll KC, Magruder CC: The role of analgesics and sedatives in the management of pain and agitation during weaning from mechanical ventilation, *Crit Care Nurs Q* 15(4):68-77, 1993.

Catterall W, Mackie K: Local anesthetics. In Hardman JG, Limbird LE, editors: *Goodman and Gilman's the pharmacological basis of therapeutics*, ed 9, pp 331-347, New York, 1996, McGraw-Hill.

Choiniere M: Pain of burns. In Wall PD, Melzack R, editors: *Textbook of pain*, New York, 1994, Churchill Livingstone.

Covino G, Wildsmith JAW: Clinical pharmacology of local anesthetic agents. In Cousins MJ, Bridenbaugh PO, editors: *Neural blockade*, Philadelphia, 1998, Lippincott-Raven.

Deglin JH, Vallerand AH: *Davis's drug guide for nurses*, ed 5, Philadelphia, 1995, FA Davis.

Driscoll PA, Gwinnutt CL, Nancarrow J: Analgesia in the emergency department, *Pain Rev* 2(3):187-202, 1995.

Drug facts and comparisons, St. Louis, 1996, Wolters Kluwer.

Ducharme J: Emergency pain management: a Canadian association of emergency physicians (CAEP) consensus document, *J Emerg Med* 12(6):855-866, 1994.

Eriksson M, Englesson S, Niklasson F et al.: Effect of lignocaine and pH on propofol-induced pain, *Br J Anaesth* 78:502-506, 1997.

Ernst AA, Marvez E, Nick T et al.: Lidocaine adrenaline tetracaine gel versus tetracaine adrenaline cocaine gel for topical anesthesia in linear scalp and facial lacerations in children aged 5 to 17 years, *Pediatrics* 95(2):255-258, 1995.

Feldman HR: Practice may make perfect but research makes a difference, *Nursing* 87(3):47-48, 1987.

Fitzgerald M, Millard C, McIntosh N: Cutaneous hypersensitivity following peripheral tissue damage in newborn infants and its reversal with topical anaesthesia, *Pain* 39:31-39, 1989.

Franck LS, Gregory GA: Clinical evaluation and treatment of infant pain in the neonatal intensive care unit. In Schechter N, Berde CB, Yaster M, editors: *Pain in infants, children, and adolescents*, pp 519-535, Baltimore, 1993, Williams & Wilkins.

Gedaly-Duff V, Burns C: Reducing children's pain-distress associated with injections using cold: a pilot study, *J Am Acad Nurse Practitioners* 4(3):95-100, 1992.

Goodfriend B: Slap down injection discomfort, *Consultant* 27:154, March 1987.

Grass JA, Sakima NT, Valley M et al.: Assessment of ketorolac as an adjuvant to fentanyl patient-controlled epidural analgesia after radical retropubic prostatectomy, *Anesthesiology* 78:642-648, 1993.

Graves JR, Moran TJ, Porter BR et al.: Propofol as an adjunct in the treatment of cancer-related pain, *Pain Digest* 6:371-373, 1996.

Gronert BJ, Motoyama EK: Induction of anesthesia and endotracheal intubation. In Motoyama EK, Davis PJ, editors: *Smith's anesthesia for infants and children*, pp 281-312, St. Louis, 1996, Mosby.

Hayward CJ, Nafziger AN, Kohlhepp SJ et al.: Investigation of bioequivalence and tolerability of intramuscular ceftriaxone injections by using 1% lidocaine, buffered lidocaine, and sterile water diluents, *Antimicrob Agents Chemother* 40(2):485-487, 1996.

Heitz L, Symreng T, Scamman FL: Effects of music therapy in the postanesthesia care unit: a nursing intervention, *J Post Anesth Nurs* 7(1):22-31, 1992.

Hillman H, Jarman D: Freezing skin, *Nurs Times* 82:40-41, 1986.

Hobbs WR, Rall TW, Verdoorn TA: Hypnotics and sedatives; ethanol. In Hardman JG, Limbird LE, editors: *Goodman and Gilman's the pharmacological basis of therapeutics*, ed 9, pp 361-396, New York, 1996, McGraw-Hill.

Houry D: Topical lidocaine adrenaline tetracaine (LAT) gel, *West J Med* 167(2):79-81, 1997.

Hudziak B: Contralateral ice massage during bone marrow aspiration, *PRN Forum* 2:5, 1983.

Illingworth KA, Simpson KH: *Anaesthesia and analgesia in emergency medicine*, New York, 1994, Oxford University Press.

IOMED, Inc: Iontocaine package insert, Salt Lake City, Utah, 1996, IOMED, Inc.

Irwin MG, Thompson N, Kenny GNC: Patient-maintained propofol sedation, *Anaesthesia* 52:525-530, 1997.

Jacox A, Carr DB, Payne R et al.: *Management of cancer pain: clinical practice guideline* No. 9, AHCPR Publication No. 94-0592, Rockville, Md, Agency for Health Care Policy and Research, U.S. Department of Health and Human Services, Public Health Service, March 1994.

Johnson KO, editor, Johns Hopkins Hospital: *The Harriet Lane handbook*, ed 13, St. Louis, 1993, Mosby.

Kain ZN, Mayes LC, Caramico MD et al.: Parenteral presence during induction of anesthesia, *Anesthesiology* 84:1060-1067, 1996.

Keen MF: Comparison of intramuscular injection techniques to reduce site discomfort and lesions, *Nurs Res* 35:207-210, 1986.

Klafta JM, Klock A, Young CJ et al.: The effects of propofol on induced pain in humans, *Anesthesiology* 83(3A):A1, September 1995 (abstract).

Krane EJ, Davis PJ, Smith RM: Preoperative preparation. In Motoyama EK, Davis PJ, editors: *Smith's anesthesia for infants and children*, pp 213-228, St. Louis, 1996, Mosby.

Krasner D: Managing pain from pressure ulcers, *Am J Nurs* 95(6):22, 24, June 1995.

Lander J, Brady-Fryer B, Metcalfe JB et al.: Comparison of ring block, dorsal penile nerve block, and topical anesthesia for neonatal circumcision, *JAMA* 278(24):2157-2162, 1997.

Lee MG, Hanna W, Harding H: Sedation for upper gastrointestinal endoscopy: a comparative study of midazolam and diazepam, *Gastrointest Endosc* 35(2):82-84, 1989.

Locsin RG: Pinch-grasp technique, *PRN Forum* 4:4-5, 1985.

Lugo R, Fishbein M, Nahata MC et al.: Complication to intranasal midazolam, *Pediatrics* 92(4):638, October 1993 (letter).

Lugo-Janer G, Padial M, Sanchez JL: Less painful alternatives for local anesthesia, *J Dermat Surg Oncol* 19(3):237-240, 1993.

Mader TJ, Playe SJ, Garb JL: Reducing the pain of local anesthetic infiltration: warming and buffering have a synergistic effect, *Ann Emerg Med* 23(3):550-554, 1994.

Marshall BE, Longnecker DE: General anesthetics. In Hardman JG, Limbird LE, editors: *Goodman and Gilman's the pharmacological basis of therapeutics*, ed 9, pp 307-330, New York, 1996, McGraw-Hill.

Martinez S, Achauer B, Dobkin de Rios M: Ketamine use in a burn center: hallucinogen or debridement facilitator? *J Psychoactive Drugs* 17(2):45-48, 1985.

Maxwell LG, Yaster M, Wetzel RC et al.: Penile nerve block for newborn circumcision, *Obstet Gynecol* 70:415, 1987.

McCafferty DF, Woolfson AD, Boston V: In vivo assessment of percutaneous local anaesthetic preparations, *Br J Anaesth* 62:17-21, 1989.

McCafferty DF, Woolfson AD, Handley J et al.: Effect of percutaneous local anaesthetics on pain reduction during pulse dye laser treatment of portwine stains, *Br J Anaesth* 78:286-289, 1997.

McCaul KD, Malott JM: Distraction and coping with pain, *Psychol Bull* 95(3):516-533, 1984.

McGlone R, Bodenham A: Reducing the pain of intradermal lignocaine injection by pH buffering, *Arch Emerg Med* 9:147-148, 1990.

Meissner JE: Using the vastus lateralis for injections, *Nursing* 87(7):82, 1987.

Mitchell V, Grange C, Black A et al.: A comparison of midazolam with trimeprazine as an oral premedicant for children, *Anaesthesia* 52:416-421, 1997.

Moroi SE, Lichter PR: Ocular pharmacology. In Hardman JG, Limbird LE, editors: *Goodman and Gilman's the pharmacological basis of therapeutics,* ed 9, pp 1619-1645, New York, 1996, McGraw-Hill.

Morrill GB, Katz MD: The use of lidocaine to reduce the pain induced by potassium chloride infusion, *J Intravenous Nurs* 11(2):105-108, 1988.

Morton NS: Abolition of injection pain due to propofol in children, *Anaesthesia* 45:70, 1990 (letter).

Moyle J: The use of propofol in palliative medicine, *J Pain Symptom Manage* 10(8):643-646, 1995.

Notcutt WG: Transporting patients with overwhelming pain, *Anaesthesia* 49:149-147, 1994.

Ochsenreither JM: Better topical anesthetic, *Am J Nurs* 96(5):21-22, May 1996.

Ohmeda Pharmaceutical Products Division, Inc: Revex (nalmefene HCL injection) package insert, Liberty Corner, NJ, 1995.

Osmond MH, Klassen TP, Quinn JV: Economic comparison of a tissue adhesive and suturing in the repair of pediatric facial lacerations, *J Pediatr* 126(6):892-895, 1995.

Pasero C: *Acute pain management service policy and procedure guideline manual,* Rolling Hills Estates, Calif, 1994, Academy Medical Systems.

Pasero C, Bennett P: Combining analgesia with sedation on the unit, *Am J Nurs* 96(11);17, 19, 1996.

Pasero C, McCaffery M: Avoiding opioid-induced respiratory depression, *Am J Nurs* 94(4):25-31, April 1994.

Pooler-Lunse C, Barkman A, Bock BF et al.: Effects of modified positioning and mobilization to back pain and delayed bleeding in patients who had received heparin and undergone angiography: a pilot study, *Heart Lung* 25(2):117-123, 1996.

Puntillo KA: Pain experiences of intensive care unit patients, *Heart Lung* 19:526-533, 1990.

Puntillo KA: Effects of interpleural bupivacaine on pleural chest tube removal pain: a randomized controlled trial, *Am J Crit Care* 5(2):102-108, 1996.

Reisine T, Pasternak G: Opioid analgesics and antagonists. In Hardman JG, Limbird LE, editors: *Goodman and Gilman's the pharmacological basis of therapeutics,* ed 9, pp 521-555, New York, 1996, McGraw-Hill.

Rettig FM, Southby J: Using different body positions to reduce discomfort from dorsogluteal injection, *Nurs Res* 31:219, July/August 1982.

Rice LJ: Regional anesthesia and analgesia. In Motoyama EK, Davis PJ, editors: *Smith's anesthesia for infants and children,* pp 403-442, St. Louis, 1996, Mosby.

Richtsmeier AJ, Hatcher JW: Buffered lidocaine for skin infiltration prior to hemodialysis, *J Pain Symptom Manage* 10(3):198-203, 1995.

Rust D: Noninvasive, needle-free dermal anesthesia now available, *Oncol Nurs Forum* (Product Information) 24(3):589-590, 1997.

Schichor A, Bernstein B, Weinerman H et al.: Lidocaine as a diluent for ceftriaxone in the treatment of gonorrhea, *Arch Pediatr Adolesc Med* 148(1):72-75, 1994.

Schilling CG, Bank DE, Borchert BA et al.: Tetracaine, epinephrine (adrenalin), and cocaine (TAC) versus lidocaine, epinephrine, and tetracaine (LET) for anesthesia of lacerations in children, *Ann Emerg Med* 25(2):203-208, 1995.

Scott AA: Analgesia with nitrous oxide/oxygen mixtures, *Can Med Assoc J* 125:810, October 15, 1981.

Serour F, Mori J, Barr J: Optimal regional anesthesia for circumcision, *Anesth Analg* 79:129-131, 1994.

Shapiro BA, Warren J, Egol AB et al.: Practice parameters for intravenous analgesia and sedation for adult patients in the intensive care unit: an executive summary, *Crit Care Med* 23(9):1596-1600, 1995.

Siddique NI, D'Alessio JG, Dmochowski RM: A comparative study of topical eutectic mixture of local anesthetics (EMLA) cream and dorsal nerve block for circumcision in adult males, *Reg Anesth* 22(2S):94, March-April 1997.

Sitbon P, Laffron M, Lesage V et al.: Lidocaine plasma concentrations in pediatric patients providing airway topical anesthesia from a calibrated device, *Anesth Analg* 82:1003-1006, 1996.

Smith GA, Strausbaugh SD, Harbeck-Weber C et al.: Comparison of topical anesthetics without cocaine to tetracaine-adrenaline-cocaine and lidocaine infiltration during repair of lacerations: bupivacaine-norepinephrine is an effective new topical anesthetic agent, *Pediatrics* 97:301-307, 1996.

Smith GA, Strausbaugh SD, Harbeck-Weber C et al.: New non-cocaine-containing topical anesthetics compared with tetracaine-adrenaline-cocaine during repair of lacerations, *Pediatrics* 100(5):825-830, 1997.

Smith NK, Pasero C, McCaffery M: Using nondrug methods during procedures, *Am J Nurs* 97(8):18-20, August 1997.

Smith R: Propofol sedation protocol, Bangor, Maine, 1995, Eastern Maine Medical Center Pain Program.

Somerson SJ, Husted CW, Sicilia MR: Insights into conscious sedation, *Am J Nurs* 95(6):26-33, June 1995.

Spencer DM, Miller KA, O'Quin M et al.: Dorsal penile nerve block in neonatal circumcision: chloroprocaine versus lidocaine, *Am J Perinatol* 9(3):214-218, 1992.

Streisand JB, Varvel JR, Stanski DR: Absorption and bioavailability of oral transmucosal fentanyl citrate, *Anesthesiology* 75(2):223-229, 1991.

Syrjala KL: Integrating medical and psychological treatments for cancer pain. In Chapman CR, Foley KM, editors: *Current and emerging issues in cancer pain: research and practice,* pp 393-408, New York, 1993, Raven Press.

Taddio A, Ohlsson A, Einarson TR: A systematic review of lidocaine-prilocaine cream (EMLA) in the treatment of acute pain in neonates (abstract), *Pediatrics* 101(2), 1998.

Taddio A, Stevens B, Craig K et al.: Efficacy and safety of lidocaine-prilocaine cream for pain during circumcision, *N Engl J Med* 336(17):1197-1201, 1997.

Thorpe SJ, Balakrishnan VR, Cook LB: The safety of patient-controlled sedation, *Anesthesia* 52:1144-1150, 1997.

Uhari M: A eutectic mixture of lidocaine and prilocaine for alleviating vaccination pain in infants, *Pediatrics* 92:719-720, 1993.

University of Wisconsin Hospital and Clinics: Guidelines for continuous opioid intravenous infusions (for inpatients), 1997.

Valvano MN, Leffler S: Comparison of bupivacaine and lidocaine/bupivacaine for local anesthesia/digital nerve block, *Ann Emerg Med* 27(4):490-492, 1996.

Varrassi G, Panella l, Piroli A et al.: The effects of perioperative ketorolac infusion on postoperative pain and endocrine-metabolic response, *Anesth Analg* 78:514-519, 1994.

Waldbilling DK, Quinn JV, Stiell IG et al.: Randomized double blind controlled trial comparing room temperature and heated lidocaine for digital nerve block, *Ann Emerg Med* 26:677-681, December 1995.

Wallace J: Patient-controlled sedation enables greater patient participation, *Anesthesiol News* 23(3):2, 1997.

Wattenmaker I, Kasser JR, McGravey A: Self-administered nitrous oxide for fracture reduction in children in an emergency room setting, *J Orthop Trauma* 4(1):35-38, 1990.

Weinreb N: Pain management in special situations. In Salerno E, Willens JS, editors: *Pain management handbook: an interdisciplinary approach,* pp 465-523, St. Louis, 1996, Mosby.

Welborn LG: Pediatric outpatient anesthesia. In Motoyama EK, Davis PJ, editors: *Smith's anesthesia for infants and children,* pp 709-725, St. Louis, 1996, Mosby.

Welch J: Starting painless IVs is easy, *Oncol Nurs Forum* 23(6):973, 1996.

Williamson ML: Circumcision anesthesia: a study of nursing implications for dorsal penile nerve block, *Pediatr Nurs* 23(1):59-63, 1997.

Williamson PS, Williamson ML: Physiologic stress reduction by a local anesthetic during newborn circumcision, *Pediatrics* 71(1):36-40, 1983.

Wong D: Overcoming 'needle phobia' with EMLA, *Am J Nurs* 95(2):24, February 1995a.

Wong D: EMLA's safety for small infants, *Am J Nurs* 95(8):18-19, August 1995b (response to letter to the editor).

Wong D: *Wong and Whaley's clinical manual of pediatric nursing,* ed 4, St. Louis, 1996a, Mosby.

Wong, Donna, RN, PhD, Nursing Consultant at the Children's Hospital at Saint Francis, Tulsa, OK, personal communication with Chris Pasero regarding use of anesthetic refrigerant sprays, October 8, 1996b.

Wong, D: DPT pedi-cocktail: not a good mix, *Am J Nurs* 94(6):14-15, June 1996c.

Wong D: *Wong and Whaley's essentials of pediatric nursing,* ed 5, St. Louis, 1997, Mosby.

Zeltzer LK, Jay SM, Fisher DM: The management of pain associated with pediatric procedures, *Pediatr Clin North Am* 36(4):941-964, 1989.

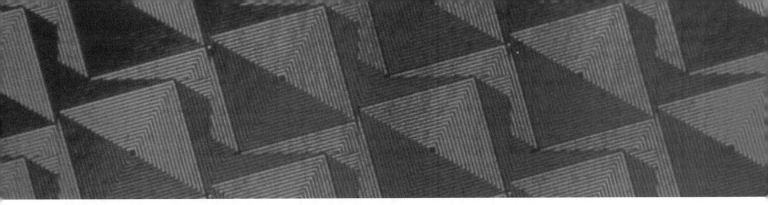

chapter nine

PRACTICAL NONDRUG APPROACHES TO PAIN

Margo McCaffery and Chris Pasero

CHAPTER OUTLINE

TERMINOLOGY

Standardized definitions and classifications of non-drug pain treatments are lacking. The following describe how the terms are used in this chapter.

Cutaneous stimulation: Stimulation of the skin by such methods as heat, cold, and vibration.

Distraction: Sometimes referred to as cognitive refocusing. Attention and concentration are directed at stimuli other than pain.

Imagery: Mental pictures imagined by the patient or suggested by a clinician. Imagery may be used for relaxation or for distraction, depending on the content of the imagery. A peaceful scene may relax, whereas a humorous memory may distract. Some types of imagery are designed to reduce pain, such as imagining that the pain is becoming smaller or floating away.

Nondrug pain treatments: Nonmedicine intervention or treatment for pain management, not necessarily pain relief. Benefits may also include improved sleep, anxiety reduction, improved mood, or increased sense of control.

Relaxation: A state of relative freedom from both anxiety and skeletal muscle tension.

Nondrug measures for pain management refer to a variety of nonmedication treatments. The term "nondrug pain *relief* measures" has been used by authors in previous publications, but we have stopped using the term "relief" because we believe it is misleading. As discussed in the following, these methods do not necessarily relieve pain.

Other terms often used interchangeably with nondrug include nonpharmacologic, alternative, complementary, unconventional, and noninvasive therapies. No uniformly accepted classification system exists for the many categories of nondrug methods. Examples of categories used by various authors include cognitive strategies such as distraction, behavioral approaches such as biofeedback and rehearsal of the painful event, physical interventions such as heat and cold, interpersonal/spiritual measures such as therapeutic touch, and environmental approaches such as music (Fernandez, 1986; Spross, Wolff, 1995). To complicate matters further, some techniques fall into more than one category. Thus the lack of a satisfactory classification system and the absence of standardized definitions tend to produce confusion when this topic is discussed. Terminology and Table 9.1, misconceptions about nondrug approaches to pain, are provided at the beginning of this chapter as an overview of the chapter topic.

The nondrug approaches to pain addressed in this chapter are limited to three categories: cutaneous stimulation, distraction, and relaxation. As with other attempts at categorizing, some techniques fall into more than one category. For example, music may be used as a distraction or as a relaxation technique. Massage may be used as a method of cutaneous stimulation or as a relaxation technique.

Compared with the first edition of this book, limited space is devoted to nondrug approaches to pain management because of the lack of scientific evidence to support their use. Furthermore, no studies to date have identified that the undertreatment of pain is caused by failure to use nondrug approaches. Rather, undertreatment of pain is related to failures in assessment and use of analgesics, topics that are covered extensively in this revision.

The specific nondrug interventions included in this chapter are limited to those that appear to appeal to many members of this society and that are usually easily, quickly, and inexpensively implemented. Before discussing these, the role of nondrug pain treatment will be explored.

ROLE OF NONDRUG PAIN TREATMENTS

Analgesics are the mainstay of pain relief, especially acute pain (e.g., postoperative pain), cancer pain, and pain in the terminally ill. Increasingly, analgesics, including opioids, are also the mainstay of pain relief for patients with chronic nonmalignant pain. However, even with the optimal use of analgesics, most pain is best treated with a combination of drug (analgesic) and nondrug approaches. For some types of mild to moderate pain, nondrug approaches alone may provide sufficient relief.

Over the past several decades numerous nondrug treatments, such as relaxation, physical therapy, transcutaneous electrical stimulation (TENS), and acupuncture, have been integrated into the treatment of chronic nonmalignant pain. These are less likely to be used in the care of patients with acute pain or cancer pain, but efforts are being made to encourage the identification and use of appropriate nondrug techniques in these populations. For example, clinical practice guidelines for cancer pain management include simple nondrug approaches to pain such as relaxation (Jacox, Carr, Payne et al., 1994a,b)

Rationale for Use: Benefits and Limitations

Spross and Wolff's (1995) review of the literature regarding the benefits and rationale for use of nondrug approaches to pain revealed a number of reasons to encourage their use. Although they are not a substitute for analgesics, nondrug methods of pain management may

TABLE 9.1 ● ● ● ● ●

Misconceptions   **Nondrug Approaches to Pain**

MISCONCEPTION	CORRECTION
1. Most nondrug methods reduce the intensity of pain for most patients.	Pain reduction is not a predictable outcome of many nondrug techniques for pain management. Most nondrug techniques do, however, have other benefits, such as making pain more bearable, improving mood, reducing distress, giving the patient a sense of control, and sometimes aiding with sleep.
2. The effectiveness of nondrug approaches to pain management has been well established through research.	Research is limited, and results are conflicting and inconclusive. Most nondrug approaches to pain are promoted on the basis of patient testimonials and clinicians' favorable experiences with the techniques.
3. Nondrug measures should be used instead of analgesics or to extend the interval between doses of analgesics.	Nondrug approaches to pain management are never a substitute for appropriate analgesia and anesthesia. They are used in addition to analgesics, after the analgesics have been tailored to the patient's needs.
4. Many nondrug techniques for pain management relieve pain by increasing endorphin levels, the body's natural opioids.	This is mere speculation. No research has been able to show an increase in endorphins as a result of nondrug pain relief measures. Even if endorphin release occurred, it would provide analgesia for only a very short time.
5. Cutaneous stimulation techniques must be used over the site of pain.	Cutaneous stimulation techniques such as heat, cold, and vibration may be effective when used at sites quite distant from the pain (e.g., contralaterally—on the opposite side of the body).
6. The patient who can be distracted from pain does not have very severe pain, or the pain is not as severe as the patient says.	Although distraction may be difficult to use when pain is severe, those who can use it may find that it makes severe pain more bearable or gives them a sense of control. Severe pain cannot be discounted simply because the patient is able to use distraction.

May be duplicated for use in clinical practice. From McCaffery M, Pasero C: *Pain: Clinical manual*, p. 401. Copyright © 1999, Mosby, Inc.

---

diminish the emotional components of pain, strengthen coping abilities, reduce perceived threat, give the patient and family a sense of control, change expectations, enhance comfort, contribute to pain relief, decrease fatigue, restore hope, promote sleep, and improve quality of life.

Note that reduction in pain intensity is only one of the benefits of nondrug methods, and it is not expected to occur with all techniques. Furthermore, when a specific technique is used, such as relaxation or distraction, pain reduction may occur in some patients but not in others.

Nondrug techniques also may have physiologic effects. Some may decrease stimulation of the sympathetic nervous system, produce muscle relaxation, lower heart rate, improve oxygenation, lower blood pressure, and possibly release endogenous pain-relieving substances. Because the effectiveness of nondrug methods is often explained on the basis of endorphin release, it is important to note that very little evidence supports this. It is mere speculation. Even if endorphin release occurred, this would provide only brief pain relief because endorphins are degraded rapidly (Wallace, 1992).

In a meta-analysis of noninvasive treatment for chronic cancer and noncancer pain, researchers concluded that various techniques seem to be uniformly effective despite differences in types of pain treated and other variables (Malone, Strube, 1988). This raises the possibility that nondrug interventions are effective because they require clinicians to interact with the patient in a manner that includes identifying psychologic factors related to pain, offering hope of relief, establishing an empathic relationship, and spending time working directly with the patient. One may then ask, is the effectiveness of the nondrug intervention any more than a nonspecific placebo effect? It may be the *interpersonal process* of using the technique rather than the specific technique that produces any positive effects.

The unpredictability of outcomes when nondrug techniques are used is clearly one of their disadvantages. In health care, emphasis on outcomes is increasingly important as attempts are made to improve the quality of care but also decrease the cost of care. Health care practices will be determined on the basis of outcomes. It is not possible to devote staff time and institutional financing to the provision of treatments that have not yet been researched and found to be effective. More rigorous research on nondrug approaches to pain is desperately needed to provide guidelines for patient selection and to demonstrate the usefulness of these therapies. The literature on nondrug approaches is littered with testimonials from users and selected patient examples of success. These must be replaced with scientific data.

Avoid Abuse of Nondrug Pain Treatments

In today's society people tend to have a negative attitude toward drugs and an open, if not positive, view of nondrug approaches to treating illness and maintaining health. A potential danger in using nondrug methods of pain management is that they will be substituted for the more effective and appropriate use of analgesics and other medical treatments. The fact that many nondrug methods of pain management are very low risk, inexpensive, easy to do, and readily available may lull clinicians into complacency. However, these methods do have the potential for being abused. For example, rather than combine distraction with appropriate analgesia/anesthesia for a painful procedure, the patient and/or clinician may expect that distraction alone is sufficient. Or, once a patient with cancer pain learns a relaxation technique, the patient may try to endure pain without analgesics. To ensure that nondrug methods of pain management are used appropriately, clinicians must be aware of how both drug and nondrug approaches are regarded by the public—the patients and their families—and health care professionals.

Public attitudes about drug and nondrug methods of pain management

In a telephone interview survey of 1539 adults conducted in 1991, 34% reported using at least one unconventional therapy in the past year (Eisenberg, Kessler, Foster et al., 1993). Back problems and chronic pain were among the most common conditions treated with unconventional methods. Relaxation techniques, chiropractic, and massage were the most common therapies used. Overall the researchers concluded that the use of unconventional therapy in the United States is far greater than previously reported.

In a national telephone survey of 1000 Americans conducted in 1993, 77% said that when they had pain they preferred to try "natural" techniques before turning to medication (Mayday Fund, 1993). Respondents seemed to believe that pain is often psychologic and that will power is the best way to overcome it. Almost all the respondents (95%) agreed with the statement that "stress makes pain worse," and 56% strongly agreed with this. Although 93% put prescription pain medicine at the top of the list of effective methods of pain relief, they were also enthusiastic about massage (72%) and relaxation (70%).

Despite the widespread belief that Americans too readily take "pills" for pain relief, this survey data revealed that the public has many concerns about analgesics. For example, 41% thought physicians tend to overprescribe, 87% were fearful of becoming overreliant on pain medication, and 82% were concerned about becoming addicted. Many (72%) worried that pain medication would lose its effectiveness with continued use.

Interestingly, conflicts between personal values and actions were suggested by some of the respondents' answers. Apparently many people want to view themselves as withstanding pain without quickly resorting to medication. Only 30% said that in general they acted quickly to relieve pain. However, later in the interview when they were asked about a specific recent experience with severe pain, 64% admitted they had acted quickly to relieve it. Of those who acted quickly, most took a nonprescription pain reliever.

Patient's and families' attitudes about drug and nondrug methods of pain management

Public attitudes about pain relievers and nondrug pain treatments are similar to those found in patients with pain. A survey of 270 patients with cancer pain revealed a reluctance to report pain and to use analgesics, resulting in poor pain relief (Ward, Goldberg, Miller-McCauley, 1993). Poor pain relief was associated with concerns about addiction, side effects, injections, tolerance, believing that "good" patients do not complain, and believing that pain is inevitable. Respondents tended to agree with statements such as "Pain medicine cannot really control pain," "People get addicted to pain medicine easily," and "Good patients avoid talking about pain."

Not surprisingly, family members of patients with pain have similar concerns about addiction. A study of 85 family caregivers of patients with cancer pain revealed that caregivers believed it was their responsibility to try to avoid addiction by limiting the amount of medication used (Ferrell, Cohen, Grant, 1991).

Implications for clinicians' attitudes toward use of nondrug pain treatments

Clinicians need to remember that the general public tends to endorse and value a "grin and bear it" approach to pain, wanting to avoid the use of pain medication and to rely on "natural" methods of pain management. Furthermore, the public is fearful of pain medication, particularly "narcotics" and addiction. Finally, the public has very little confidence in the effectiveness of pain medication.

Patients' and families' exaggerated fears about "narcotics" and their skepticism about the ability of health care professionals to relieve pain may increase their interest in and openness to nondrug pain methods. Paralleling this are clinicians' fears of opioids because of lack of knowledge about pain management. This suggests the unfortunate possibility that nondrug pain treatments might be promoted by clinicians and accepted by patients because of unfounded fears of analgesics. Obviously, clinicians must guard against this.

Whenever clinicians introduce nondrug pain treatments to patients and families, the appropriate use of analgesics should be emphasized. Clinicians must be careful to assess whether patients are using nondrug methods because they or their family members have unwarranted fears of analgesics.

The attitudes of clinicians who discuss nondrug treatments with patients deserve careful scrutiny. Very enthusiastic clinicians who emphasize experiences of patients who were exceptionally successful in using nondrug techniques may easily mislead patients in several ways. Patients may expect that the technique is invariably effective. When patients do not benefit from the technique, they may believe that they, rather than the technique, have failed. This scenario was very typical of women in the 1960s and 1970s who tried unsuccessfully to have a painless childbirth or avoid analgesics by using certain methods of childbirth such as the Lamaze method.

Advocates of nondrug pain treatment also may unintentionally convey to patients that if they are not willing to try the technique, then they are close minded or not truly committed to doing their best to manage their pain. Worse yet, such patients may be labeled uncooperative and unmotivated.

Advocates of nondrug pain treatments need to balance their own enthusiasm against the fact that society is more approving of nondrug than drug treatments. Patients may be easily coerced into using nondrug methods against their will and then feel that they must report success even when it does not occur. Because many nondrug treatments involve increased clinician-patient contact, patients may be prone to say that the nondrug treatments are effective merely as a way of expressing gratitude to clinicians for their efforts to help. Careful evaluation of the effectiveness of nondrug treatments is essential.

Considerations in Selecting and Using Nondrug Pain Treatments

Following are guidelines for selecting among the wide variety of nondrug methods available for pain management and considerations for integrating them into the total plan of care. These are summarized in Box 9.1.

1. The relationship between nondrug pain management and use of analgesics. This must be clarified for the patient, family, and health care providers.

    When analgesics are appropriate, the first priority is to individualize them for the patient. Nondrug pain methods are then used in addition to analgesics. Nondrug treatments should not be used instead of analgesics or in an effort to increase the interval between doses. Usually the nondrug methods are used only after pain is reasonably well controlled with analgesics.

    Patients who have been taking analgesics may mistakenly assume that when clinicians suggest a nondrug pain treatment, the purpose is to avoid or reduce analgesics. Patients then may be reluctant to try the method or to admit that it was effective to any extent, thinking that if the nondrug intervention is even partially successful, the analgesic will be discontinued. Therefore when nondrug methods are offered, clinicians must clarify to patients how the nondrug methods are to be used in relation to analgesics (Ferrell, Rhiner, 1994).

    If the goal is to reduce analgesic use and substitute nondrug treatment, clinicians must be sure that the rationale for this is sound and that it is explained carefully to the patient. Analgesic doses should be reduced gradually while the patient learns how to use nondrug methods and evaluates the effectiveness of them. Gradual reduction of opioids is especially important to prevent withdrawal syndrome. Sensitivity to pain increases during opioid withdrawal, and failure to suppress withdrawal may cause the clinician and patient to conclude that the nondrug method makes pain worse.

2. Patient's previous experience and present attitude. Is the patient interested in nondrug pain methods? Has the patient tried any nondrug strategies? If so, what happened? Is the patient using nondrug methods because of unfounded fears about analgesics?

    Willingness and interest are important to the use of nondrug treatments. However, as mentioned earlier, patients may fear taking analgesics that clearly are indicated for their pain, such as NSAIDs for an inflammatory painful condition. Their use of nondrug pain treatments may be an inappropriate substitution for analgesics, and education about pain medicines may be necessary.

    Other patients may have tried many nondrug methods before resorting to the health care system, and now they may expect a distinctly different type of care such as medication or surgery. Some patients, for cultural or personal reasons, prefer to explore nontraditional techniques such

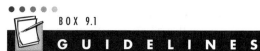

BOX 9.1

GUIDELINES

SELECTION AND USE OF NONDRUG PAIN TREATMENTS

1. Clarify the relationship between the use of nondrug pain treatments and the use of analgesics.
   - In most clinical situations (e.g., postoperative pain or cancer pain) nondrug pain treatments should be used in addition to analgesics.
   - Emphasize to the patient that nondrug therapies do not replace analgesics.

2. Assess the patient's attitude toward and experience with nondrug pain treatments.
   - If the patient has used nondrug methods, find out whether they were successful and what, if any, problems were encountered.
   - Find out whether the patient feels that personal attempts at nondrug therapies have been exhausted and that more conventional pain therapies are now appropriate.
   - Find out whether the patient is using nondrug methods to avoid using analgesics. If analgesics are appropriate, discuss the patient's concerns.

3. Ask the patient what, besides taking pain medicine, usually helps with the pain.
   - Try to identify nondrug treatments that are similar to the patient's coping style.
   - Some patients simply want more information about pain or its management, whereas others want to divert their attention away from pain.
   - Many patients naturally use distraction to cope with pain. For these patients, providing a selection of music or videotapes may be helpful.

4. Assess the patient's level of fatigue, cognitive status, and ability to concentrate and follow instructions.
   - Optimal functioning in these areas is desirable to learn and to use a technique such as relaxation imagery but is unnecessary if a cold pack is used.
   - Some patients barely have enough time to perform required activities of daily living. Adding a lengthy relaxation technique may simply increase stress and decrease the patient's sense of control.

5. Ask the patient's family/friends if they wish to be involved in nondrug pain treatments.
   - In home care the primary caregiver may already be overburdened and have no time or energy to help the patient with a technique such as massage.
   - Some family/friends may welcome a technique like massage that allows them to touch the patient and "do something." However, not all patients or family members are comfortable with techniques that involve touch.

6. Provide the patient and family with adequate support materials.
   - Whenever possible, supply written or audiotaped instructions for even the simplest techniques.
   - Determine whether the appropriate equipment is available. If not, can the patient afford to purchase it? If not, identify less expensive nondrug materials or therapies.

as acupuncture, chiropractic, meditation, or herbs before turning to traditional Western medicine. When such a patient finally seeks medical attention, the patient may expect prescriptions for opioid or nonopioid analgesics and certainly may not want to be introduced to yet another unconventional method of pain relief such as a relaxation technique. Whenever possible, the patient's expectations should be met or addressed. If nondrug pain treatments are indicated, perhaps analgesics can be used first along with an explanation that the nondrug therapies should be added soon. Meeting the patient's expectations first probably will facilitate obtaining the patient's cooperation with other therapies.

Some patients have made unsuccessful attempts at using nondrug techniques. Negative experiences with nondrug methods of pain management or disinterest in them do not necessarily rule out their use. With more discussion and explanation a patient may be willing to try what the clinician recommends. For example, if the patient has had no success with a relaxation technique, the clinician may describe a very different approach to relaxation that the patient may be willing to consider. However, nondrug methods should never be forced on the patient, nor should the patient be made to feel guilty about refusing such interventions. As discussed in the following, mismatched interventions (those that are not consistent with the patient's natural coping style) may increase pain or distress associated with pain.

3. Patient preferences and coping styles. Patients differ considerably in the type of nondrug pain treatments they wish to try. Encouraging patients to choose from a variety of techniques allows them to match the technique to their own coping styles. When it is not possible to offer a variety of tech-

niques because of limited time, the patient's decision to refuse what may be available should at least be respected. For example, cold may be the nondrug technique chosen to be offered routinely to patients in ambulatory surgery. Some patients may refuse because of a preference for heat, which might not be an alternative because it could increase bleeding.

Asking patients how they usually cope with pain is another way to determine what may interest them and be effective for them. Mismatching, or having patients use nondrug methods that are contrary to their usual coping styles, can cause pain to increase. For example, in a small study of children, those who usually coped with pain by distracting themselves exhibited a substantial increase in pain ratings when they were asked to attend to the discomfort and try to change the quality of the sensation (Fanurik, Zeltzer, Roberts et al., 1993).

Similar results were obtained in a study of elderly patients with chronic knee pain (Fry, Wong, 1991). Findings suggested that patients were more willing to learn coping skills that are consistent with their preferred styles and that interventions that are contrary to their coping style are likely to be ineffective. Hence, patient preferences are an important consideration in the selection and use of nondrug pain treatments.

Research on use of nondrug interventions for pain in cancer patients ($n = 40$) cared for at home sheds some light on potential preferences (Rhiner, Ferrell, Ferrell et al., 1993). The patients' ages were 60 years or older, with a mean age of 66. They were offered five forms of nondrug pain management: heat, cold, massage/vibration, distraction, and relaxation imagery. On average, three nondrug methods were used by each patient. The two most popular methods were heat and massage/vibration; relaxation imagery and cold were seldom selected. Heat and massage/vibration were also rated by the patients as the most effective methods. The authors noted that anxious patients seemed to prefer physical nondrug methods such as heat over cognitive ones such as imagery.

Cultural or religious taboos must be considered because some may prohibit the patient from using certain nondrug approaches to pain. For example, some groups may object to hypnosis, others to massage. For relaxation, some may prefer religious rather than popular music. (Refer to Box 9.8 on p. 415 for more on use of music to relax.)

4. Patient's physical and mental abilities. Does the patient have the physical and mental abilities necessary for using the nondrug treatment? Does the patient have sufficient energy to learn and perform the tasks involved? Some nondrug approaches to pain management require that the patient be actively involved, able to concentrate, and provide feedback.

Physical and mental fatigue may interfere with some techniques such as distraction or relaxation imagery. Patients who are confused or unable to concentrate obviously will have difficulty learning new techniques. For patients who are already experiencing considerable stress, learning even a simple nondrug strategy may increase their stress.

Nondrug therapies that are time-consuming (such as a 20-minute relaxation technique) often are not appealing to patients who already are unable to complete what they want or need to do. In such instances nondrug therapies such as application of heat or cold may be far more suitable.

5. Involvement of family/friends. Do others want to be involved in helping the patient? Is the method a potential vehicle for improving relationships between the patient and others?

Nondrug methods that patients cannot do for themselves, such as massage, may be a burden to some caregivers in the home, whereas other caregivers may welcome that opportunity to be physically close to a loved one. Some nondrug methods, such as relaxation, may be used simultaneously by both patients and family members, benefiting both and giving them an opportunity to share an activity. Distraction techniques that use family photo albums may be a source of pleasure to both patient and family.

6. Support materials/patient education. Many nondrug approaches to pain can be provided at minimal cost, such as a cold pack made with a plastic bag, alcohol, and water (see p. 407) as opposed to purchasing a gel pack. Some nondrug methods such as cold also require little if any formal education of the patient/family. However, no matter how simple the technique, it is wise to provide written or audiotaped instructions. Various "Patient Information" sheets (pp. 410, 415, 417, 420) about nondrug pain treatments are included in this chapter and may be duplicated and left with the patient.

CUTANEOUS STIMULATION

The types of cutaneous stimulation presented here are superficial heating and cooling and vibration. (Superficial massage is also a form of cutaneous stimulation and is discussed later in this chapter as a method of inducing relaxation.) The potentially beneficial effects of cutaneous stimulation techniques are numerous and range from making pain more tolerable to actual reduction of pain. The focus in this chapter is on their use as methods of pain relief or comfort rather than on their use for therapeutic purposes (such as the use of cold for lowering body temperature).

Patients tend to be receptive to the use of cutaneous stimulation techniques, as mentioned previously. In a study of patients with cancer pain, the two most popular methods of nondrug pain relief were heat and massage/vibration (Rhiner, Ferrell, Ferrell et al., 1993). For vibration, patients most often chose the vibrator with heat.

The mechanisms underlying pain relief that may result from these and other types of cutaneous stimulation are unclear. Historically, the gate control theory (Melzack, Wall, 1965) has been used as a way of explaining the effectiveness of cutaneous stimulation. This theory suggests that stimulation of the skin may activate the large diameter fibers. In turn, that activation may provoke an inhibition of the "pain messages" carried by the smaller fibers, that is, close the gate to the transmission of impulses felt as painful (Newton, 1990). This theory, however, has been replaced in large part by more factual information about the mechanisms underlying pain; unfortunately, these mechanisms do not yet offer a proven explanation for the effects of superficial heat and cold (see Chapter 2).

The cutaneous stimulation techniques discussed here are most often applied to the site of pain. However, several studies indicate that stimulation of a wide variety of sites other than the pain site may produce pain relief (Ekblom, Hansson, 1985; Thorsteinsson, Stonnington, Stillwell et al., 1978). For example, after lidocaine injection of osteoarthritic knees, patients have reported some pain relief in the opposite knee (Creamer, Hunt, Dieppe, 1996). Because stimulation of sites other than the site of pain may be effective, trial and error combined with open-mindedness is needed. Following are easily located sites that may be stimulated in an effort to relieve pain (Figure 9.1):

- Directly over or around pain. This is usually, but not always, the best site (Bini, Cruccu, Schady et al., 1984).
- Proximal to pain—"between pain and brain" (Shere, Cleeland, O'Sullivan et al., 1986).
- Distal to pain—"beyond the pain" (Shere, Cleeland, O'Sullivan et al., 1986).
- Contralateral to pain—"opposite side" (Collins, 1985; Creamer, Hunt, Dieppe, 1996; Lehman, Strain, 1985; Melzack, Schecter, 1965; Yarnitsky, Kunin, Brik et al., 1997).

Acupuncture or acupressure points, as well as trigger points, may be stimulated to relieve pain, but instructions regarding their locations are beyond the scope of this chapter. (Refer to Figure 12.12, p. 571, for location of trigger points associated with myofascial pain syndrome.)

The mechanisms underlying pain relief produced by stimulation of sites distant to pain are not fully understood. Cutaneous stimulation at one site may produce at least mild effects at distant sites in the body, called the

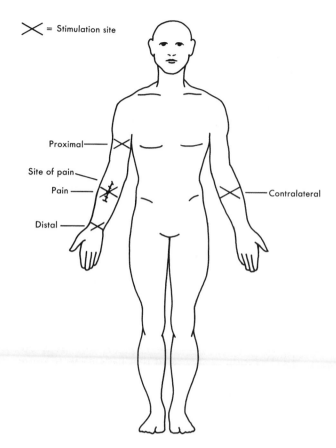

FIGURE 9.1   Sites for cutaneous stimulation. Examples of four possible sites: site of pain, proximal to pain, distal to pain, and contralateral.

consensual response (Lehman, de Lateur, 1982b). For example, heat applied to one site increases blood flow in other parts of the body such as the contralateral limb (Michlovitz, 1990a). It also seems possible that distraction may play a role. For example, a cold pack placed at a site distant from the site of pain may divert the patient's attention away from pain.

Superficial Heating and Cooling

Superficial heating and cooling techniques described in this chapter are for pain relief or comfort, not for therapeutic or curative purposes. Therapeutic uses of heat include increasing the blood supply to an area, whereas cold may be used for the opposite effect. Directions for therapeutic use differ slightly from those presented here for symptomatic relief of pain or for general comfort.

The underlying mechanisms of pain relief from heating and cooling are uncertain. Both heat and cold cause decreased sensitivity to pain (Lehmann, de Lateur, 1982 a, b). The effects of cold may progress to partial or complete anesthesia or numbness of the skin (Michovitz, 1990b). Some of the effects of heat and cold may be similar, but the mechanisms underlying the effects may be different. For example, either heating or cooling may decrease muscle spasm, but for different reasons (Lehman, de Lateur, 1982b; Michlovitz, 1990b).

Methods of superficial heating and cooling

The following are ways of supplying superficial heating or cooling for the purpose of providing general comfort or relieving pain. Keep these points in mind when a patient wishes to try heat or cold, and use the information in Boxes 9.2 and 9.3 on p. 410 to assist patients with heat/cold pain management.

Convenient methods of superficial *heat* commonly available in the home or hospital setting include the following:

- Hot pack, such as rubber hot water bottle, electric heating pad (dry or moist), hot moist compress, and hydrocolator. The latter two are inconvenient to prepare. For all types of hot packs, care must be taken to wrap the pack well to prevent burns. In most cases, the protection of one towel between the skin and the heating device is sufficient. However, hydroculators may require 8 to 12 layers of cloth. If the patient has decreased skin sensation or lies on top of a hot pack, more layers of cloth will be needed for skin protection (McCaffery, Wolff, 1992).
- Immersion in water (e.g., tub, basin, whirlpool).
- Retention of body heat with plastic wrap (e.g., Saran Wrap, plastic dry cleaner bag taped to itself).

Convenient, relatively safe, and readily available methods of *cold* application include:

- Waterproof bags (e.g., rubber or plastic) filled with ice melting in water.
- Terry cloth (e.g., towel) dipped in water with ice shavings and wrung out. The need for frequent reapplication is an inconvenience.
- Gel packs may be kept in the refrigerator and are very convenient.
- Homemade cold packs that are comfortable, quick, and inexpensive:
  - Sealed plastic container (e.g., plastic bag) with one third alcohol and two thirds water placed in the freezer produces a flexible, unfrozen slush.
  - Damp cloth or towel, folded in the desired shape, sealed in a plastic bag, and placed in the freezer produces a flexible cold pack.
  - One pound bag of frozen green peas or kernels of corn (hit gently to separate contents).

Ideally, cold packs should be sealed to prevent dripping and flexible so that they conform to body contours. Cold packs must be adequately wrapped to prevent skin irritation and to ensure a comfortable intensity of cold.

For added convenience, especially for the active or ambulatory patient, applications of heat or cold can be secured in place with elastic bandages or cloth pocket holders with Velcro straps.

Electrically operated aqua pads may be used as a source of either heat or cold. Water is circulated through a pad that is placed on a body part, such as over the abdomen for incisional pain. Water temperature may be set and maintained at any one of a wide range of settings.

Appropriate and inappropriate uses of heat and cold

The following recommendations are based on both research and anecdotal reports. Because heat and cold are physical modalities with well-defined parameters, such as measurable temperature ranges, it is tempting to think that precise information is available about which one should be used for certain conditions, how often, how long, and where. However, well-controlled research is lacking. Ideas about uses of heat or cold are more likely to be derived from what we see used within our own specific culture and from our personal experiences than from scientific information (McCaffery, Wolff, 1992).

Guidelines for use of heat or cold have changed over the years. For example, traditionally, heat was recommended for joint pain. Now it is recognized that cold is also very effective for relief of arthritic pain (*Cold may ease arthritis pain,* 1982; *Cooling more effective,* 1982). For many types of pain, heating and cooling can be used interchangeably unless there are contraindications. Contrary to popular opinion, either superficial heating or cooling may be used for muscle spasms, joint stiffness, low back pain, itching, or aching muscles. Cold is often more effective than heat. However, although cooling is often recommended for the treatment of musculoskeletal pain and many patients say they benefit, little scientific evidence supports its effectiveness (Ernst, Fialka, 1994).

Uses of Heat

Situations in which superficial heat is usually preferred to cold for pain relief include decubiti, superficial boils, superficial thrombophlebitis, anorectal pain, and hematoma resolution after the acute phase of bleeding has ceased. Nipple pain associated with breastfeeding also seems to be responsive to superficial heat. In a study of 65 women who were breastfeeding and had everted nipples, application of tea bags, warm water compresses, or no treatment were compared. Water compresses or tea bags were applied to the nipple for 15 minutes and the nipple was allowed to dry. Findings revealed that warm water compresses or tea bags effectively reduced nipple pain during the early postpartum period (Lavergne, 1997).

Superficial heating to large areas of the body (e.g., warm whirlpool) should be used with caution in patients prone to orthostatic hypotension. Heat should not be applied over the topical application of menthol-containing products because of the tissue damage that may occur (Heng, 1987). Cold, however, can be used.

Superficial heating probably should be avoided over skin where a patient is receiving radiation therapy. Because the patient's skin is more sensitive, heat can feel hotter to the skin and could cause tissue damage. Of course, heat is almost always contraindicated if bleeding is occurring.

Patients with musculoskeletal pain such as arthritis may find that they are able to get out of bed and ambulate more comfortably if warmth is applied to the affected area before getting out of bed in the morning. A convenient arrangement may be to have an electric heating pad plugged into a timer that turns on the heating pad 5 minutes or so before the patient usually awakens. Care must be taken to avoid tissue damage by covering the pad and using a low setting.

Uses of Cold

Cold is preferred to heat for pain relief in the presence of acute trauma, bleeding, swelling, an acute state of rheumatoid arthritis, and tissues with an irreversible inadequate vascular supply (heat may increase metabolic demand and cause necrosis). One study revealed that cold was more effective than warmth for episiotomy pain (Ramler, Roberts, 1986). Headache, especially migraine, may be very responsive to cooling methods. Figure 9.2 illustrates the uses of cold packs.

A common misconception is that heat is invariably appropriate 24 to 48 hours after an acute soft tissue injury. However, application of cold rather than heat is recommended, especially before therapeutic exercise. This reduces edema that commonly occurs when active exercise is used early in the recovery period, as is often done with athletes (Hillman, Delforge, 1985).

Superficial cold should not be used if the patient is allergic to cold (a rare condition) and should be avoided in patients with peripheral vascular diseases such as Raynaud's disease. Cold should be discontinued immediately if a "hunting reaction" occurs, that is, when the skin alternately blanches and turns red after application of cold. This signifies that the temperature is low enough to be potentially destructive to tissues.

Guidelines for selecting and using heating/cooling

Once contraindications for the use of heat and cold have been considered, the basic approach to selection and use is trial and error. Heat and/or cold probably work best for well-localized pain. Heating or cooling measures are especially appropriate at bedtime and for patients with limited physical and mental energy (McCaffery, Wolff, 1992). In the hospital, applications of heat or cold require a physician's prescription or a protocol.

In clinical practice, when the intent of heating or cooling methods is to bring comfort or pain relief, the temperature of the hot or cold application is rarely measured. The best guide probably is patient preference and regular assessment of the skin for redness and other signs of irritation.

If measurement of temperature is indicated, such as in a cognitively impaired patient, the following serve as guidelines. Superficial heating methods are usually at a temperature of 40° to 45° C (104° to 113° F) at point of contact with skin. Ordinarily, this warms only the skin. Muscles and other deeper tissues usually are not affected because they are insulated by the subcutaneous fat. Methods of cooling are usually at temperatures around 15° C (59° F) at skin contact. This cools the skin and, if applied long enough, the muscles. Cold application drops the muscle temperature in slender people after about 10 minutes and in obese people after about 30 minutes (McCaffery, Wolff, 1992). Moisture or water increases the intensity of the heating or cooling sensation more than dry wrappings. This may or may not be desirable, depending on patient preference or avoidance of tissue damage (McCaffery, Wolff, 1992).

With both heating and cooling methods, care must be taken to avoid tissue damage. Unwanted side effects, such as burns, bleeding, and swelling, are more frequent with heating than with cooling. However, at very low temperatures, cooling may cause blistering or excessive redness that does not subside between uses. Both heat and cold must be used with caution in patients who are unconscious or who have impaired sensation in the area of application.

The duration and frequency of using heating or cooling methods is determined by trial and error in addition to what is convenient and practical. Probably the most frequent period of time suggested for heating or cooling is 20 to 30 minutes. However, to a certain extent, the longer stimulation is used, the longer pain relief will last after the stimulation is stopped. The minimum effective time is about 5 to 10 minutes (McCaffery, Wolff, 1992). If the heating or cooling method is kept at a comfortable level of intensity and if the skin is carefully protected, heat or cold may be applied indefinitely (24 hours a day) if desired.

Whenever possible, cutaneous modalities should be used before pain occurs or increases. Stimulation should be discontinued if pain or skin irritation (e.g., rash or blistering) occurs or if the patient asks that it be discontinued. Patient information on use of cold and heat is presented in Boxes 9.2 and 9.3 respectively on p. 410.

Encouraging the Use of Cold

When cold relieves pain, it tends to be more effective than heat. Research has shown that cold works better than heat for many conditions traditionally treated with

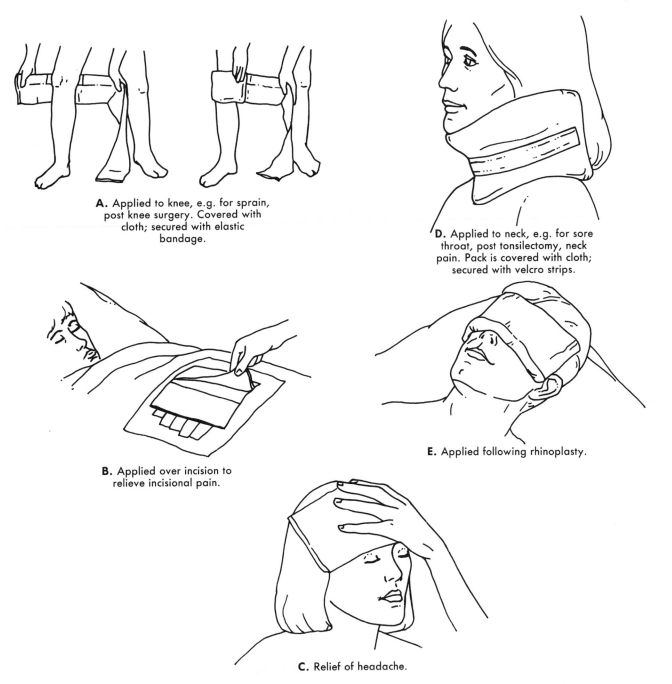

A. Applied to knee, e.g. for sprain, post knee surgery. Covered with cloth; secured with elastic bandage.

B. Applied over incision to relieve incisional pain.

C. Relief of headache.

D. Applied to neck, e.g. for sore throat, post tonsilectomy, neck pain. Pack is covered with cloth; secured with velcro strips.

E. Applied following rhinoplasty.

FIGURE 9.2   Uses of flexible cold gel packs. Some may also be used for heat by warming them in water. Notice that the pack is covered with cloth.

heat, such as arthritis (Michlovitz, 1990b) or episiotomy pain (Ramler, Roberts, 1986). When cold is compared with heat for pain relief:

- Cold usually relieves more pain than heat.
- Cold usually relieves pain faster than heat.
- Pain relief from cold lasts longer than relief from heat.

Effects of cold last longer than the effects of heat because the vessels remain constricted after cold application is removed, and rewarming of tissue from inside is delayed accordingly along with delayed warming from the outside. When cold penetrates deep enough to cool the muscle, rewarming of the muscle is further prolonged because of the insulating fat layer. The effects of heating do not last as long as the effects of cold because, after the heat source is removed, the increased blood flow accompanying heating rapidly cools the tissues to a normal temperature.

• • • • •

BOX 9.2   Patient Information: Use of Cold

Cold may relieve the following types of pain, and it often works better than heat:
- Muscle aches or spasms, such as neck or low back pain
- Joint pain
- Headache
- Surgical incision
- Itching

Precautions:
- Do not use cold over areas of poor circulation or skin being treated with radiation therapy.
- Do not use cold if pain increases.
- Think cool, not cold. Keep the sensation of cold at a cool, comfortable level.
- Cover the cold pack with a towel.
- Remember that moisture increases the intensity of cold.
- Remove the cold pack if your skin becomes numb.
- Do not freeze your skin.

Equipment for cold can be any of the following:
- Ice bag
- Gel pack
- Ice and water in a plastic bag

- A bag of frozen peas or frozen corn kernels (Hit the bag on the countertop to break up the frozen vegetables so it will mold to your skin.)
- Slush pack made by freezing in a sealed plastic container (e.g., plastic bag) 1/3 alcohol and 2/3 water
- Towel soaked in water and ice chips and wrung out
- Flexible cold pack made with a damp cloth or towel, folded in the desired shape, sealed in a plastic bag, and placed in the freezer

Application of cold:
- Cover ice pack with a pillowcase or one or more towels.
- Keep it at a comfortably cool intensity.
- Apply to painful area for 10 to 20 min. You may use cold for any length of time if it remains at a comfortable level of coolness that does not irritate your skin.
- If you cannot get to the area that hurts, apply the cold pack to any or all of the following sites:
  - Opposite side of body corresponding to the pain (e.g., left leg if the right leg hurts)
  - Above the pain (e.g., over upper arm if your lower arm hurts)
  - Below the pain (e.g., over the lower arm if your upper arm hurts)

• • • • •

BOX 9.3   Patient Information: Use of Heat

Heat may relieve the following types of pain:
- Muscle aches or spasms, such as neck or low back pain
- Joint pain
- Itching
- Rectal pain

Precautions:
- Do not use heat if pain increases.
- Think warm, not hot. Keep the sensation at a warm, comfortable level.
- Cover the heat source with a towel.
- Remember that moisture increases the intensity of heat.
- Do not use heat over skin where menthol ointment or an oily substance has been applied.
- Do not use over an area that is bleeding or recently injured.

Equipment for heat application can be any of the following:
- Hot water bottle
- Electric heating pad
- Hot moist compresses (e.g., towel)

- Immersion in water (e.g., tub, basin, whirlpool)
- Retention of body heat with plastic wrap (e.g., Saran Wrap, plastic dry cleaner bag taped to itself). Be careful to wash and dry your skin well at least once a day if you are using this method.

Application of heat:
- Cover heat source with a pillowcase or one or more towels.
- Keep it at a comfortably warm intensity.
- Do not fall asleep on top of an electric heating pad.
- Apply to painful area for 10 to 20 min. You may use warmth for any length of time if it remains at a comfortable level that does not irritate your skin.
- If you cannot get to the area that hurts, apply the heat pack to any or all of the following sites:
  - Opposite side of body corresponding to the pain (e.g., left leg if the right leg hurts)
  - Above the pain (e.g., over upper arm if your lower arm hurts)
  - Below the pain (e.g., over the lower arm if your upper arm hurts)

Patients are often reluctant to try cold. However, because cold applications have the potential for relieving more pain than heating methods, the clinician may wish to encourage the patient to experiment with cold. Box 9.4 lists some approaches to persuading patients to try cold.

Alternating Heat and Cold

Alternating heat and cold (e.g., every few seconds or minutes) probably is more effective than either one alone. The patient may simply develop his or her own rhythm. Intervals may be as short as 5 to 10 seconds. This technique has been shown to be extremely effective even for severe pain (Gammon, Staff, 1941). Alternating cold and heat has been used for stump pain after amputation and other forms of deafferentation pain (Rana, 1987).

Methods of alternating heat and cold include alternating a heating pack and a cold pack. Or, simply the use of intermittent heat will produce a heating and cooling

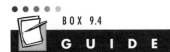
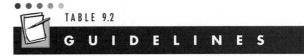

G U I D E L I N E S

ENCOURAGING THE PATIENT TO TRY COLD

If use of cold for pain relief appears to be indicated but the patient is reluctant, the following may help persuade the patient to give it a try:
- Explain the potential benefits of cold:
  - It may be more effective than heat.
  - Pain relief from cold lasts longer than pain relief from heat.
- Provide a gradual onset of cold by one of the following methods:
  - Wrap the cold pack with many layers of cloth so that initially it feels only slightly cool. Remove layers slowly, one at a time, over a long enough period that the skin gradually becomes accustomed to the cold.
  - Begin with a warm moist cloth between the skin and cold pack.
- Use a cold pack that has the following features:
  - Soft
  - Lightweight
  - Conforms to body contours
  - Does not leak
- Protect the patient against generalized chilling by being sure the patient is warm at the start. Add warmth by providing additional cover such as an electric blanket, heating pad, or sweater.

TABLE 9.2

G U I D E L I N E S

CONTRAST BATHING: COMBINED HEAT AND COLD

Uses: on extremities with severe pain, pain that responds to both heat and cold, or joint stiffness (results in increased blood flow)
Supplies: 2 containers of water
- Cold water at approximately 15° C (59° F)
- Hot water at approximately 40° C (104° F)
Method: Immerse the limb for a total of 30 min, alternating as follows:

Time (Min) in Hot Water	Time (Min) in Cold Water
10	
	1
4	
	1
4	
	1
4	
	1
4	
(Total of 30 min)	

effect. For example, heat may be applied for 30 seconds and removed for 30 seconds. The increased blood flow that accompanies heating will allow the part to cool rapidly after removing the heating pad.

Contrast bathing is another method of alternating heat and cold and may be especially useful for painful conditions of the extremities, such as joint pain in the legs or arms or reflex sympathetic dystrophy of the limbs. Placing the painful part alternately in two containers of hot and cold water for a period of approximately 30 minutes may bring lasting relief. Directions are given in Table 9.2. Patients may follow these suggestions for timing or develop their own rhythm of alternating heat and cold.

Vibration

Vibration is a form of electric massage. Research suggests that it may be an effective substitute for TENS (Ekblom, Hansson, 1985; Guieu, Tardy-Grevet, Roll, 1991).

When vibration is applied lightly, it may have a soothing effect similar to massage. Vibration applied with moderate pressure may relieve pain by causing numb-

ness, paresthesia, and/or anesthesia of the area stimulated. If this type of vibration is continued for 30 minutes or longer, pain relief may last for several hours afterward (Ekblom, Hansson, 1985; Lundeberg, Ottoson, Hakansson et al., 1983). Vibration may also change the character of the sensation from sharp to dull (Bini, Cruccu, Schady et al., 1984).

Types of vibrating devices

A number of vibrating devices are available commercially, and many have two or more adjustable speeds. Some also have an optional heating element. Common types of vibrators are:
- Handheld vibrators: These may be operated with batteries or house current. Pressure and movements are provided by the operator. Frequencies and amplitudes vary widely, coarser movement oscillating at 10 to 50 Hz and finer movements at 100 to 200 Hz, the latter probably being more common and comfortable. High-frequency vibration, 100 Hz, tends to be the most effective (Lundeberg, Nordemar, Ottoson, 1984; Spross, Wolff, 1995).

  Many handheld vibrators have interchangeable applicators of different shapes and sizes made of plastic or rubber. Those with rounded tips (e.g., shaped like a phallus) are particularly good for stimulating certain acupuncture or trigger points.

Some small vibrators are strapped to the dorsum of the hand, allowing the human hand to be in contact with the patient's skin. This type allows better adaptation to the contours of the body.

- Stationary vibrators: Body parts are held against these devices. Vibrating pads may be a contoured back pad or may resemble a seat cushion. Vibrating elements may be incorporated into an armchair or bed mattress. These are probably best suited for providing superficial massage. The body part, such as the back, is placed against the surface. Some are constructed especially for massaging the feet.

Appropriate and inappropriate situations for vibrating devices

Appropriate situations for using vibration for comfort or pain relief include the following:
- Muscle pain or spasm, acute or chronic (e.g., back or neck pain)
- Tension headache
- Itch
- Near an injection site (e.g., during IM injection) (Wachter-Shikora, 1982)
- Neuropathic pain (e.g., postherpetic neuralgia; surrounding the area if the site of pain is too sensitive) (Russell, Espir, Morganstern, 1957)
- Phantom limb pain, stump pain (Russell, Espir, Morganstern, 1957)
- Chronic orofacial pain (Lundeberg, Ottoson, Hakansson et al., 1983)
- Tooth extraction (Hansson, Ekblom, Thomasson et al., 1986)
- Acute tendinitis
- As a substitute for TENS (Ekblom, Hansson, 1985; Guieu, Tardy-Grevet, Roll, 1991)
- Various types of chronic nonmalignant neuropathic or musculoskeletal pain (Lundeberg, 1984; Lundeberg, Nordemar, Ottoson, 1984)

Inappropriate situations for vibrating devices include the following:
- Patients who bruise easily
- Areas of thrombophlebitis
- Sites where skin has been injured (e.g., burned or cut)
- Migraine headache or any headache that worsens with movement or sound

Guidelines for using handheld vibrating devices

A trial and error approach is necessary. By use of a handheld device, vibration may be applied for about 1 minute to various sites to determine which site results in the best pain relief. Because producing numbness is one of the ways that vibration relieves pain, the best results may be obtained by using a handheld vibrator with moderate pressure at the site of pain. The duration of application can vary from 20 seconds to 15 minutes. However, the longer the duration of vibration, the longer pain relief lasts afterward. Findings of one study revealed that vibration at 100 Hz applied for 1 to 15 minutes produced very brief poststimulatory pain relief (Lundeberg, Ottoson, Hakansson et al., 1983). However, pain relief lasted up to 10 hours when vibration was used for 30 minutes. This type of stimulation caused redness, but no tissue damage was reported. For some patients use of vibration for 30 minutes two to three times a day may be indicated.

If there is a choice of speeds, high-frequency vibration should be tried because it tends to be the most effective. Initially the patient may note a sensation of warmth, and this may change to numbness. If vibration is uncomfortable, it should be discontinued (Spross, Wolff, 1995).

Vibration may be a practical nondrug method of pain management for outpatient use, provided the device is available or affordable. Vibration is easily administered and, depending on the site of pain, may be done by the patient. In the hospital a physician's prescription is necessary.

DISTRACTION

Distraction is sometimes referred to as cognitive refocusing and consists of directing attention away from pain. The mechanisms underlying the effectiveness of distraction as a method of handling pain are unclear. The major theoretical explanation is the resources or limited capacity model of attention (Johnson, Petrie, 1997). Theoretically, a person's capacity for processing information is limited, so that allocation of attention to one task limits the attention that may be given to another (Kahneman, 1973). Thus if the patient with pain pays attention to a television program, less attention is available for focusing on pain.

In simple terms distraction may be thought of as a kind of sensory shielding; that is, the patient is shielded from the sensation of pain by increased sensory input from other sources. By focusing attention and concentration on stimuli other than pain, pain is placed on the periphery of awareness. This stimuli may be from internal or external sources. For internal stimuli, or mental distraction, patients may imagine something distracting (distraction imagery) such as a happy event or "hear" themselves singing silently. External sources of stimuli might include an audio tape of music.

The beneficial effects of distraction as a method of pain management are unpredictable but may include decreased intensity of pain, increased pain tolerance, a more acceptable pain sensation (such as less sharp and more dull), and improved or positive mood (such as increased feelings of happiness). Thus for some patients distraction may decrease pain; for others, distraction may make the pain more bearable but have no effect on actual pain intensity. Distraction strategies may also provide the patient with a sense of control over the painful experience.

In a study of 80 male volunteers, distraction was compared with relaxation for experimentally induced finger pressure pain (Bruehl, Carlson, McCubbin, 1993). Patients using distraction were asked to relive a happy moment, and those using relaxation were instructed to breathe slowly and regularly. The findings revealed that the distraction strategy was more effective than relaxation. Distraction reduced pain, fear, and anxiety, but the relaxation instruction did not. This study was limited to use of only one type of relaxation, and the results certainly do not suggest that all relaxation techniques are less effective than distraction overall. However, the findings do support the benefits of distraction.

Use of distraction is accompanied by some negative aspects. When patients use distraction for pain management, they do not "look like" they are in pain. This may result in family and clinicians doubting that pain is as severe as reported, leading to failure to provide appropriate analgesics or other methods of pain relief. Another "side effect" of distraction reported by many patients is that after the distraction is over, the awareness of pain is increased, fatigue is increased, and the patient may be irritable. After distraction, many patients need a pain relief measure such as an analgesic that allows them to rest. The benefits and limitations of distraction for pain management are summarized in Box 9.5.

> ● ● ● ● ●
>
> | BOX 9.5 | **Distraction for Pain Management: Benefits and Limitations** |
>
> Possible benefits of distraction:
> ↑ Pain tolerance
> ↑ Self-control
> ↓ Pain intensity
> Positive mood
> Changes quality of pain to more acceptable sensation (e.g., changes from sharp to dull)
> Potential limitations of distraction:
> During use of distraction, others doubt the existence or severity of pain because patient does not "look like" he is in pain.
> After the distraction is over:
> Irritability
> ↑ Awareness of pain
> ↑ Fatigue
> Patient needs a pain relief measure that allows him to rest (e.g., analgesic), and staff may be reluctant to administer because patient previously did not "look like" he had pain.

May be duplicated for use in clinical practice. From McCaffery M, Pasero C: *Pain: Clinical manual*, p. 413. Copyright © 1999, Mosby, Inc.

Many patients seem to be receptive to the use of distraction as a nondrug method of pain management. In a study of patients with cancer pain, 50% selected distraction as a nondrug approach to pain (Rhiner, Ferrell, Ferrell et al., 1993). Music as a distraction was chosen more often than humor. Distraction is often a self-initiated method of handling pain. Without any instruction to do so, patients may engage in a distraction such as visiting with friends, reading, and watching television.

Indications for Distraction

The distraction strategies described in this chapter are most appropriate for use over a brief period of time, such as minutes up to an hour, and for pain that is mild to moderate in intensity. They are especially useful for brief painful procedures such as lumbar puncture, bone marrow aspiration, burn debridement, suture removal, painful injection such as hydroxyzine IM, difficult venipuncture, and uterine contractions during childbirth.

Distraction may also be used for brief periods of time for patients who have chronic pain (Johnson, Petrie, 1997). However, more evidence supports the use of distraction for brief episodes of pain than supports its use over prolonged periods of time for chronic pain. In fact, the value of distraction as a major coping mechanism for chronic pain is questionable. Although studies reveal that many patients with chronic pain use distraction, these patients also often experience more intense pain (Jensen, Turner, Romano et al., 1991; Keefe, Crisson, Urban et al., 1990; Rosenstiel, Keefe, 1983; Turner, Clancy, 1986). Several possibilities have been proposed as to why distraction may increase pain. Distraction may require so much of the patient's attention that the patient fails to heed warning signals that a certain activity is causing more pain and should be stopped. For example, the patient may fail to pace activities and continue to engage in a behavior, such as sitting at a computer for a long time, that increases pain. Distraction may also leave the patient so fatigued that other helpful strategies such as appropriate exercise or relaxation techniques are not performed.

Although distraction may be effective for intense pain, it may be most effective for mild to moderate pain. When the patient has intense pain, it may be difficult to divert attention from pain and concentrate on a distraction.

Appropriate candidates for a distraction strategy include both adults and children who are interested in using distraction and can understand the instructions. Patients also need to have the mental capacity to concentrate, and they need the physical agility and energy to perform the distraction activities.

Patients who meet the above criteria and who are about to experience pain from a brief procedure should be given the option of using a distraction strategy in addition to appropriate analgesia and anesthesia. However, before diverting attention away from the procedure, patients should be provided with information about the procedure, such as what will be done, length of time, and sensations that may occur. Although it is probably more effective to use distraction preventively, that is, before pain begins, initially patients may want to observe the painful procedure. Their sense of safety may be increased by seeing what is happening before they divert their attention away from it.

Distraction probably is not suitable for patients who continue to show a need to be vigilant during a painful procedure. Techniques that focus on pain and try to change the nature of the pain into something less painful may be more helpful for such patients. For example, the patient may try to make a sharp sensation feel more dull.

Characteristics of Effective Distraction Strategies

Both patients and nurses spontaneously devise effective distraction techniques for pain. During a painful procedure, a nurse may begin asking the patient about a topic of interest to the patient, such as a ball game. Or, the patient may do mental math or sing silently. Watching television and making telephone calls are other common, self-initiated distractions. The distraction strategies described here are more structured attempts to divert attention.

The effectiveness of a distraction strategy is determined in part by the degree to which it is either active or passive redirection of attention. Relatively passive distraction strategies include simply listening to music, whereas playing a video game is more active redirection of attention. In a review of the literature, McCaul and Malott (1984) concluded that those distraction strategies that demand the most patient involvement are the most effective ones. They also, of course, tend to require the most mental and physical ability and will not be possible for all patients.

Once a distraction strategy becomes easy to perform or boring, its effectiveness diminishes. Something can be added to increase the complexity of the technique, or another strategy may be needed to replace the easy one. Increasing the complexity of a distraction strategy is also helpful in dealing with pain that increases during a procedure. This may be as simple as being able to turn up the volume of music when pain increases.

Returning to the idea just mentioned that distraction is a form of sensory shielding, it makes sense to provide as much sensory input as possible. Therefore distraction strategies are likely to be more effective if they include sensory input for all the major sensory modalities—auditory, visual, tactile, kinesthetic (movement), and perhaps olfactory (smell). Incorporating rhythm in the presentation of some stimuli probably

---

• • • • •

> **BOX 9.6** **Characteristics of Effective Distraction Strategies for Brief Episodes of Pain**
>
> 1. Interesting to the patient
> 2. Consistent with patient's energy level and ability to concentrate
> 3. Rhythm is included and emphasized (e.g., keeping time to music)
> 4. Stimulates the major sensory modalities:
>   • Hearing
>   • Vision
>   • Touch
>   • Movement
> 5. Capable of providing a change in stimuli when the pain changes (e.g., ↑ stimuli for ↑ pain)

May be duplicated for use in clinical practice. From McCaffery M, Pasero C: *Pain: Clinical manual,* p. 414. Copyright © 1999, Mosby, Inc.

---

helps the patient maintain concentration. For example, the patient will attend more closely to music if asked to tap out the rhythm of the tune.

Ordinarily distraction strategies are chosen that are of interest to the patient. However, some patients find that attending to and complaining about something they do not like is a very effective distraction during pain. Box 9.6 summarizes characteristics of effective distraction strategies for brief episodes of pain.

Specific Structured Distraction Strategies

Whenever possible, patients should be given written directions for distraction strategies that are fairly complex. Directions for two structured strategies using music for distraction are presented in Boxes 9.7 and 9.8. Figure 9.3 illustrates the components of active listening to recorded music as presented in Box 9.8. Directions for using pictures for distraction are provided in Box 9.9 on p. 417.

The beneficial effects of music as a distraction during painful events are suggested in several studies. Research by Eland (reported by Cook, 1986) using music with headsets for children during lumbar puncture, bone marrow aspiration, and other painful procedures revealed that children found this method to be very effective for pain management. Patients with painful neurologic diseases and headaches who listened periodically to 20 minutes of symphonic music required fewer sedatives and analgesics than patients who did not listen to the music (Brody, 1984). In a 6-month study of patients who listened to music while in pain, a 30% reduction was noted in pain medication (Herth, 1978). Preferred music every 2 hours for 30 minutes over a 48-hour period to gynecology/obstetric patients resulted in less use of pain medication (Locsin, 1981). In a small study of 15 patients,

• • • • •

BOX 9.7 **Patient Information: Sing and Tap Rhythm for Distraction**

TO: _____ (patient's name)

DATE: _____

1. Keep your **eyes open and focus** steadily on one stationary spot or object. If you wish to close your eyes, picture something about the song you will be singing.
2. **Select a song** that you know the words to (at least four or more lines), such as a hymn, nursery rhyme, popular song, or commercial jingle.
3. **Sing the song.** To avoid disturbing others or feeling self-conscious, most adults choose to sing silently. You may emphatically mouth the words silently or whisper the words.
4. **Mark time to the song** (e.g., tap out the rhythm with your finger or nod your head). This helps you concentrate on the song instead of your discomfort.
5. Begin singing slowly. **Sing faster if the pain increases;** sing slower when the pain decreases.
6. If this is **not effective enough, try adding or changing** one or more of the following: massage your body in rhythm to the song; try another song; ask someone to sing with you; or mark time to the song in more than one manner (e.g., nod your head at the same time you tap your finger).

Additional points: This technique is easy to learn, but if you are already tired, you may find it physically exhausting if you do it for more than a few minutes. You may also feel self-conscious when you first do this, but you may find you do not mind as long as the technique helps you get through your discomfort.

From: _____ (nurse's name)

Phone: _____

May be duplicated for use in clinical practice. From McCaffery M, Pasero C: *Pain: Clinical manual,* p. 415. Copyright © 1999, Mosby, Inc.

• • • • •

BOX 9.8 **Patient Information: Active Listening to Recorded Music for Distraction**

Use:
• The following suggestions may help you with a brief period of pain, that is, pain that lasts from a few minutes up to an hour.
• Use these suggestions along with your pain medicine.
Instructions:
1. Obtain the following:
   • A cassette player or tape recorder. (Small, battery-operated ones are more convenient.)
   • Earphone or headset. (This is a more demanding stimulus than a speaker a few feet away, and it avoids disturbing others.)
   • Cassette of music you like. (Most people prefer fast, lively music, but some select relaxing music. Other options are comedy routines, sporting events, old radio shows, or stories.)
2. **Listen to the music** at a comfortable volume. **If the discomfort increases, try increasing the volume;** decrease the volume when the discomfort decreases.
3. **Mark time to the music** (e.g., tap out the rhythm with your finger or nod your head). This helps you concentrate on the music rather than your discomfort.
4. Keep your **eyes open and focus** steadily on one stationary spot or object. If you wish to close your eyes, picture something about the music.
5. If this is **not effective enough, try adding or changing** one or more of the following: massage your body in rhythm to the music; try other music; mark time to the music in more than one manner (e.g., tap your foot and finger at the same time).

Additional points: Many patients have found this technique helpful. It tends to be very popular among patients, probably because the equipment is usually readily available and is a part of daily life—you see many people exercising and listening to a recording through a headset. Other advantages are that it is easy to learn and is not physically or mentally demanding. For these reasons, it may be used for up to an hour. If you are very tired, you may simply listen to the music and omit marking time or focusing on a spot.

May be duplicated for use in clinical practice. From McCaffery M, Pasero C: *Pain: Clinical manual,* p. 415. Copyright © 1999, Mosby, Inc.

music reduced pain in 75%; 47% had a moderate to great reduction in pain (Beck, 1991). In another study of patients with chronic cancer pain, music lowered the pain intensity (Zimmerman, Pozehl, Duncan et al., 1989). Other studies have also suggested that music can increase pain tolerance or lower pain intensity (Bailey, 1983; Whipple, Glynn, 1992).

These studies suggest possible positive effects of music on pain, but they have several limitations. It is difficult to ascertain from the research whether the music actually distracted the patients or helped them relax. Another limitation of some of these studies is that pain ratings were not systematically obtained, and it is dangerous to assume that a decrease in analgesic use actually reflects decreased pain. Many patients endure pain rather than request medication. If patients knew the purposes of the studies, they may have tried to cooperate by not requesting analgesics or by reporting less pain.

No instructions are given here for using humor as distraction, but simple methods include providing audio tapes and video tapes of the patient's favorite comedians.

Preferences for humor differ from one individual to another. Fortunately, the availability of VCRs and videotapes makes different sources of humor easily accessible. Situation comedies may be videotaped and played at a convenient time for the patient. Video stores rent a variety of humorous tapes including movies and performances by stand-up comedians.

In a study of elderly patients with cancer pain, researchers noted that sources of humor should be selected with the patient's age in mind (Rhiner, Ferrell, Ferrell et al., 1993). These elderly patients preferred tapes of Will Rogers, Jack Benny, Erma Bombeck, and W.C. Fields over contemporary comedians. In the resource section,

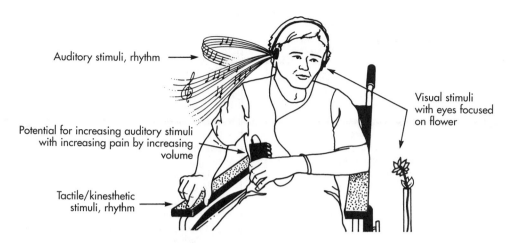

Auditory stimuli, rhythm

Potential for increasing auditory stimuli
with increasing pain by increasing
volume

Tactile/kinesthetic
stimuli, rhythm

Visual stimuli
with eyes focused
on flower

FIGURE 9.3   Active listening to recorded music illustrates the distraction strategy described in Box 9.8. By listening to music through a headset, tapping out the rhythm, and focusing on the flower, the patient is making his pain more tolerable. Using the headset helps keep his attention focused on the music, helps him tune out other things in his environment, and prevents the music from disturbing others.

note that videos of *Candid Camera* can be obtained by patients at home. Children, of course, may have entirely different preferences for humor.

Preliminary research suggests that humor may have positive effects on immune function (Martin, Dobbin, 1988). The effectiveness of laughter has often been explained on the basis of increased endorphin level, but research has failed to show an increase in endorphin levels after laughter (Berk, Tan, Fry et al., 1989).

Nevertheless, the belief that humor can help in coping with pain is widespread. Norman Cousins (1979) wrote an entire book testifying to his own experience with the positive effects of humor during a painful illness. Research, although limited, suggests that humor is an enjoyable and often effective method of distraction for many patients with pain. Fritz (1988) conducted a questionnaire survey of 53 patients with chronic cancer pain, asking them to identify and rate the effectiveness of self-initiated, nondrug measures that they used to cope with their pain. Patients rated laughter as the most effective. Patients have reported that humorous anecdotes before application of painful topical medications are helpful (Ditlow, 1993). The results of a comparison of the effects on pain of humorous versus documentary tapes showed that no differences were found between the effects of the two tapes on subjects' pain tolerance, but subjects thought that humor had been more effective (Nevo, Keinan, Teshimovsky-Arditi, 1993). In other words no significant difference was found in the length of time they tolerated pain while they watched the humorous tape compared with the documentary, but they believed they had tolerated pain longer when they watched the humorous tape.

Humor may be particularly useful before a painful procedure because it appears to have some carryover effects. Cogan and others (1987) conducted two experiments in a laboratory setting by using human subjects to measure pressure-induced discomfort thresholds before and 10 minutes after listening to 20 minutes of audio tapes. The first experiment compared effects of laughter-inducing, relaxation-inducing, dull-narrative, and no tape. Discomfort thresholds were higher for the laughter and relaxation tapes. In other words it took more intense stimuli to cause pain in subjects who had used distraction or relaxation. The second experiment compared effects of laughter-inducing, interesting narrative, or uninteresting narrative audio tapes, multiplication tasks, or no intervention. This showed that only laughter significantly increased discomfort thresholds. In conclusion, it appears that laughter may be more effective than other types of distraction and that the effects continue for at least 10 minutes after laughter subsides.

Another study also found that subjects tolerated pain longer after exposure to humorous versus nonhumorous conditions (Hudak, Dale, Hudak et al., 1991). Still another study supported the finding of increased pain tolerance after exposure to humor but found that exposure to a video of tragedy was equally effective (Zillmann, Rockwell, Schweitzer et al., 1993). One study found that men, but not women, exhibited increased pain endurance after exposure to comedy and tragedy, with comedy being more effective than tragedy (Weaver, Zillmann, 1994).

Ordinarily distraction is effective only during the time it is used, and afterward pain may seem even more intense. Distraction with humor that induces laughter or distraction with a story of tragedy may be the exception.

BOX 9.9 Patient Information: Describing Pictures for Distraction

Use:
- The use of pictures may help with a brief period of pain, that is, pain that lasts a few minutes up to an hour.
- Use this activity along with your pain medicine.

Instructions:
1. **Obtain pictures** that interest you.
   - Types of pictures, such as pictures from magazines; photographs of friends, family, or a vacation; merchandise catalogs; or books with pictures of a specific subject such as airplanes or the civil war. You may want pictures on the same subject or different subjects. Avoid any pictures that you find disturbing or that remind you of your discomfort.
   - Number of pictures. The number of pictures you need will depend on several factors, such as how long your discomfort will last, how much detail you describe, and how fast you talk.
2. You may need **assistance.** If you do not have much time or energy, you may consider asking a friend to obtain the pictures for you (e.g., cut out magazine pictures). You may also want someone to hold the pictures up for you to see as you describe them and help you with your descriptions by asking you for some of the details discussed below.
3. **Look at the pictures and describe them** in any manner that interests you. Usually it is best to continue looking at the pictures while you describe them (as opposed to looking at the picture briefly, hiding it, and then trying to remember the details of the picture). Ways of describing or talking about the pictures include the following—to help you keep your attention focused on the pictures, you may want a friend to have this list and ask you about these items:
   - Pretend you are in the picture. What would you do?
   - Count the number of items in the picture.
   - Name each item in the picture.
   - Name the colors.
   - What is happening in the picture? Make up a story about the picture.

   As soon as you are no longer interested in the picture, put it away and look at another picture. Proceed from one picture to another as rapidly as you wish. If the picture reminds you of something you would like to describe or discuss, try doing so. What the picture reminds you of may be more distracting than the actual picture.
4. If this is **not effective enough, try adding or changing** one or more of the following: try different pictures or different questions; reverse the procedure and ask questions of the person who is assisting you; include at random some surprise pictures that may be difficult to describe but have novel value (e.g., simple cartoons or scantily clad figures); if the discomfort increases, try changing the pictures more rapidly; if you feel self-conscious talking aloud, try describing the pictures to yourself silently.

   This technique may be an ideal way to involve someone who has extra time and wants to help you with your pain. A friend or nurse may gather pictures in his or her spare time and give them to you before a painful event, or the person might be there to show you the pictures and ask questions.

These studies, however, were conducted on volunteers who were exposed to experimental pain. Results in the clinical setting may differ.

RELAXATION

Relaxation was conceived of in the 1930s, and initially it was used as a technique for reducing muscle tension and anxiety (Syrjala, 1990). When relaxation techniques are used for patients with pain, anxiety is often reduced and sometimes, but not always, pain is lessened. The mechanisms underlying pain relief resulting from relaxation techniques are unclear. Obviously, in some types of pain, such as tension headaches, pain relief may be due to reduced muscle tension.

To achieve the maximum stress-reducing response from relaxation, researchers have suggested that a 20-minute technique be used three times a day (Benson, Beary, Carol, 1974). None of the studies cited in the following used relaxation techniques to this extent. In fact, many of the techniques were very brief, raising the possibility that a state of relaxation was not achieved and that relaxation was not the underlying mechanism for some of the positive results. Because physiologic measures of relaxation such as decreased heart rate and oxygen consumption are not included in most research on relaxation for pain control, it is not clear whether the effects of the techniques studied are due to relaxation, distraction, or some other mechanism. For example, thinking about something pleasant clearly diverts attention away from pain.

Relaxation may be defined as a state of relative freedom from both anxiety and skeletal muscle tension. Relaxation techniques discussed in this chapter focus on brief techniques and include a variety of potential approaches to achieving relaxation, such as music, massage, and the traditional slow breathing method. There is overlap with other techniques, since massage may be used as a cutaneous stimulation technique and music may be used for distraction.

Relaxation techniques also include relaxing imagery such as remembering a pleasant or peaceful experience. In reviewing the literature, however, confusion arises with these terms because relaxation imagery is sometimes considered separately from other relaxation techniques. As mentioned at the beginning of this chapter, nondrug approaches to pain management suffer from lack of universally accepted definitions and categorizing.

In this chapter relaxation is recommended as adjunctive (additional) treatment for pain. Relaxation is not considered a pain relief measure per se because it does not always reduce the intensity of pain. Also, it is never a substitute for other appropriate pain relief measures such as analgesics. Usually relaxation reduces distress associated with pain and is taught as a coping skill in response to stress.

In addition to reduced anxiety and possible pain reduction, potential benefits of relaxation may include promotion of sleep, improved ability to problem solve, reduced skeletal muscle tension, decreased fatigue, and increased confidence in the ability to handle pain.

Research Evidence of Relaxation as a Method of Pain Management

The National Institutes of Health (NIH) Technology Assessment Panel on Integration of Behavioral and Relaxation Approaches Into the Treatment of Chronic Pain and Insomnia (1996) concluded that there is strong evidence for the use of relaxation techniques in reducing chronic pain in a variety of medical conditions. Relaxation was also found to be effective for insomnia, a common problem in patients with chronic pain. The data, however, are insufficient to conclude which technique is likely to be more effective than another for a given condition. Trial and error must be used to determine which is most effective for the individual patient.

The need for more research was illustrated in a review of the literature from 1982-1995 regarding use of relaxation and imagery for cancer pain (Wallace, 1997). Only nine clinical studies could be identified. Most had small sample sizes and could not demonstrate significant effects of relaxation and imagery. Only three studies (Ferrell, Ferrell, Ahn et al., 1994; Graffam, Johnson, 1987; Sloman, Brown, Aldana et al., 1994) found a significant decrease in pain intensity as a result of patients using relaxation techniques.

One of the studies involved 67 patients with chronic cancer pain (Sloman, Brown, Aldana et al., 1994). A group receiving no relaxation intervention was compared with groups receiving relaxation by either audio tapes or by direct live teaching by nurses. Relaxation sessions were conducted twice a week for 3 weeks and consisted of deep breathing, muscle relaxation, and imagery. Pain ratings were lower for both groups receiving relaxation than for those who received no relaxation intervention, and instances of breakthrough pain appeared to decrease.

A later study was conducted with cancer patients (*n* = 94) who had oral mucositis pain related to bone marrow transplants (Syrjala, Donaldson, Davis et al., 1995). Results revealed that relaxation with imagery reduced pain. For achieving pain reduction, this study and others (Fernandez, Turk, 1989) suggest that imagery is a powerful component of a relaxation strategy. This is supported by a study of acute pain in 126 postthoracotomy patients who spontaneously used pleasant imaging as a way of coping with pain (Bachiocco, Bragaglia, Carli, 1994). Compared with other coping strategies such as external distraction, pleasant imaging was clearly the most effective. This study is an example, however, of the confusion that exists in the literature regarding what is relaxation and what is imagery.

The researchers had a category of coping techniques labeled as relaxation that did not include the pleasant imagining.

In support of these findings regarding the importance of imagery, the results of a study of experimentally induced pain revealed that imagery using a pleasant memory reduced pain ratings, but pain ratings were not reduced when subjects used a brief relaxation intervention lasting 3 to 5 minutes and involving slow, deep breathing (Bruehl, Carlson, McCubbin, 1993). However, imagery was not referred to as relaxation. This lack of consistent categorizing of nondrug pain interventions adds to confusion about what is effective.

The effect of relaxation on acute pain is less clear than it is for chronic pain. For postoperative pain the findings of one study revealed that relaxation resulted in less distress but had no effect on pain (Morgan, Wells, Robertson, 1985). In another study of pain associated with open heart surgery, researchers also reported that relaxation reduced distress but not pain (Horowitz, Fitzpatrick, Flaherty, 1984). These results were supported in a study of experimental ischemic pain where relaxation did not reduce pain (Clum, Luscomb, Scott, 1982). On the other hand, two studies of postoperative pain found that jaw relaxation taught preoperatively reduced pain when used postoperatively (Ceccio, 1984; Flaherty, Fitzpatrick, 1978). Results are inconclusive but somewhat suggestive of the benefits of relaxation for acute pain, at least in terms of reduced distress.

The failure of relaxation to reduce acute pain may be due in part to the tendency to use brief relaxation techniques for this type of pain. Often the circumstances of acute pain preclude the use of lengthy techniques. It may be difficult to find time to teach patients in advance, and patients may not have the energy and ability to concentrate.

Indications for Use of Relaxation

Relaxation may be appropriate for almost any type of pain. The goals of relaxation usually are to reduce muscle tension and anxiety. Chronic pain may be especially responsive to the use of relaxation techniques. Patients who report being anxious or who have sleep difficulties are good candidates for trying relaxation. Patients who have tense or aching muscles related to painful conditions such as temporomandibular joint disorder are also likely to benefit from relaxation.

However, one study of patients with chronic cancer pain found that introduction of a time-consuming relaxation technique was viewed by patients as another source of stress (Kaempfer, 1982). When patients are already debilitated and burdened with many treatment activities such as clinic appointments, relaxation may appear to be indicated but may simply drain the patient's already limited time and energy.

This is supported to some degree in a study of elderly patients with chronic cancer pain who had the opportunity to choose from a variety of nondrug approaches to pain (Rhiner, Ferrell, Ferrell et al., 1993). Relaxation imagery was seldom selected. The researchers noted that the anxious patients seemed to benefit more from a physical intervention such as heat or massage. Relaxation techniques that allow the patient to be more passive, such as listening to music or having a massage, may be more appropriate for many patients with progressive disease. These are also appropriate for patients who are cognitively impaired.

For a patient who is already tense and in pain, a brief and simple technique such as one that centers around slow, deep breathing is probably appropriate. For patients with chronic pain, a more involved technique such as a combination of rhythmic breathing and peaceful imagery may be indicated.

For patients who have difficulty ridding themselves of intrusive thoughts, relaxation imagery may be difficult. One study found that such patients preferred the progressive muscle relaxation technique (tensing and relaxing muscle groups) to imagery (Graffam, Johnson, 1987). This technique, like slowed breathing, gives the patient something physical to do and holds the patient's attention more easily.

Relaxation techniques may be learned and practiced by anyone interested in and capable of doing so. Relaxation techniques, especially brief ones, are relatively free of adverse effects. However, they should be used with caution in patients with a history of significant psychiatric problems such as having hallucinations. Meditative techniques probably should be avoided in depressed patients because they may become more withdrawn. Quick and easy relaxation techniques such as brief use of slow, deep breathing could be used with these patients. However, patients with respiratory disease such as emphysema may have difficulty with those relaxation techniques that include a focus on breathing.

Care should be taken with patients who view the use of relaxation as an indication that clinicians think the pain is "all in my head." Such patients may feel that their report of pain is being discounted if relaxation is suggested.

Theoretically, if a technique elicits the relaxation response, it could precipitate adverse physiologic events such as hypotension. Apparently this is rare because only one such instance was found in the literature (Spross, Wolff, 1995).

Characteristics of Effective Relaxation Techniques

Relaxation techniques tend to have a narrow focus on the repetition of one thing such as a word, sound, phrase, or physical activity, particularly slow, deep breathing. Ef-

fective relaxation techniques also usually rely to some extent on classical conditioning, that is, behavior already paired with relaxation, such as a deep breath, abdominal breathing, yawning, or past peaceful experiences. Whereas distraction strategies are most effective if they are changing and novel, relaxation techniques tend to be more effective if the same one is used each time. Practice with the technique is recommended to help establish the conditioned response of relaxation. If relaxing imagery is included, repetition and practice also improve the patient's mental ability to construct the imagery. Ask patients if they have used relaxation techniques for other purposes such as childbirth. If the technique was effective, it probably should be used again rather than introducing a new one.

The effectiveness of the more lengthy relaxation techniques is enhanced by a quiet environment and having the patient assume a comfortable, well-supported position. When the environment is noisy, using a headset to listen to a taped relaxation technique helps the patient focus.

When brief relaxation techniques are used under stressful circumstances, the word "relax" probably should be avoided. Certainly one would want to resist telling the patient who is experiencing acute distress and pain, "Relax. Everything will be OK." In other words try to tell the patient *how* to relax. Give the patient directions to perform a behavior that usually produces relaxation, such as taking a deep breath and letting it out slowly.

Specific Relaxation Techniques: Active Patient Involvement

Active patient involvement obviously requires that the patient be able to understand the instructions and physically perform the tasks. Numerous audiotapes of relaxation techniques are available commercially, including progressive relaxation (tensing and relaxing various muscle groups) and a wide variety of relaxation images (e.g., contact Academy for Guided Imagery listed in the resource section). Limited instructions for relaxation are included here, and the reader is urged to take advantage of the many tapes that already exist.

Following is an example of a relaxation technique that can be taught quickly and easily to most patients and takes advantage of the possibility that relaxation is conditioned to follow certain behaviors. Tell the patient to:

1. Clench your fists, breathe in deeply, and hold it a moment.
2. Breathe out and let yourself go limp.
3. Start yawning.

Deep breathing is probably one of the most rapidly learned of the relaxation techniques. Written instructions to help the patient learn this are presented in Box 9.10. Because research shows that imagery is among the more effective approaches to relaxation that reduces pain intensity, one of the additional points for the patient to

●●●●●

BOX 9.10	**Patient Information: Deep Breathing for Relaxation With the Option of Peaceful Imagining**

1. Breathe in slowly and deeply.
2. As you breathe out slowly, feel yourself beginning to relax; feel the tension leaving your body.
3. Now breathe in and out slowly and regularly, at whatever rate is comfortable for you.
4. To help you focus on your breathing and breathe slowly and rhythmically:
   Breathe in as you say silently to yourself, "in, two, three."
   Breathe out as you say silently to yourself, "out, two, three."
   or
   Each time you breathe out, say silently to yourself a word such as peace or relax.
5. You may imagine that you are doing this in a place you have found very calming and relaxing for you, such as laying in the sun at the beach.
6. Do steps 1 through 4 only once or repeat steps 3 and 4 for up to 20 minutes.
7. End with a slow, deep breath. As you breathe out you may say to yourself, "I feel alert and relaxed."

Additional points:

- This technique for relaxation has the advantage of being very adaptable. You may use it for only a few seconds or for up to 20 minutes. For example, you may do this regularly for 10 minutes twice a day. You may also use it for one or two complete breaths any time you need it throughout the day or when you awaken in the middle of the night.
- If you use this technique for more than a few seconds, try to get in a comfortable position in a quiet environment.
- A very effective way to relax is to add peaceful images once you have performed steps 1 through 4 above. Following are some ideas about finding your own peaceful memories.

  Something may have happened to you a while ago that can be of use to you now. Something may have brought you deep joy or peace. You may be able to draw on that past experience to bring you peace or comfort now. Think about these questions.

  Can you remember any situation, even when you were a child, when you felt calm, peaceful, secure, hopeful, or comfortable?

  Have you ever laid back, kicked off your shoes, and daydreamed about something peaceful? What were you thinking of?

  Do you get a dreamy feeling when you listen to music?
  Do you have any favorite music?

  Do you have any favorite poetry that you find uplifting or reassuring?

  Are you now or have you ever been religiously active? Do you have favorite readings, hymns, or prayers? Even if you haven't heard or thought of them for many years, childhood religious experiences may still be very soothing.

  Very likely some of the things you think of in answer to these questions can be tape recorded for you, such as your favorite music or a prayer read by your clergyman. Then you can listen to the tape whenever you wish. Or, if your memory is strong, you may simply close your eyes and recall the events or words.

consider is to combine slow breathing with imagining a peaceful experience.

Specific Relaxation Techniques: The Patient as Passive Recipient

When patients are fatigued or lack the physical or mental ability to participate actively in relaxation strategies, massage, music, or even animal companions may be effective alternatives.

Superficial massage

The effects of superficial body massage are usually soothing and relaxing, both physically and mentally. Almost everyone likes a massage, although touch may be unacceptable to some patients. Massage is one method of helping patients relax that has the advantage of requiring little if any effort on the patient's part. Massage may also decrease pain, perhaps mainly by relaxing muscles. In addition, massage may be used as a sleep aid.

Research suggests that brief massage is safe and effective. When a 6-minute, slow stroke back massage was given 2 to 3 days after acute myocardial infarction, no significant changes in cardiovascular response were observed (Bauer, Dracup, 1987). A 3-minute, slow stroke back rub for terminally ill patients (average age 71) lowered blood pressure, indicating relaxation (Meek, 1993). A 1-minute back rub on critically ill adults was mildly stimulating but well tolerated by most (Tyler, Winslow, Clark et al., 1990). A meta-analysis of the effects of effleurage (long, slow gliding strokes) backrubs supports the use of a simple 3-minute backrub to enhance comfort and relaxation and suggests that it may have a positive effect on cardiovascular parameters such as blood pressure (Labyak, Metzger, 1997). The findings of a study of postoperative patients reveals significantly lower pain ratings in patients who had received massage (Nixon, Teschendorff, Finney et al., 1997). In this study there was some indication that the longer the massage, the more effective it was.

A study of patients with cancer revealed that a 10-minute massage significantly decreased pain in men (Weinrich, Weinrich, 1990). Unexplainably, the same reduction in pain was not achieved in the women. Massage seemed especially helpful when pain was at high levels. The conclusion emphasized the simultaneous use of massage and medication. If an analgesic is administered at the same time that massage is provided, the patient seems to achieve immediate pain relief from massage and pain relief later from the medication.

Probably the most common areas of the body to massage are the back and shoulders. Extremities may be added. When it is inconvenient to do a backrub, massage of both hands or both feet may be equally or more effective (Cyriax, 1985; Day, Mason, Chesrown, 1987). Instructions for massage are presented in Box 9.11 and

● ● ● ● ●

> **BOX 9.11** **Massage for Relaxation**
>
> Massage is an age-old method of helping someone relax. Some examples are:
> 1. Brief touch or massage (e.g., handholding or briefly touching or rubbing a person's shoulder). These are so common and quickly done that we sometimes forget they are methods of helping someone relax.
> 2. Warm foot soak in a basin of warm water, or wrap the feet in a warm, wet towel.
> 3. Massage (3 to 10 minutes) may consist of whole body or be restricted to back, feet, or hands. If the patient is modest or cannot move or turn easily in bed, consider massage of the hands or feet.
>
>   Use a warm lubricant (e.g., a small bowl of hand lotion may be warmed in the microwave oven, or a bottle of lotion may be warmed by placing it in a sink of hot water for about 10 minutes).
>
>   Massage for relaxation is usually done with smooth, long, slow strokes. (Rapid strokes, circular movements, and squeezing of tissues tends to stimulate circulation and increase arousal.) However, try several degrees of pressure along with different types of massage (e.g., kneading, stroking, and circling). Determine which is preferred.
>
>   Especially for the elderly person, a back rub that effectively produces relaxation may consist of no more than 3 minutes of slow, rhythmic stroking (about 60 strokes/minute) on both sides of the spinous process from the crown of the head to the lower back. Continuous hand contact is maintained by starting one hand down the back as the other hand stops at the lower back and is raised.
>
>   Set aside a regular time for the massage. This gives the patient something to look forward to and depend on.

May be duplicated for use in clinical practice. From McCaffery M, Pasero C: *Pain: Clinical manual*, p. 421. Copyright © 1999, Mosby, Inc.

may be given to family or friends of the patient with the patient's permission.

Massage also may be used to create an acceptable method of touch for a patient who experiences limited physical contact with others, such as a patient who is away from family. Or, massage may be used to communicate care and concern when verbal communication is limited or impossible, such as when a patient speaks another language, has impaired hearing, or is cognitively impaired. Family caregivers may welcome the use of massage as a method of providing comfort for a loved one, especially when the patient is terminally or critically ill (Juarez, Ferrell, 1996; Leiber, Plumb, Gerstenzang et al., 1976).

Music

Music may be used for relaxation for some patients. Background music or headsets for individual listening have been used in various clinical settings, including chronic and cancer pain care centers, preoperative holding areas, outpatient surgery, pediatric units, and postanesthesia care units. Positive effects have been

noted and may be a result of music producing relaxation. For example, in a study of patients who listened to music in the postanesthesia care unit, patients reported their experience as significantly more pleasant than those who did not listen to music (Heitz, Symreng, Scamman, 1992).

In a study of 96 postoperative patients, the effects of 30-minute sessions of music video, music alone, and rest were compared (Zimmerman, Nieveen, Barnason et al., 1996). Although pain scores for the three groups over a 3-day period showed no differences, pain scores immediately after the sessions improved for all three groups. Sleep improved in both groups exposed to music. These results show that rest or music tends to reduce pain temporarily. Also, the findings suggest that music can be a valuable sleep aid. Perhaps patients could select relaxing music and practice with it preoperatively. Patients could then use this at their own discretion postoperatively, especially before bedtime, to promote sleep.

Patient preference should be respected when music is used, especially for relaxation purposes. Music can be an unpleasant experience if patients are not allowed to choose the type of music they enjoy (see Box 8.8, p.391).

Animals

Companion animals are also a method of providing relaxation and can be used for patients, including children, who are unable to engage in more involved relaxation techniques. A study in one hospice setting revealed that dog visits were found by patients to be relaxing (Phear, 1996). Animal visitation information is included in the resource section at the end of the chapter.

NONDRUG APPROACHES TO PAIN MANAGEMENT FOR CHILDREN

Many of the nondrug approaches to pain management discussed in this chapter can be used without modification for adolescents. Suggestions for young children are listed in Box 9.12.

INTEGRATING NONDRUG PAIN TREATMENT INTO CLINICAL PRACTICE

Unfortunately, nurses rarely discuss nondrug methods with patients (e.g., Donovan, Dillon, 1987). This may be due to lack of education about when such therapies are appropriate, which ones are most likely to be acceptable to patients, and exactly what the technique involves. Simply offering a cold pack to a patient postoperatively can be awkward if the clinician has no knowledge of the potential benefits and just how the cold pack should be prepared. In many clinical settings clinicians are also extremely busy and unable to take the extra time to locate and prepare something as seemingly easy as a cold pack.

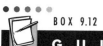

BOX 9.12

G U I D E L I N E S

NONDRUG APPROACHES TO PAIN MANAGEMENT IN CHILDREN

General Strategies

Form a trusting relationship with child and family.
- Express concern regarding their reports of pain.
- Take an active role in seeking effective pain management strategies.

Prepare child before potentially painful procedures but avoid "planting" the idea of pain. For example, instead of saying, "This is going to (or may) hurt," say, "Sometimes this feels like pushing, sticking, or pinching, and sometimes it doesn't bother people. Tell me what it feels like to you."

Stay with child during a painful procedure.
- Encourage parents to stay with child if child and parent desire; encourage parent to talk softly to child and to remain near child's head.
- Involve parents in learning specific nonpharmacologic strategies and assisting child in their use.

Educate child about the pain, especially when explanation may lessen anxiety (e.g., that child's pain is expected after surgery and does not indicate something is wrong; reassure child that he or she is not responsible for the pain).

For long-term pain control, give child a doll, which becomes "the patient," and allow child to do everything to the doll that is done to the child; pain control can be emphasized through the doll by stating, "Dolly feels better after the medicine."

Teach procedures to child and family for later use.

Specific Strategies

Distraction
- Involve parent and child in identifying strong distractors.
- Involve child in play; use radio, tape recorder, record player; have child sing or use rhythmic breathing.
- Have child take a deep breath and blow it out until told to stop (French, Painter, Coury, 1994).
- Have child blow bubbles to "blow the hurt away."
- Have child concentrate on yelling or saying "ouch" by focusing on "yelling loud or soft as you feel it hurt; that way I know what's happening."

- Have child look through kaleidoscope (type with glitter suspended in fluid-filled tube) and encourage to concentrate by asking, "Do you see the different designs?" (Vessey, Carlson, McGill, 1994).
- Use humor, such as watching cartoons, telling jokes or funny stories, or acting silly with child.
- Have child read, play games, or visit with friends.

Relaxation

With an infant or young child:
- Hold in a comfortable, well-supported position, such as vertically against the chest and shoulder.
- Rock in a wide, rhythmic arc in a rocking chair or sway back and forth, rather than bouncing child.
- Repeat one or two words softly, such as "Mommy's here."

With a slightly older child:
- Ask child to take a deep breath and "go limp as a rag doll" while exhaling slowly, then ask child to yawn (demonstrate if needed).
- Suggest that the child pretend to float like a balloon.

Imagery for Distraction or Relaxation
- Have child identify some highly pleasurable real or pretend experience.
- Have child describe details of the event, including as many senses as possible (e.g., "feel the cool breezes," "see the beautiful colors," "hear the pleasant music").
- Have child write down or record script.
- Encourage child to concentrate only on the pleasurable event during the painful time; enhance the image by recalling specific details, such as reading the script or playing the record.
- Combine with relaxation.

Cutaneous Stimulation

Includes simple rhythmic rubbing; use of pressure, electric vibrator; massage with hand lotion, powder, or menthol cream; application of heat or cold, such as an ice cube on the site before giving injection or application of ice to the site opposite the painful area (e.g., if right knee hurts, place ice on left knee).

May be duplicated for use in clinical practice. As appears in McCaffery M, Pasero C: *Pain: Clinical manual*, p. 422, 1999, Mosby, Inc.

Modified from Wong DL: *Whaley & Wong's essentials of pediatric nursing*, ed 5, p 634, St. Louis, 1997, Mosby.

Information from French GM, Painater EC, Courty DL: Blowing away shot pain: A technique for pain management during immunization, *Pediatrics* 93:384-388, 1994; Vessey JA, Carlson KL, McGill J: Use of distraction with children during an acute pain experience, *Nurs Res* 43:369, 1994.

For these reasons, practical plans for integrating nondrug pain therapies probably should be founded on easy access. When nondrug pain management is not as high a priority as analgesic management, the nondrug therapy may be coordinated with activities related to providing analgesics.

Nondrug pain treatment can also be incorporated into the routine patient teaching that precedes painful procedures, including surgery (e.g., preadmission testing). Specific nondrug methods can be listed in the "preoperative checklist." (See Form 6.2, p. 273, for a pain management teaching checklist.) A method of superficial cooling could be introduced to the patient along with how to use a PCA button. If possible, the patient could be shown a lightweight cold pack and told that it can be wrapped to provide a comfortable degree of coolness.

Although patients tend to be reluctant to try cold, cold relieves pain rapidly and also has the beneficial therapeutic effect of vasoconstriction to reduce bleeding and edema. Therefore promoting the use of cold postoperatively seems to have several advantages.

In the emergency department (ED) cold packs could become a routine offering, especially to young children with fractures or lacerations. A refrigerator containing cold packs could be placed in a central area. Reminders of simple nondrug methods, such as taking a deep breath to relax, could be posted in treatment rooms, or audiocassettes for distraction might be placed in each room.

Simple instructions, prepared in advance, for patients and clinicians may encourage use of nondrug methods. Many are contained in this chapter and may be duplicated for use in clinical practice. In the hospital a physician's prescription is necessary for the use of heat or cold. To facilitate the nurse's use of heat or cold, preprinted admission orders may include a section that the physician may check for use of heat and/or cold as needed for relief of discomfort. A policy can be written that guides the nurse's use of heat and cold.

Clinical practice guidelines published by the Agency for Health Care Policy and Research recommend integrating nondrug measures into acute and cancer pain management, and its patient guides contain some simple examples of nondrug strategies (AHCPR, 1992a,b; Jacox, Carr, Payne et al., 1994a,b). These guides may be given to patients, along with a brief explanation of what the booklet suggests for nondrug treatment.

Some health care facilities have developed resources for nondrug treatment. In hospital settings the equipment and instructions for a variety of nondrug treatments may be placed on a cart that is brought to the patient's room. In home care the same items may be placed in a suitcase that is taken to the patient's home (Rhiner, Ferrell, Ferrell et al., 1993). A "lending library" of nondrug pain treatments can be developed.

Suggestions for these portable resource carts or suitcases include gel packs for heat or cold, cassette players with a variety of audiotapes of comedy and different types of music, a cross section of videotapes, joke books, art books, tinker toys, a vibrating/heating device, relaxation audio and video tapes, various ointments such as menthol, and small bottles containing different smells such as chocolate and perfumes. Audio and video tapes should be selected on the basis of the patients' ages. For elderly patients, comedians such as Jack Benny may be more appealing than Jay Leno. Music popular in the 1930s and 1940s is likely to be more desirable than hard rock.

One of the drawbacks to using some of the nondrug interventions such as music may be the cost of equipment. In some instances hospital volunteers or community charity groups have adopted this as a project and raised money for the health care agency to purchase items such as cassette players, portable tape recorders, headphones, and compact discs.

Resources

Organizations

- Academy for Guided Imagery
  Provides training, certifications, and numerous audiotapes of imagery.
  To contact:
  P.O. Box 2070
  Mill Valley, CA 94942
  Phone: (415) 389-9324
  Fax: (415) 389-9342

- American Alliance of Aromatherapy (AAOA)
  AAOA is a nonprofit organization established as a resource center and voice for aromatherapy. Purpose: resource center, education, advocate further enhancement and development of aromatherapy.
  Membership benefits: Quarterly newsletter, listing in AAOA resource database, and complimentary issue of *The International Journal of Aromatherapy*. To contact:
  P.O. Box 309
  Depoe Bay, OR 97341
  Phone: (800) 809-9850
  Fax: (800) 809-9808

- American Holistic Medical Association
  4101 Lake Boone Trail, Suite #201
  Raleigh, NC 27607
  Phone: (919) 787-5146

- American Holistic Nurses Association
  4101 Lake Boone Trail, Suite 201
  Raleigh, NC 27607
  Phone: (919) 389-9324
  Fax: (919) 787-4916
  Web site: *http://www.wholenurse.com*
  "Whole Nurse: Holistic Nursing on the Web" provided by the AHNA consists of information regarding acupuncture, massage, healing touch, guided imagery, and aromatherapy.

- Healing Touch International
  198 Union Blvd. #204
  Lakewood, CO 80228
  Phone: (303) 989-0581

- Nurse Healers—Professional Associate, Inc.
  A nonprofit cooperative of health care professionals for the promotion of healing. The mission of NHPA is to lead, inspire, and advance therapeutic touch, other healing modalities, and healing lifeways for the world community. To contact:
  1211 Locust St.
  Philadelphia, PA 19107
  Fax: (215) 545-8107
  E-mail: *nhpa@nursecominc.com*

- Office of Alternative Medicine (OAM): In 1992, NIH created the Office of Alternative Medicine (OAM) to evaluate alternative medical treatment modalities such as visual imagery and healing touch. It has released an exhaustive report titled "Alternative Medicine: Expanding Medical Horizons." To obtain fact sheets or more information, write:

9000 Rockville Pike
Building 31, Room 5B-38
Bethesda, MD 20892
Phone: (301) 402-2466
Fax: (301) 402-4741
or
OAM Clearinghouse
P.O. Box 8218
Silver Spring, MD 20907-8218
Phone: (888) 644-6226

A journal, *Complementary and Alternative Medicine at the NIH,* is published by the Office of Alternative Medicine Clearinghouse.

Animal Resources

- The Delta Society
  Provides information and educational conferences on animal visit programs for health care facilities. To contact:
  289 Perimeter Road E.
  Renton, WA 98055-1329
  Phone: (800) 869-6898 or (206) 226-7357
  Web site: *http://www2.deltasociety.org/deltasociety/*

- Therapy Dog International
  Provides information on animal visit programs and the names of health care facilities that participate in dog visitation programs. To contact:
  Phone: (973) 252-9800
  Fax: (973) 252-7171

Humor

- American Association for Therapeutic Humor
  Purpose: The advancement of knowledge and understanding of humor and laughter as they relate to healing and well-being. AATH provides a networking source for application of humor in care giving professions, bimonthly newsletter, humor bibliography, annual conference, and speakers bureau. To contact:
  222 Meramec, Suite 303
  St. Louis, MO 63105
  Phone: (314) 863-6232
  Fax: (314) 863-6457

- Healing Through Laughter and Play Conferences
  Institute for the Advancement of Human Behavior
  P.O. Box 7226
  Stanford, CA 94309
  Phone: (415) 851-8411

- Humor & Health Institute
  Publishes a bimonthly newsletter, *Humor and Health Letter,* about laughter research and applications. To contact:
  P.O. Box 16814
  Jackson, MS 39326-6814
  Phone: (601) 957-0075
  Fax: (601) 977-0423
  E-mail: *jrdunn@intop.net*
  Web site: *http://www.introp.net/rjdunn*

- Humor Project (Publishes *Laughing Matters,* a quarterly journal; sponsors an annual conference.)
  110 Spring Street
  Saratoga Springs, NY 12866
  Phone: (518) 587-8770
  Web site: *http://www.wizvax.net/humor*

- Jest for the Health of It Services
  Offers seminars and presentations on the topics of health, humor, and how to provide and promote humor in health care settings. To contact:
  c/o Patty Wooten
  P.O. Box 4040
  Davis, CA 95617
  Phone: (916) 758-3826
  E-mail: *JestPatty@mother.com*

- *Journal of Nursing Jocularity*
  Sponsors an annual spring conference on humor. Provides a speakers bureau and publishes a journal focusing on humor in the medical profession. To contact:
  P.O. Box 40416
  Mesa, AZ 85274
  Phone: (602) 835-6165
  Web site: *Jocularity.com*

Music

- American Music Therapy Association
  Purpose: The progressive development of the therapeutic uses of music in rehabilitation, special education, and community settings. The AMTA is committed to the advancement of education, training, professional standards, credentialing, and research in support of the music therapy profession. Membership: Categories include professional, associate, and student. Quarterly research-oriented journal and bimonthly newsletter provided with membership. Has certification program. To contact:
  AMTA
  8455 Colesville Rd., Suite 1000
  Silver Springs, MD 20910
  Phone: (301) 589-3300
  Fax: (301) 589-5175
  E-mail: *info@namt.com*
  Web site: *http://www.namt.com/NAMT.htm1*

- The Bonny Foundation
  A nonprofit institute for music-centered therapies. To contact:
  2020 Simmons St.
  Salina, KS 67401
  Phone: (913) 827-1497

- Institute for Consciousness and Music
  7027 Bellona Ave.
  Baltimore, MD 21212

- Institute for Music, Health, and Education
  P.O. Box 1244
  Boulder, CO 80306
  Phone: (303) 443-8484

- Music RX
  Music designed for hospital use. To contact:
  P.O. Box 173
  Port Townsend, WA 98368
  Phone: (206) 385-6160
- Steven Halpern (Hospital Suite)
  Music designed for hospital use. To contact:
  P.O. Box 1439
  San Rafael, CA 94915
  Phone: (415) 491-1930

Resources Especially for Patients

- American Massage Therapy Association
  820 Davis St., Suite 100
  Evanston, IL 60201-4444
  Phone: (847) 864-0123
  Fax: (847) 864-1178
  E-mail: info@amtamassage.org
  Web site: *http://www.amtamassage.org*
  This organization can be contacted for the names of certi-
  fied massage therapists in specific geographic locations.
- "The Cancer Pain Education Program" is a patient educa-
  tion kit designed for use in home care. It contains two cas-
  sette tapes about drug and nondrug pain relief along with
  a booklet to reinforce the audio tapes, instructions for 16
  nondrug pain relief methods, and a self-care log. Send
  $45.00 (this includes sales tax, shipping and handling) to:
  Marketing Dept.
  City of Hope Medical Center
  1500 E. Duarte Rd.
  Duarte, CA 91010
  Based on: Rhiner M, Ferrell BR, Ferrell BA, Grant MM: A
  structured non-drug intervention program for cancer pain,
  Cancer Pract 1(2):137-143, July/August 1993.
- "Coping Skills for Bone Marrow Transplantation" by Karen
  Syrjala, Ben Danis, Janet Abrams, and Rosemarie Keenan,
  is written for the patient. Topics include relaxation, imagery,
  focusing attention (e.g., distraction), and conversations with
  yourself (e.g., positive thoughts). These nondrug ap-
  proaches to pain management would be helpful for many
  patients with painful experiences other than bone marrow
  transplantation. To order the booklet and accompanying
  audio tape for relaxation (approximately $15.00):
  Biobehavioral Sciences
  Fred Hutchinson Cancer Research Center
  1100 Fairview Avenue N., FM815
  Seattle, WA 98109-1024
  Phone: (206) 667-5022
- Educational booklets
  Pain control after surgery: A patient's guide, AHCPR Pub.
  No. 92-0021.
  Management of cancer pain: Patient guide, AHCPR Pub.
  No. 94-0595.
  These contain some examples of nondrug pain methods. To
  order free copies:
  AHCPR, Publications Clearinghouse
  P.O. Box 8547
  Silver Spring, MD 20907
  Phone: (800) 358-9295 (from outside the United States,
  [410] 381-3150)

Hearing impaired TDD service (888) 586-6340.
To get copies off Web site: *http//www.ahcpr.gov/guide/*

- Laughter Therapy. The **individual** with the illness (or
  his/her representative) must write a letter explaining the na-
  ture of the illness. (Because of copyright laws, requests from
  organizations and institutions cannot be accommodated.)
  Then the first of four *Candid Camera* videos is mailed to the
  individual. When the individual returns the tape, the second
  video is sent. The process continues until all four have been
  viewed and returned.
  Laughter Therapy (founded by Allen Funt)
  Candid Camera, Inc.
  P.O. Box 827
  Monterey, CA 93942
  Phone: (408) 625-3788
  Fax: (408) 625-3835

References

Agency for Health Care Policy and Research (AHCPR): *Acute pain man-agement in adults: operative procedures. Quick reference guide for clinicians,* AHCPR Pub. No. 92-0019, Rockville, Md, Agency for Health Care Policy and Research, Public Health Service, U.S. De-partment of Health and Human Services, 1992a.

Agency for Health Care Policy and Research (AHCPR): *Pain control af-ter surgery: a patient's guide,* AHCPR Pub. No. 92-0021, Rockville, Md, Agency for Health Care Policy and Research, Public Health Ser-vice, U.S. Department of Health and Human Services, 1992b.

Aronoff GM: Ice massage for pain, *Aches Pains* 3:33-36, 1982.

Bachiocco V, Bragaglia R, Carli G: Antalgic positions in alleviating post-thoracotomy pain: their introduction in a pain relief program, *Chest* 105:1299, 1994.

Bailey L: The effects of life music versus tape-recorded music on hospi-talized cancer patients, *Music Ther* 2:17-28, 1983.

Bauer WC, Dracup KA: Physiological effects of back massage in pa-tients with acute myocardial infarctions, *Focus Crit Care* 14(6):42-46, 1987.

Beck S: The therapeutic use of music for cancer-related pain, *Oncol Nurs Forum* 18:1327-1337, 1991.

Benson H, Beary J, Carol M: The relaxation response, *Psychiatry* 37:3746, 1974.

Berk LS, Tan SA, Fry WF et al.: Neuroendocrine and stress hormone changes during mirthful laughter, *Am J Med Sci* 296:390-396, 1989.

Bini G, Cruccu K-E H, Schady W et al.: Analgesic effect of vibration and cooling on pain induced by intraneural electrical stimulation, *Pain* 18, 239-248, 1984.

Brody R: Music medicine, *Omni* 6:24, 110, 1984.

Bruehl S, Carlson CR, McCubbin JA: Two brief interventions for acute pain, *Pain* 54:29-36, 1993.

Ceccio CM: Postoperative pain relief through relaxation in elderly pa-tients with fractured hips, *Orthop Nurs* 3:11-19, May-June 1984.

Cleeland CS: Nonpharmacological management of cancer pain, *J Pain Symptom Manage* 2:S23-S28, Spring 1987.

Clum GA, Luscomb RL, Scott L: Relaxation training and cognitive redi-rection strategies in the treatment of acute pain, *Pain* 12:175-183, 1982.

Cogan R, Cogan D, Waltz W et al.: Effects of laughter and relaxation on discomfort thresholds, *J Behav Med* 10:139-144, 1987.

Collins PM: *Contralateral ice massage during bone marrow aspiration,* Masters thesis, University of Miami, June 1985.

Cook JD: Music as an intervention in the oncology setting, *Cancer Nurs* 9:23-28, 1986.

Cold may ease arthritis pain, *J Gerontol Nurs* 8:471, Aug 1982.

Cooling more effective, *Aches Pains* 3:37, 1982.

Cousins N: *Anatomy of an illness as perceived by the patient,* New York, 1979, Norton.

Creamer P, Hunt M, Dieppe P: Pain mechanisms in osteoarthritis of the knee: effect of intraarticular anesthetic, *J Rheumatol* 23:1031-1036, 1996.

Cyriax JH: Clinical applications of massage. In Basmajian JB, editor: *Manipulation, traction and massage,* ed 3, pp. 270-288. Baltimore, 1985, Williams & Wilkins.

Day JA, Mason RR, Chesrown SE: Effect of massage on serum level of β-endorphin and β-lipotropin in healthy adults, *Phys Ther* 67:926-930, 1987.

Ditlow F: The missing element in health care: humor as a form of creativity, *J Holistic Nurs* 11:66-79, 1993.

Donovan M, Dillon P: Incidence and characteristics of pain in a sample of hospitalized cancer patients, *Cancer Nurs* 10:85-92, 1987.

Eisenberg DM, Kessler RC, Foster C et al.: Unconventional medicine in the United States: prevalence, costs, and patterns of use, *N Engl J Med* 328(4)246-252, 1993.

Ekblom A, Hansson P: Extrasegmental transcutaneous electrical nerve stimulation and mechanical vibratory stimulation as compared to placebo for the relief of acute oro-facial pain, *Pain* 23:223-229, 1985.

Ernst E, Fialka V: Ice freezes pain? A review of the clinical effectiveness of analgesic cold therapy, *J Pain Symptom Manage* 9:56-59, 1994.

Fanurik D, Zeltzer LK, Roberts MC et al.: The relationship between children's coping styles and psychological interventions for cold pressor pain, *Pain* 53:213-222, 1993.

Fernandez E: A classification system of cognitive coping strategies for pain, *Pain* 26:141-151, 1986.

Fernandez E, Turk DC: The utility of cognitive coping strategies for altering pain perception: a meta-analysis, *Pain* 38:123-135, 1989.

Ferrell BR, Cohen MZ, Grant M: Pain as a metaphor for illness. II. Family caregivers' management of pain, *Oncol Nurs Forum* 18(8):1315-1321, 1991.

Ferrell BR, Ferrell BA, Ahn C et al.: Pain management for elderly patients with cancer at home, *Cancer* 74(suppl):2139-1246, 1994.

Ferrell BR, Rhiner M: Managing cancer pain: a three-step approach, *Nursing* 24(7):56-59, 1994.

Flaherty GD, Fitzpatrick JJ: Relaxation technique to increase comfort level of postoperative patients: a preliminary study, *Nurs Res* 27: 3522-3355, 1978.

Fritz DJ: Noninvasive pain control methods used by cancer outpatients, *Oncol Nurs Forum* suppl:108, 1988 (abstract).

Fry PS, Wong PTP: Pain management training in the elderly: matching interventions with subjects' coping styles, *Stress Med* 7:93-98, 1991.

Gammon GD, Staff I: Studies on the relief of pain by counterirritation, *J Clin Invest* 120:13-20, 1941.

Good M: Relaxation techniques for surgical patients, *Am J Nurs* 95(5):38-42, 1995.

Graffam SJ, Johnson A: A comparison of two relaxation strategies for the relief of pain and its distress, *J Pain Symptom Manage* 2:229-231, 1987.

Guieu R, Tardy-Gevert M-F, Roll J-P: Analgesic effects of vibration and transcutaneous electrical nerve stimulation applied separately and simultaneously to patients with chronic pain, *Can J Neurol Sci* 18:113-119, 1991.

Hansson P, Ekblom A, Thomasson M et al.: Influence of naloxone on relief of acute oro-facila pain by transcutaneous electrical nerve stimulation (TENS) or vibration, *Pain* 24:323-329, 1986.

Heitz L, Symreng T, Scamman FL: Effects of music therapy in the postanesthesia care unit: a nursing intervention, *J Post Anesth Nurs* 7:22-31, 1992.

Heng MCY: Local necrosis and interstitial nephritis due to topical methyl salicylate and menthol, *Cutis* 39:442-444, 1987.

Herth K: The therapeutic use of music, *Supervisor Nurse* 9:22-23, 1978.

Hillman SK, Delforge G: The use of physical agents in rehabilitation of athletic injuries, *Clin Sports Med* 4:431-438, 1985.

Horowitz BF, Fitzpatrick JJ, Flaherty GG: Relaxation techniques for pain relief after open heart surgery, *Dimens Crit Care Nurs* 3:364-371, 1984.

Hudak DA, Dale A, Hudak MA et al.: Effects of humorous stimuli and sense of humor on discomfort, *Psychol Rep* 69:779-786, 1991.

Jacox A, Carr DB, Payne R et al.: *Management of cancer pain: adults: quick reference for clinicians: clinical practice guideline No. 9,* AHCPR Pub. No. 94-0593, Rockville, Md, Agency for Health Care Policy and Research, Public Health Service, U.S. Department of Health and Human Services, 1994a.

Jacox A, Carr DB, Payne R et al.: *Management of cancer pain: patient guide: clinical practice guideline No 9,* AHCPR Pub. No. 94-0595, Rockville, Md, Agency for Health Care Policy and Research, Public Health Service, U.S. Department of Health and Human Services, 1994a.

Jensen MP, Turner JA, Romano JM et al.: Coping with chronic pain: a critical review of the literature, *Pain* 47:249-283, 1991.

Johnson MH, Petrie SM: The effects of distraction on exercise and cold pressor tolerance for chronic low back pain sufferers, *Pain* 69:43-48, 1997.

Juarez G, Ferrell BR: Family and caregiver involvement in pain management, *Clin Geriatr Med* 12:531-547, 1996.

Kaempfer SH: Relaxation training reconsidered, *Oncol Nurs Forum* 9:15-19, Spring 1982.

Kahneman D: *Attention and effort,* Englewood Cliffs, NJ, 1973, Prentice-Hall.

Keefe FJ, Crisson J, Urban BJ et al.: Analyzing chronic low back pain: the relative contribution of pain coping strategies, *Pain* 40:293-301, 1990.

Labyak SE, Metzger EL: The effects of effleurage backrub on the physiological components of relaxation: a meta-analysis, *Nurs Res* 46:59-62, 1997.

Lavergne NA: Does application of tea bags to sore nipples while breast-feeding provide effective relief? *J Obstet Gynecol Neonatal Nurs* 26(1):53, 1997.

Lehmann JF, de Lateur BJ: Cryotherapy. In Lehmann JF, editor: *Therapeutic heat and cold,* ed 3, pp 563-602, Baltimore, 1982a, Williams & Wilkins.

Lehmann JF, de Lateur BJ. Therapeutic heat. In Lehmann JF, editor: *Therapeutic heat and cold,* ed 3, pp 404-562, Baltimore, 1982b, Williams & Wilkins.

Lehmann WP, Strain F: Comparative effects of ipsilateral and contralateral TENS on subjective sensitization to tonic heat, *Clin J Pain* 1:211-216, 1985.

Leiber L, Plumb M, Gerstenzang M et al.: The communication of affection between cancer patients and their spouses, *Psychosom Med* 38:379-389, 1976.

Locsin R: The effect of music on the pain of selected postoperative patients, *J Adv Nurs* 6:19-25, 1981.

Lundeberg T: Long-term results of vibratory stimulation as a pain relieving measure for chronic pain, *Pain* 20:13-23, 1984.

Lundeberg T, Nordemar R, Ottoson D: Pain alleviation by vibratory stimulation, *Pain* 20:25-44, 1984.

Lundeberg T, Ottoson D, Hakansson S et al.: Vibratory stimulation for the control of intractable chronic orofacial pain, *Adv Pain Res Ther* 5:555-561, 1983.

Malone M, Strube M: Meta-analysis of non-medical treatments for chronic pain, *Pain* 34:231-244, 1988.

Martin F, Dobbin J: Sense of humor, hassles, and immunoglobulin A: evidence for a stress-moderating effect of humor, *Int J Psychiatry* 18:93-105, 1988.

The Mayday Fund: *1993 pain survey,* New York, 1993, Author.

McCaffery M, Wolff M: Pain relief using cutaneous modalities, positioning, and movement. In Turk DC, Feldman CS, editors: *Noninvasive approaches to pain management in the terminally ill,* New York, 1992, Haworth Press.

McCaul KD, Malott JM: Distraction and coping with pain, *Psychol Bull* 95:516-533, 1984.

Meek SS: Effects of slow stroke back massage on relaxation in hospice clients, *Image* 25:17-21, 1993.

Melzack R, Schecter B: Itch and vibration, *Science* 147:1047-1048, 1965.

Melzack R, Wall PD: Pain mechanisms: a new theory, *Science* 150:971-979, 1965.

Michlovitz SL: Biophysical principles of heating and superficial heat agents. In Michlovitz SL, editor: *Thermal agents in rehabilitation,* pp 88-108, Philadelphia: 1990a, FA Davis.

Michlovitz SL, Cryotherapy: The use of cold as a therapeutic agent. In Michlovitz SL, editor: *Thermal agents in rehabilitation,* pp 63-87, Philadelphia, 1990b, FA Davis.

Mogan J, Wells N, Robertson E: Effects of preoperative teaching on postoperative pain: a replication and expansion, *Int J Nurs Stud* 22:267-280, 1985.

Nevo O, Keinan G, Teshimovsky-Arditi M: Humor and pain tolerance, *Humor* 6:71-88, 1993.

Newton RA: Contemporary views on pain and the role played by thermal agents in managing pain symptoms. In Michlovitz SL, editor: *Thermal agents in rehabilitation,* pp 18-42, Philadelphia, 1990, FA Davis.

NIH Technology Assessment Panel on Integration of Behavioral and Relaxation Approaches In the Treatment of Chronic Pain and Insomnia: integration of behavioral and relaxation approaches into the treatment of chronic pain and insomnia, *JAMA* 276:313-318, 1996.

Nixon M, Teschendorff J, Finney J et al.: Expanding the nursing repertoire: the effect of massage on post-operative pain, *Aust J Adv Nurs* 14(3):21-26, 1997.

Phear DN: A study of animal companionship in a day hospice, *Palliative Med* 10:336-338, 1996.

Ramler D, Roberts J: A comparison of cold and warm sitz baths for relief of postpartum perineal pain, *J Obstet Gynecol Neonatal Nurs* 15:471-474, 1986.

Rana S: Pain: a subject ignored, *Pediatrics* 79:309, 1987.

Rhiner M, Ferrell, BR, Ferrell BA et al.: A structured non-drug intervention program for cancer pain, *Cancer Pract* 1:137-143, 1993.

Rosentiel AK, Keefe FJ: The use of coping strategies in chronic low back pain patients: relationship to patient characteristics and current adjustment, *Pain* 17:33-44, 1983.

Russell WR, Espir MLE, Morganstern FS: Treatment of post-herpetic neuralgia, *Lancet* 1:242, 1957.

Shere CL, Cleeland JA, O'Sullivan P et al.: The effect of two sites of high frequency vibration on cutaneous pain threshold, *Pain* 25:133-138, 1986.

Sloman JR, Brown P, Aldana E et al.: The use of relaxation for the promotion of comfort and pain relief in persons with advanced cancer, *Contemp Nurse* 3:6-12, 1994.

Spross JA, Wolff M: Nonpharmacological management of cancer pain. In McGuire DB, Yarbro CH, Ferrell BR, editors: *Cancer pain management,* ed 2, pp 159-205, Boston, 1995, Jones and Bartelett.

Syrjala KL: Relaxation techniques. In Bonica JJ: *The management of pain,* pp 1742-1750, Philadelphia, 1990, Lea & Febiger.

Syrjala KL, Donaldson GW, Davis MW et al.: Relaxation and imagery and cognitive-behavioral training reduce pain during cancer treatment: a controlled clinical trial, *Pain* 63:189-198, 1995.

Thorsteinsson G, Stonnington HH, Stillwell GK et al.: The placebo effect of transcutaneous electrical stimulation, *Pain* 5:31-41, 1978.

Turner JA, Clancy S: Strategies for coping with chronic low back pain: relationship to pain and disability, *Pain* 24:355-364, 1986.

Tyler DO, Winslow EH, Clark AP et al.: Effects of a 1-minute back rub on mixed venous oxygen saturation and heart rate in critically ill patients, *Heart Lung* 19 (5, pt.2):562-565, Sept. 1990.

Wachter-Shikora HL: Does mechanostimulation control pain? *Am J Nurs* 82:81, 1982.

Wallace K: The pathophysiology of pain, *Crit Care Nurs Q* 15(2):1-13, 1992.

Wallace KG: Analysis of recent literature concerning relaxation and imagery interventions for cancer pain, *Cancer Nurs* 20:79-87, 1997.

Ward SE, Goldberg N, Miller-McCauley V et al.: Patient-related barriers to management of cancer pain, *Pain* 52:319-324, 1993.

Weaver J, Zillmann D: Effect of humor and tragedy on discomfort tolerance, *Percept Mot Skills* 78:632-634, 1994.

Weinrich SP, Weinrich MC: The effect of massage on pain in cancer patients, *Applied Nurs Res* 3:140-145, 1990.

Whipple B, Glynn NJ: Quantification of the effects of listening to music as a noninvasive method of pain control, *Scholarly Inquiry Nurs Pract* 6(1):43-58, 1992.

Yarnitsky D, Kunin M, Brik R et al.: Vibration reduces thermal pain in adjacent dermatomes, *Pain* 69:75-77, 1997.

Zillmann D, Rockwell S, Schweitzer K et al.: Does humor facilitate coping with physical discomfort? *Motivation Emotion* 17:1-21, 1993.

Zimmerman L, Nieveen J, Barnason S et al.: The effects of music interventions on postoperative pain and sleep in coronary artery bypass graft patients, *Scholarly Inquiry Nurs Practice* 10:153-170, 1996.

Zimmerman L, Pozehl B, Duncan K et al.: Effects of music in patients who had chronic cancer pain, *West J Nurs Res* 11:298-309, 1989.

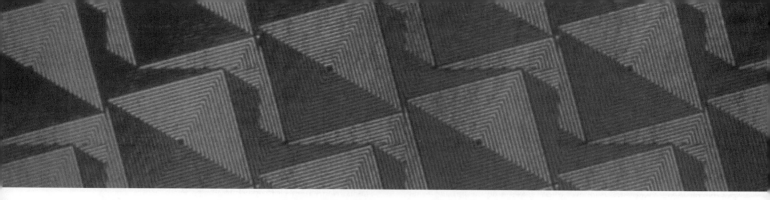

chapter ten
SUBSTANCE ABUSE

Peggy Compton

TERMINOLOGY

Addiction: An acquired, chronic disease of subcortical brain structures; equivalent to *substance dependence* as defined in DSM-IV (APA, 1994). Characterized by a persistent pattern of dysfunctional drug use (use for nonmedical reasons) and aberrant behavior involving loss of control over use and continued use despite adverse physiologic, psychologic, and/ or social consequences (see also Box 10.10). More specifically, opioid addiction is a pattern of compulsive drug use characterized by a continued craving for the opioid and the need to use the opioid for effects other than pain relief.

Chemical dependence: *Physical dependence* on a drug or medication (see following).

"Drug seeking": A set of behaviors in which an individual makes a directed and concerted effort to obtain a medication. Regarding opioid analgesics, behaviors may include "clock watching," frequent requests for early refills, or hoarding opioid analgesics. These behaviors do not, in themselves, constitute addiction. When these behaviors are for the purpose of obtaining adequate pain relief, this is called pseudoaddiction (Weissman, Haddox, 1989). If the behaviors are for the purpose of using the drug for non-medical purposes, they are suggestive of abuse or addiction.

Hyperalgesia: An increased response to a stimulus that is normally painful (i.e., increased pain).

Narcotic: Legal, not pharmacologic, term used in reference to all substances covered by the 1961 Single Convention on Narcotic Drugs, including synthetic and naturally occurring opioids and cocaine. Because the term covers a variety of substances with abuse potential, it is considered an obsolete term in the fields of addiction and pain management.

Opioid: Generic term used to refer to all agents either natural or synthetic, endogenous or exogenous, that bind to opioid receptor sites in the central and peripheral nervous system.

Physical dependence: A neuroadaptive state resulting from chronic drug administration in which abrupt cessation of the drug, or administration of an antagonist to the drug, results in a drug-specific withdrawal syndrome. Physical dependency is an expected physiologic occurrence in all individuals in the presence of continuous use of certain drugs, such as opioid analgesics, for therapeutic or nontherapeutic purposes. It does not in and of itself imply addiction and does not cause addiction (see also Box 10.10).

Substance abuse: The DSM-IV term for a less severe form, and often a predecessor to, addiction or substance dependence distinguished by a shorter duration of impairment and the absence of neurophysiologic symptoms (see Box 10.2).

Substance dependence: The DSM-IV term for *addiction* to a drug or medication (see earlier and Box 10.1) defined as a "maladaptive pattern of substance use, leading to clinically significant impairment or distress" (APA, 1994, p. 108).

Tolerance: A neuroadaptive state resulting from chronic drug administration that results in diminution of drug effect over time, requiring increasing amounts of drug to induce the same effect as obtained with the original dose (see also Box 10.10). Tolerance is an expected physiologic occurrence in all individuals in the presence of continuous use of certain drugs, such as opioid analgesics, for therapeutic or nontherapeutic purposes. It does not in and of itself imply addiction and does not cause addiction.

It is reasonable to question why a chapter devoted to substance abuse and addiction is included in a clinical manual on the assessment and management of pain. Clinicians confuse addiction and opioid-induced pain relief, and this adversely affects the care of both patients with substance abuse disorders and those with pain. Fears, misconceptions, and a general lack of knowledge about the nature and course of addiction have profoundly affected the provision of opioid analgesics to persons in pain.

Surveys in two separate states, Wisconsin and North Carolina, found that only 16% and 17% of nurses, respectively, correctly identified the likelihood of addiction as less than 1% when patients with cancer receive opioid analgesics for pain relief (O'Brien, Dalton, Konsler et al., 1996; Votherms, Ryan, Ward, 1992). The length of time on opioid analgesics appears to be a critical factor influencing nurses' concerns about addiction. In another survey, 34.8% of nurses believed that addiction would occur in 25% or more of patients who received opioids for 3 months or longer, whereas less than 4% of nurses thought addiction would occur in the same percentage

of patients receiving opioid analgesics for between 1 and 3 days (McCaffery, Ferrell, 1997). Irrational and simplistic concerns that the liberal use of opioids to relieve pain will inevitably cause or worsen addictive disease have resulted in what one expert terms "opiophobia" (Morgan, 1986) and left untold millions of persons suffering pain unnecessarily (Joranson, Colleau, 1996; Melzack, 1990; Zenz, 1991).

Clinically, pain and addiction intersect on several levels. As noted, fears of causing or inducing addiction make clinicians reticent or conservative in their prescription of opioid analgesics, especially to persons with ongoing or nonmalignant pain conditions (Academy of Pain Medicine and the American Pain Society, 1997; Ferrell, McCaffery, Rhiner, 1992; Perry, 1984; Portnow, Strassman, 1985; Savage, 1996; Schuster, 1989; Siwek, 1989). Confusion about what constitutes addiction results in patients with pain who receive opioid analgesics on a chronic basis to be mistakenly labeled "addicted" (Clark, Sees, 1993; Friedman, 1990; Wesson, Ling, Smith, 1993). These issues become exaggerated in the case of providing pain management to a person with active or remitted addictive disease and are complicated by criminal justice and moral responses to addiction (Perry, 1985; Stimmel, 1989). Furthermore, complicating the problem is accumulating scientific evidence that the phenomena of addiction and pain share common neurophysiologic bases, thus the presence of one may affect the expression of the other.

Addiction, whether it is suspected or actually present in the individual patient, shapes and is reflected in current patterns of pain management, which do not consistently ensure that adequate relief is provided. An overriding theme of this chapter is that neither pain nor addiction can be adequately treated without a good understanding of how the presence of addiction (or the fear of its presence) influences the expression and management of pain.

The chapter begins with information about the disease of addiction because an accurate and clear understanding of the disorder is necessary to distinguish between (1) the stigmatizing labels of addiction (i.e., "drug seeking"), (2) the actual disease of addiction, and (3) patients seeking drugs for the legitimate purpose of pain relief. Information on alcohol and drug abuse treatment is then provided to enable clinicians to appreciate the complexity of the addiction recovery process and to provide tools to intervene more effectively. These concepts are then examined within the context of pain, with empirically based guidelines for the clinician to enable the provision of appropriate analgesia for those individuals who may be addicted and also have pain. Terminology and common misconceptions (Table 10.1) related to this content are listed at the beginning of this chapter.

ADDICTION

In his many speeches to public and political and scientific audiences, Alan Leshner, director of the National Institute on Drug Abuse, refers to what he calls the "Great Disconnect" in addiction. He is referring to the general public's ignorance or lack of endorsement of the impressive body of empirical and rigorous knowledge

TABLE 10.1 ● ● ● ●

Misconceptions | Addiction

MISCONCEPTION	CORRECTION
1. Drug treatment does not work for addicts.	Although a single treatment episode may be unsuccessful (because of the chronic, relapsing nature of addictive disease), drug abuse treatment has been demonstrated to have excellent efficacy, not only with respect to decreased drug use but also along health, psychologic, and social domains. Patients, as a rule, require more than one treatment episode to recover from the disease.
2. If a patient relapses to drug use, he or she is a treatment failure.	Relapse is a defining characteristic of addictive disease, and, more often than not, a critical step in the recovery process. The relapse experience enables the patient and clinician to refine and renew recovery efforts.
3. Exposure to addictive drugs results in addiction.	Many more people are exposed to substances with abuse potential (i.e., through experimental, recreational, or social use) than have addictive disease develop; in fact, addiction is an unlikely outcome of drug exposure.
4. Drug detoxification is a method of treating addiction.	Detoxification refers to the process of removing drug from the body, typically in a controlled and medically monitored way. Although detoxification may be a component of drug treatment, it does not treat addictive disease.
5. Most chronic pain patients on opioid analgesics are addicts.	Although patients with chronic pain receiving opioid analgesia may be physically dependent and tolerant, they are no more likely than the general adult population to have addictive disease.
6. Opioids should not be used for the treatment of chronic pain because the patient will become tolerant to the analgesic effects.	Although analgesic tolerance has been demonstrated to occur in pain-free individuals, no good evidence exists that tolerance develops in the context of acute or chronic pain. In the patient with pain, increased analgesic need appears to be a reflection of increased or progressing pathology as opposed to tolerance.
7. Persons in pain receiving opioid analgesia are at increased risk for addiction.	No evidence exists that persons receiving opioid analgesia for the treatment of pain are at risk for developing addictive disease. On the basis of large surveys, rates of iatrogenic addiction have been estimated to be less than 1%.

that details the etiologic factors for addictive disease; its biologic, psychologic, and social indicators and sequelae; and principles of effective treatment. For reasons that will be described, most people, including politicians, societal leaders, and well-meaning care providers, are not "connected" to this scientific understanding of addiction. Although widespread recognition exists that addiction is a disease, persons continue to understand and respond to addiction from other than scientific viewpoints.

Models of Addiction

The discrepancy arises from two broad models or general views of addiction that are at odds with the empirically validated disease perspective, referred to as the *moral model* and the *criminal model* of addiction (Table 10.2). Taken to its extreme, the moral model of addiction views substance abuse as a reprehensible and shameful behavior or a behavior in which good and moral persons do not participate. It is seen as a behavior that an individual can freely choose to do or not do, and persons who do not stop problematic drug or alcohol use have insufficient moral fortitude or resolution. Because addicts in this model appear unwilling or unable to adhere to the so-called virtuous path, they are viewed as at fault for any negative consequences arising from their drug use and, frequently, as less worthy of our care and concern than the patient suffering a "faultless" disease (Malone, 1996).

Somewhat different, but resulting in the same negative, judgmental view of addiction, is the criminal or criminal justice model. It is illegal in this country and many others around the world to use certain drugs for the purpose of experiencing their psychoactive effects, thus persons possessing or ingesting drugs are criminals and subject to punishment and imprisonment. The predominance of the criminal justice view of addiction is reflected in large percentages of Americans incarcerated in federal (59.5%) and state prisons (22.3%) for drug offenses (Office of National Drug Control Policy [ONDCP], 1997). It has been estimated that recent increases in the number of drug offenders in American prisons accounts for nearly three quarters of the total

growth in federal prison inmates since 1980 (ONDCP, 1997), a period of time when "Zero Tolerance" and "Just Say No" dominated governmental strategies to deal with addiction. Although use of alcohol is legal, laws against drunk driving and public intoxication criminalize excessive alcohol use too. Interestingly, addiction is the only recognized disease for which its sufferers risk arrest for being impaired by its symptoms. In fact, the United States has an entire agency (the Drug Enforcement Agency, [DEA]) devoted to finding and prosecuting persons suffering from the disease. Thus, in the criminal justice model, like the moral model, persons suffering addictive disease are characterized as bad, unethical, and deserving of criminal justice and/or social sanctions. The pervasiveness of these societal views is evident in patients' general fear or avoidance of taking opioids for pain relief, even when clearly indicated (Fins, 1997; Ward, Goldberg, Miller-McCauley et al., 1993).

Unlike the moral or criminal justice models, the medical model views addiction as a disease, specifically, as an acquired disease of the brain. Like any disease, addiction has identifiable risk factors and a demonstrated pathophysiologic basis, can be diagnosed according to a well-described cluster of signs and symptoms, follows a predictable pattern of progression, and can be managed and treated with interventions of known efficacy. Also, as with other diseases, its ultimate expression in the individual patient is unique and varied, and its negative effects protract on to psychologic and social domains. Unlike the moral or criminal justice models, the medical model of addiction imbues no blame or negative social value to the sufferer. The focus is rather on understanding the characteristics of the host (the patient), the vector (drug of abuse), and the conditions of exposure (setting, route of administration, stress level) that result in disease development and progression, and on evaluating methods of prevention and treatment. Punishing and stigmatizing the addicted individual are not viewed as effective methods of intervention for addiction in the disease model, whereas treatment approaches including pharmacotherapy, cognitive-behavioral skill training, group support, and lifestyle change are.

● ● ● ● ●

TABLE 10.2 **Models of Addiction**

	MORAL MODEL	CRIMINAL MODEL	DISEASE MODEL
Etiology	Moral weakness, lack of willpower	Bad or evil character	Acquired brain disease
Treatment goal	Increase moral strength/fortitude	Rehabilitation	Normalize brain disruption
Treatment strategies	Religious conversion	Incarceration	Pharmacotherapy, cognitive-behavioral therapy

May be duplicated for use in clinical practice. From McCaffery M, Pasero C: *Pain: Clinical manual,* p. 431. Copyright © 1999, Mosby, Inc.

Addiction is an acquired disease because people are not born with the condition but may have the disease develop on a given physiologic exposure to a substance of abuse (including alcohol, nicotine, and caffeine); thus addictive drugs can be considered the necessary vector to which the individual must be exposed to acquire the disease. Yet many more people are exposed to these substances (i.e., through experimental or recreational use) than actually have the disease develop, implying that certain individuals, either through inherited or environmental factors, are more likely than others to have the disease develop on exposure to the drug.

Addiction is clearly a disease of the brain, much like Parkinson's disease, schizophrenia, and depression. Diseases such as these are increasingly understood to be related to either inefficient, overactive, or poorly regulated transmission of certain neurochemicals in specific pathways in the brain. The pathways affected in these diseases tend to be in structures of the brain termed "subcortical," areas not involved in higher (cortical) cognitive processing and responding to stimuli.

It is known that the subcortical area of the brain, with respect to evolution, is the oldest part of the human brain and that part of our brain we share with lower animals. It is the area of the brain that motivates and mediates instinctual, drive-based, or emotionally-charged behaviors, particularly those behaviors compatible with species survival (i.e., eating, sexual behavior, response to threat). By means of the *h*ypothalamus, these structures are chemically wired to the *p*ituitary and *a*drenal glands (the so-called *HPA* axis), which together mediate the more slower acting hormonal, chronic stress, and immune responses. Because addiction arises from structures that motivate and fine-tune highly instinctual and emotional behaviors, the predominant symptoms of the disease are seen as aberrant patterns of behavior.

Drugs of Abuse

What are these vectors of the disease of addiction, addictive drugs? Of the thousands of different chemical compounds in the world there are actually only a few that laboratory animals will self-administer and to which certain humans will become addicted (Gardner, 1997). Drugs with a demonstrated human addiction liability are listed in Table 10.3. Although pharmacologically speaking, alcohol (ETOH) is a "drug" (a central nervous system [CNS] depressant), it is typically not categorized as one in the substance abuse literature. Not only does ETOH have no therapeutic indications, its use is legal and socially sanctioned, making it distinct from most other prescribed or abused drugs.

The pharmacologic effects of these listed drugs encompass a wide range of sites and mechanisms of action. Included are drugs that stimulate the CNS, drugs

● ● ● ● ● ●
TABLE 10.3

ADDICTIVE DRUGS BY CLASS	
Class	**Examples**
Opioids	Heroin, methadone, morphine, hydromorphone
Cocaine	Crack, freebase cocaine
CNS stimulants	Methamphetamine, amphetamine
Alcohol	
CNS depressants	Barbiturate
Sedative-hypnotics	Benzodiazepine
Marijuana	
Hallucinogens	LSD, mescaline, psilocybin

May be duplicated for use in clinical practice. From McCaffery M, Pasero C: *Pain: Clinical manual*, p. 432. Copyright © 1999, Mosby, Inc.

that depress the CNS, drugs that provide analgesia, and drugs that calm anxiety. Table 10.4 lists some of the important acute and chronic pharmacologic effects of these addictive drugs; chronic drug effects are evident in the withdrawal syndrome associated with each drug of abuse.

Despite their varied pharmacologic actions, drugs of abuse all share one key action believed to underlie their "addictive" properties: all drugs of abuse activate a specific neuronal pathway in the subcortical area of the brain, the so-called mesolimbic dopamine pathway, located in the "reward center" (Figure 10.1 on p. 434) of the brain (DiChiara, Imperato, 1988; Wise, 1980; Wise, Rompre, 1989). Either by direct or indirect activation of this pathway, the use of all drugs of abuse effectively results in increased release of a specific neurotransmitter, dopamine, in this pathway, which in turn stimulates some of the brain's own endogenous opioid systems. Release of these chemicals in this reward pathway appears to underlie the profound euphoria and elevated mood associated with drug intoxication, a feeling so reinforcing that certain laboratory animals and humans will actively seek to repeat it (Gardner, 1997).

The reward pathway in our head serves a functional purpose; under normal conditions, this pathway is activated when we are engaged in activities that are beneficial to ourselves with respect to survival of the species (eating, drinking, having sex, nursing infants), thus increasing the likelihood that we will repeat them. Drugs of abuse bypass these normal, somewhat diffuse or muted, sources of reward by activating the reward pathway in a direct chemical way. The amount of reward a drug of abuse provides varies with the class of drug, route of drug administration, and, as will be discussed, the in-

● ● ● ● ●
TABLE 10.4

ACUTE AND CHRONIC EFFECTS OF DRUGS OF ABUSE

Drug Class	Acute Effects	Chronic Effects Evident on Cessation of Use; Withdrawal
Opioids (heroin, methadone, morphine)	Analgesia, drowsiness, euphoria, mental clouding, miosis (constricted pupils), depressed cough reflex, nausea and vomiting, respiratory depression	Lacrimation and rhinorrhea, yawning, pupillary dilatation, gooseflesh, tremor, insomnia, diarrhea, vomiting, anorexia, irritability, elevated blood pressure, muscle cramps/spasm, dysphoria and drug craving
Alcohol and the CNS depressants	Dysarthria (slurred speech), ataxia, hyperreflexia (increased reflexes), nystagmus and/or diploplia, impaired cognition, anterograde amnesia, intoxication, stupor to coma, decreased respirations	Tremor, insomnia, impaired cognition, hypereflexia, hallucinations (primarily visual), delirium, generalized seizures, autonomic hyperactivity, anxiety, drug craving
Cocaine and the CNS stimulants	Euphoria, hypervigilance, anxiety, psychomotor agitation, tremor, tachycardia, pupillary dilatation, increased blood pressure, anorexia, cardiac arrhythmia, generalized seizure, psychotic, delirium, transient movement disorders	Dysphoria, drug craving, anhedonia (inability to gain pleasure from environmental stimuli), affective disorder
Hallucinogens (LSD, mescaline, psilocybin)	Pupillary dilatation, tachycardia, perceptual alterations, tremor, acute anxiety, depersonalization	None reported
Sedative hypnotics (benzodiazepine)	Anxiolysis, sedation, ataxia, dysarthria, impaired cognition, nystagmus, respiratory depression	Anxiety, tremor, insomnia, anorexia, vomiting, hallucinations, generalized seizures, delirium, hyperpyrexia
Marijuana	Perceptual alteration, impaired time orientation, mild euphoria, decreased reaction time, decreased attention span, incoordination	Mild anxiety, mild tremor, to none reported

May be duplicated for use in clinical practice. From McCaffery M, Pasero C: *Pain: Clinical manual*, p. 433. Copyright © 1999, Mosby, Inc.

dividual characteristics of the user and the environmental context. It is believed that changes that occur in this reward pathway with chronic drug administration account for the dysphoric and drug-craving components common to withdrawal from all drugs of abuse (Koob, Bloom, 1988). In that the effect of cocaine or methamphetamine is to directly activate brain reward pathways, the predominant symptoms of withdrawal from these drugs reflect reward pathway withdrawal (Miller, Gold, 1993).

What Is Addiction?

Viewing addiction from different and sometimes competing points of view contributes to confusion on both the part of lay people and clinicians about whether addictive disease is present in a given individual. To clar-

ify what addiction is, it may be easier to review first what addiction is not.

Addiction is not drug tolerance

As noted in Chapter 6, (pp. 171-173) tolerance is a pharmacodynamic response at the neurophysiologic level to chronic drug administration, evident as a reduction in response to a given dose of a drug after repeated administration. Tolerance to some of the effects of opioids is expected and is not the same as addiction. Tolerance develops to the effects of many classes of drugs (e.g., cortisone), not just drugs of abuse, and it does not develop uniformly with all addictive drugs (i.e., across use episodes, cocaine appears to produce reverse tolerance or have a "kindling" effect). Thus a person can be tolerant to the effects of a drug but not be addicted, and not all

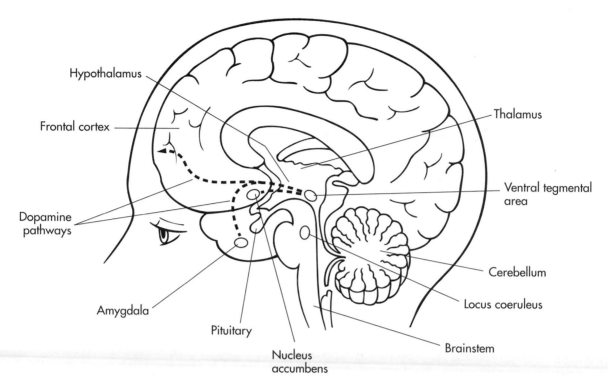

May be duplicated for use in clinical practice. From McCaffery M, Pasero C: *Pain: Clinical manual,* p. 434. Copyright © 1999, Mosby, Inc.

● ● ● ● ●
FIGURE 10.1 **Dopamine Pathway.** All drugs of abuse activate a specific neuronal pathway in the subcortical area of the brain, the so-called mesolimbic dopamine pathway, located in the "reward center" of the brain. Drugs of abuse increase the release of dopamine, which in turn stimulates some of the brain's own endogenous opioid systems. Release of these appears to underlie the profound euphoria and elevated mood associated with drug intoxication.

addicts demonstrate tolerance to their drug of abuse. Although the two may coexist, addiction is not equivalent to drug tolerance (Friedman, 1990; Portenoy, Payne, 1997; Wesson, Ling, Smith, 1993).

Addiction is not physical dependence

Like tolerance, physical dependence is a neurophysiologic response to the chronic presence of a drug. Over repeated drug administrations, the nervous system develops mechanisms or patterns of functioning to overcome, counteract, or adapt to the drug effects, thereby maintaining homeostasis at the level of the organism. As would be expected, many of these changes are the same as those responsible for tolerance, which functionally attenuate drug effect. Physical dependence becomes evident when the drug is withdrawn or reversed and drug blood levels fall below a critical level. Suddenly unopposed by drug effects, neuroadaptive changes made in response to chronic drug presence become profoundly nonadaptive and emerge as the drug-specific withdrawal syndrome (see Table 10.4). Physical dependence on a drug is neither a necessary nor defining condition of addiction (Friedman, 1990; Schnoll, Finch, 1994); the withdrawal syndrome associated with certain drugs of abuse

(e.g., marijuana) is arguably minimal if existent, even in individuals who are clearly addicted, whereas patients with diabetes "physically dependent" on insulin (i.e., discontinuation results in a "withdrawal" response) exhibit no symptoms of addiction.

Addiction is not drug-seeking

Individuals seek and obtain drugs for a myriad of reasons, only one of which is because they are addicted. The distinction between appropriate drug-seeking and addiction is clear in the case of drugs that have no psychoactive effect (e.g., antibiotics, nonopioid analgesics), but becomes less apparent when a drug with a known abuse potential (e.g., an opioid analgesic) is sought by the patient, regardless of the apparent validity of the complaint. The confusion is exemplified by the case of opioid analgesic-seeking by the person in pain because the severity of pain suffered cannot be objectively quantified but only subjectively reported.

Patients with pain may take what appear to be extraordinary steps to ensure adequate medication supply, but, rather than indicating addictive disease, may in fact be appropriate responses to either underrelieved or well-relieved pain. In the case of inadequate analgesia, drug-seeking behaviors arise when a patient cannot obtain tolerable relief with the prescribed dose of analgesic and seeks alternate sources or increased doses of analgesic, a phenomenon called *pseudoaddiction* (Weissman, Haddox, 1989). Alternately, patients receiving good pain relief may evidence drug-seeking behaviors because they understandably fear not only the reemergence of pain but perhaps also the emergence of withdrawal symptoms. Rather than indicative of addictive disease, such behaviors, termed *therapeutic dependence* (Portenoy, 1994), are actually the efforts of an anxious patient to maintain a tolerable level of comfort. Clearly, even in the case of highly addictive drugs, drug-seeking may not indicate addiction. Unfortunately, such behaviors continue to be used to suggest abuse or addiction in patients who are seeking opioid analgesics for pain relief (Miotto, Compton, Ling et al., 1996; Schnoll, Finch, 1994).

What addiction is

Several sets of standardized diagnostic criteria exist to enable reliable, empirically based identification of addictive disease. Probably the most widely used and accepted criteria in the United States are those specified by the American Psychiatric Association in the fourth edition of the *Diagnostic and Statistical Manual* (*DSM-IV,* 1994) (problems associated with applying these criteria to patients with chronic pain are discussed later in this chapter). The term *addiction,* as it has thus far been used in this chapter, corresponds to what the *DSM-IV* calls *substance dependence,* a "maladaptive pattern of substance use, leading to clinically significant impairment or distress" (APA, 1994, p. 108) (Box 10.1). Note these criteria identify addiction across classes of addictive drug, provide a temporal context for the disease (symptoms must be present for at least a year), and require only the presence of any three indicators to arrive at the diagnosis of substance dependence or addictive disease.

It is of diagnostic significance that only two of the criteria (No. 1 and No. 2) for addiction refer to the neurophysiologic responses to chronic drug use discussed earlier, tolerance and physical dependence. The presence of both alone is not enough to meet diagnostic criteria, although addiction can exist without the presence of either if at least three of the remaining criteria are met. Evident is an emphasis on the essentially behavioral nature of addictive disease; indicators of addiction reflect effects on psychologic and social functioning of the individual. Being a disease of brain structures that initiate and shape behavior, it follows that signs and symptoms associated with the disease be manifest in behavioral realms.

Adhering to a disease model of addiction, the *DSM-IV* also recognizes an earlier or less severe form of addictive disease, termed *substance abuse.* The criteria for substance abuse are listed in Box 10.2 and can be distinguished from those of addiction by the shorter duration

---

BOX 10.1 *DSM-IV* **Diagnostic Criteria for Substance Dependence***

A maladaptive pattern of substance use, leading to clinically significant impairment or distress, as manifested by three (or more) of the following, occurring at any time in the same 12-month period:

1. Tolerance, as defined by either of the following:
   a. A need for markedly increased amounts of the substance to achieve intoxication or desired effect
   b. Markedly diminished effect with continued use of the same amount of the substance
2. Withdrawal, as manifested by either of the following:
   a. The characteristic withdrawal syndrome for the substance
   b. The same (or a closely related) substance is taken to relieve or avoid withdrawal symptoms
3. The substance is often taken in larger amounts over a longer period than was intended
4. A persistent desire or unsuccessful efforts to cut down or control substance use are present
5. A great deal of time is spent in activities necessary to obtain the substance (e.g., visiting multiple doctors or driving long distances), use the substance (e.g., chain-smoking), or recover from its effects
6. Important social, occupational, or recreational activities are given up or reduced because of substance use
7. The substance use is continued despite knowledge of having a persistent or recurrent physical or psychologic problem that is likely to have been caused or exacerbated by the substance (e.g., current cocaine use despite recognition of cocaine-induced depression, or continued drinking despite recognition that an ulcer was made worse by alcohol consumption)

*The term "substance dependence" means addiction.

Modified from American Psychiatric Association: *Diagnostic and statistical manual of mental disorders,* ed 4, Washington, DC, 1994, APA.

---

of impairment and the absence of neurophysiologic symptoms. It is pertinent to note that abuse and substance dependence (addiction) are only 2 of 12 disorders the American Psychiatric Association (1994) recognizes as substance related. Addiction is only one of many neuropsychiatric disorders associated with the use of drugs of abuse.

The *DSM-IV* further provides diagnostic criteria for the intoxication and withdrawal syndromes associated with each class of abused drug listed in Table 10.3. Knowledge of these is helpful in structuring assessment or treatment for problems with a particular drug of abuse, but substance abusers in the 1990s tend to exhibit patterns of use characterized by *polysubstance* abuse, or the concurrent or sequential use of several different types of drugs or drug classes. In practice it is often impossible to attribute physical findings to the effects of one drug versus another; typically the user is under the influence of/or withdrawing from more than one substance, with alcohol being one of the most common.

BOX 10.2 *DSM-IV* Diagnostic Criteria for Substance Abuse

A maladaptive pattern of substance use leading to clinically significant impairment or distress, as manifested by one (or more) of the following, occurring within a 12-month period:

1. Recurrent substance use, resulting in a failure to fulfill major role obligations at work, school, or home (e.g., repeated absences or poor work performance related to substance use; substance-related absences, suspensions, or expulsions from school; neglect of children or household).
2. Recurrent substance use in situations in which it is physically hazardous (e.g., driving an automobile or operating a machine when impaired by substance use) or recurrent substance-related legal problems (e.g., arrests for substance-related disorderly conduct).
3. Continued substance use despite having persistent or recurrent social or interpersonal problems caused or exacerbated by the effects of the substance (e.g., arguments with spouse about consequences of intoxication, physical fights).

The symptoms have never met the criteria for Substance Dependence for this class of substance.

Modified from American Psychiatric Association: *Diagnostic and statistical manual of mental disorders*, ed 4, Washington, DC, 1994, APA.

TABLE 10.5 **Alcohol and Drug Disorders in Different Types of Psychiatric Disorders**

MENTAL DISORDER	ALCOHOL ABUSE/ ADDICTION (%)	DRUG ABUSE/ ADDICTION (%)
Schizophrenia	33.7	27.5
Antisocial personality	73.6	42.0
Anxiety disorder	17.9	11.9
Obsessive compulsive	24.0	18.4
Bipolar	43.6	40.7
Major depression	16.5	18.0

May be duplicated for use in clinical practice. From McCaffery M, Pasero C: *Pain: Clinical manual*, p. 436. Copyright © 1999, Mosby, Inc.

Information from Regier DA, Farmer ME, Rae DS et al.: Comorbidity of mental disorders with alcohol and other drug abuse: Results of the Epidemiologic Catchment Area Study, *JAMA* 264:2511-2518, 1990.

Finally, evident in these diagnostic criteria for addiction is the multidimensionality of the syndrome. Addiction, perhaps more so than any other disease and similar to pain, has manifestations in the biologic, psychologic, social, and spiritual life of the individual. A quintessential human condition, the distress and morbidity associated with addictive disease is expressed along all domains of human functioning. The syndromal nature of addiction requires that effective treatment include interventions aimed beyond the pathophysiology of the disease to include psychologic, social, and spiritual healing.

Phenomenology of Addiction

Beyond having standardized diagnostic criteria, the nature and course of addictive disease have been well characterized. Specifically, addiction is a chronic disease that tends to occur with psychiatric and medical illness and to run in certain families. It is characterized by relapse, often coexists with criminality, and decreases the individual's ability to cope with stress. A good understanding of the phenomenology of addiction is needed to structure appropriate assessment and effective interventions.

Psychiatric comorbidity

It is extremely common that the sufferer of addictive disease also suffers from a concurrent psychiatric illness or disorder. It has been estimated that up to 72% of persons meeting diagnostic criteria for an alcohol or drug

disorder (abuse or addiction) at some point during their lifetime also meet diagnostic criteria for a psychiatric disorder (Regier, Farmer, Rae et al., 1990). Table 10.5 provides the prevalence of alcohol and drug disorders among persons suffering from various psychiatric disorders, whereas Table 10.6 lists the prevalence rates of certain comorbid psychiatric illnesses in persons with alcohol and other drug use disorders. Note that anxiety and affective disorders each occur in fully one quarter of drug abusers, which clearly complicates addiction treatment. Also note that almost one half of drug abusers meet diagnostic criteria for an alcohol abuse or dependence disorder, illustrating the prevalence of polysubstance abuse.

Patients with both a psychiatric illness and addictive disease are referred to in the literature as "dual-diagnosis" patients (Raskin, Miller, 1993; Weiss, Mirin, 1989). A central treatment issue becomes determining the temporal relationship of the two conditions (i.e., did the psychiatric illness precede the addiction, or is it a consequence of addictive drug use?). Both scenarios are tenable; persons suffering uncomfortable or disruptive feelings or mood states find they can effectively "self-medicate" these symptoms with abused drugs (Khantzian, 1985). Conversely, the use of drugs of abuse, both acutely and chronically, disrupts neurotransmission in key subcortical brain pathways and can, in certain individuals, result in the new onset of a psychiatric disorder. It is becoming apparent from large epidemiologic studies that anxiety disorders tend to precede substance use disorders, whereas depression tends to be secondary (Kessler, Nelson, McGonagle et al, 1996). Recent work by Brady

● ● ● ● ●

TABLE 10.6	**Psychiatric Disorders in Drug and Alcohol Abusers**				
	ANY MENTAL DISORDER	SCHIZOPHRENIA	ANY AFFECTIVE DISORDER	ANY ANXIETY DISORDER	ALCOHOL ABUSE/ ADDICTION
Alcohol abuse/ addiction (%)	36.6	3.8	13.4	19.4	
Drug abuse/ addiction (%)	53.1	6.8	26.4	28.3	47.3

May be duplicated for use in clinical practice. From McCaffery M, Pasero C: *Pain: Clinical manual*, p. 437. Copyright © 1999, Mosby, Inc.

Information from Regier DA, Farmer ME, Rae DS et al.: Comorbidity of mental disorders with alcohol and other drug abuse: Results of the Epidemiologic Catchment Area Study, *JAMA* 264:2511-2518, 1990.

and colleagues (1993) reveals gender differences in disease onset; for women, depression tends to precede substance abuse, whereas it follows substance abuse for men. To order the correlational relationship between addiction and psychiatric illness in the clinical setting, it is ideal to evaluate the subject after at least 6 weeks of abstinence to determine whether psychiatric morbidity persists. Unfortunately, in reality, 6 weeks of abstinence is difficult for a patient to achieve, especially in the presence of psychiatric symptoms and within current outpatient models of care, thus practitioners usually begin to treat the psychiatric symptoms before addictive drug use is fully resolved.

Medical morbidity

The health consequences of chronic substance use are substantial, and it is important to keep in mind that the two largest sources of addiction morbidity are due to the abuse of legal addictive drugs, ETOH and nicotine (Dans, Matricciani, Otter et al., 1990; Hser, Anglin, Powers, 1993; Moos, Brennan, Mertens, 1994; Soderstrom, Smith, Dischinger et al., 1997; Tonnessen, Petersen, Hojgaard et al., 1992). A recent epidemiologic study (Fox, Merril, Chang et al., 1995) identifies more than 60 medical conditions involving 110 diagnoses that are, at least in part, attributable to substance abuse. These same investigators found that 1 of 5 hospital days were for substance abuse-related conditions, amounting to more than $8 billion in Medicaid expenses in 1994.

Substance-induced illnesses, as well as the inability of the addicted individual to engage in a healthy lifestyle, result in drug abusers being a relatively ill population. Furthermore, the criminality associated with illicit drug use is a significant contributor to addiction-related morbidity; trauma, infection, and poor perinatal outcomes are health consequences of the illegality of drug use. Persons with addictive disease tend to be unemployed or less than fully employed and may lack health care insurance or have limited access to health care, particularly preven-

tive care. They may also be reluctant to seek health care for fear their abuse problem will be detected; thus they tend to present late and in a more debilitated state.

A chronic, relapsing condition

A common societal misconception is that addictive disease can be effectively treated in a single treatment episode, and if a patient relapses to addictive drug use, it is due to his or her lack of moral fortitude, motivation, desire to change, or some other failure or weakness on the part of the patient. Such beliefs ignore what is known about the natural history of addictive disease (Cotton, 1994; Hser, Anglin, Powers, 1993) and, worse, serve to diminish the hopes and real achievements of the patient who has struggled with addiction and failed.

Most patients do not achieve long-term abstinence after a single treatment episode, which should not be surprising to the average reader who has tried to initiate and maintain a significant change in lifestyle. Anyone who has gone on a diet or started a new exercise program knows that giving up old habits and adopting new ones is difficult. Change may be maintained for the short run, but to sustain change for longer periods of time (i.e., >6 months) is rare. The behaviors a substance abuser must change to become drug free are typically much more complex, deeply ingrained, and physiologically and socially reinforced than adherence to an exercise plan, for example, making abstinence after a single treatment intervention an unlikely outcome.

Addiction therefore is characterized, and can be recognized, by relapse. Approximately 60% of abusers of alcohol, tobacco, or heroin relapse to use within 1 year of stopping (Marlatt, Gordon, 1985). Effective models of drug treatment anticipate relapse and use the relapse experience as a learning tool to help patients identify their own affective, situational, and interpersonal risks for resuming drug use (see Cognitive-behavioral treatment, p. 445). In these treatment programs it is expected that remaining drug free is extremely difficult for the newly abstinent patient, thus relapse is not equated with failure but as a part of the process of recovery. Although the risk of relapse decreases over time, it remains a lifelong potential for the sufferer, especially under conditions of stress (Marlatt, Gordon, 1985). Recovery-oriented habits and behaviors require long-term reinforcement.

The fact that an ex-substance abuser is always at risk for relapse reflects the chronicity of the disease. Like many chronic conditions, addiction is a disease of exacerbations and remissions, with periods of time when the individual is able to remain drug-free and other times when abstinence cannot be maintained. Again, resuming drug use is not conceptualized as a failure but as evidence of disease progression and an indication that treatment interventions need to be modified or reinforced.

It is important to emphasize that relapse to drug use may involve the abuse of a different substance from the one(s) initially involved. It is not unusual for an individual initially to suffer a heroin addiction, but at a certain age or under a certain set of environmental conditions, heroin use falls off while alcohol consumption rises to problematic levels (see Hser, Anglin, Powers, 1993). Addiction generalizes across drugs of abuse; although a particular patient can easily identify his or her "drug of choice," any drug providing psychoactive reinforcement is likely to be abused by the patient with addictive disease. As noted, polysubstance abuse is the normative pattern of drug consumption for most addicted individuals.

A family disorder

Addiction is a familial disease. A positive family history of substance abuse, whether for alcohol or other prescribed or illicit drugs, is a risk factor for addictive disease in all clinical populations (Annis, 1974; Cadoret, Troughton, O'Gorman et al., 1986; Cotton, 1979). Best studied in the case of alcoholism (alcohol being a particularly prevalent drug of abuse across populations and generations), large surveys of adoptees and twins reared apart from their biologic family of origin indicate that heredity is a stronger predictor of alcoholism than environment (Buchloz, Heath, Reich et al., 1996; Slutske, Heath, Madden et al., 1996). Children of alcoholics and certain ethnic groups evidence patterned differences in their physiologic responses to alcohol (Schuckit, Smith, 1996, 1997; Schuckit, Tsuang, Anthenelli et al., 1996). This speaks to increasingly appreciated genetic markers for addiction or genes that are demonstrated to predict individual differences in drug reinforcement, metabolism, or physiologic effects. Individual variation in each of these types of drug responses can clearly contribute to the addiction potential of a drug of abuse (Schuster, 1990-91). An emerging science in the addiction literature is *pharmacogenetics,* which uses strains of animals with inherited differences in drug responses to learn how these may predict the development of substance dependence (Crabbe, Belknap, Buck, 1994; George, 1993).

Yet the importance of the family environment in predicting adult drug and alcohol dependence cannot be minimized. Patterns of learning and coping developed by children who grow up with an addicted parent(s), in an often highly dysfunctional family system, have been long-recognized as good predictors of problematic substance use in adolescents (Bergman, Smith, Hoffman, 1995; Trachtenberg, Fleming, 1994). Supporting the profound effect of environment on drug use patterns is interesting recent preclinical evidence showing that under conditions of environmental stress, the pharmacologic reinforcing effects of several drugs of abuse are significantly increased (Shaham, Alvarez, Nespor et al., 1992; Shaham, Klein, Alvarez et al., 1993). In other words, first exposure to a drug that might only be mildly rewarding in a neutral or comfortable environment becomes highly rewarding when the individual is experiencing significant or chronic stress, conditions that are likely to be present in the "alcoholic" or "addicted" family. Whether caused by genetic factors, environmental influences, or a combination of the two, a predisposition to problematic substance use is evident in certain families.

A primary coping response

As persons become increasingly dependent on drugs of abuse, their repertoire of adaptive coping responses to stress narrows, with drug use eventually becoming the sole stress management strategy available to the addicted patient. Certainly, a glass of wine at the end of day provides a stress-reducing effect for many of us, but we have also developed alternate and much more effective coping responses for situations that require these. Asking that someone give up their most used and reliable mechanism for dealing with stress (drug use) when their lives have become very stress filled, is difficult and, understandably, quite scary for the patient. Until alternate, nondrug coping strategies are learned, relearned, available, or adopted, the addicted individual cannot begin to face the stresses involved in becoming drug free. Stress is a primary precipitator of relapse (Marlatt, Gordon, 1985); strong psychologic reliance on drug use in the addicted individual functions to maintain the behavior.

Consequences of illegality

In discussing key and defining attributes of addiction, it is important to keep in mind that most abused drugs are illegal to possess or ingest, except under medically prescribed conditions (e.g., morphine for analgesia, cocaine for ophthalmic surgery, benzodiazepine for anxiety disorder, marijuana for glaucoma). Other drugs of abuse and formulations of drugs of abuse have no medically defined indications and thus are never legal to produce, possess, or ingest (e.g., methamphetamine). It follows that for most persons addicted to substances other than those that are legal to purchase and self-administer (alcohol, nicotine, caffeine), they must break the law to engage in the very behaviors that characterize the disease. Of the 1.14 million arrests for drug law violations made in this country in 1994, 75.1% were for drug possession (ONDCP, 1997), and most of these were individual users possessing drugs for their own consumption. In other words, simply by being addicted to an illegal drug, an individual becomes a criminal; in fact, it is a diagnostic criterion for substance abuse in *DSM-IV* (APA, 1994) (see Box 10.2, No. 2).

Because illicit drugs rely on a black market economy, persons who are dependent on them often resort to criminal activity to obtain the capital (either money or services) to purchase them. Between 1994 and 1996, 66% of arrestees in the State of California had the metabolites of at least one abused drug in their urine when booked on arrest for nondrug-related charges (California Department of Alcohol and Drug Programs [CDADP], 1997). In 1991, between 10% and 17% of federal and state prison inmates reported committing criminal offenses to pay for drugs (ONDCP, 1997), and between 1994 and 1997, 30% of California arrestees were charged with so-called "income-generating crimes" (i.e., burglary, commercial sex, forgery, stolen property), the types of crimes engaged in by persons supporting an addiction (CDADP, 1997). These data highlight how the life of a person suffering addiction is very likely to be complicated by criminal involvement and legal problems.

As noted, the criminality of this disease brings with it many of the health (and often pain-producing) consequences of illicit drug use: Traumatic violence occurs in the context of drug trafficking; infection with sexually transmitted diseases (STD), including HIV, occurs through commercial sex work (prostitution for money or drugs); bloodborne disease (i.e., HIV, hepatitis) is transmitted by shared injection supplies (obtaining sterile injection equipment remains illegal in many communities); and poor or absent prenatal health care results from feared sanctions from child protection agencies.

It is instructive to consider how the prevalence of criminal activity might increase among current law-abiding Americans if alcohol or nicotine, for example, were to suddenly become illegal. Prohibition in the 1920s illustrated clearly the overnight development of a black market for alcohol, with increases in violence and criminal activity associated with alcohol "trafficking." Because the defining symptom of their disease (taking an illegal substance) is in fact illegal, criminality and its consequences frequently complicate addiction.

Common misconceptions

Drug Exposure Leads to Drug Addiction

As has been recently publicized in political and media forums, young people in this country are using drugs at the highest rate in years. In 1995, almost 11% of adolescents reported having used an illicit substance (illegal drug, not including alcohol) in the past 30 days (ONDCP, 1997). This rate had jumped by more than 2.5% from 1994 reports and doubled since 1992, being the highest rate of drug use since 1979 (16.3%). A large 1996 high school survey showed that more than half the students had used an illegal drug by the time they graduated from high school, primarily marijuana (ONDCP, 1997). Alcohol is the drug most often used by adolescents; one third of 12th graders report having had five or more drinks on at least one occasion within 2 weeks of being surveyed. Thus by conservative estimates, more than 65% of high school graduates have used an addictive substance before graduation. These data do not survey drug use of non-high school graduates; neither does it follow nondrug users into college. It is likely that if alcohol and drug use were tapped in these additional samples, the population prevalence of drug exposure would approach 90%.

Yet epidemiologic surveys find that only 17% of the general US population suffer from a substance dependence disorder over the course of their lifetime. In other words, very few of the persons exposed to an addictive drug actually develop addictive disease. Although the vector (drug) is endemic in our environment, only certain individuals become affected. Some of the known susceptibility factors or correlates of the disease have been described earlier and include genetics, family dysfunction, chronic stress, and psychiatric illness. Yet the odds are against problematic drug use being the outcome of the interaction between an individual and an addictive drug; the data indicate that addiction is the unlikely response.

Further evidence that addiction is an idiosyncratic drug response is illustrated in historical data on addiction. Although the relative use of alcohol or other drugs has increased and decreased over historical eras, the overall prevalence of addictive disease has remained remarkably stable (Musto, 1997). Drug availability in society has had little impact on the incidence of addiction. Addiction is likely to be a problem in a subgroup of individuals, and on the basis of recent historical evidence, this percentage will be expressed in society regardless of the popular or available drug of the time.

Drug Treatment Does Not Work

Another unfortunate misconception about addiction related to high relapse rates is that addiction treatment "doesn't work." On the contrary, good evidence exists that treatment in many forms is effective, especially treatments of longer duration that keep the patient engaged in treatment by providing services that meet his or her individual needs (see Cotton, 1994). The single best predictor of good treatment outcome is the amount of time the patient spends in drug treatment; the longer a patient stays in treatment the better he or she will do in terms of drug use, as well as other prosocial behaviors. Younger substance abusers or those with less lengthy and/or severe addiction histories are also more likely to have positive treatment responses (Hubbard, 1997).

Rather than focusing on response to treatment at the individual level, the efficacy of drug treatment may be better appreciated at the aggregate level. In the national "Treatment Outcome Prospective Survey," (Hubbard, Marsden, Rachal et al., 1989) that followed 10,000 patients receiving treatment in 1 of 37 different treatment programs over a 5-year period, an overall 71% decrease in alcohol and drug use was found. After a year of treatment, 75% of patients in outpatient treatment and 56% in residential treatment had stopped using heroin or cocaine. Beneficial effects of treatment extend beyond drug use; in the same study employment rates among the patients surveyed doubled. Furthermore, 70% of the outpatients and 97% of residential clients, who had committed at least one predatory crime in the year before treatment entry, had no criminal activity during the first 6 months of treatment.

Treatment is also a highly cost-effective method of addressing substance dependence. It has been estimated that the societal costs of illicit drugs related to drug-related morbidity, mortality, and crime to the nation total approximately $66.9 billion per year (ONDCP, 1997). The National Institute of Drug Abuse (1993) estimates that the 6-month costs to society of an untreated or incarcerated addict is more than double of what it costs to provide residential drug treatment, which is a rather expensive form of drug treatment (see Figure 10.2). A study in the mid-1980s found that for every dollar invested in drug treatment programs, taxpayers enjoy a $4 return in the reduction of drug-related costs (Hubbard, Marsden, Rachal et al., 1989); a more recent study in California calculated that the financial return had increased to $7 per $1 invested (State of California Department of Alcohol and Drug Problems, 1994). Thus treatment works for society in general, substance abusers in the aggregate, and at the level of the individual client. Neither clinicians nor the lay public should be pessimistic about the efficacy of drug treatment.

Treatments for Addiction

Characteristics of drug treatment

Having established that addiction treatment is effective, an overview of the major models and strategies of drug treatment will now be provided. Several points about drug treatment in general must be made. First, *wide* variation exists in the range and quality of services provided across programs of treatment. Being a relatively unregulated system of care, drug treatment programs can adopt whichever treatment strategies and delivery methods they deem important or necessary; with the exception of those programs that provide significant medical services and pharmacotherapy, no overriding governing or regulating body monitors the components or quality of care in drug treatment. The diversity of available types of programs may benefit patients in that if one program or approach does not work, others are available, and that innovative new programs and strategies are free to develop. Unfortunately, the relative lack of system-level oversight occasionally results in the presence of programs with ineffective care or unscrupulous practices. Before referring to a particular program, it is in the patient's best interest that the clinician has some knowledge of the program methods and effectiveness.

As a result of its rather unregulated status and the fact that it serves a relatively stigmatized or marginalized population, drug abuse treatment has historically been provided in a separate or fragmented way from more traditional health care (Silverman, 1985). Rarely are high-quality (or any) health care or mental health services available in drug treatment programs. It is therefore incumbent on the clinician to provide case management to the patient in need of drug treatment; when health or psychiatric morbidity complicate addiction, resources to meet these additional needs should be actively recruited.

As a system, drug abuse treatment is rather unorganized and disjointed. Little or no integration or overlap of services exists across program type; neither is there a unifying framework to structure which addict will get what treatment and in what stage of the disease (Glaser, 1990; Gostin, 1990). There is no centralized or standard system of triage or treatment entry, no ordered progression through type or intensity of treatment programs, and a lack of consensus on what are believed to be the critical components to an effective drug treatment program. The program within which a patient finds himself or herself is as likely to be based on circumstantial and availability issues rather than on logical or empirical grounds that it is the best program for the patient. Finding the ideal treatment program in the unorganized maze of treatment providers is, at best, a complex task for the patient; it is critical that the clinician serve as patient advocate and actively seek and refer to the best treatment environment available to the patient.

Increasingly, the type of drug treatment a particular patient receives is dictated by his or her managed care provider. Currently, most managed care organizations do not provide their own drug treatment services but "carve" or contract out for these from a drug treatment provider(s) in the community. Patients with addiction within a managed care context are limited in the type(s) and duration of treatment they will receive. Although the chronic and relapsing nature of addiction is increasingly appreciated by scientists and clinicians, current systems of reimbursement still focus on episodic models of care, which are limited both in the duration of a single treatment episode and the number of treatment episodes a patient may receive in a given time period.

Finally, it must be acknowledged that the predominant societal response to addiction is incarceration and that formalized drug treatment within the prisons and jails is frequently nonexistent. Inmates typically detoxify

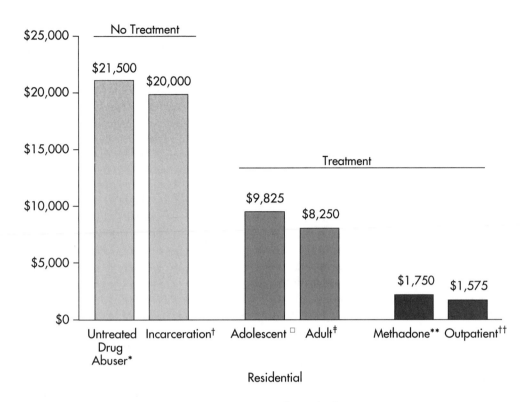

All Costs Are For a 6-Month Period, Per Person

Information from:

* *Estimated social and governmental costs of an untreated drug abuser,* 1985, New York State Division of Substance Abuse Services.

† Godshaw G, Koppel R, Pancoast R: *Anti-drug law enforcement efforts and their impact,* Washington, DC, 1987, U.S. Customs Services, Department of the Treasury.

□ Butynski W: Paper presented at Research Analysis Utilization System (RAUS) Review Meeting of National Institute on Drug Abuse, Washington, DC, August 1989.

‡ Gerstein DR, Harwood HJ, editors: *Treating drug problems,* vol 1, p. 189, Washington, DC, 1990, National Academy Press. Average treatment costs for adult residential drug-free treatment range from $6500 to $10,000.

** Gerstein DR, Harwood HJ, editors: *Treating drug problems,* vol 1, p. 188, Washington, DC, 1990, National Academy Press. Average outpatient methadone treatment costs range from $1500 to $2000.

†† Gerstein DR, Harwood HJ, editors: *Treating drug problems,* vol 1, p. 189, Washington, DC, 1990, National Academy Press. Average treatment costs for outpatient drug-free treatment range from $1350 to $1800.

FIGURE 10.2 **Compare the Costs.**

From National Institute on Drug Abuse (NIDA): *Drug abuse treatment: An economical approach addressing the drug problem in America,* Compare the costs, p. 4, Rockville, Md, 1993, NIDA.

with little to no medical management, certainly no comfort interventions, and have relatively easy access to drugs of abuse while in jail. They are then released with a drug problem that is inadequately addressed, if addressed at all. As is evident in Figure 10.2, straight criminal justice approaches to addiction are expensive and ineffective. A trend toward strong research and funding exists to examine how drug treatment for the incarcerated population can be structured and made more effective.

Models of Treatment

Multiple models or types of drug treatment exist (see Brower, Blow, Beresford, 1989), which for the outside observer can be difficult to distinguish from one another. Few programs actually advertise the specific types of

services provided, and it is not uncommon to find components of several models combined within a single program. Four predominant types of substance abuse treatment, twelve-step, pharmacotherapy, cognitive-behavioral, and residential, will be described, prefaced by a discussion of a common intervention too often mistakenly assumed to be a treatment for addiction, detoxification.

Detoxification: The treatment that is not a treatment

Detoxification from a drug on which a patient is physically dependent in and of itself is not an addiction treatment. All detoxification provides is a drug-free person with addictive disease, not a disease-free person.

During detoxification, the drug is removed from the body, usually while withdrawal symptoms are minimized and overall health status is maximized (see Boxes 10.5, 10.6, 10.7, pp. 456, 458, 459). Yet, the behavioral, psychologic and social indicators of addiction are not addressed by detoxification, nor can they be; detoxification programs typically last no more than 21 days, and while actively detoxifying, few patients are cognitively composed enough to participate in recovery efforts. Thus once the detoxified patient returns to natural conditions and lifestyle, without new skills or resources to maintain abstinence, relapse is the overwhelmingly likely outcome. Unless integrated with an intensive aftercare component, detoxification cannot be considered an addiction treatment.

This is not to imply that detoxification may not be an integral component to drug treatment. Withdrawal from the sedative-hypnotic drugs and CNS depressants (i.e., alcohol) can be life-threatening, thus the patient may require pharmacologic tapering and medical oversight to attain abstinence. Even for drugs of abuse with less toxic withdrawal symptoms (i.e., opioids, nicotine), providing pharmacologic adjuncts and social support as the patient tapers use makes the abstinence process more humane and leaves the patient more likely to trust and work with treatment providers. When indicated, detoxification must be provided, yet should never be considered a drug treatment intervention; it is simply a first step in preparing certain patients for participating in drug treatment.

Although historically done as an inpatient procedure, detoxification is increasingly done on an outpatient basis, where the patient comes to the program daily for assessment, counseling, and medication provision as necessary but returns home for the remainder of the day. Profound medical or psychiatric instability or a previous history of severe withdrawal remain the only clear indications for inpatient detoxification (see Making Drug Treatment Referrals, p. 446).

As noted, four major models of addiction treatment will be described. Table 10.7 differentiates the major assumptions and components associated with each of these models. The separation between these types of programs is more instructive than reality based; again, many treatment programs combine elements of several models, and there are certainly programs in which all four are used (see Brower, Blow, Beresford, 1989).

Twelve-step treatment

Probably one of the most recognized and used models of drug and alcohol treatment is the 12-step or self-help model. Twelve-step programs are formalized support groups, or fellowships, of persons with the same or similar types of addictive disease who come together on a regular basis to study the principles, traditions, and steps to recovery as described by Alcoholics Anonymous (AA) (Box 10.3).

AA is a nonprofessional group; no counselors or psychiatrists are present, and group leaders arise from the membership. No health or social services are provided. It is a self-supporting, autonomous organization, is freely available to all patients, and neither follows nor teaches a particular political or denominational perspective. Accepting one's own weaknesses and powerlessness over drug use are central to the AA philosophy. Although the belief in a "higher power" is necessary to the program, it is not a religious organization; the sole mission of members of AA is "to stay sober and help other alcoholics to achieve sobriety" (AA, 1976, p. 383).

A key element of AA is sponsorship. On joining, each member is provided a sponsor, a person in the group who has achieved some extended sobriety time and is learned in the 12-step tradition and program. The spon-

TABLE 10.7   **Comparison of the Major Models of Drug Treatment**

MODEL OF TREATMENT	ETIOLOGY OF ADDICTION	DESIRED TREATMENT OUTCOME	TREATMENT STRATEGY
AA	Lack of moral strength	Increased willpower	Spiritual awakening, fellowship
Pharmacotherapy	Disrupted subcortical neurotransmitter systems	Normalized subcortical neurotransmitter function	Prescription of medications with activity at addiction-relevant receptors
Cognitive-behavioral	Lack of needed skills and coping strategies	Self-control by means of new learning	Cognitive restructuring, skill rehearsal
Residential	Poor socialization	Behavior consistent with societal norms	Community responsibility, punishment

May be duplicated for use in clinical practice. As appears in McCaffery M, Pasero C: *Pain: Clinical manual*, p. 442, 1999, Mosby, Inc.

Modified from Brower KJ, Blow FC, Beresford TP: Treatment implications of chemical dependency models: An integrative approach, *J Substance Abuse Treatment* 6:147-157, 1989.

sor serves as a personal support system to work with and assist the new member achieve and maintain a drug-free lifestyle and is intended to be a qualitatively different relationship than that which exists between a professional therapist and patient, principally because the sponsor lives with the disease the patient has.

Twelve-step meetings may be open or closed meetings, with the former being open to nonaddicted persons, and the latter open only to members or interested addicted individuals. At meetings, which typically last 1 hour, selected members may speak to the group about their addiction and recovery, discussions on certain topics related to recovery may take place, or one of the 12-steps may be studied. Attendance is not taken, and members are free to enter and leave different groups as they so choose (Nace, 1997).

Despite its popularity, the effectiveness of AA has never been rigorously studied, thus its ultimate effect on the treatment of addiction is unknown. Because of the anonymity provided its membership and the lack of objective measures of sobriety, the 12-step model is not amenable to empirical evaluation. The most outspoken proponents of AA are those persons for whom it has worked; numbers of addicted individuals do not find 12-step meetings helpful. This is not to minimize the successes and benefits of 12-step programs; each of the other models of treatment presented in this chapter, recommend, if not provide on-site, 12-step meetings for patients. If nothing else, AA has an augmenting or reinforcing effect on other forms of treatment for many addicted persons.

Pharmacotherapy

For a limited number of drugs of abuse, medications are used to treat addictive disease in an attempt to substitute for or counteract the abused drug's actions. Yet, even the most powerful and effective medications are seen only as adjuncts to treatment or a tool to maximize the individual's ability to participate in recovery efforts. In that the focus of this section is addiction treatment, pharmacotherapies discussed will be limited to those prescribed to treat the addiction rather than medications that may be used to treat concurrent psychiatric illness (i.e., antidepressants, mood stabilizers) or treat withdrawal symptoms during planned detoxification (see Boxes 10.5, 10.6, 10.7, pp. 456, 458, 459).

Addiction pharmacotherapies are currently available to persons with opioid and alcohol addiction. Considerable federal and drug company medication development dollars are being spent to find medications that can treat cocaine and methamphetamine addiction—diseases that have thus far been relatively drug resistant. A cocaine "vaccine" and several "anticraving" agents are currently being evaluated in clinical trials (Cotton, 1994).

Opioid Addiction Pharmacotherapy

Opioid addiction pharmacotherapies can be classified as either *substitution* or *blocking* agents. The former, methadone and levo-alpha-acetylmethadol (LAAM), consist of long-acting opioids that take the place of the abused agent, preventing the emergence of withdrawal symptoms and drug craving. Because they occupy the opioid receptors with great affinity, they further prevent other abused opioids from providing subjective effects in opiate-addicted persons. The patient in pain, though, can still benefit from opioid analgesic effects, even with methadone or LAAM therapy. Substitution pharmacotherapies for heroin addiction developed during a period of tremendous proliferation of pharmacotherapies for a variety of psychiatric disorders. Methadone was introduced as a long-acting, orally administered opioid substitution medication that blocked the psychoactive effects of subsequently administered doses of heroin (Dole, Nyswander, Kreek, 1966) and for almost 35 years has

---

BOX 10.3	**The Twelve Steps**

1. We admitted we were powerless over alcohol—that our lives had become unmanageable.
2. Came to believe that a Power greater than ourselves could restore us to sanity.
3. Made a decision to turn our will and our lives over to the care of God *as we understood him.*
4. Made a searching and fearless moral inventory of ourselves.
5. Admitted to God, to ourselves, and to another human being the exact nature of our wrongs.
6. We're entirely ready to have God remove all these defects of character.
7. Humbly asked Him to remove our shortcomings.
8. Made a list of all persons we had harmed and became willing to make amends to them all.
9. Made direct amends to such people wherever possible, except when to do so would injure them or others.
10. Continued to take a personal inventory, and when we were wrong, promptly admitted it.
11. Sought through prayer and meditation to improve our conscious contact with God *as we understood Him,* praying only for knowledge of His will for us and the power to carry that out.
12. Having had a spiritual awakening as the result of these steps, we tried to carry this message to alcoholics and to practice these principles in all our affairs.

From Alcoholics Anonymous: *Alcoholics Anonymous: The big book,* pp 59-60, New York, 1976, AA World Services Incorporated.

The Twelve Steps are reprinted with permission of Alcoholics Anonymous World Services, Inc. Permission to reprint the Twelve Steps does not mean that A.A. has reviewed or approved the contents of this publication, nor that A.A. agrees with the views expressed herein. A.A. is a program of recovery from alcoholism *only*—use of the Twelve Steps in connection with programs and activities which are patterned after A.A., but which address other problems, or in any other non-A.A. context, does not imply otherwise.

remained the prototypic opioid substitution therapy available for American opioid addicts. It allowed heroin addicts to discontinue their four to six intravenous administrations of heroin per day and their participation in activities to obtain the drug.

The benefits of opioid substitution treatment, such as decreased illicit opioid use, retention in treatment, and improved social functioning, have been clearly demonstrated within the methadone maintenance model (see reviews Ball, Ross, 1993; Hubbard, Marsden, 1986; Senay, Uchtenhagen, 1990). Furthermore, methadone maintenance therapy for opioid addiction has been shown to decrease the mortality and morbidity associated with illicit drug use (Ball, Ross, 1993; Grönbladh, Ohlund, Gunne, 1990; Segest, Mygind, Bay, 1990), dramatically diminish the transfer of HIV (Ball, Lange, Myers et al, 1988; Cooper, 1989; Des Jarlais, Friedman, Hopkins, 1985; Dole, 1989; Drucker, 1986), profoundly reduce criminal activity associated with drug abuse in general (Anglin, Speckart, Booth et al., 1989; Dole, Robinson, Orraca et al., 1969; Hubbard, Marsden, Rachal et al., 1989; Hubbard, French, 1991), and normalize disruptions in immune and endocrine function caused by episodic drug use (Kreek, 1991).

A single dose of methadone suppresses opioid withdrawal for 24 to 36 hours in the stabilized patient without producing euphoria or sedation; thus the patient must take it daily. Relapse rates significantly decrease when methadone is provided on a long-term (maintenance) basis; short-term detoxification with methadone has generally been unsuccessful (Kreek, 1991). High-dose (70 to 100 mg) methadone maintenance, which adequately prevents withdrawal symptoms and blocks the effects of illicit opioids, results in better treatment outcome than low-dose (20 to 50 mg) maintenance. Methadone is dispensed within a system of highly regulated clinics set apart from the mainstream health care system, where counseling, health care, and educational services may be provided to varying degrees. Yet methadone has not provided a pharmacologic panacea for all opioid addicts; recent estimates from the Institute of Medicine (Gerstein, Harwood, 1990) indicate that of 500,000 to 1 million heroin addicts in the United States, approximately 100,000 patients, receive methadone maintenance in between 750 and 800 clinics across the country.

In 1993, LAAM was approved for use in the United States, being the first opioid substitution alternative to methadone, which, like methadone, is legislated to be dispensed solely at government-approved treatment programs for the treatment of addiction (Ling, Rawson, Compton, 1994). Unlike methadone, LAAM is not approved for use as an analgesic. Although it is often referred to as "long-acting methadone," the comparison with methadone is misleading. LAAM is a pro-drug, which itself has little opioid effect, but is metabolized in the liver into two long-acting metabolites with opioid activity. Patient acceptance and treatment response have been found to be similar for LAAM and methadone (Tennant, Rawson, Pumphrey et al 1986; Trueblood, Judson, Goldstein, 1978). LAAM appears to be most effective for patients who benefit from a reduced frequency of clinic visits and less so for patients perceived as needing the intense support of daily clinic visits. Categories of patients who find LAAM particularly useful include persons with transportation or scheduling problems, persons with past history of methadone failure, and persons who do not want methadone maintenance. It is hoped that the option of LAAM will attract currently untreated heroin addicts to opioid substitution treatment.

The opioid effect that occurs when LAAM is administered is slower in onset and longer in duration (up to 72 hours) than that of methadone, which is administered every 24 hours. The relatively more stable pharmacokinetic profile of LAAM provides patients with a smoother drug response and less daily fluctuation of drug effects. Its extended duration of action allows for three times per week administration. Repeated oral administration of 70 to 100 mg of LAAM three times weekly blocks the subjective "effects" of a 25 mg dose of intravenous heroin for up to 72 hours; maintenance on lower doses of LAAM (50 mg) produces partial blockade of the same heroin dose for the same period. In general, any patient addicted to opioids and/or previously stabilized on methadone maintenance can be treated with LAAM, although current regulations prohibit dispensing LAAM to pregnant women, nursing mothers, and persons less than 18 years old.

Side effects of opioid substitution medications are generally those observed with opioids and include reports of nausea, vomiting, constipation, excessive sweating, decreased sexual interest, and delayed ejaculation. All but a few cases of methadone or LAAM overdose have involved multiple drugs; when encountered, opioid overdose should be treated with naloxone (Narcan) once a patent airway is established. Because of the long-acting nature of both, continuous or repeated naloxone administration to treat overdose is preferred to oral naltrexone (see below), which may precipitate prolonged opioid withdrawal symptoms. Consideration of gradual discontinuation of methadone or LAAM maintenance is made part of a comprehensive treatment plan and depends on the patient's readiness to adopt a drug-free lifestyle. Stable long-term opioid substitution therapy is preferable to repeated cycles of premature discontinuation of medication followed by relapse to uncontrolled addiction.

In the 1970s, the opioid antagonist, naltrexone, became available as a treatment for opioid addiction. It blocks the effects of opioids so that when the patient attempts to maintain abstinence, an impulsive return to opioid use will not produce the usual effect. Naltrexone is a long-acting, orally administered form of naloxone

(Narcan), which appears to have no pharmacologic effect in the nonopioid-dependent individual. It can only be given to a patient who is completely detoxified from opioids because it will precipitate a prolonged withdrawal syndrome, thus its usefulness is limited in the large number of addicts who are unsuccessful in detoxification. The medication is typically prescribed at 50 mg/day, with the patient taking it on a 3-day per week dosing schedule (100 mg Monday, 100 mg Wednesday, 150 mg Friday) during clinic visits when counseling, group, or education services are provided. Not being a controlled substance, naltrexone can be provided by any drug treatment facility or private physician.

Although naltrexone appears to be the "ideal" pharmacotherapy for opioid addiction (it blocks the effects of the abused drug with essentially no side effects), its clinical success has been limited. Naltrexone treatment is highly dependent on patient compliance, and unless the patient has participated in adequate psychosocial recovery efforts, has excellent social supports, or has a powerful reason to stop using (i.e., loss of professional licensure), he or she tends to stop taking the medication and relapse. As with all treatment pharmacotherapies, naltrexone is most successful when delivered on a long-term basis and within the context of psychosocial and educational services.

Alcohol Addiction Pharmacotherapies

Probably the best known pharmacotherapy for alcohol addiction is disulfiram (Antabuse), which produces a severe adverse reaction when alcohol is consumed. Disulfiram irreversibly inactivates acetaldehyde dehydrogenase, an enzyme necessary to the metabolism of alcohol, resulting in the accumulation of the relatively toxic metabolite acetaldehyde. The resulting disulfiram-alcohol reaction is characterized by flushing, throbbing headache, nausea, vomiting, sweating, chest pain, tachycardia, confusion, and agitation. This reaction can occur with alcohol blood levels as low as 50 to 100 mg/dl and last between 30 and 60 minutes. When severe, respiratory depression and cardiac collapse can occur, making it a potentially dangerous pharmacotherapy in the active alcoholic. Daily doses between 250 mg and 500 mg are effective for up to 72 hours. Much individual variability is noted in the disulfiram response; some patients have little reaction to frank alcohol intake, whereas others become ill with inadvertent ingestion of over-the-counter medications or foods containing small amounts of alcohol.

Recently approved for the treatment of alcoholism is naltrexone, the same medication described above for the treatment of opioid addiction. In that naltrexone blocks opioid receptors in the brain, neither exogenously administered nor endogenous opioids can have an effect. As previously discussed (p. 432), endogenous opioids are involved in the reinforcing effects of all drugs of abuse, including alcohol. Blocking these receptors appears to decrease the subjective reward that an individual receives from alcohol. Two recent human clinical trials have shown that patients receiving naltrexone in the context of comprehensive treatment programs had lower rates of relapse, fewer drinking episodes, longer time to relapse, and were less likely to suffer a full-blown relapse when they "slipped" (O'Malley, Jaffe, Chang et al., 1992; Volpicelli, Alterman, Hayashida et al., 1992).

Cognitive-behavioral treatment

Cognitive-behavioral interventions for the treatment of addictive disease are predicated on the assumption that much of addiction is learned and socially reinforced. The overall goals of this model of treatment are to facilitate the acquisition of (1) specific skills for resisting substance use and (2) more general coping skills for dealing with negative feeling states, social pressures, and interpersonal conflicts that serve to maintain problematic substance use. It is believed that the key difficulty in stopping drug use is a lack of feelings of self-efficacy, which results in low self-esteem or feelings of inadequacy.

With respect to the first set of skills, patients are taught to focus in-depth on and track the thoughts, feelings, and environmental contexts associated with drug use episodes in an effort to identify for the given individual the key addiction-sustaining or exacerbating factors. Once these are identified, the patient and counselor together devise strategies to avoid or to manage these precipitators of use and practice implementing these strategies. To improve more general coping skills, patients are assisted to engage or to improve social supports (i.e., 12-step group), make lifestyle changes, and learn stress-management techniques, with positive effects expected in all aspects of patient functioning, not just substance use.

A mainstay of the cognitive-behavioral approach is a set of practical techniques collectively known as *relapse prevention* (Marlatt, Gordon, 1985). Relapse is a cardinal characteristic of addiction (see p. 437); critical to achieving abstinence is preventing or minimizing relapse episodes. In this conceptualization of relapse, the risk of relapse significantly increases when the patient encounters a high-risk situation that might consist of a feeling state, an interpersonal conflict, an environment associated with drug use, or increased drug availability/access. Such so-called cues for drug use vary between individuals but always result in subjective craving for the drug.

Without skills and resources to manage or avoid these cues when present, the patient is likely to feel unable to keep from using (decreased self-efficacy) and to expect that drug use will improve the uncomfortable situation. Initial use of the substance (termed a "slip" in this model) results in the abstinence violation effect, which is that cognitive attribution the patient makes that because he or she has used, treatment is a failure and he or she might as well return to addictive drug use. Any of us who have "slipped" on a diet by eating a few potato chips and then proceed to eat the whole bag because the diet is "ruined" understand this violation effect. The negative feeling states and low self-worth that accompany the slip make it extremely likely that the patient will relapse to addictive drug use. Thus the goal of relapse prevention techniques is to provide patients with well-rehearsed coping skills to use in the face of cues, such that they will not slip and thereby have increased feelings of self-efficacy around their ability to control drug use.

Residential treatment

Residential treatment, as the name implies, has traditionally referred to relatively long-term ($\geq$ 6 months) intensive treatment where the patient actually resides with other patients in a living or boarding home–type setting. These programs are also referred to as *therapeutic communities,* or sober living homes, with some of the better known being Daytop Village and Pheonix House. Treatment in these facilities is based on a social learning model; it is expected that with intensive, peer-based, and somewhat confrontational group work, behavioral and attitudinal change will occur (McDermott, Matthews, 1994). In addition to addiction treatment-specific activities, patients are expected to participate in the tasks necessary for the day-to-day maintenance of the community (i.e., housework, cooking), thus fostering cooperative and prosocial interactions. Typically, the roles of patients within the community follow a hierarchical or military structure, with those patients having more drug-free time, exhibiting more prosocial behavior, or participating more fully in recovery efforts, assuming leadership roles and enjoying more privileges (i.e., trips outside the community, less housework) than those earlier or less stable in the recovery process.

In the past, therapeutic communities were heavily used as an alternative to juvenile delinquency facilities, thus program components were most relevant to male adolescents and young adults (O'Brien, Delvin, 1997). Today, the scope of these programs has broadened and includes services for women, dually diagnosed patients, HIV-positive patients, and the homeless. Alliances with the criminal justice system remain strong, though, and many programs serve as alternatives to incarceration for the drug offender, or to treat individuals on parole or probation in an effort to reduce recidivism to crime (Lipton, Wexler, 1988).

Commonalties Across Treatment Models

As noted, although different models of treatment are designed to intervene with different aspects of the disease and are based on different conceptualizations of what

addiction is, certain commonalties to implementing or providing drug treatment exist that generalize across specific treatment models. Specifically, the use of *group therapy* is critical to the provision of many types of services; patients benefit from interacting with peers who also suffer the disease and sharing experiences, successes, problems, and the social support the group provides. Similarly, addiction counselors and group leaders are frequently themselves *recovered addicts,* either laypersons or paraprofessionals, who serve as role models and provide directed support to patients attempting to become drug free. The use of *urine toxicology,* collected on a regular and sometimes random basis, frequently provides an objective indication of drug use, gauges treatment response, and provides feedback to the patient to help him or her improve abstinence strategies. Becoming standard in drug treatment today is an appreciation of the specific and unique treatment needs of female addicts, thus provision of *women-specific services* is an increasingly common aspect to all treatment models.

Newer trends, based on empirical data on treatment effectiveness, are becoming evident in the practice arena. A commonly held belief has been that an addict will not get better until he or she is "ready" to enter treatment, yet newer data indicate that *coerced treatment* can be extremely effective (Lawental, McLellan, Grisson et al., 1996), thus the current trend toward alternative-to-incarceration or prison-based treatment. Although always suspected to improve treatment outcomes, the inclusion of *psychosocial services* (i.e., housing, parenting, family counseling, psychiatric, vocational training) clearly demonstrate dose-related improvements in treatment outcome (the more intensive these services, the better patients do) (McLellan, Arndt, Metzger et al., 1993), thus in programs where it is feasible, a broader array of on-site services are being provided. Finally, *contingency-based treatment* or treatment that rewards the patient with material or financial benefits for remaining abstinent has been shown to be extremely successful with certain cocaine-abusing and heroin-abusing populations (Iguchi, Stitzer, Bigelow et al., 1988), thus overt strategies to reward the patient for "clean time" may be a component of treatment.

Making Drug Treatment Referrals
Motivational interviewing

Although not a requisite of successful drug treatment outcome, it is helpful if before referring a patient to drug treatment, the patient himself or herself acknowledges that drug use has become problematic and that treatment is necessary. A powerful strategy the clinician can use for preparing a patient for drug treatment is an interpersonal technique known as *motivational interviewing* (Miller, Rollnick, 1991). Motivational interviewing consists of a set of formalized, theory-based, and empirically-evaluated interpersonal communication techniques designed to help patients identify and acknowledge substance-abusing behaviors and to move toward cessation of these. It relies on nonconfrontational approaches that ideally result in the patient, rather than the clinician, eliciting concerns about alcohol or drug use and expressing the need to reduce or cease substance intake. With the use of these techniques, the reality of relapse in addictive disease is acknowledged and again, rather than considered a roadblock, is viewed as a potential opportunity to move the patient toward more healthful outcomes. The techniques central to motivational interviewing are consistent with those demonstrated to be effective in brief intervention settings, making motivational interviewing an ideal intervention for the relatively short and episodic patterns of care characteristic of health care in managed care and cost-conscious environments.

The strategies of motivational interviewing rest on the primary assumption that motivation is a variable state rather than static trait, and thus the amount of motivation a patient possesses at a particular point in time is fluid and can be increased or decreased by forces and influences external to the patient. In this view the clinician is responsible for motivating or increasing the likelihood that the patient will follow a course of action toward change. The role of the clinician is not to point out problematic substance use or to advise the patient to stop using but, through purposeful interaction, to enhance the patient's *motivation* to change problematic alcohol or drug use. The actual changing of addictive behaviors can only be accomplished by the patient, and such change will not be attempted or maintained without an adequate level of motivation. Knowledgeably moving persons toward change and supporting them in this decision is the purpose of motivational interviewing. Only after the decision to change has been made can the need for more formalized or intensive alcohol or drug treatment be assessed.

Stages of Change

Motivational interviewing techniques take into account what is known about the stages of behavioral change as described by Prochaska and DiClemente (1982). Acknowledging that persons proceed through a predictable sequence of stages (listed in Table 10.8) in achieving and maintaining a behavioral change, Miller and Rollnick (1991) devised a "wheel of change" illustrating the steps individuals go through toward changing problematic drug or alcohol use. In this conceptualization, five stages (described in the following) are shown on the wheel, with a sixth, the precontemplation stage, lying outside the wheel as the entry point to change. The circular nature of these stages reflects the revolving nature of change and the fact that persons typically have to go around the wheel multiple times (average between four and seven times) before change is maintained. Thus relapse to alcohol or drug use is recognized as a distinct stage of change and not a failure to change; if approached appropriately, relapse should result in a renewed and refined change effort.

Critical to these stages is the understanding that different skills and interpersonal techniques are required at different stages; patients just beginning to accept that they may have a problem with alcohol intake (in the precontemplation or contemplation stages) require different motivational approaches than do persons engaging in activities to bring about change (action stage). If techniques appropriate for one stage are applied at another, the likely response on the part of the patient is resistance to change, commonly interpreted as a "lack of motivation." In fact, if resistance is encountered, it is likely that the stage of change has been misidentified and requires reassessment.

Precontemplation

Precontemplation is the entry stage to the process of change. In this stage the patient may not even recognize that his or her use of alcohol or drugs is problematic, thus is not even considering a behavioral change. These

TABLE 10.8 **Motivational Task by Stage of Change**

CLIENT STAGE	CLINICIAN'S MOTIVATIONAL TASKS
Precontemplation	Raise doubt: increase the client's perception of risks and problems with current behavior.
Contemplation	Tip the balance: evoke reasons to change, risks of not changing; strengthen the client's self-efficacy for change of current behavior.
Determination	Help the client to determine the best course of action to take in seeking change.
Action	Help the client to take steps toward change.
Maintenance	Help the client to identify and use strategies to prevent relapse.
Relapse	Help the client to renew the processes of contemplation, determination, and action, without becoming stuck or demoralized because of relapse.

May be duplicated for use in clinical practice. From McCaffery M, Pasero C: *Pain: Clinical manual*, p. 447. Copyright © 1999, Mosby, Inc.

Information from Miller WR, Rollnick S: *Motivational interviewing: Preparing people to change addictive behavior*, New York, 1991, The Guilford Press.

patients are commonly picked up in routine medical examination or on hospital rounds and, by definition, do not appear for drug or alcohol addiction treatment. A patient in this stage needs information and feedback delivered in a nonconfrontational manner to raise his or her awareness of a problem and the possibility of change. For example, the clinician might share with the patient an observation that his sinus problems may be related to his cocaine use or that her alcohol intake in the evening likely underlies her difficulties with sleep, and that changing drug use behaviors might improve well-being. Providing advice or options for treatment referral will be counterproductive at this stage because the patient is not yet secure in the belief that a problem exists.

Contemplation

Contemplation is the first stage of change because here the patient is willing to consider that his or her use of drugs or alcohol may constitute a problem and that changing this behavior may be necessary. But contemplation of change is not commitment for change. Persons in this stage can easily get "stuck," going back and forth between feeling motivated to change and motivated not to change, and the primary task of the clinician is to recognize and work with this ambivalence. Miller and Rollnick (1991) describe ambivalence not as a lack of motivation to change, but rather, as the expected cognitive response to the prospect of giving up a behavior to which the patient is strongly attached. By virtue of being in the contemplation stage, problems associated with and reasons to change substance use behaviors are appreciated by the individual, but so are the very salient and strong reasons to continue drug or alcohol use. Physical and psychologic dependence, learned and conditioned responses, and social fellowship constitute some of the many powerful attachments persons have to substance use.

The primary task of the clinician working with the ambivalent patient is to attempt to tip the patient's decisional balance in favor of changing drug or alcohol use behaviors. It is critical that the clinician not expound on the costs of continued use or consistently take the "you should change" stance in the decisional balance. Doing so will only result in the patient defending (and feeling more strongly about) the alternate view and preclude the patient working through the ambivalence, which is critical in coalescing determination for change. Thus in addition to pointing out problems associated with continued drug use, the clinician should verbally acknowledge the positive aspects of his or her drug use (i.e., increased sociability, stress relief, feeling "high"). Not only does such affirmation enable the patient to freely consider change, it also highlights personal incentives for drug use that can be addressed in the action phase.

Determination

Determination is the outcome of contemplation and occurs when the patient expresses a commitment to take action and decides to take steps to stop the problem behavior. Determination may be transient, and if not capitalized on, the patient can slip back into the contemplation stage. Here the clinician's task is not so much to motivate but to help the patient find the most appropriate and effective strategies to achieve change. These may include helping the patient devise a realistic tapering schedule, providing ways to manage withdrawal discomforts and stresses or engaging the patient in a formalized treatment program. It is helpful to keep in mind that although a first attempt at matching a determined client with a particular action strategy may not be successful, such matching becomes more refined and appropriate each time the patient cycles through the wheel of change.

Action

In the action stage the agreed on change strategy is implemented and the role of the clinician is to enhance or maintain the patient's sense of self-efficacy, praise accomplishments, and attribute successes to the capabilities of the patient. Over the course of the action stage, the clinician should remain alert to the need to modify the action plan as needed. It is in this stage when formal addiction treatment or pharmacotherapy is used.

Maintenance

The action stage usually lasts between 3 and 6 months with most addicted patients (DiClemente, 1991). Once the new behavior patterns initiated in this stage become firmly established, the patient is described as having entered the maintenance stage. To maintain the change a new set of skills and behavior patterns must be adopted by the patient; as Miller and Rollnick (1991) point out, the behaviors needed to initiate a change are different from those needed to maintain a change. This point is probably best illustrated in the case of losing weight; it is well accepted that quite a different set of strategies are required to keep weight off once lost. To be successful, these behaviors must include strategies to prevent relapse; emphasis is placed on practicing relapse prevention skills and testing these by relapse "rehearsal" (Marlatt, Gordon, 1985).

Relapse

Finally, if (and, for the first few times around the wheel, when) a relapse to drug or alcohol use occurs, it is the responsibility of the clinician to help the patient get back on the wheel and become determined to change again. As noted, relapses are normal and expected as individuals attempt to change a long-standing behavior to which they have multiple and powerful attachments. On the basis of the reasons precipitating the relapse episode, the clinician and patient together can refine the action plan and improve on maintenance skills so that efforts to change are increasingly successful.

Motivational Approaches

What specifically are the interaction techniques demonstrated to motivate persons to change? Miller and

Rollnick (1991) list eight specific strategies to be used in the motivational interviewing context.

1. *Giving Advice:* Although confrontational or directive techniques are not advocated in interacting with substance-abusing patients, the motivating effect of well-timed and level-headed advice is not minimized. Such advice should clearly and in a nonjudgmental manner identify the problem, explain why the change is important, and recommend behavior change. Such advice can be used to raise awareness of a problem, such as in the precontemplation stage, or to help the patient select an appropriate action plan in the determination stage. For example, in the case of the alcohol-abusing patient with sleeping difficulties, the clinician might say, "Alcohol use in the evening is known to disrupt restful sleep. Your inability to sleep is clearly causing you fatigue during the day and affecting your ability to work, thus I suggest that you refrain from drinking alcohol after dinner." When the patient finds that she is unable to control or limit her drinking as advised, the addictive nature of her alcohol use will become more salient to her.

2. *Removing Barriers:* Effective motivational counseling helps patients to identify barriers to changing drug-using or alcohol-using behaviors and to creatively problem solve to overcome these barriers. Some barriers may be practical in nature and have to do with obtaining access to treatment or other change strategies (e.g., how to arrange transportation and childcare so as to attend 12-step meetings); others are more complex and require assessing the role of spouses, employment, or social interaction in maintaining the problematic behavior. Providing assistance in negotiating through treatment systems and involving concerned individuals in the change process are examples of ways the clinician may overcome barriers to change.

3. *Providing Choices:* Persons facing a difficult change generally feel threatened and do not like being told what to do. As noted, directing what the patient should do may actually move him or her further away from recovery. Providing patients with a set of alternatives to address the problematic behavior enables them to choose the strategy that is most appropriate and accessible to them and provides them a sense of ownership over the action plan. For example, the clinician can list three alternate ways the patient might address problematic crack cocaine use, such as limit cocaine use to once per month by the intranasal route of administration only, stop cocaine use entirely, or attend three Cocaine Anonymous meetings in the next 2 weeks. Because a specific plan of action is not imposed, resistance to that plan is likely to be minimized.

4. *Decreasing Desirability:* In dealing with the powerful ambivalence plaguing the patient contemplating change, the patient must be helped to weigh the pros and cons of the desired change without being pushed too hard in the direction of change, or the risk of raising resistance and decreasing motivation to change is incurred. It is important that the clinician carefully decrease the perceived desirability of the current behavior, keeping in mind the positive incentives or personal reinforcers underlying drug or alcohol use and knowledgeably minimizing, undermining, or counterbalancing these. Increasing the salience of adverse consequences of use (describing in detail the clinical significance of abnormal liver function test results, for example), providing alternative reinforcers, and providing positive incentives for alternate behaviors are ways the clinician can decrease the desirability of continued drug and alcohol use.

5. *Practicing Empathy:* A well-established characteristic of effective therapists and counselors is the ability to accurately empathize with what the patient is experiencing. Empathy is not so much an ability to identify with the experiences of the patient or a personality style but a learned skill enabling full understanding of the meaning of these experiences to the patient. Accurate empathy requires careful attention to what the patient says and does and skilled reflective listening. If the patient feels secure that the clinician appreciates the difficulties inherent in change, the efforts of the clinician to motivate and sustain change are more likely to be accepted and acted on.

6. *Providing Feedback:* To sustain the change process, patients need to know, on an ongoing basis, how they are doing with respect to the change they are attempting to achieve. Clear and accurate feedback can come in the form of results from health assessments or objective tests of drug or alcohol use (i.e., urine toxicology, liver function tests), reviewing substance use diaries or contracts at regular intervals, and even expressions of concern when it is clear that the patient is struggling with change.

7. *Clarifying Goals:* Individuals facing change need clear goals against which to compare their current behavior to appreciate when progress is being made and to make adjustments in behavior when needed. Goals set must be realistic, attainable, and desirable to the patient to sustain the motivation necessary to work toward these. For example, the clinician might state, "Your goal was to refrain from all cocaine use over the past 2 weeks, yet your urine toxicology results indicate that you have used cocaine recently. Maybe we should try for a shorter period of abstinence or see if attending some 12-step

meetings might help you reach this goal of 14 consecutive 'clean' days." By reemphasizing goals at each visit and modifying these as necessary, the clinician can ensure that behaviors are consistent with those needed to reach these desired end points.

8. *Active Helping:* Finally, to help patients through the change process, they need to feel that the clinician is genuinely interested in their progress. This is accomplished by taking an active role in the patient's work and showing professional commitment to helping the patient through the stages of change. Thus rather than simply referring the patient to treatment to follow-up on, calls to the referral program would be made for the patient, the clinician might attend a treatment meeting or two with the patient, or in general do whatever is required to facilitate treatment engagement. Feeling that the clinician is committed to helping the patient change encourages commitment to change on the part of the patient.

Importance of the Interpersonal Context

Integral to motivational interviewing strategies is the development of a caring, therapeutic interpersonal relationship between the clinician and patient. Being a variable state influenced by external factors, it is only through interpersonal interaction that the clinician can actively affect motivation. Thus the clinician is not a passive observer of the patient's motivational state, but rather an important determinant of this state through his or her deliberate interaction with the patient. Motivational intervention is predicated on interpersonal, face-to-face communication between the patient and clinician; it is the relationship that provides the context in which motivation can be effectively altered and the energy sustained to achieve change.

Guidelines for treatment referral

As noted, the drug treatment system in most communities tends to be rather disjointed and poorly integrated with mainstream health and mental health care, thus knowing the best program and model of treatment to which a patient with an identified substance use disorder should be referred is a challenging task for most nonaddiction specialists. To simplify this process and assist clinicians to make knowledgeable referrals, the American Society of Addiction Medicine has developed *patient placement criteria* (Hoffman, Halikas, Mee-Lee et al., 1991) that specify the level of care required by addicted patients on the basis of six patient-related and disease-related variables (Table 10.9).

On the basis of these criteria, only the patient for whom a severe withdrawal syndrome is likely or who has an unstable mental or medical condition is inpatient treatment indicated; most patients with addictive disease can be successfully treated in outpatient programs. Note that high levels of treatment resistance, high potential for relapse, or a nonsupportive living environment do not qualify persons for medically managed treatment; this most costly form of treatment is reserved for persons with significant health problems or at risk of these developing.

RELIEVING PAIN IN THE CONTEXT OF ADDICTION

As noted in the introduction of this chapter, the actual or feared presence of addictive disease makes a profound impact on the provision of adequate opioid analgesia to people with pain (Friedman, 1990; Lander, 1990; Melzack, 1990; Morgan, 1985-86, Schuster, 1989). Clinicians understandably want to avoid inducing addictive disease in patients with pain for whom they provide care, as well as scrutiny from the Drug Enforcement Agency (DEA), so become uncomfortable when patients request more opioid medication than seems to be necessary or continue to take opioid analgesics for an extended period of time (Bressler, Geraci, Schatz, 1991; Hill, 1993; Krick, Lindley, Bennett, 1994; Perry, 1984). Two situations in which clinicians have been particularly reticent to provide opioid analgesia are for the patient suffering from a chronic nonmalignant pain condition and the patient with a current or remote history of addictive disease. Although the latter situation is the focus of this chapter, the two conditions can and do co-occur in the same individual (see p. 461), making pain management particularly challenging.

Complicating pain management for the person with a past or current history of addiction are exaggerated concerns that exposure to opioid medications, even in the presence of well-documented pain, will reinduce or worsen addictive disease. In this case, clinicians may actually believe they are helping the patient by withholding opioids. The prescription of opioids to known opioid addicts for the purpose of maintaining the addiction is illegal in this country, which further inhibits opioid prescription for these patients (Clark, Sees, 1993; Stimmel, 1989). Although prescribed for pain, physicians report that they are reticent to do so for fear of DEA and regulatory sanctions (Cooper, Czechowicz, Petersen et al., 1992; Joranson, 1993; Perry, 1985; Shapiro, 1994). Furthermore, moral and criminal views of the addicted patient, so prevalent in societal responses to these individuals, are frequently reflected in the belief system of the treating clinician or facility, resulting in an attribution that the patient is a "bad" person and therefore undeserving or unworthy of aggressive and complete pain relief. Conceptualizing addiction as a disease, complete with known

TABLE 10.9 **Patient Placement Criteria**

CRITERIA DIMENSIONS	LEVELS OF CARE			
	LEVEL I OUTPATIENT TREATMENT	LEVEL II INTENSIVE OUTPATIENT TREATMENT	LEVEL III MEDICALLY MONITORED INTENSIVE INPATIENT TREATMENT	LEVEL IV MEDICALLY MANAGED INTENSIVE INPATIENT TREATMENT
1. Acute intoxication or withdrawal potential or both	No withdrawal risk	Minimal withdrawal risk	Severe withdrawal risk but manageable in Level III	Severe withdrawal risk
2. Biomedical condition and complications	None or very stable	None or nondistracting from addiction treatment and manageable in Level II	Require medical monitoring but not intensive treatment	Require 24-h medical/ nursing care
3. Emotional or behavioral conditions or complications	None or very stable	Mild severity with potential to distract from recovery	Moderate severity needing a 24-h structured setting	Severe problems requiring 24-h psychiatric care with concomitant addiction treatment
4. Treatment acceptance or resistance	Willing to cooperate but needs motivating and monitoring strategies	Resistance high enough to require structured program but not so high as to render outpatient treatment ineffective	Resistance high enough despite negative consequences and needs intensive motivating strategies in 24-h structure	Problems in this dimension do not qualify patient for Level IV
5. Relapse potential	Able to maintain abstinence and recovery goals with minimal support	Intensification of addiction symptoms and high likelihood of relapse without close monitoring and support	Unable to control use despite active participation in less intensive care and needs 24-h structure	Problems in this dimension do not qualify patient for Level IV
6. Recovery environment	Supportive recovery environment or patient has skills to cope	Environment unsupportive but with structure or support patient can cope	Environment dangerous for recovery necessitating removal from the environment: logistical impediments to outpatient treatment	Problems in this dimension do not qualify patient for Level IV

May be duplicated for use in clinical practice. As appears in McCaffery M, Pasero C: *Pain: Clinical manual*, p. 451, 1999, Mosby, Inc.

From Hoffman NG, Halikas J, Mee-Lee Y et al.: *Patient placement criteria for the treatment of psychoactive substance use disorders*, Chevy Chase, Md, 1991, American Society of Addiction Medicine.

risk factors, a predictable pattern of progression, and effective treatment interventions, serves to simplify and provide direction for the provision of appropriate and effective opioid analgesia to these patients.

Accepting that pain relief is a primary goal in caring for all patients with pain, regardless of how they have used or currently do use drugs of abuse, is critical to implementing the guidelines presented later. As described in Chapter 2, clear health consequences are associated with unrelieved pain. Physical stasis, prolonged postoperative recovery time, and even increased tumor growth are demonstrated correlates of ongoing pain. An additional consequence of unrelieved pain in the recovering addict may be relapse. Although poorly studied, the emotional and physiologic responses to unrelieved pain may serve as powerful "cues" for drug use. Patients with a history of addictive disease know very well what will provide them instantaneous "relief," and under conditions in which their pain is not being aggressively treated, will be very likely to turn to these substances.

While an actively using addict has unrelieved pain it is *never* the appropriate time to introduce or attempt aggressive addiction interventions. The patient learns no "lesson" by having opioid analgesics withheld when clearly indicated; punishment is not an effective treatment for addictive disease as relapse rates after incarceration indicate. As noted earlier, drugs of abuse may appear even *more* desirable under conditions of physical and psychologic suffering. The first priority in treating these patients is to ensure that they are comfortable; only then can addictive disease be effectively addressed. If patients trust that their health care provider genuinely wants to make them comfortable, they are more likely to be open to the clinician's efforts to address and initiate addiction treatment.

Sources of Overlap Between Pain and Addiction

Before describing specific guidelines for the management of pain when addictive disease is or has been present, it must be appreciated that pain and addiction are not unrelated phenomena. Multiple sources of potential overlap between these conditions exist in both psychologic and physiologic domains. Evidence exists that the presence of pain and addiction affect the expression of each other.

Nonspecific effects of addiction on pain

Relatively nonspecific consequences of addictive disease serve to increase the experience of pain, regardless of the specific drug(s) abused (Savage, 1994). Drug intoxication and withdrawal carry with them activation of the sympathetic nervous system, which is a known contributor to the pain experience. Specifically, intoxication with cocaine and CNS stimulants increases central noradrenergic activity, whereas withdrawal from opioids, CNS depressants, and/or sedative hypnotics has the same effect (see Table 10.4) (Miller, Gold, 1993). The resultant increased muscle tension, anxiety, and irritability noted during intoxication or withdrawal from these drugs serve to augment discomfort.

As noted on p. 432, the "high" or reward associated with all drugs of abuse depends on endogenous opioid system activation in the subcortical structures of the brain. Although not definitively demonstrated, it is reasonable to suspect that changes occurring in these endogenous opioid pathways caused by addictive drug use might alter pain perception. For example, in a small sample of cocaine addicts, active cocaine addicts ($n = 21$) tolerated cold-pressor pain approximately one third less time than did ex-cocaine addicts ($n = 32$) whose performance was comparable with that of published norms

(Compton, 1994). Addictive drug use, regardless of specific drug of abuse, may alter endogenous opioid activity and result in increased pain.

Neurophysiologic adaptations to opioid addiction

Recent evidence indicates that molecular changes occurring with the development of opioid tolerance specifically may decrease tolerance for painful stimuli (see Basbaum, 1995). Again, although tolerance is not addiction, it is present in opioid addiction, and thus can affect pain responses. With animal models, investigators found that opioid-tolerant animals were less tolerant of pain (Mao, Price, Mayer, 1995). These results are similar to those in a study of pain tolerance in opioid addicts on methadone maintenance pharmacotherapy. These data showed that methadone-maintained individuals ($n = 43$) tolerated cold-pressor pain on an average of 30 seconds less than matched ex-addict drug-free controls ($n = 26$), with methadone dose being inversely related to cold-pressor pain tolerance ($r = -.25$, $p = 0.05$) (Compton, 1994).

Individual differences in pain and addiction

It is important to consider whether individuals with a genetic propensity for addictive disease may not also possess characteristic responses to pain (i.e., high versus low pain tolerance). For example, it is well known that certain individuals metabolize opioids more quickly than others (Gonzalez, 1991; Ingelman-Sundberg, Johansson, Persson et al., 1994; Otton, Schadel, Cheung et al., 1993), thus theoretically putting them at decreased risk for addiction (i.e., they get less drug "reward") but at increased risk for undermanagement of pain. Interestingly, preliminary data indicate that persons who extensively metabolize opioids are less tolerant of experimental pain, which has been ascribed to theorized problems in their ability to synthesize endogenous opioids (Sindrup, Poulsen, Brosen et al., 1993).

More intriguing may be the presence of heritable differences in both the reward and pain processing systems between individuals. Although as yet unexplored in clinical samples, good evidence exists that certain strains of rodents, demonstrated to differ in level of activity within their endogenous opioid systems, also differ in the amount of reward and analgesia they receive from a given dose of opioid, as well as on their baseline tolerance for painful stimuli (see Berrettini, Alexander, Ferraro et al., 1994; Crabbe, Belknap, Buck, 1994; Frischknecht, Siegfried, Waser, 1988; Marley, Elmer, Goldberg, 1992; Mogil, Marek, O'Toole et al., 1994; Mogil, Sternberg, Marek et al., 1996; Schuster, 1990-91). The well-known individual variation in humans with respect to tolerance for pain, opioid analgesia (Buschbaum,

Davis, Coppola et al., 1981; Galer, Coyle, Pasternak et al., 1992; Portenoy, 1994), and drug reward indicates that heritable differences in endogenous opioid activity might account for these differences.

Does pain affect drug reward?

What remains to be demonstrated is how the presence of pain might alter or attenuate the amount of reward provided by a given substance of abuse. Although extensive pharmacologic studies have not been able to separate the rewarding effects of opioids from their analgesic effects (see Woods, Winger, France, 1992), it is possible that the latter predominate in the pain state. Clinical lore states that patients in pain taking opioid analgesics receive little "brain reward," at least not to the degree that they begin drug-seeking once the painful condition has resolved, with iatrogenic opioid addiction rates at less than 1% if present at all (Medina, Diamond, 1977; Perry, Heidrich, 1982; Porter, Jick, 1980). Zacny and colleagues (1996) found that under experimental conditions, human subjects reported less opioid reward from a dose of opioid paired with a painful stimulus than that reported during the same opioid challenge without pain.

Similarly, while in pain, it is not clear that opioid tolerance and physical dependence develop to the same degree as demonstrated in pain-free individuals. Vaccarino and colleagues (1993) provide interesting preclinical evidence that rats chronically receiving morphine paired with acute formalin-induced pain demonstrated less analgesic tolerance and naloxone-precipitated withdrawal than rats with the same chronic exposure to opioids without pain. These data parallel the anecdotal experience of many pain clinicians who report that they do not encounter opioid tolerance when providing chronic opioid analgesia to persons with malignant or nonmalignant pain syndromes and find that doses only need be increased when pathology progresses (Collin, Poulain, Gauvain-Piquard et al., 1993; Portenoy, 1990; Portenoy, Payne, 1997).

Clinical Management of Patients With Pain and Addiction

The combined presence of pain and addiction result in two interrelated clinical challenges: (1) how to best provide analgesia to persons with a current or past history of addiction, and (2) how to assess for and identify addictive disease in pain patients on opioid analgesic maintenance therapy. After a discussion of the general principles for treating the pain of persons suffering addiction, the specific pain management for patients actively abusing drugs, patients in recovery, and patients on pharmacotherapy for the treatment of addictive disease will be reviewed. Difficulties inherent in assessing for ad-

diction in the presence of chronic opioid analgesia will be reviewed, and guidelines for detecting addictive disease in this context will be presented.

All management principles are based on the premise that addicted individuals comprise a group of patients whose pain is quite likely to be mismanaged or undermanaged, yet are a group for whom adequate pain relief can provide great benefit. To withhold appropriate pain assessment and relief from a person with current or past addictive disease is a form of discrimination, a double standard of practice, and an unethical position. As mentioned throughout this book, clinical practice guidelines state that *all* patients deserve the best possible pain relief that may safely be provided (Acute Pain Management Guideline Panel, 1992).

General principles

Before treatment for pain is initiated for the patient with a current or past history of addiction, it is incumbent on the clinician to acknowledge his or her own personal biases about addictive disease and make a conscious effort to effectively put them aside (Liaschenko, 1994). Being a member of society and likely coming to the clinical setting with his or her own personal experiences with addiction (in family, friends, or even self), it is expected that the clinician will hold value judgments about the disease reflecting moral or criminal societal perspectives (Chappel, Schnoll, 1977; Stimmel, 1989). Yet, the health care *professional* is charged with providing effective and compassionate care to all patients without bias. Personal beliefs about addiction are irrelevant when treating pain in the addicted patient; instead, care should be provided on the basis of a scientific understanding of pain and addictive disease.

Still, biases do interfere with clinical care, with these patients described in the literature as "hateful" (Groves, 1978), "demanding," (Carroll, 1993) and "difficult" (Podrasky, Sexton, 1988). In a survey examining nurses' assessments and analgesic choices, McCaffery and colleagues (1992) found that responses differed for two hypothetical patients: (1) a patient described as a "risk taker," a consumer of alcohol, and unemployed, and (2) a patient described as typically middle-class. Nurses in this sample responded that although they themselves would provide the same care for both patients, they believed their colleagues would treat the patients differently, with a tendency to disbelieve and undertreat the "irresponsible" patient. As a group, these nurses indicated that they did not want personal values to interfere with the quality of care provided and felt that they could benefit from discussion (and permission to say they do not like certain patients) to prevent these from affecting care.

As with any other patient, the clinician must accept the addict's report of pain. Provision of adequate analgesia is the primary goal, which in this population carries with it the additional benefits of averting relapse or making the patient more receptive to addiction interventions. Evidence reviewed above indicates that persons with addictive disease may actually be less pain tolerant than their nonaddicted peers, which may be due to preexisting individual differences or drug-induced neuroadaptations. Yet, these are the very patients whose pain is likely to be undermanaged related to staff attributions and misconceptions about addictive disease and fears of being "duped" (see McCaffery, Vourakis, 1992). The clinician must remember that addiction is a treatable disease; it is better to err on the side of providing adequate pain relief than to let patients suffer for fear of promoting addiction.

Disputing or not aggressively treating the patient's report of pain produces an adversarial relationship that invites the patient to retaliate with anger and manipulations. Problems arise when the special needs of the patient with a history of addiction are not addressed. The goal of the clinician is to provide help on the basis of a scientific understanding of the disease, not punish for immoral or criminal behavior. Providing adequate pain relief to the addicted patient presents an opportunity to have a positive, even motivational (see Motivational Interviewing, p. 446), interaction with the individual, which can be the first step in moving an addicted person toward recovery.

Pain relief for the active addict on inpatient and outpatient bases

Active drug abuse complicates pain management in several ways. Addicted patients have difficulty adhering to a pain management regimen, and ongoing drug intoxication or withdrawal complicate the pain experience. Hyperalgesia, for example, is an identifying characteristic of opioid withdrawal; if the patient is an active opioid abuser, the emergence of subtle withdrawal symptoms will exacerbate the pain condition.

Pain management for a patient with addiction differs according to the temporal nature and treatment setting of the pain. Specifically, is the pain acute or chronic in nature (see Chapter 11) and thus primarily treated on an inpatient or outpatient basis? Inpatient interventions for acute pain (i.e., postoperative pain, labor pain) are simplified by the fact that the nature and quality of pain is relatively predictable, the source of the pain is known, and the duration of opioid exposure is likely to be brief. With chronic pain, physiologic and psychologic responses to the pain, as well as to repeated opioid exposure (tolerance and physical dependence), complicate outpatient management. In the case of an addict with chronic nonmalignant pain, the cause of the pain is sometimes unclear, making clinicians even more reluctant to accept the patient's report of pain. Although pain can never be proven or disproven, treating pain in an addicted patient is often

more acceptable to clinicians when a physical cause for the pain can be readily identified.

Guidelines for the management of pain in a patient with addictive disease, on an inpatient or outpatient basis, are provided in Box 10.4.

Inpatient Management

To manage acute pain, it is important to establish specifically the types of drugs to which the patient is addicted. Although not well-researched, it is logical to suspect that when an opioid analgesic is used, a heroin addict would be at greater risk for medication misuse than an alcoholic who had never abused opioids; although addiction generalizes across substances, the heroin addict is being exposed to his or her drug of choice. Dunbar and Katz (1996) provide evidence that among substance abusers, primary alcoholics are the least likely to abuse opioid analgesics, and Bruera and colleagues (1995) found alcoholic cancer patients used no more opioid analgesia than did nonalcoholic cancer patients.

The many nonopioid and adjuvant analgesics for providing pain relief (see Chapters 5 and 7) should be explored and implemented with these patients (Savage, Schofferman, 1995; Schofferman, Savage, 1994), but appropriate use of opioids should not be delayed. When facing pain management for the patient with addictive disease, clinicians tend to focus on the problems associated with providing opioid analgesics without always fully exploiting alternate nonopioid and adjuvant analgesic interventions. Pharmacologic analgesia still tends to be the first line pain intervention in tertiary health care settings. As should be done with all patients, nondrug interventions also should be implemented to keep opioid requirements to a minimum (Aston, 1987; Savage, 1994).

As noted earlier, psychologic and physiologic aspects of drug withdrawal syndromes can exacerbate the pain experience, thus to the extent possible, withdrawal should be avoided or aggressively managed in these patients. No need exists to contribute to discomfort while the patient has acute pain, and during this time of acute stress detoxification should be avoided. Physical dependence should be treated with long-acting formulations of the abused drug (Fishbain, Rosomoff, Rosomoff, 1992; Fultz, Senay, 1975; Fultz, Senay, Pray et al., 1980; Payne, 1989) and, if attempted, detoxification should proceed very gradually following established protocols (see Boxes 10.5, 10.6, and 10.7 on pp. 456, 458, and 459) to prevent the emergence of pain-intensifying withdrawal symptoms. Note that pharmacologic detoxification is not indicated for withdrawal from CNS stimulants, cocaine, hallucinogens, and marijuana because accompanying physiologic instability is minimal. Environmental, behavioral, and pharmacologic management of other potentially pain-augmenting symptoms, for example anxiety, depression, and sleep disturbance, should be instituted.

BOX 10.4

GUIDELINES

MANAGEMENT OF PAIN IN PATIENTS WITH ACTIVE ADDICTION

General Guidelines That Apply to All Clinical Settings

1. If the patient acknowledges addiction or use of substances for nonmedical reasons, openly discuss this and encourage the patient to express any fears of how this may affect pain management and treatment by staff.
2. Accept and act on the patient's report of pain with appropriate assessment and treatment.
3. Aggressively manage pain: addiction treatment is not a priority when the patient has unrelieved pain.
4. Reassure the patient that staff is committed to providing aggressive and effective pain relief.
5. Develop with the patient a treatment plan for pain management. If feasible, provide the patient with a written copy.
6. Remind staff that (a) prescription of opioids to a known addict for the management of pain is not illegal, (b) persons with addictive disease may be relatively pain intolerant, and (c) that detoxification is an ineffective treatment for addictive disease.
7. Request consultation from an addiction specialist and a pain specialist so that both patient and staff know that support and guidance are available if needed.
8. Begin with nondrug or nonopioid analgesia. However, if pain relief is inadequate, add opioids. Begin with opioids when pain is moderate to severe.
9. If the patient is physically dependent on opioids, *do not* administer mixed opioid agonist/antagonists for analgesia (e.g., nalbuphine) because withdrawal will be precipitated.
10. Assess patient's motivation for drug treatment; implement motivational interviewing strategies, and have treatment referral references on hand.

Inpatient Setting

1. Consider IV PCA as a method of administering opioid analgesics. PCA gives the patient more control and may reduce potentially confrontational interactions with staff. Monitor and adjust pump parameters because active addicts may require and safely receive larger doses than other patients.
2. For persons physically dependent on alcohol, sedative-hypnotics, or opioids, provide long-acting formulations of substitution medications (see Boxes 10.5, 10.6, and 10.7) to prevent emergence of withdrawal symptoms.
3. Monitor at least q4h for emergence of withdrawal symptoms from all drugs potentially abused by the patient, including alcohol, and treat aggressively and symptomatically.
4. When opioids are no longer needed for analgesia, taper them very slowly to minimize emergence of withdrawal symptoms; assess for presence of withdrawal symptoms at least q4h during analgesic taper; treat symptomatically.

Outpatient Setting

1. When opioid analgesics are required, select long-acting formulations such as transdermal fentanyl or controlled-release morphine. Less frequent dosing may increase the patient's adherence to the treatment plan. Also, drugs with a slow onset tend to have a low street value.
2. Administer analgesics ATC, giving the patient the specific times for taking medication, rather than saying three times a day.
3. Carefully document the treatment plan and provide the patient with a copy.
4. Provide the patient with whatever written information is available such as hours of operation, policies, methods of obtaining refills, and phone number, especially when the facility is not open.
5. At each visit, include the patient's analgesic use, pain severity and quality, level of function, and side effects. Record and discuss with the patient any behavior suggestive of inappropriate opioid use.

May be duplicated for use in clinical practice. From McCaffery M, Pasero C: *Pain: Clinical manual,* p. 455. Copyright © 1999, Mosby, Inc.

Opioids must not be withheld from persons with pain who are suffering addictive disease. No scientific evidence exists that providing opioid analgesia to these patients in any way worsens the disease, or conversely, that withholding opioid analgesia increases the likelihood of recovery (McCaffery, Vourakis, 1992). When indicated, long-acting opioid agents, with slower onset and less psychoactive effect, are desirable (Newshan, 1996). When possible, a single opioid agent should be used. Mixed opioid agonist-antagonists should never be used in the opioid-dependent patient because these will precipitate withdrawal (Payne, 1989). Analgesics should be ordered on an around-the-clock basis to avoid de-creased opioid blood levels with associated breakthrough pain and withdrawal because both are risks for increased drug use. As acute pain decreases, opioids prescribed for analgesia should be tapered on a gradual schedule to prevent the emergence of subtle opioid withdrawal symptoms. Addicts are extremely sensitive to symptoms indicative of withdrawal, and these can serve as a powerful cue for inappropriate drug use (e.g., obtaining drugs from visitors).

Written agreements and treatment plans are helpful in providing pain relief for addicted patients (Wesson, Ling, Smith, 1993). If available, the same written agreements can be given to patients with pain to reenforce

BOX 10.5

GUIDELINES

ALCOHOL DETOXIFICATION PROTOCOL

Overview: The current state of the art for alcohol detoxification is to use a symptom-triggered approach with a long-acting benzodiazepine to treat alcohol withdrawal symptoms (see Table 10.4) on the basis of Clinical Institute Withdrawal Assessment (CIWA; Sullivan, Sykora, Schneiderman et al., 1989) score (Form 10.1) (CSAT, 1995; Lohr, 1995). This approach has been demonstrated to minimize the total amount of medication needed and to shorten the overall detoxification period (Saitz, Mayo-Smith, Roberts, 1994). Because it is difficult to predict which alcoholic will have severe withdrawal symptoms develop, it is safer to provide treatment to patients who may not need it than to withhold medication until severe symptoms develop. Withdrawal severity appears to depend less on absolute amount of alcohol intake, but increases with the number of times a patient has detoxified. Although most detoxifications are still done on an inpatient basis, day hospital and ambulatory alcohol detoxifications are increasingly and safely done in certain patients (i.e., younger patients, those without a history of withdrawal seizures or DTs, fewer previous withdrawal episodes, good compliance and social support) (see also Table 10.9). *Remember, detoxification alone is an ineffective treatment for addiction.*

1. Assess CIWA score immediately on admission or decision to detoxify and q4h. Mild withdrawal symptoms typically emerge between 6 and 24 h after last drink. The key is to treat symptoms *before* they become severe.
2. A CIWA score of less than 10 requires no pharmacologic treatment; a score of 10 to 20 requires increased assessment frequency and low-dose pharmacotherapy; and a score greater than 20 merits full pharmacologic treatment and assessment at 1- to 2-h intervals. The goal is to keep CIWA score ≤ 12.
3. Long-acting oral benzodiazepines (Librium, Valium) are the drugs of choice; shorter-acting agents (Serax, Ativan) are indicated in the elderly and those with impaired hepatic function. Doses used are higher than anxiolytic doses.
4. Watch degree of sedation with dosing; do not repeat doses in overly sedated patients.
5. With long-acting benzodiazepines, taper over 3 to 6 days with QD dosing; with shorter acting agents, taper over 4 to 8 days and do not deviate from QID dosing.
6. Haldol, .05 to 2.0 mg PO q4 prn, for delirium psychosis.
7. Thiamine, 100 mg PO QD × 2, to prevent Wernicke-Korsakoff syndrome.

Equivalent benzodiazepine doses for treating CIWA scores > 20; for scores between 10 and 20, use half or quarter doses

Medication	Administration Route	
	Oral (mg)	Intravenous (mg)
Librium (chlordiazepoxide)	100	—
Valium (diazepam)	20	5-10
★Ativan (lorazepam)	4	1-2
★Serax (oxazepam)	120	—

*Short-acting formulations.

May be duplicated for use in clinical practice. From McCaffery M, Pasero C: *Pain: Clinical manual,* p. 456. Copyright © 1999, Mosby, Inc.

Information from Center for Substance Abuse Treatment: *Detoxification from alcohol and other drugs, Treatment improvement protocol series No. 19,* Rockville, Md, 1994, CSAT; Lohr RH: Treatment of alcohol withdrawal in hospitalized patients, *Mayo Clinic Procs* 70:777-782, 1995; Saitz R, Mayo-Smith MF, Roberts MS: Individualized treatment for alcohol withdrawal: A randomized double-blind controlled trial, *JAMA* 272:519-523, 1994; Sullivan JT, Sykora K, Schneiderman J et al.: Assessment of alcohol withdrawal: The revised Clinical Institute Withdrawal Assessment for Alcohol Scale (CIAW-Ar), *Br J Addiction* 84:1353-1357, 1989.

---

pain treatment plans. See Appendix B for a discussion of agreements.

Although patient-controlled analgesia (PCA) is widely used for the management of postoperative and traumatic pain, controversy exists as to whether it is appropriate for patients with addiction. Although demonstrated to provide better analgesia and to obviate drug-seeking behavior, some clinicians are not comfortable with addicted patients having relatively "free access" to an abusable drug, especially since a lack of control over drug use is a defining characteristic of addiction. With IV PCA, the patient does not have to ask the nurse for each dose of analgesic. Thus use of PCA decreases the number of potentially confrontational interactions between the patient and staff and minimizes the tendency to develop manipulative behavior to obtain analgesic doses.

A small study by Paige and colleagues (1994) found no differences in PCA analgesic use between active drug-abusing (opioid, cocaine) patients and normal controls, indicating that addicted patients can use PCA responsibly. See Appendix B for a sample treatment agreement for PCA use with the addicted patient.

Outpatient Management

As with any patient, when the actively addicted patient is discharged with chronic pain of malignant or nonmalignant origin, less invasive routes of administration are used, if possible, such as oral or transdermal opioid analgesics. Doses should be aggressively titrated to meet analgesic need. At each patient visit, it is critical that the clinician assess and chart on each of the following: severity and quality of pain, the patient's level of

FORM 10.1 Addiction Research Foundation Clinical Institute Withdrawal Assessment—Alcohol (CIWA-Ar) This scale is not copyrighted and may be used freely.

Patient: _____   Date: /____ /____ /____   Time: ____ : ____
                                                  y   m   d   (24-hour clock, midnight = 00:00)

Pulse or heart rate, taken for one minute: _____   Blood pressure: ____ /____

NAUSEA AND VOMITING—Ask "Do you feel sick to your stomach? Have you vomited?" Observation.
0 No nausea and no vomiting
1 Mild nausea with no vomiting
2
3
4 Intermittent nausea with dry heaves
5
6
7 Constant nausea, frequent dry heaves and vomiting

TREMOR—Arms extended and fingers spread apart. Observation.
0 No tremor
1 Not visible, but can be felt fingertip to fingertip
2
3
4 Moderate, with patient's arms extended
5
6
7 Severe, even with arms not extended

PAROXYSMAL SWEATS—Observation.
0 No sweat visible
1 Barely perceptible sweating, palms moist
2
3
4 Beads of sweat obvious on forehead
5
6
7 Drenching sweats

ANXIETY—Ask "Do you feel nervous?" Observation.
0 No anxiety, at ease
1 Mildly anxious
2
3
4 Moderately anxious, or guarded, so anxiety is inferred
5
6
7 Equivalent to acute panic states as seen in severe delirium or acute schizophrenic reactions

AGITATION—Observation.
0 Normal activity
1 Somewhat more than normal activity
2
3
4 Moderately fidgety and restless
5
6
7 Paces back and forth during most of the interview, or constantly thrashes about

TACTILE DISTURBANCES—Ask "Have you any itching, pins and needles sensations, any burning, any numbness, or do you feel bugs crawling on or under your skin?" Observation.
0 None
1 Mild itching, pins and needles, burning or numbness
2 Mild itching, pins and needles, burning or numbness
3 Moderate itching, pins and needles, burning or numbness
4 Moderately severe hallucinations
5 Severe hallucinations
6 Extremely severe hallucinations
7 Continuous hallucinations

AUDITORY DISTURBANCES—Ask "Are you more aware of sounds around you? Are they harsh? Do they frighten you? Are you hearing anything that is disturbing to you? Are you hearing things you know are not there?" Observation.
0 Not present
1 Very mild harshness or ability to frighten
2 Mild harshness or ability to frighten
3 Moderate harshness or ability to frighten
4 Moderately severe hallucinations
5 Severe hallucinations
6 Extremely severe hallucinations
7 Continuous hallucinations

VISUAL DISTURBANCES—Ask "Does the light appear to be too bright? Is its color different? Does it hurt your eyes? Are you seeing anything that is disturbing to you? Are you seeing things you know are not there?" Observation.
0 Not present
1 Very mild sensitivity
2 Mild sensitivity
3 Moderate sensitivity
4 Moderately severe hallucinations
5 Severe hallucinations
6 Extremely severe hallucinations
7 Continuous hallucinations

HEADACHE, FULLNESS IN HEAD—Ask "Does your head feel different? Does it feel like there is a band around your head?" Do not rate for dizziness or lightheadedness. Otherwise, rate severity.
0 Not present
1 Very mild
2 Mild
3 Moderate
4 Moderately severe
5 Severe
6 Very severe
7 Extremely severe

ORIENTATION AND CLOUDING OF SENSORIUM—Ask "What day is this? Where are you? Who am I?"
0 Oriented and can do serial additions
1 Cannot do serial additions or is uncertain about date
2 Disoriented for date by no more than 2 calendar days
3 Disoriented for date by more than 2 calendar days
4 Disoriented for place and/or person

Total CIWA-A Score ____
Rater's Initials ____
Maximum Possible Score   67

May be duplicated for use in clinical practice. From McCaffery M, Pasero C: *Pain: Clinical manual*, p. 457. Copyright © 1999, Mosby, Inc.

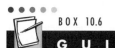

GUIDELINES

SEDATIVE-HYPNOTIC/BENZODIAZEPINE DETOXIFICATION PROTOCOL

Overview: Physical dependence on these classes of medications does not necessarily constitute addiction (i.e., may be prescribed for panic or anxiety disorder), thus detoxification is not strictly indicated. Detoxification typically proceeds on an inpatient basis, although ambulatory treatment is increasingly used with certain patients (see Table 10.9 and Box 10.5). Two general types of detoxification are used: either (1) gradual tapering of abused medication, or (2) conversion to phenobarbital equivalents and gradual tapering of phenobarbital (CSAT, 1994). Phenobarbital is a long-acting barbiturate that produces little psychoactive effect and has smooth dimunition of action. Dose of treatment medication and choice of detoxification method vary with daily dose and formulation of abused agent; time after last dose when withdrawal symptoms (see Table 10.4) emerge varies with agent half-life. *Remember, detoxification alone is an ineffective treatment for addiction.*

1. Consider gradual taper of medication if patient taking Librium, Valium, or other long-acting benzodiazepine, is compliant, is not concurrently abusing alcohol or other drugs, and is in good general state of health (see Table 10.9). Decrease total daily dose gradually over a 10-day to 2-week period, slowing taper if withdrawal symptoms become evident.

2. Use phenobarbital conversion approach for all other cases. Convert patient's average total daily dose of benzodiazepine or sedative-hypnotic into phenobarbital equivalents and divide into three doses for tid PO administra-

tion. Decrease by 30 mg of phenobarbital per day, slowing taper if withdrawal symptoms become evident.

a. Hold phenobarbital dose if nystagmus is present. If nystagmus is accompanied by slurred speech and ataxia, hold next two doses, and reduce daily dosage by half.

Phenobarbital Withdrawal Equivalents

Medication	Dose equivalent to 30 mg Phenobarbital PO
Benzodiazepines	
Xanax	1 mg
Librium	25 mg
Klonopin	2 mg
Tranxene	7.5 mg
Valium	10 mg
Dalmane	15 mg
Ativan	2 mg
Serax	10 mg
Restoril	15 mg
Halcion	0.25 mg
Sedative-hypnotics	
Amytal	100 mg
Fiorinal	100 mg
Nembutal	100 mg
Seconal	100 mg
Placidyl	500 mg

function, the amount of analgesic being used, and any evidence of opiate misuse (see Box 10.8, p. 459). Doing so ensures that pain is being adequately managed and that medication misuse will be caught early. It also provides adequate documentation of the pain condition and appropriate opioid prescription for regulatory audits (Medical Board of California, 1996).

It should be noted that diagnosis with a terminal disease can be a powerful motivator for recovery from addiction, and significant steps toward the treatment of addictive disease can occur in the presence of opioid analgesic maintenance. Every effort should be made to facilitate recovery efforts of the dying patient.

Outpatient management of the discomfort for the patient suffering nonmalignant pain is complicated, even in patients without addictive disease, by difficulties in discerning the source and progression of the pain and the exaggerated concerns about providing ongoing opioid

exposure (Trachtenberg, 1994). For all patients with chronic nonmalignant pain, a treatment plan should be developed, ideally in writing, and agreed to by the staff and the patient. It should become a permanent part of the patient's chart (Weinstein, Cunningham, 1994). Patients discharged on an opioid analgesic should be instructed on specific dosing times (i.e., not "tid"), and the use of an alternate dispenser of medication (i.e., spouse, community health nurse, pharmacy) should be considered. Opioid agents with less street value (i.e., codeine, controlled-release morphine) should be selected (Brookoff, 1993). Ongoing consultation from an addiction specialist should be sought to help monitor for the progression or worsening of addictive disease and to be available for the patient, should he or she decide to seek treatment. If drug treatment is desired, this should be part of the treatment plan, along with whether the patient is willing to submit to random urine screens.

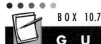

BOX 10.7

GUIDELINES

OPIOID DETOXIFICATION PROTOCOL

Overview: Physical dependence on opioids does not necessarily constitute addiction (i.e., may be prescribed for chronic pain management), thus detoxification is not strictly indicated. Although extremely uncomfortable, opioid withdrawal alone is never life-threatening (see Table 10.4), thus detoxification typically proceeds on an outpatient basis. Medications are used to (1) treat autonomic symptoms associated with withdrawal, and/or (2) substitute for the abused opioid and enable gradual tapering. Time after last opioid dose when withdrawal symptoms emerge varies with the half-life of the drug. *Remember, detoxification alone is an ineffective treatment for addiction.*

1. Clonidine 0.1 to 0.2 mg PO q 4-6 h to treat symptoms associated with autonomic hyperactivity; does not treat insomnia or drug craving.
   a. Monitor for orthostatic hypotension
   b. Alternatively may be administered by transdermal patch
   c. May be used in conjunction with opioid substitution treatment
2. Methadone, a long-acting opioid, is the substitution drug of choice for opioid detoxification. If known, convert pa-

tient's average total daily dose of opioid into methadone equivalents (see Equianalgesic Dose Chart, pp. 241-243) and administer in bid or qd doses. If illicit opioids of unknown purity have been abused, begin with daily methadone dose of 40 to 60 mg. Gradually decrease dose by 2.5 to 5 mg methadone qd, slowing taper if withdrawal symptoms become evident.

a. Methadone detoxification can only be provided in licensed inpatient or outpatient programs.
b. Methadone detoxification is typically offered over 30 or 120 day periods; in both the patient is required to meet with a counselor and receive minimal psychosocial services.
c. Opioid-dependent inpatients diagnosed as addicted and being treated for an acute medical illness can receive methadone if it is documented that opioid withdrawal would complicate the medical condition.
d. If the clinician cannot verify patient's claim to be addicted, it is best to start with low doses of methadone (i.e., 5-10 mg) on emergence of signs of withdrawal (Fultz, Senay, 1975).

May be duplicated for use in clinical practice. From McCaffery M, Pasero C: *Pain: Clinical manual,* p. 459. Copyright © 1999, Mosby, Inc.
Information from Fultz JM, Senay EC: Guidelines for the management of hospitalized narcotic addicts, *Ann Intern Med* 82:815-818, 1975.

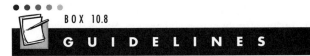

BOX 10.8

GUIDELINES

DOCUMENTATION OF ADDICTION AND PAIN RESPONSES

A. Pain severity and quality
B. Level of function
C. Opiate analgesic use
D. Evidence of opiate misuse
E. Evaluation and plan

May be duplicated for use in clinical practice. From McCaffery M, Pasero C: *Pain: Clinical manual,* p. 459. Copyright © 1999, Mosby, Inc.

Pain relief for persons recovering from addictive disease

For persons in drug treatment or recovery, concern about adhering to a drug-free philosophy will affect acceptance of opioids for pain relief. Even patients who have been drug free for years may be extremely fearful of

taking opioids (Aston, 1987; Gonzales, Coyle, 1992; Newshan, 1996), although available data indicate that patients with a more remote history of substance abuse are unlikely to abuse analgesics (Dunbar, Katz, 1996). Usually the patient's family is also very concerned. It is important that the patient be made aware of the health risks associated with unrelieved pain, with one of the most important being the increased likelihood of relapse. Nonopioid interventions should be offered, and the decision whether to use PCA should depend on the patient's comfort level with the self-administration method. If the patient is concerned about loss of control over analgesic use, alternate administration methods should be offered.

During this period of vulnerability to relapse, recovery supports should be used or intensified by the patient; increased contact with a sponsor or counselor are extremely helpful (Stock, 1991). As with the active addict, referral to an addiction medicine psychiatrist or clinical nurse specialist should be initiated to enable ongoing assessment of addictive disease and to let the patient know that adequate drug treatment supports are available if needed (Wesson, Ling, Smith, 1993). If addiction is treated as a known risk when providing opioid analgesia to a patient in recovery, its development can be minimized while pain relief is provided. A pain specialist also should be consulted to identify appropriate options for analgesia.

Traditionally AA has advised persons in recovery not to use psychoactive substances even when medically indicated, including the use of opioids for pain relief. Not all AA members are aware of a change in this position. When the patient is considering options for analgesia, it is helpful for the patient to know that an AA publication states, "Some members have taken the position that no one in A.A. should take any medication. While this position has undoubtedly prevented relapses for some, it has meant disaster for others. . . . Just as it is wrong to enable or support any alcoholic to become readdicted to any drug, it's equally wrong to deprive any alcoholic of medication which can alleviate or control other disabling physical and/or emotional problems." (Alcoholics Anonymous World Services, p. 13). A copy of this booklet may be obtained from AA (see Resources).

With respect to relapse, the clinician needs to keep in mind the chronic nature of addictive disease. *All* patients with addiction are prone to relapse, regardless of the presence of pain. It is critical to acknowledge that the risk of relapse exists, but is manageable, and to assure the patient that the clinician and staff will make every effort to minimize this risk and aggressively treat any evidence of relapse. If relapse occurs, it should be treated as an exacerbation of the addictive disease, not a reason to stop treating pain, and addiction treatment efforts reworked or intensified.

If the patient is maintained on methadone or LAAM for the treatment of opioid addiction, the usual daily maintenance dose should be provided in methadone equivalents as possible, with analgesic doses administered on top of these to manage reports of pain (Payne, 1989; Payte, Khuri, Joseph, et al., 1994). Significant opioid tolerance exists in these patients, making the risk of opioid overdose unlikely but not impossible; opioid toxicity must be consistently assessed for and managed. Increased opioid exposure in the context of pain does not appear to affect the progression of addictive disease; a small study of surgical methadone maintenance patients found no escalation or progression of addictive disease after liberal postoperative opioid analgesic administration (Kantor, Cantor, Tom, 1980). Box 10.9 provides guidelines for managing pain in persons recovering from addictive disease.

Pain relief for the patient receiving naltrexone: Suggestions

Patients taking naltrexone for the treatment of opioid or alcohol addiction pose a special challenge because of the medication's antagonistic effect at the receptors to

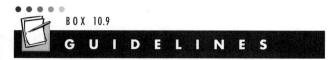

BOX 10.9

GUIDELINES

MANAGEMENT OF PAIN IN THE PATIENT RECOVERING FROM ADDICTION

1. Openly acknowledge patient's history of addiction and allow patient to discuss fears of readdiction.
2. Explain any intent to use opioids or other psychoactive medications.
3. Explain health risks associated with unrelieved pain, including increased risk for relapse.
4. Offer nonpharmacologic and nonopioid analgesia alternatives.
5. Respect the patient's right to decide whether to take opioid analgesics.
6. Explain to patient that the known risk for addiction to opioids in the context of pain is minimal.
7. Ensure that patient understands differences between addiction and physical dependence.
8. Suggest to patient that he or she contact or strengthen contact with recovery program and/or sponsor for advice, information, and support. Reassure patient that even in programs with a "drug-free" philosophy, it is acceptable to take medications for medical reasons.
9. Request consultation from in-house addiction medicine specialist, so that patient knows that professional support is available if needed.
10. Taper opioid analgesics *very* slowly to minimize emergence of withdrawal symptoms.
11. Assess for presence of withdrawal symptoms at least q4h during analgesic taper; treat symptomatically.
12. If patient is on methadone, first cover with daily methadone dose, then order analgesic.
13. Include family in these discussions; family members are typically as concerned as patients about relapse.
14. If relapse occurs, intensify recovery efforts; *do not* terminate pain care.

May be duplicated for use in clinical practice. From McCaffery M, Pasero C: *Pain: Clinical manual,* p. 460. Copyright © 1999, Mosby, Inc.

which the opioid analgesics must bind. Patients should be advised to stop taking naltrexone for 1 to 3 days before a scheduled procedure as possible; if needed emergently, higher doses of opioid analgesics can overcome the blockade (Swift, 1996). Although little research has been done in this area, these patients must be *carefully monitored* over the course of opioid exposure. The rate at which naltrexone disassociates from the opioid receptor in the presence of opioid analgesic is highly variable. In addition, it appears likely that patients with recent naltrexone exposure may be more pain sensitive (Compton, 1998) and *overly sensitive* to opioid medications. Preclinical studies have shown that opioid receptors actually become upregulated or more sensitive to opioid effect, in the presence of chronic naltrexone, an effect that may persist for up to a week after the last dose (Hollt, Przewlocki, Herz, 1978; Lee, Panerai, Bellabarba et al., 1980; Neisewander, Nonneman, Rowlett, 1994; Pert, Snyder, 1976; Ragavan, Wardlaw, Kreek et al., 1983; Romualdi, Lesa, Donatini et al., 1995). Careful titration of dose with respect to opioid response, frequent monitoring of respiratory rate and sedation level, mental status, and naloxone (Narcan) availability are principles for provision of opioid analgesia to patients being treated for addiction with either an opioid agonist or antagonist.

Assessment for addiction in patients with chronic pain

One of the most challenging tasks faced by general practitioners, pain specialists, and addiction specialists alike, is determining whether a patient with chronic pain and taking opioid analgesics is, in fact, addicted to opioid medications. In that physical dependence on, and tolerance to, opioids does not constitute addiction, the dilemma then becomes in the context of prescribed opioid maintenance, how can addiction be identified? In other words, how does addictive disease present in the individual who suffers from chronic pain and takes opioids on a regular basis in an attempt to relieve this pain?

Recent literature supports the difficulties inherent in diagnosing addictive disease in this patient population (Covington, Kotz, 1994; Sees, Clark, 1993; Vallerand, 1994; Wesson, Ling, Smith, 1993). In an important examination of the issue, Sees and Clark (1993) illustrate how persons maintained on opioids for the treatment of chronic nonmalignant pain could meet *DSM-IIIR* criteria for substance dependence (the predecessor to *DSM-IV*, see Box 10.1) without actually being addicted. Reliance on the presence of neurophysiologic adaptations to chronic drug use (physical dependence and tolerance), putative responses in virtually any individual taking opioid medications on a chronic basis, increases the risk that the patient with chronic pain who complains about the analgesic regimen will be misdiagnosed as addicted.

Yet in applying the *DSM-IV* (APA, 1994) diagnostic criteria to opioid-maintained pain patients, clinicians have also found the converse to be true: Persons who are clearly suffering from addictive disease *do not* consistently meet these standardized criteria. False-negative situations stem from two sources: (1) the source of the opioid medications is neither illicit nor illegal and, (2) the behavioral sequelae of chronic pain are not unlike those found with addictive disease (Miotto, Compton, Ling et al., 1996). The detrimental effects of drug use on lifestyle and psychosocial functioning are less evident in this population and are likely to be ascribed to pain rather than drug use.

For example, chronic pain patients with addictive disease taking legally prescribed opioids for analgesia are not necessarily likely to "spend inordinate amounts of time obtaining the drug, using the drug, or recovering from it's effects" (APA, 1994, p. 108): They frequently have an ample and legal supply of medication ordered to be taken on an around-the-clock basis, and, always being under the influence, do not spend inordinate amounts of time recovering from drug effects. Important social occupational and recreational activities may be curtailed because of unrelieved pain rather than drug effects, and it is not drug use but the pain condition that is ascribed a contributory role in ongoing physical or psychologic problems.

Further complicating assessment, as noted on p. 434, "drug-seeking" behaviors, such as obtaining medication from multiple providers, repeated episodes of prescription loss, multiple requests for early refills, and even prescription forgery (Pancratz, Hickman, Toth, 1989; Portenoy, 1994), are frequently confused with addiction. Yet, as noted, such behaviors may, in fact, be appropriate responses to either underrelieved or well-relieved pain in the patient with chronic pain and are more correctly termed *pseudoaddiction* (Weissman, Haddox, 1989) or *therapeutic dependence* (Portenoy, 1994).

Clinicians struggling with the task of identifying addictive disease in opioid-maintained patients with pain should realize that it is a challenge even for experts in the field of addiction and pain. And it is not uncommon that these experts approach assessment with very different philosophical and clinical perspectives on opioid use patterns and behaviors.

Because of this diagnostic confusion, the Committee on Pain of the American Society of Addiction Medicine has developed definitions for physical dependence, tolerance, and addiction specific to assessing the use of opioids in the context of pain treatment (Box 10.10). Note that in this situation, addiction is identified by the presence of adverse consequences associated with, and loss of control of over, opioid use, as well as a noted preoccupation with obtaining opioids (drug-seeking) despite the presence of adequate analgesia. The physiologic responses to chronic opioid ingestion (i.e., physical dependence and tolerance) become irrelevant in identifying addiction in these individuals.

Recently published is an assessment tool designed to be used with these indicators to help the clinician determine whether addictive disease is complicating maintenance opioid analgesia (Miotto, Compton, Ling et al., 1996). Evaluated are the pain condition, opioid use patterns, social and family factors, family history of pain and substance abuse syndromes, patient history of substance abuse, and psychiatric history, which together provide a comprehensive picture of the patient's opioid use patterns. Despite the tool's putative usefulness, it is not

• • • • •

| BOX 10.10 | **Definitions Related to the Use of Opioids in Pain Treatment** |

The Committee on Pain of the American Society of Addiction Medicine recognizes the following definitions as appropriate and clinically useful definitions and recommends their use when assessing the use of opioids in the context of pain treatment.

PHYSICAL DEPENDENCE

Physical dependence on an opioid is a physiologic state in which abrupt cessation of the opioid, or administration of an opioid antagonist, results in a withdrawal syndrome. Physical dependency on opioids is an expected occurrence in all individuals in the presence of continuous use of opioids for therapeutic on for nontherapeutic purposes. It does not, in and of itself, imply addiction.

TOLERANCE

Tolerance is a form of neuroadaptation to the effects of chronically administered opioids (or other medications), which is indicated by the need for increasing or more frequent doses of the medication to achieve the initial effects of the drug. Tolerance may occur both to the analgesic effects of opioids and to the unwanted side effects such as respiratory depression, sedation or nausea. The occurrence of tolerance is variable, but it does not, in and of itself, imply addiction.

ADDICTION

Addiction in the context of pain treatment with opioids is characterized by a persistent pattern of dysfunctional opioid use that may involve any or all of the following:
- Adverse consequences associated with the use of opioids
- Loss of control over the use of opioids
- Preoccupation with obtaining opioids despite the presence of adequate analgesia

May be duplicated for use in clinical practice. As appears in McCaffery M, Pasero C: *Pain: Clinical manual,* p. 462, 1999, Mosby, Inc.

Modified from Hoffman NG, Halikas J, Mee-Lee Y: *Patient placement criteria for the treatment of psychoactive substance use disorders,* Chevy Chase, Md, 1991, American Society of Addiction Medicine.

intended to be used in isolation. Gathering information from multiple sources is necessary to validate patient responses and complete a thorough assessment. Multiple assessment episodes with the patient with chronic pain may be required to establish the diagnosis.

CHALLENGES FACED

Providing humane and high-quality care to patients with addictive disease presents a challenge for the health care professional. Such care necessarily occurs within the larger societal context in which moral and criminal perspectives of addiction prevail, and thus influence the nature and intensity of treatment provided. In no situation is this challenge more evident than in the provision of pain management to a person with addiction because a primary relief intervention involves the administration of

medications (opioids) with known abuse liability. Opiophobia (Morgan, 1985-86), which compromises aggressive opioid analgesia for persons without addictive disease, becomes the overwhelming and emotionally charged response when the addict reports pain.

This response persists despite a virtual absence of sound empirical data to indicate that providing opioid analgesia to persons with addictive disease within the context of pain in any way promotes or worsens addictive disease. In fact, the available data reviewed in this chapter suggest that the presence of addiction portends an increased pain experience for the individual, and that inadequately relieved pain is the more likely culprit of disease progression. No defensible, professional excuse exists for not managing the pain of an addict as aggressively as that suffered by the patient without addictive disease. Addictive disease occurs in a given percentage of human beings for reasons that appear to be entirely unrelated to pain experiences or opioid exposure; clinicians need not worry that providing opioid analgesics in this context will appreciably alter the state of addictive disease.

This is not to imply that the clinician should ignore the presence of addictive disease, either active or in remission, in the patient requiring pain relief. These patients have special needs, pharmacologic and otherwise, that must be addressed to ensure adequate and safe provision of analgesia and to minimize the complicating effects of addictive disease. Guidelines have been presented to assist the clinician to meet these goals, which begin with nonjudgmental acknowledgment of the presence of the disease, and to recognize that every interaction with the patient provides an opportunity to introduce or facilitate recovery. Rather than approach the patient with moral and criminal perspectives on behaviors that are essentially reflections of brain disease, it is incumbent on the clinician to treat the patient from a scientific base of knowledge when addictive disease complicates pain.

Resources and Web Sites

Alcoholics Anonymous World Services: The A.A. member: Medications and other drugs, New York, 1984. To Order: AA Box 459, Grand Central Stations, New York, NY 10163.

American Society of Addiction Medicine, 4601 North Park Avenue, Suite 101, Chevy Chase, MD 20815.

Center for Substance Abuse Treatment, Rockwall II Building, 10th Floor, 5600 Fishers Lane, Rockville, MD, 20852-9949 (publishes a series of Treatment Improvement Protocols, or TIPS).

National Institute on Drug Abuse Infofax: (888) 644-6432.

National Nurses Society on Addiction, 4101 Lake Boone Trail, Suite 201, Raleigh, NC 27607.

Addiction treatment centers and resources: *http://www. nida.nih.gov/TreatmentIndex.html*

Articles and books on addictions: *http://www.arf.org/ isd/hint/html*

Links to other Web sites related to addictions: *http:// www.well.com/user/woa/aodsites.htm*

National Clearinghouse for Alcohol and Drug Abuse Information: *http://www.health.org/.*

National Institute on Alcohol Abuse and Alcoholism: *http://www.niaaa.nih.gov/.*

National Institute on Drug Abuse: *http://www.nida. nih.gov/.*

National Nurses Society on Addictions: *http://www. nnsa.org.*

Substance Abuse and Mental Health Services Administration: *http://www.samhsa.gov/.*

References

Academy of Pain Medicine and the American Pain Society: The use of opioids for the treatment of chronic pain, *Clin J Pain* 13:6-8, 1997.

Acute Pain Management Guideline Panel: *Acute pain management in adults: operative procedures, quick reference guide for clinicians,* AHCPR Pub. No. 92-0019, Rockville, MD, 1992, Agency for Health Care Policy and Research, Public Health Service, U.S. Department of Health and Human Services.

Alcoholics Anonymous: *Alcoholics anonymous: the big book,* New York, 1976, AA World Services Incorporated.

American Psychiatric Association: *Diagnostic and statistical manual of mental disorders,* ed 4, Washington DC 1994, APA.

Anglin MD, Speckart GR, Booth MW, Ryan TM: Consequences and costs of shutting off methadone, *Addict Behav* 14:307-326, 1989.

Annis HM: Patterns of intrafamilial drug abuse, *Br J Addiction* 69:361-369, 1974.

Aston R: Treating pain and anxiety in the reformed substance abuser, *J Michi Dent Assoc* 69:279-280, 1987.

Ball JC, Lange WR, Myers CP et al.: Reducing the risk of AIDS through methadone maintenance treatment, *J Health Soc Behav* 29:214-226, 1988.

Ball JC, Ross A: *The effectiveness of methadone maintenance treatment: patients, programs, services and outcome,* New York, 1993, Springer-Verlag.

Basbaum AI: Insights into the development of opioid tolerance, *Pain* 61:349-352, 1995.

Bergman PE, Smith MB, Hoffman NG: Adolescent treatment: implications for assessment, practice guidelines, and outcome management, *Pediatr Clin North Am* 42:453-472, 1995.

Berrettini WH, Alexander R, Ferraro TN et al.: A study of oral morphine preference in inbred mouse strains, *Psychiat Genet* 4:81-86, 1994.

Brady KT, Grice DE, Dustan L et al.: Gender differences in substance use disorders, *Am J Psychiatry* 150:1707-1711, 1993.

Bressler LR, Geraci MC, Schatz BS: Misperceptions and inadequate pain management in cancer patients, *DICP, Annals of Pharmacotherapy* 25:1225-1230, 1991.

Brookoff D: Abuse potential of various opioid medications, *J Gen Intern Med* 8:688-690, 1993.

Brower KJ, Blow FC, Beresford TP: Treatment implications of chemical dependency models: an integrative approach, *J Substance Abuse Treatment* 6:147-157, 1989.

Bruera E, Moyano J, Seifert L et al.: The frequency of alcoholism among patients with pain due to terminal cancer, *J Pain Symptom Manage* 10:599-603, 1995.

Bucholz KK, Heath AC, Reich T et al.: Can we subtype alcoholism? A latent class analysis of data from relatives of alcoholics in a multicenter family study of alcoholism, *Alcoholism, Clin Exp Res* 20:1462-1471, 1996.

Buschbaum MS, Davis GC, Coppola R et al.: Opioid pharmacology and individual differences. I. Psychophysical pain measurements, *Pain* 10:357-366, 1981.

Cadoret RJ, Troughton E, O'Gorman TW et al.: An adoption study of genetic and environmental factors in drug abuse, *Arch Gen Psychiatry* 43:1131-1136, 1986.

California Department of Alcohol and Drug Programs: *State demand and treatment needs assessment study: dependence and abuse of alcohol and other drugs among California arrestees,* Sacramento, 1997, State of California.

Carroll J: Attitudes of professionals to drug abusers, *Br J Nurs* 2:705-711, 1993.

Center for Substance Abuse Treatment: *Detoxification from alcohol and other drugs, Treatment Improvement Protocol Series No. 19,* Rockville, MD 1994, CSAT.

Chappel JN, Schnoll SH: Physicians attitudes: effect on the treatment of chemically dependent patients, *JAMA* 237:2318-2319, 1977.

Clark HW, Sees KL: Opioids, chronic pain, and the law, *J Pain Symptom Manage* 8:297-305, 1993.

Collin E, Poulain P, Gauvain-Piquard A et al.: Is disease progression the major factor in morphine `tolerance' in cancer pain treatment? *Pain* 55:319-326, 1993.

Compton MA: Cold-pressor pain tolerance in opiate and cocaine abusers: correlates of drug type and use status, *J Pain Symptom Manage* 9:462-473, 1994.

Compton PA: Pain tolerance in opiate addicts ON and OFF naltrexone pharmacotherapy: a pilot study, *J Pain Symptom Manage* 16:21-28, 1998.

Cooper J, Czechowicz DJ, Petersen RC et al.: Prescription drug diversion control and medical practice, *JAMA* 268:1306-1310, 1992.

Cooper JR: Methadone treatment and acquired immunodeficiency syndrome, *JAMA* 262:1664-1668, 1989.

Cotton NS: The familial incidence of alcoholism, *J Stud Alcohol* 40:89-115, 1979.

Cotton, P: `Harm reduction' approach may be middle ground, *JAMA* 271:1641-1645, 1994.

Covington EC, Kotz MM: Psychological interventions: *principles of addictive medicine,* pp 1-11, Chevy Chase, Md, 1994, American Society of Addiction Medicine.

Crabbe JC, Belknap JK, Buck KJ: Genetic animal models of alcohol and drug abuse, *Science* 264:1715-1723, 1994.

Dans PE, Matricciani RM, Otter SE et al.: Intravenous drug abuse and one academic health center, *JAMA* 263:3173-3176, 1990.

Des Jarlis DC, Friedman SR, Hopkins W: Risk reduction for acquired immunodeficiency syndrome among intravenous drug users, *Ann Intern Med* 103:755-759, 1985.

DiChiara G, Imperato A: Drugs abused by humans preferentially increase synaptic dopamine concentrations in the mesolimbic system of freely moving rats, *Proc Natl Acad Sci* 85:5274-5278, 1988.

DiClemente C: Motivational interviewing and the stages of change. In Miller WR, Rollnick S, editors: *Motivational interviewing: preparing people to change addictive behavior,* pp 191-202, New York, 1991, The Guilford Press.

Dole VP: Methadone treatment and the acquired immunodeficiency syndrome epidemic, *JAMA* 262:1681-1682, 1989.

Dole VP, Nyswander ME, Kreek MJ: Narcotic blockade, *Arch Intern Med* 118:304-309, 1966.

Dole VP, Robinson JW, Orraca J et al.: Methadone treatment of randomly selected criminal addicts, *N Engl J Med* 280:1372-1375, 1969.

Drucker E: AIDS and addiction in New York City, *Am J Drug Alcohol Abuse* 12:165-181, 1986.

Dunbar SA, Katz NP: Chronic opioid therapy for nonmalignant pain in patients with a history of substance abuse: report of 20 cases, *J Pain Symptom Manage* 11:163-171, 1996.

Ferrell BR, McCaffery M, Rhiner M: Pain and addiction: an urgent need for change in nursing education, *J Pain Symptom Manage* 7:117-124, 1992.

Fins JJ: Public attitudes about pain and analgesics: clinical implications, *J Pain Symptom Manage* 13:169-171, 1997.

Fishbain DA, Rosomoff HL, Rosomoff RS: Detoxification of nonopiate drugs in the chronic pain setting and clonidine opiate detoxification, *Clin J Pain* 8:191-203, 1992.

Fishbain DA, Rosomoff HL, Rosomoff RS: Drug abuse, dependence, and addiction in chronic pain patients, *Clin J Pain* 8:77-85, 1992.

Fox K, Merrill JC, Chang HH et al.: Estimating the costs of substance abuse to the Medicaid hospital care program, *Am J Public Health* 85:48-53, 1995.

Friedman DP: Perspectives on the medical use of drugs of abuse, *J Pain Symptom Manage* 5(Suppl):S2-S5, 1990.

Frischknecht HR, Siegfried B, Waser PG: Opioids and behavior: genetic aspects, *Experientia* 44:473-481, 1988.

Fultz JM, Senay EC: Guidelines for the management of hospitalized narcotic addicts, *Ann Intern Med* 82:815-818, 1975.

Fultz JM, Senay EC, Pray BJ et al.: When a narcotic addict is hospitalized, *Am J Nurs* 80:478-481, 1980.

Galer BS, Coyle N, Pasternak GW et al.: Individual variability in the response to different opioids: report of five cases, *Pain* 49:87-91, 1992.

Gardner EL: Brain reward mechanisms, In Lowinson JH et al., editors: *Substance abuse: a comprehensive textbook,* ed 3, pp 51-84, Baltimore, 1997, Williams & Wilkins.

George FR: Genetic models in the study of alcoholism and substance abuse mechanisms, *Neuro-Psychophamacol Biol Psychiat* 17:345-361, 1993.

Gerstein DR, Harwood HJ: *Treating drug abuse problems,* Washington, DC, 1990, National Academy Press.

Glaser FB: From theory to practice: the planned treatment of drug users, *Int J Addictions* 25:307-343, 1990.

Gonzalez FJ: Human cytochrome P450: possible roles of drug-metabolizing enzymes and polymorphic drug oxidation in addiction, *NIDA Research Monograph Series* 111:202-213, 1991.

Gonzales GR, Coyle N: Treatment of cancer pain in a former opioid abuser: fears of the patient and staff and their influence on care, *J Pain Symptom Manage* 4:246-249, 1992.

Gostin L: Waging a war on drug users: an alternative public health vision, *Law Medicine Health Care* 18:385-394, 1990.

Gronbladh L, Ohlund LS, Gunne LM: Mortality in heroin addiction: impact of methadone maintenance treatment, *Acta Psychiatrica Scandinavica* 82:223-227, 1990.

Groves JE: Taking care of the hateful patient, *N Engl J Med* 16:883-887, 1978.

Hill CS: The barriers to adequate pain management with opioids analgesics, *Semin Oncology* 20(Suppl):1-5, 1993.

Hoffman NG, Halikas J, Mee-Lee Y et al.: *Patient placement criteria for the treatment of psychoactive substance use disorders,* Chevy Chase, Md, 1991, American Society of Addiction Medicine.

Hollt V, Przewlocki R, Herz A: b-endorphin-like immunoreactivity in plasma, pituitary and hypothalamus of rats following treatment with opiates, *Life Sci* 23:1057-1066, 1978.

Hser YI, Anglin MD, Powers K: A 24-year follow-up of California narcotics addicts, *Arch Gen Psychiatry* 50:577-584, 1993.

Hubbard RL: Evaluation and outcome of treatment. In Lowinson JH et al., editors: *Substance abuse: a comprehensive textbook,* ed 3, pp 499-511, Baltimore, 1997, Williams & Wilkins.

Hubbard RL, Marsden ME, Rachal JV et al.: *Drug abuse treatment: a national study of effectiveness,* Chapel Hill, NC, 1989, University of North Carolina Press.

Hubbard RL, French MT: New perspectives on the benefit-cost and cost-effectiveness of drug abuse treatment. In Cartwright WS, Kaple JM, editors: *Economic costs, cost-effectiveness, financing and community-based drug treatment,* NIDA Research Monograph 113, Rockville, Md, 1991, GPO.

Hubbard RL, Marsden ME: Relapse to use of heroin, cocaine and other drugs the first year after treatment. In Tims FM, Leukfeld CG, editors: *Relapse and recovery in drug abuse,* NIDA Research Monograph 72, DHHS Publication No. ADM89-151963, Washington DC, 1986, GPO.

Iguchi MY, Stitzer ML, Bigelow GE et al.: Contingency management in methadone maintenance: effects of reinforcing and aversive consequences on illicit polydrug use, *Drug Alcohol Dependence* 22:1-7, 1988.

Ingelman-Sundberg M, Johansson I, Persson I et al.: Genetic polymorphism of cytochrome P450: functional consequences and possible relationship to disease and alcohol toxicity. In Jansson B et al., editors: *Toward a molecular basis of alcohol use and abuse,* pp 197-207, Basel, Switzerland, 1994, Birkhauser Verlag.

Joranson DE: Regulatory influence on pain management: real or imagined? *J Pharmaceut Care Pain Symptom Control* 1:113-118, 1993.

Joranson DE, Colleau SM: Highlights of the International Narcotics Control Board report, *Cancer Pain Release* 9(Suppl): 1-3, 1996.

Kantor TG, Cantor R, Tom E: A study of hospitalized surgical patients on methadone maintenance, *Drug Alcohol Dependence* 6:163-173, 1980.

Kessler RC, Nelson CB, McGonagle KA et al.: Comorbidity of DSM-III-R major depressive disorder in the general population: results from the U.S. National Comorbidity Survey, *Br J Psychiatry* 168 (Suppl 30):17-30, 1996.

Khantzian EJ: The self medication hypothesis of addictive disorders: focus on heroin and cocaine dependence, *Am J Psychiatry* 142:1259-1264, 1985.

Koob GF, Bloom FE: Cellular and molecular mechanisms of drug dependence, *Science* 242:715-723, 1988.

Kreek MJ: Using methadone effectively: achieving goals by application of laboratory, clinical and evaluation research and by development of innovative programs. In Pickens RW, Leukfeld CG, Schuster CR, editors: *Improving drug abuse treatment,* NIDA Research Monograph 106, Rockville, Md, 1991, GPO.

Krick SE, Lindley CM, Bennett M: Pharmacy-perceived barriers to cancer pain control: results of the North Carolina cancer pain initiative pharmacist survey, *Ann Pharmacotherapy* 28:857-862, 1994.

Lander J: Fallacies and phobias about addiction and pain, *Br J Addiction* 85:803-809, 1990.

Lawental E, McLellan AT, Grissom GR et al.: Coerced treatment for substance abuse problems detected through workplace urine surveillance: is it effective? *J Substance Abuse* 8:115-128, 1996.

Lee S, Panerai AE, Bellabarba D et al.: Effect of endocrine modifications and pharmacological treatments on brain and pituitary concentrations of β-endorphin, *Endocrinology* 107:245-248, 1980.

Liaschenko J: Making a bridge: the moral work with patients we do not like, *J Palliative Care* 10:83-89, 1994.

Ling W, Rawson RA, Compton, MA: Substitution pharmacotherapies for opioid addiction: from methadone to LAAM and buprenorphine, *J Psychoactive Drugs* 26:119-128, 1994.

Lipton DS, Wexler HK: The drug -crime connection: rehabilitation shows promise, *Corrections Today* 50:144-147, 1988.

Lohr RH: Treatment of alcohol withdrawal in hospitalized patients, *Mayo Clinic Proc* 70:777-782, 1995.

Malone RE: Almost `like family': emergency nurses and `frequent flyers', *J Emerg Nurs* 22:176-183, 1996.

Mao J, Price DD, Mayer DJ: Mechanisms of hyperalgesia and morphine tolerance: a current view of their possible interactions, *Pain* 62:259-274, 1995.

Marlatt GA, Gordon JR: *Relapse prevention,* New York, 1985, The Guilford Press.

Marley RJ, Elmer GI, Goldberg SR: The use of pharmacogenetic techniques in drug abuse research, *Pharmacol Ther* 53:217-237, 1992.

McCaffery M, Ferrell BR: Nurses' knowledge of pain assessment and management: how much progress have we made? *J Pain Symptom Manage* 14:175-188, 1997.

McCaffery M, Ferrell BR, O'Neil-Page E: Does life-style affect your pain-control decisions? *Nursing 92* 22:58-61, 1992.

McCaffery M, Vourakis C: Assessment and relief of pain in chemically dependent patients, *Orthop Nurs* 11:13-27, 1992.

McDermott N, Matthews S: *Residential treatment guidelines: a collaboration of ten therapeutic communities,* New York, 1994, Therapeutic Communities of New York.

McLellan AT, Arndt IO, Metzger DS et al.: The effects of psychosocial services in substance abuse treatment, *JAMA* 269:1953-1959, 1993.

Medical Board of California: Treatment of intractable pain: a guideline, *Action Rep* Sacramento, 1996, The Board.

Medina JL, Diamond S: Drug dependency in patients with chronic headache, *Headache* 17:12-14, 1977.

Melzack R: The tragedy of needless pain, *Sci Am* 262:27-33, 1990.

Miller NS, Gold MS: A hypothesis for a common neurochemical basis for alcohol and drug disorders, *Psychiat Clin North Am* 16:105-117, 1993.

Miller WR, Rollnick S: *Motivational interviewing: preparing people to change addictive behavior,* New York, 1991, The Guilford Press.

Miotto K, Compton P, Ling W et al.: Diagnosing addictive disease in chronic pain patients, *Psychosomatics* 37:223-235, 1996.

Mogil JS, Marek P, O'Toole LA et al.: Mu-opiate receptor binding is up-regulated in mice selectively bred for high stress-induced analgesia, *Brain Res* 653:16-22, 1994.

Mogil JS, Sternberg WF, Marek P et al.: The genetics of pain and pain inhibition, *Proc Natl Acad Sci* 93:3048-3055, 1996.

Moos RH, Breenan PL, Mertens JR: Mortality rates and predictors of mortality among late-middle-aged and older substance abuse patients, *Alcoholism Clin Exp Res* 18:187-195, 1994.

Morgan JP: American opiophobia: customary underutilization of opioid analgesics, *Adv Alcohol Substance Abuse* 5:163-173, 1985-86.

Musto DF: Historical perspectives. In Lowinson JH et al., editors: *Substance abuse: a comprehensive textbook,* ed 3, pp 1-10, Baltimore, 1997, Williams & Wilkins.

Nace EP: Alcoholics Anonymous. In Lowinson JH et al., editors: *Substance abuse: a comprehensive textbook,* ed 3, pp 383-390, Baltimore, 1997, Williams & Wilkins.

National Institute on Drug Abuse: *Drug abuse treatment: an economical approach to addressing the drug problem in America,* Rockville, Md, 1993, NIDA.

Neisewander JL, Nonneman AJ, Rowlett JK et al.: Impaired supersensitivity to morphine following chronic naltrexone treatment in senescent rats, *Neurobiology Aging* 15:91-97, 1994.

Newshan G: Considerations in pain management for chemically dependent patients, *Faculty Newsletter* 2:1,3, 1996.

O'Brien S, Dalton JA, Konsler G et al.: The knowledge and attitudes of experienced oncology nurses regarding the management of cancer-related pain, *Oncol Nurs Forum* 23:515-521, 1996.

O'Brien W, Delvin CJ: The therapeutic community. In Lowinson JH et al., editors: *Substance abuse: a comprehensive textbook,* ed 3, pp 400-405, Baltimore, 1997, Williams & Wilkins.

Office of Drug Control Policy: *The national drug control strategy, 1997,* Washington, DC 1997, GPO.

O'Malley SS, Jaffe AJ, Chang G et al.: Naltrexone and coping skills therapy of alcohol dependence, *Arch Gen Psychiatry* 49:881-887, 1992.

Otton SV, Schadel M, Cheung SW et al.: CYP2D6 phenotype determines the metabolic conversion of hydrocodone to hydromorphone, *Clin Pharmacol Ther* 54:463-472, 1993.

Paige DA, Preble LM, Watrous GA et al.: PCA use in cocaine using patients: a pilot study, *Am J Pain Manage* 4:101-105, 1994.

Pankratz L, Hickam D, Toth S: The identification and management of drug-seeking behavior in a medical center, *Drug Alcohol Dependence* 24:115-118, 1989.

Payne RM: Pain in the drug abuser. In Foley KM, Payne RM, editors: *Current therapy of pain,* pp 46-54, Toronto, 1989, BC Deker.

Payte JT, Khuri E, Joseph H et al.: Methadone patients and the treatment of pain. In *Methadone treatment works: a compendium for methadone maintenance treatment. Part 1,* pp 38-42 New York, 1994, NYS Office of Alcoholism and Substance Abuse Services.

Perry S, Heidrich G: Management of pain during debridement: a survey of U.S. burn units, *Pain* 13:267-280, 1982.

Perry, SW: The undermedication for pain, *Psychiatr Ann* 14:808-811, 1984.

Perry SW: Irrational attitudes toward addicts and narcotics, *Bull NY Acad Med* 61:706-726, 1985.

Pert CB, Snyder SH: Opiate receptor binding: enhancement by opiate administration in Vivo, *Biochem Pharmacol* 25:847-853, 1976.

Podrasky DL, Sexton DL: Nurses' reactions to difficult patients, *IMAGE* 20:16-21, 1988.

Portenoy RK: Chronic opioid therapy in nonmalignant pain, *J Pain Symptom Manage* 5(Suppl):S46-S62, 1990.

Portenoy RK: Opioid therapy for chronic non-malignant pain: current status. In Fields HL, Liebeskind JC: *Progress in pain research and management, Vol 1,* pp 247-287, Seattle, 1994, IASP Press.

Portenoy RK, Payne R: Acute and chronic Pain. In Lowinson JH et al., editors: *Substance abuse: a comprehensive textbook,* ed 3, pp 563-589, Baltimore, 1997, Williams & Wilkins.

Porter J, Jick H: Addiction rare in patients treated with narcotics, *N Eng. J Med.* 302:123, 1980.

Portnow JM, Strassman HD: Medically induced drug addiction, *Int J Addictions* 20:605-611, 1985.

Prochaska JO, DiClemente CC: Transtheoretical therapy: toward a more integrative model of change, *Psychotherapy: theory, research and practice* 19:276-288, 1982.

Ragavan VV, Wardlaw SL, Kreek MJ et al.: Effect of chronic naltrexone and methadone administration on brain immunoreactive β-endorphin in the rat, *Neuroendocrinology* 37:266-268, 1983.

Raskin VD, Miller NS: The epidemiology of the comorbidity of psychiatric and addictive disorders: a critical review, *J Addict Dis* 12:45-57, 1993.

Regier DA, Farmer ME, Rae DS et al.: Comorbidity of mental disorders with alcohol and other drug abuse: results of the Epidemiologic Catchment Area Study, *JAMA* 264:2511-2518, 1990.

Romualdi P, Lesa G, Donatini A et al.: Long-term exposure to opioid antagonists up-regulates prodynorphin gene expression in rat brain, *Brain Res* 672:42-47, 1995.

Saitz R, Mayo-Smith MF, Roberts MS: Individualized treatment for alcohol withdrawal: a randomized double-blind controlled trial, *JAMA* 272:519-523, 1994.

Savage SR: Management of acute pain, chronic pain and cancer pain in the addicted patient. In *Principles of addictive medicine,* pp 1-16, Chevy Chase, Md, 1994, American Society of Addiction Medicine.

Savage SR: Long-term opioid therapy: assessment of consequences and risks, *J Pain Symptom Manage* 11:274-286, 1996.

Savage SR, Schofferman J: Pharmacological therapies of pain in drug and alcohol addictions. In Miller NS, Gold MS, editors: *Pharmacological therapies for drug and alcohol addiction,* pp 373-409, New York, 1995, Marcel Decker.

Schnoll SH, Finch J: Medical education for pain and addiction: making progress toward answering a need, *J Law, Medicine Ethics* 22:252-256, 1994.

Schofferman J, Savage SR: Pharmacological treatments. In *Principles of addictive medicine,* pp 1-12, Chevy Chase, Md, 1994, American Society of Addiction Medicine.

Schuckit MA, Smith TL: An 8-year follow-up of 450 sons of alcoholic and control subjects, *Arch Gen Psychiatry* 53:202-210, 1996.

Schuckit MA, Smith TL: Assessing the risk for alcoholism among sons of alcoholics, *J Studies Alcohol* 58:141-145, 1997.

Schuckit MA, Tsuang JW, Anthenelli RM et al.: Alcohol challenges in young men from alcoholic pedigrees and control families: a report form the COGA project, *J Studies Alcohol* 57:368-377, 1996.

Schuster CR: Does treatment of cancer pain with narcotics produce junkies? *Adv Pain Res Therapy* 11:1-3, 1989.

Schuster L: Genetics of responses to drugs of abuse, *Int J Addictions* 25:57-79, 1990-91.

Sees KL, Clark HW: Opioid use in the treatment of chronic pain: assessment of addiction, *J Pain Symptom Manage* 8:257-264, 1993.

Segest E, Mygind O, Bay H: The influence of prolonged stable methadone maintenance treatment on mortality and employment: an 8-year follow-up, *Int J Addictions* 25:53-63, 1990.

Senay EC, Uchtenhagen A: Methadone in the treatment of opioid dependence: a review of the world literature. In Westermeyer J, Arif A, editors: *Methadone maintenance in the management of opioid dependence: an international review,* New York, 1990, Praeger.

Shaham Y, Alvarez K, Nespor SM et al.: Effect of stress on oral morphine and fentanyl self-administration in rats, *Pharmacol Biochem Behav* 41:615-619, 1992.

Shaham Y, Klein LC, Alvarez K et al.: Effect of stress on oral fentanyl consumption in rats in an operant self-administration paradigm, *Pharmacol Biochem Behav* 46:315-322, 1993.

Shapiro RS: Legal bases for the control of analgesic drugs, *J Pain Symptom Manage* 9:153-159, 1994.

Silverman I: Addiction intervention: treatment models and public policy, *Int J Addictions* 20:183-201, 1985.

Sindrup SH, Poulsen L, Brosen K et al.: Are poor metabolizers of sparteine/debrisuquine less pain tolerant than extensive metabolizers? *Pain* 53:335-339, 1993.

Siwek J: The politics of pain relief, *Am Fam Physician* 40:90-91, 1989.

Slutske WS, Heath AC, Madden PA et al.: Reliability and reporting biases for perceived parental history of alcohol-related problems: agreement between twins and differences between discordant pairs, *J Studies Alcoholism* 57:387-395, 1996.

Soderstrom CA, Smith GS, Dischinger PC et al.: Psychoactive substance use disorders among seriously injured trauma center patients, *JAMA* 277:1769-1774, 1997.

State of California Department of Alcohol and Drug Problems: *The California drug and alcohol treatment assessment,* Sacramento, 1994, State of California.

Stimmel B: Adequate analgesia in narcotic dependency, *Adv Pain Res Therapy* 11:131-138, 1989.

Stock CJ: Safe use of codeine in the recovering alcoholic or addict, *DICP, Ann Pharmacother* 25:49-53, 1991.

Sullivan JT, Sykora K, Schneiderman J et al.: Assessment of alcohol withdrawal: the revised Clinical Institute Withdrawal Assessment for Alcohol Scale (CIAW-Ar), *Br J Addiction* 84:1353-1357, 1989.

Swift RM: Pain management for patients taking opioid antagonists, Paper presented at the *Pain Management and Chemical Dependency Conference,* New York, November, 1996.

Tennant FS, Rawson RA, Pumphrey E et al.: Clinical experience with 959 opioid-dependent patients treated with LAAM, *J Substance Abuse Treatment* 3:195-202, 1986.

Tonessen H, Petersen KR, Hojgaard L et al.: Postoperative morbidity among symptom-free alcohol misusers, *Lancet* 340:334-337, 1992.

Trachtenberg AI: Opiates for pain: patients' tolerance and society's intolerance, *JAMA* 271:427, 1994.

Trachtenberg AI, Fleming MF: Diagnosis and treatment of drug abuse in family practice, *Am Fam Physician Monograph,* 1994.

Trueblood B, Judson BA, Goldstein A: Acceptability of LAAM as compared with methadone in a treatment program for heroin addicts, *Drug Alcohol Dependence* 3:125-132, 1978.

Vaccarino AL, Marek P, Kest B et al.: Morphine fails to produce tolerance when administered in the presence of formalin pain in rats, *Brain Res* 627:287-290, 1993.

Vallerand AH: Street addicts and patients with pain: similarities and differences, *Clin Nurse Specialist* 8:11-15, 1994.

Volpicelli JR, Alterman AI, Hayashida M et al.: Naltrexone in the treatment of alcohol dependence, *Arch Gen Psychiatry* 49:876-880, 1992.

Votherms R, Ryan P, Ward S: Knowledge of, attitudes toward, and barriers to pharmacologic management of cancer pain in a statewide random sample of nurses, *Res Nurs Health* 15:459-466, 1992.

Ward SE, Goldberg N, Miller-McCauley V et al.: Patient-related barriers to management of cancer pain, *Pain* 52:319-324, 1993.

Weinstein SM, Cunningham M: Written contracts facilitate cancer pain treatment in the patient with substance use disorder, *American Pain Society Annual Meeting Poster Presentation,* November 1994.

Weiss RD, Mirin SM: The dual diagnosis alcoholic: evaluation and treatment, *Psychiatric Ann* 19:261, 1989.

Weissman DE, Haddox JD: Opioid pseudoaddiction-an iatrogenic syndrome, *Pain* 36:363-366, 1989.

Wesson DR, Ling W, Smith DE: Prescription of opioids for treatment of pain in patients with addictive disease, *J Pain Symptom Manage* 8:289-296, 1993.

Wise RA: Action of drugs of abuse on brain reward systems, *Pharmacol Biochem Behav* 13:213-223, 1980.

Wise RA, Rompre PP: Brain dopamine and reward, *Annu Rev Psychol* 40:191-225, 1989.

Woods JH, Winger G, France CP: Use of in vivo apparent pA2 analysis in assessment of opioid abuse liability, *TIPS* 13:282-286, 1992.

Zacny JP, McKay MA, Toledano AY et al.: The effects of a cold-water immersion stressor on the reinforcing and subjective effects of fentanyl in healthy volunteers, *Drug Alcohol Dependence* 42:133-142, 1996.

Zenz M: Morphine myths: sedation, tolerance, addiction, *Postgrad Med J* 67(Suppl 5):S100-S102, 1991.

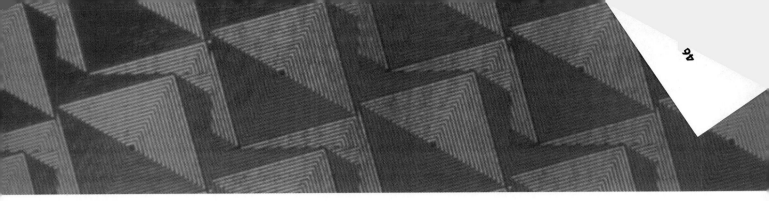

chapter eleven
CHRONIC NONMALIGNANT PAIN

Linda Dunajcik

CHAPTER OUTLINE

TERMINOLOGY

Anxiety: Anxiety is characterized by excessive worrying or some of the following symptoms: restlessness, irritability, muscle tension, disturbed sleep, feeling easily fatigued, and having difficulty concentrating.

Chronic nonmalignant pain: This pain has lasted 6 months or longer, is ongoing, is due to non–life-threatening causes, has not responded to current available treatment methods, and may continue for the remainder of the patient's life.

Chronic pain syndrome: Chronic pain syndrome is a psychosocial disorder. Pain and suffering become the central focus for the patient and may exist without known organic pathology or known objective findings that are congruent with the pain reported. It can result in an endless pursuit of diagnoses and treatments, overuse of the medical system, and surgeries or procedures of questionable value. The patient's social situation typically supports him or her in these pursuits. The patient also may be depressed, anxious, consumed by pain problems, and no longer functioning in work, personal life, or society.

Depression: Depression is a loss of interest or pleasure in activities that can also be characterized by some of the following symptoms: a sense of worthlessness or guilt, a change in appetite or weight, insomnia or hypersomnia, decreased energy, tiredness, fatigue without activity, observable restlessness or "slowed down" movements, increased irritability, difficulty thinking or concentrating, and recurrent thoughts of death, including suicidal plans or attempts.

Posttraumatic stress: Symptoms of posttraumatic stress occur after exposure to a traumatic event that leads to seeing or being threatened by death or a serious injury. It can also occur after learning about an unexpected violent death or harm of a close person. The symptoms include persistent reexperiencing of the traumatic event, persistent avoidance of reminders, and "numbing" to the external world (decreased responsiveness). Persistent increased arousal is present and may be characterized by difficulty with sleep, irritability or anger, difficulty concentrating, and hypervigilance or an exaggerated startle response. To be classified as posttraumatic stress disorder, symptoms must be present for more than 1 month and cause distress or impairment in important areas of functioning.

Somatization: Somatization is the expression of emotional or psychosocial discomfort in the physical language of body symptoms.

TABLE 11.1 ● ● ● ● ●

Misconceptions Chronic Nonmalignant Pain (CNP)

MISCONCEPTION	CORRECTION
1. Because of the chronicity of pain, patients are less sensitive and better able to tolerate pain.	Patients with CNP may be *more* sensitive to pain or other stimuli because of alterations in the neurotransmitters that help modulate pain, mood, and sleep (Ward, Bloom, Dworkin et al., 1982). Along with this, they may have declines in their natural endorphin levels and changes in the neuroplasticity of pain structures (Sinatra, 1992), all of which may increase their sensitivity to pain. Unrelieved chronic pain is not better tolerated over time. Instead a tendency toward decreased functioning and increased isolation, depression, anxiety, frustration, and sleep disturbance exists.
2. Pain for which there is no known organic cause is a symptom of psychologic disturbance (i.e., psychogenic pain).	The scientific basis of pain management is new. It is presumptuous to assume we know all the causes of pain, know all the individual responses, and have perfected diagnostic testing. The health care teams' inability to identify a physical cause for pain should not lead to a label of "psychogenic pain." Even psychiatric diagnoses (e.g., pain associated with psychologic factors, hypochrondriasis, or somatization disorder) have specific *DSM-IV* (American Psychiatric Association, 1994) criteria to fulfill, and these do not exclude the role of medical conditions in the onset or the maintenance of pain. Rather than view pain as a dichotomy, it is more productive to view the body and brain as sharing the same environment. Each contributes varying levels of input to pain perception. Also, a patient whose pain reports do not fit our known scheme should periodically be reexamined for the emergence of new symptoms that may warrant further testing.
3. If the patient's pain occurs or increases soon after a traumatic life event (e.g., a divorce or death in the family), this stress is probably what caused or increased the pain.	To say that stress directly causes pain is neither correct nor very helpful. Although it is true that traumatic life events may trigger a stress response, not all people react strongly to traumatic life events. Indeed, the way we judge and cope with stressful situations determines the consequences for our health and well-being (Lazarus, Folkman, 1984). When a combination of triggering events and poor coping skills evokes a sympathetic nervous system response, it can influence pain perception and control. Undoubtedly, someone who has poor coping skills would find a chronic situation even more difficult. Evidence also exists that the ability to cope with "daily hassles" of living may be just as important to an individual's healthy outcomes, if not more so, than the ability to cope with major life changes.
4. Patients who are awaiting litigation after an injury or who receive worker's compensation are very likely to exaggerate their pain for financial gain or may be malingerers.	Numerous studies have failed to support this claim. Solomon and Tunks (1991) found no differences in the amount of medication used, hours/day spent resting, or the number of people who returned to work when they compared litigant with nonlitigant patients with CNP. Melzack, Katz, and Jeans (1985) found that patients who receive compensation do not report higher levels of pain than patients who do not receive compensation. These authors say, "Compensation is not a *cause* of pain . . . This does not mean that malingerers or neurotics do not exist. It suggests instead that they may be relatively rare and unfortunately patients have been misdiagnosed, mistreated and allowed to suffer under the shroud of unfair labels instead of receiving appropriate therapy" (p. 111).

Continued.

TABLE 11.1 ● ● ● ● ●

Misconceptions	Chronic Nonmalignant Pain (CNP)—cont'd
MISCONCEPTION	CORRECTION
5. A patient who "exaggerates" his or her pain and/or has a greater decrease in function than can be explained by the physical cause is consciously trying to manipulate others or obtain secondary gains.	It is extremely rare to have outright fabrication of pain (e.g., malingering or factitious disorder) (Eisendrath, 1995). According to operant principles, maladaptive pain behaviors exist because they have been reinforced at some point in patients' social environments. Maladaptive pain behaviors are those that functionally impair or put clients at further risk for problems with pain (e.g., "doctor shopping," having questionable surgeries, or decreasing activities). These are learned behaviors and not behaviors contrived to fool others. An operant behavioral approach may support or restore healthy behavior by providing the patient and family with education about the painful condition, appropriate activities, and self-management skills. The goal is to increase the patient's support from the family for healthier behaviors and to decrease reinforcement for maladaptive behaviors (e.g., staying in bed or not participating in activities of daily living or work) (Fordyce, Roberts, Sternbach, 1985).
6. If the patient is depressed, especially if there is no known physical cause for pain, then depression is causing his or her pain. The pain would subside if the depression could be effectively treated.	Depression and inadequate coping skills may interfere with pain control; this is true regardless of whether the pain predated the depression or vice versa. Significant symptoms of depression occur in 12% to 36% of patients with a general medical condition (Depression Guideline Panel, 1993), and the incidence of depression in CNP is even higher, ranging from 31% to 100% (Romano, Turner, 1985). Depression in patients with CNP is treated concurrently with their chronic pain condition to optimize the outcomes in both disorders.
7. Opioids are totally inappropriate for all patients with CNP. People with chronic pain who have been taking opioids for months or years are narcotic addicts.	"Addicts" seek opioids for psychologic reasons and accelerate their use to the extent the drugs are available. Their pursuit and use of drugs over time lead to declines in their overall functioning. Patients with CNP who have failed other treatments may benefit from opioid therapy when they meet certain criteria. Patients with stable conditions generally do not increase their opioid use over time. Furthermore, their functioning increases as better pain control allows them to do more activities or return to work (Portenoy, 1996).
8. When patients with CNP are non-compliant, it is probably because they do not want to give up their pain.	Patients with chronic pain, just like patients with other chronic disorders, may not adhere to a treatment plan. Sclar, Tartaglione, and Fine (1994) found that compliance was the exception versus the rule in adults taking medications, and that noncompliance for all medications ranged from 13% to 93%. Turk and Rudy (1991) emphasize that not enough is known about relapse, noncompliance, and adherence to self-maintenance skills in the treatment of patients with chronic pain. To increase compliance, involve the patient in treatment choices and offer pain relief alternatives that are realistic. Expensive medications that the patient would not purchase, relaxation techniques that are not appealing, and PT exercises that are not understood will not be used.

May be duplicated for use in clinical practice. From McCaffery M, Pasero C: *Pain: Clinical manual,* pp. 469-470. Copyright © 1999, Mosby, Inc. Information from American Psychiatric Association: *Diagnostic and statistical manual of mental disorders,* ed 4, Washington, DC, 1994, Author; Depression Guideline Panel: *Depression in primary care. Vol. 1. Detection and diagnosis,* AHCPR Publication No. 93-0550, Rockville, Md, April 1993, U.S. Department of Health and Human Services; Eisendrath SJ: Psychiatric aspects of chronic pain, *Neurology* 45(12 Supp 9):S26-S34, 1995; Fordyce WE, Roberts AH, Sternbach RA: The behavioral management of chronic pain: A response to critics, *Pain* 22:113-125, 1985; Lazarus RS, Folkman S: *Stress, appraisal, and coping,* New York, 1984, Springer; Melzack R, Katz J, Jeans ME: The role of compensation in chronic pain: Analysis using a new method of scoring the McGill pain questionnaire, *Pain* 23:101-112, 1985; Portenoy RK: Opioid analgesics. In Portenoy RK, Kanner RM, editors: *Pain management: Theory and practice,* pp 248-276, Philadelphia, 1996, FA Davis; Romano JM, Turner JA: Chronic pain and depression: Does the evidence support a relationship? *Psychol Bull* 97(1):18-34, 1985; Sclar DA, Tartaglione TA, Fine MJ: Overview of issues related to medical compliance with implications for the outpatient management of infectious diseases, *Infect Agents Dis* 3:266-273, 1994; Sinatra RS: Pathophysiology of acute pain. In Sinatra RS, Hord AH, Ginsberg B et al., editors: *Acute pain mechanisms and management,* pp 44-57, St. Louis, 1992, Mosby; Solomon P, Tunks E: The role of litigation in predicting disability outcomes in chronic pain patients, *Clin J Pain* 7:300-304, 1991; Turk DC, Rudy TE: Neglected topics in the treatment of chronic pain patients: Relapse, noncompliance, and adherence enhancement, *Pain* 44:5-28, 1991; Ward NG, Bloom VL, Dworkin S et al.: Psychobiological markers in coexisting pain and depression: Toward a unified theory, *J Clin Psychiatry* 43:32-39, 1982. See text for further references.

The saddest story in all of pain management may well be about chronic nonmalignant pain (CNP). More people have CNP than any other type of pain. The people who have it have suffered a long time, sometimes years. The health care professionals providing care for them may feel powerless as they fail in their repeated efforts to help.

MISCONCEPTIONS

Appropriate care of patients with CNP is often hampered by misconceptions. There are many misconceptions about CNP and patients' motives or legitimacy. Unlike other chronic disorders, CNP requires the health care team to depend on the patient's self-report as one of the most important measures of relief. Team members cannot quantify the successes of their treatments like they can with other chronic conditions such as hypertension (blood pressure readings) and diabetes (blood sugar checks). Feeling vulnerable about the possibility of being deceived by the patient, clinicians may become suspicious of patients for illogical reasons.

For example, clinicians want patients with chronic illnesses to learn about their conditions and self-management skills. However, when a patient is knowledgeable about pain medications and dosages and reminds the staff of when they are due, the staff sometimes reacts differently than if it were a diabetic patient asking for his or her insulin. When the patient with chronic pain has the same self-maintenance information and has learned to use it to manage pain, ironically this tends to upset the health team.

In one study of 268 registered nurses' responses to descriptions of patients with various types of pain, findings showed that many nurses have a negative stereotype of the patient with chronic pain. They tend to believe that pain is less intense in patients with chronic versus acute pain, especially if no signs of pathology are evident. Nurses are particularly likely to have negative attitudes about patients with chronic low back pain compared with their attitudes toward patients with headache or joint pain. A tendency also exists for nurses to believe that pain relief measures are less effective when the patient is depressed; these nurses fail to appreciate that the pain may contribute to the depression (Taylor, Skelton, Butcher, 1984). For other common misconceptions, review Table 11.1 at the beginning of this chapter.

SCOPE OF THE PROBLEM

Definition of Chronic Nonmalignant Pain

A truly satisfactory or generally agreed on definition of CNP does not exist. In fact, some clinicians do not use the phrase, preferring other terminology such as chronic benign pain or chronic intractable benign pain syndrome.

The term "nonmalignant" pain rather than "benign" pain is used in this chapter because benign tends to suggest a mild condition, which CNP certainly is not. Malignant refers to conditions that are potentially life-threatening. The word nonmalignant is used in this chapter to describe pain that results from causes that are not life-threatening. Nonetheless, the pain and its resulting problems are serious.

For purposes of this chapter the *working definition* of CNP is *pain that has lasted 6 months or longer, is ongoing, is due to non–life-threatening causes, has not responded to currently available treatment methods, and may continue for the remainder of the patient's life.*

A diagnosis of *chronic pain syndrome* can be made when patients' CNP symptoms consume and incapacitate them to the point that their pain and suffering have become their sole focus. Frequently these patients seek endless consults and procedures by physicians and others, and they may have numerous diagnostic tests with negative results or results that are not congruent with known pathology. In recent years this criterion has been reexamined because it is now recognized that the cause for some types of pain such as neuropathic pain cannot always be identified with current tests, and we are reliant on the patient's subjective descriptions to assess it. In addition to the preceding criteria, patients with chronic pain syndrome are typically depressed or anxious and are no longer functioning in their work roles, personal lives, or society (Fordyce, 1976).

Conditions, Prevalence, and Cost of Chronic Nonmalignant Pain

CNP encompasses diverse types of pain that may occur in virtually any area of the body. The pain can be intermittent or constant and can vary in intensity from mild to excruciating. It can be a symptom that results from a variety of diseases or injuries. Some of these diseases are organically based and have well-defined pain patterns and characteristics. Other diseases are more insidious, with poorly understood organic causes and more diffuse patterns of pain. However, the most difficult type of CNP to comprehend is that which occurs without an association with a known pathologic disease process or a past injury. Most of these types of pain are neuropathic or myofascial.

CNP exacts a high price from the sufferer and his or her family or other caregivers. To society in general in the United States it literally represents a yearly cost well in excess of $100 billion (Sternbach, 1986).

The prevalence of CNP in the general population is speculative, although some insight about persistent pain can be gleaned from past survey information. Lou Harris and Associates were commissioned in 1985 to conduct a nationwide survey of pain in adults for the Nuprin Pain

Report (Sternbach, 1986). A representative sample of 1254 U.S. adults were asked in a telephone interview about the presence and severity of seven types of pain. More than 30% reported having persistent pain, and the top four categories of pain that were reported to occur for 101 or more days out of the previous year were joint pains (10% of sample), backaches (9%), muscle pains (5%), and headaches (5%).

More recently the National Headache Foundation estimated that 45 million Americans have recurring painful headaches. Guo, Tanaka, and Cameron (1995) found that 18% of a random sample of working adults in the United States age 18 years or older had back pain lasting a week or longer. Carey, Evans, Hadler and others (1996) found the prevalence of back pain to be lower in their random survey of North Carolina adults 21 years or older. Only 7.6% of their sample had back pain in the previous year that limited their activities between 1 day and 3 months. Crook, Rideout, and Browne (1984) found that 11% of a sample of the general United States adult population reported some persistent pain condition. In total, these surveys suggest the prevalence of chronic pain in the general population of adults in the United States is greater than previously suspected, and ranges from 11% (Crook, Rideout, Browne, 1984) to about 30% (Sternbach, 1986).

The survey data also concur closely with the common types of CNP problems that are referred to pain clinics and obtained by patient surveys. Box 11.1 provides other examples of CNP; see Chapter 12 for a discussion of some of the types of pain. The most common types of CNP problems in a national survey of 204 members of a chronic pain self-help organization (Hitchcock, Ferrell, McCaffery, 1994) were back/neck (47%), myofascial/fibromyalgia (20%), headaches (8%), arthritis (6%), and neuropathic (5%) pains.

BOX 11.1 Examples of Chronic Nonmalignant Pain

Arthritis—rheumatoid or osteoarthritis
Causalgia, neuralgia (e.g., postherpetic neuralgia, trigeminal neuralgia)
Chronic abdominal pain (e.g., chronic pancreatitis, Crohn's disease, irritable bowel syndrome)
Fibromyalgia
Headaches (e.g., cluster, migraine, tension)
Low back pain (e.g., ankylosing spondylitis, arachnoiditis, failed back syndrome)
Myofascial pain (e.g., neck pain from whiplash injury)
Peripheral neuropathy (e.g., resulting from diabetes, AIDS, or Raynaud's disease)
Phantom limb pain
Reflex sympathetic dystrophy
Sickle cell disease
Temporal mandibular joint dysfunction

Information from Bonica JJ: *The management of pain, Vols I and II,* ed 2, Philadelphia, 1990, Lea & Febiger.

Treatment Challenges

People with CNP can be especially difficult for many practitioners to accept and treat because they do not fit the traditional "cause and cure" model of medicine. Many times they respond poorly or in unexpected ways to treatments that are successful for more acute situations. Unfortunately, in their desperation to seek relief, people with CNP may aggressively pursue and overuse acute care services. This increases the likelihood of their obtaining inappropriate interventions. Ironically, approaching CNP problems with acute care solutions can frequently complicate patients' circumstances with iatrogenic effects. Questionable surgeries, medications inappropriate for long-term use, or unwarranted restrictions on activities can further impede patients' efforts to effectively manage their ongoing problems.

Because of its chronicity and impact on patients' functioning and psychosocial states, CNP may be accompanied by many other problems (Holzberg, Robinson, Geisser, 1996). Along with unrelenting pain, some people with CNP may become physically deconditioned and intolerant of activities. They may have changes in their parenting or work roles, and they may be socially isolated or alienated in their relationships. Because of chronic pain they may be frustrated, depressed, suicidal, anxious, or angry and suffer from sleep deprivation because of their chronic pain (Eisendrath, 1995). Some may have poor coping skills or confounding psychologic disorders. Still others may live in social situations with families or friends who unknowingly contribute to their pain problems in their best efforts to help. When these symptoms remain untreated, they may lead to chronic pain syndrome, a disorder in which patients can be consumed and incapacitated by their pain to the point that it becomes their sole focus and they are no longer effectively functioning in life. Foremost, patients may have a poor understanding about useful self-management skills for handling their chronic condition.

Appropriate treatment of chronic pain problems requires a rehabilitative focus with patient participation and coordination of practitioners knowledgeable in treating chronic conditions. When a patient has a chronic pain condition that is uncomplicated, the primary care practitioner may easily coordinate care, such as planning a physical therapy (PT) stretch program with a physical therapist to treat a patient's muscle spasms. However, in complex chronic pain situations coordinating care can become much more complicated and time-consuming. Referral to other specialists increases the risk of inappropriate acute intervention that may involve overuse of expensive diagnostic resources such as CT scans, MRIs, and surgery (Carey, Evans, Hadler et al., 1995). Acute interventions may also contribute to prescribing of inappropriate medications such as muscle relaxants, which are not suitable for long-term management, and recommendations to restrict activities, which over time contribute to disuse and a decrease in patients' functioning.

Multidisciplinary chronic pain facilities may be considered for such complex situations, especially if the patient has chronic pain syndrome. In a meta-analysis of 65 articles addressing the multidisciplinary management of pain, Flor, Fyrich, and Turk (1992) found that multidisciplinary programs are more effective than unimodal (medical only) treatment programs or no treatment for chronic pain management. Patients who had received care in multidisciplinary programs used fewer medical resources, were more likely to return to work, and had greater improvements in pain and mood scores than patients receiving only medical treatments. Limitations of this meta-analysis were the low internal validities of the articles used (57 of the 65 articles received a low score for internal validity), the lack of control groups, and the sampling methods when control groups were used (convenience sampling). More rigorous studies are needed not only on patient outcomes but also on the cost/benefit ratio, the patient selection, and the makeup of multidisciplinary pain management programs.

PURPOSE AND LIMITATIONS OF CHAPTER

The purpose of this chapter is to discuss the principles related to the assessment and comprehensive treatment of pain in patients with CNP. By definition, CNP has not responded to efforts to eliminate it. Therefore approaches suggested are not expected to put an end to CNP. Rather, the hope is to suggest ways the health care team can collaborate and assist the patient in learning to manage the chronic condition. CNP requires daily management, very much like other chronic illnesses such as diabetes or hypertension. The goals of patient care are twofold: (1) decreasing the pain intensity to the extent possible, but not expecting that it will disappear, and (2) helping the patient obtain an optimal quality of life and level of function.

To accomplish these goals, the purposes of this chapter are as follows:

- To improve the quality of the interaction between the practitioner and the person with CNP by addressing the common misconceptions that hamper this and suggesting some approaches to collaborating with, or working with, patients.
- To present guidelines for establishing realistic goals and identifying appropriate interventions to help the patient with CNP in various settings, including teaching self-management skills.
- To identify professional and self-help resources the practitioner may suggest for the patient with CNP, including pointers on selecting a pain management program.

This chapter does not, however, discuss guidelines for establishing a pain management program, although re-

sources throughout the chapter are helpful for practitioners who work in those settings.

CLINICAL SETTINGS PROVIDING CARE

Pain is the most common presenting symptom when people seek help from their physicians. Patients with CNP may be seen in any clinical setting. Far more pain problems are seen and treated in physicians' offices than in specialized pain management programs. Most of the CNP problems are treated in primary and specialty care office practices.

Acute Care Settings and Emergency Departments

Patients with CNP frequently access help through acute care settings. The patient with chronic pain syndrome can be particularly frustrating to work with in this setting. Typically the patient returns again and again to the acute health care setting, whether it is the physician's or surgeon's office, the emergency department, or an urgent care center. When the patient repeatedly seeks help for unrelieved problems, this may result in multiple referrals to subspecialists with resulting diagnostic tests that often show insignificant or negative findings. The patients may also receive and use multiple or overlapping treatments or medications from different practitioners and accumulate different diagnoses. Eventually, through a line of referrals, the patient can end up in a surgeon's office and be channeled into surgeries of questionable value that actually may contribute to iatrogenic problems. A preponderance of patients have back pain, and many of them are eventually seen in orthopedic or neurosurgeons' offices.

Patient Example

Mr. E. comes self-referred to a neurosurgeon for a second opinion about surgery to help relieve his back pain. The first surgeon, who performed several of his previous surgeries, does not recommend additional surgery. Mr. E. has continued, unrelieved pain despite taking eight analgesics, including three opioid medications and two muscle relaxants. To get relief from his pain and muscle spasms, he combines analgesics from practitioners he sporadically sees. He is depressed, anxious, and understandably focused on his symptoms. He spends most of his day lying in bed or on a couch, and he is concerned that even with limited movement his back might "pop out." Despite repeated surgeries that he admits helped only temporarily, he strongly believes he needs another surgery to improve his problems. The most recent MRI of his back shows no changes compared with a scan done 1 year ago. He has a history of nine back surgeries, including laminectomies, diskectomies, rod placements, and rod removals.

Until this point, Mr. E. has not had a single practitioner to coordinate his overall care. He organizes his care and seeks surgeries and medications from different practitioners that provide him some temporary relief. He has poor knowledge of chronic illness maintenance, and despite his nine surgeries, he is still searching for the "magic" surgery or medication to cure him. He continues to search for help in the only way that he knows possible by going to doctors and nurses.

Mr. E.'s CNP has been poorly managed by the various health care providers he has contacted. He has had inadequate assessment of his pain and medication use, and he has received no education about CNP and the resources for its treatment. This is not his fault, and he should not be blamed for trying to get relief in the only means that have been offered to him by health care professionals.

Mr. E. demonstrates the iatrogenic risks that patients with CNP face, not only with multiple surgeries but also with medications, when their care is not coordinated by one practitioner knowledgeable about CNP. At the time of his consultation with the neurosurgeon, his combined prescribed medications from three practitioners included oxycodone, 5 mg, and acetaminophen, 325 mg (Percocet), 3 to 4/day; hydrocodone, 5 mg, and acetaminophen, 500 mg (Vicodin), 2 to 3/day; propoxyphene napsylate, 100 mg, and acetaminophen, 650 mg (Darvocet-N 100), up to 8/day; cyclobenzaprine (Flexeril), 10 mg bid; carisoprodol (Soma), 350 mg tid; naproxen, 250 mg 1 to 2 bid; buspirone hydrochloride (BuSpar), 5 mg tid; and over-the-counter ibuprofen, 200 mg up to 3/day.

Mr. E. faces iatrogenic risks related to lack of coordination in relation to his medications. He receives three opioids instead of one at an effective dose. He is at risk for liver failure because of the toxic dose of acetaminophen from his combined doses of Percocet, Vicodin, and Darvocet (up to 8000 mg/day of acetaminophen). Taking two NSAIDs, naproxen and ibuprofen, places him at risk for GI bleeding. He has been taking two "muscle relaxants" for more than a year, neither of which has been proven helpful for long-term treatment of spasms. Finally, a side effect of most of his medications is sedation, which increases his fatigue and depression. Although muscle spasms have been a problem for a while, he has not seen a physical therapist—nor has he been directed to other rehabilitative or nonpharmacologic means of managing his spasms. He spends up to 20 hours per day either in bed or lying on his couch because he fears that activity will provoke his pain. Because of his fatigue, fears, depression, and pain, he seldom leaves home.

Outcome

The neurosurgeon did not recommend surgery and explained that further surgery was statistically less likely to reduce Mr. E.'s pain than his first surgery. He went over results from his physical examination and the MRI and assured Mr. E. that his physical condition was stable, although admittedly painful. He referred Mr. E. to a multidisciplinary pain facility with the specialists he needed.

Mr. E. was evaluated by a neurologist and a psychiatrist at the multidisciplinary pain management facility, and the psychiatrist coordinated his care by other practitioners. He was diagnosed with failed back syndrome with neuropathic and myofascial pain and depression. His prescriptions were adjusted over time to controlled-release oxycodone (OxyContin), 10 mg bid, gabapentin (Neurontin, an anticonvulsant with analgesic activity), 3000 mg/day; sertraline (Zoloft), 100 mg; and amitriptyline (Elavil, an antidepressant with analgesic activity), 50 mg hs. (Gabapentin and amitriptyline are adjuvant analgesics; see Chapter 7.)

Mr. E. rates his pain at 3 to 4/10 (a level acceptable for him), his depression is well controlled, he is sleeping 9 to 10 hours per night, he attends a therapeutic pool program, and he has increased his activities up to 10 hours of active time per day. He continues a daily stretch and walking program, and he continues to receive follow-up support, education, and encouragement for CNP management from the clinic programs and staff.

The patient with CNP may also seek treatment in emergency departments (EDs) during a pain flare-up period. The patient with chronic pain syndrome may routinely seek care in the ED, and this patient may be particularly stressful for staff. Such a patient may be called a "repeater" or "frequent flyer," and the staff may keep his name in a card file along with the other people that they suspect are abusing medications. (See Chapter 3 on mistaking "pain relief seeking" for "drug seeking.") The patient may report that his pain is excruciating but have no objective test findings to prove that he has the migraine or the back pain that he claims. He may have been in pain for so long that he no longer acts like he is in pain because he takes pride in functioning despite his pain or because he is simply exhausted. However, he may be frustrated, depressed, anxious, angry, and demanding of staff. Unfortunately, many times practitioners reinforce the patient's repeated search for a cure by again obliging with short-term interventions to discharge him. These interventions may treat immediate symptoms, but bedrest, muscle relaxants, and short-acting opioids are not appropriate for long-term management.

Patient Example

Mr. S. was referred to the pain management facility by his insurance plan. He presumably went to EDs in three separate states over a holiday weekend seeking treatment for migraine headaches. He states he was desperate for someone to help. He is angry and believes his insurance company is unfairly picking on him. He laments that the staff in the EDs did not know what they were doing because of the various medications he has been given. He states, "I always tell them what works best for me, but they almost never listen to me." He identifies IM meperidine (Demerol) as the best medication to abort his migraines. He has prophylactic migraine medications that he inconsistently uses, reasoning, "Why take them if I'm just going to get a headache anyway?" He recently lost his job as a security guard because of time off from work (60 days in the past year), and he believes his headaches are taking over his life. He states he's so irritated that if he cannot get relief, he'd just as soon die. He says he has gone to EDs a couple times a week, and his insurance company substantiates that with a list of 52 ED visits over the past 4 months. Most of his visits did result in medication prescriptions, recommendations to use ice, recommendations for detoxification, and referrals to neurologists. Only one doctor, in all the records obtained, documented recommendations for other methods of management, such as a multidisciplinary pain program, biofeedback, and physical therapy.

Outcome

Mr. S. had filled out daily diary cards that showed he had a clear rebound pattern when the therapeutic blood level of his medications decreased. (See Chapter 12, p. 559, regarding rebound headache.) His medications were very inconsistent and were made up of various combinations of those he obtained from EDs or sporadic visits to various practitioners. His medications included sumatriptan (Imitrex) 25 mg PO up to 100 mg; oxycodone hydrochloride, 4.5 mg; oxycodone terephthalate, 0.38 mg, and aspirin, 325 mg (Percodan); oxycodone, 5 mg, and acetaminophen, 325 mg (Percocet); codeine, 30 mg, and acetaminophen, 300 mg (Tylenol No. 3); acetaminophen, 325 mg, butalbital, 50 mg, and caffeine, 40 mg (Fioricet); aspirin, 325 mg, butalbital, 50 mg, and caffeine, 40 mg (Fiorinal); hydrocodone, 5 mg, and acetaminophen, 500 mg (Vicodin); butorphanol (Stadol) nasal spray; meperidine (Demerol); prochlorperazine (Compazine); carisoprodol (Soma); methocarbamol (Robaxin); isometheptene, 65 mg, acetaminophen, 325 mg, and dichloralphenazone, 100 mg (Midrin); and several NSAIDs. His sleep was inconsistent, and he said that he slept only when his medications helped his headache and made him tired. He was not taking any prophylactic medications at that time. It was unclear from his account and past records whether prophylactic medications such as tricyclic antidepressants, calcium channel blockers, or betablockers, had been tried long enough to determine effectiveness.

In consultation with a comprehensive headache program, hospitalization was recommended to Mr. S. on its medical unit for purposes of tapering his medications in a safe environment to control withdrawal and to monitor his headaches, depression, and sleep problems. Prophylactic therapies would also be initiated in a controlled manner, and PT, biofeedback, and group therapy for chronic headache management, education, and support would be a part of his program. A careful assessment could be documented in his record to develop plans for long-term management at home and recommendations for immediate abortive therapies for flares treated in the acute care setting. This would include a consistent practitioner for prescribing his medications, a daily plan for managing his headaches, and a consistent plan for treating his acute headaches in an identified ED, if needed.

Psychiatric Settings

Patients with CNP who have severe psychologic problems may be receiving care in a day treatment program or on a psychiatric unit because of threatening psychopathology, ongoing suicidal thoughts, or suicidal attempts. In a recent survey (Hitchcock, Ferrell, McCaffery, 1994), an alarming 50% of patients with CNP belonging to a self-help group admitted to feeling hopeless enough to contemplate suicide. In patients with CNP, research has documented an increased incidence of depression, somatization, anxiety, substance abuse, and personality disorders (Eisendrath, 1995). These emotional disturbances may occur either before or after the onset of chronic pain. In one study of patients with chronic low back pain (CLBP), depression was equally likely to occur before or after the onset of pain. Thus depression may predispose a patient to CNP, but it is equally likely to be a consequence of CNP. On the other hand, substance abuse not only occurred at a higher rate in patients with CLBP than the general population, but it also almost always occurred before, not after, the onset of pain, suggesting that substance abuse may contribute to the development of CNP (Polatin, Kinney, Gatchel et al., 1993).

Chronic pain disorders can coexist with other psychiatric problems such as posttraumatic stress disorder and sexual abuse. Studies show a clear relationship between self-reported sexual abuse and the increased occurrence of chronic conditions such as pelvic and gastrointestinal pain (Drossman, Leserman, Nachman et al., 1990; Fry, 1993) and musculoskeletal pain and back pain (Linton, 1997; Wurtele, Kaplan, Keairnes, 1990). (Other psychiatric conditions that may have a relationship with chronic pain disorders are listed in Box 11.2.) It is important that mental health professionals and other practitioners knowledgeable about chronic pain problems consult with each other about difficult cases. This is true whether patients with psychologic disturbances have complaints of unrelieved pain or whether patients' pain relief does not seem to improve their psychologic status.

Patient Example

Ms. P. is referred by an anesthesiologist to a psychiatrist for depression and stress. Ms. P.'s hands were damaged quite extensively 6 years ago in a crushing punch press accident. Since that time she has had 15 hand or lower arm surgeries and her hands are quite deformed with several amputated digits. Ms. P. is a fidgety female who appears sad and anxious. She denies any current suicidal thoughts, intentions, or plans. However, she cries easily and has other signs of depression, such as decreased sleep, decreased energy, loss of appetite, and a 5% weight loss in a month. She has difficulty falling asleep and sleeps an average of 5 hours a night with four to five interruptions. She states that before getting medication and treatment from her anesthesiologist to help manage her pain, she did have thoughts of suicide and 6 months ago wrote a suicide note. She says her bilateral hand/lower arm pain is much worse with stressful situations or when she feels tense.

Pain and bad dreams wake her up. Many times, she says, the pain causes her to dream about her accident. She is reluctant to describe her dreams, other than to say that they are about her hands caught in the punch press and feelings that she is going to die. She admits to feeling anxious and depressed, and says certain "factory sounds and smells" make her feel nauseous and panicky. In fact, she describes going to great lengths to avoid factories that are close to her home. She once heard the sound of punch presses coming from one of the factories and "it made me feel nuts." (She smelled and reexperienced her accident.) The biggest stressors she identifies are her ongoing dreams about her accident.

Outcome

Ms. P. was diagnosed with depression, posttraumatic stress disorder (PTSD), and neuropathic and myofascial pain. She was referred to the pain management facility's psychologist and psychiatrist for her depression and PTSD. Her counseling sessions with the psychologist help her understand her PTSD symptoms, and she states she feels like she has some control over "smaller"

> ### BOX 11.2 Coexistence of Chronic Nonmalignant Pain and Psychiatric Disorders*
>
> Major depressive disorder
> Dysthymic disorder
> Generalized anxiety disorder
> Posttraumatic stress disorder
> Panic disorders
> Sexual abuse
> Pain disorder associated with both psychologic factors and a general medical condition
> Borderline personality disorder
> Histrionic personality disorder
> Dependent personality disorder

*There is an established relationship with the coexistence of some specific and general chronic pain disorders and these diagnoses. That is, their coexistence is greater than what you would expect by chance. Both the chronic pain and the psychiatric diagnoses are treated together for optimal results.

NOTE: In rare psychiatric disorders, pain reports can be a presenting symptom. These are uncommon and not listed.

Information from American Psychiatric Association: *Diagnostic and statistical manual of mental disorders*, ed 4, Washington, DC, 1994, APA; Eisendrath SJ: Psychiatric aspects of chronic pain, *Neurology* 45(12 Suppl 9):S26-S34, 1995.

---

anxieties by using some of the distraction, stress management, deep breathing, and other relaxation and coping techniques she has learned. The psychiatrist started her on an antidepressant and an anxiolytic medication PRN. (Note that only under certain circumstances should anxiolytics be prescribed for patients who have CNP and anxiety or panic disorders.) After trials of various types of antidepressants, an effective one was identified. Her crying and other symptoms of depression have cleared up, and she is more optimistic. She is sleeping 6 to 7 hours at night without as many interruptions, and her anxiety and panic symptoms have decreased.

Other treatments she received were several sets of trigger point injections done by the anesthesiologist in the muscles of her arms and shoulders, which helped her "ache" type pain. She was also referred to PT for a home stretch program and reconditioning, and an ergonomic evaluation was done of her office work site. Modifications were made at her work site to help her maintain good posture with her office and computer tasks.

Ms. P. was also titrated up on gabapentin (Neurontin), which she found to be very helpful for her burning pain in her right hand. She had several trials with sustained-released, longer-acting opioids, and a transdermal fentanyl patch, but she had problems with nausea, rashes, itching, and drowsiness. She wanted to manage with minimal medications, so she tried only antihistamines for a short period of time, which she found helpful for her side effects, but she decided to discontinue the antihistamines and her long-acting opioid medication.

Her current medications are mirtazapine (Remeron), 15 mg/day; alprazolam (Xanax), 0.5 mg ½ to 1 PRN up to qid; gabapentin, 2400 mg/day; and propoxyphene napsylate 100 mg and acetaminophen, 600 mg (Darvocet-N100), 2/day.

She currently rates her pain as 2 to 3/10, which is acceptable to her. She has returned to part-time work after a short leave of absence in an office where she answers phones and does some typing on a computer. She has recently started to date and hopes to remarry someday.

If a patient has pain for which there is no known cause, it should not be assumed that pain is a symptom of psychologic disturbance. It is relatively rare to have psychiatric disorders in which pain is the presenting symptom (American Psychiatric Association, 1994). Unfortunately, it is not uncommon for patients with CNP to be suspected of malingering, hypochondriasis, and histrionic behavior because of pain that persists in the absence of physical findings. Research, on the other hand, supports the view that chronic pain reflects numerous complex issues including a sense of victimization from such sources as the adversarial nature of workers' compensation system (Tait, Chibnall, Richardson, 1990) or a history of physical or sexual abuse (Fry, 1993; Linton, 1997; Wurtle, Kaplan, Keaimes, 1990). Many power struggles develop along the course of chronic pain because of multiple physician contacts, legal entanglements, and insurance company delays, all promoting a sense of helplessness and loss of control over one's life.

Whether physical findings explain the persistent pain or not may have very little relevance. Regarding patients treated in a chronic pain program, Hubbard, Tracy, Morgan and others (1996) found no significant difference in outcome between patients with objective medical findings and those with no objective findings. Despite the emphasis that health care professionals tend to place on identifying the physical cause of the pain, the presence or absence of physical findings may play only a minor role in the recovery of many patients. There is considerable controversy over what constitutes an adequate organic finding to explain the pain and at what point pain reports are considered excessive. Thus diagnosing the patient with CNP with a psychologic disorder involves considerable subjectivity. Furthermore, in the past many types of pain could not be explained by a known medical condition but now have an explanation (e.g., the neuropathic origin of some types of pelvic pain and the central mechanisms involved in phantom limb pain). Because pain is a new science, it is inevitable that some types of pain remain unexplained, not because no physical reason exists, but because research has not yet revealed that reason. We should expect that we will not know the causes of all types of pain. Unknown cause does not equal no cause or no pain. Clinicians may say, "There is no reason for the patient to hurt," when the truth is simply, "We do not know why the patient hurts."

Dual Diagnostic and Addiction Treatment Centers

As a special note, the most regrettable health care treatment for patients with CNP is that offered in psychiatric dual diagnostic or addiction treatment centers that have little understanding of chronic pain treatment. Patients with CNP may be referred inappropriately to these centers by practitioners who are unfamiliar with their chronic pain condition or treatment. The referral frequently results from a practitioner's alarm that the patient is addicted to his or her prescribed medications when, in fact, the patient is simply taking prescribed medications for a medical reason—pain relief. The ensuing care in these centers can be demeaning and confusing for the patient and frequently lacks other methods of pain control or physical therapy rehabilitation. During detoxification, patients predictably have exacerbations of the chronic condition.

Under very limited circumstances (e.g., the patient who is diagnosed with addictive disease) and with appropriate supports (e.g., physical therapy and alternative pain management practices), an addiction treatment center may be considered for a patient. However, most patients who need to be tapered off medications and switched to other regimens can do this in an outpatient setting with a practitioner knowledgeable about their chronic pain condition. The practitioner should be able to monitor the taper and offer alternative rehabilitation or other pain therapies in a supportive environment.

ASSESSMENT OF CHRONIC NONMALIGNANT PAIN

Elements of the Assessment

To establish a treatment plan for the patient with CNP, a thorough assessment is required, including physical and psychosocial examinations. To facilitate routine comprehensive assessments, a chronic pain questionnaire can be developed and sent to patients ahead of time to help gather information (see example, Form 11.1). Records should also be requested and obtained from any referring or treating practitioners before the patient is seen. Along with past medical records, any diagnostic tests, x-ray films, or scans, as well as medication and treatment histories, are important. Frequently, patients with CNP have been referred to different specialists, and they have a wealth of diagnostic information.

Text continued on p. 486.

FORM 11.1 **Patient Questionnaire**

Thank you for taking the time to answer this questionnaire. Please bring it with you to your appointment. It will be reviewed with you at that time.

Name: _____ Nickname: _____

Address: _____ SS#: _____

City, State, ZIP Code: _____

Home Phone: ( ) _____ Work Phone: ( ) _____

Date of Birth: _____ Age: _____ Sex: _____

1. Who referred you to the pain clinic? _____

2. What is his/her phone number? _____

3. Who is your primary doctor? _____

4. What is his/her phone number? _____

5. Are you allergic to anything? If so, please list. _____

   _____

   _____

Nurse's Notes:

Date: _____ Time: _____ T= _____ P= _____ R= _____ BP= _____

Height: _____ Weight: _____

_____

_____

NPO since: _____ Driver available: _____

_____ Signature: _____ , RN

---

6. When did your pain problem begin? Month _____ Year _____

7. Describe your pain problem: _____

   _____

   _____

   _____

8. Describe when your pain problem occurs. (i.e., Is it constant, intermittent, only at night, etc.?) _____

   _____

9. How did your pain problem first start? (Car accident? Fall? Job-related injury?, etc.) _____

   _____

   _____

10. Do you think a treatment can help the type of pain you have?   ( ) Yes   ( ) No   ( ) Unsure

11. Estimate the number of visits to health care providers for your pain problem you have made in the last year.

   _____

   Continued.

12. Have you been hospitalized for your pain in the past? ( ) Yes ( ) No

    If yes, how many times this year? _____

13. Are you involved in legal action related to your pain problem or considering it in the future?

    ( ) Yes ( ) No   If yes, describe the current state of litigation. _____

    _____

14. Please circle the level of your primary pain from 0 (no pain) to 10 (worst pain imaginable) for the following:

    PRESENT level of pain:

               0   1   2   3   4   5   6   7   8   9   10
           (No pain)   (Worst pain imaginable)

    WORST pain you've had:

               0   1   2   3   4   5   6   7   8   9   10
           (No pain)   (Worst pain imaginable)

    LEAST pain you've had:

               0   1   2   3   4   5   6   7   8   9   10
           (No pain)   (Worst pain imaginable)

15. Using the same scale, what level of pain is ACCEPTABLE for you?

               0   1   2   3   4   5   6   7   8   9   10
           (No pain)   (Worst pain imaginable)

16. Use the figures below to shade in the areas where you have pain. If your pain moves around, put an "X" where it starts and draw an arrow to where it spreads.

Nurse's Notes: _____

_____

Continued.

17. Look at the following categories of words used to describe pain. From each group of words circle the one word that best describes your primary pain. If there is no word in a numbered group that seems to describe your pain, then skip that group.*

1.
Flickering
Quivering
Pulsing
Throbbing
Beating
Pounding

2.
Jumping
Flashing
Shooting

3.
Pricking
Boring
Drilling
Stabbing
Lancinating

4.
Sharp
Cutting
Lacerating

5.
Pinching
Pressing
Gnawing
Cramping
Crushing

6.
Tugging
Pulling
Wrenching

7.
Hot
Burning
Scalding
Searing

8.
Tingling
Itchy
Smarting
Stinging

9.
Dull
Sore
Hurting
Aching
Heavy

10.
Tender
Taut
Rasping
Splitting

11.
Tiring
Exhausting

12.
Sickening
Suffocating

13.
Fearful
Frightful
Terrifying

14.
Punishing
Grueling
Cruel
Vicious
Killing

15.
Wretched
Blinding

16.
Annoying
Troublesome
Miserable
Intense
Unbearable

17.
Spreading
Radiating
Penetrating
Piercing

18.
Tight
Numb
Drawing
Squeezing
Tearing

19.
Cool
Cold
Freezing

20.
Nagging
Nauseating
Agonizing
Dreadful
Torturing

18. If the above words do not describe your pain, describe in your own words what your pain is like.

_____

_____

_____

_____

Nurse's Notes: _____

_____

Continued.

19. Are there things that influence your pain? Please check all that apply.

TREATMENT	RELIEVES	WORSENS	NO DIFFERENCE	COMMENTS
Exercise				
Walking				
Massage				
Sitting				
Standing				
Touch				
Heat pack				
Ice pack				
Temperature (hot)				
Temperature (cold)				
Weather				
Bright lights				
Eating				
Alcohol				
Emotional stress				
Urination				
Defecation				
Noise				
People				
Music				
Sleeping				
Sexual activity				
Menstrual cycle				
Medicines				
Rolling in bed				
Moving from sitting to standing				
Stairs				
Other				

Continued.

20. What treatments have you received for pain in the past? Please check if treatment was helpful or not helpful.

TREATMENT	HELPFUL	NOT HELPFUL	COMMENTS
Surgery			
Nerve block			
Steroid injection			
Acupuncture			
Trigger point injection			
TENS unit			
Heat/ice treatment			
Biofeedback			
Hypnosis			
Relaxation training			
Counseling			
Physical therapy			
Traction			
Chiropractic treatment			
Occupational therapy			
Other (explain)			

Nurse's Notes: _____

_____

_____

_____

_____

 Continued.

FORM 11.1 Patient Questionnaire—cont'd

21. Are there areas of your life that have been affected by your pain problem? Check all that apply:

   a. ( ) Sleep _____

   b. ( ) Appetite _____

   c. ( ) Relationships _____

   d. ( ) Work _____

   e. ( ) Finances _____

   f. ( ) Physical activity _____

   g. ( ) Use of alcohol _____

   h. ( ) Use of recreational drugs _____

   i. ( ) Emotions _____

   j. ( ) Concentration _____

   k. ( ) Other, describe: _____

22. Please list all of your current medications, both prescription and "over-the-counter" medications, that you take:

MEDICATION	DAILY AMOUNT	EFFECTIVENESS	SIDE EFFECTS	ORDERING DOCTOR

Nurse's Notes: _____

_____

_____

23. What best describes your present use of pain medications?

   a. ( ) Definitely increasing

   b. ( ) Increasing slightly

   c. ( ) Same as always

   d. ( ) Decreasing slightly

   e. ( ) Definitely decreasing

   f. ( ) Not applicable

 Continued.

24. List all past medications you have taken for your pain problem:

_____

_____

_____

_____

_____

_____

_____

25. Please check any of the following conditions you have had or presently have:

( ) Diabetes   ( ) Arthritis
( ) Cancer   ( ) Ulcer
( ) Heart problems   ( ) Kidney problems
( ) Respiratory problems   ( ) Bleeding problems
      (e.g., asthma, emphysema)   ( ) Seizures
( ) Infectious disease   ( ) Neurogenic disease
( ) High blood pressure
( ) Other _____

26. Please list all past surgeries and hospitalizations:

DATE	PROCEDURE	DOCTOR	FACILITY

27. Have you had any of the following tests performed within the past 24 months?

TEST	DATE	FACILITY WHERE TEST WAS DONE	RESULTS
X-ray film			
CT Scan			
MRI			
Laboratory			
EMG			
Myelogram			
Other			

 Continued.

28. Are you pregnant or planning to become pregnant?   ( ) Yes   ( ) No

29. What is your current marital status?
    a. ( ) Single
    b. ( ) Living with significant other
    c. ( ) Married
    d. ( ) Divorced
    e. ( ) Widowed
    f. ( ) Separated

30. What was your marital status when your pain problem began?
    a. ( ) Single
    b. ( ) Living with significant other
    c. ( ) Married
    d. ( ) Divorced
    e. ( ) Widowed

31. What is the highest level of education you've finished? _____

32. List the names and ages of all the people who live with you: _____
    _____

33. Are you currently working?   ( ) Yes   ( ) No   ( ) Retired   If yes, describe your occupation:
    _____

34. Is this the same occupation you had before your pain started?   ( ) Yes   ( ) No
    If you answered "yes" to the above, skip to question No. 36

35. If you are not working, has pain forced you to stop working?   ( ) Yes   ( ) No

36. If you are not working, what type of work did you do before your pain became a problem? _____
    _____

37. Does your spouse work? ( ) Yes   ( ) No   If yes, what is your spouse's occupation? _____

38. Are you being treated under Worker's Compensation?   ( ) Yes   ( ) No

39. Are you currently receiving disability benefits?   ( ) Yes   ( ) No

40. Do you smoke? ( ) Yes   ( ) No   If yes, how many packs per day? _____

41. Do you drink alcoholic beverages? ( ) Yes ( ) No   If yes, how many ounces for average daily use?____

42. Do you drink beverages with caffeine (i.e., coffee, tea, soda, hot chocolate, etc.)? ( ) Yes   ( ) No
    If yes, how many 8-oz glasses for average daily use? _____

43. Do you exercise on a regular basis? ( ) Yes   ( ) No
    If yes, what type of exercise and how many times per week? _____

44. Is there anything else that you can think of that will help us with your treatments? _____
    _____
    _____

    Signature: _____ , RN

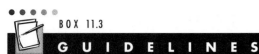

BOX 11.3

G U I D E L I N E S

ASSESSMENT OF A PATIENT WITH CHRONIC NONMALIGNANT PAIN

I. History
   A. Past general health history
   B. Pain assessment/history
      1. Location, intensity, and quality
      2. Onset, duration, and patterns
      3. Coping with or expression of pain
      4. Past treatments and their effectiveness
      5. Triggers or precipitants of pain
   C. Family health and pain history
   D. Current and past medication use
   E. Use of alcohol or recreational drugs
   F. Social and work history
   G. Mental health history
   H. Lifestyle factors: smoking, caffeine use, and exercise
   I. Treatment history
      1. Review of past medical records, including clinical laboratory results, complete radiographic examinations (x-ray films, myelograms, CT scans, MRIs)
      2. Health care use (especially inappropriate doctor shopping, ED visits, combining medications, etc.)
II. Physical examination
   A. Regional examination of pain problem
   B. General, neurologic, and orthopedic examinations as needed
   C. Functional limitations
III. Psychosocial evaluation
   A. Effects of pain on emotions, relationships, sleep, and activities
   B. Family member interview
      1. Patient's functioning
      2. Family coping
   C. Psychiatric interview, when needed for assessing
      1. Coping skills, adjustment to chronic pain
      2. Coexisting and primary psychiatric disorders
      3. Overall effectiveness, autonomy, and satisfaction in life and relationships
   D. Psychometric tests as needed for information on pain, related pain problems, and psychopathology
      1. Pain-related symptom assessment instruments*
         a. Beck Depression Inventory
         b. Chronic Illness Problem Inventory
         c. Illness Behavior Questionnaire
         d. McGill Pain Questionnaire
         e. Multidimensional Pain Inventory
         f. Sickness Impact Profile
      2. Common personality assessment instruments*
         a. Coping Strategies Questionnaire
         b. Millon Clinical Multiaxial Inventory
         c. Minnesota Multiphasic Personality Inventory-2 (MMPI-2)
         d. Symptom Checklist-90R
IV. Diagnostic tests as needed
   A. Clinical laboratory studies
   B. Radiographic examinations (x-ray films, myelograms, CT scans, MRIs)
   C. Electromyography
   D. Diagnostic pain blocks
V. Review results and recommendations with patient and family

May be duplicated for use in clinical practice. From McCaffery M, Pasero C: *Pain: Clinical manual*, p. 486. Copyright © 1999, Mosby, Inc.

*For more information, see resource section.

Assessment of the patient with CNP consists of many elements (summarized in Box 11.3). A pain history should also be obtained from patients. Patients should be asked to describe the nature, location, and onset of pain and any qualitative characteristics and patterns of exacerbation or relief of pain. A description of the activities, medications, or therapies and treatments that relieve pain and a description of those that do nothing or make pain worse are also needed. Contributing lifestyle factors should also be explored, such as smoking, caffeine consumption, and lack of exercise.

A physical examination is needed to compare the present pain report with previously documented disease processes or past traumatic injuries. Depending on the patient, the examination could be a regional examination of the pain problem along with general, neurologic, or orthopedic examinations as needed. The examination should also include an evaluation of functional physical status. This may be done by the practitioner during the examination, or it may be done at a later time by a physical therapist.

In total, this evaluation determines whether a new symptom is present that needs further diagnostic workup or whether a referral is needed for treatment of an underlying pathologic process causing or contributing to the patient's pain symptoms. It also determines whether physical rehabilitation is needed to help the patient regain function so commonly lost through the deconditioning effects of chronic pain.

A psychosocial assessment is as important as the physical examination for an understanding of the pain problem. This gives the clinician a comprehensive view of how the pain affects the patient's life and helps determine whether the patient has chronic pain syndrome. A psychosocial interview with the patient and a family member or friend can determine the patient's level of functioning, coping skills or responses to stressors, fulfillment of role responsibilities, and use of health care resources. A good baseline assessment of these factors can help determine the patient's response to treatment when future outcome measures of functioning are compared with the baseline measurements.

Psychiatric conditions may coexist or be primary to the patient's chronic pain problem and are important in determining treatment options. A large percentage of patients with chronic pain have concurrent psychologic disturbances, and a routine part of an evaluation should include assessment for psychopathology, especially depression and anxiety and the symptoms that go along with these disorders (e.g., sadness, irritability, frustrated feelings, sleep disturbance, weight gain or loss, and suicidal thoughts). Sometimes psychometric tools (see p. 519) may be used to obtain information on the patient's pain, related pain problems, and psychopathology. However, if these tools are used, they should be interpreted by someone trained in their interpretation and knowledgeable about the common problems associated with CNP. To do otherwise risks the chance of mislabeling the patient or using the information detrimentally or in a manner in which it was not meant to be applied.

Assessment of Suicidal Risk

Depression should always be assessed with chronic conditions. Not only do patients with CNP have a higher rate of depression, but suicide potential is also a serious concern for this population. As previously mentioned, in one survey of patients with CNP, 50% indicated that they had contemplated suicide because of their pain (Hitchcock, Ferrell, McCaffery, 1994). The risk for depression and suicidal ideas is much higher compared with the general population (Eisendrath, 1995; Romano, Turner, 1985). A suicide risk assessment should be done whenever a patient indicates depression or has signs of depression. (Questions to ask in a suicide risk assessment are provided in Box 11.4.) Again, a good baseline assessment of these factors is important in determining treatment interventions and in comparing future responses to treatments prescribed.

REHABILITATIVE TREATMENT GOALS

Treatment of the patient with CNP begins with a review of the evaluation. It is important that the patient and family understand the diagnostic workup. If no recommendations for further diagnostic studies or invasive procedures are made, this needs to be clearly explained. Reviewing x-ray films, scans, or other diagnostic tests with the patient and family is helpful. To become involved in

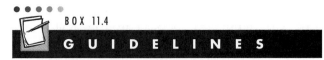

BOX 11.4

GUIDELINES

ASSESSMENT OF SUICIDAL RISK

Does the patient have the INTENTION to kill himself?
Assessment questions: "Have you ever thought that your pain and other problems could make it impossible to go on living?" If the patient answers "yes," then continue. "Have you thought of ending your life? Are you worried that you might actually do it?" Or, "Have you ever had thoughts of harming or killing yourself?"

If the patient has vague thoughts of harming or killing himself without any definite plans, or if he expresses not caring if he would just die, his immediate suicide risk is lower than someone who expresses more direct intentions, such as "Yes, I plan to end this suffering soon by . . ."

Does the patient have an ACCESSIBLE METHOD to kill himself easily?
Assessment questions: "How have you thought of harming or killing yourself?" Or, "How do you plan to kill yourself?"

The patient's risk is high if he has a definite plan he could easily carry out, such as, "I plan to kill myself by taking all my pills." Or, "I plan to shoot myself with my gun."

What is the IMMEDIACY of the plan?
Assessment questions: "When do you plan to kill yourself?" Or, "Is this something you are planning on doing soon?"

The patient's risk is higher if the plan is immediate, such as, "I'm shooting myself when I go home from here today." Or, "I'll jump off the bridge tonight." If he is indefinite about the time, such as, "I don't know. I haven't thought about it" and he has future plans for other activities in his life, his risk is lower than that of someone who has expressed more immediate intentions.

When a patient expresses immediate intentions of killing himself and he has an easily accessible plan to do so, he is at high risk for committing suicide. Stay with the patient and notify emergency services. The patient should be transported by ambulance to a psychiatric facility or emergency department that has mental health professionals who can perform a suicide risk assessment and assist with an admission or commitment for the patient's safety, if needed.

Patients who do not meet all three criteria for emergency psychiatric services should be provided with information on crisis services in the community along with a 24-hour hotline number or telephone number for emergency psychiatric services. The patient's suicide risk should be reassessed in future contacts.

the recommended treatment, the patient needs to understand when no surgeries or quick fixes are available for the problem. It is also vital to assure the patient and family that there are ways of managing the pain problems and to discuss with them the overall goals and the rationale for CNP treatment.

The goals in treating CNP are best understood in a rehabilitative model. As summarized in Box 11.5, the goals are to reduce the patient's level of pain whenever possible; to restore function and prevent future injuries; to develop self-help and maintenance skills for managing pain or the associated problems; to improve depression, anxiety, or psychopathology; and to improve relationships with family and health care providers. This also includes teaching the patient how to access the health care system in a manner that is helpful for his or her chronic condition and not detrimental to long-term maintenance (e.g., establish a consistent ED treatment plan with the patient who has acute migraine headache exacerbations, or establish a coping plan with the patient that lists in order of priority the techniques, coping skills, and medications that are helpful for managing pain exacerbations). This meets the patient's needs for having techniques or responsive services that effectively treat the chronic pain problems. It also prevents overuse of inappropriate resources, and it prevents iatrogenic effects of debatable acute treatments. The treatment plan should take into account the physical, psychologic, and social elements that interact in CNP problems.

Communicating and Coordinating Treatment

Effective treatment depends on setting specific, realistic goals with the patient that are congruent with the overall treatment goals of CNP management. Communicating and coordinating these treatment goals with other members of the health care team are equally important.

Patient Example

Ms. L. is referred by her primary care practitioner to a nurse for biofeedback for her migraine headaches. She is currently taking atenolol (Tenormin, a beta blocker), 100 mg daily, as a prophylactic medication and sumatriptan, 50 mg PO PRN, as an abortive medication. She is also taking birth control pills.

Ms. L. has a goal of tapering off her medications and becoming pregnant. This goal was communicated to her practitioners who prescribe her medications, including her primary care practitioner, her neurologist, and her gynecologist. Through education and biofeedback sessions Ms. L. learned how to manage her headaches with nonpharmacologic means such as stretch exercises, posture control, relaxation and coping techniques, pacing known stressors, adhering to regular sleep

<table>
<tr><td colspan="2">● ● ● ● ●
BOX 11.5 Overall Goals in the Treatment of CNP</td></tr>
<tr><td>
1. Reduce pain, whenever possible.
2. Restore or improve functioning.
3. Develop self-help and maintenance skills for managing CNP and its related problems.
4. Improve depression, anxiety, or psychopathology.
5. Improve relationships with family members and health care professionals. This includes accessing the health care system in an appropriate manner to meet chronic pain and other health care needs.
</td></tr>
</table>

May be duplicated for use in clinical practice. From McCaffery M, Pasero C: *Pain: Clinical manual*, p. 488. Copyright © 1999, Mosby, Inc.

and awake cycles, diet control, and ice. Should she require medication for a migraine headache after becoming pregnant, a backup plan for acetaminophen with codeine was established in consultation with her gynecologist. A taper schedule for her atenolol was arranged with her neurologist and initiated once she was proficient in the nonpharmacologic means of managing her headaches.

Outcome

By the completion of her biofeedback sessions, Ms. L. was successfully tapered off her atenolol. Once she managed headaches with nonpharmacologic means, she was taken off her contraceptive. She had an exacerbation of headaches for several days, which was diminished once she started the recommended PT. A coping strategies plan was developed with her in anticipation of managing headaches. It outlined her strategies and also listed phone numbers of her biofeedback therapist, physical therapist, and physicians. A copy of the plan was given to her and mailed to all her practitioners.

Ms. L. became pregnant 3 months later and continues nonpharmacologic management of her headaches, which occur once a month. Before starting atenolol she had daily headaches with exacerbations of acute migraines three to four times each month for which she used sumatriptan, but she has not had to resort to medications during her pregnancy. Ms. L. considers her treatment a success for meeting her goals and plans to continue her treatment plan after her baby is born so that she can breast feed.

Larger multidisciplinary pain programs may have case managers who are responsible for coordinating the patient's care with providers. However, this ideal situation does not exist for most clinical locations that provide care for patients with CNP problems. In these instances, one practitioner should take charge of prescribing the patient's analgesics and, whenever possible, should do the overall coordinating of the patient's treatment, such as ordering PT, communicating with other providers, and referring for counseling. A summary sheet (Form 11.2)

FORM 11.2 **Treatment/Medication for Chronic Pain Conditions: Patient Example**

Client name: _Mr. X_   DOB: _1/27/43_

Allergies: _NKA_

Diagnosis/Other conditions: _Chronic myofascial pain neck/upper trapezius muscles,_

? neuropathic pain (L) arm

Surgeries/Invasive procedures: _status post cervical fxs. C5-C7 c̄ anterior fusion/halo 1994,_

spontaneous collapsed lung 1969

Date	Problem	Treatment Recommendations	MD/PT RN/Other	Response/ Comments
5/22/97	Sharp, knife pain (L) arm	Neurontin 300 mg PO # 45 c̄ ī refill ī qd × 2d → ī bid × 2d → ī tid	J. Bonner, MD	5/29/97 Pt. calls, no change in pain c̄ Neurontin bid. Begins tid dose today. Will call back 1 wk. Denies side effects. K. Gackstatter, RN
6/19/97	Sharp, knife pain (L) arm	Neurontin 300 mg # 150 c̄ ī refill ī qid × 1 wk → ī qid and HS × 1 wk → īī tid	J. Bonner, MD	6/19/97 No change in pain c̄ tid dose. Rates sharp, stabbing pain in (L) arm 9/10. K. Gackstatter, RN
		Stop Tylenol #3 OxyContin 10 mg ī PO bid, #15	J. Bonner, MD	
6/26/97	Sleep disturb. Myofascial pain	6/26/97 Trazodone 100 mg ī PO q̄ hs, #30 Biofeedback eval for myofascial pain.	J. Bonner, MD	6/25/97 Sharp pain in (L) arm better. Rates 4/10. Sleep is a problem—sleeps 3° @ time, total—6 h/night. Rainy weather ↑ in shoulder aches, rates 4-5/10. L. Dunajcik, RN
7/03/97	Myofascial pain Postural deviations Asymmetric muscle tension traps.	7/03/97 Biofeedback eval done, see note. Follow up 1 wk.	L. Dunajcik, RN	7/03/97 Sleep better. Sleeps 4-5° s̄ awakening, total 8-9 h/ night. No side effects. Rec. PT eval to Dr. Bonner due to ↑ muscle tension (L) trap. L. Dunajcik, RN

May be duplicated for use in clinical practice. As appears in McCaffery M, Pasero C: *Pain: Clinical manual*, p. 489, 1999, Mosby, Inc.
Courtesy St. John's Mercy Pain Therapy Center, St. Louis, 1998.

can be used wherever the patient is treated by multiple team members. Not only does the summary sheet provide a quick review for practitioners, but it also meets Joint Commission on Accreditation of Healthcare Organizations (JCAHO) outpatient facility requirements to provide a summary of treatment with results for patients who are receiving ongoing treatment for chronic conditions.

Setting Realistic Patient Goals

Setting realistic expectations for helping the patient in varied clinical settings is far from simple. It is essential that the goals be attainable for the patient, caregivers, and health care providers. Pursuing unattainable goals or expecting the patient to do something he or she does not value becomes a negative and frustrating experience for all concerned. Care requires an educated practitioner with time to teach the patient new pain management skills and to support the patient in unfamiliar or previously aversive skills (e.g., increasing physical activity). To set realistic expectations, clinicians must take into consideration that patient's willingness to take part in change and to try new methods of managing pain. Goals may be more ambitious for some patients than for others. Goals for increasing activities should be set below the patient's current baseline, and a gradual increase in quotas should be used to help the patient successfully increase activities (Fordyce, 1976).

Three practical considerations in setting goals are (1) the patient's stage of acceptance of the condition and motivation for treatment, (2) the patient's ability to follow through independently with recommendations, and (3) the time and available resources. Sometimes despite clinicians' efforts to motivate a patient, the patient may not value a rehabilitative approach and may still pursue an immediate solution. In these cases clinicians are left with providing whatever appropriate care they can, such as prescribing medications that are suitable for long-term chronic pain management; teaching the application of heat, ice, or other nonpharmacologic interventions; confining iatrogenic effects (e.g., in most instances not recommending bedrest or questionable invasive procedures); and providing information on chronic pain resources (e.g., lay organizations or multidisciplinary pain clinics) that the patient can access in the future.

Likewise, whenever the patient is unable to follow through independently with setting or attaining goals, the patient and situation should be reassessed. Is the patient resistant to change or reliant on others to provide his or her care, or is there some other barrier? If the patient is resistant to change, the former suggestions would be used to direct him or her to appropriate treatment and to give suitable resources for use in the future. If the patient depends on others for care, interventions must be explained not only to the patient but also to the care-

givers. A caregiver is an essential person in such a patient's rehabilitation, and whenever possible, the routine caregiver should attend appointments with the patient, be given a contact number for questions, and be offered lay or professional resources that can provide information and support.

PATIENT CARE GUIDELINES FOR GENERAL CLINICAL PRACTICE

Finally, when the clinical site itself does not allow the time or resources for addressing the long-term management of a chronic problem, the practitioner should provide whatever appropriate care is possible, again congruent with the overall goals of CNP treatment. Specific care guidelines are summarized in Box 11.6 and are listed in somewhat of a hierarchy, from the simple to the more complex interventions. These guidelines can be used in any setting, although it is normally not possible to follow all the suggestions in every setting. In general, following these guidelines introduces sound principles of chronic pain management that have helped countless patients attain goals of reducing pain, improving functioning, and developing skills that can be used to more independently manage their pain problems.

The clinicians in the ED may be able to work only on steps involved with the patient's medication management and in their limited interactions provide the patient with some appropriate resources for chronic pain management. A health care provider in an outpatient office may have repeated contacts with the patient, allowing more time for assessing and introducing other ways of managing the patient's pain, which may include pharmacologic and nonpharmacologic methods. These care guidelines are introduced as a way to address the goals of chronic pain management in a variety of settings.

In acute care and outpatient settings, taking care of the patient with complex CNP problems is often frustrating. Such patients, especially those with chronic pain syndrome, are commonly referred to as difficult. However, the guidelines that follow may help prevent difficulties. If the patient is already angry, complaining, dissatisfied, ordering staff around, or threatening staff, it still is not too late to use these guidelines to help meet goals. The suggestions may not result in instant success, but consistent persistence usually succeeds.

Meanwhile, remember that the patient's initial reaction to you is probably formed on the basis of countless unsatisfying and perhaps adversarial encounters with caregivers. Most patients who have had pain for very long have been told some of the following: "It can't hurt that much," "It's all in your head," "You're just using your pain," "You're getting addicted," or "You'll just have to learn how to live with this." So the patient is likely to be upset at the outset.

The care guidelines that follow are one of the few places in this book where the word "never" is used repeatedly. This is probably because more misconceptions exist about the treatment of CNP than other types of pain.

Respect for the Individual

Never argue with the patient over whether he or she has the degree of pain that is reported. Arguing in this way sets up an adversarial relationship rather than a partnership. Treat with respect whatever the patient says

BOX 11.6

G U I D E L I N E S

OVERALL CARE OF THE PATIENT WITH CNP

1. Never argue with the patient about the pain the patient reports.
2. Never refer to the patient as a "narcotic addict."
3. Never use a placebo to try to determine whether the patient has "real" pain, has a physical cause for pain, or is lying about the pain.
4. Be especially alert to any changes in the patient's condition and any advances in treating the patient's pain.
5. Recognize and treat acute pain or exacerbations of chronic pain differently from ongoing CNP.
6. Be sure the patient believes that an adequate explanation of the cause of pain has been provided by an appropriate person. Explain pain management rationale underlying treatment options so the patient can be motivated and involved in selecting and carrying out self-management treatments.
7. Avoid sudden withdrawal of opioid, sedative, hypnotic, anxiolytic, muscle relaxant, or other medication that results in physical dependency. These medications should be reduced gradually. When medication reduction is indicated, give priority first to tapering the medication that is causing the most problems with functioning. Arrange for follow-up on medication tapering schedules.
8. When analgesics are appropriate, administer them orally, if at all possible, at high enough doses to provide satisfactory pain relief and often enough on a regular ATC schedule to prevent the return of pain.
9. For long-term management of complex pain problems, a combination of different medications and therapies may be needed to maximize pain relief. This should be done on the basis of the assessment of the patient, the pain problem(s), and risk factors.
10. Offer pain relief alternatives that are realistic for the patient. Management of a chronic condition involves active participation and motivation on the patient's part, but expensive medications that will not be purchased, relaxation techniques that are not appealing, and PT exercises that are not understood will not be used.
11. Assess for common mood or associated problems such as depression, *suicidal risk,* anxiety, or sleep disturbance. Consult with a psychiatrist or other mental health professional if needed. Evaluate the appropriateness of psychotropic medications and/or psychosocial interventions (e.g., relaxation, stress management, or sleep management techniques).
12. Help the patient learn and plan to use helpful coping strategies, especially relaxation, distraction, and those strategies that refute negative thoughts or avoid catastrophizing.
13. Assess the patient's activity level. How is the patient spending most of the day (e.g., in bed or on a couch)? Does the patient worry about injury? Evaluate posture or exaggerated gait, limping, guarding, or splinting. Determine the need for consultation with a physical therapist or an occupational therapist who works with increasing functioning in patients with CNP.
14. Assess disturbances in social or work role activities. Is the patient unemployed because of pain? Does the patient go to outside events and have a support system outside family, or is the patient overreliant on family? Does the patient have chronic pain syndrome? Help the patient develop a daily commitment to specific activities (e.g., physical and/or social), especially a return to employment of any type, if appropriate. Determine the need for consulting with a social worker, a vocational counselor, or a multidisciplinary chronic pain facility.
15. The use of opioids for CNP is considered when other appropriate pharmacologic and nonpharmacologic methods have failed. The patient should meet certain criteria and be informed of the risks and side effects. Medication contracts are not routinely needed and should be considered only in selected situations.
16. Refer patients with chronic pain syndrome or complex, unresolved pain problems; or those needing evaluation for advanced pain management techniques (e.g., implantation of intrathecal pumps or spinal cord stimulators) to a multidisciplinary pain management facility.
17. Help those living with the patient, especially the spouse, to work with the patient to establish expectations and limitations regarding the activities of the patient and others in relation to the patient's pain.
18. All recommendations to the patient regarding management of chronic pain need to be specific and detailed in writing with a copy for the patient and the health care team. Include when the patient will return for treatment (e.g., to an outpatient clinic), develop a summary of the present treatment, and evaluate the effectiveness of each specific recommendation made for pain management. Consider having the patient track outcomes with written daily diaries.

about pain and be prepared to intervene on the basis of what the patient reports. There are many differences among people in the way they perceive and describe their pain (see Chapter 3). Given identical painful injuries, individuals will respond in unique ways, depending on a variety of moderating variables, such as physiologic, psychologic, and social factors.

Avoiding Mislabeling Appropriate Opioid Use

Never refer to the patient as a "narcotic addict" or as "drug seeking." Pain relief is a legal, medical reason for the use of opioids. When a patient is taking opioids for pain, no matter how long or how much, he or she is not an addict (American Pain Society, 1992). Even if a patient requires an increase in opioid dose because of tolerance to analgesia or a change in the chronic condition, this does not mean the patient is an addict. Likewise, if the patient develops withdrawal syndrome when opioids are abruptly stopped, this is not the same as addiction (see Chapters 3 and 10 for definitions and distinctions between these terms).

Not only is it inaccurate to refer to the patient who takes opioids for CNP as an addict, it is also degrading to the patient. Considerable stigma is attached to the term. In our society, to be an addict is to be a "bad" person.

No Placebos for Treatment

Never use a placebo to try to determine whether the patient has "real" pain, has a physical cause for pain, or is lying about his or her pain. The American Society of Pain Management Nurses in their position statement on the use of placebos for pain management (1997) adamantly opposes the use of placebos in the clinical practice of assessing and treating pain. Placebos are defined as "inactive substances (e.g., normal saline injections), subtherapeutic doses of active substances (e.g., injection of 0.5 mg morphine in 1 ml of saline for an adult), or a sham procedure (electrodes with no therapeutic value)." Placebo use is deceptive, it violates the milieu of trust between the patient and his or her health care practitioners, and it raises ethical concerns.

Pain relief from a placebo proves nothing. It merely confirms the pharmacologic fact that approximately 36% or more of patients with obvious physical causes for pain of moderate to severe intensity will report adequate pain relief after placebo injections (Goodwin, Goodwin, Vogel, 1979) (see Chapter 3 for further discussion of placebos). The only proper use of placebos is with patients participating in controlled research studies who have been informed and agree to the potential use of placebos.

Reevaluating at Each Admission

Be alert to any changes in the patient's condition and any advances in diagnosing and treating chronic pain

problems. Changes in a patient's underlying condition may go unnoticed when practitioners tune out reports of persistent pain without really listening to what the patient is saying. Just like anyone else, patients with CNP may have new physical illnesses develop, such as malignancies or cardiac ischemia. For this reason, the patients must be carefully assessed at each encounter, and new symptoms require a thorough examination.

The elements in a chronic pain assessment (see Box 11.3, p. 486) can be used as a quick guide for reassessing. However, ongoing assessment of some of the major concerns in CNP management (e.g., pain level, medication use, mood, sleep, and activities or functioning) should be communicated succinctly in office notes to allow clinicians to compare past assessments with the current patient situation (Box 11.7).

Progress is also being made in many areas of pain control. Some new treatment may be indicated for the patient's pain. For example, adjuvant analgesics (see Chapter 7) have been found effective with certain types of pain. Anticonvulsants are now used for phantom limb pain or trigeminal neuralgia. Certain medications can complement existing treatments, such as capsaicin cream for arthritic joints along with a NSAID medication and a PT stretch program. Other new medications may have reduced side effects and toxicity, such as gabapentin instead of carbamazepine. There are also newer time-released preparations of NSAIDs and opioids that require less frequent dosing (see Chapters 5 and 6). Certain medications have also been found to be highly selective for treating particular conditions, such as sumatriptan or zolmitriptan for migraine headaches.

Developments in understanding underlying mechanisms of pain no doubt will lead to the development of even more specific medications and treatments. Staying abreast of these changes along with listening to our patients will lead to better pain management care.

BOX 11.7 Charting Example—Office Visit

46-YEAR-OLD PATIENT WITH MULTIPLE SCLEROSIS
96.7, 76, 18, 110/80
Current pain: Back = 8/10. Ribs—new, 10+/10 because of recent fall.
Meds: OxyContin, 20 mg bid, Vicodin PRN for breakthrough pain up to 3/day since fall, Elavil 100 mg, Prozac 20 mg, baclofen 10 mg, methotrexate, Coumadin, ibuprofen 600 mg tid per primary care doctor.
Sleep: "Not bad before fall, bad after." Decreased from 8 h to 5-6 h, frequent waking because of pain.
Appetite: "Bad since fall"—no weight loss.
Activity: "Decreased"—was walking with walker in living room, lost balance and fell against padded arm of chair hitting ribs on left side. Currently using wheelchair.
Mood: "Bad since fall," no suicidal ideation.

Patient Example

Ms. S. initially came to the multidisciplinary pain center with complaints of total body pain that shifted around and worsened under stress, especially at work. She was referred by her internist with a recent MRI and CT scan of her head and back, which were normal. She had previous negative workups by a neurologist and a rheumatologist.

Ms. S. was evaluated by the pain center's psychiatrist and anesthesiologist and diagnosed with myofascial pain, depression, and sleep disturbance. Her depression and sleep disturbance started with her total body pain. Her treatment included a PT reconditioning and stretch program, and she obtained a TENS unit, which relieved some of her back pain. She also began taking nortriptyline, a tricyclic antidepressant, to treat her depression and sleep disturbance, and ibuprofen, a NSAID, that she found helpful in the past for her various pains. She was concurrently tapered down on her opioid medication from six to three tablets a day with an improvement in her energy level.

Over the next several months, Ms. S. made frequent calls to the nursing staff with various incessant reports of pain. She was anxious and depressed. She was placed on case management, and the clinical specialist worked with her to initiate a change in her antidepressant; she was taken off her nortriptyline and switched to sertraline, 100 mg. She was also referred to a pain psychologist for counseling. Her depression and sleep disturbance improved, her somatic ruminations decreased, and she began to use some coping, pacing, and relaxation skills in her work situation. She also reported acceptable pain levels and more enjoyment of life. She returned to doing activities she liked, such as knitting and reading. She was stable on her pain management plan for well over a year.

One day the clinical specialist received a call from Ms. S. She reported increased total body pain and fatigue, difficulty feeling and working with her knitting needles, and vision problems (e.g., driving and reading were difficult because of blurred vision). Ms. S. attributed these changes to the recent stress of being laid off from work. The nurse, recognizing these as very different from her previous symptoms, recommended she see an ophthalmologist, consulted with her psychiatrist, and scheduled her with the pain management center's neurologist. Later that week, the ophthalmologist's office called to report that Ms. S. had ocular changes, optic neuritis, consistent with multiple sclerosis (MS). The pain center's neurologist ordered a repeat MRI of her head, almost 2 years from her first one, and this time it showed changes also consistent with MS. This was confirmed later with laboratory tests.

Ms. S. was referred to a primary neurologist for the management of her MS, and because of her rapidly deteriorating visual and now ambulatory status she was put on short-term steroid treatment. Her ongoing treatment now includes routine follow-up with her primary neurologist for the management of her MS, continued support through the pain center's programs (e.g., education and support groups, psychotherapy, and medication management for pain and depression), and coordination of treatments between the pain center's staff and her primary neurologist. She is again stable on her pain management plan.

Acute Versus Chronic Pain Treatment

Recognize and treat acute pain or exacerbations of pain differently from CNP. This requires careful assessment to distinguish between the two types of pain. Unfortunately, it is common for some types of acute pain to be mistaken for CNP. When acute pain is prolonged (e.g., lasting weeks or months), is recurrent (e.g., weekly or monthly episodes for a few days), or is an exacerbation of pain, these situations may be misunderstood as CNP. Examples of acute pain in chronic situations are sickle cell crisis, acute burn pain that occurs periodically over an extended period (e.g., that which accompanies debridements, grafting, and dressing changes), weeks or months of pain related to multiple orthopedic injuries after an accident (e.g., unhealed fractures, infected wounds), and postoperative pain (e.g., a patient with chronic low back pain recovering from a total hip replacement). Increased analgesics or opioids and limited activity may be indicated temporarily for the acute pain situation, keeping in mind that the long-term goal is to increase the chronic pain patient's functioning and to enhance his or her self-maintenance skills.

Unfortunately, in an acute pain situation, the patient with CNP may be undertreated with analgesics, especially opioids. Fear of causing addiction by adding or increasing opioid doses to accommodate for the acute pain situation (a very common concern) or fear of allowing the patient to become "accustomed" to the relief of yet stronger analgesics often results in inadequate treatment of acute pain in patients with concurrent CNP conditions. However, an intravenous opioid is entirely appropriate for sickle cell crisis, postoperative pain, or burn tanking and debridement. On the other hand, in the same patient, an intravenous opioid is obviously not the answer for treatment for daily CNP. High doses of oral opioids on a regular basis are appropriate while complicated orthopedic injuries heal. At the same time, techniques often recommended for CNP may be useful for the patient with concurrent acute pain (e.g., methods such as passive muscle or imagery relaxation, distraction, deep breathing exercises, reducing catastrophizing thoughts, and pacing, see p. 504).

The difference between acute and chronic pain must be clear to both the patient and the clinicians. Just because pain is prolonged and not life-threatening is not justification for treating it as CNP as defined in this chapter. For pain to be classified and treated as CNP, it must have also failed to respond to appropriate treatment, further medical and surgical interventions to cure the cause of the pain should not be indicated, and pain must be expected to continue indefinitely. This is not the case with the preceding examples. Either the pain will subside as healing takes place (e.g., orthopedic injuries) or the pain is a time-limited episode (e.g., postoperative pain, or sickle cell crisis).

Education as a Therapeutic Tool

Be sure the patients receive what they believe is an adequate explanation from the appropriate person of why they have pain. Ask patients to describe what they believe causes the pain or why they have pain. Patients may have false beliefs about the causes and the continuation of pain, fears about unfounded diseases or malignancies, or fears of reinjury. All these may stand in the way of rehabilitation. Any misunderstandings patients have about pain should be discussed and a clear explanation offered.

Certainly a nurse knowledgeable about CNP and a particular patient's case is well qualified for providing information and answering questions. However, it is also important to identify if anyone else, such as a physician, could help clarify results from diagnostic workups, answer questions about continuing pain, or go over the rationale for recommended treatments. Every attempt needs to be made to provide a clear explanation to the patient. This increases the patient's satisfaction with care, reduces requests for additional diagnostic tests, decreases overuse of health care services, and stabilizes changes from one agency or physician to another (Deyo, Diehl, 1986).

The explanation of why the patient has continuing pain need not be complicated. Many times the patient with CNP is interested in the anatomic or physical reasons for his or her pain and shuns away from psychologic determinants. A safe way to introduce these ideas is through a simple discussion of why the perception of pain in one person is not the same as it is in another person with similar injuries. That is, chronic pain sensation is influenced by physical (e.g., genetics and physical injury), psychologic (e.g., coping strengths, motivation, affect, and judgment), and social factors (e.g., culture and support systems). The patient can also be introduced to the pain models that support these reasons, and the rationale for a multidisciplinary approach to CNP management. A good explanation helps set up the rationale for treatment approaches with different team members. As suggested by self-efficacy theory (see page 501), there

is also a possibility for better outcomes when patients understand their diagnoses and outlooks in management (Bandura, 1992). This is especially important for patients with chronic conditions who will select and carry out self-management activities.

Medication Management
Avoiding sudden withdrawal

Avoid sudden withdrawal of opioid, sedative, hypnotic, anxiolytic, muscle relaxant, or other medication capable of producing physical dependency. Some patients have tried the "grandstand" approach of suddenly stopping all medications. The results are often devastating for them. Not only do they face the sudden return of pain, insomnia, anxiety, or other disturbances, but they also frequently stop medication without safe precautions or alternative medical or self-management treatment choices. A patient can experience "super-flu" with opioid withdrawal (e.g., runny nose, abdominal cramping, diarrhea, and "goose flesh"). Benzodiazepine withdrawal symptoms include insomnia, anxiety, agitation, muscle twitching or tremors, headaches, and nausea. Furthermore, life-threatening grand mal seizures may occur with abrupt discontinuation of benzodiazepines and barbiturates (Pap, Gorman, 1993).

A patient is tapered off a medication for a variety of reasons that should be determined on the basis of individual assessment. First, a taper may be done to eliminate a medication such as a muscle relaxant that is not appropriate for a particular chronic pain condition. Concurrently, more appropriate medication(s) and/or self-management technique(s) may be initiated with the patient. Second, a taper may also be done when a medication, although appropriate for chronic pain management, causes side effects that are detrimental to the patient's level of functioning. A third consideration for tapering is the patient's personal preference to eliminate a medication.

The medications that are most frequently overprescribed or misprescribed for patients with CNP are sedatives, hypnotics, muscle relaxants, anxiolytics (e.g., benzodiazepines or barbiturates), and short-acting opioids. Frequently these medications, especially benzodiazepines, are tapered in pain management programs and more pertinent therapies are begun. Short-acting opioids may be tapered or converted to sustained or longer-acting opioids, depending on the patient's assessment and circumstances.

Benzodiazepines are commonly prescribed and have virtually replaced barbiturates as a treatment for anxiety. With few exceptions, such as clonazepam for lancinating neuropathic pain, benzodiazepines are not analgesic. According to a 1981 survey (Pap, Gorman, 1993), about 1 of 10 American adults have taken a benzodiazepine. (A list of common benzodiazepines is provided in Box 11.8.)

They are typically prescribed for anxiety, although other common indications include insomnia, seizures, muscle spasms, and anesthesia induction. It is easy to see how patients with CNP who may have concurrent problems such as anxiety, sleep disturbances, or muscle spasms are readily prescribed benzodiazepines. Benzodiazepines may be beneficial for short-term use, but will, in long-term use, impede recovery because of sedative properties. Evidence also exists that benzodiazepines interfere with relief obtained from opioids in acute pain situations (Gear, Miaskowski, Heller et al., 1997). However, further research is needed to determine whether this negative interaction holds up for CNP patients who concurrently take opioids and benzodiazepines.

Muscle relaxants should be used with caution because their effectiveness when taken orally is questionable and they often cause sedation (see Chapter 7). Thus they are usually used on a time-limited basis, sometimes for an acute injury or exacerbation or in conjunction with active PT until the patient is able to do exercises that keep the muscles from contracting.

Tapering

A gradual reduction of the aforementioned medications should be suggested for patients who wish to discontinue their use and who have been taking them for 3 weeks or longer. With benzodiazepines and barbiturates, it is best to err on the side of slow detoxification. For benzodiazepines the dose should be reduced by less than 10% every 3 days (Pap, Gorman, 1993). Opioids can be tapered at a higher percentage of 20% every other day. Gradual reduction over periods ranging from as short as 1 week for opioids to as long as 8 weeks for benzodiazepines helps prevent significant withdrawal symptoms.

If the reduction of more than one medication is indicated and contacts with the patient are limited, it is probably wisest to decrease only one at a time. First eliminate the medication that causes the most detrimental effects on functioning, especially one that causes sedation and/or contributes to depression. Provide the patient with a daily taper schedule and ask the patient to call periodically with an update.

To ensure a more successful taper, find out from the patient what symptoms are treated by the medication or consult with the prescribing practitioner about the rationale for the medication. Discuss with the patient and the treatment team the pros and cons of the current medication regimen and the alternatives for treating the symptoms for which the medication was prescribed (e.g., relaxation, sleep techniques, and a low-dose tricyclic antidepressant for insomnia instead of a sedative; PT or warm water pool therapy for muscle spasms instead of a muscle relaxant). Whenever possible arrange for the alternative therapies to start before the taper to allow the patient to practice with new self-management skills before the elimination of medication.

Exceptions to Tapering

Also keep in mind that circumstances exist where it may be better for the patient with CNP to continue the medication. Reddy and Patt (1994) state that a role for benzodiazepines may exist in the following situations: (1) acute muscle spasms, given for limited duration; (2) concomitant chronic pain and anxiety, under the management of a multidisciplinary setting that has neuropsychiatric and rehabilitation components; and (3) neuropathic pain that is lancinating, in which case they recommend clonazepam and alprazolam as medications of choice. These would be used after failure of first-line and in many cases second-line treatments.

Research on opioids also shows that when other treatment strategies have failed, patients meeting certain criteria have been successfully maintained on oral opioids for long periods and that opioid use increased their functioning and enabled them to return to work (Portenoy, 1996; Portenoy, Foley, 1986; Tennant, Robinson, Sagherian et al., 1988). To ensure that patients meet criteria for chronic opioid maintenance, guidelines have been suggested for the selection and maintenance of patients; these will be discussed later in the chapter (Portenoy, 1996; Saper, 1996; Turk, 1996).

● ● ● ● ●
BOX 11.8

COMMON BENZODIAZEPINES*	
Generic Name	**Trade Name**
Alprazolam	Xanax
Chlordiazepoxide	Librium, Limbitrol†, Librax†
Clonazepam	Klonopin
Clorazepate	Tranxene
Diazepam	Valium
Estazolam	ProSom
Flurazepam	Dalmane
Lorazepam	Ativan
Midazolam	Versed
Oxazepam	Serax
Quazepam	Doral
Temazepam	Restoril
Triazolam	Halcion

May be duplicated for use in clinical practice. From McCaffery M, Pasero C: *Pain: Clinical manual*, p. 495. Copyright © 1999, Mosby, Inc.

*NOTE: Benzodiazepines can be classified as anticonvulsants, sedatives, hypnotics or sleeping aids, and antianxiety agents. When possible, benzodiazepines should be tapered and eliminated as a long-term medication for treating nonmalignant pain with the exception of clonazepam, which has some benefits for certain neuropathic pains.

†Combination products that contain the medication.

Information from *Physician's Desk Reference*, ed 52, Montvale, NJ, 1998, Medical Economics.

Oral medications in safe combinations

Whenever analgesics are required, give them orally, if at all possible, at high enough doses to provide satisfactory pain relief and often enough on a regular ATC schedule to prevent the return of pain. For long-term management of complicated pain problems, a combination of different medications and therapies may maximize pain relief efforts, while minimizing doses of each medication. A patient may benefit from a NSAID, an opioid, and one or more adjuvant analgesics. Emphasize to the patient that medication management is just one part of CNP management and frequently it is more effective when combined with other techniques (e.g., biofeedback and physical therapy for migraine headaches in addition to a prophylactic tricyclic antidepressant and an abortive migraine medication, or counseling on coping strategies and therapeutic water exercise for an anxious, depressed patient with fibromyalgia who is taking a selective serotonin reuptake inhibitor [SSRI]).

Different medications that act on separate components of the pain pathway may in concert provide better pain control, especially in complicated pain situations (e.g., neuropathic pain) (Virani, Mailis, Shapiro et al., 1997). For example, desipramine may be particularly helpful for continuous burning pain, and carbamazepine may relieve episodes of intermittent lancinating pain.

Patient Example

Mr. W., a man with failed back syndrome with neuropathic and musculoskeletal pain components, is on a combination of medications that includes amitriptyline (antidepressant with analgesic activity), gabapentin (anticonvulsant with analgesic activity), nabumetone (NSAID), and controlled-release oxycodone (opioid). He also uses a TENS unit and occasional heat, paces his activities, attends local support groups with his wife, does his home PT, and participates in volunteer work with his church board and in therapeutic pool programs.

More than one medication may be necessary not only to treat multiple pain symptoms originating from different areas of the pain pathway but also to treat the commonly associated psychiatric or other symptoms that may occur with CNP (e.g., depression, anxiety, fatigue, and insomnia). Combination analgesic treatment for pain relief may also be beneficial because of its dose-sparing effect. For example, adding a NSAID to an opioid may allow for smaller doses of the opioid.

Smaller doses in turn can also lessen the long-term side effects of chronic drug administration at higher doses. Griffin, Piper, Daugherty and others (1991) in their 2-year review of elderly Tennessee Medicaid enrollees who were hospitalized for peptic ulcer disease or GI hemorrhage noted that the risk for serious ulcer disease associated with nonaspirin NSAIDs increased significantly as the dose increased. Elderly people maintained on lower doses of nonaspirin NSAIDs had significantly less GI effects than those maintained on higher doses, although they were still at a greater risk for GI problems than the elderly population not taking NSAIDs at all.

In a clinical review of NSAIDs, Amadio, Cummings, and Amadio (1993) found that the elderly were more at risk for GI, renal, and hemovascular effects and more likely to die from gastroduodenal complications than any other age group. They state that the elderly appear to be the least likely to have warning symptoms of GI damage, further putting them at risk.

In addition to age risk factors, additional circumstances may exist in which it would not be appropriate to try additive medications. These include the patient's medical condition and potential interaction with medications the patient may be taking for problems other than pain (Amadio, Cummings, Amadio, 1993; Griffin, Piper, Daugherty et al., 1991; Virani, Mailis, Shapiro et al., 1997; Yost, Morgan, 1994). The decision to use several medications should always be made on the basis of the assessment of the patient. Although smaller doses can lessen long-term side effects, the combination of medications can increase the number of side effects and the potential for interaction with other medications. For some elderly patients, the combination of an opioid and a NSAID could be more dangerous than relying on the opioid alone.

Chronic opioid maintenance therapy

The use of opioids for CNP is a recognized form of treatment when other appropriate pharmacologic and nonpharmacologic methods of therapy have been tried and have failed. Recently the American Academy of Pain Medicine and the American Pain Society (1997) jointly released a statement supporting the use of opioids in selected patients with CNP. In the past 10 years, many states have also adopted intractable pain treatment acts that address the prescribing of opioids for chronic pain conditions (Joranson, Gilson, 1997).

The policies adopted by states fall under three basic categories: state laws (statutes), administrative regulations, and medical board guidelines. Statutes and regulations are enacted through the state legislation, and as such they are subject to influence by different political interests that are not based on medical practice. Medical board guidelines, on the other hand, are approved by the state's medical board. Medical board guidelines are easier to change and they can more readily reflect current medical practice. However, they can be less consistent because they are open to change whenever the membership of the medical board changes. Medical board guidelines also do not carry the force of the law, and they are not effective if they are not implemented in medical board policy.

Most states have intractable pain treatment policies in the form of medical board guidelines, and complementary guidelines have been adopted by some boards of nursing and boards of pharmacy in states such as California (Joranson, Gilson, 1997).

In general, intractable pain treatment policies recognize that prescribing opioid therapy for chronic pain conditions is acceptable medical practice. They may also specify the parameters for prescribing or expectations of prescribers. The intractable pain treatment acts can provide immunity from discipline for physicians who prescribe opioids for pain management. However, they may not offer protection to practitioners from investigations by regulatory agencies (e.g., a licensing body, a state Bureau of Narcotics and Dangerous Drugs [BNDD], or a regional Federal Drug Enforcement Agency [DEA]) or the costs of those investigations (Joranson, Gilson, 1997).

Practitioners who prescribe opioids should be aware of the terms of their state's intractable pain management policy. Pain management practitioners are encouraged to get to know their state licensing board members and to offer assistance in reviewing or revising intractable pain management policies that reflect current medical practice (Joranson, Gilson, 1997). Assistance in the form of participation or education from pain management organizations and practitioners helps base intractable pain treatment policies on current practice and avoids unjustifiable restrictions on pain management practice.

Before initiating chronic opioid maintenance therapy, appropriate classes of nonopioid medications should be optimized along with nonpharmacologic treatments. A trial of opioids may be considered appropriate when other reasonable treatment options fail and patients are appropriate candidates. Portenoy (1996) suggests that in certain cases opioid therapy can add to some patients' problems by contributing to their disability. On the other hand, for some patients opioid therapy can give some of the same benefits of improved quality of life and functioning that are seen in cancer populations. Until appropriate controlled clinical trials are performed, Portenoy suggests a balanced perspective. He proposes that if clinicians accept that different outcomes may result from the same therapy, then the clinical stance should shift from one of overall rejection of opioid therapy to one of more appropriate patient selection and guidelines for the administration of opioids. Several clinicians have presented or published guidelines for chronic opioid maintenance therapy (Biondi, 1997; Portenoy, 1994; Portenoy, 1996; Saper, 1996; Turk, 1996). Those suggested by Portenoy (1994) are presented in Box 11.9 and discussed in the following text.

Patients should be informed of the risks of opioid therapy just as they should be informed of risks for any therapy. A discussion of risks includes informing patients of side effects, physical dependence, and the potential for withdrawal symptoms with the abrupt discontinuation of therapy. Opioid therapy for CNP should be put into the total therapeutic context of providing functional restoration, and this should be discussed with the patient. There is an expectation that along with the opioid treatment, patients will engage in other aspects of treatment (e.g., psychologic and rehabilitative therapies) that can lead to improving function. In general, a trial of opioids should result in improvement in quality of life and functioning to consider extending it to longer-term therapy.

An agreement should also be made about how medications will be routinely provided (see items 3, 6, 8, 9, 10, and 11 in Box 11.9), as well as the number of rescue doses or adjustments that can be made for exacerbations of pain. One practitioner should be primarily responsible for coordinating and prescribing pain management, and an identified pharmacy should be used for refilling medications. Medications should be prescribed ATC on a set schedule. Enough medication should be prescribed until the next regular routine appointment the patient has with the practitioner. Portenoy (1996) suggests initially scheduling appointments no less frequently than a month apart.

Patients should demonstrate responsible use of medications. Some intractable pain treatment acts exclude patients who use medications "for nontherapeutic purposes" (Joranson, Gilson, 1997). Practitioners should explain to patients the reality of regulatory concerns and under what circumstances opioids will cease to be prescribed. Circumstances that cause concern about prescribing opioids include selling or giving medications to others, repeatedly losing or spilling medications, and repeatedly reporting prescriptions as stolen. Portenoy (1996) suggests that ongoing documentation should address the patient's comfort level, functioning, side effects, and the occurrence of any aberrant drug-taking behaviors. Opioid prescribing may also need to be reassessed in situations of uncontrolled medication escalations without consulting the clinician or against the advice of the prescribing practitioner or in situations where the patient is taking additional opioids prescribed by others. In certain situations the practitioner may discontinue opioid treatment. In other instances more stringent guidelines or a written contract may be implemented.

If a decision is made to use opioids, controlled-release opioids offer extended periods of analgesia and fewer doses. This can help prevent pain from interrupting sleep and minimize skipped doses, thereby reducing the likelihood of withdrawal symptoms. Controlled-release formulations of opioids include morphine (MS Contin, Oramorph SR, Kadian), oxycodone (OxyContin), and transdermal fentanyl (Duragesic patch). Controlled-release formulations of other opioids soon will be available. Although methadone has been classified as a long-acting opioid, it is not chosen as a first-line treatment. It is reserved for those situations in which other opioids have not helped.

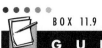

BOX 11.9

G U I D E L I N E S

MANAGEMENT OF OPIOID THERAPY FOR CHRONIC NONMALIGNANT PAIN

1. Opioid therapy should be considered only after all other reasonable analgesic therapies have failed.

2. A history of substance abuse, severe character pathology, or chaotic home environment should be viewed as relative contraindications.

3. A single practitioner should take primary responsibility for treatment.

4. Patients should give informed consent before the start of therapy; points to be covered include the following:
   a. Recognition of the low risk of true addiction as an outcome
   b. Potential for cognitive impairment from the drug alone or from the combination of the drug with other centrally acting drugs
   c. Potential for other side effects
   d. Likelihood that physical dependence will occur (abstinence syndrome possible with acute discontinuation)
   e. Need for responsible drug-taking behavior (e.g., no unsanctioned dose escalation and no prescriptions from other physicians)

5. The use of a written contract to inform patient of his or her responsibilities should be considered but is not mandatory.

6. Except in rare circumstances, therapy should be administered by the oral route.

7. The use of a long-acting opioid (e.g., controlled-release morphine or methadone) may be preferable because of ease of administration, but it is not mandatory.

8. Dosing on a fixed-schedule basis ("around the clock") is preferable if the patient experiences continuous or frequently recurring pain.

9. In addition to the daily dose determined initially, most patients should be permitted to escalate dose transiently on days of increased pain; the following two methods are acceptable:
   a. Prescription of an additional 4-6 "rescue doses" to be taken as needed during the month
   b. Instruction that one or two extra doses may be taken on any day but must be followed by an equal reduction of dose on subsequent days

10. Initially, patients must be seen and drugs prescribed at least monthly; when stable, less frequent visits may be acceptable.

11. Several weeks should be agreed on as the period of initial dose titration; although improvement in function should be continually stressed, at least partial analgesia should be viewed as the primary goal of therapy.

12. Failure to achieve at least partial analgesia at relatively low initial doses in the patient with limited prior opioid consumption should raise questions about the potential treatability of the pain syndrome with opioids and lead to reassessment.

13. Emphasis should be given to attempts to capitalize on improved analgesia by gains in physical and psychosocial function; opioid therapy should be considered complementary to other analgesic and rehabilitative approaches.

14. Exacerbations of pain not effectively treated by transient and small increases in dose are best managed in the hospital, where dose escalation, if appropriate, can be observed closely and return to baseline doses can be accomplished in a controlled environment.

15. Evidence of drug hoarding, acquisition of drugs from other physicians, uncontrolled dose escalation, or other aberrant behaviors must be carefully assessed. In some cases tapering and discontinuation of opioid therapy will be necessary. Other patients may appropriately continue therapy with rigid guidelines. Consideration should be given to consultation with an addiction medicine specialist.

16. At each visit, assessment should specifically address the following:
   a. Comfort (degree of analgesia)
   b. Opioid-related side effects
   c. Functional status (physical and psychosocial)
   d. Existence of aberrant drug-related behaviors

17. Use of self-report instruments may be helpful in documenting pain relief and functional status but is not mandatory.

18. Documentation is essential; the medical record should specifically address comfort, function, side effects, and the occurrence of aberrant behaviors repeatedly during the course of therapy.

Modified from Portenoy RK: Opioid therapy for chronic nonmalignant pain: Current status. In Fields HL, Liebeskind JC, editors: *Progress in pain research and management. Vol 1. Pharmacologic approaches to the treatment of chronic pain: New concepts and critical issues*, pp. 274-275, Seattle, 1994, IASP Press.

Doses should be titrated for the individual and should be a balance between optimal analgesia and side effects. Therapy for the management of side effects such as constipation should also be planned when opioids are prescribed. No set dose of opioid will be safe and effective for all patients. Some patients require far higher doses than others. If a practitioner is uncomfortable with the dose required for pain relief, he or she should consult a pain management specialist.

In the event a decision is made to initiate a trial of long-acting opioid with a patient, concurrent benzodiazepine therapy should be evaluated and eliminated when possible because it may hinder the full effectiveness of the opioid. Benzodiazepines may antagonize opioid-induced analgesia by enhancing the inhibitory neurotransmitter, GABA, at the GABA-A receptors in the descending pain modulation system. In a double-blind, placebo-controlled study, 71 dental patients underwent standardized surgery for the removal of at least one bony impacted mandibular third molar (Gear, Miaskowski, Heller et al., 1997). They were given an IV injection of diazepam for sedation before surgery, and after surgery they were given an IV injection of 6 mg of morphine sulfate. Patients then received either placebo IV or IV flumazenil, a benzodiazepine antagonist, 40 minutes after receiving the morphine sulfate. Those who received IV flumazenil required less postoperative analgesic medication.

Although contracts are not widely used when opioids are prescribed, some chronic pain facilities will use them with selected patients. If a decision is made to use contracts, legal review of the document should be considered. (See Appendix B for discussion of contracts and agreements related to chronic opioid maintenance therapy.) Contracts are not required by state intractable pain treatment acts, although a select number of states do require that the prescribing physician obtain signed informed consent from the patient. Keep in mind, clinicians do not routinely contract for other controlled substances, some of which may be more sedating and have a greater impact on functioning (e.g., benzodiazepines). Many decisions about treatment are verbally agreed on and documented in patients' records. A contract is not needed to provide good, prudent care, nor does it necessarily demonstrate such care. A contract also is not needed to discontinue a patient from a treatment that is not helpful or healthy for him or her. A clinician who contracts with patients taking opioids may convey mistrust and insult to someone who is seeking treatment for his or her pain problems.

Psychosocial Considerations

Psychosocial considerations are also important when planning treatment for most patients with CNP. These patients have an increased incidence of depression, anxiety, somatization, sleep disturbances, substance abuse, and personality disorders (Eisendrath, 1995). Emotional disturbances can occur before or after the start of chronic pain (see Box 11.2 for psychiatric disorders that may be associated with CNP). Sexual abuse and trauma can also be precursors to some chronic pain conditions (Drossman, Leserman, Nachman et al., 1990; Fry, 1993; Linton, 1997).

People with CNP may also have significant role changes because of their actual limitations, their coping, or their families' enabling of their sick role. This may affect their work and family roles, and their financial well-being. They are more likely to experience unemployment, separation, and divorce.

Depression management

Assess for common mood or associated problems such as depression, suicidal risk, anxiety, or sleep disturbance. Depression is estimated to occur in 31% to 100% of people who experience chronic pain (Romano, Turner, 1985). The causal relationship is unclear. However, as mentioned previously, patients with CNP are at greater risk for depression and suicidal thoughts than the general population.

People with CNP and depression also have poorer outcomes than do those who are not depressed. Research by Haythornthwaite, Sieber, and Kerns (1991) revealed that depressed patients with CNP were more likely to report higher pain levels, more pain behaviors (although not greater disability), and greater obstacles than nondepressed patients. However, Averill, Novy, Nelson et al. (1996) found no relationship between depression and self-reported pain intensity or the number of pain-related surgeries in their study of 254 chronic pain patients. Interestingly, both studies found no significant difference in the number of pain medications in depressed versus nondepressed patients with CNP. Overall, though, the poorer outcomes reported in studies are typically related to poorer physical and psychosocial functioning (Averill, Novy, Nelson et al., 1996; Holzberg, Robinson, Geisser et al., 1996).

The first priority in treating patients with depression is to assess suicidal risk. Most important is to assess whether they have the intentions and a plan for killing themselves (see Box 11.4 for assessing suicidal risk). If the patient is in danger of committing suicide, hospitalization in a protective environment may be needed, along with antidepressant and supportive therapies. A patient who is depressed will require antidepressants at levels that are therapeutic to treat depression. A pain practitioner may select antidepressants that have known pain relief benefits, such as tricyclic antidepressants and some of the SSRIs.

Sleep management

Sleep disturbances are also common for patients with CNP, and their continuation may have an increasing detrimental effect on patients' efforts to manage their pain. A poor night's sleep contributes to depression, muscle soreness, difficulty thinking, and decreased motivation. Sedatives or hypnotic medications to which the patient may become tolerant, especially benzodiazepines and barbiturates, should be avoided. Tricyclic antidepressants, especially amitriptyline at subtherapeutic doses for depression, are often excellent bedtime aids that have the added benefit of pain relief for some types of neuropathic pain. Of course, if sleep disturbance occurs with depression, using antidepressants at levels therapeutic for depression will help the depression, sleep, and many times the pain. If the patient has hypersomnia, an antidepressant with nonsedating qualities, such as fluoxetine (Prozac), should be selected.

If the patient has insomnia, offer to teach the patient relaxation (see Chapter 9) and sleep hygiene techniques that may help him or her get to sleep faster and get back to sleep if he or she awakens during the night. According to a NIH panel report, relaxation techniques and biofeedback are effective in alleviating insomnia by improving sleep onset and total sleep time (NIH Technology Assessment Panel on Integration of Behavioral and Relaxation Approaches into the Treatment of Chronic Pain and Insomnia, 1996). Cognitive forms of relaxation like meditation are more effective than progressive muscle relaxation. Sleep restriction, stimulus control, and multimodality treatments are the most effective ways of decreasing insomnia. Biofeedback and relaxation techniques may decrease sympathetic activity (DeGood, 1993), whereas behavioral techniques (e.g., sleep restriction and stimulus control) may reduce arousal and shift circadian rhythms to improve poor sleep habits (Jacobs, Rosenberg, Friedman et al., 1993a,b). Cognitive approaches can also change dysfunctional beliefs and decrease arousal, thereby contributing to improved sleep.

Anxiety management

If the patient is having difficulty sleeping because of anxiety, using the nonpharmacologic techniques mentioned is beneficial. However, the patient may also benefit from some brief methods of relaxation that can be used throughout the day. This may include paced, deep breathing, which teaches the patient to maintain relaxed breathing when anxiety threatens (see Chapter 9). An abbreviated form of progressive muscle relaxation can help him or her relax tense muscles, and a short version of autogenic training with thoughts of warming extremities can also decrease arousal. If anxiety is such that the patient has panic attacks, distraction techniques and desensitization programs with biofeedback or relaxation training with a trained therapist may be beneficial.

When medication management is needed, consult with a psychiatrist. Some of the antidepressant agents that are helpful with the management of symptoms of obsessive compulsive disorders or anxiety conditions may help (e.g., sertraline, nefazodone, and paroxetine). In the event that a benzodiazepine is used, follow-up should be done with a practitioner knowledgeable in neuropsychiatric and rehabilitation pain practices, such as practitioners who work in a comprehensive pain facility (Reddy, Patt, 1994).

Assess the need for requesting a consultation to treat depression, anxiety, or PTSD. Discuss the rationale for the patient's consulting with a mental health professional. Frequently, patients can misinterpret a psychiatric consult as an accusation that pain is all in the head. Try to approach this by clarifying that pain often causes depression and anxiety that make it more difficult to handle pain. Reassure the patient that after even a few weeks of pain, it would be abnormal if no depression or anxiety was present.

Finally, recognition is growing that pain incurred as a result of unexpected trauma, such as an accident, may lead to PTSD. This may have a paralyzing effect on the patient, but it may be treated with therapy that gradually desensitizes the patient to fearful aspects. A referral to a psychologist or a counselor who works with PTSDs may be helpful as an adjunct to pain management treatment. Those patients whose pain may be related to past abuse may benefit from insight-oriented psychotherapy.

Cognitive behavioral therapy

Cognitive behavioral therapies help change negative attitudes and thoughts. They also teach healthy, adaptive thoughts and may positively influence emotions and behaviors. This is done through education, "skills acquisition," practice of new cognitive behavior skills in a safe environment, generalization of the new skills to the overall environment, and maintenance of the gains through relapse prevention.

In general, patients should be considered and referred for cognitive behavioral techniques if they have maladaptive beliefs and behaviors that may include inappropriate health-seeking behaviors, ongoing depression or anxiety, or poor coping skills. Cognitive behavioral techniques are taught by therapists such as mental health practitioners or trained clinicians in a multidisciplinary pain clinic or center.

Relaxation

Relaxation techniques are usually a part of the cognitive behavioral skills taught for a variety of pain problems (Syrjala, 1990) in pain treatment facilities. Hypnosis, a form of deep relaxation, has been shown to be effective in reducing pain perception, such as in the treatment of cancer-related pain (Syrjala, Cummings, Donaldson, 1992). Unfortunately, people vary widely in their susceptibility and ability to be hypnotized. Hypnotizing patients for pain control typically takes the form of focusing on relaxation, ignoring intrusive thoughts, and introducing the idea of analgesia to the painful area. Hypnosis is done only by specially trained clinicians.

Biofeedback (BF) techniques provide patients with physiologic information that is displayed on a computer screen and/or in sound. BF is a form of psychophysiologic feedback that gives people insight into responses they normally do not see. Through relaxation and other cognitive behavior techniques patients can learn how to control responses not ordinarily under voluntary control, and they can recognize disregulation (e.g., very tense muscles displayed on a screen that were not tense in their conscious awareness). In a study of three types of treatment for chronic musculoskeletal pain, 57 patients with chronic back pain and 21 patients with temporomandibular pain were randomly assigned to electromyography (EMG) BF treatment, cognitive-behavioral therapy, or medical treatment (Flor, Birbaumer, 1993). All three groups showed improvement immediately after treatment, with the BF group demonstrating the most improvement. The BF group was the only group, however, that maintained significant reductions in pain severity, affective distress, and pain-related use of the health care system at 6- and 24-month follow-ups.

Types of common BF technologies used are EMG BF for reducing muscle tension, thermal BF for autogenic training, electrodermal BF for reducing hyperaroused states, and pneumograph and plethysmograph BF for teaching deep breathing skills. BF is effective in teaching skills to patients with headaches or myofascial pain (Flor, Birbaumer, 1993). It is also helpful for patients who are anxious or who have autonomic symptoms of being hyperaroused. Biofeedback should not be recommended for the severely depressed, cognitively impaired, or psychotic patients, until their underlying psychopathology is managed (Schwartz, 1987).

Self-Efficacy Theory and Coping Strategies

Bandura's (1977) cognitive theory of self-efficacy is helpful in understanding coping in the chronic pain experience (Bandura, Adams, Beyer, 1977). Self-efficacy is one's beliefs about his or her ability to perform behaviors that will yield certain outcomes. Bandura hypothesizes that one's expectation of self-efficacy determines whether the person will initiate coping behavior, the amount of effort that the person will put into it, and how long the person will persist in the face of obstacles. In general, people become involved in activities they think they have the skills to handle. People fear and avoid threatening situations that they believe to be beyond their coping skills.

How would a practitioner change these maladaptive ways of coping with pain by changing self-efficacy?

Bandura found through research that participant methods of learning can bring about more generalized, lasting changes in self-efficacy and behavior. Thus it would be important to demonstrate pain control methods to the patient and practice them together. If available, another patient who successfully uses some of the pain control methods may function as a stronger model. Supportive group education and practicing new techniques under conditions in which the patient is likely to succeed will help develop new skills and increase confidence in being able to do new activities. When the patient is comfortable practicing the skills in a learning situation, encourage the patient to practice in other locations.

Patient Example

Mr. S. has myofascial pain in his neck and upper back from a whiplash injury and participates in PT treatments. His physical therapist demonstrates exercises to him, practices the initial set with him, and has him return demonstrations until he feels comfortable. Posture techniques are also taught to him in this manner along with methods to check himself periodically during the day.

Mr. S. does exercise sessions along with other patients who have chronic pain, and he attends group educational meetings. During an educational session, former participants of the program explain the benefits of their exercises in managing their chronic conditions. Educational sessions also address how to maintain exercise and other gains during pain flare-up periods.

Finally, to help Mr. S. generalize his program his therapist has him record on a card the assigned exercises he does at home and the posture checks he does periodically throughout the day. He is reinforced for the practices he accomplishes, and as he feels better, he feels further motivated and more in control of managing his pain condition on his own.

Cognitive Theory of Stress and Coping

Coping, as described by Lazarus (1967), occurs as a cognitive mediating process when stress is appraised. This "cognitive appraisal" determines how an individual views, reacts to, and handles a situation (Folkman, Lazarus, 1980; Lazarus, Folkman, 1986). In other words, the way a person interprets a situation helps determine the emotional reaction. These appraisals and emotions in turn influence the choice of coping strategies. Thus a person who perceives a stressful event will apply coping processes. Some coping strategies may increase the risk of pain, illness, or maladaption, whereas others decrease it. An increasing number of studies address coping strategies related to positive or negative outcomes with people who have pain problems.

Some coping strategies such as catastrophizing and passivity are related to poorer outcome measures and self-efficacy. These strategies may also stand in the way of developing healthier styles of coping. Chaves and Brown (1987) found that catastrophizing thoughts were the most common maladaptive cognitions in a population of 75 adult clients undergoing dental procedures. Catastrophizing took the form of negative self-statements or catastrophizing thoughts or imagery. Thirty-seven percent of this population engaged in catastrophizing during their procedures, resulting in higher levels of reported stress.

Passivity is a way of coping with pain that is also related to poorer outcomes. Brown and Nicassio (1987) assessed coping strategies in a chronic pain population of 361 rheumatoid arthritic patients and identified two main groups through factor analysis. One group was identified as active copers and the other as passive copers. The Passive Coping Scale was "correlated with reports of greater depression, greater pain and flare-up activity, greater functional impairment, and lower general self-efficacy" (Brown, Nicassio, 1987, p. 53). The Passive Coping Scale assessed strategies such as wish-fulfilling thoughts, restricting activities, and depending on others for help.

Conversely, coping strategies are also related to positive pain management outcomes. Keefe, Caldwell, Queen et al. (1987) investigated the pain-coping strategies used by a population of osteoarthritic patients as measured by the Coping Strategies Questionnaire (CSQ). Pain Control and Rational Thinking coping strategies were related to lower reported levels of pain, increased health status, and decreased psychologic distress. Turner and Clancy (1986) in a study involving 74 patients with low back pain found that increased use of praying and hoping strategies decreased pain intensity. Decreased catastrophizing was also related to decreased pain intensity and decreases in physical and psychosocial impairment.

In conclusion, effective coping strategies associated with improved outcomes are those that impart a sense of control (e.g., rational thinking and pain control) (Keefe, Caldwell, Queen et al., 1987), those associated with distraction (e.g., praying and hoping strategies), or those that decrease catastrophizing (Turner, Clancy, 1986). It is also suggested that successful outcomes may not be related to specific strategies but to how often strategies are used in nonpain states. Strategies may be effective because they interfere with catastrophizing (Turner, Clancy, 1986).

Coping strategies that are maladaptive, such as negative thoughts and catastrophizing, can be targeted for change. Patients can be given tools to identify their negative, catastrophizing thoughts that make them feel sad, frustrated, or angry. Techniques such as "thought stopping" (Davis, Eshelman, McKay, 1988) or refuting negative beliefs can be taught (Ellis, Harper, 1978). In thought stopping a patient is taught to replace a negative or unproductive thought with a quick, positive response designed to stop the thought, such as "I can cope with this pain, I have before" or "I am relaxed, I can manage."

In an ABCD model of refuting irrational ideas (Ellis, Harper, 1978), the patient is encouraged to confront his or her negative thoughts and change them. This is done by listing the activating event, describing beliefs about the event, listing consequences or feelings attached to the original beliefs, and then disputing the negative thinking with new thoughts that are positive or neutral and healthier.

Patient Example

Mr. E., who has chronic low back pain, has been working with his therapist to stay active and pace activities. His tendency in the past has been to lie down as soon as his back is stressed or hurting. At the beginning of his treatment he was only getting out of bed to eat, go to doctor appointments, and go to the bathroom. He has worked with his therapist to decrease some of the catastrophizing thoughts he has about his pain when he hurts, and he has learned different ways of viewing painful incidents so he can maintain a healthier functioning level.

A. **Activating event:** (Ask the patient to write down the facts of the event.)
   "I twisted and hurt my back picking up a book from the floor."

B. **Belief:** (Ask the patient to write down his beliefs about the event. This can include subjective assumptions, values, or worries.)
   "I can't live with this pain. I don't deserve this."
   "I'm so stupid for getting out of bed; now I've really injured my back."
   "I'll never be able to do things I like to do; I'll be bed-bound by the time I'm 40."

C. **Consequence:** (Have the patient focus on his emotional response.)
   "I feel bad about myself. I feel depressed and hopeless about my situation."

D. **Dispute:** (Help the patient challenge and change his beliefs about the initial event by substituting alternative ideas.)
   1. Write down the faulty or irrational belief.
      "I can't live with this pain. I don't deserve this."
   2. Is there support for this belief?
      No.
   3. What supports that this is a faulty belief?
      "I live every day with pain; some days are better than others. Life is not fair. Some events of living may be pleasurable; others may be painful."
   4. Is there any evidence that supports the original belief?

"No, only that I've made myself feel hopeless about my situation."

5. What is the worst that can happen in this situation?

"My pain can get worse. I may end up taking extra pain medication. I may end up lying down."

6. What are the good things that might happen?

"I might try some of the relaxation techniques, stretch exercises, or some ice. I might try managing my pain without going to bed. I might feel like I had more control, and I could do more if I didn't go to bed."

E. The alternative thoughts and emotions can then be listed.

"I can do some things to try to decrease my pain. If I don't go to bed, I can talk to a friend. I'm disappointed that I hurt, but I can manage."

This sequence of steps has workbook techniques as its basis (Davis, Eshelman, McKay, 1988) and can be repeated with each one of the negative or catastrophizing thoughts, teaching the patient different ways of looking at and responding to negative and catastrophizing thoughts.

Physical Rehabilitation

Functional activities

Patients with CNP should be assessed for physical deconditioning and disuse, poor posture, or abnormal gait. Poor physical functioning may be due to activity restrictions and muscle splinting or guarding. Splinting frequently occurs as a protective reaction to safeguard a previously injured area, a spasming muscle, or a painful area. Restrictions on activities may be self-initiated by patients because of their increased pain with activities or because of their fears of reinjury. Inappropriate restrictions also may have been recommended previously by well-meaning professionals (e.g., bedrest or prescribed time off of work for a strained back). Guidelines for acute low back problems (Bigos, Bowyer, Braen et al., 1994) support 2 to 4 days of bedrest for severe radiculopathy; however, bedrest lasting longer than 4 days is not recommended.

Patients with CNP who restrict their activities can also end up isolated and removed from socially gratifying situations. This in combination with loneliness can contribute to depression. Narrowly confined activities such as lying in bed, on a recliner, or on a couch most of the day can lead to napping, interrupted circadian cycles, and sleep disturbances. Patients with limited activities do not have the natural benefits of exercise such as muscle tone, weight control, and higher endorphin levels with aerobic activity; the added aches and pains from muscle disuse can make pain management even more difficult.

Some clinicians recommend that physical agents be considered as first-line treatments in managing patients with pain (Vasudevan, 1997). Therapeutic exercises are the most important part of physical rehabilitation. Stretching and strengthening exercises may improve poor posture that contributes to pain, increase range of motion and flexibility, and strengthen muscles, thereby preventing reinjury to an area. Aerobic exercise increases general cardiovascular conditioning. Proper exercise increases patients' physical capabilities and functioning, reduces their pain, and increases their endurance. Range of motion exercises and stretch exercises can be done at home. An application of heat and use of a relaxation technique before the exercises may make them easier to do. Specific strengthening exercises can be taught by a physical therapist for home use, too, and aerobic exercises can be done by engaging in low-impact activities such as mall walking, bicycle riding, or swimming. Pacing activities may be helpful for patients who have an exacerbation of their chronic pain with activity (Box 11.10).

Physical rehabilitation interventions may also include heat, cold (see Chapter 9), TENS units, or other electrical devices. A physical therapist can teach the patient ice massage, which may be particularly helpful in numbing trigger points to aid in stretching muscles. Supportive orthotics such as braces, corsets, and splints may be helpful in specific cases such as footdrop, but evaluation for their use must be done by a therapist knowledgeable about chronic conditions. The goal is to increase functioning by increasing and improving activities.

Other rehabilitative treatment may involve traction or manual techniques such as mobilization, massage, or manipulation. Massage can be taught to patients and family members and used at home. Different types of massage can decrease edema, break down intramuscular adhesions, and reduce stiffness and pain. Massage can be helpful in managing myofascial trigger points. Mobilization techniques such as myofascial release are done by trained professionals such as physical or occupational therapists. Family members can be taught massage or simple myofascial release techniques. Manipulation, however, is done by professionals such as osteopathic physicians, chiropractors, or physical therapists, not family.

An extensive review of physical therapy and physical modalities for the control of chronic musculoskeletal pain (Feine, Lund, 1997) concludes that patient symptoms improve during treatment with most forms of physical therapy. Although little evidence exists thus far that any specific therapy has long-term benefits greater than placebo, this is probably due to the lack of scientific studies and should not be interpreted to mean that no long-term benefits are possible.

Treatment was always found to be better than no treatment, and the group that received the most physical therapy treatments seemed to do the best. Allegrante

● ● ● ● ●

| BOX 11.10 | **Patient Information: Pace Yourself** |

To: _____ (Patient's name)   Date: _____

What is pacing? It is doing things throughout the day for periods of time that do not make your pain worse. Many people with chronic pain push or force themselves for a day or so, and then end up with much worse pain and are unable to do much for several days. Pacing is the opposite of this. The purpose of pacing is to make it possible for you to be active every day. Pacing and the big push are compared below.

Pacing: Take a break before you need it.

Benefits:
1. Pain stays manageable.
2. Able to maintain a certain level of activity day after day. No need to take time off.
3. Every day you are able to accomplish something you want or need to do.

Big Push: Force yourself.

Results:
1. Pain increases significantly. Medication intake increases. Irritability increases.
2. Must take time off to recover. Recovery may be slow and depressing.
3. You accomplish your goal, but while you are recovering, you cannot do much at all.

By trial and error you can find out what you can do and for how long without your pain increasing or returning. For example, you may find that you can work at a certain activity for 30-minute periods, taking off 5 minutes every half hour. Setting a timer helps you remember. At the end of the day you may discover that you have worked productively for a total of 5 hours without increasing your pain. However, if you had pushed yourself to work 3 hours straight without a break, you might have increased pain and gotten less done and ended up spending time in bed.

From: _____ (Clinician's name)

Phone: _____

(1996) also found that interventions that combine exercise with patient education regarding the cause of pain and training in coping skills, such as relaxation and distraction, result in overall improvements in pain outcomes that include functional gains.

Social and work roles

Physical or mental activity is important for all patients who must cope with pain daily, but it seems especially important for the depressed patient (consider using Box 11.11 as a guide). Help the patient develop his or her own daily commitment to specific activities, such as physical and/or social, especially a return to employment of any type.

A return to some level of employment is helpful in many ways, ranging from earning money to increasing feelings of worthiness; however, this is not always appropriate. The patient may be far too disabled to return to his former employment, and reeducation for a new job may not be feasible. The patient may have been retired from work for some years and have no desire to return, or the female patient may never have worked outside the home. Volunteer work is an alternative and may increase feelings of being capable and adequate because of making some contribution to others.

Support is an important factor in improving activities. In a study of 181 patients with chronic pain, those who had supportive families reported significantly reduced pain intensity, less reliance on medications, and more activity than those who had nonsupportive families (Jamison, Verts, 1990). Two studies also demonstrate that one socially supportive phone call a month made by lay personnel can help reduce pain and improve functional status (Rene, Weinberger, Mazzuca et al., 1992; Weinberger, Tierney, Booker et al., 1989).

Long-Term Planning and Measuring Outcomes

Discharge from hospital

When patients with CNP are discharged from an acute care setting, plan ahead for outpatient follow-up. Within the constraints of time, try the following:

- About 24 hours before discharge, make a list of all pain relief measures used during this hospitalization, such as analgesics and muscle relaxants, noninvasive pain relief measures, and PT. Involve the physical therapist, if possible, or at least obtain specific information about what was done and what exercises are recommended now.
- Review this list with the patient and ask for any additions.
- On the basis of the patient's answers, identify with the patient what seems to be a logical plan of treatment on return. Findings may suggest a revision of the previous plan. For example, if the patient had both opioids and nonopioids ordered but they were never given together, the future plan may be to try this combination.
- Integrate this plan with medications, exercises, and any other approaches for pain control after discharge.

Box 11.12 may be copied and used for this purpose. This form may be completed by both patient and nurse. One copy is given to the patient and another kept in the patient's record by the agency or facility treating the patient.

Outpatient follow-up

Whether the discharge recommendations involve medication adjustments, relaxation, PT, or some other specialized approach, make specific plans for an outpatient appointment with a practitioner who will be managing the pain. Ask the patient to take the plan to the practitioner.

If a period of days or weeks goes by, the patient is likely to have difficulty remembering exactly what happened in relation to pain. Memory may be adversely affected by many factors, such as pain, medications, and a desire to forget or deny how severe the pain has been. In the outpatient setting a standard pain scale should be used to evaluate pain at each contact. When the patient is unable to give a specific or complete history of pain and its management, a daily diary may be indicated.

Assessing the results of treatment with each outpatient visit allows comparisons for improvements in care. Not only is it important to assess an individual's response to treatment, but the argument has been made that it is also essential to assess the quality of your practice. Box 11.13, *A, B, C,* is an example of a simple tool that can assess individual patient visits and the population's response to treatment.

ADVANCED PAIN MANAGEMENT TECHNIQUES

Choices in the management of CNP are made on a continuum from less invasive to more aggressive treatments. Patients are typically started with nonopioid medications and PT for reconditioning. Adjuvant medications are added on the basis of their appropriateness for the pain symptoms. Cognitive behavioral therapies and relaxation techniques are taught to enhance coping skills.

The patient may also be considered for nerve block therapy for either diagnostic or therapeutic indications. (Table 11.2 lists pain blocks that reduce pain.) Trigger point and epidural steroid injections are the most frequent types of pain blocks done for people with CNP. However, recent guidelines on acute low back problems

Text continued on p. 510.

● ● ● ● ●

BOX 11.11   Patient Information: Overall Daily Plan

To: _____ (Patient's name)   Date: _____

As a general rule, keep your pain under control by using your approaches to coping with pain before you really need them. Plan a daily schedule that includes each of the following to some extent in some way. Keep your pain under control. Do not wait until your pain is severe before you use something like relaxation, coping skills, short rest periods, ice or heat packs, realistic goal setting, or medication.

1. **Pacing:** Plan short periods of rest before your pain increases and before you get tired.
2. **Exercises:** One to two times per day, perform exercises that are appropriate for you. You may need advice from a physical therapist. The main purposes of the exercises are as follows:
   - Stretch muscles to reduce soreness and muscle spasm
   - Strengthen muscles
   - Increase range of motion and flexibility, reduce stiffness
   - General physical fitness (this helps avoid further injury)
   - Increase ability to perform other activities; increase aerobic activity to stimulate natural endorphins
3. **Relaxation:** Allow yourself to relax completely at intervals throughout your day. Practice at least one longer period of 10-15 minutes of relaxation once a day. You may use a relaxation tape, prayer, listening to music, or anything else that brings you peace of mind and contentment. Pain is stressful and frustrating, so you need to give yourself a real break from stress by truly relaxing. Just sitting down and watching TV is not really profound relaxation. You may want to ask your nurse about short relaxation techniques such as deep breathing and body scanning for muscle tension that you can use throughout your day. You may want to get relaxation tapes or receive instruction on longer techniques. Relaxation is a way to recharge yourself. Afterward you will feel more energetic and more able to think clearly.
4. **Coping techniques:** Passively accepting, or worse yet, catastrophizing about your pain problem will only increase your sense of helplessness, depression, and stress. Use coping techniques that will distract you, stop catastrophizing thoughts, and refute negative ideas. Remember, if you do a healthy activity, you stand a greater chance of feeling a sense of control and hope than if you simply give up.
5. **Nondrug methods:** Other things to consider are cold and/or heating packs, 15 minutes on, then off. You can use either one or the other, or you can alternate between cold and heat. Try massage and acupressure. If you go to a massage therapist, see one who is certified and inform him or her of your chronic pain problems. Consider signing up for lessons on massage techniques with your spouse. This has the potential to be fun, and you can each benefit from exchanging massages. Use humor or some interesting activity for distraction. Try a TENS unit.
6. **Plan and set realistic goals:** Set goals that are realistic—if you have been inactive, do not start exercising by walking a mile. Walk your usual distance, then gradually increase the distance a small amount each day, such as one block longer. Make plans that allow you to pace yourself or to leave early from planned events if needed. Allow your family to stay active and attend an event or a planned activity without you.
7. **Medications:** Medications for pain should be taken regularly by the clock or at least before pain begins or increases.
8. **Things to do every day:** Do something every day that involves the following three things:
   - Work (for wages, volunteer work, or study). Do activities you are capable of.
   - Contact family or close friends. Be sure you hug somebody or give back positive feelings.
   - Fun. Be sure you laugh.

From: _____ (Clinician's name)

Phone: _____

● ● ● ● ●

| BOX 11.12 | **Patient Information: Planning for the Future—Review of Pain Relief Measures** |

To: _____ (Patient's name)   Date: _____

Purpose: To use the information available from a recent episode of pain to plan the best possible pain relief for any future occurrence of similar pain. This is accomplished by identifying the effect of pain relief measures used for a recent episode of pain.

Nature of pain: _____ From (date): _____ to _____.

Medications used in relation to problem of pain (e.g., opioid and nonopioid analgesics, antidepressants, anticonvulsants, other adjuvants, and/or muscle relaxants):

Medication name, dose, frequency: Helpful? Other comments:

Nonpharmacologic (nondrug) pain relief measures (e.g., relaxation, distraction, TENS, ice, heat, and/or stretch exercises):

Method, frequency: Helpful? Other comments:

Summary of what did help: **Summary of what did not help:**

Plans for pain relief if situation occurs again (e.g., at home, follow-up outpatient visit, readmit to hospital, or return to emergency department):

Plans for pain relief at home or in immediate future, if applicable:

From: _____ (Clinician's name)

Phone: _____

May be duplicated for use in clinical practice. From McCaffery M, Pasero C: *Pain: Clinical manual*, p. 507. Copyright © 1999, Mosby, Inc.

●●●●●

BOX 11.13A **Example of Survey Tool for Return Visits to Pain Management Program**

SURVEY: RETURN VISIT

1. Which practitioners do you currently see at the Pain Therapy Center?

    _____

    _____

2. Have you seen practitioners other than those at the Pain Therapy Center for your pain problem since your last visit?   Yes _____   No _____

3. What was your level of pain on your first visit here?

    0 1 2 3 4 5 6 7 8 9 10

4. How would you currently rate your level of pain?

    0 1 2 3 4 5 6 7 8 9 10

5. What would be an acceptable level of pain for you to attain?

    0 1 2 3 4 5 6 7 8 9 10

6. Have you experienced any additional stressors that could influence your level of pain?   Yes ____   No ____

7. If you answered "yes," please describe: _____

    _____

    _____

8. Since your initial visit to the Pain Therapy Center, how would you rate the following?

	Improved	No Change	Worse
Pain level			
Ability to manage pain and related problems			
Sleep			
Relationships with others			
Ability to do housework or job			
Mood			

May be duplicated for use in clinical practice. As appears in McCaffery M, Pasero C: *Pain: Clinical manual*, p. 508, 1999, Mosby, Inc.
Courtesy St. John's Mercy Pain Therapy Center, St. Louis, 1998.

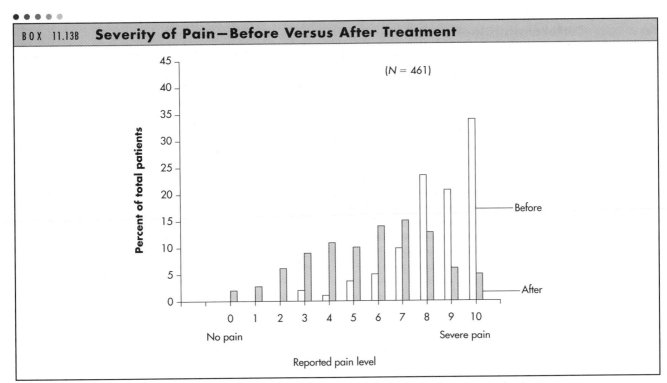

BOX 11.13B **Severity of Pain—Before Versus After Treatment**

May be duplicated for use in clinical practice. As appears in McCaffery M, Pasero C: *Pain: Clinical manual*, p. 509, 1999, Mosby, Inc.

Boxes 11.13B., C. Example of results from survey tool.

Box 11.13.B. Before initial visit, white bar; after, return visit, blue bar. In a convenience sample of 461 patients who filled out the survey, it can be deduced that pain levels did decrease for some. Thirty-four percent of patients rated their pain as a 10 on a scale of 0-10 at their initial visit. Only 5% rated pain at the "10 level" at return visits. There is a general downward shifting of pain levels from the 8-10 level to lower levels.

Courtesy St. John's Mercy Pain Therapy Center, St. Louis, 1998.

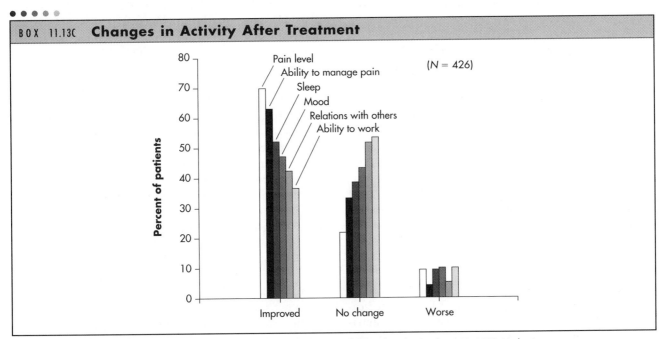

BOX 11.13C **Changes in Activity After Treatment**

May be duplicated for use in clinical practice. As appears in McCaffery M, Pasero C: *Pain: Clinical manual*, p. 509, 1999, Mosby, Inc.

Box 11.13.C. Improvements occurred for many patients who completed the survey. The most dramatic improvements were in pain levels (70% improved) and the ability to manage pain (64% improved). Surveys over time at this center have shown between 5% and 10% of people returning for treatment indicate that they are "worse" on some of the measures. It is not known why this is so. A focused group session with practitioners and patients suggested that new stressors may be an intervening factor in pain levels and managing pain. An open-ended question is now asked about stressors that influence pain levels (see questions 6 and 7 in Box 11.13 **A**). So far, a little greater than 30% of patients state that they have stressors that influence pain levels. Currently topics for patient education classes are planned to focus on stressors commonly listed by patients.

Courtesy St. John's Mercy Pain Therapy Center, St. Louis, 1998.

● ● ● ● ●

TABLE 11.2 **Differential Blocks**

PAIN SITES	TYPE OF BLOCK REDUCING PAIN	PATHOPHYSIOLOGY OF PAIN
Head and neck pain	Upper and middle cervical ganglion block Deep and superficial cervical plexus block Peripheral somatic nerve block Trigger point injections to individual muscles in head and neck	Sympathetic-mediated pain Somatic nerve–mediated pain Somatic nerve–mediated pain Myofascial pain
Upper extremities	Stellate block Brachial plexus block	Sympathetic-mediated pain Somatic nerve–mediated pain
Thoracic pain	Intercostal nerve block Thoracic epidural with sensory block Thoracic epidural sympathetic block	Somatic nerve–mediated pain Somatic nerve–mediated pain Sympathetic-mediated pain
Abdominal pain	Intercostal nerve block (T10-12) Celiac plexus block	Abdominal wall pain Abdominal visceral pain
Pelvic and perianal pain	Intrathecal/epidural somatic block Presacral plexus block	Somatic nerve–mediated pain Sympathetic/visceral pain
Lower extremities	Lumbar epidural/intrathecal block Paravertebral somatic nerve block Lumbar sympathetic block	Somatic nerve–mediated pain Somatic nerve–mediated pain Sympathetic-mediated pain

May be duplicated for use in clinical practice. As appears in McCaffery M, Pasero C: *Pain: Clinical manual*, p. 510, 1999, Mosby, Inc.
Modified from Ferrer-Brechner T: Regional anesthesia: Local anesthetics and neurolytic agents. In Raj PP: *Practical management of pain*, ed 2, p 471, St. Louis, 1992, Mosby.

(Bigos, Bowyer, Braen et al., 1994) and a current study (Carette, Legiaire, Marcoux et al., 1997) indicate that benefits to receiving epidural steroid injections for back pain or sciatica may be questionable. A randomized, double-blind trial (Carette, Legiaire, Marcoux et al., 1997) of 158 patients with sciatica caused by a herniated nucleus pulposus was conducted with half the patients receiving three injections of epidural methylprednisolone and the other half receiving three injections of epidural saline. The epidural steroid injections offered some short-term improvements in leg pain and sensory deficits; however, they did not offer significant functional improvement, and they did not reduce the need for back surgery. Again, assessment and documentation of patients' outcomes are essential. Form 11.3, *A,* is an example of a form for documenting during a procedure, and Form 11.3, *B,* provides a patient example. Pain records not only result in better pain relief (Faries, Mills, Goldsmith et al., 1991), but they can also compile information about outcomes that is useful for future comparisons of pain relief efforts.

When adequate sequential trials of medications are done with NSAIDs and appropriate adjuvant medications (see Chapters 5 and 7, respectively) and combination medication therapies are not helpful, opioid analgesia may be considered for patients who are appropriate candidates and who meet the criteria (see Box 11.9).

Sometimes despite these aggressive methods, the patient's pain may remain uncontrolled or aversive side effects may occur. After all reasonable and available non-pharmacologic and pharmacologic techniques are tried, the patient may be a candidate for invasive procedures such as spinal cord stimulators (North, 1997) or implantable spinal infusions (Krames, 1996). These are therapies of last resort and are done only before neuroablative and neurodestructive procedures are considered.

What types of pain syndromes would be appropriate for neurostimulator or implantable spinal infusion therapies? As described by Krames (1996), nociceptive pain is produced by damage to the body and is usually responsive to opioids. Neuropathic pain, on the other hand, is produced by damaged or pathologically changed central or peripheral nerve mechanisms. Neuropathic pain is not as responsive to opioids; however, it appears to be responsive to some of the newer therapies under investigation for spinal administration (e.g., medications such as alpha$_2$-adrenergic agonists, somatostatin, and NMDA receptor antagonists) (Krames, 1996).

Neuropathic pain from failed back syndrome has been the most common indication for spinal cord stimulation (North, Campbell, Names et al., 1991); however, there are other indications such as peripheral vascular disease, angina pectoris, spinal cord–injured patients with segmental pain, postamputation syndromes, and peripheral nerve injuries, neuralgia, causalgia, and reflex sympathetic dystrophy (North, 1997). Krames (1996) recommends that spinal cord stimulation be tried before spinal infusion because it has been used longer, it is considered

FORM 11.3A **Anesthesia Nerve Block Record**

Date

			Sex	Age		Location of pain or trigger points
Patient Name						
Patient No.	Anesthesiologist					
Diagnosis			Code			
Procedure			Code			

Time

Oxygen ___ L/min

Totals

Propofol (mg)

Versed (mg)

100	200
% O₂ SAT	
90	180
80	160	IV site

☐ RT   ☐ LT

Gauge

BP < >	140
HR •	
R o	120
Tourniquet ↑	
Tourniquet ↓	100

Position

☐ Supine
☐ Sitting
☐ Prone
☐ Lateral

Pressure ___	80
Location ___	
O₂ SAT ____	
	60

Prep Sol

☐ Betadine
☐ Alcohol

	40
	20
	10
	0

Symbols		Total Fluids
LR		
D₅LR		

Medications

	Amount		Route	Location	Needle type	Size
Marcaine	%	ml	☐ Epidural	Level	☐ Crawford	☐ 18-gauge
Lidocaine	%	ml	☐ Intrathecal	Level	☐ Touhey Schiff	☐ 22-gauge
Depo-Medrol	mg	ml	☐ Trigger point		☐ Regional	☐ 3" ☐ 5"
Triamcinolone	%	ml	☐ Intercostal	Level	☐ Spinal	
Phenol	%	ml	☐ Stellate	☐ RT ☐ LT	☐ Other	
Alcohol	%	ml	☐ Brachial plexus		☐ RT ☐ LT	
Other	%	ml	☐ Sympathetic	Level		
Local infiltration			☐ Other			

	Amount		Size of needle			
Marcaine	%	ml	☐ 27-gauge			
Lidocaine	%	ml	☐ 30-gauge			

Nurse's Notes	Discharge Orders
	Discharge when VS stable, the patient is ambulatory, and drinking liquids.
	Give instruction sheet to patient.
	Photocopy of prescription

Signature   RN   Signature   MD

May be duplicated for use in clinical practice. As appears in McCaffery M, Pasero C: *Pain: Clinical manual*, p. 511, 1999, Mosby, Inc.
Courtesy St. John's Mercy Pain Therapy Center, St. Louis, 1998.

FORM 11.3B Patient Example of Anesthesia Nerve Block Record

Date 1-14-98

Patient Name Stella Snow		Sex f	Age 47

Patient No. 4922701-1	Anesthesiologist	

Diagnosis Lumbar spinal stenosis	Code

Procedure Lumbar epidural steroid injection	Code

Location of pain or trigger points

Time		10^{00}	10^{10}	10^{12}	10^{22}			
Oxygen ____ L/min								

Totals

Propofol (mg)	
Versed (mg)	

100	200	98%	98%	98%	97%	
% O₂ SAT						
90	180					
80	160					

IV site
☐ RT   ☐ LT
Gauge

BP <>	140
HR •	
R o	120
Tourniquet ↑	
Tourniquet ↓	100
Pressure ____	
Location ____	80
O₂ SAT ----	
	60

Position
☐ Supine
☐ Sitting
☐ Prone
☒ Lateral R
Side down
Prep Sol
☒ Betadine
☐ Alcohol

98.1

Pain Ratings

	40
	20
	10
	0

3/10   4/10

npo 8°
Steady gait
Driver here

Symbols	Pre	Post	Total Fluids
LR			
D₅LR			

Medications

	Amount		Route	Location	Needle type	Size
Marcaine	%	ml	☒ Epidural	Level Lumbar	☐ Crawford	☒ 18-gauge
Lidocaine	%	ml	☐ Intrathecal	Level	☒ Tuohy	☐ 22-gauge
Depo-Medrol	120 mg	1½ ml	☐ Trigger point		☐ Regional	☒ 3" ☐ 5"
Triamcinolone	%	ml	☐ Intercostal	Level	☐ Spinal	
Phenol	%	ml	☐ Stellate	☐ RT ☐ LT	☐ Other	
Alcohol	%	ml	☐ Brachial plexus		☐ RT ☐ LT	
Other Saline	0.9%	7 ml	☐ Sympathetic	Level		
Local infiltration			☐ Other			

	Amount		Size of needle			
Marcaine	%	ml	☒ 27-gauge			
Lidocaine	1%	3 ml	☐ 30-gauge			

Nurse's Notes

10^{00} Permit signed and monitors placed.

10^{12} Tolerated procedure well.

10^{15} Repositioned and given juice.

10^{30} Instructions given.

10^{35} Discharged ambulating well.

Discharge Orders

Discharge when VS stable, the patient is ambulatory, and drinking liquids.

Give instruction sheet to patient.

*Photocopy of prescription

Signature Wools LaVelle, CCRN   RN   Signature H Brey   MD reversible, and the long-term effects of spinal infusions are not known.

Clinicians (Krames, 1996; North, 1997) are in agreement that before implanting devices the following conditions should be met: the patient should be psychologically screened as appropriate for the procedure, other conservative therapies have failed, no further surgery is indicated, and no contraindications to implantations exist. A trial of the chosen implantable device should be successful before permanent placement is done, and clinicians with the expertise to manage them must be available afterward.

It has also been demonstrated that although they have expensive up-front fees, the intrathecal devices can save costs over other treatments for cancer patients at 3 months and for patients with CNP at 22 months (Hassenbusch, Paice, Patt et al., 1997). The cost-effectiveness of spinal cord stimulation in the treatment of patients with failed back syndrome pays for itself in 2.2 years in those individuals in which it is successful by reducing the demand for medical care. Factoring costs in all cases, both successful and unsuccessful, the therapy pays for itself in 5.5 years (Bell, Kidd, North, 1997).

REFERRAL TO A PAIN MANAGEMENT PROGRAM

A specialized program in pain management is not necessary for every person with CNP. However, when pain becomes the central feature of a person's life, some type of special help is indicated. Effective treatment and management may be offered by a concerned and knowledgeable health care professional. Sometimes the primary care physician can do this in conjunction with appropriate consultations and referrals. The more disabled patients are by their pain problems, however, the more likely they are to need a referral to a comprehensive pain management center or clinic.

Pain management programs are extremely varied. At present, there is no comprehensive listing of such programs, and no group or agency is empowered to license or accredit all pain programs. There are some credentialing mechanisms for physicians in pain medicine through the American Academy of Pain Medicine and the American Board of Anesthesiology, but at present no credentialing mechanisms are available for other disciplines in pain management practice. Determining the need for a pain program and finding qualified professionals is a complicated matter. General information about pain programs can be obtained from the American Pain Society (p. 516) and the Commission on Accreditation of Rehabilitative Facilities (CARF, 1995) (p. 517), from which pain programs may voluntarily request and pay for certification.

One way to distinguish between the various types of pain programs is to ask the following four questions:

1. What types of pain are treated? Some pain programs treat only certain types of patients, such as those with cancer, headache, neck and spine problems, or arthritis.

2. How are services offered? Some pain programs offer services on an individual level, possibly with some group involvement, such as group therapy. Others have a rather structured program in which the patient is treated in a group of patients and receives some individual attention. Most programs are outpatient based. Some programs may be structured to involve specific blocks of time, such as 2 to 6 weeks, during which the patient, and usually the family, is intensively involved in the program.

3. Which services are offered? Some programs offer only a few treatment approaches, whereas others offer a wide variety of strategies. The restricted ones are sometimes referred to as modality oriented and may mainly offer BF for relaxation or stress reduction, TENS, acupuncture, or nerve blocks. The more comprehensive programs are referred to as multidisciplinary (Box 11.14). A services checklist is provided in Box 11.15.

4. What type of follow-up is offered by the program? Do the staff communicate with the primary care physician, other health care professionals, or an ED about the pain management plan or adjustments to that plan, if needed? What type of coverage is offered for after-hours services? Is follow-up care provided after the completion of a time-limited program?

Text continued on p. 516.

● ● ● ● ●

| BOX 11.14 | **International Association for the Study of Pain Classifications of Pain Facilities** |

MULTIDISCIPLINARY PAIN CENTER

- This is the largest, most complex organization and is composed of health care professionals and basic scientists who do research and teach about the care of acute and chronic pain. Typically it is a component of a medical school or a teaching hospital, and the clinical programs are supervised by an appropriately trained and licensed clinical director. If the clinical director is not a physician, a director of medical services should be responsible for monitoring medical services.
- Pain services are integrated and based on interdisciplinary assessment and management, with regular communication between practitioners about individual patients and programs.
- It offers both inpatient and outpatient programs.
- A wide array of specialists are required, and at least three medical specialties must be a part of the staff. If one of the physicians is not a psychiatrist, the minimum required are two physicians from different specialties and a clinical psychologist. Other essential staff include nurses; social workers; and physical, occupational, or vocational therapists.

MULTIDISCIPLINARY PAIN CLINIC

- This facility specializes in multidisciplinary diagnosis and treatment of patients with chronic pain. It does not include research and teaching facilities. The clinical programs must be supervised by an appropriately trained and licensed clinical director with similar requirements as those of the director of the multidisciplinary pain center.
- It may have diagnostic and treatment facilities that are inpatient, outpatient, or both.
- Pain services are integrated and based on interdisciplinary assessment and management, with regular communication between practitioners about individual patients and programs.
- It is also staffed by physicians of different specialties and other health care practitioners, similar to a multidisciplinary pain center.

PAIN CLINIC

- This facility focuses on diagnosis and management of patients with chronic pain and may specialize in diagnoses or pain management related to a specific region of the body, such as low back pain or headache.
- The practitioners do not provide interdisciplinary assessment or treatment.
- An isolated, solo practitioner could never call his or her practice a pain clinic; however, a single physician functioning within a complex health care institution that offers appropriate consultative and therapeutic services would qualify.

MODALITY-ORIENTED CLINIC

- This facility provides a specific type of treatment, such as nerve blocks, transcutaneous electrical nerve stimulation, acupuncture, or biofeedback.
- The practitioners do not provide a comprehensive assessment or an integrated, comprehensive approach to treatment.
- There may be one or more health care providers with different professional training backgrounds.

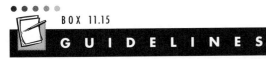

BOX 11.15

G U I D E L I N E S

GATHERING INFORMATION ABOUT A PAIN MANAGEMENT PROGRAM

Program name: _____ Telephone: _____

Address: _____

General Information

Name of person giving initial information about the program (e.g., the person on the telephone): _____

Date: _____

Director of program: _____

Other staff members met or talked with: _____

Specific Questions

1. What types of pain problems are treated? (Describe the pain problem and ask if it is treated here; if not, do they have a recommendation?)
2. What are the training and subspecialties of the practitioners you will see? (e.g., neurologist, anesthesiologist, psychiatrist, physiatrist, nurse practitioner)
3. How are services offered? (e.g., individual appointments, in groups, inpatient, outpatient, structured, specific period of time such as a 2-week program)
4. Which services are offered? For convenience, the following may be used as a checklist (probably not all will be included, and some may not be desired):
   ____ Thorough initial assessment to determine need for further medical or surgical approaches.
   ____ Team of health professionals (i.e., more than one person available as needed, e.g., physician, physical therapist, psychologist, nurses).
   ____ Medication adjustments, tapering. (If so, which drugs? _____)
   ____ Nerve block services.
   ____ Physical therapy. (How often? _____ Hours/day? _____ Therapeutic pool? _____ Written exercise program? _____)
   ____ TENS (transcutaneous electrical nerve stimulation).
   ____ Massage therapy, acupressure.
   ____ Acupuncture.
   ____ Relaxation skills training. (Biofeedback? _____)
   ____ Individual psychotherapy or counseling.
   ____ Family group therapy or counseling. (When? _____)
   ____ Educational groups. (Coping skills training _____ , assertiveness training _____ , anger management _____ , stress management _____ , goal setting _____ , other _____)
   ____ Recreational therapy. (Types _____)
   ____ Occupational therapy. (Types _____)
   ____ Vocational counseling. (Training? _____)
   ____ Nutritional counseling. (Weight loss required? _____)
   ____ Expressive therapies. (e.g., art, dance, music)
   ____ Support groups.
   ____ Follow-up care after completion of program. (By whom? _____ How often? _____ Alumni group? _____)
   ____ Mechanisms for working with those involved or affected by participation in the program (e.g., present physician, worker's compensation case worker).
5. What are the goals or benefits for the patient who completes the program? (e.g., Are the goals the same for every patient? Are the goals established by the program or by the individual patient? Are these goals congruent with your goals? Is tapering required?)
6. Exactly what is expected of persons who participate in the program? (e.g., participation in certain activities or all activities, hospitalization, weekly appointments, no smoking, special diet)
7. Exactly what is expected of the patient's family? (e.g., accompany patient on the initial visit, weekly therapy)
8. What are other sources of information about the program?
   ____ Brochures, videotapes.
   ____ Names and telephone numbers of "graduates" of the program who may be contacted.
   ____ Journals or magazines with articles about the program or articles written by health team members who staff the program.
9. How long has the program been in operation? Especially if the program is new, ask what other programs the director and staff have been associated with.
10. Has the pain program been certified or accredited? (e.g., Commission of Accreditation of Rehabilitation Facilities (CARF), Joint Commission on Accreditation of Healthcare Organizations [JCAHO])
11. How much does the program cost? Are there incidental expenses? Does insurance or Medicare pay for any of this? Can you get an estimate for your third-party payment? What will be your out-of-pocket expenses?
12. What is the earliest date open for an initial appointment? If this is a structured group program, what is the earliest date the person could expect to be admitted?

CHRONIC NONMALIGNANT PAIN RESOURCES FOR PATIENTS/CLINICIANS

Following is a list of various resources that may be helpful to clinicians interested in CNP and to patients with CNP and their families. Resources related to selected CNP problems are also included in Chapter 12. To avoid duplication, they are not listed again here.

Organizations

- American Academy of Head, Facial and Neck Pain, and TMJ Orthopedics
  520 W. Pipeline Road
  Hurst, TX 76053
  (817) 282-1501
  Fax: (812) 282-8012
  Web site: www.aahnfp.org
  E-mail: central@aahnfp.org
  Provides information on the diagnosis and treatment of temporomandibular disorders and seeks specialty status for those professionals interested in the clinical treatment of head, neck, and face pain patients.

- American Academy of Physical Medicine and Rehabilitation
  One IBM Plaza, Suite 2500
  Chicago, IL 60611
  (312) 464-9700
  Fax: (312) 464-0227
  Web site: www.aapmr.org
  E-mail: aapmrl.aol.com
  Members are physiatrists (MDs and DOs). Its goal is to upgrade practice through seminars, workshops, and work studies.

- American Amputee Foundation (AAF)
  P.O. Box 250218
  Little Rock, AR 72225
  (501) 666-2523
  Fax: (501) 666-8367
  Members include amputees, professionals, and family members. It offers free information for adults and children on phantom limb pain and advice on self-help, support groups, and referrals. Membership includes *Active Living,* a quarterly magazine, and periodic updates. AAF funds the "give-a-limb" program, which provides prostheses to those who are uninsured and cannot afford the cost of a prosthetic device.

- American Board of Pain Medicine (ABPM)
  4700 W. Lake Avenue
  Glenview, IL 60025-1485
  Evaluates and certifies physicians as Diplomats in Pain Medicine. The ABPM seeks to improve the quality of graduate medical education in pain medicine by collaborating with related organizations. It also provides information about the specialty of pain medicine to the public.

- American Chiropractic Association
  1701 Clarendon Boulevard
  Arlington, VA 22209
  (703) 276-8880
  Information line: (800) 986-INFO
  Fax: (703) 243-2593
  Web site: http://www.amerchiro.org/shared/aboutaca.htm
  Members are chiropractors. The goal is to advance chiropractic standards of ethics and patient care for the profession. It is also active in education and research.

- American Chronic Pain Association (ACPA)
  P.O. Box 850
  Rocklin, CA 95677
  (916) 632-0922
  Fax: (916) 632-3208
  E-mail: ACPA@pacbell.net
  A self-help organization that provides individual and group support through local chapters offered nationwide. It offers an informational manual to help people with chronic pain and guidelines for what to look for in a pain clinic.

- American Counsel for Headache Education (ACHE)
  19 Mantua Road
  Mt. Royal, NJ 08061
  (609) 423-0258
  Fax: (609) 423-0082
  E-mail: achehq@ache.smarthub.com
  Web site: http://www.achenet.org/index.html
  ACHE is a national nonprofit patient/physician partnership that supports sufferers of chronic headaches while working to educate the public about this painful condition. Membership includes a quarterly newsletter, brochures, and other educational materials provided free or at a discount to ACHE members. ACHE sponsors support groups nationwide and a variety of information and support services online.

- American Foundation for Pain Research (AFPR) (Interstitial Cystitis)
  120 S. Spalding Dr., #210
  Beverly Hills, CA 90212
  (310) 274-6294
  Fax: NONE
  E-mail: NONE
  Web site: http://www.social.com/health/nhic/data/hr2300/hr2313.html
  AFPR's goal is to promote research into the field of interstitial cystitis and other women's urogynecologic diseases. It provides up-to-date information on interstitial cystitis and its treatment, and information on the psychologic and physiologic needs of patients. It also publishes a cookbook, *My Body, My Diet,* for interstitial cystitis and colitis patients.

- American Pain Society (APS)
  4700 W. Lake Avenue
  Glenview, IL 60025-1485
  (847) 375-4715
  Fax: (847) 375-4777
  E-mail: info@ampainsoc.org
  Web site: http://www.ampainsoc.org/
  An interdisciplinary professional organization that provides education, research support, and advocacy through lobbying and policies in pain management. The members come from fields such as anesthesiology, psychology, nursing, physical medicine and rehabilitation, neurology, neuro-

science, and dentistry. Membership includes a bimonthly newsletter, *APS Bulletin;* a quarterly journal, *Pain Forum;* the *Pain Facilities Directory* (which lists members' pain facilities); and discounts on publications and registration at the annual scientific meeting.

- American Society of Pain Management Nurses (ASPMN)
    7794 Grow Dr.
    Pensacola, FL 32514
    (850) 473-0233
    Fax: (850) 484-8762
    E-mail: *aspmn@aol.com*

    A professional organization for registered nurses interested in pain management education, advocacy, and research. Membership includes a quarterly newsletter, *Pathways;* a directory book of members with specialty backgrounds and networking interests; and discounts on publications and registrations at the annual meeting or regional meetings.

- Association for Applied Psychophysiology and Biofeedback (AAPB)
    10200 W. 44th Avenue, Suite 304
    Wheat Ridge, CO 80033-2840
    (800) 477-8892 or (303) 422-8436
    Fax: (303) 422-8894

    AAPB is an interdisciplinary organization that provides professional education and advocacy in biofeedback and other self-regulation therapies. Members come from the fields of psychology, psychiatry, medicine, dentistry, nursing, physical and occupational therapy, social work, education, counseling, and others. Information on biofeedback training and certification can be obtained from AAPB. Membership includes a quarterly newsmagazine, *Biofeedback;* a professional journal, *Biofeedback and Self-Regulation;* and access to their Web site.

- Commission on Accreditation of Rehabilitation Facilities (CARF)
    4891 E. Grant Road
    Tucson, AZ 85712
    (520) 325-1044
    Fax: (520) 318-1129
    E-mail: *webmaster@carf.org*
    Web site: *http://www.carf.org*

    CARF provides accreditation of pain services for facilities and hospitals that voluntarily request and pay for the services. It provides various types of information including a list of facilities that have CARF-accredited chronic pain programs and a booklet titled "Program Evaluation in Chronic Pain Management Programs."

- Crohn's & Colitis Foundation of America (CCFA)
    Research queries: *research@ccfa.org*
    Chapters: *chapters@ccfa.org*
    Educational material requests: *material@ccfa.org*
    Membership information: *member@ccfa.org*
    Web site: *http://www.ccfa.org*

    Has a free Web site that offers comprehensive information about inflammatory bowel disease. Offers news updates, current research, information about special events, support groups, and an "Ask the Specialist" database, listings of speakers bureau, and listing of brochures and books.

- Crohn's & Colitis Foundation of Canada
    Web site: *http://www.ccfa.ca/site.html*

- Interstitial Cystitis Association (ICA)
    P.O. Box 1553
    Madison Square Station
    New York, NY 10159
    (212) 979-6057
    Fax: NONE
    E-mail: NONE
    Web site: *http://www.ichelp.com/contents.htm*

    Offers information and support to interstitial cystitis patients and families and educates the medical community about interstitial cystitis. It also promotes research to find effective treatment and, ultimately, a cure for interstitial cystitis.

- National Institute of Arthritis, Musculoskeletal and Skin Diseases Information Clearinghouse (NAMSIC)
    National Institute of Health
    1 Ams Circle
    Bethesda, MD 20892-3675
    (301) 495-4484
    Fax: (301) 587-4352
    TTY: (301) 565-2966

    This is a government agency that disseminates information, locates sources, creates health information materials, and participates in a national federal database on health information.

- National Neurofibromatosis Foundation, Inc.
    95 Pine St., 16th Floor
    New York, NY 10005
    (800) 323-7938
    Fax: (212) 747-0004
    E-mail: *nnff@aol.com*
    Web site: *http://www.nf.org*

    Nonprofit medical foundation. Sponsors research aimed at finding effective treatment, provides patient support and public education, and raises funds for research and education.

- National Vulvodynia Association (NVA)
    P.O. Box 19288
    Sarasota, FL 34276-2288
    (941) 927-8503
    Fax: (941) 927-8602
    Web site: *http://www.ivf.com//nvabackg.html*

    Organization's purpose is to improve the lives of individuals affected by vulvodynia. It provides information to patients and health care professionals, and encourages the exchange of ideas and research. Membership includes quarterly newsletter, a vulvodynia bibliography, and names of other organizations that offer support for related disorders.

- North American Chronic Pain Association of Canada (NACPAC)
    150 Central Park Dr., Unit 105
    Brampton, Ontario L6T2T9
    (905) 793-5230
    Fax: (905) 793-8781
    (800) 616-PAIN
    E-mail: NONE
    Web site: *http://www3.sympatico.ca/nacpac/*

A self-help organization dedicated to supporting people who are in chronic pain. It provides numerous links to pain resources in the United States and Canada.

- Osteoporosis and Related Bone Diseases National Resource Center

    1150 17th St., N.W., Suite 500
    Washington, DC 20036-4603
    (202) 223-0344
    (800) 624-BONE
    Fax: (202) 223-2237

    Provides patients, families, and health care professionals with resources and information on metabolic bone diseases. Its mission is to expand awareness and enhance the knowledge and understanding of the prevention, early detection, and treatment of these diseases. It provides information on osteoporosis, Paget's disease of the bone, osteogenesis imperfecta, primary hyperparathyroidism, and other metabolic bone diseases and disorders.

- Trigeminal Neuralgia Association (TNA)

    P.O. Box 340
    Barnegat Light, NJ 08006
    (609) 361-1014
    Fax: (609) 361-0982
    Web site: http://brain.mgh.harvard.edu:100/tna/

    TNA's purpose is to provide information, resources, material aids, and support to patients with this condition and to facilitate and promote research. Local TNA mutual support groups are available in many states.

Books

- Catalano EM: *The chronic pain control workbook: A step by step guide for coping with and overcoming your pain,* Oakland, Calif, 1987, New Harbinger Publications.
    This is written for the person with chronic pain and is a fairly comprehensive guide to understanding and coping with pain. Special sections cover specific types of pain, such as headaches, irritable bowel syndrome, and temporal mandibular joint disorders.

- Davis M, Eshelman ER, McKay M: *The relaxation and stress reduction workbook,* ed 3, Oakland, Calif, 1988, New Harbinger Publications.
    This book has step-by-step directions for different relaxation exercises such as progressive relaxation, self-hypnosis, autogenics, deep breathing, and visualization that can be helpful for people with chronic pain. It has practical stress management tools and information on such topics as refuting irrational ideas, coping skills training, thought stopping, time management, and job stress.

- Duckro PN, Richardson WD, Marshall JE: *Taking control of your headaches,* New York, 1995, Guilford Press.
    This is a self-help book for people with headache problems. It describes headaches and treatments that include a multimodality method of addressing chronic, complex headaches. Practical tools and information are given not only on headaches but also on medications, relaxation and coping skills, and other nonpharmacologic means of managing headaches such as PT.

- Hanna T: *Somatics, reawakening the mind's control of movement, flexibility, and health,* Reading, MA, 1988, Addison-Wesley.
    This book teaches flexibility through structured exercises on the basis of sensory reeducation. A helpful manual for patients with musculoskeletal disorders and chronic pain. Good model demonstrations of exercises throughout the book.

- Loring K, Fries JF: *Arthritis helpbook: A tested self-management program for coping with arthritis and fibromyalgia,* Reading, MA, 1995, Addison-Wesley.
    This book contains sections on flexibility and strengthening exercises specifically geared to those with joint problems. Other sections cover pain, fatigue, and working with your doctor.

- The Saunders Group, Inc., 4250 Norex Dr., Chaska, MN 55318 (phone [800] 654-8357) puts out several manuals written by H. Duane Saunders, MS, PT, including *For your neck, a self-help manual* and *For your back, a self-help manual.*
    The manuals discuss the disorders and their anatomy and PT treatments such as proper posture, body mechanics, and exercises. Both manuals have clear illustrations of exercises for flexibility and strengthening.

Relaxation Audiotapes

Organizations such as the Applied Psychophysiology and Biofeedback Society and the National Headache Foundation have relaxation tapes, self-help books, and other self-management resources that they sell. Call and ask for their catalogs (see numbers given earlier).

- Exceptional Cancer Patients, 1302 Chapel St., New Haven, CT 06511 (phone [203] 865-8392). This is a healing center founded by Bernie Siegel, MD, that sells self-help materials and audiotapes, including relaxation tapes developed by Dr. Siegel for cancer patients.

- New Harbinger Publications, 5674 Shattuck Avenue, Oakland, CA 94609 (phone [510] 652-0215), has a catalog of relaxation and stress management tapes and self-help books on a variety of topics that are pertinent for people with CNP, such as anxiety, habit control, communications, chronic pain, self-esteem, anger, and cognitive stress intervention. It has a wide variety of relaxation tapes. It is a good resource for cognitive behavioral tapes on assertion training, change and problem solving, and distorted thinking.

- Source, P.O. Box 6028, Auburn, CA 95604 (phone [800] 52-TAPES), has a catalog with a wide variety of relaxation and stress management tapes based on specific techniques such as autogenics, muscle tense release, breathing, visualization, and self-hypnosis. "Letting go of stress" is a good overall tape; however, other tapes on managing pain successfully, headache relief, and healing back pain are available. Its catalog helps to identify the appropriate tapes for the person's concerns.

Pain and Related Symptom Assessment Instruments

Beck Depression Inventory (BDI)

Quick and easy tool (21 items) useful in the clinical diagnosis of depression.

- Beck AT, Steer RA, Garbin MG: Psychometric properties of the Beck Depression Inventory: Twenty-five years of evaluation, *Clin Psychol Rev* 8(1):77-100, 1988.
- Beck AT, Ward CA, Mendelson M et al.: An inventory for measuring depression, *Arch Gen Psychiatry* 4:561-571, 1961.

Chronic Illness Problem Inventory (CIPI)

65-item self-report tool that measures problems in functioning associated with chronic illness.

- Kames LD, Naliboff BD, Heinrich RL et al.: The Chronic Illness Problem Inventory: Problem-oriented psychosocial assessment of patients with chronic illness, *Int J Psychiatry Med* 14:65-75, 1984.

Illness Behavior Questionnaire (IBQ)—Pilowsky

Self-report questionnaire (62 items) with seven scales for assessment of attitudes toward illness, affective behavior, and hypochondriasis.

- McFarlane AC, Brooks PM: Psychological predictors of disease course in rheumatoid arthritis, *Psychosom Res* 31:757-764, 1987.

McGill Pain Questionnaire

Popular tool useful in clinical assessment and diagnosing pain problems. Questionnaire is divided into three areas congruent with the gate theory: word descriptors, ratings of pain intensity, and drawings of pain location. Obtain from International Association for the Study of Pain, 909 NE 43rd St., Suite 306, Seattle, WA 98105-6020, (206) 547-6409.

- Holroyd KA, Holm JE, Keefe FJ et al.: A multi-center evaluation of the McGill Pain Questionnaire: Results from more than 1700 chronic pain patients, *Pain* 48(3):301-311, 1992.
- Melzack R: The McGill Pain Questionnaire: Major properties and scoring methods, *Pain* 1:277-299, 1975.

Multidimensional Pain Inventory (MPI)

Formerly the West Haven–Yale Multidimensional Pain Inventory (WHYMPI). Tool (52 items) that assesses three major areas, impact of pain on client's life, responses of significant others to client's pain, and the client's level of participation in daily activities.

- Kerns RD, Turk DC, Rudy TE: The West Haven–Yale Multidimensional Pain Inventory (WHYMPI), *Pain* 23:345-356, 1985.

Sickness Impact Profile (SIP)

Self-report questionnaire (136 items) that is scored in three scales: physical, psychosocial, and total. This tool helps assess the impact of health problems in 12 areas of functioning.

- Bergner M, Bobbitt RA, Carter WB et al.: The Sickness Impact Profile: Development and final revision of a health status measure, *Health Care* 19:787-805, 1981.

Common Personality Assessment Instruments

Coping Strategies Questionnaire (CSQ)

Questionnaire (42 items) that assesses seven different cognitive or behavioral pain coping strategies.

- Geisser ME, Robinson ME, Henson CD: The Coping Strategies Questionnaire and chronic pain adjustment: A conceptual and empirical reanalysis, *Clin J Pain* 10:98-106, 1994.
- Rosenstiel AR, Keefe FJ: The use of coping strategies in chronic low back pain patients: Relationship to patient characteristics and current adjustment, *Pain* 17:33-44, 1983.

Millon Clinical Multiaxial Inventory

Self-report questionnaire (175 items) that is used to distinguish between psychiatric and personality disorders. Computer scored. Can obtain from National Computer Systems/PAS Division, P.O. Box 1416, Minneapolis, MN 55440, (800) 627-7271.

- McCabe SP: Millon Clinical Multiaxial Inventory. In Keyser DJ and Sweetland RC, editors, *Test Critiques, vol. I*, pp. 455-465, Kansas City, Mo, 1984, Test Corporation of America.
- Millon T: *Millon Clinical Multiaxial Inventory manual*, ed 3, Minneapolis, 1983, Interpretive Scoring Systems.

Minnesota Multiphasic Personality Inventory-2 (MMPI-2)

MMPI-2 is a self-report questionnaire (567 items) that provides psychologic measurements with 10 clinical scales and four validity scales. Popular tool in clinical research; computer scored. Obtain from National Computer Systems/PAS Division, P.O. Box 1416, Minneapolis, MN 55440, (800) 627-7271.

- Duckworth JC, Anderson WP: *MMPI and MMPI-2: Interpretation manual for counselors and clinicians*, ed 4, Bristol, PA, 1995, Accelerated Development.
- Keller LS, Butcher JN: *Assessment of chronic pain patients with the MMPI-2*, Minneapolis, 1989, University of Minnesota Press.

Symptom Checklist-90R (SCL-90R)

A self-report questionnaire (90 items) that is useful for clinical psychologic screening and research. Can evaluate psychologic symptoms in nine primary symptom divisions, and give three global indices of distress (90 items). Brief Symptom Inventory (BSI) is the short version (53 items) of SCL-90R. Obtain from National Computer Systems/PAS Division, P.O. Box 1416, Minneapolis, MN 55440, (800) 627-7271.

- Derogatis LR, Rickels K, Rock AF: The SCL-90 and the MMPI: A step in the validation of a new self-report scale, *Br J Psychol* 128:280-289, 1976.
- Tennen H, Affleck G, Herberger S: SCL-90R. In Keyser DJ, Sweetland RC, editors: *Test critiques, vol. III*, pp 583-594, Kansas City, Mo, 1985, Test Corporation of America.

REFERENCES FOR FURTHER ASSESSMENT/ PSYCHOMETRIC TESTS

- Conoley JC, Kramer JJ, editors: *The tenth mental measurements yearbook,* Lincoln, Neb, 1989, The University of Nebraska Press.

- Keyser DJ, Sweetland RC: *Test critiques, Vol. VIII,* Kansas City, Mo, 1991, Test Corporation of America.

- Krug SE: *Psychware sourcebook 1987-1988,* ed 2, Kansas City, Mo, 1987, Test Corporation of America.

- Sweetland RC, Keyser DJ, editors: *Tests,* ed 3, Austin, Tex, 1991, PRO-ED.

References

Allegrante JP: The role of adjunctive therapy in the management of chronic nonmalignant pain, *Am J Med* 101(Suppl 1A):33S-39S, 1996.

Amadio Jr P, Cummings DM, Amadio P: Nonsteroidal antiinflammatory drugs: tailoring therapy to achieve results and avoid toxicity, *Postgrad Med* 93(4):73-97, 1993.

American Academy of Pain Medicine, American Pain Society: *The use of opioids for the treatment of chronic pain: a consensus statement from the American Academy of Pain Medicine and the American Pain Society,* Glenview, Ill, 1997, Author.

American Pain Society: *Principles of analgesic use in the treatment of acute pain and cancer pain,* ed 3, Skokie, Ill, 1992, Author.

American Psychiatric Association: *Diagnostic and statistical manual of mental disorders,* ed 4, Washington, DC, 1994, Author.

American Society of Pain Management Nurses: *ASPMN position statement: use of placebos for pain management,* Pensacola, Fla, 1997, Author.

Averill PM, Novy DM, Nelson DV et al.: Correlates of depression in chronic pain patients: a comprehensive examination, *Pain* 65:93-100, 1996.

Bandura A: Self-efficacy: toward a unifying theory of behavior change, *Psychol Rev* 84(2):191-215, 1977.

Bandura A: Psychological aspects of prognostic judgments. In Evans RW, Baskin DS, Yatsu FM, editors: *Prognosis of neurological disorders,* p 13, New York, 1992, Oxford University Press.

Bandura A, Adams NE, Beyer J: Cognitive processes mediating behavioral change, *Personality Social Psychol* 35(3):125-139, 1977.

Bell GK, Kidd D, North R: Cost-effectiveness analysis of spinal cord stimulation in the treatment of failed back syndrome, *J Pain Symptom Manage* 13:286-295, 1997.

Bigos S, Bowyer O, Braen G et al.: *Acute low back problems in adults,* Clinical practice guideline, Quick reference guide No. 14, Rockville, Md; U.S. Department of Health and Human Services, Public Health Service, Agency for Health Care Policy and Research, AHCPR Pub. No. 95-0643, Dec 1994.

Biondi DM: Scheduled opiates for chronic refractory headache: guidelines for appropriate patient and medication selection. Paper presented at the American Pain Society's 16th Annual Meeting, New Orleans, Oct 25, 1997.

Brown GK, Nicassio PM: Development of a questionnaire for the assessment of active and passive coping strategies in chronic pain patients, *Pain* 31:53-64, 1987.

Carette S, Legiaire R, Marcoux S et al.: Epidural corticosteroid injections for sciatica due to herniated nucleus pulposus, *N Engl J Med* 336(23):1634-1640, 1997.

Carey TS, Evans AT, Hadler NM et al.: Care-seeking among individuals with chronic low back pain, *Spine* 20:312-317, 1995.

Carey TS, Evans AT, Hadler NM et al.: Acute severe low back pain: a population based survey of prevalence and care seeking, *Spine* 21, 339-344, 1996.

Chaves JF, Brown JM: Spontaneous coping strategies for the control of clinical pain and stress, *J Behav Med* 10(3):263-276, 1987.

Commission on Accreditation of Rehabilitative Facilities: *Standards manual for organizations serving people with disabilities,* Tucson, Ariz, 1995, Author.

Crook J, Rideout D, Browne G: The prevalence of pain complaints in the general population, *Pain* 18:299-314, 1984.

Davis M, Eshelman ER, McKay M: *The relaxation and stress reduction workbook,* ed 3, Oakland, Calif, 1988, New Harbinger Publications.

DeGood DE: What is the role of biofeedback in the treatment of chronic pain patients? *APS Bull* 3(3):1-2,4-6, 1993.

Deyo RA, Diehl AK: Patient satisfaction with medical care for low-back pain, *Spine* 11:28-30, Jan-Feb 1986.

Drossman DA, Leserman J, Nachman G et al.: Sexual and physical abuse in women with functional or organic gastrointestinal disorders, *Ann Intern Med* 113:828-833, 1990.

Eisendrath SJ: Psychiatric aspects of chronic pain, *Neurology* 45(12 Suppl 9):S26-S34, 1995.

Ellis AE, Harper RA: *A new guide to rational living,* Hollywood, Calif, 1978, Wilshire Book Company.

Faries JE, Mills DS, Goldsmith KW et al.: Systematic pain records and their impact on pain control: a pilot study, *Cancer Nurs* 14(6):306-313, 1991.

Feine JS, Lund JP: An assessment of efficacy of physical therapy and physical modalities for the control of chronic musculoskeletal pain, *Pain* 71:5-23, 1997.

Flor H, Birbaumer N: Comparison of the efficacy of electromyographic biofeedback, cognitive-behavioral therapy, and conservative medical interventions in the treatment of chronic musculoskeletal pain, *J Consult Clin Psychol* 61(4):653-658, 1993.

Flor H, Fyrich T, Turk DC: Efficacy of multidisciplinary pain treatment centers: a meta-analytic review, *Pain* 49:221-230, 1992.

Folkman S, Lazarus RS: An analysis of coping in a middle-aged community sample, *J Health Soc Behav* 21:219-239, 1980.

Fordyce WE: *Behavioral methods for chronic pain and illness,* St. Louis, 1976, Mosby.

Fry R: Adult physical illness and childhood sexual abuse, *J Psychosom Res* 37:89-103, 1993.

Gear RW, Miaskowski C, Heller PH et al.: Benzodiazepine mediated antagonism of opioid analgesia, *Pain* 71:25-29, 1997.

Goodwin JS, Goodwin JM, Vogel AA: Knowledge and use of placebos by house officers and nurses, *Ann Intern Med* 91:106-110, 1979.

Griffin MR, Piper JM, Daugherty JR et al.: Nonsteroidal anti-inflammatory drug use and increased risk for peptic ulcer disease in elderly persons, *Ann Intern Med* 114(4):257-263, 1991.

Guo HR, Tanaka S, Cameron LL: Back pain among workers in the United States: national estimates and workers at high risk, *Am J Ind Med* 28:591-602, 1995.

Hassenbusch SJ, Paice JA, Patt RB et al.: Clinical realities and economic considerations: economics of intrathecal therapy, *J Pain Symptom Manage* 14:S36-S48, 1997.

Haythornthwaite JA, Sieber WJ, Kerns RD: Depression and the chronic pain experience, *Pain* 46:177-184, 1991.

Hitchcock LS, Ferrell BR, McCaffery M: The experience of chronic nonmalignant pain, *J Pain Symptom Manage* 9:312-318, 1994.

Holzberg AD, Robinson ME, Geisser ME et al.: The effects of depression and chronic pain on psychosocial and physical functioning, *Clin J Pain* 12:330-337, 1996.

Hubbard JE, Tracy J, Morgan SF et al.: Outcome measures of a chronic pain program: a prospective statistical study, *Clin J Pain* 12:330-337, 1996.

International Association for the Study of Pain: *Desirable characteristics for pain treatment facilities,* Seattle, 1990, Author.

Jacobs GD, Rosenberg PA, Friedman R et al.: Multifactor behavioral treatment of chronic sleep-onset insomnia using stimulus control and the relaxation response: a preliminary study, *Behav Modif* 17(4):498-509, 1993a.

Jacobs GD, Rosenberg PA, Friedman R et al.: Multifactor behavioral treatment of chronic sleep-onset insomnia using stimulus control and the relaxation response, *Behav Modif* 17:498-509, 1993b.

Jamison RN, Verts KL: The influence of family support on chronic pain, *Behav Res Ther* 28:283-287, 1990.

Joranson DE, Gilson AM: State intractable pain policy: current status, *APS Bull* 7(2):7-9, 1997.

Keefe FJ, Caldwell DS, Queen KT et al.: Pain coping strategies in osteoarthritis patients, *J Consult Clin Psychol* 55(2):208-212, 1987.

Krames ES: The role of implantable pain management technologies: an algorithm for decision-making. In Waldman SW, Winnie AP, editors: *Interventional pain management,* pp 501-510, Philadelphia, 1996, WB Saunders.

Lazarus RS: Cognitive and personality factors underlying threat and coping. In Appley MH, Trumbell R, editors: *Psychological stress issues in research,* pp 151-181, New York, 1967, Appleton-Century-Crofts.

Lazarus RS, Folkman S: Cognitive theories of stress and the issue of circularity. In Appley MH, Trumbell R, editors: *Dynamics of stress,* pp 63-79, New York, 1986, Plenum.

Linton SJ: A population based study of the relationship between sexual abuse and back pain: establishing a link, *Pain* 73:47-53, 1997.

NIH Technology Assessment Panel on Integration of Behavioral and Relaxation Approaches into the Treatment of Chronic Pain and Insomnia: Integration of behavioral and relaxation approaches into the treatment of chronic pain and insomnia, *JAMA* 276:313-318, 1996.

North RB: Spinal cord stimulation. In North RB, Levy RM, editors: *Neurosurgical management of pain,* pp 271-282, New York, 1997, Springer-Verlag.

North RB, Campbell JN, Names CS et al.: Failed back surgery syndrome: five year follow-up in 102 patients undergoing repeated operation, *Neurosurgery* 28:685-691, 1991.

Pap LA, Gorman JM: Pharmacological approach to the management of stress and anxiety disorders. In Lehrer PM, Woolfolk RL, editors: *Principles and practice of stress management,* ed 2, pp 463-478, New York, 1993, Guilford Press.

Polatin PB, Kinney FK, Gatchel RJ et al.: Psychiatric illness and chronic low-back pain: the mind and the spine—which goes first? *Spine* 18: 66-71, 1993.

Portenoy RK: Opioid therapy for chronic nonmalignant pain: current status. In Fields HL, Liebeskind JC, editors: *Progress in pain research and management. Vol 1. Pharmacologic approaches to the treatment of chronic pain: new concepts and critical issues,* pp 247-287, Seattle, 1994, IASP Press.

Portenoy RK: Opioid analgesics. In Portenoy RK, Kanner RM, editors: *Pain management: theory and practice,* pp 248-276, Philadelphia, 1996, FA Davis.

Portenoy RK, Foley K: Chronic use of opioid analgesics in non-malignant pain: report of 38 cases, *Pain* 25:171-186, 1986.

Reddy S, Patt RB: The benzodiazepines as adjuvant analgesics, *J Pain Symptom Manage* 9(8):510-514, 1994.

Rene J, Weinberger M, Mazzuca SA et al.: Reduction of joint pain in patients with knee osteoarthritis who have received monthly telephone calls from lay personnel and whose medical treatment regimens have remained stable, *Arthritis Rheum* 35:511-515, 1992.

Romano JM, Turner JA: Chronic pain and depression: does the evidence support a relationship? *Psychol Bull* 97(1):18-34, 1985.

Saper JR: Proposed initial guidelines for the selection and use of opioids in the treatment of non-malignant pain, *Top Pain Manage* 11(12):45-46, 1996.

Schwartz MS: Selected problems associated with relaxation therapies and guidelines for coping with problems. In Schwartz MS: *Biofeedback: a practitioner's guide,* pp 163-172, New York, 1987, Guilford Press.

Sternbach RA: Survey of pain in the United States: the Nuprin pain report, *Clin J Pain* 2:49-53, 1986.

Syrjala K: Relaxation techniques. In Bonica JJ, editor: *The management of pain,* vol 2, pp 1742-1750, Malvern, Pa, 1990, Lea & Febiger.

Syrjala KL, Cummings C, Donaldson GW: Hypnosis or cognitive behavioral training for the reduction of pain and nausea during cancer treatment: a controlled clinical trial, *Pain* 48(2):137-146, 1992.

Tait RC, Chibnall JT, Richardson WD: Litigation and employment status: effects on patients with chronic pain, *Pain* 43:37-46, 1990.

Taylor AG, Skelton JA, Butcher J: Duration of pain condition and physical pathology as determinants of nurses' assessments of patients in pain, *Nurs Res* 33:4-8, Jan-Feb 1984.

Tennant FS, Robinson D, Sagherian A et al.: Chronic opioid treatment of intractable, nonmalignant pain, *Pain Manage* p 18-26, Jan-Feb 1988.

Turk DC: Clinicians' attitudes about prolonged use of opioids and the issue of patient heterogeneity, *J Pain Symptom Manage* 11(4): 218-230, 1996.

Turner JA, Clancy C: Strategies for coping with chronic low back pain: relationship to pain and disability, *Pain* 24:355-364, 1986.

Vasudevan SV: Physical rehabilitation in managing pain, *Pain: Clin Updates* 5(3):1-4, 1997.

Virani A, Mailis A, Shapiro LE et al.: Drug interactions in human neuropathic pain pharmacotherapy, *Pain* 73:3-13, 1997.

Weinberger M, Tierney WM, Booker P et al.: Can the provision of information to patients with osteoarthritis improve functional status? A randomized, controlled trial, *Arthritis Rheum* 32:1577-1583, 1989.

Wurtele SK, Kaplan GM, Keairnes M: Childhood sexual abuse among chronic pain patients, *Clin J Pain* 6:110-113, 1990.

Yost JH, Morgan CG: Cardiovascular effects of NSAIDs, *J Musculoskeletal Med* 11(10):22-34, 1994.

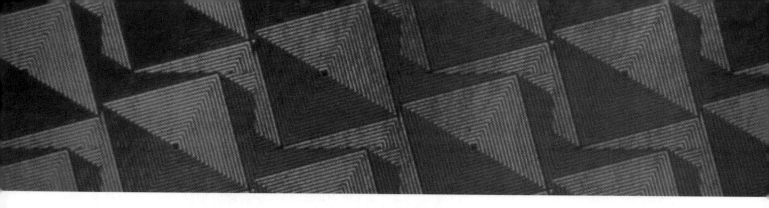

chapter twelve
SELECTED PAIN PROBLEMS

Editor: Margo McCaffery

This chapter provides brief introductions to various pain problems selected on the basis of frequency of inquiries from our colleagues. Often the pain problem, although prevalent in some settings, is encountered only rarely in others. Such is the case with sickle cell disease-related pain. Or the pain problem is stigmatized and poorly understood, such as is the case with fibromyalgia syndrome. Others, such as arthritis and osteoporosis, are very common but tend to be ignored, especially in the elderly. These selected pain problem overviews are for the purpose of helping the clinician become quickly oriented to the pain management needs of the patient.

section 1
QUICK GUIDES TO SELECTED PAIN PROBLEMS

ARTHRITIS: OSTEOARTHRITIS AND RHEUMATOID ARTHRITIS

Barbara Reed and Karen P. Kettelman

Description

Arthritis is the inflammation of a joint. The two major types of arthritis are osteoarthritis (OA) and rheumatoid arthritis (RA) (Krug, 1997) (Figure 12.1).

Osteoarthritis

OA is the most common form of arthritis, affecting almost 16 million people in the United States. It is also known as "degenerative joint disease" or "degenerative arthritis." The breakdown and abrasion of joint cartilage, with the formation of new bone at the joint surfaces, lead to joint pain and stiffness (Eliopoulos, 1997). OA, although painful when the affected joint is moved, does not cause inflammation, deformity, or crippling. It is thought that the wear and tear on the joints as a person ages is the major cause. Weight-bearing joints are most often affected (i.e., knees, hips, and vertebrae) (Figure 12.2). It also affects the finger joints, the joint at the base of the thumb, and the joint at the base of the great toe (*Arthritis Fact Sheet,* 1997). Classic symptoms of this progressive disease are aching, stiffness, and limited range of motion of the joint. OA is the leading cause of disability in the elderly.

Rheumatoid arthritis

RA is the most common inflammatory arthritis. It is usually considered a disease of joints, but it has characteristics of systemic disease. RA affects approximately 1% of the world's population. Approximately one fourth of all patients referred to rheumatologists are those with RA. The actual cause of RA is still unclear, but it is believed that a combination of genetic and environmental factors is responsible. Women are affected with RA two times as often as men. The deformity and disability associated with the disease begin during early adulthood and peak during middle age, but systemic involvement occurs in old age (Eliopoulos, 1997).

The cause of pain in RA, a progressive polyarticular disease, varies depending on the duration and severity of the disease. Initially pain results from the inflammation causing tenderness and swelling of the joint. As the disease progresses, erosion of cartilage and bone contributes to the pain (Pisetsky, 1997).

The joints affected by RA are extremely painful, stiff, swollen, red, and warm to the touch. Joint pain is present during both rest and activity. Multiple joints are usually inflamed in a symmetric pattern. The joints most commonly affected are the small bones of the hands and feet, knees, shoulders, ankles, wrists, and elbows (Figure 12.3). The cervical spine is also often affected with pain that radiates down both arms. The hips are often spared from the progression of the disease. There may be subcutaneous nodules over bony prominences, and bursae may be present, as well as deforming flexion contractures. Systemic symptoms of RA may include fatigue, malaise, weakness, weight loss, wasting, fever, and anemia (*www.medicinenet. com,* 1997). (NOTE: "Rheumatism" does not refer exclusively to RA. It is a general term for acute and chronic conditions characterized by inflammation, soreness, and stiffness of muscles and pain in joints and associated structures.)

Pain Characteristics

Osteoarthritis

The pain of OA may be described as a "deep, aching pain" and may become severe as the disease progresses. Pain is felt not only in the affected joints but may also be referred to the adjacent muscle groups. The pain usually increases in proportion to the use of the joint (Merskey, Bogduk, 1994).

Because osteoarthritis is noninflammatory, onset may be subtle and gradual, involving one or only a few joints. Pain is usually the first symptom and is made worse by exercise. Acute flare-ups may be episodic in the beginning, but as the disease progresses, joint motion becomes

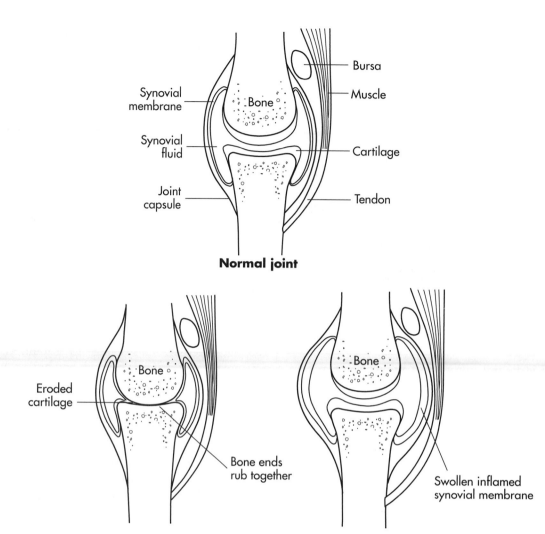

May be duplicated for use in clinical practice. From McCaffery M, Pasero C: *Pain: Clinical manual*, p. 524. Copyright © 1999, Mosby, Inc.

● ● ● ● ●
FIGURE 12.1   *Characteristics of normal and arthritic joints. In osteoarthritis, a major cause of pain is rubbing of bone upon bone. In rheumatoid arthritis, inflammation of surrounding tissues such as synovial membrane is a major source of pain.*

diminished and tenderness and crepitus (grating sound) occur. Joint enlargement and chronic synovial proliferation and inflammation ultimately occur. In some cases morning stiffness may follow inactivity but improves with exercise (Merskey, Bogduk, 1994).

Rheumatoid arthritis

The pain of RA may be described as an "aching, burning joint pain" (Merskey, Bogduk, 1994). This pain is usually moderately severe with exacerbations and remissions.

RA has a slow onset and usually affects large and small joints in a symmetric pattern. Patients with RA experience enlargement of the affected joints, which may be very painful initially. Later after the synovium is damaged

in advanced disease, joints may be only minimally tender. Morning stiffness (sometimes referred to as the "gel phenomenon") or stiffness after a period of restricted movement is common (Pisetsky, 1997).

A "flare," or a painful exacerbation of RA, may occur at any time, with a dramatic increase in inflammation. These flares usually involve multiple joints. The degree of joint involvement does not necessarily determine the severity of the pain (Pisetsky, 1997).

When body tissues are inflamed, the disease is considered active. When the inflammation subsides, the disease is inactive. When the disease is active, symptoms may include fatigue, lack of appetite, low-grade fever, muscle and joint aches, and stiffness. Muscle and joint stiffness is most noticeable in the morning and after long periods of

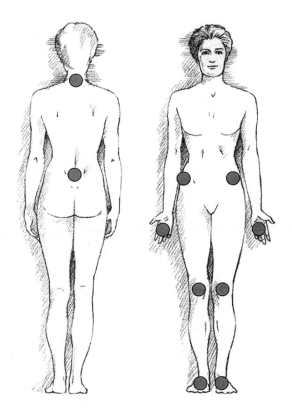

May be duplicated for use in clinical practice. As appears in McCaffery M, Pasero C: *Pain: Clinical manual,* p. 525, 1999, Mosby, Inc.

● ● ● ● ●
F I G U R E 12.2 Joints usually affected by osteoarthritis.

From the brochure "Osteoarthritis," © 1997. Used by permission of the Arthritis Foundation. For more information, please call the Arthritis Foundation's information line, (800) 283-7800.

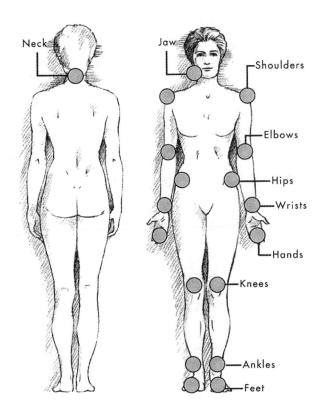

May be duplicated for use in clinical practice. As appears in McCaffery M, Pasero C: *Pain: Clinical manual,* p. 525, 1999, Mosby, Inc.

● ● ● ● ●
F I G U R E 12.3 Joints that may be affected by rheumatoid arthritis.

From the brochure "Rheumatoid arthritis," © 1998. Used by permission of the Arthritis Foundation. For more information, please call the Arthritis Foundation's information line, (800) 283-7800.

inactivity. The inflammation of the joint lining causes deterioration of the joint, limited motion, and pain. Joint stiffness and pain are often the first indication to the patient that a medical problem exists. These symptoms, and the accompanying fatigue, may be the reason many patients seek medical attention (Belza, Henke, Yelin et al., 1993).

Assessment

Making a distinction between RA and OA may be difficult. The major differences between the two are the inflammatory nature and the symmetric polyarticular characteristics of RA. OA may involve only a single joint and is caused by degeneration of the articular cartilage, not inflammation. Ruling out other diseases that share symptoms of joint pain and swelling is important. For example, in the patient with pain and swelling in a single joint, septic arthritis should also be ruled out before making the diagnosis of RA.

Osteoarthritis

No official diagnostic criteria exist for OA, although criteria have been proposed for OA of the knee joint. Typically, OA is diagnosed if the patient exhibits nonin-

flammatory arthritis of one or more joints in the absence of any known predisposing cause, with loss of cartilage and/or osteophyte formation demonstrated by x-ray films (Merskey, Bogduk, 1994). The presence of Bouchard's nodes or Heberden's nodes is also characteristic of OA (Krug, 1997).

Rheumatoid arthritis

Diagnosis of RA depends primarily on physical findings and history. The presence of rheumatoid factor supports the diagnosis of RA, but only about 80% of patients are positive for rheumatoid factor. Other laboratory values include increased sedimentation rate, anemia, and thrombocytosis. Deformities of the hands and feet and the presence of rheumatoid nodules are also indicative of RA (Pisetsky, 1997).

Pain Management

Osteoarthritis

The goal of treatment in OA is to reduce joint pain and inflammation, and to improve and maintain joint function and mobility. Several methods of pain control may be combined to give the best result.

Physical Methods

Because overuse of the joint will increase pain, the patient is encouraged to decrease the intensity and/or frequency of activities that cause joint pain. Exercises can strengthen muscular support around joints and maintain joint mobility (when performed at levels that do not cause joint pain). Application of local heat before exercise can soothe and relax muscles, and cold packs after exercise cause a numbing effect and decrease swelling and pain. Joint mobility may be maintained with walking, stationary cycling, and light weight training.

Physical and occupational therapists may recommend support devices such as splints, canes, walkers, and braces for assistance and safety. Paraffin wax dips, warm water soaks, and nighttime cotton gloves may relieve hand pain, and a neck collar, lumbar corset, or firm mattress can improve spine symptoms.

Pharmacologic Methods

OTC pain relievers such as aspirin and acetaminophen, either in tablet form or creams applied to the skin over affected joints, may be sufficient treatment for some cases of OA. NSAIDs may reduce pain and inflammation of the joints. Many NSAIDs are OTC and may be effective in treating mild to severe pain.

Oral cortisone is not usually used in treating OA, but injection into inflamed joints may rapidly decrease pain and restore function. The number of injections that can be done without harming tissue and bones is limited, so they are reserved for patients with pronounced symptoms (*www.medicinenet.com, 1997*).

Surgery

Surgery may be indicated for patients who have severe disease that is unresponsive to conservative treatments. Total joint replacement, especially of the hip and knee, may offer the patient dramatic pain relief and improved function. Arthroscopy may be helpful in cartilage tears, osteotomy can help realign a deformity, and fusion may improve function and stability of severely degenerated joints.

Rheumatoid arthritis

The goal of treatment for RA is to reduce joint inflammation and pain, maximize joint function, and prevent joint destruction and deformity. Early in the disease process, treatment of RA and its related pain involves the use of NSAIDs, including aspirin, patient education about self-care and how to protect joints, and physical therapy to maintain muscle tone and range of motion. Early intervention assists in a better long-term outcome for the patient with RA.

Physical Methods

The same physical methods that were outlined under OA (e.g., rest and joint protection, proper exercise, support devices, and heat and cold) are also helpful for patients with RA. As the disease progresses, the use of assistive devices such as canes, splints, and walkers can relieve pain and provide support for mobility.

Pharmacologic Methods

"First-line" drugs are aspirin, acetaminophen, and other NSAIDs. Some patients with mild disease may obtain adequate pain relief with these drugs. Topical preparations may provide symptomatic pain relief when rubbed over affected joints. Corticosteroids may be given orally or injected into affected joints but are useful only for short periods of severe flares. They are not indicated for long-term use.

"Second-line" drugs are used in patients with an aggressively destructive form of RA that is unresponsive to NSAIDs and corticosteroids. Oral drugs include hydroxychloroquine and sulfasalazine. Gold salts are given by injection, initially on a weekly basis, for months to years. Gold may also be given orally. D-penicillamine is an oral agent that affects the immune system by decreasing IgM rheumatoid factor. Immunosuppressive drugs such as methotrexate, azathioprine, cyclophosphamide, chlorambucil, and cyclosporine may provide pain relief by suppressing the inflammation of RA (*www.medicinenet.com, 1997*).

Opioids are used when NSAIDs and the other therapies are not providing adequate pain relief. The use of opioids is especially common in patients awaiting a surgical intervention such as joint replacement.

Surgery

Surgical intervention is sometimes indicated to relieve pain and improve function. Procedures include synovectomy, cervical spine fusion, fusion at the base of the thumb, tendon repairs, osteotomies, and hip and knee arthroplasty or replacement. Surgical approaches are reserved for patients not responding to more conservative measures or when function is at risk (Kelley, Ruddy, Harris et al., 1997).

SUMMARY

Characteristics of OA and RA include the following:
- OA is progressive and worsens with age.
- RA is inflammatory and has exacerbations and remissions.
- Pain of OA is "deep, aching pain."
- Pain of RA is "aching, burning joint pain."
- Episodes of acute pain superimposed on chronic pain occur with both.
- The goal for both OA and RA is reduced joint pain and inflammation.

Pain management is a critical aspect of care for patients with either OA or RA. Teach patients how to rest, exercise, adapt their lifestyle, maintain adequate nutrition, recognize and treat fatigue, and take advantage of community resources. Care and education of the patient with OA or RA are multifaceted, multidisciplinary tasks, involving a combination of pharmacologic, physical, surgical, and other approaches.

Resources

Arthritis Foundation
National Office
1330 West Peachtree St.
Atlanta, GA 30309
(404) 872-7100
Arthritis Answers: (800) 283-7800
Web site: *http://www.arthritis.org*

National Arthritis and Musculoskeletal and Skin Diseases
Clearinghouse
Box AMS
Bethesda, MD 20892
(301) 495-4484

National Institute of Arthritis and Musculoskeletal and Skin
Diseases
Building 31, Room 4C05
Bethesda, MD 20892-2350
(301) 496-8190

The Arthritis Foundation offers a variety of programs that can help people with arthritis make life easier and less painful. These services include self-help courses, water- and land-based exercise classes, support groups, instructional videotapes, educational brochures and booklets, and a bimonthly consumer magazine called *Arthritis Today*.

References

Arthritis Fact Sheet: 1997, Atlanta, Ga, Arthritis Foundation.
Belza B, Henke C, Yelin E et al.: Correlates of fatigue in older adults with rheumatoid arthritis, *Nurs Res* 42:93-99, 1993.
Eliopoulos C: *Gerontological nursing*, Philadelphia, 1997, JB Lippincott.
Kelley WN, Ruddy S, Harris ED et al., editors: *Textbook of rheumatology*, ed 5, Philadelphia, 1997, WB Saunders.
Krug B: Rheumatoid arthritis and osteoarthritis: a basic comparison, *Orthop Nurs* 16:73-75, 1997.
Merskey H, Bogduk N: *Classification of chronic pain*, ed 2, pp 47-49, Seattle, 1994, IASP Press.
Pisetsky DS: Pain in rheumatoid arthritis and osteoarthritis. In Kanner R, editor: *Pain management secrets*, pp 113-121, Philadelphia, 1997, Hanley & Belfus.
www.medicinenet.com, 1997.

BURN PAIN

Sharon Lauterbach and Russell George

Description

Burn patients sustain insults to the skin from various sources, including hot liquids, chemical agents, electric current, frostbite, and exfoliating disorders such as Stevens-Johnson syndrome. Each year 2.25 million people are burned in the United States and Canada (National Center for Health Statistics, 1990). Of these, approximately 6000 die (National Fire Protection Association, 1990) and 75,000 require hospitalization (American Burn Association, 1991; National Center for Health Statistics, 1992). Males outnumber females 2:1 in the burn population. This is related to male household and job roles, which increase the risk for burn injury. Furthermore, males more commonly engage in risk-taking behaviors involving chemicals, flammable materials, or electricity. The burn population exhibits a higher incidence of factors that contribute to the risk for injury, such as substance abuse, psychiatric history, mental retardation, family disruption, and history of thrill seeking (Maaser, 1995; Tucker, 1986).

Burns are classified according to depth of injury as depicted in Figure 12.4: first degree (superficial burn), second degree (partial-thickness burn), third degree, and fourth degree (full-thickness burn). A patient may have more than one depth of burn. The surface appearance of the burn wound may be indicative of the depth. The appearance of the wound may be red or pink with blisters (partial thickness); cherry red eschar, white or brown leathery eschar (full thickness); or a charred eschar (full thickness).

The extent of the injury is usually expressed in percent of total body surface area (TBSA). The extent of injury varies from one person to the next. Extent can be determined by a number of methods including the Rule of 9's, Berkow's chart, or a patient's hand size, which is approximately 1% TBSA (Kowalske, Tanelian, 1997).

The American Burn Association has classified burns into two categories: major and minor. Seriousness of the burn injury is determined in part by the depth and extent of injury. For example, a person with a 20% TBSA partial-thickness burn is less seriously injured than a person with a 60% TBSA full-thickness burn. Preburn conditions (e.g., diabetes and congestive heart failure) and concurrent trauma (e.g., head injury and inhalation injury) also increase the seriousness of the burn injury.

Treatment progresses through three distinct phases: emergent, healing, and rehabilitation (Ready, Edwards, 1992). Length of these phases varies enormously from 1 day to years of hospitalization and up to months or years of rehabilitation. Factors that affect treatment are patient cooperation, patient age, depth and location of burn, and burn size.

Pain Characteristics and Assessment

Overall, patients report that burn pain is the worst pain imaginable (Charlton, Klein, Gagliardi et al., 1983; Fagerhaugh, 1974; Mannon, 1985). In one study of burn patients, 84% reported that their worst pain was severe or excruciating, 100% experienced pain every day, and 92% were awakened by pain every night (Perry, Heidrich, Ramos, 1981). Pain often varies throughout the day, vacillating from mild to the worst possible pain.

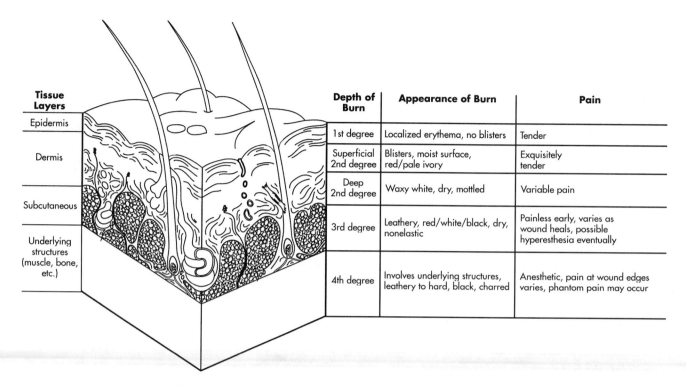

Depth of Burn	Appearance of Burn	Pain
1st degree	Localized erythema, no blisters	Tender
Superficial 2nd degree	Blisters, moist surface, red/pale ivory	Exquisitely tender
Deep 2nd degree	Waxy white, dry, mottled	Variable pain
3rd degree	Leathery, red/white/black, dry, nonelastic	Painless early, varies as wound heals, possible hyperesthesia eventually
4th degree	Involves underlying structures, leathery to hard, black, charred	Anesthetic, pain at wound edges varies, phantom pain may occur

May be duplicated for use in clinical practice. As appears in McCaffery M, Pasero C: *Pain: Clinical manual*, p. 528, 1999, Mosby, Inc.

FIGURE 12.4   Depth of burns and associated appearance and pain.
From Lifeart Collections, Professional Medical Computer Graphics Super Anatomy. © Tech Pool Corp. By permission of Williams & Wilkins.

The intensity of burn pain cannot be predicted. Burn size does not correlate with pain intensity (Perry, Heidrich, Ramos, 1981) because a 3% TBSA burn can hurt as much as a 60% TBSA burn. Depth of the burn may be somewhat related to pain intensity. The deeper the burn, the more damage to the nerve endings, and a full-thickness (third-degree) burn is considered painless. However, patients rarely have only one depth of burn. It is more common for burn depth to be variable throughout the wound bed (Kowalske, Tanelian, 1997). Fourth-degree burns are anesthetic, but phantom pain may occur. Burn pain also cannot be predicted on the basis of other factors such as age, sex, ethnicity, education, occupation, or socioeconomic status (Atchison, Osgood, Carr, 1991; Choiniere, Melzack, Rondeau et al., 1989; Perry, Heidrich, Ramos, 1981).

Burn pain may intensify over time instead of steadily declining (Choiniere, 1994). Increased pain levels may be attributed to several factors, including repeated dressing changes, occurrences of cellulitis or wound infection, procedures such as skin grafting, donor sites, and range of motion exercises (Choiniere, 1994). The healing process is also painful. As wounds heal, skin buds form with a proliferation of new nerve endings that are often exquisitely tender. Usually the burn patient's pain resolves when no open wounds are present and the scars have totally healed (Kowalske, Tanelian, 1997).

Patients describe burn pain as burning and aching, with intermittent sharp pain, especially after dressing changes and exercises. Some patients also experience neuropathic pain, described as burning, tingling, shooting, or numbing (Kowalske, Tanelian, 1997).

As listed in column one of Table 12.1, burn patients typically experience three types of pain on a daily basis: background, breakthrough, and procedural. Background pain is the constant pain that exists on a 24-hour basis. Breakthrough pain occurs when blood levels of pain medications drop below what is needed to control background pain. Procedural pain is caused by procedures such as wound care or range of motion exercises. Pain ratings for all three types of pain must be obtained throughout each day because each is different. A pain flow sheet (see p. 79 or 87) might be modified to include a pain rating column for each of these three types of pain. Pain flow sheets may be kept at the bedside along with vital sign records, and patients who are able to do so may record on the pain flow sheet.

Posttraumatic stress disorder (PTSD) commonly occurs after a burn injury, and this may complicate pain assessment. PTSD is manifested by recurring nightmares concerning the traumatic event, insomnia, exaggerated startle response, flat affect, memory impairment related to the event, and irritability (Maaser, 1995; Ptacek, Patterson, Montgomery et al., 1995). The patient

TABLE 12.1 Parkland Burn Acute Care Unit Adult Pain Management Pathway

Critical elements	STAGE 1	STAGE 2 WOUND MANAGEMENT			STAGE 3
	Stage 1 (1-3 days) Admission/resuscitation Stabilization/postoperative	Planned LOS short term <3 days	Planned LOS short term >3 days	Planned LOS long term	Predischarge 3 days before discharge
Medications	MS via PCA pump	Lorcet 10	MS drops PO	MS Contin	
Background pain	*Loading dose:* MS, 5 mg before first tanking Option: may repeat × 2 PRN during tanking Continuous infusion MS, 0.5-2 mg q1h	*Lorcet 10 one PO q4h ATC*	*MS drops PO q4h ATC* Take previous 24 h IV MS usage (minus tanking dose). And convert to: >90 mg in 24 h 2:1 ratio <90 mg in 24 h 3:1 ratio *Discontinue PCA	MS Contin q8h ATC Convert dosage in the same way as the MS drops except give the first dose 4 h before discontinuing PCA *Stop before last surgery	*Wean MS drops* ½ ATC dose 72 h before Stop ATC dose 48 h before Stop procedural dose last *Stop all MS 24 h before discharge
Breakthrough pain	*PCA dose:* MS, 2 mg q10min with 30 mg q4h lockout *Dosage varies depending on patient's requirements	MS drops q4h PRN: MS drops calculated to ⅙ of total 24-h MS dose *Increase background dose if patient requires >3 times/day	MS drops q4h PRN: MS drops calculated to ⅙ of total 24-h MS dose *Increase background dose if patient requires >3 times per day	MS drops q4h PRN: MS drops calculated to ⅙ of total 24-h MS dose *Increase background dose if patient requires >3 times per day	*Discontinue all MS 24 h before discharge Lorcet 10 one PO q4h PRN Motrin, 600 mg PO q6h PRN with food
Procedural pain	*Dressing changes:* MS, 5-10 mg *Dosage varies depending on patient's requirements	Dressing changes: MS, 20-60 mg PO	Dressing changes: MS, 20-60 mg PO	Dressing changes: MS, 20-60 mg PO	*Discharge order:* Lorcet 10 Motrin, 600 mg ordered if pain not controlled by Lorcet 10
Anxiety/procedural	Ativan, 1 mg IV for initial tanking Ativan, 1 mg PO for subsequent dressing changes Nitrous oxide PRN for dressing changes only	Ativan, 1 mg PO with option to refuse Nitrous oxide PRN for dressing changes only	Ativan, 1 mg PO with option to refuse Nitrous oxide PRN for dressing changes only	Ativan, 1 mg PO with option to refuse Nitrous oxide PRN for dressing changes only	Ativan, 1 mg may be used for anxiety for the first week after discharge
Sleep	Restoril, 15-30 mg at hs PRN	Restoril, 15-30 mg at hs PRN	Restoril, 15-30 mg at hs PRN	Restoril, 15-30 mg at hs PRN	Restoril may be used PRN after discharge
Constipation	Colace, 100 mg PO bid	Colace, 100 mg PO bid Dulcolax, 10 mg PO/PR PRN if no BM for 3 days	Colace, 100 mg PO bid Dulcolax, 10 mg PO/PR PRN if no BM for 3 days	Colace, 100 mg PO bid Dulcolax, 10 mg PO/PR PRN if no BM for 3 days	Colace may be used PRN after discharge

*Please note.
Courtesy Parkland Health & Hospital System, Dallas.

has reduced involvement with the external world but at the same time is hyperalert to it. One study suggests that patients with PTSD are more sensitive to pain than those without PTSD but less likely to report it or to express it behaviorally. They appear to be detached. Flattened affect may cause the clinician to perceive the patient's pain as being under control, but patients must be asked to rate their pain for an accurate assessment (Perry, Cella, Falkenberg, 1987).

Pain Management

Like other types of pain, burn pain tends to be undertreated. Procedure-related pain is particularly likely to be undertreated (Ashburn, 1995). In one survey of burn facilities, 17% of respondents would not use opioid analgesics for wound debridement in a 3-year-old child (Perry, Heidrich, 1982).

Management of burn pain varies from one institution to the next. The diversity of styles used by health care providers to manage burn pain reflects differences in burn treatment and a variety of misconceptions. A common misconception is the unfounded fear of causing addiction by administering opioids for pain relief or of making addiction worse if the patient is already addicted. Lack of understanding of how to monitor sedation levels to prevent respiratory depression also contributes to undertreated pain. Furthermore, clinicians often lack knowledge about opioid analgesics, such as the need to avoid meperidine because of its active metabolite, to avoid IM administration because of delayed and unreliable absorption, and the fact that no evidence has been found that benzodiazepines reduce pain or opioid requirement. Clinicians may not realize that tolerance to analgesia is expected and may be safely and easily handled by titration. These and other misconceptions about opioids are discussed in Chapter 6.

An adult pain management pathway (Table 12.1) was developed at the Burn Acute Care Unit at Parkland Health and Hospital System, Dallas, Texas. The pathway was devised for spontaneously breathing, conscious adult patients with 40% or less TBSA burn wound. This pathway serves as a consistent guideline for evaluating the effectiveness of pain management. The efficacy of the pathway has been assessed since November 1994, and several revisions have been made on the basis of experience.

Care of patients with burn pain will be discussed with this pathway as an example. The columns of the pathway reflect the phases of healing and the decreasing levels of pain expected as a person progresses through these phases. The first column lists the types of situations that will require medication for most patients. This discussion will focus on three of the items: background, breakthrough, and procedural pain.

Stage 1 addresses the admission and postoperative period, during which the first doses of opioid analgesic are given. We use morphine, although other opioids such as hydromorphone (Dilaudid), fentanyl, and methadone are acceptable alternatives.

Morphine is administered IV (not IM) using a PCA pump. If the patient is unable to activate the pump, it may be nurse activated. Starting with loading doses, pain is brought under control, and a dose for continuous infusion is established for background pain. Doses are titrated up or down on the basis of pain ratings and safety parameters.

For breakthrough pain, a bolus dose is determined and then administered by the patient when needed. A typical dose for our patients is morphine, 2 mg q10 minutes, with a 30 mg 4-hour limit set.

For procedural pain, such as dressing changes, doses of 5 to 10 mg morphine are administered IV by the nurse. Ativan, 1 mg, is used for preprocedural anxiety only, not pain.

Stage 2, wound management, is divided into three columns that are based on length of stay. During this phase the patient is converted from IV to PO morphine to facilitate independence and ambulation. If the patient's pain is not well controlled with oral analgesics, nurses should return to Stage 1. The conversion ratios shown on the pathway are different from most recommendations, but we have found them to effectively control pain without interfering with the patient's ability to perform rehabilitation therapies such as range of motion exercises. Higher ratios tend to make patients too somnolent to participate in therapies.

Nitrous oxide is an effective adjunct to morphine for dressing changes. Patients self-administer the gas and report minimal problems. Dizziness and nausea rarely occur. Restrictions to using this gas exist, such as age of less than 6 years, pregnancy, and presence of disease or traumatic injury affecting the head or chest (Helvig, Heimback, 1992).

Stage 3 addresses pain management within 3 days before discharge. Patients are weaned from morphine to Lorcet 10 (hydrocodone 10 mg and acetaminophen 650 mg). Occasionally ibuprofen is used as an adjunct to Lorcet 10. One of the limitations with Lorcet 10 is the amount of acetaminophen in each tablet. The authors discuss with the patient that the limit is six tablets in a 24-hour period because more tablets would exceed the maximum recommended daily dose of 4000 mg of acetaminophen.

Neuropathic pain is not often identified during hospitalization but becomes more prevalent in the outpatient phase. The main adjuvant analgesics the authors use are antidepressants, such as amitriptyline (Elavil) and fluoxetine (Prozac). Others have reported the usefulness of anticonvulsants (Ready, Edwards, 1992). In addition, IV lidocaine by continuous infusion has reportedly been effective (Jonsson, Cassuto, Hanson, 1991), but research is lacking.

Some clinicians have attempted pain control with topical anesthetics (e.g., lidocaine cream, 5%; spray, 1%; or gel, 2%) applied to the burn wound or donor sites (Brofeldt, Cornwell, Doherty et al., 1989; Freund, Marvin, 1990;

Owen, Dye, 1990). Further research is needed to establish the safety and efficacy of these modalities.

Hypnosis and other nondrug pain relief measures have been used with burn patients. The effectiveness and practicality of these interventions, however, are limited by how well the patient's pain is controlled with analgesics, allocation of staff, and the willingness of the patient to participate.

Assessment, treatment, and effects of depression in the burn patient have not been well researched. However, study results indicate that depression, especially in a burn wound size greater than 25% TBSA, needs to be addressed (Ulmer, 1997).

SUMMARY

The overall treatment and care of the burn patient is very complex and multifaceted. Challenges arise when trying to maintain a balance between the physiologic needs and the psychologic needs of the patient. Resuscitative research and defined treatment modalities have reduced the incidence of burn shock. Hopefully, one day the patient's pain will be as well managed.

Resources

American Burn Association
New York Hospital—Cornell Medical Center
    521 E. 68th St., Room L-706
    New York, NY 10021
    (800) 548-2876

The Phoenix Society for Burn Survivors
    33 Main St., Suite 304
    Nashua, NH 03060
    (800) 888-2876
    Fax: (603) 889-4688
    Web sites:
        http://www.lewisville.com/nporgs/phoenix.html
        http://tallahassee.net/~Tbr/phoenix.html

    Provides referral to an area coordinator who can give information about local resources, such as support groups, family groups, and burn camps.

Reviewed by John L. Hunt, MD, co-director, Burn Unit; Gary F. Purdue, MD, co-director, Burn Unit; Phala A. Helm, retired director, Physical Medicine and Rehabilitation; Karen J. Kowalske, director, Physical Medicine and Rehabilitation, Parkland Hospital, University of Texas Southwestern Medical School, Dallas, Texas.

References

American Burn Association: *Annual burn facility survey data,* 1991 (unpublished).

Ashburn M: Burn pain: the management of procedure-related pain, *J Burn Care Rehabil* 16:365-371, 1995.

Atchison NE, Osgood PF, Carr DB: Pain during burn dressing changes in children: relationship to burn area, depth and analgesic regimen, *pain* 47:41-47, 1991.

Brofeldt BT, Cornwell P, Doherty D et al.: Topical lidocaine in the treatment of partial thickness burns, *J Burn Care Rehabil* 10:63-68, 1989.

Charlton JF, Klein R, Gagliardi G et al.: Factors affecting pain in burned patients—a preliminary report, *Postgrad Med J* 59:604-607, 1983.

Choiniere M: Pain of burns. In *Textbook of pain,* pp 523-537, New York, 1994, Churchill Livingstone.

Choiniere M, Melzack R, Rondeau J et al.: The pain of burns, characteristics and correlates, *J Trauma* 29:1531-1539, 1989.

Fagerhaugh SY: Pain expression and control on a burn care unit, *Nurs Outlook* 22:645-650, 1974.

Freund PR, Marvin JA: Postburn pain. In Bonica JJ, editor: *The management of pain,* ed 2, pp 481-489, Philadelphia, 1990, Lea & Febiger.

Helvig E, Heimbach D: Nitrous oxide in the management of burn pain. In *Pain management in the burn patient: a workshop review,* pp 15-18, 1992, Seattle.

Jonsson A, Cassuto J, Hanson B: Inhibition of burn pain by intravenous lignocaine infusion, *Lancet* 338:151-152, 1991.

Kowalske K, Tanelian DL: Burn pain evaluation, *Anesthesiol Clin North Am* 15:269-283, 1997.

Maaser B: Early psychological interventions with adult burn survivors and their families, *Top Emerg Med* 17(1):50-56, 1995.

Mannon JM: Caring for the burned: life and death in a hospital burn center, Springfield, Ill, 1985, Charles C Thomas.

National Center for Health Statistics: *National health interview survey,* Hyattsville, Md, 1990, The Center.

National Center for Health Statistics: *Hospital discharge abstract survey,* Avon, Mass, 1992, The Center.

National Fire Protection Association: *Fire incident report system data,* 1990, The Association.

Owen TD, Dye D: The value of topical lidocaine gel in pain relief on skin graft donor sites, *Br J Plast Surg* 43:480-482, 1990.

Perry S, Heidrich G: Management of pain during debridement: a survey of U.S. burn units, *Pain* 13:267-280, 1982.

Perry S, Heidrich G, Ramos E: Assessment of pain in burned patients, *J Burn Care Rehabil* 2:322-326, 1981.

Perry SW, Cella DF, Falkenberg J: Pain perception in burn patents with stress disorder, *J Pain Symptom Manage* 2:29-33, 1987.

Ptacek JT, Patterson DR, Montgomery BK et al.: Pain, coping, and adjustment in patients with burns: preliminary findings from a prospective study, *J Pain Symptom Manage* 10:446-455, 1995.

Ready LB, Edwards WT: *Management of acute pain: a practical guide,* Seattle, 1992, IASP.

Tucker P: The burn victim: a review of psychosocial issues, *Aust NZ J Psychiatry* 20:413-420, 1986.

Ulmer JF: An exploratory study of pain, coping, and depressed mood following burn injury, *J Pain Symptom Manage* 13:148-157, 1997.

CANCER-RELATED PAIN

Mary Layman Goldstein

Description

In 1997 approximately 560,000 Americans died of cancer, most often cancers of the lung and bronchus, prostate, breast, and colon and rectum (Table 12.2) (Parker, Tony, Bolden et al., 1997). Two thirds had pain at some point during their disease. The following three types of pain tend to occur in patients with cancer:

1. Tumor involvement: local, regional, and metastatic spread of disease, estimated to occur in approximately 65% to 85% of patients.
2. Cancer-related procedures and treatment effects, estimated to occur in approximately 15% to 25% of adults. Children with cancer have a higher percentage of procedural pain.
3. Causes unrelated to cancer, estimated in approximately 3% to 10% of patients. This includes such

● ● ● ● ●

TABLE 12.2 **Estimated Summary for 1997 of the Three Most Common Newly Diagnosed Cases of Cancer and Cancer Deaths in the United States for Males and Females***

	MEN	WOMEN
Estimated new cancer cases	1. Prostate, 43% 2. Lung and bronchus, 13% 3. Colon and rectum, 8%	1. Breast, 30% 2. Lung and bronchus, 13% 3. Colon and rectum, 11%
Estimated cancer deaths	1. Lung and bronchus, 32% 2. Prostate, 14% 3. Colon and rectum, 9%	1. Lung and bronchus, 25% 2. Breast, 17% 3. Colon and rectum, 10%

*Excludes basal and squamous cell cancer and carcinoma in situ except bladder. Based on American Cancer Society estimations.
Information from Parker SL, Tony T, Bolden S et al.: Cancer statistics, 1997, *CA Cancer J Clin* 47(1):5-27, 1997.

● ● ● ● ●

TABLE 12.3 **Common Sites of Pain Associated With Disease Involvement for Patients With Cancer of Lung and Bronchus, Breast, Prostate, and Colon and Rectum**

TUMOR TYPE	COMMON SITES OF PAINFUL DISEASE INVOLVEMENT	PAIN MANAGEMENT CONSIDERATIONS
Lung and bronchus	• Local to regional spread (including chest wall infiltration) • Bones: long bones, vertebrae (may progress to ESCC)	• Brain involvement (may make patient more susceptible to CNS effects of opioids) • Early recognition of increased back pain as a sign of pending ESCC (see text for discussion of ESCC treatment)
Breast	• Chest wall infiltration • Lymph nodes • Pleura • Skin • Bones: long bones, vertebrae (may progress to ESCC)	• Brain involvement (may make patient more susceptible to CNS effects of opioids) • Early recognition of increased back pain as a sign of pending ESCC (see text for discussion of ESCC treatment)
Prostate	• Local to regional spread • Liver • Bones: long bones, vertebrae (may progress to ESCC)	• Early recognition of increased back pain as a sign of pending ESCC (see text for discussion of ESCC treatment)
Colon and rectum	• Bowel (local extension and deeper, which may progress to obstruction) • Liver • Bones: pelvis, hips, vertebrae (may progress to ESCC)	• Early recognition of increased back pain as a sign of pending ESCC (see text for discussion of ESCC treatment)

Information from Caraceni A: Clinical correlates of common cancer pain syndromes, *Hematology/Oncol Clin North Am* 10(1):57-78, 1996; Coyle N, Foley KM: Prevalence and profile of pain syndromes in cancer patients. In McGuire D, Henke Yarbro C, editors: *Cancer pain management,* pp 21-46, New York, 1987, Grune & Stratton; Elliott K, Foley KM: Neurologic pain syndromes in patients with cancer, *Crit Care Clin* 6(2):393-420, 1990; Foley KM: Pain assessment and cancer pain syndromes. In Doyle D, Hanks GH, McDonald N, editors: *Oxford textbook of palliative medicine,* pp 148-165, Oxford, 1993, Oxford University Press; Foley KM: Supportive care and quality of life. In DeVita VT, Hellman S, Rosenberg SA, editors: *Cancer: Principles and practice of oncology,* ed 5, pp 2807-2841, Philadelphia, 1997, Lippincott-Raven; Parker SL, Tony T, Bolden S et al.: Cancer statistics, 1997, *CA Cancer J Clin* 47(1):5-27, 1997; Rogers AG: *Therapeutic management of cancer pain,* illustrated cards 1-5, 1987, MRA Publications, Inc. (Sponsored by an educational grant from The Purdue Frederick Company, Norwalk, Conn.)

things as chronic low back pain, diabetic neuropathies, and rheumatoid arthritis.

Frequently patients have a combination of all three types of pain (Caraceni, 1996; Coyle, Foley, 1987; Elliott, Foley, 1990; Foley, 1993, 1997).

Pain Characteristics and Assessment

Depending on the cause of the pain, it can be chronic or acute. A patient with chronic pain may have acute episodes of pain superimposed on his or her chronic pain (Adelhardt, Byrnes, Derby et al., 1995).

● ● ● ● ●

TABLE 12.4 Pain Related to Musculoskeletal Tumor Involvement

AREA INVOLVED (TUMOR FREQUENTLY INVOLVED)*	PATIENT MAY REPORT PAIN AS	PAIN MANAGEMENT CONSIDERATIONS
General bony involvement: • Long bones (P, B, L & B, C & R) • Shoulder (B, L & B) • Pelvis (P, C & R) • Hip (P, C & R)	• Sharp, throbbing, achy, or pressure-like	• Well localized • Worsened by movement and weight bearing • Potential for fracture • Plane x-ray film may be helpful followed by a bone scan if necessary
First cervical vertebra (B) *Multiple myeloma; metastasis to bone from breast*	• Sharp neck pain	• May radiate to posterior skull • May have sensory or motor loss in upper extremities
Chest wall (B, L & B)	• Sharp, throbbing, achy, or pressure-like	• Local pain • May experience hyperalgesia (extreme sensitivity to pain) • Tumor may progress to invade ribs, intercostal nerves, vertebrae, and brachial plexus

May be duplicated for use in clinical practice. As appears in McCaffery M, Pasero C: *Pain: Clinical manual,* p. 533, 1999, Mosby, Inc.

*B, breast; P, prostate; L & B, lung and bronchus; C & R, colon and rectum.

Information from Caraceni A: Clinical correlates of common cancer pain syndromes, *Hematol/Oncol Clin North Am,* 10(1):57-78, 1996; Coyle N, Foley KM: Prevalence and profile of pain syndromes in cancer patients. In McGuire D, Henke Yarbro C, editors: *Cancer pain management,* pp 21-46, New York, 1987, Grune & Stratton; Elliott K, Foley KM: Neurologic pain syndromes in patients with cancer, *Crit Care Clin* 6(2):393-420, 1990; Foley KM: Pain assessment and cancer pain syndromes. In Doyle D, Hanks GH, McDonald N, editors: *Oxford textbook of palliative medicine,* pp 148-165, Oxford, 1993, Oxford University Press; Foley KM: Supportive care and quality of life. In DeVita VT, Hellman S, Rosenberg SA, editors: *Cancer: Principles and practice of oncology,* ed 5, pp 2807-2841, Philadelphia, 1997, Lippincott-Raven.

Illustration from Rogers AG: *Therapeutic management of cancer pain,* illustrated cards 1-5, 1987, MRA Publications, Inc. Used with permission, Family Practice Recertification, MRA Publications, an MWC Company, Jamesburg, NJ.

Pain sites

Pain may be experienced at the site of tumor involvement or referred to a more distant site. Neurotoxic drugs such as vincristine can cause pain that occurs in the hands and feet. Patients frequently experience more than one site of pain (Caraceni, 1996; Coyle, Foley, 1987; Elliott, Foley, 1990; Foley, 1993, 1997; Rogers, 1987). New reports of pain need to be investigated because they may represent new treatable sites of disease (Gonzales, Elliott, Portenoy et al., 1991).

Pain intensity

Pain intensity can vary and is often a barometer of what is occurring with the disease. For example, a person experiencing spinal cord compression may find that pain severity is rapidly increasing as the compression progresses.

Pain syndromes

Cancer-related pain syndromes can be characterized as nociceptive, neuropathic, or mixed. Many dis-

tinct pain syndromes related to cancer are possible. Tumors involving the breast, prostate, lung and bronchus, and colon and rectum frequently involve painful sites of disease involvement (Table 12.3). Tables 12.4 to 12.6 review some of the syndromes that are commonly seen in these tumors. These same pain syndromes may also occur in patients with other types of primary cancer. Other primary cancers with specific pain syndromes include pancreatic cancer and head and neck cancers (Caraceni, 1996; Coyle, Foley, 1987; Elliott, Foley, 1990; Foley, 1993, 1997; Rogers, 1987).

• Nociceptive pain: results from the activation of nociceptors in somatic or visceral structures and often relates to tissue damage.

  • Somatic pain caused by damage to the musculoskeletal, cutaneous, or deep tissues is often reported as sharp, throbbing, aching, or pressure-like in well-localized locations. Frequently experienced examples include bone pain (see Table 12.4) or postsurgical pain (Table 12.7).

Text continued on p. 537.

● ● ● ● ●

TABLE 12.5   **Pain Associated With Tumor Involvement of Viscera**

AREA INVOLVED (TUMOR FREQUENTLY INVOLVED)*	PATIENT MAY REPORT PAIN AS	PAIN MANAGEMENT CONSIDERATIONS
Abdomen (P, C & R) 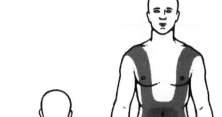 Advanced cancer of pancreas, colon, uterus, ovaries; intestinal obstruction.	• Cramping	• May radiate to groin, shoulder, or back • With retroperitoneal involvement, bending over or curling up may lessen pain severity
Abdomen, resulting in intestinal obstruction and peritoneal carcinomatosis (P, C & R) 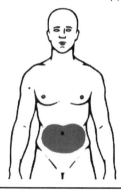	• Colicky, cramping, dull, aching	• May be accompanied by abdominal distention, ascites, diarrhea, constipation, nausea, vomiting, and bowel obstruction

May be duplicated for use in clinical practice. As appears in McCaffery M, Pasero C: *Pain: Clinical manual*, p. 534, 1999, Mosby, Inc.

*B, breast; P, prostate; L & B, lung and bronchus; C & R, colon and rectum.

Information from Caraceni A: Clinical correlates of common cancer pain syndromes, *Hematol/Oncol Clin North Am* 10(1):57-78, 1996; Coyle N, Foley KM: Prevalence and profile of pain syndromes in cancer patients. In McGuire D, Henke Yarbro C, editors: *Cancer pain management*, pp 21-46, New York, 1987, Grune & Stratton; Elliott K, Foley KM: Neurologic pain syndromes in patients with cancer, *Crit Care Clin* 6(2):393-420, 1990; Foley KM: Pain assessment and cancer pain syndromes. In Doyle D, Hanks GH, McDonald N, editors: *Oxford textbook of palliative medicine*, pp 148-165, Oxford, 1993, Oxford University Press; Foley KM: Supportive care and quality of life. In DeVita VT, Hellman S, Rosenberg SA, editors: *Cancer: Principles and practice of oncology*, ed 5, pp 2807-2841, Philadelphia, 1997, Lippincott-Raven.

Illustrations from Rogers AG: *Therapeutic management of cancer pain*, illustrated cards 1-5, 1987, MRA Publications, Inc. Used with permission, Family Practice Recertification, MRA Publications, an MWC Company, Jamesburg, NJ.

TABLE 12.6 **Pain Associated With Peripheral or Central Nervous System Tumor Involvement (Neuropathic Pain)**

AREA INVOLVED (TUMOR FREQUENTLY INVOLVED)*	PATIENT MAY REPORT PAIN AS	PAIN MANAGEMENT CONSIDERATIONS
Ribs/intercostal nerves (B, L & B) *Tumor infiltration of peripheral nerves (most commonly, paravertebral or retroperitoneal tumors)* 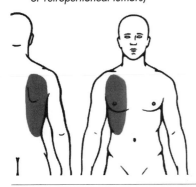	• Burning, shooting, shock-like	• May radiate along nerve root • May be worsened by deep breathing or moving • May experience sensory loss distal to area of nerve compression
Brachial plexus (B, L & B) *Superior sulcus tumors of lung* 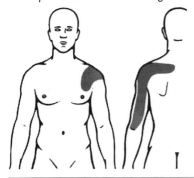	• Burning, shooting, shock-like	• Located in shoulder and arm and radiates down arm • Caused by compression or infiltration of plexus by tumor • May experience numbness, paresthesias (burning, tingling), hyperalgesia (extreme sensitivity to touch), and allodynia (distress from painful stimuli) • Tumor may progress to epidural space *(increasing risk of spinal cord compression)* • Depending on status of disease and goals of care, may need evaluation of plexus with CT or MRI
Lumbar plexus (P, C & R) 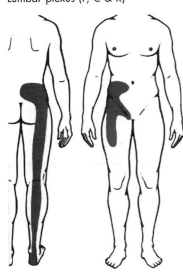	• Burning, shooting, shock-like, aching, pressure-like	• Radiates down anterior thigh and groin or posterior aspect of thigh • Can be caused by local extension of nodular metastasis • May experience numbness (not relieved by analgesics), paresthesias (burning, tingling, prickling), weakness, and later, leg edema

Continued.

TABLE 12.6   **Pain Associated With Peripheral or Central Nervous System Tumor Involvement (Neuropathic Pain)—cont'd**

AREA INVOLVED (TUMOR FREQUENTLY INVOLVED)*	PATIENT MAY REPORT PAIN AS	PAIN MANAGEMENT CONSIDERATIONS
Sacral plexus (P, C & R) Genitourinary, gynecological, and colonic cancers.	• Burning, shooting, shock-like, dull, aching	• Midline of lower back • May experience perianal sensory loss, difficulty sitting, impotency, bowel and bladder dysfunction
Spinal cord: cervical, thoracic, and lumbosacral vertebrae (B, L & B, P, C & R) *Spinal cord compression after metastasis to bone from breast, lung, kidney, or prostate; bone and soft-tissue cancers without bone metastasis (lymphoma sarcoma); gastrointestinal tumors; myeloma*	• Dull, aching, sharp with movement, tight, band-like	• Back pain worse with lying down, coughing, sneezing, or weight bearing • May experience local pain over involved vertebrae • Posterior extension from a vertebral body *can lead to this oncologic emergency, ESCC* • Untreated, ESCC can lead to paraplegia or quadriplegia (depending on location of involvement) • Diagnosis and treatment before development of sensory or motor weakness can lead to a better functional outcome • Neurologic findings before treatment are not usually reversible • ESCC can rapidly progress from reports of pain to sensory loss to loss of motor function and loss of bowel or bladder control • All reports of back pain must be taken seriously and evaluated • MRI most sensitive, noninvasive way to evaluate for ESCC

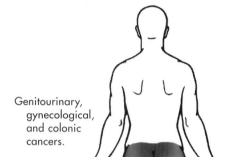
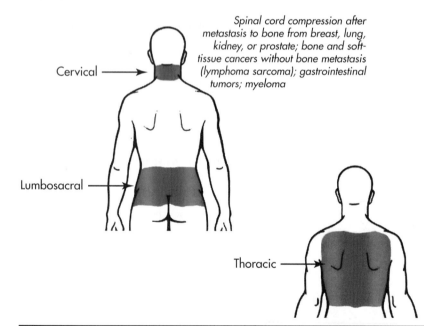

May be duplicated for use in clinical practice. As appears in McCaffery M, Pasero C: *Pain: Clinical manual,* pp. 535-536, 1999, Mosby, Inc.

NOTE: These individuals may also experience nociceptive pain.

*B, breast; P, prostate; L & B, lung and bronchus; C & R, colon and rectum.

Information from Caraceni A: Clinical correlates of common cancer pain syndromes, *Hematol/Oncol Clin North Am* 10(1):57-78, 1996; Coyle N, Foley KM: Prevalence and profile of pain syndromes in cancer patients. In McGuire D, Henke Yarbro C, editors: *Cancer pain management,* pp. 21-46, New York, 1987, Grune & Stratton; Elliott K, Foley KM: Neurologic pain syndromes in patients with cancer, *Crit Care Clin* 6(2):393-420, 1990; Foley KM: Pain assessment and cancer pain syndromes. In Doyle D, Hanks GH, McDonald N, editors: *Oxford textbook of palliative medicine,* pp 148-165, Oxford, 1993, Oxford University Press; Foley KM: Supportive care and quality of life. In DeVita VT, Hellman S, Rosenberg SA, editors: *Cancer: Principles and practice of oncology,* ed 5, pp 2807-2841, Philadelphia, 1997, Lippincott-Raven.

Illustrations modified from Rogers AG: *Therapeutic management of cancer pain,* illustrated cards 1-5, 1987, MRA Publications, Inc. Used with permission, Family Practice Recertification, MRA Publications, an MWC Company, Jamesburg, NJ.

● ● ● ● ●

TABLE 12.7   **Postsurgical Pain Associated With Cancer Treatment**

PAIN SYNDROME (TUMOR FREQUENTLY INVOLVED)*	AREA INVOLVED	PATIENT MAY REPORT PAIN AS	PAIN MANAGEMENT CONSIDERATIONS
Postmastectomy pain syndrome (B) 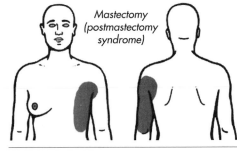 *Mastectomy (postmastectomy syndrome)*	• Posterior arm, axilla, anterior chest wall	• Tight, constricting, burning (= neuropathic pain)	• Usually begins 1 to 2 mo after surgery or as late as 6 mo • Worse with movement, may lead to a frozen shoulder
Postthoracotomy pain syndrome (L & B) 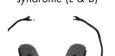 *Thoracotomy (postthoracotomy syndrome)*	• Chest wall	• Constant, aching, burning, occasionally shock-like (= neuropathic pain)	• May experience numbness • Worse with movement, may lead to a frozen shoulder • May experience extreme tenderness at most medial and apical points of scar • Persistent or recurrent pain in the thoracotomy scar area is often associated with recurrent tumor

May be duplicated for use in clinical practice. As appears in McCaffery M, Pasero C: *Pain: Clinical manual,* p. 537, 1999, Mosby, Inc.

*B, breast; P, prostate; L & B, lung and bronchus; C & R, colon and rectum.

Information from Caraceni A: Clinical correlates of common cancer pain syndromes, *Hematol/Oncol Clin North Am* 10(1):57-78, 1996; Coyle N, Foley KM: Prevalence and profile of pain syndromes in cancer patients. In McGuire D, Henke Yarbro C, editors: *Cancer pain management,* pp 21-46, New York, 1987, Grune & Stratton; Elliott K, Foley KM: Neurologic pain syndromes in patients with cancer, *Crit Care Clin* 6(2):393-420, 1990; Foley KM: Pain assessment and cancer pain syndromes. In Doyle D, Hanks GH, McDonald N, editors: *Oxford textbook of palliative medicine,* pp 148-165, Oxford, 1993, Oxford University Press; Foley KM: Supportive care and quality of life. In DeVita VT, Hellman S, Rosenberg SA, editors: *Cancer: Principles and practice of oncology,* ed 5, pp 2807-2841, Philadelphia, 1997, Lippincott-Raven.

Illustrations from Rogers AG: *Therapeutic management of cancer pain,* illustrated cards 1-5, 1987, MRA Publications, Inc. Used with permission, Family Practice Recertification, MRA Publications, an MWC Company, Jamesburg, NJ.

• Visceral pain, originating from stretching or distention of the thoracic or abdominal viscera, can be described as cramping or gnawing or deep aching, is often poorly localized, and may be referred from other sites. In the cancer population examples include bowel obstruction or distention of the liver capsule (see Table 12.5).

• Neuropathic pain: often described as burning, shooting, "pins and needles," or shock-like sensations and comes from peripheral or central nervous system damage (see Table 12.6). Neuropathic pain can be referred to areas of the body innervated by the affected nerve root. For example, a lesion in the back may refer to a distant site such as the groin, knee, or ankle. The actual site of referred pain will depend on the nerve root

involved. Vinca alkaloid chemotherapeutic agents can cause painful treatment-related peripheral neuropathies (Table 12.8).

Procedural and treatment-related pain

Children are most vulnerable to procedural pain. Acute pain can be caused by surgery (postoperative pain), chemotherapy (e.g., mucositis, gastrointestinal distress, joint pain, or extravasation), and radiation (e.g., skin burn, mucositis, or proctitis). Examples of chronic treatment-related pain for patients with lung and bronchus, breast, prostate, and colon and rectal cancer are described in Tables 12.7 to 12.9 (Adelhardt, Byrnes, Derby et al., 1995; Caraceni, 1996; Coyle, Foley, 1987; Elliott, Foley, 1990; Foley, 1993, 1997; Martin, Hagen, 1997; Rogers, 1987).

● ● ● ● ●

TABLE 12.8   **Postchemotherapy Pain Associated With Cancer Treatment**

PAIN SYNDROME (TUMOR FREQUENTLY INVOLVED)*	AREA INVOLVED	PATIENT MAY REPORT PAIN AS	PAIN MANAGEMENT CONSIDERATIONS
Painful peripheral neuropathy (B, P, L & B, C & R) 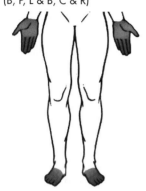	• Hands and feet	• Burning, tingling	• Neuropathic-like pain • Worsened by minor stimuli • May experience loss of reflexes • Pain may resolve as neuropathy resolves
Corticosteroid-associated pain (B, P, L & B, C & R) 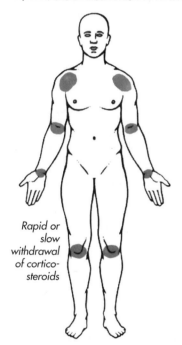 *Rapid or slow withdrawal of cortico-steroids*	• Muscles and joints	• Tenderness, aching	• Transient • May also experience fatigue and malaise • Can occur with rapid or slow taper of steroids • Relieved by reinstitution of steroid and a slower, more gradual taper

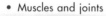

May be duplicated for use in clinical practice. As appears in McCaffery M, Pasero C: *Pain: Clinical manual*, pp. 538-539, 1999, Mosby, Inc.   *Continued.*

● ● ● ● ●

TABLE 12.8 **Postchemotherapy Pain Associated With Cancer Treatment—cont'd**

PAIN SYNDROME (TUMOR FREQUENTLY INVOLVED)*	AREA INVOLVED	PATIENT MAY REPORT PAIN AS	PAIN MANAGEMENT CONSIDERATIONS
Aseptic necrosis of femoral or humoral head from chronic corticosteroid therapy (B, P, L & B, C & R)	• Humoral (shoulder) and femoral head (knee or leg)	• Throbbing, aching	• Joint movement limitation and sometimes joint tenderness • Worsened by movement and relieved by rest • Bone scan and MRI helpful in diagnosis • Treat pain and decrease/discontinue steroids • If severe, depending on status of disease and goals of care, may necessitate joint replacement

Chronic corticosteroid therapy (aseptic necrosis of bone)

May be duplicated for use in clinical practice. As appears in McCaffery M, Pasero C: *Pain: Clinical manual*, pp. 538-539, 1999, Mosby, Inc.

*B, breast; P, prostate; L & B, lung and bronchus; C & R, colon and rectum.

Information from Caraceni A: Clinical correlates of common cancer pain syndromes, *Hematol/Oncol Clin North Am* 10(1):57-78, 1996; Coyle N, Foley KM: Prevalence and profile of pain syndromes in cancer patients. In McGuire D, Henke Yarbro C, editors: *Cancer pain management*, pp 21-46, New York, 1987, Grune & Stratton; Elliott K, Foley KM: Neurologic pain syndromes in patients with cancer, *Crit Care Clin* 6(2):393-420, 1990; Foley KM: Pain assessment and cancer pain syndromes. In Doyle D, Hanks GH, McDonald N, editors: *Oxford textbook of palliative medicine*, pp 148-165, Oxford, 1993, Oxford University Press; Foley KM: Supportive care and quality of life. In DeVita VT, Hellman S, Rosenberg SA, editors: *Cancer: Principles and practice of oncology*, ed 5, pp 2807-2841, Philadelphia, 1997, Lippincott-Raven.

Illustration from Rogers AG: *Therapeutic management of cancer pain*, illustrated cards 1-5, 1987, MRA Publications, Inc. Used with permission, Family Practice Recertification, MRA Publications, an MWC Company, Jamesburg, NJ.

Pain Management

If possible, one treats the underlying cause of the pain, *always in addition to treating the pain itself.* This includes the following:

- Surgery to decrease the tumor burden
- Radiation therapy to decrease the tumor burden
- Chemotherapy to decrease the tumor burden
- Antibiotics to treat infection (e.g., patients with head and neck cancers or gynecologic cancers can experience an increase in pain with infection that decreases as the infection clears)

When caring for cancer patients, it is important to be alert to increasing back pain because this may be a sign of pending epidural spinal cord compression (ESCC), an oncologic emergency (see Table 12.6). Early diagnosis and treatment of ESCC (before loss of sensory or motor function) can lead to a better func-tional outcome. Treatment of ESCC involves high-dose steroid administration (usually dexamethasone, 10 to 100 mg intravenously) followed by a lower dose every 6 hours. The patient also receives radiation to the area of the ESCC and the two adjacent vertebrae above and below this site. The steroids are continued throughout the treatment and then tapered as the radiation is completed.

Patients who have already received the maximum dose of radiation to this area or who experience progression of neurologic symptoms during radiation treatment are evaluated for emergency surgery to relieve the cord compression.

Treatment of the symptom of pain

- Pharmacotherapy: The World Health Organization (WHO) ladder, using opioids, nonopioids, and adjuvant

TABLE 12.9   **Postradiation Pain Associated With Cancer Treatment**

PAIN SYNDROME (TUMOR FREQUENTLY INVOLVED)*	AREA INVOLVED	PATIENT MAY REPORT PAIN AS	PAIN MANAGEMENT CONSIDERATIONS
Radiation fibrosis of brachial plexus (B, L & B) 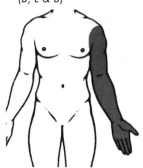	• Shoulder and arm	• Burning	• Occurs 6 mo to 20 yr after radiation therapy caused by fibrosis of the surrounding connective tissue and secondary damage to nerve • May experience numbness, tingling, and progressive neurologic deficits • Difficult to distinguish from tumor infiltration
Radiation fibrosis of lumbosacral plexus (P, C & R) 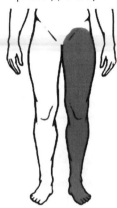	• Leg and buttocks or perineum	• Aching, pulling, burning	• Occurs 1 to 30 yr after treatment • May experience numbness, tingling, and progress to weakness in legs • May include necrosis of bone
Radiation myelopathy 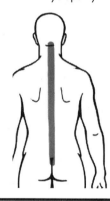	• Localized to spine or referred	• Aching	• Occurs 5 to 30 mo after treatment • Must be carefully assessed to rule out ESCC and other diagnosis • Pain can be managed, but myelopathy is not reversible

May be duplicated for use in clinical practice. As appears in McCaffery M, Pasero C: *Pain: Clinical manual*, p. 540, 1999, Mosby, Inc.

*B, breast; P, prostate; L & B, lung and bronchus; C & R, colon and rectum.

Information from Caraceni A: Clinical correlates of common cancer pain syndromes, *Hematol/Oncol Clin North Am* 10(1):57-78, 1996; Coyle N, Foley KM: Prevalence and profile of pain syndromes in cancer patients. In McGuire D, Henke Yarbro C, editors: *Cancer pain management*, pp 21-46, New York, 1987, Grune & Stratton; Elliott K, Foley KM: Neurologic pain syndromes in patients with cancer, *Crit Care Clin* 6(2):393-420, 1990; Foley KM: Pain assessment and cancer pain syndromes. In Doyle D, Hanks GH, McDonald N, editors: *Oxford textbook of palliative medicine*, pp 148-165, Oxford, 1993, Oxford University Press; Foley KM: Supportive care and quality of life. In DeVita VT, Hellman S, Rosenberg SA, editors: *Cancer: Principles and practice of oncology*, ed 5, pp 2807-2841, Philadelphia, 1997, Lippincott-Raven.

Illustrations from Rogers AG: *Therapeutic management of cancer pain*, illustrated cards 1-5, 1987, MRA Publications, Inc. Used with permission, Family Practice Recertification, MRA Publications, an MWC Company, Jamesburg, NJ.

analgesics, is the mainstay of the pharmacologic approach (see discussion in Chapters 4, 5, 6, and 7).

- Opioids and nonopioids are used for the treatment of nociceptive pain.
- For bone-related pain, in addition to opioids, consider the use of adjuvant medications such as corticosteroids, bisphoshonates, gallium nitrate, calcitonin, and strontium-89. Some adjuvant analgesics may be contraindicated for patients receiving certain primary cancer treatments. For example, a patient with multiple myeloma who is receiving steroids as a chemotherapeutic agent would probably not be able to receive additional steroids for pain treatment. The patient's primary physician is best able to address this issue.
- For neuropathic pain, in addition to opioids, adjuvant analgesics, such as antidepressants, anticonvulsants, oral and cutaneous local anesthetics, corticosteroids, clonidine, benzodiazepines, neuroleptics, and NMDA antagonists, can be helpful depending on the specific pain syndrome.
- Cognitive behavioral techniques: can be useful as an adjunct to other cancer pain treatments to promote a sense of control, physical comfort, relaxation, and distraction (see discussion in Chapters 8 and 11).
- Invasive techniques: For some selected specific pain syndromes in the hands of skilled, experienced practitioners, invasive techniques are of value, such as epidural analgesics or various nerve blocks (Adelhardt, Byrnes, Derby et al., 1995; Cherny, Portenoy, 1994; Foley, 1997; Management of Cancer Pain Guideline Panel, 1994; Martin, Hagen, 1997).

Considerations for management of chronic cancer-related pain

- Confirm that sufficient ATC and PRN analgesics are ordered and available.
- Make certain that the patients can obtain prescribed analgesics at their usual pharmacy or that an alternate source is found.
- Instruct patients receiving chronic opioid therapy to carry written documentation of their current analgesic regimen (drug, dose, frequency, and route) and treating physician (with phone number) when leaving their home. This information can be essential should an emergency arise.
- Be aware of the analgesic effect of corticosteroids. If they are tapered, it may necessitate increasing opioids to provide the same analgesia. Also, the reverse may be true; if steroids are added, it may be necessary to decrease the opioids administered to prevent side effects (Rogers, 1987).
- Increasing pain or decreasing analgesic effectiveness, without change in analgesic regimen, frequently means

advancing disease, not tolerance (Cherny, Portenoy, 1994). Additional assessment of the cause of pain is necessary. This may result in diagnosis of treatable conditions (Gonzales, Elliott, Portenoy et al., 1991).

- With the primary physician, develop a plan to be used in the case of a pain crisis (sudden escalation of pain).
- As cancer progresses, continually assess whether pain is being controlled and the patient is satisfied with the method of control.
- Avoid the IM route. Consider the use of an indwelling subcutaneous needle should repeated injections become necessary (Adelhardt, Byrnes, Derby et al., 1995).
- Educate the patient and caregiver to identify situations that require professional intervention (e.g., unrelieved pain, acute changes in severity, location, or duration of pain, or unrelieved complications of the pain management regimen).
- Educate the patient, caregiver, and other health care professionals as to the purpose of specific adjuvant analgesics to ensure that they will not be inadvertently discontinued.
- Understand that the use of morphine, methadone, or the IV route may have special meaning to a patient or family. For example, use of morphine or the IV route may be interpreted that the patient is close to death when in fact the patient may not be, or the use of methadone may be interpreted that the patient is a drug addict when in fact methadone may be an effective analgesic for that particular patient.
- Individuals with chronic cancer-related pain who experience acute pain episodes (such as surgery) will need continued treatment of their chronic cancer-related pain in addition to treatment of the acute pain.
- Be aware of a patient's goals of care. Goals of care can include any one or combination of the following: maximizing survival, maximizing function, and maximizing comfort. Knowledge of goals of care is necessary when evaluating the risk/benefit ratio of pain treatments. For example, in an opioid-naive, fragile patient whose only goal is to maximize survival, it may be necessary to limit the use of opioids. In the dying patient, it may not be possible to maximize function and comfort. A decision will need to be made as to what the primary goal is to ensure appropriate treatment.
- Some health care professionals mistakenly believe that if a cancer patient is dying, the opioid used for pain relief should be changed to morphine. This is not necessary as long as the prescribed analgesic controls the pain without dose-limiting side effects.
- Be very cautious about the use of naloxone in opioid-tolerant patients. Be aware of the goals of care. Rule out progression of disease and other medications as the cause of deteriorating respiratory status.

If administration of naloxone is appropriate, administer slowly, titrating to effect to avoid precipitating withdrawal and severe pain.

Considerations related to settings where patient receives care

Inpatient Care

- Instruct patients on admission to send home any analgesics they may have brought with them.
- Early on if a possibility exists that the patient will be discharged or transferred with a PCA pump, epidural catheter, or other high-tech analgesic intervention, evaluate patient's home situation and insurance coverage to determine whether this will be a safe and insurance-covered situation (Whedon, Ferrell, 1991).

Home Care

- Become comfortable with telephone assessment. Use documentation forms that reflect a systematic assessment. Be alert to the development of new pains.
- Encourage patient and/or caregiver to use a pain control record (e.g., p. 87) to keep track of medication use, especially use of PRN doses and pain ratings after pain relief measures.
- Encourage patient and/or caregiver to notify primary physician that medication supply is getting low in enough time to have prescriptions renewed without an interruption in analgesic regimen. It is often a good idea to have a separate 3-day to 4-day supply kept for use in emergencies.
- Encourage patients to take a sufficient supply of pain medications with them whenever they leave home.
- Consider the need for parenteral medications in the home, and identify and educate the caregiver who could administer this medication should the need arise.
- Make sure that the patient and caregiver know who is to be contacted should a situation arise that requires professional intervention. This should cover situations arising 24 hours a day, 7 days a week.

Emergency Department Care

- Quickly identify the extent of disease, goals of care, DNR status, and present analgesic regimen (especially specific analgesic use and effectiveness in the last 48 hours). Is this patient opioid naive or tolerant? Has this patient been able to take analgesics by the route prescribed?
- Be very cautious about the use of naloxone. See previous discussion pp. 541-542.

SUMMARY

Almost two thirds of patients with cancer will have pain at some point during their illness. Cancer pain may be a result of tumor involvement or cancer-related procedures and treatments. The pain may be acute, chronic, or both. Pain syndromes may be nociceptive, neuropathic, or mixed. The mainstay of cancer pain relief is aggressive use of analgesics, including opioids. For neuropathic pain, adjuvant analgesics may be a valuable addition. A knowledge of the syndromes commonly seen with specific tumors aids the clinician in assessment and treatment choices.

Resources

1. Clinical practice guidelines from the Agency for Health Care Policy and Research (AHCPR): Several versions exist to meet different informational needs. Included are the following:

   Management of Cancer Pain Guideline Panel: *Management of cancer pain. Clinical practice guideline,* AHCPR Pub. No. 94-0592, Rockville, Md, Agency for Health Care Policy and Research, Public Health Service, U.S. Department of Health and Human Services, 1994.

   Management of Cancer Pain Guideline Panel: *Management of cancer pain. Clinical practice guideline and quick reference guide,* AHCPR Pub. No. 94-0593, Rockville, Md, Agency for Health Care Policy and Research, Public Health Service, U.S. Department of Health and Human Services, 1994.

   Management of Cancer Pain Guideline Panel: *Management of cancer pain. Patient's guide,* AHCPR Pub. No. 94-0595, Rockville, Md, Agency for Health Care Policy and Research, Public Health Service, U.S. Department of Health and Human Services, 1994. Available in English and Spanish.

   To order or to obtain information regarding guideline availability, call (800) 4-CANCER or write to:

   AHCPR Clearinghouse
   Cancer Pain Guideline
   P.O. Box 8547
   Silver Spring, MD 20907

2. Educational guidelines for health care professionals:

   Ad Hoc Committee on Cancer Pain of the American Society of Clinical Oncology: Cancer pain assessment and treatment curriculum guidelines, *J Clin Oncol* 10:1976-1982, 1992.

   Spross JA, McGuire DB, Schmitt RM: Oncology Nursing Society position paper on cancer pain, part I, *Oncol Nurs Forum* 17(4):595-614, 1990.

   Spross JA, McGuire DB, Schmitt RM: Oncology Nursing Society position paper on cancer pain, part II, *Oncol Nurs Forum* 17(5):751-760, 1990.

   Spross JA, McGuire DB, Schmitt RM: Oncology Nursing Society position paper on cancer pain, part III, *Oncol Nurs Forum* 17(6):943-955, 1990.

References

Adelhardt J, Byrnes M, Derby S et al.: Care of the patient in pain: standard of oncology nursing practice. In Layman Goldstein M, editor: *Pain resource notebook*, New York, 1995, Division of Nursing, Memorial Sloan-Kettering Cancer Center.

Caraceni A: Clinical correlates of common cancer pain syndromes, *Hematol/Oncol Clin North Am* 10(1):57-78, 1996.

Cherny N, Portenoy RK: Practical issues in the management of cancer pain. In Wall PD, Melzack R, editors: *Textbook of pain*, ed 3, pp 1437-1467, Edinburgh, 1994, Churchill Livingstone.

Coyle N, Foley KM: Prevalence and profile of pain syndromes in cancer patients. In McGuire D, Henke Yarbro C, editors: *Cancer pain management*, pp 21-46, New York, 1987, Grune & Stratton.

Elliott K, Foley KM: Neurologic pain syndromes in patients with cancer, *Crit Care Clin* 6(2):393-420, 1990.

Foley KM: Pain assessment and cancer pain syndromes. In Doyle D, Hanks GH, McDonald N, editors: *Oxford textbook of palliative medicine*, pp 148-165, Oxford, 1993, Oxford University Press.

Foley KM: Supportive care and quality of life. In DeVita VT, Hellman S, Rosenberg SA, editors: *Cancer: principles and practice of oncology*, ed 5, pp 2807-2841, Philadelphia, 1997, Lippincott-Raven.

Gonzales GR, Elliott KJ, Portenoy RK et al.: Impact of a comprehensive evaluation in the management of cancer pain, *Pain* 47:141-144, 1991.

Management of Cancer Pain Guideline Panel: *Management of cancer pain. Clinical practice guideline*, AHCPR Pub. No. 94-0592, pp i-xvii, 1-257, Rockville, Md, Agency for Health Care Policy and Research, Public Health Service, U.S. Department of Health and Human Services, 1994.

Martin LA, Hagen N: Neuropathic pain in cancer patients: mechanisms, syndromes, and clinical controversies, *J Pain Symptom Manage* 14(2):99-117, 1997.

Parker SL, Tony T, Bolden S et al.: Cancer statistics, 1997, *CA Cancer J Clin* 47(1):5-27, 1997.

Rogers AG: *Therapeutic management of cancer pain*, illustrated cards 1-5, 1987, MRA Publications, Inc. (Sponsored by an educational grant from The Perdue Frederick Company, Norwalk, Conn.)

Whedon M, Ferrell BR: Professional and ethical considerations in the use of high-tech pain management, *Oncol Nurs Forum* 18(7):1135-1143, 1991.

EHLERS-DANLOS SYNDROME

Kathryn Hagen and Linda Neumann-Potash

Description

Ehlers-Danlos syndrome (EDS) is actually a group of variable genetic connective tissue disorders characterized by joint hypermobility, tissue fragility, and skin extensibility (Beighton, De Paepe, Steinmann et al., 1998). Abnormalities in the formation of collagen molecules lead to these hallmark signs, as well as easy bruising, abnormal scarring, poor wound healing, and a bleeding tendency. Prevalence is estimated to be approximately 1:10,000 births, but EDS may be difficult to identify and is no doubt underdiagnosed. Although pain is an important component of the EDS, little research has been conducted about its management (Sacheti, Szemere, Bernstein et al., 1997).

Most individuals with EDS will have a normal lifespan. This may not be the case with the vascular type of EDS (previously called EDS type IV): death may result from arterial, intestinal, or uterine rupture.

Pain Characteristics

Individuals with EDS often experience both acute and chronic discomfort or pain related to a variety of causes. By adolescence they have generally experienced onset of chronic pain in at least one body area, and this pain interferes with sleep or activities of daily living. Patients report the pain as usually moderate to severe, yet x-ray films and MRIs show no abnormalities. It may be constant yet changeable in quality throughout the day (Sacheti, Szemere, Bernstein et al., 1997). Many adults are on disability because no pain management techniques have proven effective for them.

Acute discomfort often results from trauma, such as fractures, dislocations, subluxations, bruising after falls, and subcutaneous bleeding. Postoperative pain from joint surgeries or other repairs is another possible cause.

Chronic pain may result from joint, muscle, or soft tissue damage, lower extremity discomfort, pain from repeated or failed joint surgeries, early osteoarthritis resulting from unstable joints, generalized pain accompanied by fatigue, nerve injury, abdominal pain, or chest pain if mitral valve prolapse is present. Possible sites of chronic pain are numerous (Figure 12.5).

Some of the pain sites EDS patients report include or relate to the following:

- *Musculoskeletal:* joint pain; joint instability leading to spontaneous dislocations or subluxations; flat feet; temporal mandibular joint syndrome; back pain; scoliosis; fibromyalgia; joint hypermobility (Ainsworth, Aulicino, 1993); chronic joint and limb pain with normal skeletal x-ray films (Beighton, De Paepe, Steinmann et al., 1998).
- *Dermatologic:* easy bruising; spontaneous ecchymosis; connective tissue fragility; stretchy or soft, doughy skin; visible veins; dystrophic scarring; impaired wound healing; wound dehiscence; tendency for prolonged bleeding despite normal coagulation studies (Beighton, 1993).
- *Neurologic:* chronic headaches.
- *Gastrointestinal:* intestinal cramping; bowel perforation; other GI complaints (Smith, Snyder, 1993; Stillman, Painter, Hollister, 1991).
- *Obstetric/gynecologic:* increased menstrual bleeding; dyspareunia; increased joint laxity while pregnant; early labor; postpartum complications (Sakala, Harding, 1991; Sorokin, Johnson, Rogowski et al., 1994).
- *Cardiovascular:* tachycardia; mitral valve prolapse; vascular fragility; aneurysm.
- *Eye:* cone-shaped corneas; other ocular defects.

Assessment

No laboratory tests confirm or rule out EDS. Symptoms, such as chronic pain, may precede radiographic

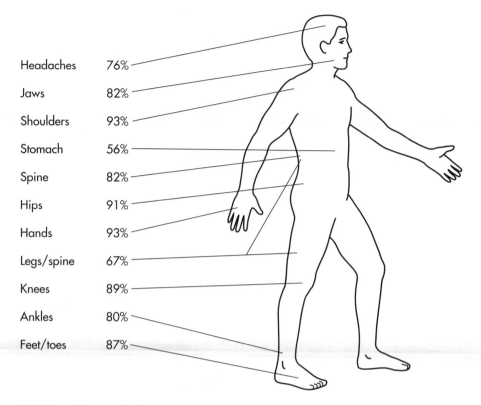

Headaches	76%
Jaws	82%
Shoulders	93%
Stomach	56%
Spine	82%
Hips	91%
Hands	93%
Legs/spine	67%
Knees	89%
Ankles	80%
Feet/toes	87%

May be duplicated for use in clinical practice. From McCaffery M, Pasero C: *Pain: Clinical manual*, p. 544. Copyright ©
1999, Mosby, Inc.

F I G U R E   12.5   Distribution of chronic pain in individuals with Ehlers-Danlos syndrome. % patients reporting chronic pain
occurring at that site at some time in their lives beginning in childhood.

Information from Sacheti A, Szemere J, Bernstein B et al.: *Chronic pain is a manifestation of the Ehlers-Danlos syndrome, J Pain Sympt Manage* 14(2)
88-93, 1997.

abnormalities by years. Clues may come from the patient's family history, although manifestations of EDS and their severity can vary among family members. Consultation with a geneticist familiar with EDS may be helpful.

Patients often become frustrated because of the difficulty of diagnosing EDS. Some clinicians may be familiar with only one or two manifestations of the disorder and believe their adult patient has multiple sclerosis, rheumatoid arthritis, or lupus. However, lupus involves an antigen-antibody reaction within connective tissue, whereas EDS results when a genetic change causes collagen molecules to be abnormally formed. EDS is in the same category of disorders as osteogenesis imperfecta and Marfan syndrome.

Because EDS generally affects multiple sites, a pain assessment tool that allows multiple assessments may prove most satisfactory. Patients may be familiar with rating their pain level on a scale of 0 to 10 and be satisfied with this method. However, when multiple sites with differing pain intensities are involved, a body outline (see p. 60) is also useful.

Patients may find it helpful to keep a pain control record (see p. 87), listing each affected site along with a description of the type and intensity of pain, a list of the day's activities, and pain ratings before and after medications (Sacheti, Szemere, Bernstein et al., 1997).

Pain Management

Because multiple sites with differing types and intensities of pain are such a part of EDS, the ongoing pain management program must use a combination of modalities. Some possibilities include the following:

- Medications: NSAIDs (must be used with care for individuals with bleeding tendency); opioids; opioids in combination with antidepressant therapy; nonprescription analgesics; muscle relaxants; sumatriptan (Imitrex) for migraines; anticonvulsants.
- Surgery (generally last resort): joint fusions; stabilizations; replacements.
- Other treatments: heat; cold; warm water exercise; splinting; bracing; pacing of activities; resting in position of comfort supported by pillows; physical and

occupational therapies; relaxation; biofeedback; diversional activities.

Preventing Pain in Various Patient Care Settings

- Home: Remove throw rugs and avoid clutter. Encourage patient to consider one-story home or one with elevator. Recommend safety bars in bathroom and aids for activities of daily living, such as jar openers.
- Emergency department: Avoid applying tape directly to skin because skin may tear when tape is removed. Sutures may not hold; depending on type of wound, staples or Steri-Strips may help. Sutures may need to be left in longer because of poor wound healing (Blair, 1990). Some individuals show decreased response to local lidocaine anesthetic (Arendt-Nielsen, 1990). IVs may be difficult to place or maintain.
- Inpatient: Mouth care must be gentle or lesions may result. Skin is generally sensitive; use special care. Move patients carefully.
- Physical therapy: Patient may be unwilling or unable to continue with treatment if it leads to increased pain, dislocations, or subluxations. Water therapy may be an option (Blair, 1990; Huey, 1991).
- General considerations: Preventing falls is important in all settings. Also, avoid asking patients to extend their joints past a normal range of motion (i.e., "parlor tricks") and encourage them not to do so at home or school.

SUMMARY

Patients with EDS are often undiagnosed or misdiagnosed for years. They may be told they are merely seeking attention or pain medications. Clinicians may attribute their difficulties to "depression" and refer them to psychiatrists (Lumley, Jordan, Rubenstein et al., 1994). When they seek an answer regarding their child's pain or other symptoms, parents may hear they are simply "overprotective" of their undiagnosed child or may be suspected of child abuse because of frequent bruising or dislocations.

Because management of EDS-related pain has not been studied in depth, no treatment protocols exist. Even after correct diagnosis, unsuccessful trials of multiple medications or modalities may take their toll on patients and those who support them physically, emotionally, and financially.

Resources

The Ehlers-Danlos National Foundation
6399 Wilshire Boulevard, Suite 510
Los Angeles, CA 90048
(213) 651-3038
Web sites: U.S.: *www.ednf.org*

Canada: *www.interlog.com/~ceda*
U.K.: *ourworld/compuserve.com/homepages/ EDS_UK/Ehlers.htm*

NOTE: *Loose Connections* is the official newsletter of the Ehlers-Danlos National Foundation.

National Organization for Rare Disorders
P.O. Box 8923
New Fairfield, CT 06812-8923
(203) 746-6518
Web site: *www.pcnet.com/~orphan*

References

Ainsworth S, Aulicino P: A survey of patients with Ehlers-Danlos syndrome, *Clin Orthop Rel Res* 286:250-256, 1993.

Arendt-Nielsen L: Insufficient effect of local analgesics in Ehlers-Danlos type III patients, *Loose Connections* 8(2):7, 1990.

Beighton P: The Ehlers-Danlos syndromes. In Beighton P, editor: *Heritable disorders of connective tissue*, pp 189-251, St. Louis, 1993, Mosby-Year Book.

Beighton P, De Paepe A, Steinmann B et al.: Ehlers-Danlos syndrome: revised nosology, *Am J Genet* 77:31-37, 1998.

Blair T: The emergency room and Ehlers-Danlos syndrome, *Loose Connections* 5(4):1-5, 1990.

Huey L, Neumann-Potash L: Water training and Ehlers-Danlos syndrome, *Loose Connections* 6(4):4-5, 1991.

Lumley M, Jordan M, Rubenstein R et al.: Psychosocial functioning in the Ehlers-Danlos syndrome, *Am J Med Genet* 53:149-152, 1994.

Sacheti A, Szemere J, Bernstein B et al.: Chronic pain is a manifestation of the Ehlers-Danlos syndrome, *J Pain Sympt Manage* 14(2):88-93, 1997.

Sakala E, Harding M: Ehlers-Danlos syndrome type III and pregnancy: a case report, *J Reprod Manage* 36(8):622-624, 1991.

Smith L, Snyder M: Gastrointestinal considerations in people suffering from the Ehlers-Danlos syndrome, *Loose Connections* 8(2):1-4, 1993.

Sorokin Y, Johnson M, Rogowski N et al.: Obstetric and gynecologic dysfunction in the Ehlers-Danlos syndrome, *J Reprod Med* 39(4):281-284, 1994.

Stillman A, Painter R, Hollister D: Ehlers-Danlos syndrome type IV: diagnosis and therapy of associated bowel perforation, *Am J Gastroenterol* 86(3):360-362, 1991.

FIBROMYALGIA SYNDROME

Jaynie St. Pierre

Description

Fibromyalgia syndrome (FMS) is characterized by generalized pain and musculoskeletal tenderness, fatigue, nonrestorative sleep, and morning stiffness (Wolfe, 1996). The condition has been given such labels as "rheumatism," fibromyositis, and myositis, the latter two being misnomers given the lack of evidence of inflammation.

Fibromyalgia syndrome has been called an invisible illness, often denied or misunderstood. Because patients with the syndrome do not "look sick," they are often treated without empathy by clinicians, family, and friends. This situation can lead over time to self-doubt and diminished self-esteem.

No known definitive laboratory test is diagnostic for FMS, and most patients suffer more than 6 years before

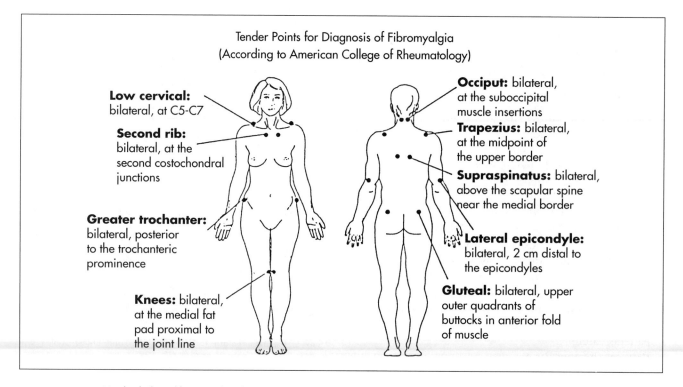

Tender Points for Diagnosis of Fibromyalgia
(According to American College of Rheumatology)

Low cervical: bilateral, at C5-C7

Second rib: bilateral, at the second costochondral junctions

Greater trochanter: bilateral, posterior to the trochanteric prominence

Knees: bilateral, at the medial fat pad proximal to the joint line

Occiput: bilateral, at the suboccipital muscle insertions

Trapezius: bilateral, at the midpoint of the upper border

Supraspinatus: bilateral, above the scapular spine near the medial border

Lateral epicondyle: bilateral, 2 cm distal to the epicondyles

Gluteal: bilateral, upper outer quadrants of buttocks in anterior fold of muscle

May be duplicated for use in clinical practice. As appears in McCaffery M, Pasero C: *Pain: Clinical manual,* p. 546, 1999, Mosby, Inc.

● ● ● ● ●
F I G U R E   12.6   Identification of fibromyalgia tender points.

From Sahley BJ: *Malic acid and magnesium for fibromyalgia and chronic pain syndrome,* San Antonio, Tex, 1996, Pain & Stress Publications; information from Wolfe F, Smythe HA, Yunus MB et al.: The American College of Rheumatology 1990 criteria for the classification of fibromyalgia: Report of the Multicenter Criteria Committee, *Arthritis Rheum* 6(45):160-172, 1990.

their illness is correctly diagnosed. However, diagnostic criteria have been established that allow a skilled rheumatologist to diagnose FMS when local tenderness is elicited in 11 or more of 18 "tender points" on digital examination, widespread pain of at least 3 months' duration in all four quadrants of the body exists, and the patient experiences nonrestorative sleep (Wolfe, Smythe, Yunus et al., 1990) (Figure 12.6 and Box 12.1).

Fibromyalgia has been observed in association with various other clinically defined disorders, including irritable bowel syndrome, irritable bladder, chronic migraine and tension headache, primary dysmenorrhea, chronic fatigue syndrome, temporomandibular joint dysfunction, restless legs syndrome, periodic limb movement disorder, and myofascial pain syndrome (MPS). These diseases consistently have been found to be more common in patients with primary FMS than in individuals with rheumatoid arthritis or in healthy controls (Yunus, Masi, 1993; Yunus, Masi, Aldag, 1989).

Signs and symptoms of FMS besides pain are dry eyes and mouth, subjective sensations of swelling, sleep myoclonus, costochondritis, paresthesias, poor posture or "guarding," weight gain, cold sensitivity, exercise intol-erance, difficulty with concentration and attention span, forgetfulness, dizziness, visual and balance disturbances, and anxiety. Associated nonrestorative sleep may result in lethargy and cognitive difficulties.

Patients report that certain factors may precipitate and intensify symptoms: febrile illnesses, physical and emotional trauma, cold or damp weather, cold drafts, changes in barometric pressure, and acute or chronic stress (Starlanyl, Copeland, 1996).

Possible causes/theories

The cause or causes of FMS are unknown, but there are several theories. Most etiologic hypotheses have focused on psychologic factors, muscle abnormalities, or neurologic defects.

A psychologic origin for FMS was suggested by studies showing that anxiety and depression are common in patients with the syndrome. Recent research findings, however, argue against a psychogenic or somatoform origin. Anxiety and depression are likely the results of the disorder, not the causes (Goldenberg, 1989; Yunus, Ahles, Aldag et al., 1991). In studies of FMS patients in the community rather than the clinic, a high prevalence of psychologic distress has not been found, suggesting

● ● ● ● ●

| BOX 12.1 | **The American College of Rheumatology 1990 Criteria for the Classification of Fibromyalgia***

1. History of widespread pain.
   Definition. Pain is considered widespread when all of the following are present: pain in the left side of the body, pain in the right side of the body, pain above the waist, and pain below the waist. In addition, axial skeletal pain (cervical spine or anterior chest or thoracic spine or low back) must be present. In this definition, shoulder and buttock pain is considered as pain for each involved side. "Low back" pain is considered lower segment pain.
2. Pain in 11 of 18 tender point sites on digital palpation.
   Definition. Pain, on digital palpation, must be present in at least 11 of the following 18 tender point sites:
   Occiput: bilateral, at the suboccipital muscle insertions.
   Low cervical: bilateral, at the anterior aspects of the intertransverse spaces at C5-C7.
   Trapezius: bilateral, at the midpoint of the upper border.

Supraspinatus: bilateral, at origins, above the scapula spine near the medial border.
Second rib: bilateral, at the second costochondral junctions, just lateral to the junctions on upper surfaces.
Lateral epicondyle: bilateral, 2 cm distal to the epicondyles.
Gluteal: bilateral, in upper outer quadrants of buttocks in anterior fold of muscle.
Greater trochanter: bilateral, posterior to the trochanteric prominence.
Knee: bilateral, at the medial fat pad proximal to the joint line.
Digital palpation should be performed with an approximate force of 4 kg.
For a tender point to be considered "positive" the subject must state that the palpation was painful. "Tender" is not to be considered "painful."

May be duplicated for use in clinical practice. As appears in McCaffery M, Pasero C: *Pain: Clinical manual*, p. 547, 1999, Mosby, Inc.

* For classification purposes, patients will be said to have fibromyalgia if both criteria are satisfied. Widespread pain must have been present for at least 3 months. The presence of a second clinical disorder does not exclude the diagnosis of fibromyalgia.

From Wolfe F, Smythe HA, Yunus MB et al.: The American College of Rheumatology 1990 criteria for the classification of fibromyalgia: Report of the Multicenter Criteria Committee, *Arthritis Rheum* 6(45):160-172, 1990.

that it is the increasing severity of FMS that leads to psychologic symptoms.

The myogenic hypothesis is based in part on findings of reduced levels of adenosine diphosphate, adenosine triphosphate, and phosphoryl creatinine in FMS tender points, which can be caused by hypoxia or a metabolic defect in the muscle (Bengstsson, Henriksson, Larsson, 1986). Also, poor cellular energy production from mitochondrial poisoning or "muscle toxicity" caused by endotoxins or exotoxins has been linked to FMS (Bland, 1997). The problem with the myogenic hypothesis is that it does not account for all the diverse manifestations of FMS (e.g., pain in joints and other organs such as the GI tract and bladder) (Wolfe, 1996).

Central metabolic or neurochemical hypotheses hold more promise. An interpretative defect in the central nervous system that could be responsible for abnormal pain perception (Russell, 1994) and low serum serotonin that could increase pain perception and impair stage-four sleep (Russell, 1996) are two postulated causes. Theories of a neurogenic cause are supported by research findings that cerebrospinal fluid levels of substance P in FMS patients are three times the normal (Russell, Orr, Littman et al., 1994).

Prevalence

The Arthritis Foundation (1996) has reported that FMS affects some 5 million Americans, or approximately 2% of the population. A consensus of rheumatologists holds that FMS is the second most common ailment for which patients seek their care, second only to rheumatoid arthritis (Fransen, Russell, 1996).

The syndrome is approximately 8 to 10 times more common among women than among men. The average age at diagnosis is in the mid-forties, but FMS has been found at all ages.

Pain Characteristics

The cardinal features of FMS are widespread pain and tenderness. Patients report that they "hurt all over." Although pain intensity varies, it is often more severe than that reported by patients with rheumatoid arthritis or osteoarthritis (Wolfe, 1996). Many patients describe pain as aching, exhausting, or nagging (Leavitt, Katz, Golden et al., 1986). Unlike stiffness associated with rheumatoid arthritis, pain from FMS does not diminish with activity (Bland, 1997). Pain is most commonly associated with tender points in the occiput, neck, shoulders, chest wall, elbows, knees, hips, and back. The patient may report only the most bothersome area unless questioned about other sites. Tenderness, like pain, is generalized; tender points are those areas with greater sensitivity (Wolfe, 1996).

Although FMS is classified as a chronic pain syndrome, "flares" of acute pain often occur. The pain of these flares has been described by patients as an "all-over" deep aching, like a bad case of the flu. Pain can become so severe that it limits range of motion and functional ability.

Muscle cramping and spasms are common. They are usually more frequent in the evening and can contribute to nonrestorative sleep. Because more than 80% of FMS patients experience alpha-delta sleep disturbance, they often wake up with muscle pain and fatigue. The repair of daily muscle microtrauma cannot occur under these conditions (Fransen, Russell, 1996). In addition, patients sometimes experience secondary joint pain.

Often accompanying pain and tenderness is stiffness. Individuals with FMS rarely can sit or stand in one position for very long without having to reposition or get up and move around. Prolonged sitting or standing can aggravate FMS symptoms, as can repetitive movements (Starlanyl, Copeland, 1996).

Fibromyalgia syndrome and MPS are two distinct conditions, but they often coexist and perpetuate and reinforce each other. In MPS, "trigger points" refer pain to distal sites and can occur as single or multiple points, can manifest as acute MPS, or even worsen to become a part of the FMS/MPS complex. Treatment of FMS/MPS complex can be complicated because MPS trigger points can be magnified by FMS, which can amplify pain (Starlanyl, Copeland, 1996).

Assessment

Patience and empathy, as well as skill, are key to pain and symptom assessment in the FMS patient. Long-term assessment should include use of a health status questionnaire and a pain rating scale. A short instrument developed specifically for FMS, the Fibromyalgia Impact Questionnaire, evaluates pain and stiffness, sleep disturbance, functional and work capabilities, and psychologic distress (Burckhardt, Clark, Bennett, 1991).

Other information important to obtain in assessing the patient includes the following:
- Which factors contribute to increased pain or "flares" and which alleviate symptoms
- Sleep quality and quantity
- Stress levels at work and at home
- Posture and body mechanics
- Nutritional status
- Social, emotional, spiritual, and environmental circumstances that may influence the patient's symptoms and overall well-being, including lack of family or social support, illness or recent death in the family, and financial burdens

Physical assessment of the FMS patient should be left to a rheumatologist or physiatrist skilled in the location and digital examination of tender points.

Pain Management

Often the first step in management once the diagnosis is finally made is explaining the syndrome to the patient. Educating the patient and significant others about this disorder is vitally important. In particular, great care should be taken to reassure them that FMS is not life-threatening and does not cause deformity or destroy the joints. Also, the patient (and family) should be instructed that FMS is a real illness, not "all in your head."

Other important first steps in managing the pain and symptoms of FMS are lifestyle changes. The patient should attempt to balance activity with rest, improving the quality and quantity of sleep. Avoiding emotional and physical stress is necessary to prevent or minimize the occurrence of flares. Patients who push themselves beyond their physical limits will end up in a flare nearly every time. Even worse, not "giving in" to a flare prolongs and complicates recovery.

In the workplace, patients can minimize stress by working fewer hours, taking frequent breaks, modifying deadlines, or transferring to a position that is less physically and emotionally demanding. Other basic measures include improving posture and body mechanics, eating nutritiously, learning to "listen to" and respect one's body, building a strong support system, and developing and maintaining a positive attitude. Unfortunately, probably the greater stressors to patients are family members who do not respect their limitations and continue to expect them to maintain the same pace they previously held in home and family activities.

Pharmacologic treatment

The tricyclic antidepressant amitriptyline (Elavil) and the muscle relaxant cyclobenzaprine (Flexeril) have been shown to be efficacious against FMS in clinical trials (Wolfe, 1996). Cyclobenzaprine has been found to be especially helpful in relieving muscle tightness, spasms, and twitches, and in promoting stage-four sleep (Starlanyl, Copeland, 1996). However, data suggest that only some, not all, patients benefit from tricyclic drugs and that the benefits are limited.

Amitriptyline, which inhibits reuptake of both serotonin and epinephrine, is believed to increase the availability of serotonin in neuromuscular synapses, promote stage-four sleep, and enhance the effects of endorphins and enkephalins (Fransen, Russell, 1996). It is also thought to provide some analgesia in the periphery by an unknown mechanism. The properties are important in reducing pain and improving well-being.

Selective serotonin reuptake inhibitors, such as sertraline (Zoloft) and paroxetine (Paxil), have been used under the rationale that they might offer efficacy comparable with that of amitriptyline without that drug's daytime sedation and other troublesome side effects. Fluoxetine (Prozac) has been effective when combined with amitriptyline (Goldenberg, Mayskiy, Mossey et al., 1996). The combination has led to improvement in pain relief, well-being, sleep, and function, and the two drugs' side effects, rather than being additive, may negate each other, such as with effects on body weight and sedation. The two drugs together may provide a better balance of serotonin, epinephrine, and norepinephrine reuptake inhibition than either drug alone.

Although a consensus exists that NSAIDs are usually not effective, some patients do find them helpful (Fransen,

Russell, 1996). Moreover, although most authorities on FMS treatment believe opioid analgesics and cortisone are ineffective and should be avoided, some favor considering them for occasional rescue doses when pain of "flares" cannot be controlled through other means (Starlanyl, Copeland, 1996).

Nonpharmacologic measures

The benefit of gentle aerobic exercise is limited, and not all patients find it effective. Given the lack of adequate treatment for FMS, however, it should be tried in nearly all patients (McCain, 1989). Recommended low or nonimpact aerobic exercises include walking, swimming and water aerobics, and stationary bicycling. Weight training is not recommended.

Many patients, Bennett (1993) observes, are reluctant to exercise because of their muscle pain and fatigue. When they do, they seem to suffer more postexercise pain than do persons without FMS, and after unusual exertion they may experience malaise for several days. Bennett suggests beginning slowly and progressing in intensity and duration gradually to prevent flares. Similarly, Sharon Clark, an exercise physiologist experienced in FMS, stresses that the patient start at a level of exertion he or she is capable of at present, not at one he or she may have achieved before his or her illness (Thorson, 1997). Other recommendations by Clark to patients include the following (Thorson, 1997):

- Gently stretching and warming muscles before and after exercising to minimize soreness and microtrauma
- Avoiding cold water and cold or damp air
- Breaking up 20- to 30-minute sessions into six 5-minute walks per day, if this can make exercise easier to tolerate
- Avoiding eccentric muscle movements (contracting the muscle while moving the ends farther apart), which can lead to microtrauma and pain
- Maintaining correct posture and working over a balanced center of gravity to minimize strain
- Protecting the neck and shoulder muscles from strain

Physical therapy has not been evaluated in clinical trials. However, anecdotal evidence suggests it can be of great benefit for relieving pain and stiffness and improving strength and range of motion.

Combining heat, massage, and stretching has been a time-honored approach to treating FMS (Bennett, 1993). Massage therapy by licensed practitioners skilled in trigger point treatment can be prescribed to perform myofascial release and acupressure. This has been reported by many patients to be even more beneficial than physical therapy in relieving pain, restoring range of motion, and improving sleep.

Nonpharmacologic pain management and stress reduction techniques are very effective in FMS treatment (Fransen, Russell, 1996; Starlanyl, Copeland, 1996). Psy-

chologic therapy has not been clearly established as beneficial, but some FMS treatment centers include it in their care (Wolfe, 1996). Occupational therapy may be prescribed to assist patients in adapting to their environment and learning how to use various adaptive aids.

Acupuncture and injection of trigger points with lidocaine, which have been evaluated in a limited number of studies, are usually reserved for those patients with FMS/MPS complex who do not find adequate relief with other modalities. Rarely a stellate ganglion block for severe upper extremity pain has been used with apparent success (Bennett, 1993).

Patients who do not benefit from standard measures may be helped by referral to a chronic pain management clinic, which may provide such treatments as trigger point injections, nerve blocks, and medication trials. In most cases, however, FMS can be managed adequately by a rheumatologist, especially if the patient takes an active role in care.

Some patients are quite eager to try a variety of treatment modalities and supplemental nutrients that offer hope of relief. However, some alternative measures are controversial and still need more study to establish their effectiveness and safety. It is very important that the patient consult the primary physician and rheumatologist before starting any physical activity, diet, or supplement program.

SUMMARY

The cardinal features of FMS are widespread pain and tenderness along with nonrestorative sleep. Many other disorders such as irritable bowel syndrome may accompany FMS. Pain associated with FMS is chronic with intermittent "flares" of acute pain. Patients describe ongoing pain as aching and flares as being like a bad case of the flu. Diagnostic criteria for FMS include tenderness at 11 of 18 "tender points." The cause of FMS is unknown, but one hypothesis is that it is due to metabolic or neurochemical abnormalities. Pain management may include medications such as amitriptyline (Elavil), cyclobenzaprine (Flexeril), and NSAIDs. Many patients find that a combination of heat, massage, and stretching is also beneficial.

Resources

American Association for Chronic Fatigue Syndrome, P.O. Box 895, Olney, MD 20830.

American College of Rheumatology, 60 Executive Park South #150, Atlanta, GA 30329, (404) 633-3777.

American FMS Association, Inc., P.O. Box 9699, Bakersfield, CA 93389, (805) 633-3777.

American Sleep Disorders Association, 604 Second St., S.W., Rochester, MN 55902.

Chronic Fatigue Immune Deficiency Syndrome Association of America, P.O. Box 220398, Charlotte, NC 28222-0398, (800) 442-3437.

Fibromyalgia/Fibromyalgia Management Association, Inc. (FM/FMA), P.O. Box 8119, Minneapolis, MN 55408-0119, (800) 362-4151.

Fibromyalgia Alliance of America, P.O. Box 21990, Columbus, OH 43221-0990, (614) 457-4222.

Fibromyalgia Network, P.O. Box 31750, Tucson, AZ 85752-1750, (800) 853-2929.

National Fibromyalgia Research Association, P.O. Box 500, Salem, OR 97308.

National Foundation of Fibromyalgia, P.O. Box 3429, San Diego, CA 92163-1429, (800) 251-9528.

NIH/National Arthritis and Musculoskeletal and Skin Diseases Information Clearinghouse, 9000 Rockville Pike, Bethesda, MD 20892, (301) 495-4484.

References

Arthritis Foundation: *Fibromyalgia syndrome*, pp 1-2, Atlanta, 1996, The Foundation (brochure).

Bengtsson A, Henriksson KG, Larsson J: Reduced high energy phosphate levels in the painful muscles of patients with primary fibromyalgia, *Arthritis Rheum* 299:817-821, 1986.

Bennett RM: The fibromyalgia syndrome: myofascial pain and the chronic fatigue syndrome. In Kelly WN, Harris ED, Ruddy S et al., editors: *Textbook of rheumatology*, ed 4, vol 1, pp 471-479, Philadelphia, 1993, WB Saunders.

Bland JS: *The 20 day rejuvenation diet program*, New Canaan, Conn, 1997, Keats Pub.

Burckhardt CS, Clark SR, Bennett RM: The fibromyalgia impact questionnaire: development and validation, *J Rheumatol* 18:728-733, 1991.

Fransen J, Russell IJ: *The fibromyalgia help book: practical guide to living better with fibromyalgia*, St. Paul, Minn, 1996, Smith House Press.

Goldenberg DL: Psychological symptoms and psychiatric diagnoses in patients with fibromyalgia, *J Rheumatol* 16 (Suppl 19):127-130, 1989.

Goldenberg D, Mayskiy M, Mossey C et al.: A randomized, double-blind crossover trial of fluoxetine and amytriptyline in the treatment of fibromyalgia, *Arthritis Rheum* 39(11):1852-1859, 1996.

Leavitt F, Katz RS, Golden HE et al.: Comparison of pain properties in fibromyalgia patients and rheumatoid arthritis patients, *Arthritis Rheum* 29:775-781, 1986.

McCain GA: Nonmedicinal treatments in primary fibromyalgia, *Rheum Dis Clin North Am* 15:73-90, 1989.

Russell IJ: Biochemical abnormalities in fibromyalgia syndrome. In Pillemer SR, editor: *The fibromyalgia syndrome: current research and future directions in epidemiology, pathogenesis, and treatment*, New York, 1994, Haworth Medical Press.

Russell IJ: Neurochemical pathogenesis of fibromyalgia syndrome, *J Musculoskeletal Pain* 4:61-93, 1996.

Russell IJ, Orr MD, Littman B et al.: Elevated cerebrospinal fluid levels of substance P in patients with the fibromyalgia syndrome, *Arthritis Rheum* 37:1593-1601, 1994.

Starlanyl D, Copeland ME: *Fibromyalgia and chronic myofascial pain syndrome: a survival manual*, Oakland, Calif, 1996, New Harbinger Pub.

Thorson K: The right approach to exercise . . . without taking three steps forward and ten steps back, *Fibromyalgia network: a newsletter for people with fibromyalgia/chronic fatigue* (Tucson, Health Information Network, Inc., Tucson, Ariz), ed 38, pp 3-6, July 1997.

Wolfe F: Fibromyalgia and myofascial pain syndrome. In Portenoy RK, Kanner RM: *Pain management: theory and practice*, pp 145-169, Philadelphia, 1996, FA Davis.

Wolfe F, Smythe HA, Yunus MB et al.: The American College of Rheumatology 1990 criteria for the classification of fibromyalgia: report of the Multicenter Criteria Committee, *Arthritis Rheum* 6(45):160-172, 1990.

Yunus MB, Ahles TA, Aldag JC et al.: Relationship of clinical features with psychological status in primary fibromyalgia, *Arthritis Rheum* 34(1):15-21, 1991.

Yunus MB, Masi AT: Fibromyalgia, restless legs syndrome, periodic limb movement disorder, and psychogenic pain. In McCarty DJ, Koopman WJ, editors: *Arthritis and allied conditions: a textbook of rheumatology*, ed 12, vol 2, pp 1383-1401, Philadelphia, 1993, Lea & Febiger.

Yunus MB, Masi AT, Aldag JC: A controlled study of primary fibro-myalgia syndrome: clinical features and association with other functional syndromes, *J Rheumatol* 16(Suppl 19):62-71, 1989.

HEADACHE

Lora McGuire

Description

"Not tonight, dear, I have a headache." This statement sounds like an overused excuse, but for 45 million Americans, this pain is a major health problem. Headache is the most common of all types of pain (Solomon, 1993). Approximately 15% of the U.S. population suffer from chronic headaches.

As with all types of pain, patients with headache frequently suffer unnecessarily because of misdiagnosis and mistreatment. Often these patients do not even consult with their physicians, and they frequently self-treat their headaches. More than $4 billion a year is spent on OTC analgesics, many of which are ineffective for headache (National Headache Foundation, ND). Many patients who have sought professional help have gone to extremes to obtain relief. Surgeries such as temporomandibular joint (TMJ), sinus, and nasal/septal repairs; neck manipulations; and psychiatric hospitalizations are only a few of the desperate measures patients have taken to alleviate their pain.

Fortunately, headache research is progressing rapidly. The new medications that are now available, particularly for migraines, are milestones in relief from headache pain. In addition, the headache classifications published in 1988 by the International Headache Society (IHS) (Headache Classification Committee of the International Headache Society, 1988) have made it easier for clinicians to diagnose the most common types of headaches.

Guidelines for all types of headaches are presented followed by a discussion of four major headache types: migraine, tension–type, cluster, and rebound headaches.

Assessment and Treatment Guide: All Types of Headaches

As with all pain assessment, careful histories are necessary to accurately diagnose headache. Most primary headache disorders can be diagnosed by completing a thorough interview and following the IHS criteria. A complete headache history should include the following: family history of headaches, age headaches first started, site, pain characteristics, frequency, duration, intensity, any signs and symptoms preceding or during the headache, aggravating or precipitating factors, what usually helps, medication use, and any other interventions. Good questions to ask are, "How are the headaches interfering with your daily life?" and "What are they preventing you from doing?" A headache diary (Form 12.1, *A*, and Form 12.1, *B*)

FORM 12.1A Headache Diary

Date and time started	Time ended	Site or location of pain	Quality or description	Pain intensity 0-10 scale	Associated symptoms/ aura present? Yes/No	Trigger Factors					Meds taken and time	Pain intensity 0-10 scale	Other relieving factors
						Environmental	Foods	Stress	Menses	Other			

May be duplicated for use in clinical practice. From McCaffery M, Pasero C: *Pain: Clinical manual,* p. 551. Copyright © 1999, Mosby, Inc.

FORM 12.1B Headache Diary: Patient Example

Date and time started	Time ended	Site or location of pain	Quality or description	Pain intensity 0-10 scale	Associated symptoms/ aura present? Yes/No	Trigger Factors					Meds taken and time	Pain intensity 0-10 scale	Other relieving factors
						Environmental	Foods	Stress	Menses	Other			
9-16-97 1:30 PM	7:00 PM	Behind eyes and forehead	pressure	7	No aura					✓ sinus	Fiorinal 4:30	2	sleeping for about 1-1/2 h
9-17-97 8:00 PM	9-18-97 7:00 AM	Left temple	throbbing pounding	started at a 5 and by 9:00 it was about 7-8	No aura present. Did have nausea, photophobia					✓ no cause, it just started	Excedrin 3 tablets @ 8:15 PM; Compazine 5 mg	7—no relief; awoke during PM; still had it. When I woke up at 7:00 AM, it was gone.	ice bag— went to sleep; apply pressure to affected side
9-28-97 7:30 AM	12:00 PM	Left temple	pounding	4	No aura					✓	Excedrin 3 tablets	2	none

May be duplicated for use in clinical practice. From McCaffery M, Pasero C: *Pain: Clinical manual,* p. 551. Copyright © 1999, Mosby, Inc.

is very helpful for assessing and treating patients with chronic headaches. Particular attention should be paid to dietary triggers and the relationship to menses and hormones.

As with many patients with chronic pain, patients with headaches often are not believed. They literally are told the pain is "all in your head." Highly educated people, professionals, and the general public have said headaches are simply due to stress. Patients are made to think that if they could just get control of their lives, their headaches would abate. Yet it has been known for some time that psychologic and emotional problems do not *cause* headaches, but stress may *bring on* a migraine or tension-type headache in those individuals who are prone to headaches.

The National Headache Foundation (see Patient Resources) has offered general guidelines for headache sufferers. Some of these suggestions include the importance of waking up at the exact same time every day, even on weekends; stopping smoking; not skipping meals; moderating caffeine intake; and trying to identify triggers that bring on headaches.

Migraine Headache

Description: Migraine

Even with recent advances in headache research, migraine headache is underdiagnosed and undertreated. Twenty-three million Americans suffer from migraine headaches (Stewart, Lipton, Celentano et al., 1992). Adult migraine is approximately three times more likely to occur in women than men. It affects about 18% of women and 6% of men during their lifespan, peaking between the ages of 25 and 55 (Lipton, 1997). Not only do women have an increased prevalence of migraine, but they also have more frequent attacks.

Many patients with migraine have never been diagnosed. It is estimated that 59% of women and 71% of men with headaches have undiagnosed migraines (Lipton, Stewart, Celentano et al., 1992). One reason may be that patients do not consult their physicians about headache pain.

In 10% to 20% of migraine sufferers, a warning or aura occurs lasting 10 to 20 minutes before the headache's onset (Silberstein, Lipton, 1994). The characteristics of the aura vary greatly but usually include some kind of visual disturbance, weakness, dizziness, or other vague neurologic symptom. When IHS (Headache Classification Committee of the International Headache Society, 1988) developed the new headache classification system, migraine without aura was changed to common migraine. Migraine with aura is now called classic migraine. Figure 12.7 gives the IHS criteria for diagnosing common and classic migraines. Because it may be difficult to distinguish a migraine attack from other types of headache, a patient must suffer at least five attacks before the migraine diagnosis can be made (Headache Classification Committee of the International Headache Society, 1988).

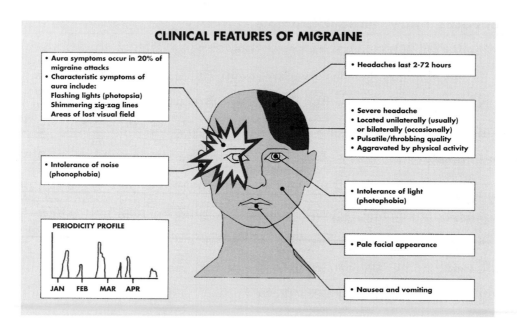

CLINICAL FEATURES OF MIGRAINE

- Aura symptoms occur in 20% of migraine attacks
- Characteristic symptoms of aura include:
  Flashing lights (photopsia)
  Shimmering zig-zag lines
  Areas of lost visual field

- Intolerance of noise (phonophobia)

PERIODICITY PROFILE
JAN FEB MAR APR

- Headaches last 2-72 hours

- Severe headache
- Located unilaterally (usually) or bilaterally (occasionally)
- Pulsatile/throbbing quality
- Aggravated by physical activity

- Intolerance of light (photophobia)

- Pale facial appearance

- Nausea and vomiting

May be duplicated for use in clinical practice. As appears in McCaffery M, Pasero C: *Pain: Clinical manual*, p. 552, 1999, Mosby, Inc.

F I G U R E 12.7 **WHICH Headache? A Guide to the Diagnosis and Management of Headache.**
Published by Professional Postgraduate Services Europe Ltd, Worthing, UK, 1993, under an educational grant from Cerenex Pharmaceuticals, division of Glaxo Inc.

Known trigger factors for migraines include emotional stress, menses, certain foods or alcoholic beverages, smoking, skipping meals, sleeping too much or too little, and bright lights. Changes in weather or altitude can also bring on an attack. Although there has been much talk about following a strict diet to prevent migraines, only about 10% to 20% of migraine patients will improve. It is essential to identify triggers for each individual patient because they can vary.

For years it was thought that migraine headache was caused solely by dilated cranial blood vessels. Now it is known to be more complicated. Researchers today are not in complete agreement as to the cause of migraine, but all suggest that many complex central nervous system mechanisms are involved. The current theory of migraine is that along with vasodilatation and neurogenic inflammation, there is an abnormal metabolism of the neurotransmitter, serotonin. The change in serotonin levels in the brain stem alters the cranial circulation, which then activates the trigeminal nerve. The sensory fibers of the trigeminal nerve surround cranial arteries and release chemicals. As the blood vessels become inflamed, serotonin levels drop, which leads to a migraine attack.

More recently, findings suggest that altered levels of brain magnesium may also play a role in migraine (Mazzotta, Sarchielli, Alberti et al., 1996). Mauskop, Altura, Cracco et al. (1996) also found that the decreased levels of magnesium point to the pathogenesis of migraine. In their study of 40 patients, IV infusion of 1 g of magnesium sulfate resulted in 80% having elimination of headache within 15 minutes. Fifty-six percent had no recurrence or worsening of pain within 24 hours.

Pain characteristics: Migraine

The pain of migraine is episodic and can range from mild to severe. A recent Gallop survey of migraine sufferers found that 35% had pain so bad they wished they were dead. Migraine pain is usually unilateral and pulsating and worsens with physical activity, bright lights, and loud noise. Headaches usually last from 4 to 72 hours and often are accompanied by nausea and/or vomiting (Headache Classification Committee of the International Headache Society, 1988).

Pain management: Migraine

The goal of acute migraine treatment is for the patient to be nearly pain free in about 2 hours after drug administration, with minor side effects and no nausea. A variety of medications may be used (see Table 12.10). The breakthrough for migraine relief came in 1992 with the FDA approval of sumatriptan. Patients have called it the "miracle drug" and "the one that saved my life."

Sumatriptan is a serotonin 5HT1 receptor agonist. It stimulates the 5HT1 receptors in cerebral blood vessels, causing brief and selective vasoconstriction and decreased blood flow. The new 5HT1 agonists help migraine by selectively blocking the development of neurogenic inflammation after trigeminal stimulation (Moskowitz, 1991). They act in the brain stem to inhibit sensory nerves around cerebral blood vessels.

With the addition of serotonin-receptor agonist drugs such as sumatriptan, more drugs and routes are available. Patients can self-administer migraine medications at home, so emergency room visits have decreased.

Sumatriptan is effective in about 70% of patients. Unlike other abortive migraine drugs, sumatriptan can be taken any time during the course of a migraine attack. The manufacturer of sumatriptan suggests that it be taken for at least three separate headaches before deciding it does not work for a particular patient. Headache experts are unsure why sumatriptan is not effective in every migraine patient. Visser, DeVrienc, Jaspers and others (1996) believe that treating a migraine too early with sumatriptan is a possible reason for lack of response. Others have also observed that giving sumatriptan during the aura phase of a headache will not prevent or stop a migraine.

Ninety-five percent of migraine sufferers have nausea and vomiting during an attack (Wilkinson, 1988). It is also well documented that drug absorption in the intestines is delayed and impaired during a migraine attack (Klapper, 1993). Antiemetics should be used with other abortive agents during an acute attack. Metoclopramide (Reglan) increases GI motility and can be very effective when given with aspirin or the NSAIDs for mild to moderate pain. One Danish study found in more than 400 migraine patients, metoclopramide, 10 mg, and aspirin, 900 mg, was just as effective as 100 mg of oral sumatriptan but less costly (Tfelt-Hansen, Henry, Mulder et al., 1995).

For years ergotamine has been used effectively for moderate to severe migraines. Ergotamine works by stimulating smooth muscle and causing vasoconstriction. It also helps migraine pain by decreasing neurogenic inflammation (Silberstein, 1997). Both oral Cafergot (1 mg of ergotamine) and the rectal form (2 mg of ergotamine) contain 100 mg of caffeine. When given with ergotamine, caffeine enhances absorption. Caffeine also increases absorption of other medications (e.g., antiemetics) and has analgesic properties of its own.

Ergotamine is associated with rebound or chronic daily headaches (Mathew, Kurman, Perez, 1990). Consequently, ergotamine should be limited to no more than 2 days per week and no more than 10 mg/week (Capobianco, Cheshire, Campbell, 1996).

Prophylactic treatment of migraine should be considered when a patient has two to three migraines a month. Prophylactic medication is also indicated if a patient's medical condition is a contraindication to use of abortive

Text continued on p. 556.

GUIDE TO HEADACHE MEDICATIONS

Medication	Dose	Side effects	Comments
Migraine: Acute/Abortive			
Mild analgesics			For mild headache pain only; daily use of ASA and/or acetaminophen may lead to rebound headache. NSAIDs may help with migraine prophylaxis.
ASA	1000 mg tid-qid	GI upset and GI bleeding; tinnitus	
NSAIDs	See Chapter 5 on NSAIDs		
Acetaminophen (Tylenol)	1000 mg tid-qid	Hepatotoxicity	
Antiemetics			More helpful when given with mild analgesics.
Metoclopramide (Reglan)	PO 5-20 mg IV 10-15 mg	Sedation, confusion, hypotension, anticholinergic effects	Reglan enhances absorption. It is used for symptomatic treatment of nausea and vomiting with migraine.
Chlorpromazine (Thorazine)	12.5-25 mg IV 100-mg suppository		
Prochlorperazine (Compazine)	5-10 mg PO or IV 25-mg suppository		
5HT receptor agonists			
Sumatriptan (Imitrex)	6 mg SC; maximum SC dose 12 mg/day 25 mg and 50 mg PO; maximum PO dose 300 mg/day 5 and 20 mg nasal spray; maximum dose 40 mg/day	Flushing, tingling, warmth, numbness, tightness in chest	Pills and spray are less expensive and cause fewer side effects; 50 mg PO as effective as 100 mg PO. Contraindicated in coronary artery disease, ischemic disease, or with ergotamines. Possibility of headache recurrence.
Naratriptan (Amerge)	2.5 mg PO	Nausea, headache, paresthesias, dizziness, fatigue	Slower onset, longer acting.
Zolmitriptan (Zomig)	2.5, 5, 10 mg PO May repeat dose in 2 h Maximum dose 10 mg/day	Dizziness, asthenia, paresthesia, drowsiness, nausea, throat or neck tightness or pressure	Useful for menstrual migraines; 2.5 mg bid for duration of cycle.
Ergotamine ErgostatSL	1 tablet onset, maximum 3/day	Abdominal cramps, nausea, diarrhea	Effective, but high incidence of side effects; associated with rebound headache; contraindicated with pregnancy, cerebral, coronary, and peripheral vascular disease.
*Cafergot, Wigraine oral, rectal	2 tablets onset, maximum 6/day 1 suppository onset		
Dihydroergotamine (DHE)	IV/IM 1 mg No more than 6 mg/wk Nasal spray SC	Same as ergotamine, but less severe	Similar to ergotamine, but no rebound; less potent arterial vasoconstriction than ergotamine. Self-administration may lead to decreased ER visits. Locally compounded nasal spray. Inexpensive and convenient.
Isometheptene (Midrin) Combination drug of isometheptene, 65 mg, acetaminophen, 325 mg, dichloralphenazone, 100 mg	2 tablets at onset, 1-2 q 30-60 min, maximum 5-6 tablets/day	Dizziness, sedation	For mild-moderate migraine; weaker vasoconstriction than ergotamine, but still not to be used with coronary artery disease; not to be used with monoamine oxidase inhibitors.

From McCaffery M, Pasero C: *Pain: Clinical manual*, pp. 554-556. *Continued.*

GUIDE TO HEADACHE MEDICATIONS

Medication	Dose	Side effects	Comments
Migraine: Acute/Abortive—cont'd			
Lidocaine	Intranasal 4%		Rapid relief of migraine, lasts 10-15 min, may have headache relapse in 50%.
Corticosteroids (Prednisone)	40-100 mg/day PO and taper	Edema, hyperglycemia, weight gain, mood changes	For severe and prolonged migraines >72 h.
Dexamethasone (Decadron)	8-20 mg/day PO and taper	Cushing-like symptoms	
Migraine: Prophylactic			
Beta-blockers			
Propranolol (Inderal)	20-80 mg tid-qid	Lethargy, depression, impotence, weight gain, hypotension	First-line treatment for migraine prevention; only beta-blocker approved by FDA for migraine use.
Atenolol (Tenormin)	25-100 mg bid	Lethargy, depression, impotence, weight gain, hypotension	Do not use beta-blockers with Raynaud's disease, congestive heart failure, asthma. Do not stop drugs abruptly.
Calcium channel blockers Verapamil (Calan, Isoptin)	80-160 mg tid-qid Do not use sustained release	Constipation, hypotension, headache, weight gain	Widely used although not FDA approved for migraine or cluster prophylaxis. Treatment of choice for cluster.
Tricyclic antidepressants	See tension headache, below		
Anticonvulsants			
Valproic acid (Depakote)	250 mg bid up to 1000 mg/day	Weight gain; nausea and vomiting, diarrhea, dizziness	Recently FDA approved for migraine prophylaxis.
Serotonin antagonists Methysergide (Sansert)	2 mg 3-5 times/day, not to exceed 14 mg/day	Weight gain, hallucination, nausea, muscle aching, insomnia, dizziness, tissue fibrosis	Rare, but serious fibrotic lesions may occur; not to be used longer than 4 mo.
Tension Headache			
Mild analgesics (ASA, NSAIDs)	Same as for migraine	Same as for migraine	Same as for migraine
Tricyclic antidepressants Amitriptyline (Elavil)	10-150 mg at hs	Orthostatic hypotension, constipation, dry mouth	May take up to 5-7 days before effect is seen.
Nortriptyline (Pamelor)	10-100 mg at hs	Same as amitriptyline but less severe	May not be as effective as amitriptyline, but less side effects.
Doxepin (Sinequan)	10-150 mg at hs	Similar to amitriptyline	
Cluster Headache: Acute			
O$_2$ therapy	7-10 L/min for 10 min with patient in forward position	None	Helps 70%. Not to be used with chronic obstructive pulmonary disease patients; some patients do not like the inconvenience.
Ergotamine	Same as migraine	Same as migraine	Same as migraine
Dihydroergotamine (DHE)	Same as migraine	Same as migraine	Same as migraine
Sumatriptan (Imitrex)	Same as migraine	Same as migraine	Not indicated for cluster headache, but may benefit some patients.

Continued.

GUIDE TO HEADACHE MEDICATIONS

Medication	Dose	Side effects	Comments
Cluster Headache: Prophylactic			
Calcium–channel blockers (Verapamil)	120–160 mg tid–qid	Edema, fatigue, constipation	First choice treatment for cluster prevention.
Corticosteroids (Prednisone)	PO 40–100 mg/day and taper	Edema, hyperglycemia, decreased wound healing, mood changes	Helpful in preventing headache during exacerbations.
Dexamethasone (Decadron)	PO or IV 8–20 mg/day and taper	Edema, hyperglycemia, decreased wound healing, mood changes	Many serious side effects related to long-term use; tapering doses is essential.
Lithium	150–300 mg bid–tid	Tremors, mental changes, thirst, edema	For difficult cluster cases, because cluster headaches may by cyclic; may be effective for same reasons it helps cyclic bipolar patients; patients must avoid excessive salt intake, monitor blood levels, thyroid, and renal function.
Methysergide (Sansert)	Same as migraine	Same as migraine	Same as migraine
Valproic acid	Same as migraine	Same as migraine	Although not FDA approved for cluster prevention, some patients benefit.

May be duplicated for use in clinical practice. From McCaffery M, Pasero C: *Pain: Clinical manual*, pp. 554-556. Copyright © 1999, Mosby, Inc.
*Contain ergotamine and caffeine.
Information from Campbell JK: Diagnosis and treatment of cluster headache, *J Pain Symptom Manage* 8:155-164, 1993; Capobianco DJ, Cheshire WP, Campbell JK: An overview of the diagnosis and pharmacologic treatment of migraine, *Mayo Clin Proc* 71:1055-1066, 1996; Kudrow L: Response of cluster headache attacks to oxygen inhalation, *Headache* 21:1-4, 1981; Kuritzky A, Hering R: The treatment of cluster headache with sodium valproate: A new approach, *Headache* 27:301, 1987; Saper JR, Silberstein S, Gordon CD: *Handbook of headache management*, Baltimore, 1993, Williams & Wilkins; Silberstein SD, Lipton RB: Overview of diagnosis and treatment of migraine, *Neurology* 44(Suppl 7):S6-S16, 1994; Welch KMA: Drug therapy of migraine, *N Engl J Med* 329:1476-1483, 1993.

drugs, if the side effects of these drugs are too disabling, of if acute treatments are ineffective. See Table 12.10 for possible prophylactic medications. The goal of preventive therapy is to decrease the frequency of attacks by 50% with minor side effects. Patients who are successfully managed with prophylactic therapy may still require abortive medications during an acute attack. Patients should be advised that prophylactic migraine treatment most likely will not make the headaches disappear completely, but they should be less frequent and more tolerable.

The beta-blockers are the first-line treatment for migraine prevention. Propranolol (Inderal) is the drug of choice and the only one the FDA has approved for this use. The beta-blockers decrease frequency of attacks by 50% in 60% to 80% of patients (Saper, Silberstein, Gordon, 1993). These drugs should not be given to patients with congestive heart failure, asthma, or Raynaud's disease. They should never be stopped abruptly because this can lead to serious cardiac problems.

When patients are treated with migraine prophylactic medications, a trial-and-error approach is recommended, introducing only one drug at a time (Capobianco, Cheshire, Campbell, 1996). The clinician individualizes therapy through trial and error. The patient's headache diary is reviewed at each visit and should include number of attacks, severity, and occurrence of side effects.

Migraines that are continuous and last longer than 3 days are referred to as intractable, or status, migraines. For these severe and prolonged migraines, hospitalization may be necessary. Treatment may consist of intravenous steroids and dihydroergotamine (DHE). In one study, IV DHE given every 8 hours with metoclopramide for 2 to 3 days provided relief for 90% of patients. Strong analgesics are also needed during this time. Table 12.10 provides specific information about medications used to treat or prevent migraine.

Although no data exist to support the use of oxygen therapy for migraines, it may be useful. Seven to 10 L/min

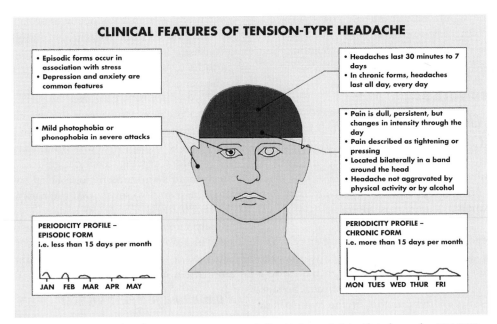

May be duplicated for use in clinical practice. As appears in McCaffery M, Pasero C: *Pain: Clinical manual*, p. 557, 1999, Mosby, Inc.

● ● ● ● ● ●
F I G U R E 12.8 WHICH Headache? A Guide to the Diagnosis and Management of Headache.

Published by Professional Postgraduate Services Europe Ltd, Worthing, UK, 1993, under an educational grant from Cerenex Pharmaceuticals, division of Glaxo Inc.

by mask for 10 minutes is known to help patients with cluster headaches.

Tension-Type Headaches

Description: Tension

The old terms for tension-type headaches were "muscle contraction," or "depressive," headache. The word "tension" in tension-type headaches misleads health care professionals and patients into believing these headaches are solely caused by stress. Psychologic factors have an impact on these headaches but are not necessarily the cause. As with migraines, more women suffer from tension-type headaches than men.

Pain characteristics: Tension

Pain characteristics of tension-type headaches according to the IHS criteria (Figure 12.8) include mild to moderate bilateral dull pain with a tightness around the head, scalp, or neck. Patients often describe the headache as a "tight band around the head." These headaches generally occur at least 15 times in 1 month. Often patients have them daily, occurring first thing on awakening. Family history of headaches, sleeping difficulties, and depression are commonly associated. It is sometimes difficult to distinguish daily tension-type headache from rebound headache.

Currently there is controversy among headache experts as to whether tension-type headaches are actually a form of migraines. Saper, Silberstein, and Gordon (1993) believe that tension-type headache is a variant of migraine. Leston (1996) also holds the view that migraine and tension-type headaches are on opposite ends of the continuum. Although no clinical data support these opinions, these experts mention that many of their patients with tension-type headache have histories of suffering intermittent episodes of migraines 5 to 10 years previously. The question still exists as to whether these daily refractory-type tension headaches are actually caused by drug-related rebound headaches.

As with migraines, the pathophysiology of tension-type headache is not completely understood. Several mechanisms are involved with tension-type headaches, with sustained muscle contraction commonly occurring. The major source of pain in these headaches is probably caused by sensitization of nociceptors in the pericranial muscles (Jensen, Olsen, 1996).

Pain management: Tension

Treatment for tension-type headache is largely symptomatic. Prophylactic medications are not effective. Nonopioid analgesics and low-dose tricyclic antidepressants are the drugs of choice (Table 12.10). Although Fiorinal, a combination drug of aspirin, caffeine, and barbiturate, is approved by the FDA for use in tension-type headache only, it is not recommended for chronic use because of the possibility of causing rebound headaches. In a study by Schachtel, Furey, and Thoden (1996), ibuprofen, 400 mg, was found to be significantly more effective than aceta-minophen, 1000 mg, for treating tension-type headaches. Table 12.10 provides more specific information about medications used to manage tension-type headaches.

Cluster Headaches

Description: Cluster

Cluster headaches, often called the "suicide" headache because of the horrendous pain, occur predominantly in men (Saper, Silberstein, Gordon, 1993). Luckily, these headaches are not very prevalent, occurring anywhere from 10 to 50 times less often than migraines (Campbell, 1993).

Cluster headaches are not associated with any familial tendencies. The average age of onset is 20 to 40 years (Saper, Silberstein, Gordon, 1993). Although the cause is unknown, the autonomic features of the headache suggest that some sort of dysfunction of the sympathetic nervous system is involved in the pathophysiology of cluster headaches (Havelius, Heuck, Milas et al., 1996). Potent vasodilators, particularly alcohol, and others such as nitroglycerin and histamine can trigger an attack in susceptible individuals (Campbell, 1993).

Pain characteristics: Cluster

Cluster headaches are intense, often excruciating headaches. The term "cluster" stems from the fact that these headaches are usually episodic, occurring in groups

or clusters. Often they occur seasonally, in spring and/or fall. These cluster attacks can extend over weeks or months, followed by remissions lasting anywhere from months to years. In approximately 10% of cluster headache patients, attacks are chronic.

Cluster headaches are one of the easiest to diagnose because the signs and symptoms are classic. Patients describe cluster pain as like having "a hot poker in the eye." The pain is unilateral, in or around the eye, accompanied by ipsilateral tearing, nasal congestion, and ptosis. Other autonomic symptoms include facial sweating and flushing. The pain is so severe that the patient paces, unable to sit still. Attacks come on suddenly, without warning, usually in the middle of the night or during a nap. The pain increases in intensity, peaking after 5 to 10 minutes. The attack lasts 45 to 90 minutes on average and leaves the patient exhausted (Campbell, 1993) (Figure 12.9).

Pain management: Cluster

Treatment of acute cluster headache requires rapid-onset medications, such as nasal (e.g., butorphanol nasal spray) or parenteral ergotamine or dihydroergotamine preparations (see Table 12.10). Intranasal applications of a local anesthetic such as lidocaine have shown promise (National Headache Foundation, ND). Campbell (1993) has found placing 1 ml of 4% topical lidocaine as far back in the nose as possible on the same side as the cluster headache may provide temporary relief in acute attacks. Opioid and nonopioid analgesics are not useful for

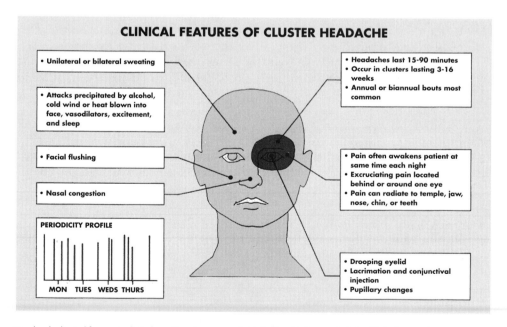

May be duplicated for use in clinical practice. As appears in McCaffery M, Pasero C: *Pain: Clinical manual*, p. 558, 1999, Mosby, Inc.

● ● ● ● ● ●
FIGURE 12.9   WHICH Headache? A Guide to the Diagnosis and Management of Headache.

Published by Professional Postgraduate Services Europe Ltd, Worthing, UK, 1993, under an educational grant from Cerenex Pharmaceuticals, division of Glaxo Inc.

the pain of acute cluster headache, unless given by a route of administration that has a rapid onset, such as parenterally.

It has been reported that oxygen therapy, if used at the onset of an attack, is effective in aborting cluster headaches in 75% of patients (Kudrow, 1981). The oxygen must be applied by mask for approximately 10 minutes at a flow rate of 7 L/min. Although somewhat inconvenient, this treatment has been extremely helpful for many patients and is usually covered by insurance if a letter is sent by the physician. Table 12.10 provides specific information about medications used to manage cluster headaches.

Rebound Headache

Description: Rebound

Rebound headaches, or headaches caused by medication withdrawal, are a result of frequent or excessive use of OTC or prescription medications. In one survey, 73% of the patients seen in headache clinics suffered from chronic, daily headache caused by overused medication (Mathew, Kurman, Perez, 1990). Typically, these patients are women with a prior history of migraines. They may have used analgesics or ergotamines for years to treat the migraines. Eventually, the headaches worsen and increase in frequency, resulting in daily, or almost daily, intake of medications that causes daily pain from withdrawal. However, another group of patients who may have no history of headache but may have rebound headaches develop are patients with posttraumatic headache caused by accidents or other incidents. They may begin to take analgesics regularly for this headache and eventually suffer rebound headache (Warner, Fenichel, 1996).

Pain characteristics: Rebound

Rebound headaches are most intense on awakening because the patient is usually drug free throughout the night (Lipton, Pfeffer, Newman et al., 1993). The pain is over the frontal area and is described as pressure or stabbing. Because of the chronicity of the pain, these patients often suffer from depression.

Frequent or daily use of analgesics, both nonopioid and opioid; ergotamines; and caffeine is the most common cause of rebound headaches (Box 12.2). The combination drugs (caffeine, barbiturates, aspirin, or acetaminophen) are even more likely to cause rebound headaches. Clinical experience has found opioid or nonopioid analgesic or ergotamine use greater than 2 days a week can lead to rebound headaches in some people.

Pain management: Rebound

After identifying whether medications are causing the daily headache, treatment consists of detoxifying the patient by tapering medications slowly. This can be very difficult for some patients who may have been on these medications for years. When medications are discontinued, initially the headaches increase in intensity. Nausea may also occur. If the patient can tolerate 3 to 5 days of this discomfort, headaches caused by rebound phenomena generally disappear. Administering one of the NSAIDs or another medication that does not cause rebound may be helpful during this period. Prophylactic medications are not effective in treating rebound headaches.

Occasionally, hospitalization is required for complete medication withdrawal. Intravenous DHE has proven to be extremely effective in treating chronic daily headache because this is one of the few headache medications that does not cause rebound (Lipton, 1997). If the patient has a history of long-term use of ergotamine, nausea is a major effect of withdrawal. IV antiemetics such as chlorpromazine (Thorazine) or prochlorperazine (Compazine) are recommended.

Silberstein, Schulman, and Hopkins (1990) found that IV DHE together with IV metoclopramide (Reglan) was very effective; 91% of 300 patients were free of headache in 2 to 3 days. Even though the success rate is high with this approach, insurance companies may refuse coverage.

SUMMARY

Headache research is progressing rapidly as illustrated by the new medications for migraines. Unfortunately, many patients with headaches are not believed or they do not consult their physicians and thereby fail to benefit from advances in treating headache. The underlying causes of migraine, tension, and cluster headaches are complex and poorly understood. One misconception is that psychologic problems cause headaches, whereas these problems only trigger headaches in some people who are prone to headaches.

• • • • •

BOX 12.2 Headache Medications That Can Lead to Rebound or Chronic Daily Headaches

Nonopioid analgesics
Opioid analgesics
Esgic (acetaminophen, butalbital, caffeine)
Fiorinal (aspirin, butalbital, caffeine)
Midrin (isometheptene, dichloralphenazone, acetaminophen)
Wigraine (ergotamine tartrate)
Caffeine

May be duplicated for use in clinical practice. From McCaffery M, Pasero C: *Pain: Clinical manual*, p. 559. Copyright © 1999, Mosby, Inc.

Information from Mathew NT, Kurman R, Perez F: Drug induced refractory headache: Clinical features and management, *Headache* 30:634-638, 1990; Saper JR, Silberstein S, Gordon CD: *Handbook of headache management*, Baltimore, 1993, Williams & Wilkins.

Four common types of headaches are as follows:

- Migraine: usually unilateral and pulsating and worsens with physical activity, bright lights, and loud noise. Usually lasts from 4 to 72 hours and is often accompanied by nausea and vomiting.
- Tension: usually described as a "tight band around the head." Occurs at least 15 times a month.
- Cluster: often called the "suicide" headache because of the severe pain. Tends to occur in clusters, such as seasonally. Pain usually lasts 45 to 90 minutes and leaves the patient exhausted.
- Rebound: caused by medication withdrawal and is a result of frequent or excessive use of nonprescription or prescription medications. Pain is usually over the frontal area and is described as pressure or stabbing.

Patient Resources

American Council for Headache Education
    19 Mantua Road
    Mt. Royal, NJ 08061
    (800) 255-ACHE (automated voice line)
    (609) 423-0258
    Fax: (609) 423-0082
    E-mail: *achehq@ache.smarthub.com*
    Web site: *www.achenet.org*

National Headache Foundation
    428 W. St. James Place
    2nd Floor
    Chicago, IL 60614-2750
    (800) 843-2256

Many pharmaceutical companies offer free information on headaches. To obtain the following, contact GlaxoWellcome by calling (800) 701-8448:

- *HeadWay:* A newsletter written especially for migraine sufferers. Each issue contains articles about managing migraine, lifestyle factors that may affect migraine, triggers, and how to develop more effective communication with your doctor. Also included are profiles and letters from other sufferers to let you know that you are not alone.
- What's Your Trigger?: A brochure that helps patients identify and avoid the factors that trigger their migraines. It explains how triggers work, lists the most common ones—dietary, emotional, and those related to activity, medications, and hormones—and tells the patient how to work with the doctor to pinpoint triggers.
- Helping Your Doctor Help You: This brochure helps patients with migraine to chart the condition by recording symptoms and providing the doctor with essential information.

Professional Resources

American Association for the Study of Headache
    19 Mantua Road
    Mt. Royal, NJ 08061

(609) 423-0043
Fax: (609) 423-0082
E-mail: *aashhq@aash.smarthub.com*
Web site: *www.aash.org*

Headache is the professional journal of this organization.

Evidenced-Based Report
    Headache AHCPR
    (800) 358-9295

References

Campbell JK: Diagnosis and treatment of cluster headache, *J Pain Symptom Manage* 8(3)155-164, 1993.

Capobianco DJ, Cheshire WP, Campbell JK: An overview of the diagnosis and pharmacologic treatment of migraine, *Mayo Clin Proc* 71:1055-1066, 1996.

Havelius U, Heuck M, Milas P et al.: Ciliospinal reflex response in cluster headache, *Headache* 36(9):568-573, 1996.

Headache Classification Committee of the International Headache Society: Society and diagnostic criteria for headache disorders, cranial neuralgias and facial pain, *Cephalagia* 8(Suppl 7):1-96, 1988.

Jensen R, Olsen J: Initiating mechanisms of experimentally induced tension-type headache, *Cephalalgia* 16(3):175-182, 1996.

Klapper J: The pharmacologic treatment of acute migraine headaches, *J Pain Symptom Manage* 8(3):140-147, 1993.

Kudrow L: Response of cluster headache attacks to oxygen inhalation, *Headache* 21:1-4, 1981.

Kuritzky A, Hering R: The treatment of cluster headache with sodium valproate: a new approach, *Headache* 27:301, 1987.

Leston JA: Migraine and tension-type headache are not separate disorders, *Cephalalgia* 16:220-222, 1996.

Lipton RB: Ergotamine tartrate and dihydroergotamine mesylate: safety profiles, *Headache* 37(Suppl 1):S33-S41, 1997.

Lipton RB, Pfeffer D, Newman LC et al.: Headaches in the elderly, *J Pain Symptom Manage* 8(2):87-97, 1993.

Lipton RB, Stewart WF, Celentano DD et al.: Undiagnosed migraine headaches: a comparison of symptom-based and reported physician diagnosis, *Arch Intern Med* 152:1273-1278, 1992.

Mathew NT, Kurman R, Perez F: Drug induced refractory headache: clinical features and management, *Headache* 30:634-638, 1990.

Mazzotta G, Sarchielli P, Alberti A et al.: Electromyographical ischemic test and intracellular and extracellular magnesium concentration in migraine and tension-type headache patients, *Headache* 36:357-361, 1996.

Moskowitz MA: The visceral organ brain: implications for the pathophysiology of vascular head pain, *Neurology* 41:182-186, 1991.

National Headache Foundation: *National Headache Foundation fact sheet*, Chicago, ND, The Foundation.

Saper JR, Silberstein S, Gordon CD: *Handbook of headache management*, Baltimore, 1993, Williams & Wilkins.

Schachtel BP, Furey SA, Thoden WR: Nonprescription ibuprofen and acetaminophen in the treatment of tension-type headache, *J Clin Pharmacol* 36:1120-1125, 1996.

Silberstein SD: The pharmacology of ergotamine and dihydroergotamine, *Headache*, 37(Suppl 1):515-525, 1997.

Silberstein SD, Lipton RB: Overview of diagnosis and treatment of migraine, *Neurology* 44(Suppl 7):S6-S16, 1994.

Silberstein S, Schulman E, Hopkins M: Repetitive intravenous DHE in the treatment of refractory headaches, *Headache* 30:334-339, 1990.

Solomon G: Treatment considerations in headache and associated medical disorders, *J Pain Symptom Manage* 8(2):73-80, 1993.

Stewart WF, Lipton RB, Celentano DD et al.: Prevalence of migraine headache in the United States: relation to age, income, race, and other sociodemographic factors, *JAMA* 267:64-69, 1992.

Tfelt-Hansen P, Henry P, Mulder LS et al.: The effectiveness of combined oral lysine acetylsalicylate and metoclopramide compared with oral sumatriptan for migraine, *Lancet* 346(8980)923, 1995.

Visser WH, DeVrienc RHM, Jaspers NHWM et al.: Sumatriptan nonresponders: a survey in 366 migraine patients, *Headache* 36:471-475, 1996.

Warner JS, Fenichel AM: Chronic post-traumatic headache often a myth? *Neurology* 46:915, 1996.

Wilkinson M: Treatment of the acute attack of migraine. In Rose F, editor: *The management of headaches*, p 75, New York, 1988, Raven.

HERPES ZOSTER AND POSTHERPETIC NEURALGIA

Pamela Stitzlein Davies

Description of Disease

Herpes zoster

Herpes zoster (HZ, or "shingles") is caused by reactivation of the varicella–zoster virus (VZV, or chickenpox virus). It occurs only in persons who previously had chickenpox, lying dormant for decades in the dorsal root ganglion (nerve cell nuclei). An unknown stimulus causes reemergence of VZV, which travels along peripheral sensory nerves to erupt in painful vesicles on the skin. These vesicles are similar in appearance to a chickenpox outbreak and have been described as "a dewdrop on a rose petal."

The rash appears in a discrete, unilateral, dermatomal pattern, most frequently on the thorax (Figure 12.10) or ophthalmic division of the trigeminal nerve (forehead).

Appearance of the typical HZ vesicles is usually preceded by a prodrome of itching, tingling, aching, or sharp pain for several days, which occasionally may be misdiagnosed as myocardial infarction, pleurisy, cholecystitis, appendicitis, or ovarian cyst. Headache, malaise, low-grade fever, and nausea often accompany the outbreak. Over several days, the HZ vesicles become pus filled, then break open and weep. The patient is highly contagious for chickenpox (but not herpes zoster) until all vesicles are crusted over, usually after 10 days to 3 weeks.

HZ occurs most frequently in adults older than 50, with 25% occurrence by age 60, increasing to 50% occurrence by age 80 (Gershon, 1996). The incidence is significantly increased in immunocompromised patients, especially those with Hodgkin's disease, non-Hodgkin's lymphoma, pediatric leukemia, bone marrow transplant, and HIV disease, and may present with a disseminated rash over the entire body. Persons with disseminated HZ

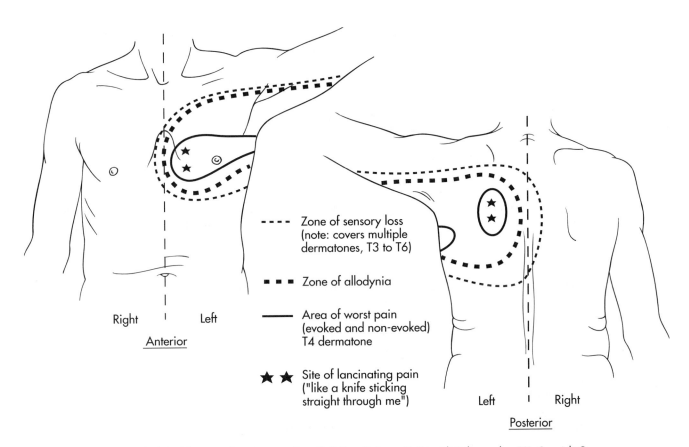

Zone of sensory loss (note: covers multiple dermatones, T3 to T6)

Zone of allodynia

Area of worst pain (evoked and non-evoked) T4 dermatone

★★ Site of lancinating pain ("like a knife sticking straight through me")

Right | Left
Anterior

Left | Right
Posterior

●●●●● F I G U R E 12.10   Postherpetic neuralgia. Following herpes zoster along the thoracic nerve, postherpetic neuralgia developed in this patient, who experienced some sensory loss and several types of pain, including allodynia (pain caused by normally non-painful stimuli such as the touch of clothing) and lancinating (knife-like) pain.

who are not known to be immunodeficient should be worked up for possible malignancy.

Complications include meningoencephalitis and zoster ophthalmicus. Persons with ophthalmic HZ must be seen by an ophthalmologist to evaluate for the latter, which could impair vision if not treated. A large study is currently in progress to evaluate whether HZ may be prevented by giving VZV immunizations to elders to boost immunity. It is hypothesized that a second outbreak of HZ is rarely seen because HZ infection provides a marked boost in VZV immunity (Oxman, 1995). With mass VZV immunizations in schoolchildren, we should start to see a decreased incidence of HZ in 4 decades.

Postherpetic neuralgia

Postherpetic neuralgia (PHN) is a chronic neuropathic pain condition occurring after an HZ outbreak. Various authors define it as pain continuing 1 to 3 months after crusting of the HZ lesions. Patients may experience a brief pain-free interval before the neuralgia starts.

It is not known why some persons have PHN after HZ and others do not. The overall incidence is 10% to 15% of all HZ patients. Advanced age is the strongest predictor of development of PHN; for example, a 60-year-old with HZ has a 50% chance of PHN developing, and an 80-year-old has an 80% chance (Rowbotham, 1994). The intractability of PHN appears to increase with age, so that an older person is less likely to spontaneously recover. Other prognostic indicators for development of PHN in immunocompetent patients include severity of HZ lesions, duration of HZ rash, and increased pain severity (Dworkin, Portenoy, 1996). Additional factors are being studied, such as degree of psychologic stress at the time of the HZ outbreak and comorbid depression, somatization, and disease conviction (Engberg, Grondahl, Thibom, 1995). The incidence of PHN is not increased in immunocompromised individuals.

Pain Characteristics

Herpes zoster

Patients with herpes zoster are miserable. The pain is severe and debilitating, and hospitalization is occasionally required for pain management. Descriptions of deep soreness, sharp, and stabbing pain are common. The pain frequently continues for several weeks after lesions are crusted, gradually fading over weeks to months.

Postherpetic neuralgia

With the development of PHN, many patients will note a definite change in pain character to that typical of neuralgia: (1) a continuous deep, burning, aching, or bruised pain; (2) paroxysmal (sudden) lancinating pain like electric shocks or sharp stabs; and (3) abnormal cutaneous (skin) sensitivity, such as allodynia (pain caused by stimuli that do not ordinarily cause pain). Patients may experience any combination of pain characteristics but typically have the continuous burning pain with some degree of allodynia.

PHN is located in the same unilateral, dermatomal distribution of the HZ outbreak. Although the HZ outbreak is described as occurring in a single dermatome, the neuralgic pain is noted in several dermatomes above and below the silver scar left after the rash heals (see Figure 12.10). It is not unusual for patients to report pain sensations in areas anatomically unrelated to the HZ outbreak. For example, one patient with right T6 PHN experienced severe allodynia when brushing his hair on the right side (C2 level). Lancinating pains may also start or end outside the area of HZ outbreak.

Some persons with PHN find they are comfortable only while sitting still or while calm and relaxed; others find constant activity and distraction needed to relieve pain. Allodynia may be so severe that an individual cannot tolerate wearing clothes, such as a bra or shirt, over the affected area. This creates obvious social difficulties, and many female PHN sufferers find themselves essentially homebound, topless, with the shades drawn. Others with severe allodynia in the axillary region find it helpful to keep a small pillow tucked firmly under their arm at all times. This prevents any stimulation of the painful skin area. Intense and unremitting itching may be the most unbearable aspect of PHN for some individuals, especially as pain resolves from either natural healing or medication management.

Assessment

Once PHN has developed, most elders of average cognitive status can excel at describing pain with a 0 to 10 scale after a little practice. Many will spontaneously offer various ratings for each of their pain subtypes, which is extremely helpful in choosing or modifying drug therapies. For example, "my burning pain is 3/10, but the electric shocks are 10/10."

A new assessment tool for neuropathic pain has been developed, which is brief yet comprehensive (see pp. 76-77) (Galer, Jensen, 1997). Using eight descriptor items specific to neuropathic pain (sharp, hot, cold, sensitive itchy, etc.), each item is rated on a 0 to 10 scale. The tool is easy for most patients to learn, takes about 5 minutes to complete, and is sensitive to treatment effect. The short form McGill Pain Questionnaire (Melzack, 1987) is useful to capture the multiple descriptions of neuropathic pain but does not provide quantification of each descriptor.

Pain Management

Herpes zoster

Aggressive pain management of HZ with opioids, antiviral agents, and nerve blocks is strongly encouraged by most experts. Research is beginning to show that patients treated with these modalities have a lower incidence of PHN, thereby decreasing overall health care costs and improving quality of life (Dworkin, Portenoy, 1996.)

Opioids are the mainstay of pain management for acute zoster attack. However, frail, opioid-naive elders may quickly become overly sedated or experience light-headedness and balance problems with the doses needed to relieve the severe pain of HZ. Short-acting opioids, such as oxycodone, should be used, starting with low doses in older adults, then slowly increasing the dose as tolerated. The patient must be warned to avoid driving and use care to prevent falls for the first several days of treatment. Patients taking opioid compounds containing acetaminophen must be instructed not to take more than 4 g of acetaminophen per day and avoid other products with this drug to protect liver function.

Some clinicians consider use of an oral or intravenous antiviral agent standard treatment for HZ. Some studies have shown that antivirals shorten the duration and severity of zoster outbreak and decrease pain if treatment is started within 48 hours of appearance of HZ skin lesions (Beutner, 1994). Because of this, many authors predict the use of antivirals will prevent development or decrease the severity of PHN. However, a recent meta-analysis of clinical trials did not support this theory (Jackson, Gibbons, Meyer et al., 1997). More studies with a variety of antiviral agents are needed to clarify this confusing picture. Oral or intravenous steroids are not currently recommended in uncomplicated cases.

A series of epidural, sympathetic, or intercostal nerve blocks are frequently used to control HZ pain. Subcutaneous injection of long-acting local anesthetic and steroids may also decrease pain and inflammation. Aluminum acetate solution (Domeboro) soaks may be soothing and aid in cleansing the weeping lesions.

Postherpetic neuralgia

As with all neuropathic pain, management is very difficult and frustrating for patient and caregiver alike. The high percentage of geriatric clients makes treating this problem especially challenging because many cannot tolerate the side effects of standard oral therapy.

Pain management includes antidepressants, anticonvulsants, topical therapy, and opioids. (See the quick guide on Painful Peripheral Neuropathies [p. 576] for a discussion of these treatments.) Following are additional comments specific to PHN.

Antidepressants and Anticonvulsants

As with other neuropathies, tricyclic antidepressants are the cornerstone of pain management. However, many practitioners are reluctant to provide these drugs to elderly clients because of the frequent incidence of un-

pleasant or potentially dangerous side effects, such as sedation, dizziness, constipation, and dry mouth. Low starting doses, gradual titration, and frequent follow-up are key to a successful trial. Desipramine is recommended as the first drug (Davies, Reisner-Keller, Rowbotham, 1996). A minimum of 50 mg for 2 weeks is considered an adequate trial before considering a switch to another drug. Because many patients report a decrease in lancinating pain with use of an antidepressant, the addition of an anticonvulsant may not be required.

Topical Therapy

The author has had a great deal of success in treating PHN allodynia and itching with Lidoderm gel and patches, a new product due for FDA approval in late 1998 (Rowbotham, Davies, Verkempinck et al., 1996). Lidocaine is delivered to the free nerve endings in the skin, and the patch has the added benefit of stabilizing the skin to prevent movement-induced pain. There are multiple reports of success with aspirin in chloroform for treatment of allodynia (King, 1993). A trial of capsaicin cream may be undertaken, but the side effect of burning is often unbearable for many patients with allodynia.

Opioids

Opioid therapy for chronic nonmalignant pain is gaining acceptance and may be very helpful in a subset of PHN patients (Pappagallo, Raja, Haythornthwaite et al., 1994). As noted earlier, dose adjustments should be made to prevent the increased incidence of side effects in the elderly.

Other Therapies

Mexiletine and clonidine are third-line therapy for recalcitrant PHN. Although serial nerve blocks are often done, the literature does not currently support this practice for well-established PHN (Rowbotham, 1994). The literature on neuroablative and surgical sectioning is sparse and inconclusive and is generally not recommended.

Nonpharmacologic Therapies

Some nonpharmacologic therapies can be very helpful in elders who cannot tolerate medication side effects. Many of the author's patients have reported ice packs to be beneficial in relieving pain and itching, especially when applied four to six times daily for 20 minutes. Psychologic therapies, such as relaxation or biofeedback, should be offered, although the author has found many geriatric clients unwilling to use these therapies despite explanations to remove misconceptions.

SUMMARY

- Herpes zoster is a reactivation of the chickenpox virus, causing painful skin lesions in a unilateral dermatomal pattern. It occurs most frequently in older adults.

- Postherpetic neuralgia is a chronic neuropathic pain syndrome occurring in up to 15% of all persons with herpes zoster and 80% of persons older than 80.
- The risk factors for postherpetic neuralgia developing after herpes zoster are increased age, increased severity and duration of zoster lesions, and increased pain severity during zoster outbreak.
- Postherpetic neuralgia may have three types of pain: deep burning pain, painful skin sensitivity, and lancinating pains.
- Medication management of herpes zoster includes opioids, antiviral therapy, and nerve blocks. Aggressive therapy may help prevent development of PHN.
- Medication management of PHN includes antidepressants, topical agents, and opioids. PHN is very difficult to manage successfully, especially given the advanced age of most sufferers.

Resources

1. VZV Research Foundation
   40 E. 72nd St.
   New York, NY 10021
   (212) 472-3181
   Fax: (212) 861-7033

   A nonprofit group for the purpose of combating VZV and the diseases it causes: chickenpox, shingles, and PNH. It supports research, publishes a newsletter, hosts annual scientific meetings, and provides literature.

   Recommended lay literature (free): *Shingles & PHN: Your questions answered.*

2. Suggested reading for clinicians:

   Neuropathic pain, *Semin Neurol* 14(3):195-280, 1994.

   An 85-page supplement on mechanisms, diagnosis, and management of neuropathic pain directed at the practicing clinician. A specific section on postherpetic neuralgia (Rowbotham) is noted below.

   Zoster in the elderly, *J Geriatr Derm* 2(Suppl A):3A-32A, 1994.

   A special supplement addressing diagnosis and management of chickenpox, herpes zoster, and postherpetic neuralgia.

References

Beutner KR: Antivirals in the treatment of pain, *J Geriatr Derm* 2(Suppl A):23A-28A, 1994.

Davies PS, Reisner-Keller L, Rowbotham MC: Randomized, double-blind comparison of fluoxetine, desipramine and amitriptyline in postherpetic neuralgia, International Association for the Study of Pain: Eighth World Congress on Pain Abstract #193, Aug 20, 1996 (abstract).

Dworkin RH, Portenoy RK: Pain and its persistence in herpes zoster, *Pain* 67(2):241-251, 1996.

Engberg IB, Grondahl GB, Thibom K: Patients' experiences of herpes zoster and postherpetic neuralgia, *J Adv Nurs* 21(3):427-433, 1995.

Galer BS, Jensen MP: Development and preliminary validation of a pain measure specific to neuropathic pain: the neuropathic pain scale, *Neurology* 48:332-338, 1997.

Gershon AA: Epidemiology and management of postherpetic neuralgia, *Semin Derm* 15(2 Suppl 1):8-13, 1996.

Jackson JL, Gibbons R, Meyer G et al.: The effect of treating herpes zoster with oral acyclovir in preventing postherpetic neuralgia: a meta-analysis, *Arch Intern Med* 157(8):909-912, 1997.

King RB: Topical aspirin in chloroform and the relief of pain due to herpes zoster and postherpetic neuralgia, *Arch Neurol* 50(10):1046-1053, 1993.

Melzack R: The short-form McGill Pain Questionnaire, *Pain* 30:191-197, 1987.

Oxman MN: Immunization to reduce the frequency and severity of herpes zoster and its complications, *Neurology* 45(Suppl 8):S41-S46, 1995.

Pappagallo M, Raja SN, Haythornthwaite JA et al.: *Analgesia* 1(1):51-55, 1994.

Rowbotham MC: Postherpetic neuralgia, *Semin Neurol* 14(3):247-254, 1994.

Rowbotham MC, Davies PS, Verkempinck C et al.: Lidocaine patch: double-blind controlled study of a new treatment method for post-herpetic neuralgia, *Pain* 65:39-44, 1996.

HIV-RELATED PAIN

Anne M. Hughes

Description

Human immunodeficiency virus (HIV) disease is a complex syndrome characterized by infection with a highly replicating retrovirus. After infection with HIV, there is a long period of clinical latency (no HIV-related symptoms) during which time the immune system is being constantly assaulted and valiantly attempts to keep the infection in check (Brennan, Porche, 1997). Eventually without effective antiretroviral therapy, the immune system is exhausted. At that time, most persons with HIV infections develop opportunistic infections, malignancies, and other conditions associated with advanced HIV disease, such as peripheral neuropathy.

A variety of infectious (e.g., cryptococcal meningitis, cytomegalovirus esophagitis) and malignant (Kaposi's sarcoma or non–Hodgkin's lymphoma) manifestations of HIV disease are associated with pain. Similar to cancer-related pain, HIV therapies may also cause pain (e.g., isoniazid (INH)–induced peripheral neuropathy). Fifty percent of pain in persons with HIV is related to HIV infection itself or its complications, 30% is related to HIV treatments or procedures, and 20% is unrelated to either the disease or its treatment (Breitbart, Lefkowitz, 1997).

Recent advances in HIV therapies along with new understandings of the pathogenesis of HIV infection have led some researchers to consider the possibility that the natural history of HIV infection can be changed (Feinberg, 1996). If this proves to be true, much of what is known about the natural history (clinical trajectory) of HIV disease, including the presence of pain or other associated signs and symptoms, will change.

At the most advanced stages, persons with HIV infection are diagnosed with AIDS according to the Centers for Disease Control and Prevention (CDC) case surveillance criteria (1992). These criteria include the diagnosis of certain opportunistic infections, HIV-related cancers, or other AIDS-defining condition (e.g., dementia, wasting syndrome, severe immunosuppression based on CD4 or T lymphocyte $< 200/mm^3$) in the presence of HIV infection.

The number of cases of AIDS in the United States exceeds 600,000 (CDC, 1997a). Estimates of HIV infection in the United States vary from 650,000 to 900,000 (CDC, 1997a, b). New infections are occurring daily at an alarming rate. In the United States it is estimated that 40,000 new HIV infections occur annually (Barrows, 1997).

Pain and HIV Disease: Scope of the Problem

Since the late 1980s the problem of pain in persons with HIV infection has received increased attention by clinicians and researchers alike (Barone, Wolkomir, Muakkassa et al., 1988; Lebovits, Lefkowitz, McCarthy et al., 1989; Newshan, Wainapel, 1993; O'Neill, Sherrard, 1993). Several studies have estimated the prevalence of pain in persons with HIV/AIDS. Singer, Zorilla, Fahy-Chandon and others (1993) studied ambulatory men with HIV infection. Surprisingly, 28% of the men who had no evidence of HIV-related problems reported pain compared with 56% of those with documented HIV-related symptoms and 80% of persons with an AIDS diagnosis. Pain in terminally ill persons with AIDS has been reported in more than 90% of those receiving supportive care in residential hospice settings (Kimball, McCormick, 1996; Singh, Fermie, Peters, 1992).

Clearly, pain in HIV disease becomes an increasing problem as the disease progresses. In the future if highly active antiretroviral therapy (HAART) effectively prevents viral replication and thus the destruction of the immune system, it is conceivable that pain may be less of a problem for persons with HIV. This prediction seems supported by a research report that noted that persons receiving antiretrovirals were less likely to have pain (Breitbart, McDonald, Rosenfeld et al., 1996).

In the meantime, however, pain remains a significant problem for many that all too often is unrecognized and, even when recognized, is undertreated (Breitbart, Rosenfeld, Passik et al., 1996; McCormack, Li, Zarowny et al., 1993; Newshan, 1997). In a study of 366 ambulatory persons with AIDS (Breitbart, Rosenfeld, Passik et al., 1996) more than 60% of the patients studied reported pain in the previous 2 weeks. Most patients had 2.5 concurrent pains; nearly 50% of those reporting pain rated its intensity as severe. However, of those with severe pain, only 7% had strong opioid analgesics

prescribed to manage the pain. Persons at greatest risk for inadequate pain management were women, injection drug users, the less educated, and those with an identified religious affiliation. The researchers concluded that 85% of the AIDS patients with pain in this study were undertreated and that this rate was even more dismal than the undertreatment reported in persons with cancer-related pain.

Pain Characteristics and Sites

The characteristics of pain and the location of pain in persons with HIV disease (Figure 12.11) are related to the cause of the pain, (i.e., disease related, treatment induced, or unrelated to the disease or its treatment) and its underlying pathophysiology (i.e., nociceptive or neuropathic; if nociceptive, it can be somatic or visceral). In a group of 151 patients with pain who underwent a neurologic examination, 71% had at least one somatic pain, 46% had one or more neuropathic pains, and 29% had visceral pain (Breitbart, Rosenfeld, Passik et al., 1996).

Pain in persons with HIV may be acute (e.g., related to onset of new opportunistic infection), chronic (e.g., related to peripheral neuropathy), or both. Knowing the patient's CD4 count assists health care providers in diagnosing the underlying condition because many complications occur at certain counts. For example, Pneumocystis carinii pneumonia is rarely diagnosed in a person whose CD4 count is more than $200/mm^3$.

Figure 12.11 identifies some of the most common pain syndromes and their likely cause. Two axioms of HIV/AIDS care are worth keeping in mind. First, persons with HIV disease can and do have infections and even malignancies develop in sites previously unknown before HIV/AIDS. Second, each person's course, the infections or complications that develop, is unique and unpredictable.

Assessment of Pain in Persons With HIV

No published pain assessment tools are specifically designed for HIV-related pain. However, a number of standardized assessment tools available are widely used by HIV clinicians (see AHCPR Management of Cancer Pain: Clinical Practice Guidelines [p. 542] for examples [Jacox, Carr, Payne et al., 1994]) and researchers (Hoyt, Nokes, Newshan et al., 1994; McCormack, Li, Zarowny et al., 1993). Assessment should include a determination of other signs and symptoms the person may be experiencing such as fatigue, fever, diarrhea, skin problems, dyspnea, anorexia, cognitive problems, and nausea. In addition, determining (1) whether the person is chemically dependent on drugs or alcohol or in recovery for

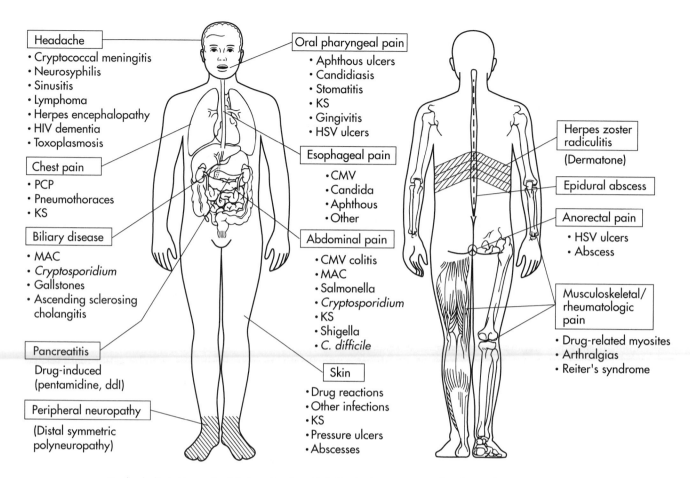

Headache
- Cryptococcal meningitis
- Neurosyphilis
- Sinusitis
- Lymphoma
- Herpes encephalopathy
- HIV dementia
- Toxoplasmosis

Chest pain
- PCP
- Pneumothoraces
- KS

Biliary disease
- MAC
- *Cryptosporidium*
- Gallstones
- Ascending sclerosing cholangitis

Pancreatitis
Drug-induced (pentamidine, ddl)

Peripheral neuropathy
(Distal symmetric polyneuropathy)

Oral pharyngeal pain
- Aphthous ulcers
- Candidiasis
- Stomatitis
- KS
- Gingivitis
- HSV ulcers

Esophageal pain
- CMV
- Candida
- Aphthous
- Other

Abdominal pain
- CMV colitis
- MAC
- Salmonella
- *Cryptosporidium*
- KS
- Shigella
- *C. difficile*

Skin
- Drug reactions
- Other infections
- KS
- Pressure ulcers
- Abscesses

Herpes zoster radiculitis
(Dermatone)

Epidural abscess

Anorectal pain
- HSV ulcers
- Abscess

Musculoskeletal/ rheumatologic pain
- Drug-related myosites
- Arthralgias
- Reiter's syndrome

May be duplicated for use in clinical practice. From McCaffery M, Pasero C: *Pain: Clinical manual*, p. 566. Copyright © 1999, Mosby, Inc.

● ● ● ● ●
FIGURE 12.11 Possible sources and locations of pain in persons with HIV disease.

chemical dependency and (2) what other prescribed medications the person is taking (to avoid drug-drug interactions or to determine any adverse reaction) will provide helpful data for planning how to manage the HIV-related pain.

Persons with neuropathic pain may deny pain but will describe burning, tingling, and pins and needles. If the person has distal symmetric polyneuropathy, the pain will generally be localized to the lower extremities. Persons with esophageal ulcers, whether CMV or aphthous, often characterize the pain as sharp and can localize the pain; it may become exquisitely painful when eating. On the other hand, persons with candidal esophagitis usually describe the sensation as having something stuck in their throat, which makes swallowing difficult. Intestinal parasitic infections (e.g., shigella, giardia) are often associated with cramping abdominal pain. Sinusitis is usually associated with frontal headaches that may be throbbing or aching in nature (Newshan, 1997).

Management of Pain in Persons With HIV

Despite the lack of clinical trials, many HIV clinicians have accepted the AHCPR's Management of Cancer Pain Clinical Guidelines endorsement of the WHO Analgesic Ladder as a useful framework for managing HIV-related pain (Breitbart, Lefkowitz, 1997; Carr, Dubois, Luu et al., 1994).

In general, given the frequency of neuropathic pain, adjuvant agents (e.g., tricyclic antidepressants, anticonvulsants, and antiarrhythmic agents) are used more frequently than in cancer-related pain. Steroids and carbamazepine, known to have immune depressive and bone marrow suppressive effects, respectively, are used with caution in persons with HIV.

Although infrequent, aphthous ulcers may be associated with severe pain. A recent report described the use of thalidomide to treat this painful condition (Jacobson, Greenspan, Spritzler et al., 1997); adverse reactions included somnolence and rash. Great care was taken to inform women considering childbearing of the teratogenic effects of thalidomide.

Adverse drug reactions (ADRs) occur more frequently in persons with AIDS who are receiving treatment or prophylaxis for opportunistic infections (Lee, 1997) than non-AIDS patients receiving these agents. Between 12% and 40% of hospitalized patients with AIDS have delirium (Breitbart, Marotta, Platt et al., 1996). Realizing this problem will help when sorting out whether a patient's altered mental status is an ADR related to an opioid or another agent just added to a regimen or whether it is unrelated.

Polypharmacy is a way of life for persons with advanced HIV disease. Many persons with AIDS are routinely taking three or four different antiretroviral agents several times a day, along with an agent to prevent Pneumocystis carinii pneumonia. Other problems such as diarrhea, fever, herpes simplex, and/or oral candidiasis will result in additional medications. Some persons with HIV may also take alternative therapies to manage distressing symptoms. Kimball and McCormick (1996) reported that on average, terminally ill persons with AIDS were prescribed 12 pharmaceutic agents.

In 1997 the CDC reported that 32% of all reported AIDS cases were associated with injection drug use (CDC, 1997a, p. 8, Table 3). This fact alone presents another complex pharmacologic pain management need in this population (see also Chapter 10 on Substance Abuse for more information on managing pain in persons who are chemically dependent). Many studies have demonstrated no differences in pain intensity or the number of pains in HIV-positive chemically dependent persons with pain compared with the HIV-positive nonchemically dependent (Breitbart, McDonald, Rosenfeld et al., 1996; Hoyt, Nokes, Newshan et al., 1994; McCormack, Li, Zarowny et al., 1993). Substance users with AIDS are at greater risk for undertreatment of pain than nonsubstance users with AIDS (Breitbart, Rosenfeld, Passik et al., 1996). Anand, Carmosino, and Glatt (1994) reported no significant analgesic dose requirements, degree of pain relief, or time to relief in patients who were past or current substance abusers compared with those who were not.

HIV disease may alter the pharmacokinetics of medications including those used to control pain (Lee, 1997). Drug absorption, metabolism, and distribution may be affected by intestinal infections with a number of pathogens that invade small bowel such as *Cryptosporidium, Isospora belli, Microsporidium,* and *Mycobacterium avium* complex. Malabsorption and malnutrition may lead to hypoproteinemia, which may result in more unbound drug and the risk of increased toxicities with analgesics or adjuvants. Diarrhea has been reported in 50% to 60% of persons with HIV at some point in their illness. Opioids may have a secondary effect in decreasing the number of stools per day; however, the rectal route of administration may not be feasible because of diarrhea and/or other rectal pathology. No pharmacokinetic studies have been published that have evaluated the efficacy of oral time-released analgesics in persons with HIV disease with severe diarrhea and/or malabsorption.

Fever increases metabolic rate. Fever was the most commonly cited presenting symptom at admission in persons with HIV followed by pain (Lebovits, Lefkowitz, McCarthy et al., 1989; Lebovits, Smith, Maignan et al., 1994). Fever surveillance may limit use of NSAIDs and acetaminophen. Increased confusion believed to be caused by bolusing transdermal fentanyl in the presence of high fevers has been reported. Duration of pain relief for some with fever with the fentanyl transdermal system was shortened to 48 hours (Newshan, 1997).

Great excitement has been generated about the new class of potent, highly active anti-HIV drugs introduced in 1996, the protease inhibitors, and their contribution to HIV combination therapy (the so-called HIV/AIDS cocktail). It is indisputable that these drugs have brought many people out of their sick beds to lead highly active and productive lives. It is also true, however, that these drugs because of an enzyme involved in the metabolism of drugs, p450, are associated with many clinically significant drug-drug interactions. The potential for drug interactions must be appreciated when starting or changing an analgesic regimen. The four currently licensed protease inhibitors are saquinavir (Invirase), ritonavir (Norvir), indinavir (Crixivan), and nelfinavir (Viracept). Ritonavir has been associated with a number of potentially lethal drug-drug interactions with meperidine (Demerol), propoxyphene (Darvon), and piroxicam (Feldene). Codeine and tricyclic antidepressants should be administered with caution (Williams, 1997). Although the drug-drug interactions are most thoroughly described for ritonavir, it is worth remembering that other drugs in this class may have similar effects and bear careful monitoring. Some persons receiving protease inhibitors have reportedly become oversedated with long-acting opioids (Lor, 1997; Newshan, 1997). Several antiretroviral agents are pain inducing (e.g., didanosine [ddI]); lamivudine (3TC) may cause pancreatitis. Indinavir is associated with nephrolithiasis. Zidovudine (AZT) and lamivudine (3TC) may cause headache. Ritonavir has been associated with abdominal pain and severe nausea and vomiting.

SUMMARY

Pain is a serious problem for persons with HIV disease and is often undertreated. The management of pain in persons with HIV is complicated by a number of factors. Pain syndromes are varied. The assessment of pain is similar to assessing pain in other populations; however, substance use history needs to be included as does a thorough medication history. Nonpharmacologic interventions, although not extensively reported in the literature, have been used with some success. Finally, the pharmacologic management of pain in this population is complicated by polypharmacy, drug-drug interactions, and adverse drug reactions.

Resources

1. Association of Nurses in AIDS Care
   11250 Roger Bacon Dr., Suite 8
   Reston, VA 20190
   (703) 925-0081
   E-mail: *AIDSNURSES@aol.com*

   Nursing specialty organization with 50 local chapters, annual conference, peer-reviewed journal, newsletter, and clinical resource directory.

2. CDC National AIDS Clearinghouse
   P.O. Box 6003
   Rockville, MD 20849-6003
   (800) 458-5231

   Provides HIV/AIDS information, resources, and publications.

3. Roxane Pain Institute
   P.O. Box 16532
   Columbus, OH 43216-6532
   (800) 335-9100
   Web site: *www.Roxane.com*

   Provides information for patients/families and professional caregivers.

4. Web sites:

   http://www.ama-assn.org/special/hivsrch.htm

   http://www.hivpositive.com

   http://www.critpath.org/aric/pwarg/contact07.htm

   http://www.partnersagainstpain.com/pro/aids.html

   http://www.hivinsite.ucsf.edu/akb/1994/4-14/ref41html

   http://www.meds.com/conrad/pmcd/breit.html

References

Anand A, Carmosino L, Glatt AE: Evaluation of recalcitrant pain in HIV-infected hospitalized patients, *J Acq Immune Defic Syndr* 7:52-57, 1994.

Barone JE, Wolkomir AF, Muakkassa FF et al.: Abdominal pain and anorectal disease in AIDS, *Gastroenterol Clin North Am* 17:631-638, 1988.

Barrows W: Personal communication, 1997.

Breitbart W, Lefkowitz M: Pain management in HIV disease, *Improv Manage HIV Dis* 5:16-20, 1997.

Breitbart W, Marotta R, Platt MM et al.: A double-blind trial of haloperidol, chlorpromazine, and lorazepam in the treatment of delirium in hospitalized AIDS patients, *Am J Psychiatry* 153:231-237, 1996.

Breitbart W, McDonald MV, Rosenfeld B et al.: Pain in ambulatory AIDS patients. I. Pain characteristics and medical correlates, *Pain* 68:315-321, 1996.

Breitbart W, Rosenfeld BD, Passik S et al.: The undertreatment of pain in ambulatory AIDS patients, *Pain* 65:243-249, 1996.

Brennan C, Porche DJ: HIV immunopathogenesis, *J Assoc Nurses AIDS Care* 8:7-22, 1997.

Carr DB, Dubois M, Luu M et al.: Pharmacotherapy of pain in HIV/AIDS. In Carr DB, editor: *Pain in HIV/AIDS: proceedings of a workshop convened by France-U.S.A. Pain Association*, pp 18-28, Washington, DC, 1994, France-U.S.A. Pain Association.

Centers for Disease Control and Prevention (CDC): 1993 revised classification system for HIV infection and expanded surveillance case definition for AIDS among adolescents and adults, *Morb Mortal Wkly Rep* 41(RR-1):1-9, 1992.

CDC: *HIV/AIDS surveillance report* 9(1):3,33-34, 1997a.

CDC: U.N. doubles estimate of new HIV cases, *San Francisco Chronicle*, Nov 26, 1997b, pg A2.

Feinberg MB: Changing the natural history of HIV disease, *Lancet* 348:239-246, 1996.

Hoyt MJ, Nokes K, Newshan G et al.: The effect of chemical dependency on pain perception in persons with AIDS, *J Assoc Nurses AIDS Care* 5:33-38, 1994.

Jacobson JM, Greenspan JS, Spritzler J et al.: Thalidomide for the treatment of oral aphthous ulcers in patients with human immunodeficiency virus infection, *N Engl J Med* 336:1487-1493, 1997.

Jacox A, Carr DB, Payne R et al.: *Management of cancer pain: clinical practice guidelines*, Rockville, Md, 1994, Agency for Health Care Policy and Research (AHCPR).

Kimball LR, McCormick WC: The pharmacologic management of pain and discomfort in persons with AIDS near the end of life: use of opioids analgesia in the hospice setting, *J Pain Symptom Manage* 11:88-94, 1996.

Lebovits AH, Lefkowitz M, McCarthy D et al.: The prevalence and management of pain in patients with AIDS: a review of 134 cases, *Clin J Pain* 5:245-248, 1989.

Lebovits AH, Smith G, Maignan M et al.: Pain in hospitalized patients with AIDS: analgesic and psychotropic medications, *Clin J Pain* 10:156-161, 1994.

Lee BL: Drug interactions and toxicities in patients with AIDS. In Sande MA, Volberding PA, editors: *The medical management of AIDS*, pp 125-142, Philadelphia, 1997, WB Saunders.

Lor E: Personal communication, 1997.

McCormack JP, Li R, Zarowny D et al.: Inadequate treatment of pain in ambulatory HIV patients, *Clin J Pain* 9:279-83, 1993.

Newshan G: Pain in human immunodeficiency virus disease, *Semin Oncol Nurs* 13:1, 36-41, 1997.

Newshan G, Wainapel SF: Pain characteristics and their management in persons with AIDS, *J Assoc Nurses AIDS Care* 4:53-59, 1993.

O'Neill WM, Sherrard JS: Pain in human immunodeficiency virus disease: a review, *Pain* 54:3-14, 1993.

Singer EJ, Zorilla C, Fahy-Chandon B et al.: Painful symptoms reported by ambulatory HIV-infected men in a longitudinal study, *Pain* 54:15-19, 1993.

Singh S, Fermie P, Peters W: Symptom control for individuals with advanced HIV infection in a subacute residential unit: which symptoms need palliating? *Proceedings of the VIII International Conference on AIDS*, Abstract PoD 5248, Amsterdam, Netherlands, 1992.

Williams A: New horizons: antiretroviral therapy in 1997, *J Assoc Nurses AIDS Care* 8:4, 26-38, 1997.

MYOFASCIAL PAIN SYNDROME
Jane Faries and Marsha Stanton

Description of Disease

Myofascial pain syndrome (MPS) is a local or regional condition caused by the presence of one or more active *trigger* points within a skeletal muscle or its fascia (Travell, Simons, 1983). A trigger point is a small, circumscribed hypersensitive area located within a tight band of muscle. Trigger points refer pain and autonomic activity in a distinctive pattern specific to the muscle called a *referred pain zone* or *zone of reference* (Travell, Simons, 1983). Suggested diagnostic criteria for MPS that describe the characteristics of trigger points are listed in Box 12.3.

BOX 12.3	**Empirical Criteria Suggested for Diagnosis of Myofascial Pain Syndrome (MPS)**

A. *Major criteria (active trigger points)*
1. Regional pain reported
2. Taut band palpable in an accessible muscle
3. Exquisite spot of tenderness in the taut band
4. Pain report or altered sensation in the expected distribution of referred pain from the tender spot
5. Some restricted range of motion, when measurable

B. *Minor criteria*
1. Reproduction of clinical pain report, or altered sensation, by pressure on the tender spot
2. Local twitch response by transverse snapping palpation of, or needle insertion into, the taut band
3. Pain alleviation by stretching the involved muscle or injecting the tender spot in it

For diagnosis of MPS, all the major criteria and at least one of the three minor criteria need to be fulfilled.

May be duplicated for use in clinical practice. As appears in McCaffery M, Pasero C: *Pain: Clinical manual,* p. 569, 1999, Mosby, Inc.

Box 12.3 identifies proposed diagnostic criteria for myofascial pain syndrome. Modified from Simons DG: Muscular pain syndromes. In Fricton JR, Awad EA, editors: *Advances in pain research and therapy,* vol 17, pp. 1-41, New York, 1990, Raven Press.

Trigger points can develop as a result of acute or chronic muscle strain and are thought to be sustained and exacerbated by predisposing and perpetuating factors (Travell, Simons, 1983). These factors are categorized as (1) mechanical stresses from muscle overuse, misuse, or disuse and (2) systemic conditions that can interfere with muscle metabolism. Mechanical stresses identified are poor posture, leg length discrepancies, short upper arms, small hemipelvis, long second metatarsal, scoliosis, trauma, repetitive motion, and muscle overload. Systemic factors identified include nutritional inadequacies, hypothyroidism, hyperuricemia, hypoglycemia, anemia, estrogen deficiency, electrolyte imbalances, psychologic disturbances, chronic infection, allergy, and poor sleep (Travell, Simons, 1983).

MPS can be as simple as an acute active trigger point in a single muscle or as complex as a chronic condition involving numerous trigger points and muscles that results in an overlap of referred pain patterns that can mimic widespread, systemic disease, such as fibromyalgia (Schneider, 1995). The characteristic referred pain zone, usually at a distance from the trigger point and also tender, can lead to confusion and misdiagnosis (Simons, 1988a). A patient with active trigger points may report headache, joint pain, backache, or sciatic-type pain and be unaware of any muscular involvement (Sola, Bonica, 1990).

Differential diagnosis is essential because trigger points are often responsive to treatment, frequently with imme-diate resolution of tenderness, referred pain, and restricted motion (Travell, Simons, 1983). Prognosis may depend on the number of perpetuating factors that must be resolved and on the skill of the clinician in identifying and treating trigger points (Simons, 1988b). MPS can also accompany other diseases such as fibromyalgia, arthritis, and myositis (Reynolds, 1981).

If MPS goes unrecognized and untreated, it can become chronic (Simons, 1988b). A study of 164 myofascial pain syndrome patients found the mean duration of pain for men was 5.8 years and 6.9 years for women, with a mean average of 4.5 clinician visits in the past for their pain (Fricton, Kroening, Haley et al., 1985). If allowed to become chronic, pain can cause disability, depression, physical deconditioning, sleep disturbances, and potentially other psychologic and behavioral disturbances.

MPS is a common but frequently unrecognized cause of pain and disability (Skootsky, Jaeger, Oye, 1989). In a prospective study of 172 consecutive patients seen in a university internal medicine clinic, Skootsky, Jaeger, and Oye (1989) found that 30% of the 54 patients whose symptoms included pain had myofascial trigger points. Among 296 patients referred to a dental clinic for chronic head and neck pain, 55.4% were found to have myofascial pain syndrome (Fricton, Kroening, Haley et al., 1985). Among 283 consecutive admissions to a comprehensive pain center, 85% were assigned a primary diagnosis of myofascial syndrome (Fishbain, Goldberg, Meagher et al., 1986). Additional controlled studies are needed to firmly establish the prevalence of this disease.

Pain Characteristics

Although MPS can affect any skeletal muscle, Sola and Bonica (1990) in a survey of 1000 patients found that postural muscles in the neck, the shoulder girdle, and the low back are most commonly involved. Exquisite tenderness is noted at the trigger point with a dull, deep aching and sometimes burning pain in the referred pain zone (Sola, Bonica, 1990; Travell, Simons, 1983). Pain may occur at rest or only with activity. The referred pain can be localized or adjacent to the trigger point, but usually is at a distance (Travell, Simons, 1983). Similar to pulling a trigger on a gun, the target (the referred pain zone) is in another location; hence the name, trigger point (Sola, Bonica, 1990).

Assessment

A careful history usually reveals either an acute onset after an activity or a gradual onset with chronic overwork of the affected muscle. Information should be obtained about daily activities at home and work that may require repetitive motion (Sola, Bonica, 1990). Travell and Simons (1992) emphasize the usefulness of precisely drawing each area of reported pain on a body form and numbering each pain area in chronologic order of appearance. The referred pain pattern, which must be learned for each muscle, is often the key to diagnosis (Simons, 1988b). In two volumes Travell and Simons (1983, 1992) have provided explicit descriptions and drawings of the characteristic referred pain patterns of all muscles in the body, as well as many caveats in the assessment and treatment of trigger points.

The most common way to identify trigger points is by manual palpation, but this requires specific skill in examination of the muscle (Gerwin, Shannon, Hong et al., 1997). In fact, four studies (Gerwin, Shannon, Hong et al., 1997; Nice, Riddle, Lamb et al., 1992; Njoo, Van der Does, 1994; Wolfe, Simons, Fricton et al., 1992), were unable to establish interrater reliability in manual detection of trigger points and all their characteristics. Despite prior experience in identifying trigger points, Gerwin, Shannon, Hong et al. (1997) found a period of training was needed to ensure consistency in defining and interpreting physical findings to achieve acceptable interrater reliability. In addition, they confirmed that the interrater reliability of various trigger point characteristics differs, with the local twitch response being the most difficult to reproduce.

Some quantifiable means can verify certain trigger point characteristics. Hand-held pressure measurement gauges, sometimes called algometers, can measure pressure threshold, the minimum force needed to induce pain, and pressure tolerance (Fischer, 1988). A tissue compliance meter measures the relative hardness of tissue by the distance a given pressure indents the skin (Fischer, 1988). These can be used to quantify findings, to demonstrate to patients the difference in the muscle, to measure changes in response to trigger point therapy (Jaeger, Reeves, 1986), for medicolegal documentation (Fischer, 1988), and for research and training (Sola, Bonica, 1990). These instruments, however, only measure the presence of two trigger point features, tenderness and taut band (Gerwin, Shannon, Hong et al., 1997), and do not identify the cause of the tenderness (Travell, Simons, 1992). Fischer and Chang (1986) used thermographic measurements to corroborate the presence of a trigger point. Thermography alone, however, cannot determine the presence of myofascial trigger points (Travell, Simons, 1992). Laboratory and imaging studies are useful only to rule out other diseases and to identify perpetuating factors (Simons, 1988a).

Pain Management

The focus of treatment is to eliminate the trigger points, prevent recurrence, and correct aggravating or perpetuating factors (McCain, 1994). The goals of treatment are to stretch the muscle to its full length and range of motion, reduce pain, and improve function. Preventing recurrence involves patient education regarding cause of pain, perpetuating factors, and self-management; an ongoing conditioning program; and control of perpetuating factors (Gerwin, Dommerholt, 1998; McCain, 1994).

Very limited studies are currently available to determine the effectiveness of different modalities commonly used to inactivate trigger points (McCain, 1994). Passive stretch is the effective component in treatment (Jaeger, Reeves, 1986), but by itself can be too painful and may cause reflex spasm that inhibits motion (Travell, Simons, 1983). Two popular treatments to inactivate trigger points are (1) spray and stretch and (2) trigger point injections followed by stretch.

Spray and stretch techniques have demonstrated effectiveness and can treat several trigger points at once (Jaeger, Reeves, 1986). Travell and Simons (1983) termed stretch the *action* and the vapocoolant spray the *distraction*. Because the commonly used vapocoolant Fluori-Methane is a chlorofluorocarbon known to damage the ozone layer, Travell and Simons (1992) have subsequently recommended the use of an alternate technique, ice stroking, to obtain a comparable effect. They suggest keeping the skin dry by wrapping the ice in thin plastic to control cooling because excessive cooling can aggravate rather than inactivate the trigger point. The patient must be in a relaxed position, one end of the muscle is anchored so that the other end can be passively stretched after stroking the length of the muscle with ice as shown in Figure 12.12. This sequence can be repeated two to three times, then the muscle warmed with the application of moist hot packs followed by several cycles of active range of motion (Travell, Simons, 1992).

Trigger point injections have been found to reduce pain and increase range of motion, exercise tolerance, and circulation in muscles, with the effects lasting minutes to months (Dorigo, Bartoli, Grisillo et al., 1979; Hameroff, Crago, Blitt et al., 1981; Jaeger, Skootsky, 1987; Lewit, 1979). Trigger point injections with local anesthetics are recommended over dry needling or injecting saline because they are less painful (Travell, Simons, 1983; McCain, 1994). Passive stretching of the muscle through its full range of motion is essential to restore the muscle to its normal resting length and to determine whether additional trigger points are present (McCain, 1994).

Other techniques that can be used to inactivate trigger points are ischemic compression (applying sustained gradual digital pressure to the trigger point), massage, acupuncture, and ultrasound (Travell, Simons, 1983). Moist heat, drug therapy, and biofeedback are useful adjuncts.

Recovery of full function requires more than inactivation of trigger points. Identification and control of perpetuating factors along with a carefully graded and

HEAD AND NECK PAIN

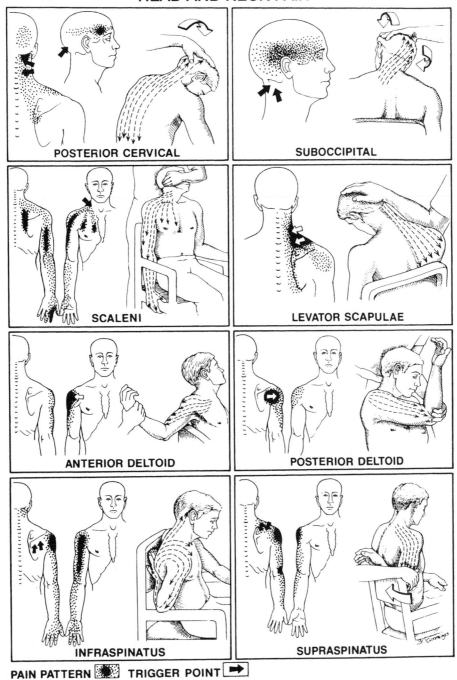

POSTERIOR CERVICAL

SUBOCCIPITAL

SCALENI

LEVATOR SCAPULAE

ANTERIOR DELTOID

POSTERIOR DELTOID

INFRASPINATUS

SUPRASPINATUS

PAIN PATTERN · TRIGGER POINT →

May be duplicated for use in clinical practice. As appears in McCaffery M, Pasero C: *Pain: Clinical manual,* p. 571, 1999, Mosby, Inc.

● ● ● ● ●
FIGURE 12.12 Illustrates the location of trigger points in MPS referred pain patterns, ice stroking, and stretch patterns for two muscles causing head and neck pain and six muscles causing shoulder and upper extremity pain. The most likely location of trigger points is noted by short, straight black and white arrows. The usual pain pattern referred by trigger points in a muscle is shown in solid black, with the stippled areas illustrating possible extended pain patterns. Dashed arrows demonstrate the ice stroking pattern, and the three-dimensional arrows emphasize the direction of the stretch.

From Simons DG: Myofascial pain syndromes. In Basmajian JV, Kirby RL, editors: *Medical rehabilitation,* Baltimore, 1984, Williams & Wilkins.

supervised program of stretching and exercise are important to long-term success (Travell, Simons, 1983). Physical therapy plays a prominent role in the successful treatment program.

Medications play a minor role. Nonsteroidal antiinflammatory drugs and/or opioids may be used temporarily for limited periods while trigger points are treated. Muscle relaxants are of limited value but can be tried briefly (Sola, Bonica, 1990; Travell, Simons, 1983). Depression and sleep disturbances should be treated if present.

SUMMARY

Although more controlled studies of prevalence are needed, MPS is a far more common cause of both acute and chronic musculoskeletal pain than is generally recognized (Simons, 1988a). Early recognition and multidisciplinary treatment will limit suffering and disability associated with chronicity.

Diagnostic criteria and treatment modalities for MPS have not been rigorously tested. Much of the literature is descriptive and relies heavily on anecdotal evidence from single investigators (McCain, 1994). The techniques of trigger point identification may be difficult to learn and may not be reliable (Wolfe, Simons, Fricton et al., 1992). Little data are currently available to support the commonly accepted perpetuating factors, and no valid clinical trials have been done comparing various proposed therapies for MPS (Wolfe, 1996). Debate remains as to the precise relationship between MPS and fibromyalgia. Clearly, a need for well-designed, multicenter clinical trials to promote early recognition and appropriate treatment for these patients exists.

Resources

Daitz B, Travell J: "Myofascial pain syndromes: The Travell trigger point tapes," Williams & Wilkins, (800) 527-5597.

Starlanyl D, Copeland ME: *Fibromyalgia and chronic myofascial pain syndrome, a survival manual,* Oakland, Calif, 1996, New Harbinger Publications.

References

Dorigo B, Bartoli V, Grisillo D et al.: Fibrositic myofascial pain in intermittent claudication: effect of anesthetic block of trigger points on exercise tolerance, *Pain* 6:183-190, 1979.

Fischer AA: Documentation of myofascial trigger points, *Arch Phys Med Rehabil* 69:286-291, 1988.

Fischer AA, Chang CH: Temperature and pressure threshold measurements in trigger points, *Thermology* 1:212-215, 1986.

Fishbain DA, Goldberg M, Meagher BR et al.: Male and female chronic pain patients categorized by DSM-III psychiatric diagnosis criteria, *Pain* 76:181-197, 1986.

Fricton JR, Kroening R, Haley D et al.: Myofascial pain syndrome of the head and neck: a review of clinical characteristics of 164 patients, *Oral Surg* 60:615-623, 1985.

Gerwin RD, Dommerholt J: Treatment of myofascial pain syndromes. In Weiner RS, editor: *Pain management: a practical guide for clinicians,* ed 5, 1:217-229, Boca Raton, Fl, St. Lucie CRC Press 1998.

Gerwin RD, Shannon S, Hong C et al.: Interrater reliability in myofascial trigger point examination, *Pain* 69:65-73, 1997.

Hameroff SR, Crago BR, Blitt CD et al.: Comparison of bupivacaine, etidocaine, and saline for trigger point therapy, *Anesth Analg* 60:752-755, 1981.

Jaeger B, Reeves JL: Quantification of changes in myofascial trigger point sensitivity with the pressure algometer following passive stretch, *Pain* 27:203-210, 1986.

Jaeger B, Skootsky SA: Male and female chronic pain patients categorized by DSM-III psychiatric criteria, *Pain* 29:263-266, 1987.

Lewit K: The needle effect in the relief of myofascial pain, *Pain* 6:83-90, 1979.

McCain GA: Fibromyalgia and myofascial pain syndromes. In Wall PD, Melzack R, editors: *Textbook of pain,* ed 3, pp 475-493, New York, 1994, Churchill Livingstone.

Nice DA, Riddle DL, Lamb RL et al.: Intertester reliability of judgments of the presence of trigger points in patients with low back pain, *Arch Phys Med Rehabil* 73:893-898, 1992.

Njoo KH, Van der Does E: The occurrence and inter-rater reliability of myofascial trigger points in the quadratus lumborum and gluteus medius: a prospective study in non-specific low back pain patients and controls in general practice, *Pain* 58:317-323, 1994.

Reynolds MD: Myofascial trigger point syndromes in the practice of rheumatology, *Arch Phys Med Rehabil* 62:111-114, 1981.

Schneider MJ: Tender points/fibromyalgia vs. trigger points/myofascial pain syndrome: a need for clarity in terminology and differential diagnosis, *J Manipulative Physiol Ther* 18(6):398-406, 1995.

Simons DG: Myofascial pain syndromes: where are we, where are we going? *Arch Phys Med Rehabil* 69(3):207-212, 1988a.

Simons DG: Myofascial pain syndrome. In Goodgold J, editor: *Rehabilitation medicine,* pp 686-723, St. Louis, 1988b, Mosby–Year Book.

Skootsky SA, Jaeger B, Oye RK: Prevalence of myofascial pain in general internal medicine practice, *West J Med* 151:157-161, 1989.

Sola AE, Bonica JJ: Myofascial pain syndromes. In Bonica JJ, editor: *The management of pain,* ed 2, 1:352-366, 1990, Philadelphia, Lea & Febiger.

Travell JG, Simons DG: *Myofascial pain and dysfunction: the trigger point manual, the upper extremities,* vol 1, Baltimore, 1983, Williams & Wilkins.

Travell JG, Simons DG: *Myofascial pain and dysfunction: the trigger point manual, the lower extremities,* vol 2, Baltimore, 1992, Williams & Wilkins.

Wolfe F, Simons DG, Fricton JR et al.: The fibromyalgia and myofascial pain syndromes: a preliminary study of tender points and trigger points in persons with fibromyalgia, myofascial pain syndrome and no disease, *J Rheumatol* 19:944-951, 1992.

Wolfe W: Fibromyalgia and myofascial pain syndrome. In Portenoy RK, Kanner RM, editors: *Pain management: theory and practice,* pp 162-169, Philadelphia, 1996, FA Davis.

OSTEOPOROSIS
Barbara Reed

Definition/Description

"Osteoporosis" literally means "porous bone." The disorder is characterized by excessive bone loss, low bone mass, and structural deterioration of skeletal tissue, leading to increased risk of bone fractures (Galsworthy, Wilson, 1996). Osteoporosis is the most common metabolic disease of the bone, affecting adults primarily in middle to later life (Eliopoulos, 1997). Primary osteoporosis is known as postmenopausal, or age–related, and secondary osteoporosis is usually the result of a preexisting medical condition or the adverse effect of drug therapy (Kessenich, 1997).

Ten million Americans have osteoporosis, and 18 million more are at high risk for the disease developing (National Osteoporosis Foundation, 1997). Eighty percent

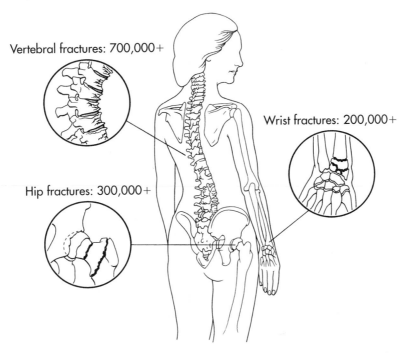

Other fractures: 300,000+

Vertebral fractures: 700,000+

Wrist fractures: 200,000+

Hip fractures: 300,000+

FIGURE 12.13 Common osteoporosis fracture sites. Each year osteoporosis leads to 1.5 million bone fractures in the United States. Common locations of bone fractures are vertebral (700,000+), hip (300,000+), and wrist (200,000+).

Courtesy National Osteoporosis Foundation, Washington, DC, 1997.

of these people are women (Galsworthy, Wilson, 1996; Habel, 1997). Every year, osteoporosis leads to 1.5 million bone fractures, including more than 700,000 vertebral fractures, 300,000 hip fractures, 200,000 wrist fractures, and 300,000 fractures of other bones (Figure 12.13) (National Osteoporosis Foundation, 1997).

One of every two women and one of every five men older than 65 probably will have an osteoporotic fracture at some time in their lives (Galsworthy, Wilson, 1996). About 40,000 women die each year from complications of osteoporotic fractures. A woman's risk of hip fracture is equal to the combined risk of developing breast, uterine, and ovarian cancers (Habel, 1997; Riggs, 1995).

Although men generally begin to start losing bone later than women, by age 65 to 70 men and women are about equally at risk for fractures. Also, although men are less likely than women to develop osteoporosis, one in three men will have it by age 75. Men older than 70 with osteoporosis account for almost one third of all hip fractures and are more likely than women to die after corrective surgery (Galsworthy, Wilson, 1996).

Pain Characteristics

Generally, osteoporosis is not painful in the absence of fractures (Kanner, 1997). However, some patients with

osteoporosis will have both acute and chronic pain. Acute pain is usually associated with a fracture. Most new fractures heal in approximately 3 months, but pain may persist after the fracture has healed. When a vertebra breaks, a few people have no pain, and other patients have excruciating pain and muscle spasms that continue long after the fracture has healed. Over time, multiple vertebral fractures result in stooped posture and continual pain (Figure 12.14).

Sudden, severe back pain may be the only symptom when the patient seeks medical care. Galindo-Ciocon, Ciocon, and Galindo (1996) studied patients older than 65 having a general examination who had back pain as a major symptom. Of 158 women, 75 had vertebral fractures and a mean pain score of 4.5 on a 0 to 5 scale. Patients with fractures reported worsening pain with activity, limiting functioning and increasing dependence in activities of daily living (Galindo-Ciocon, Ciocon, Galindo, 1996).

Assessment

Osteoporosis is considered a "silent disease" because many times the first clinical sign is the fracture, especially of the hip or spine. Typical x-ray films cannot detect osteoporosis until about 30% of bone mass has been lost.

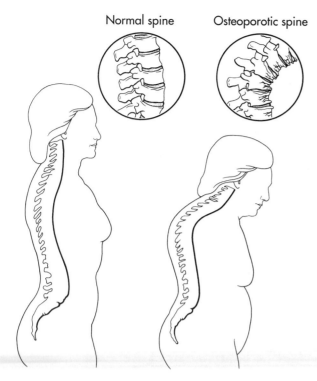

Normal spine   Osteoporotic spine

FIGURE 12.14   *Causes of stooped posture and loss of height. In osteoporosis, multiple fractures of the spine may occur over time, resulting in stooped posture, loss of height, and continual pain. The vertebral fractures heal, but the bones are flattened or may mend in a wedge shape.*
Courtesy National Osteoporosis Foundation, Washington, DC, 1997.

A more accurate test is a bone mineral density (BMD) test, such as dual-energy x-ray absorptiometry or radiographic absorptiometry (Galsworthy, Wilson, 1996). Baseline BMD studies should be done before patients are started on long-term corticosteroid therapy or very soon after because more than half of all patients on chronic steroid therapy will develop osteoporosis (Skolnick, 1997).

Analgesic Pain Management

Acute pain

Virtually all patients with vertebral fractures will experience moderate to severe back pain because of pressure on and inflammation of the nerve branches that exit in each vertebra, as well as inflammation of surrounding tissues (Galsworthy, Wilson, 1996). A combination of opioids, OTC analgesics like aspirin and acetaminophen, or NSAIDs may be necessary to obtain adequate relief in the acute phase of a vertebral fracture. If the patient experiences dizziness and drowsiness at the beginning of opioid therapy, an increased risk of falling and subsequent fractures must be considered and the patient instructed in safety measures.

Calcitonin, which inhibits bone resorption, is a naturally occurring polypeptide that may be prescribed for patients with severe osteoporosis. Although not an analgesic, it provides analgesia for fracture pain (Nguyen, 1996). It may be administered subcutaneously every day or every other day or intranasally every day. The injectable form has been associated with nausea and vomiting, facial flushing, and irritation at the injection site, whereas the nasal spray has few side effects other than occasional local irritation (Kessenich, 1997). (Calcitonin doses are covered in Chapter 7.)

Although muscle relaxants are frequently suggested as a part of pain management, no evidence exists that the drugs conventionally described in this way actually relax skeletal muscle in patients with muscle spasm or muscle tension (see Chapter 7). These drugs should not be administered in the mistaken belief that they relieve muscle spasm. They are generally well tolerated but have sedative effects that may be additive to other centrally acting drugs, including the opioids. Therefore they should be used with caution, if at all, in elderly patients.

Bedrest almost always relieves the acute pain of vertebral collapse. Initially the patient is maintained on bedrest with the therapeutic use of cold to decrease pain and swelling. Heat and gentle massage should be applied to the paravertebral muscles to control the pain of muscle spasm (Kanner, 1997). *Deep muscle massage should never be done near the spine of a patient with osteoporosis* (National Osteoporosis Foundation, 1997).

After several days of bedrest, the patient can usually tolerate short periods of sitting and walking. Approximately 10 minutes an hour out of bed should be encouraged. During this time of additional activity, an increase in the need for analgesics and for assistance in performing activities of daily living should be anticipated.

Chronic pain

Once the fracture has healed, pain may continue, requiring continuation of analgesics and further exploration of nondrug measures. When the severe acute pain subsides, the patient can usually receive adequate pain relief from aspirin, acetaminophen, and/or NSAIDs administered ATC. The NSAIDs most recommended for the elderly are choline magnesium trisalicylate (Trilisate), which does not interfere with platelet function, and nabumetone (Relafen), which has few GI side effects (Hewitt, Foley, 1997).

The use of opioids for chronic nonmalignant pain is increasing and may be appropriate for some patients with osteoporosis. The National Osteoporosis Foundation does not recommend the use of opioids for chronic pain. It states that these drugs may be ordered by the patient's physician, but it also warns of the possibility of dependence and addiction. Statements such as this may, unfortunately, increase the exaggerated concerns many patients have about taking opioid analgesics. Therefore if the physician prescribes opioids for long-term use, the patient and family should be reassured that the likelihood of addiction is minimal and that physical dependence is easily handled by gradual tapering.

Topical creams may relieve pain when rubbed directly into the painful area. These include the old standby Ben-Gay and others such as capsaicin (Zostrix) (see Chapter 7) and methyl salicylate and menthol (Theragesic).

As in other disorders, antidepressant medications will not only treat depression but also may provide pain relief to patients with osteoporosis. These drugs may also improve sleep.

Nondrug Pain Management

Transcutaneous electric nerve stimulation (TENS) can provide pain relief that lasts for several hours. However, it should be used under the supervision of health care personnel.

Spinal supports and braces reduce pain and inflammation by restricting movement. Continuous use may weaken back muscles, so these should be used in conjunction with exercises as soon as possible.

Nerve blocks occasionally may be used to provide temporary relief. The injection of local anesthetic around the nerve root affected by an osteoporotic fracture numbs the nerves and surrounding tissues. Pain relief may last from hours to months, depending on the medication used and the person's response (National Osteoporosis Foundation, 1997).

Prevention of Worsening Osteoporosis

Prevention is the best treatment for this crippling disease. Persons at high risk are postmenopausal women, men older than 80, cigarette smokers, sedentary people, those with a family history of osteoporosis, and small-framed, thin women (Eliopoulos, 1997). For the patient who already has been diagnosed with osteoporosis, the treatment should include analgesics, exercise, and therapy directed at reversing the osteoporosis (Kanner, 1997).

Adequate calcium intake is critical to maintain calcium balance and minimize bone loss. Most women consume far less than the recommended 1000 to 1500 mg/day recommended by the National Institutes of Health. Also, calcium can do its work only when taken in combination with vitamin D, which is necessary for the mineral's absorption. The recommended safe daily dose of vitamin D is 400 IU. If a person is not eating foods that provide adequate calcium and vitamin D, supplements should be ordered by the physician.

Declining sex hormones are a factor in the development of osteoporosis. Menopause is frequently related to the onset of osteoporosis in women. Estrogen replacement therapy (ERT) may be prescribed to prevent the onset of the disease; however, there is still controversy about the risk of endometrial and breast cancer. Until a risk-free version of the drug is available, the decision to use estrogen remains an individualized one for women. In men, the decrease in the male sex hormone testosterone can also result in diminished bone mass. Testosterone can be replaced by an IM injection every 2 to 3 weeks or through a transdermal scrotal patch applied every 24 hours, but questions remain about the long-term effects of this therapy (Kessenich, 1997).

Exercise, including proper weight-bearing activities, is an important part of the program to develop and maintain bone mass for a patient with osteoporosis. Examples of activities are walking, stair climbing, hiking, aerobic dancing, and weight training. Choosing an enjoyable activity, starting slowly, stretching and warming up beforehand, and gradually increasing time and effort spent can be as therapeutic as diet and medication in the prevention and treatment of osteoporosis (Kessenich, 1997).

SUMMARY

Osteoporosis increases the risk of bone fractures, and fractures in the elderly have serious consequences. Hip fractures are associated with higher mortality, morbidity, and medical costs than any other osteoporotic fracture. Almost all patients require hospitalization, and between 12% and 20% die within the first year. More than 600,000 nursing home admissions each year in the United States are associated with hip fractures. As people live longer, this "silent epidemic" will require more health care dollars and cause pain and dependency in more of our elderly patients. Prevention through education is our best hope at this time.

Resources

1. *Building Strength Together*

   Liz Stone, Manager of Support Group Services
   NOF Chicago Office
   c/o AMA
   515 N. State St.
   Chicago, IL 60610
   (312) 464-5110
   Fax: (312) 464-5863
   E-mail: *LBStone@wwa.com*

   Information on getting involved in a support group.

2. Calcium Information Center
   Clinical Nutrition and Research Unit
   Division of Nephrology, Hypertension, and Clinical Pharmacology
   Oregon Health Sciences University
   3314 SW U.S. Veterans Hospital Road
   Portland, OR 97201
   (800) 321-2681

   Information on adequate calcium intake and sources of calcium.

3. National Osteoporosis Foundation
   Dept. MQ
   P.O. Box 96616
   Washington, DC 20007-7456
   (202) 223-2226
   E-mail: *orbdnrc@nof.org*

   Information for patients and caregivers related to management of osteoporosis:

   Facts About Osteoporosis, Arthritis, and Osteoarthritis (Item #B116): Provides definitions and describes the differences between these often misunderstood diseases.

   Osteoporosis Education Catalog: A list of the multimedia materials available from the National Osteoporosis Foundation (for a free copy or multiple copies, call [202] 223-2226).

   Stand up to Osteoporosis (Item #B106): 22-page booklet providing overview of causes, diagnosis, prevention, and treatment of osteoporosis (To order 1 free copy, call [800] 223-9994).

   Strategies for People With Osteoporosis (Item #B119): Articles cover hip, vertebral, and wrist fracture recovery, fall-proofing your home, and what to do after diagnosis.

4. Older Women's League
   666 Eleventh St. NW
   Suite 700
   Washington, DC 20001
   (202) 783-6686 or (800) TAKE-OWL

   Education organization that advocates for midlife and older women. Provides patient education materials, has local chapters across the United States.

References

Coping with chronic pain: *The osteoporosis report* 12, Winter 1996.

Eliopoulos C: *Gerontological nursing*, Philadelphia, 1997, Lippincott.

Galindo-Ciocon D, Ciocon JO, Galindo D: Functional impairment among elderly women with osteoporotic vertebral fractures, *Pain Med J Club J* 2:23-24, 1996.

Galsworthy TD, Wilson PL: Osteoporosis: it steals more than bone, *Am J Nurs* 96:27-34, 1996.

Habel M: Osteoporosis: a preventable epidemic, *Nurseweek* pp 12-13, Feb 17, 1997.

Hewitt DJ, Foley KM: Pain and pain management. In Cassel CK, Cohen HJ, Larson EB et al., editors: *Geriatric medicine*, ed 3, pp 865-882, New York, 1997, Springer-Verlag.

Kanner R: Low back pain. In Kanner R: *Pain management secrets*, pp 76-83, Philadelphia, 1997, Hahley & Belfus.

Kessenich CR: Preventing and managing osteoporosis, *Am J Nurs* 97:16B-16D, Jan 1997.

National Osteoporosis Foundation: *Osteoporosis facts—1997*, Washington DC, 1997, The Foundation.

Nguyen DMT: The role of physical medicine and rehabilitation in pain management. In Ferrell BA, editor: Pain management, *Clin Geriatr Med* 12:517-529, 1996.

Skolnick AA: Rheumatologists issue guidelines for preventing and treating corticosteroid-induced osteoporosis, *JAMA* 277:98-100, 1997.

PAINFUL PERIPHERAL NEUROPATHIES
Pamela Stitzlein Davies

Description

Painful peripheral neuropathies (PPNs) are caused by a variety of conditions and are characterized by the symptom of pain in the extremities. The mechanism of nerve injury is poorly understood. The pain may present with a vast array of symptoms in patients with the same disease source (such as diabetes mellitus). Not all patients with peripheral neuropathy will have pain, but most persons with pain had a period of nonpainful peripheral neuropathy for months or years before painful symptoms developed.

The causes of PPN fall into four main categories: metabolic, drug toxicity, other causes, and idiopathic. Diabetes is the most common metabolic cause of a PPN, occurring in an estimated 10% to 32% of all diabetic patients (Ziegler, Gries, Spuler et al., 1992). Early assessment of development of a diabetic peripheral neuropathy is done by sensory testing with a fine monofilament for loss of touch sensation. The Diabetes Control and Complications Trial Research Group (1993) revealed that "tight control" of blood sugars by intensive insulin therapy resulted in a 70% reduction in neuropathy. Alcoholism is another metabolic source of PPN, resulting in a classic "burning feet syndrome." This reversible problem is due to dietary deficiencies of thiamine and B vitamins, rather than the neurotoxic effects of alcohol.

PPN from drug toxicity is most commonly due to chemotherapeutic agents. Risk factors for development of a PPN from chemotherapy include high dose, frequent dosing, preexisting neuropathic pain conditions, increased age, combination therapies with combined toxicities, and radiation treatment combined with chemotherapy. Patients who are at high risk for development of a PPN from a chemotherapeutic agent should have their deep tendon reflexes monitored routinely. Loss of the Achilles tendon reflex is a universal early symptom of development of a chemotherapy–induced neuropathy. The drug dose should be reduced to reverse or slow progression of the neuropathy. This may prevent development of a PPN.

Human immunodeficiency virus (HIV) may cause PPN by direct effect of the disease. When combined with PPN caused by HIV-related therapy and other factors, the incidence of PPN in AIDS patients reaches 15% to 50% (Hewitt, McDonald, Portenoy et al., 1997). A variety of other diseases, such as multiple sclerosis or connective tissue disorders, may be associated with

PPN. In up to one third of patients, no cause of PPN is identified (Galer, 1994).

Pain Characteristics

The pain complaint of PPN has three main categories: (1) a continuous, deep, burning, aching, or bruised pain; (2) paroxysmal (sudden) lancinating pain, like electric shocks or sharp stabs; and (3) abnormal cutaneous (skin) sensitivity, "like a bad sunburn." Patients may experience some or all of these pain descriptions. In addition, annoying paresthesias may be present, such as sensations of "bugs crawling under my skin."

A "stocking-glove" distribution is typical of PPN, with pain at more distal sites and paresthesias/dysesthesias more proximal (Figure 12.15). The typical pattern of progression is for pain to start symmetrically in the toes or feet and progress up the calf. Galer (1994) reports that once pain has reached the upper calf or knee, painful symptoms may then start in the fingers. The upper extremity symptoms may eventually become more painful than the lower extremity. Patients may report their pain is worse in the evening.

Assessment

When a patient uses words such as "burning," "pulling," "shooting," "hot," or "freezing" to describe pain, the clinician should consider neuropathic pain as the mechanism. Assessment of neuropathic pain may be accomplished with a global 0 to 10 numeric rating scale. However, many patients with PPN spontaneously offer various ratings for each of their pain subtypes. For example, "my burning pain is improved at 5/10, the skin pain is the same at 8/10, and the electric shocks are the same at 10/10 but they are occurring less frequently." This should be charted with the various categories used by the patient because it will help the prescriber in choosing or modifying drug therapies.

A new assessment tool for neuropathic pain has been developed that is brief yet comprehensive (Galer, Jensen, 1997). Using eight descriptor items specific to neuropathic pain (sharp, hot, cold, sensitive, itchy, etc.), each item is rated on a 0 to 10 scale. The tool is easy for most patients to learn, takes about 5 minutes to complete, and is sensitive to treatment effect. (See pp. 76-77 for this tool.) The short form McGill Pain Questionnaire (Melzack, 1987) is useful to capture the multiple descriptions of neuropathic pain but does not provide quantification of each descriptor.

Other assessment of peripheral neuropathy typically includes electromyography (EMG) and nerve conduction studies. However, these studies test only large nerve fiber function, and results may be normal in patients with PPN caused primarily by small nerve fiber (A-delta, C fiber) dysfunction. Negative results could lead to erroneous psy-

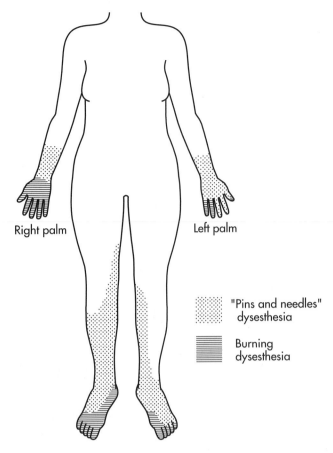

Right palm   Left palm

⬤⬤⬤ "Pins and needles" dysesthesia

≡≡≡ Burning dysesthesia

May be duplicated for use in clinical practice. From McCaffery M, Pasero C: *Pain: Clinical manual*, p. 577. Copyright © 1999, Mosby, Inc.

⬤⬤⬤⬤◦ **F I G U R E 12.15** *Painful peripheral neuropathy, showing "stocking-glove" pattern on lower legs and arms, and the characteristic burning pain distally and "pins and needles" proximally.*

chosomatic diagnosis and great frustration for the patient. Newer methods of testing thermal thresholds by quantitative sensory testing (QST) reveal changes in the small nerve fiber consistent with a diagnosis of PPN. However, QST is typically used only in research settings.

Testing in peripheral neuropathy may reveal loss of vibratory sense, increased or decreased sensation to pin prick or cold, weak finger and wrist extensors (causing loss of fine motor skills such as buttoning a shirt), and weak dorsiflexors (causing a "slapping gait"). In addition, balance and other gait disturbances may be present because of the neuropathy, increasing risk for falls.

Pain Management

Neuropathic pain such as PPN is notoriously difficult to manage, causing frustration for the patient and caregiver alike. In addition, disease progression may result in a gradual worsening of pain reports, despite excellent management.

Pain management of PPN falls into five broad categories: (1) antidepressants, (2) anticonvulsants, (3) topical therapy, (4) opioids, and (5) other therapies. The uses of these therapies in PPN are discussed below (see Chapters 6 and 7 for further details on opioid analgesics and adjuvant analgesics, respectively).

Antidepressants

Tricyclic antidepressants and anticonvulsants are the standard first-line therapy for treatment of neuropathic pain disorders. A recent meta-analysis of studies revealed that 50% to 85% of patients with painful diabetic neuropathy could achieve at least 50% reduction in pain with these drugs (McQuay, Tramer, Nye et al., 1996).

If continuous burning sensations are the main symptom, an antidepressant trial should be the first step. Amitriptyline has been well studied, but good relief with fewer side effects may be obtained from desipramine or nortriptyline. Doses should be started low and slowly titrated to pain relief or intolerable side effects. Analgesic doses are usually one third to one half of antidepressant doses. Failure of one drug to provide analgesia does not predict failure of another in the same class; therefore other drugs in the same class should be tried before moving on to another class of drugs.

Patients should be warned of typical side effects of sedation, light-headedness, dry mouth, and constipation and encouraged to "stick with it" for a minimum of 2 weeks to see whether analgesia is obtained. Sedation will usually improve with time, but patients should be cautioned that driving may be dangerous during the initial titration period. Light-headedness may be associated with orthostatic hypotension, especially in the elderly. To prevent falls, warn patients to stand up slowly and pause for a few seconds before walking. Dry mouth does not usually improve over time. Instruct patients to suck on sugar-free candies and try saliva substitutes. Good oral care and frequent dental checkups are essential. Prevention of constipation with increased water and fiber intake, regular exercise, and stool softeners may make the difference in a successful trial of these drugs.

Newer selective serotonin reuptake inhibitor (SSRI) antidepressants such as fluoxetine (Prozac) have not shown promise in relieving the pain of diabetic neuropathy but are effective for relieving depression that oftentimes accompanies a chronic pain problem (Max, Lynch, Muir et al., 1992).

Patients often have an unspoken concern that the clinician believes the "pain is all in my head" after an antidepressant is prescribed. This issue *must* be addressed to successfully use antidepressants as analgesics. Explain that animal models have consistently shown analgesic benefit of antidepressants. It may help to point out that anticonvulsant medicines are frequently used to treat this problem, even though the patient does not have epilepsy.

Anticonvulsants

If pain is predominantly lancinating, "electric shock" in nature, an anticonvulsant may be the first-line treatment or added to an antidepressant. Carbamazepine has been commonly used in the past; however, the newer drug gabapentin (Neurontin) is gaining favor among pain clinicians (Berde, 1997). Well-designed clinical trials with gabapentin are needed to assess its effectiveness in managing PPN.

Topical therapy

Topical agents have the advantage of having few side effects and little or no systemic effects, which may be advantageous in the elderly. Capsaicin (Zostrix) cream, an extract of chili peppers, has received mixed results in clinical trials but is worth a try. The chief side effect is burning at the time of application, which may be severe and unbearable in some persons. Patients must be warned to wash their hands thoroughly after application and before touching the eyes or mucous membranes to prevent severe burning. Capsaicin should be applied four times a day to the painful areas for a minimum of 2 to 4 weeks for an adequate trial. It is available without a prescription.

A new topical lidocaine preparation, Lidoderm gel and patches, has had good results in the management of painful cutaneous sensitivity from postherpetic neuralgia (Rowbotham, Davies, Verkempinck et al., 1996). Studies of this product in diabetic peripheral neuropathy are forthcoming.

Opioids

Opioids may be beneficial to patients with PPN and should certainly be considered if trials of antidepressants and anticonvulsants have failed or provided inadequate analgesia. This therapy in chronic nonmalignant pain remains controversial but is gaining acceptance (AAPM and APS, 1997; Hegarty, Portenoy, 1994). Time-contingent (ATC) dosing is preferred, with "rescue doses" available as needed for pain exacerbations. Education must be provided to patients and their families to eliminate misconceptions regarding addiction from opioids. Patients should also be warned of side effects similar to those noted for antidepressants.

In the author's experience with strong opioids in ongoing clinical trials to manage PPN and other neuropathic pain, approximately one third of patients respond well to these drugs. One patient with idiopathic PPN stands out in particular because opioids changed her life. She was once again able to pursue her hobby of ballroom dancing. Being able to tolerate long periods of standing allowed her to do the family grocery shopping again. After 6 months on moderate-dose levorphanol (an opioid), she showed no signs of tolerance or cognitive changes. Her quality of life was vastly improved with opioid therapy, whereas standard treatment had failed.

Other therapies

Other medications used for PPN include mexiletine, an antiarrhythmic agent that acts as a membrane stabilizer; and clonidine, an antihypertensive agent that is useful in sympathetically maintained pain. Many new therapies are on the horizon as continued research unveils the mystery of neuropathic pain mechanisms.

Nonpharmacologic therapies such as heat or cold packs, massage, physical therapy, biofeedback, relaxation, and psychotherapy may all be useful and should be used along with medication therapy.

Management of this difficult pain problem will be aided by a solid therapeutic relationship built on trust, patient education, and appropriate medication management.

SUMMARY

- Painful peripheral neuropathy (PPN) is caused by metabolic disorders, drug toxicity, other sources such as HIV disease, or idiopathic mechanisms.
- Pain distribution is usually in a "stocking-glove" pattern.
- Pain description falls into three categories: a continuous, deep, burning, aching, or bruised pain; paroxysmal (sudden) lancinating pain, like electric shocks or sharp stabs; and abnormal cutaneous (skin) sensitivity, "like a bad sunburn."
- Patient descriptions of sensations may be unusual or even bizarre. Accept the description without judgment; assure the patient that you believe what is said.
- Assessment tools designed specifically for neuropathic pain are useful to fully assess all aspects of patient pain complaint.
- PPNs are difficult to manage, causing great frustration for patient and caregiver alike.
- Medication management of PPN includes antidepressants, anticonvulsants, topical therapy, and opioids.

Resources

Neurology WebForums at Massachusetts General Hospital
Web site: *http://neuro-www.mgh.harvard.edu/forum/*

For online discussions and support between patients, caregivers, and doctors.

Neuropathy Association
(800) 247-6968
Web site: *www.neuropathy.org*

For articles on peripheral neuropathy, and a forum to talk to others.

Peripheral Neuropathy Support Group
20076 State St.
Corona, CA 91719

(909) 272-5877
E-mail: *mrslu@pacbell.net*

Suggested reading for clinicians:

Berde, 1997 (see reference below)

This brief but helpful discussion of anticonvulsants compares the new drug gabapentin with the old standards.

McQuay, Tramer, Nye et al., 1996 (see reference below)

An excellent review and meta-analysis of clinical trials of antidepressant in treating neuropathic pain.

Neuropathic pain, *Semin Neurol* 14(3):195-280, 1994.

An 85-page supplement on mechanisms, diagnosis, and management of neuropathic pain directed to the practicing clinician. A specific section on painful peripheral neuropathy (Galer, 1994) is noted below.

References

American Academy of Pain Medicine, American Pain Society: *Consensus statement: the use of opioids for the treatment of chronic pain*, pp 1-4, Glenview, Ill, 1997, American Pain Society.

Berde CB: New and old anticonvulsants for management of pain, *IASP Newsletter* pp 3-5, Jan/Feb 1997.

The Diabetes Control and Complications Trial Research Group: The effect of intensive treatment of diabetes on the development and progression of long-term complications in insulin-dependent diabetes mellitus, *N Engl J Med* 329:977-986, 1993.

Galer BS: Painful polyneuropathy: diagnosis, pathophysiology, and management, *Semin Neurol* 14(3):237-246, 1994.

Galer BS, Jensen MP: Development and preliminary validation of a pain measure specific to neuropathic pain: the neuropathic pain scale, *Neurology* 48:332-338, 1997.

Hegarty A, Portenoy RK: Pharmacotherapy of neuropathic pain, *Semin Neurol* 14:213-224, 1994.

Hewitt DJ, McDonald M, Portenoy RK et al.: Pain syndromes and etiologies in ambulatory AIDS patients, *Pain* 70:117-123, 1997.

Max MB, Lynch SA, Muir J et al.: Effects of desipramine, amitriptyline, and fluoxetine on pain in diabetic neuropathy, *N Engl J Med* 326:1250-1256, 1992.

McQuay HJ, Tramer M, Nye BA et al.: A systematic review of antidepressants in neuropathic pain, *Pain* 68:217-227, 1996.

Melzack R: The short-form McGill Pain Questionnaire, *Pain* 30:191-197, 1987.

Rowbotham MC, Davies PS, Verkempinck C et al.: Lidocaine patch: double-blind controlled study of a new treatment method for postherpetic neuralgia, *Pain* 65:39-44, 1996.

Ziegler D, Gries FA, Spuler M et al.: The epidemiology of diabetic neuropathy, *J Diabetes Compl* 6:49-57, 1992.

PANCREATITIS

Patrick J. Coyne

Description

Pancreatitis is an inflammatory process that destroys the ductal structures and the pancreatic parenchyma forming fibrosis (Figure 12.16). This disease is found throughout the world. The most common cause is alcohol abuse, with some estimates predicting 5% of all alcoholics will acquire this illness. There are, however, many other causes that may include idiopathic, hypertriglyceridemia, medications, hypercalcemia, lesions, trauma, infection,

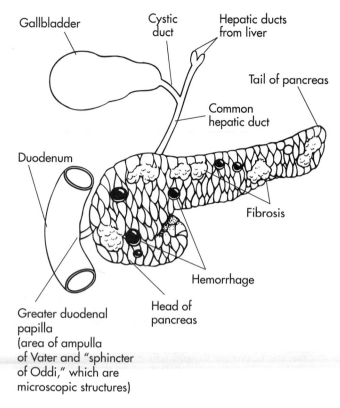

Gallbladder

Cystic duct

Hepatic ducts from liver

Tail of pancreas

Common hepatic duct

Duodenum

Fibrosis

Hemorrhage

Greater duodenal papilla (area of ampulla of Vater and "sphincter of Oddi," which are microscopic structures)

Head of pancreas

May be duplicated for use in clinical practice. From McCaffery M, Pasero C: *Pain: Clinical manual*, p. 580. Copyright © 1999, Mosby, Inc.

FIGURE 12.16 *Pancreatitis may cause autodigestion of the pancreatic cells, leading to hemorrhage and fibrosis.*

post-organ transplant, dysfunction of the sphincter of Oddi, invasive procedures, and hereditary (Toskes, Greenberger, 1994).

The pain associated with pancreatitis is varied but can be severe, occasionally refractory to opioids. The discomfort may persist for days and is commonly accompanied by nausea and vomiting. Acute pancreatitis does not typically evolve to chronic pancreatitis unless complications occur (Ambrose, Dreher, 1996). Chronic pancreatitis has many complications that can include biliary and duodenal obstruction, maldigestion, diabetes mellitus, and pancreatic cancer. (Box 12.4 lists mechanisms of pain.) At one time a belief existed that pancreatic pain would be self-limiting, but this does not appear to be true (Jansen, Kuijpers, Zitman et al., 1995).

Pain Characteristics

This pain is visceral, deep, gnawing, and typically located in the upper abdomen to the left of the midline; it frequently travels to the back, but some cases may radiate to the lower abdomen. This pain may decrease by leaning forward.

BOX 12.4 **Mechanisms of Pain in Chronic Pancreatitis**

- Ductal hypertension
- Parenchymal ischemia
- Eosinophilic perineural inflammation
- Pseudocysts—elevated intracystic pressure

From Sidhu S, Tandon R: Chronic pancreatitis: Diagnosis and treatment, *Postgrad Med J* 72:327-333, 1996, p. 329.

Assessment

An assessment of these individuals includes a comprehensive evaluation of the gastrointestinal system. Symptoms to be assessed include the following:

- Appetite
- Nausea
- Weight change
- Pain associated with meals
- Pain reduction associated with positioning, especially leaning forward
- Bloating sensation
- Dyspnea

Signs that may be found include the following:
- Rebound tenderness
- Decreased or absent bowel sounds (caused by peritoneal initiation)
- Hypotension
- Tachycardia (related to fluid sequestration)
- Decreased breath sounds (caused by pleural effusions)
- Fever
- Abdominal distention/ascites
- Steatorrhea

Laboratory findings worth examining and expected results may include increased white blood cells, increased hematocrit, decreased albumin, increased triglycerides, increased bilirubin, increased serum amylase and lipase, hypocalcemia, and hyperglycemia (NOTE: laboratory values cannot be correlated with pain intensity).

Radiographic findings can include cholelithiasis, ileus, and dilated loops of small bowel near the pancreas. Magnetic resonance imaging can define areas of obstruction/inflammation quite clearly.

Pain Management

This is a unique patient population in that the cause of the disease, specifically alcohol abuse, needs to be identified. Abstinence from alcohol in those with chronic alcoholic pancreatitis may slow or perhaps halt the progress of this disease. A diet of four or five high carbohydrates with low protein may also aid in reducing pain (Sidhu, Tandon, 1996). Pancreatic enzyme therapy has not been shown to decrease pain (Mossner, 1993).

The titration of opioids, perhaps with the aid of PCA, is clearly the place to start in managing these patients. However, many reports note that this pain is often resistant to simple techniques, and other strategies may need to be considered. Simple techniques include opioid trial accompanied by appropriate adjunct agents (Rykowski, Hilgier, 1995).

Some clinicians have perceived that meperidine does not affect the activity of the sphincter of Oddi/intrabiliary pressure. All opioids appear to increase this pressure to some degree. Perhaps meperidine effects may be less than those of other opioids (Arguelles, Franatovic, Romo-Salas et al., 1979; Coelho, Runkel, Herforth et al., 1986). Clinical studies are lacking in this area.

Promising innovations are currently being evaluated. These include the following:

- Octreotide is one such innovation. This medication is a somatostatin that may help decrease pain because of its ability to suppress pancreatic secretions. Octreotide may improve pancreatic enzyme therapy as well.
- Celiac plexus neurolytic block is a well-known, accepted, and successful intervention for pain in the pancreatic cancer population (Coyne, 1997). The use of this technique in chronic pancreatitis does not appear to offer good results. There may, however, be a role for a steroid celiac plexus block or infusion of local anesthetics to this region (Jansen, Kuijpers, Zitman et al., 1995; Sidhu, Tandon, 1996).
- The use of epidural analgesia and interpleural analgesia has been reported to be effective in some patients when other techniques fail (Reiestad, McIlvaine, Kvalhein et al., 1989).

Surgical techniques are usually aimed toward drainage of pseudocysts or ducts or stone removal but may include resection of the pancreas. Results from surgery vary both in short-term and long-term results, but for some patients this may offer a final hope. The surgical procedures associated with this illness are well beyond the scope of this section.

SUMMARY

- Pancreatitis is a common illness usually related to alcohol abuse, but other causes do exist. If the disease progresses, many complications are possible.
- Pain management may include patient education regarding diet modification and the need, if applicable, for abstinence from alcohol.
- Consider a referral to a chronic pain center for long-term management and support.

- Strategies beyond analgesic titration may need to be considered if pain is unrelieved.
- Because of the chronic nature of this disease, these individuals should be evaluated for depression caused by pain.
- A substance abuse referral may be indicated.

Resources

None known.

References

Ambrose M, Dreher H: Pancreatitis: managing a flare-up, *Nursing 96* 26(4):33-39, 1996.
Arguelles J, Franatovic Y, Romo-Salas F et al.: Intrabiliary pressure changes produced by narcotic drugs and inhalation anesthetics in guinea pigs, *Anesth Analg* 58(2):120-123, 1979.
Coelho J, Runkel N, Herforth C et al.: Effects of analgesic drugs on the electromyographic activity of the gastrointestinal tract and sphincter of Oddi and on biliary pressure, *Ann Surg* 104(1):53-58, 1986.
Coyne P: Pancreatic cancer: pain treatment and interventions, *Pathways* 6(1):14, 1997.
Jansen J, Kuijpers J, Zitman F et al.: Pain in chronic pancreatitis, *Scand J Gastroenterol* 30(Suppl 212):117-125, 1995.
Mossner J: Is there a place for pancreatic enzymes in the treatment of chronic pancreatitis? *Digestion* 54(Suppl 2):35-39, 1993.
Reiestad F, McIlvaine W, Kvalhein L et al.: Successful treatment of chronic pancreatitis pain with interpleural analgesia, *Can J Anaesth* 36(6):713-716, 1989.
Rykowski J, Hilgier M: Continuous celiac plexus block in acute pancreatitis, *Regional Anesthesia* 20(6):528-532, 1995.
Sidhu S, Tandon R: Chronic pancreatitis: diagnosis and treatment, *Postgrad Med J* 72:327-333, 1996.
Toskes P, Greenberger N: Approach to the patient with pancreatic disease. In Isselbocher K, Braunwald E, Wilson J et al., editors: *Harrison's principles of internal medicine*, New York, 1994, McGraw-Hill.

REFLEX SYMPATHETIC DYSTROPHY/CAUSALGIA

Anna DuPen and Margo McCaffery

Description

Reflex sympathetic dystrophy (RSD)/causalgia refers to a progressive and potentially severely disabling, often extremely painful, condition. It usually occurs in the distal portion of an arm or leg (more often an arm than a leg), although it may occur in any area of the body. RSD/causalgia is a multisystem syndrome, affecting nerves, skin, muscles, blood vessels, and bones. It occurs in all age groups, including children.

Terminology associated with RSD and causalgia is controversial and confusing, reflecting the complex nature of these neuropathic pains. The International Association for the Study of Pain classifies RSD as a complex regional pain syndrome I (CRPS I) and causalgia as CRPS II (Merskey, Bogduk, 1994).

The primary difference between RSD and causalgia is the inciting event. Injury to bone or soft tissue in an extremity is the most common predisposing factor for

RSD; injury to a nerve is the predisposing factor for causalgia (Portenoy, 1996). RSD/causalgia may result from relatively minor surgical or accidental injury, as well as more traumatic events such as spinal cord injury, mastectomy, or stroke. Onset may be rapid or may be delayed for a month or longer. In approximately one third of patients, no precipitating event can be identified. Incidence of RSD is often estimated at 1:5000 persons per year (Blumberg, Janig, 1994). Incidence of causalgia after injury to a peripheral nerve is estimated to be 1% to 5% (Sunderland, 1978).

For many years it was assumed that dysregulation or overactivity of the sympathetic nervous system was involved in causing the pain and dystrophy (wasting of tissues) that occur with RSD/causalgia. Now this aspect of the syndrome is referred to as sympathetically maintained pain (SMP)—pain that is maintained by sympathetic efferent innervation or by circulating catecholamines (Merskey, Bogduk, 1994). SMP may be found in association with RSD and causalgia, but it is not an essential feature. When tests show that SMP is absent, the pain is referred to as sympathetically independent pain (SIP). A patient may have both SMP and SIP.

Besides pain, which is present in most but not all patients, symptoms in the affected areas may include edema, decreased motor ability, muscle weakness leading to dystrophy or atrophy of the muscles, muscle spasm, skin changes such as scaling and increased hair growth or hair loss, nail changes, changes in skin temperature, increased or decreased sweating, bone changes with patchy osteoporosis, and joint tenderness, stiffness, and swelling. Figure 12.17 illustrates some of these symptoms.

If untreated, RSD appears to progress through roughly three stages. These stages seem to merge, and the length and symptoms of each are quite variable. Briefly, the characteristics of each stage are as follows (Blumberg, Janig, 1994; Portenoy, 1996):

Stage 1, acute stage: diffuse burning pain, edema, and warm or cool skin.

Stage 2, dystrophic stage: diffuse burning pain, cool skin, decreased hair growth, increased sweating, and trophic changes (e.g., changes in nail growth).

Stage 3, atrophic stage: diffuse burning pain that may spread, atrophy of skeletal muscles and bone, and contractures of joints. By stage 3, RSD is considered "permanent," or not likely to be completely reversible.

Pain Characteristics

Before the onset of RSD/causalgia, pain is felt in the area of the precipitating injury; with the onset of RSD, pain is diffuse and pain from the initial injury may have

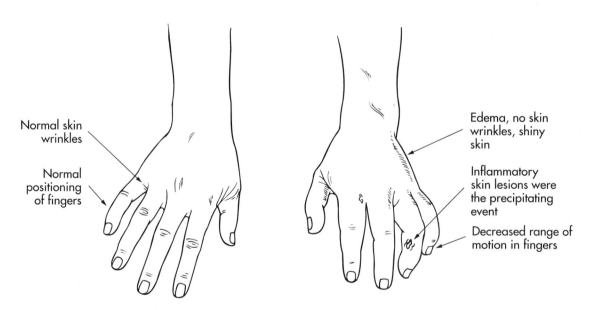

Normal skin wrinkles

Normal positioning of fingers

Edema, no skin wrinkles, shiny skin

Inflammatory skin lesions were the precipitating event

Decreased range of motion in fingers

May be duplicated for use in clinical practice. As appears in McCaffery M, Pasero C: *Pain: Clinical manual*, p. 582, 1999, Mosby, Inc.

● ● ● ● ●

F I G U R E 12.17   Example of a typical case of RSD. Patient: 51-year-old woman. The left hand has symptoms of RSD in the acute stage 1. The skin is warmer than in the right hand. Pain is diffuse and burning; some pain is throbbing. Early diagnosis, within 4 days of the onset of symptoms, and aggressive treatment (ipsilateral stellate ganglion block) resulted in full recovery. Normal use of the hand restored function without the need for physical therapy.

Modified from a case presentation. Blumberg H, Hoffmann J, Mohadjer M et al.: Clinical phenomenology and mechanisms of reflex sympathetic dystrophy: Emphasis on edema. In Gebhart GF, Hammond DL, Jensen TS, editors: *Proceedings of the seventh World Congress on Pain: Progress in pain research and management*, vol 2, pp 455-481, Seattle, 1994, IASP Press. Redrawn from a photo on page 468.

already disappeared (Blumberg, Janig, 1994). Usually, deep and diffuse burning pain along with generalized swelling occurs within minutes to hours after the inciting event (injury). Pain may also be described as throbbing, pressing, or shooting. Location of pain is usually but not always near the site of the precipitating injury. It does not follow distribution of a nerve. Pain is usually felt deep in the distal portion of an arm or leg. It may spread proximally or involve other extremities.

The pain fluctuates over time, varying from mild to excruciating, and is worse at night. Some patients have intermittent RSD/causalgia; that is, they have pain-free periods.

Pain is exacerbated by movement, mild stimulation, or stress. Even normal movement of the affected extremity is painful. Immobilization relieves the pain but contributes to worsening of the problem. Pain increases when the limb is lowered, and decreases when it is elevated. Guarding of the affected part is common because of the presence of allodynia (pain from a stimulus, e.g., touch, which does not normally cause pain) or hyperalgesia (increased pain felt from a stimulus that is normally painful). Emotional stress may contribute to pain by causing an increase in activity of the sympathetic nervous system.

Assessment

Unexplained edema, burning pain, and temperature changes in the lower part of an arm or leg should alert the clinician to the possibility of RSD or causalgia. No single laboratory or other diagnostic test establishes a diagnosis of RSD or causalgia. A diagnostic workup may include diagnostic sympathetic blocks, a phentolamine challenge test, and a three-phase bone scan (for detecting osteoporotic changes).

Early diagnosis and treatment are of paramount importance, but several factors mitigate against this. Dystrophy is included in the term but does not occur until later. Clinicians looking for this symptom will fail to recognize the syndrome in its early stages. Perhaps more importantly, patients are usually extremely anxious. The patient who is developing RSD is often agitated and suspected of being neurotic, especially because emotional stress may exacerbate the symptoms. The patient with allodynia and hyperalgesia is usually extremely protective of the affected part and appears to be overreacting. Unfortunately, RSD/causalgia may be misdiagnosed as psychogenic pain. Although many published reports discuss the profound emotional and behavioral changes associated with RSD, there is no evidence that psychologic factors predispose one to develop RSD (Bonica, 1990; Lynch, 1992).

Pain Management

The conventional approach to treatment of RSD relies on many unproved therapies often supported only by favorable anecdotes, requiring clinicians to evaluate recommendations carefully. *Although consensus is that early diagnosis and treatment—analgesia and physical therapy—are of paramount importance if normal function is to be restored, exactly how this will be accomplished is controversial.*

Two aims of treatment are pain relief and a return to normal function in the affected limb (Glynn, 1995). Pain relief alone usually will not restore function. Physical therapy is almost always necessary to overcome the restrictions imposed by edema in the acute stage and later to offset the effects of weakness and atrophy of muscle and bone. Although psychologic counseling may be helpful, it is not the primary focus of treatment. Most patients are concerned about their emotional response to the pain and disability. They should be reassured that anxiety, frustration, and anger are expected. If the emotional response interferes with physical therapy, counseling or psychotrophic medication may be required (Glynn, 1995).

The longer the patient has suffered pain and disuse of the extremity, the less favorable the outcome is likely to be. As time passes, the patient not only has the original neuropathic pain of RSD, but also has additional nociceptive pain from disuse and contractures. Both types of pain require treatment to facilitate return of normal function. Thus no single pain relief method is likely to be successful. Treatment must be multimodal and individualized, but widespread differences exist in what clinicians recommend (Glynn, 1995). Ideally, treatment should encompass all the modalities available to any patient with chronic nonmalignant pain, particularly neuropathic pain. Initially the treatment may be conservative, but if this is not effective, aggressive therapy should not be delayed.

Initial conservative therapy during the acute stage may include TENS, elevation of the affected extremity, systemic corticosteroids (e.g., high-dose prednisone for a few days and then taper), oral analgesics (NSAIDs and opioids), and tricyclic antidepressants combined with physical therapy. Physical therapy concentrates on active range of motion and must be sufficiently restrained to avoid intensifying the pain and exacerbating the problem (McLeskey, Balestrieri, Weeks, 1993).

In some patients with long-standing RSD, gabapentin (Neurontin) in doses ranging from 300 to 2400 mg/day has provided excellent pain relief (Mellick, Mellicy, 1995). If RSD is also sympathetically maintained pain, other adjuvant analgesics that may be of benefit are calcitonin, phenoxybenzamine, nifedipine, Prazosin, and propranolol (Portenoy, Kanner, 1996).

If conservative therapy fails, more aggressive therapy includes sympathetic blockade, which may also serve diagnostic purposes. Sympathetic blockade may be achieved in the following ways (Byas-Smith, 1992):

1. Paravertebral sympathetic ganglion blockade. For the arms, local anesthetic is injected into the region

of the stellate ganglion; for the legs, the lumbar sympathetic chain at L2 or L3.

2. IV regional sympathetic blockade (chemical sympathectomy, so-called Bier block). After a cuff is inflated in the upper part of the involved limb, an IV catheter is inserted in the hand or foot. The cuff remains inflated for 15 to 30 minutes while guanethidine, if available, is administered with lidocaine. Alternatives to guanethidine are bretylium or reserpine (Portenoy, 1996). IV phentolamine has also been used. Some clinicians find repetitive IV phentolamine blocks (every 7 to 21 days) a useful treatment when combined with physical therapy (Rowbotham, 1993; this reference contains a protocol for IV phentolamine).

3. Continuous sympathetic nerve blockade. To break the vicious cycle of pain in severe cases of RSD, a catheter may be placed near the paravertebral ganglion and a local anesthetic infused. Because catheter migration is common, a catheter may be placed in the epidural space to infuse dilute local anesthetic for 1 to 2 weeks.

Invasive therapy, such as dorsal column stimulation, should be used only in patients who have not responded to sympathetic blockade and conservative pharmacologic approaches and should involve consultation with practitioners who are experienced in the management of RSD/causalgia. Treatment of stage 3 refractory RSD with dorsal column stimulation has shown some promise. The safety and effectiveness of these invasive neurostimulation techniques have not been established in RSD/causalgia. Also, neurosurgical approaches such as neurectomy and cordotomy are not recommended. With the exception of sympathectomy in selected cases, surgical approaches are usually discouraged (Portenoy, 1996).

If surgery is performed to correct an abnormality that seems responsible for inciting RSD, the following vigorous pain management is recommended: (1) aggressive treatment to reduce RSD symptoms preoperatively, (2) both regional and general anesthesia for the surgery, and (3) aggressive pain management postoperatively, including opioids and possibly nerve blocks (Rowbotham, 1993).

SUMMARY

RSD/causalgia refers to a progressive and potentially severely disabling, often extremely painful, condition. The predisposing factor in RSD and causalgia is injury, often minor, in an extremity. Pain is usually deep and burning, accompanied by generalized swelling and occurring within minutes to hours after the inciting injury.

Goals of treatment are analgesia and restoration of function. Suggestions include the following:

• Provide information to the patient to correct the common misconception that pain and disability are the same thing and that the disability will disappear if the pain is relieved. Because of other symptoms such as edema and weakening of bone and muscle, physical therapy is usually necessary.

• Provide maximum analgesia for physical therapy. Failure to provide adequate pain relief for physical therapy may result in additional damage.

• Elevate the affected extremity.

• Help the patient maintain appropriate protection of the affected part. Handle affected part gently and slowly. Avoid further trauma to the affected areas (e.g., start IVs in the unaffected arm).

Resources

American Reflex Sympathetic Dystrophy Association
65 W. Valley Ridge
Ojai, CA 93023-4026

Reflex Sympathetic Dystrophy Syndrome Association of America (RSDSA)
116 Haddon Avenue, Suite D
Haddonfield, NJ 08033
(609) 795-8845
Web site: *Cyboard.com/RSDS*
Newsletter: *RSDSA Review*

Other services: self-help materials, professional membership directory, compilation of research abstracts.

References

Blumberg H, Janig W: Clinical manifestations of reflex sympathetic dystrophy and sympathetically maintained pain. In Wall PD, Melzack R, editors: *Textbook of pain*, ed 3, pp 685-698, New York, 1994, Churchill Livingstone.

Bonica JJ: Causalgia and other reflex sympathetic dystrophies. In Bonica JJ, editor: *The management of pain*, ed 2, pp 220-243, Philadelphia, 1990, Lea & Febiger.

Byas-Smith M: Management of acute exacerbations of chronic pain syndromes. In Sinatra RS, Hord AH, Ginsberg B et al., editors: *Acute pain mechanisms and management*, pp 432-444, St. Louis, 1992, Mosby.

Glynn C: Complex regional pain syndrome type I, reflex sympathetic dystrophy, and complex regional pain syndrome type II, causalgia, *Pain Rev* 2:292-297, 1995.

Lynch ME: Psychological aspects of reflex sympathetic dystrophy, *IASP Newsletter* pp 2-3, Sept/Oct 1992.

McLeskey CH, Balestrieri FJ, Weeks DB: Sympathetic dystrophies. In Warfield CA, editor: *Principles and practice of pain management*, pp 219-234, New York, 1993, McGraw-Hill.

Mellick GA, Mellicy LB: Gabapentin in the management of reflex sympathetic dystrophy, *J Pain Symptom Manage* 10(4)265-266, 1995.

Merskey H, Bogduk N, editors: *Classification of chronic pain: descriptions of chronic pain syndromes and definitions of pain terms*, ed 2, Seattle, 1994, IASP Press.

Portenoy RK: Neuropathic pain. In Portenoy RK, Kanner RM, editors: *Pain management: theory and practice*, pp 83-125, Philadelphia, 1996, FA Davis.

Portenoy RK, Kanner RM: Nonopioid and adjuvant analgesics. In Portenoy RK, Kanner RM, editors: *Pain management: theory and practice*, pp 219-247, Philadelphia, 1996, FA Davis.

Rowbotham MC: Reflex sympathetic dystrophy. In Pfeffer GB, Frey CC, editors: *Current practice in foot and ankle surgery*, vol 1, pp 175-193, New York, 1993, McGraw-Hill.

Sunderland S: *Nerves and nerve injuries*, ed 2, pp 377-420, New York, 1978, Churchill Livingstone.

SICKLE CELL DISEASE–RELATED PAIN
Margo McCaffery

Description

Sickle cell disease refers to a group of genetic disorders characterized by the inheritance of an alteration of hemoglobin (sickle hemoglobin, Hb S). The red blood cells (RBCs) are sensitive to decreases in oxygen tension, which cause them to change from flexible disks into sticky and rigid sickle shapes that clump together, clogging smaller blood vessels. Primary features are anemia, acute and chronic pain, and progressive organ failure. Sickle cell disease is a chronic, potentially life-threatening disease that is presently incurable. In the United States it is most prevalent among African-Americans and Hispanics, affecting more than 50,000 Americans (Shapiro, 1996).

Pain Characteristics

Both acute and chronic pain may result from sickle cell disease. Repeated vasoocclusive crises (acute pain) may result in progressive organ failure (chronic pain) from ischemia and infarction. (Figure 12.18 provides examples of pain.)

Acute pain

The hallmark of this disease is the sickle cell crisis, or vasoocclusive crisis. The sickle-shaped RBCs clump together to block normal blood flow, causing occlusion, hypoxia, and infarction (Shapiro, 1996). This ischemic pain is similar to that of myocardial infarction.

Painful crises may begin in infancy. Crisis pain is unpredictable as to which areas of the body are affected, severity of pain, when and how often it occurs, and how long it lasts. A crisis may be precipitated by a variety of factors, such as infection, overexertion, and dehydration. It may last from a few hours to several weeks and may occur in any tissue or structure supplied with blood vessels. Most painful crises involve musculoskeletal pain felt in the low back and extremities, involving muscles, tendons, ligaments, periosteum, bone marrow, joints, and arteries. Visceral pain may also occur, especially from vasoocclusion in the spleen, liver, and lungs. Pain during a crisis may also migrate (Shapiro, 1996).

The type of patient most likely to be seen in emergency departments or inpatient areas has frequent crises (up to 40 per year) with severe or excruciating pain lasting 4 days or longer. This patient represents about 20% of the total population of persons with sickle cell disease. The remaining 80% with this disease may never have a painful crisis or may have only one severe episode each year or several mild episodes (Shapiro, 1996). The number of painful crises per year is an indication of the severity of the disease and is correlated with early death (Platt, Thorington, Brambilla et al., 1991).

Chronic pain

Repeated vasoocclusive episodes may lead to organ or tissue damage and chronic pain. Chronic pain is often associated with bony changes, such as aseptic necrosis of the femoral head or vertebral collapse, or chronic non-healing leg ulcerations.

Assessment

As with all types of pain, assessment of intensity relies on patient self-report, using a pain-rating scale when possible. Vital signs and laboratory values such as hemoglobin, reticulocyte count, and bilirubin are not related to pain and should not be a part of pain assessment (Shapiro, Schechter, Ohene-Frempong, 1994). Patients in severe pain may show no behavioral signs of pain for a variety of reasons (e.g., exhaustion, use of effective coping strategies, or efforts to be brave in the face of pain).

Ask the patient if this pain is his or her usual sickle cell crisis pain. This is a critical distinction, and it is not always an easy one for patients and clinicians to make. It is always possible that acute pain can be due to complications of sickle cell disease, such as acute chest syndrome or bowel infarction and necrosis, or nonsickle cell-related processes, such as appendicitis or peptic ulcer disease (Beyer, Platt, Kinney et al., 1994).

Pain Management

Three main components of treating a crisis are opioids, nonopioids, and aggressive hydration. Oxygen is appropriate only in hypoxic patients; no evidence exists that oxygen reverses or shortens the crisis (Shapiro, 1996).

These patients are at high risk for undertreatment of pain. Unfortunately, there is a tendency to decrease opioid doses as the number of hospitalizations increases (Armstrong, Pegelow, Gonzalez et al., 1992), resulting in progressive undertreatment of pain. Often patients are labeled addicts. However, addiction rarely results from use of opioids to relieve pain, and no studies show that the incidence of addiction is any higher in patients with sickle cell disease than in patients with any other disease. One study reported "problems" with opioids in approximately 9% of the patients with sickle cell disease (Payne, 1989), but other studies have reported a lower incidence of problems (Brozovic, Davies, Yardumian et al., 1986; Cole, Sprinkle, Smith et al., 1986; Vichinsky, Johnson, Lubin, 1982). The fact that these patients may require frequent treatment with high doses of opioids is an indication of disease severity, not addiction.

Patients with this painful disease may become angry and manipulative because of years of dealing with health care professionals who doubted their pain, accused them

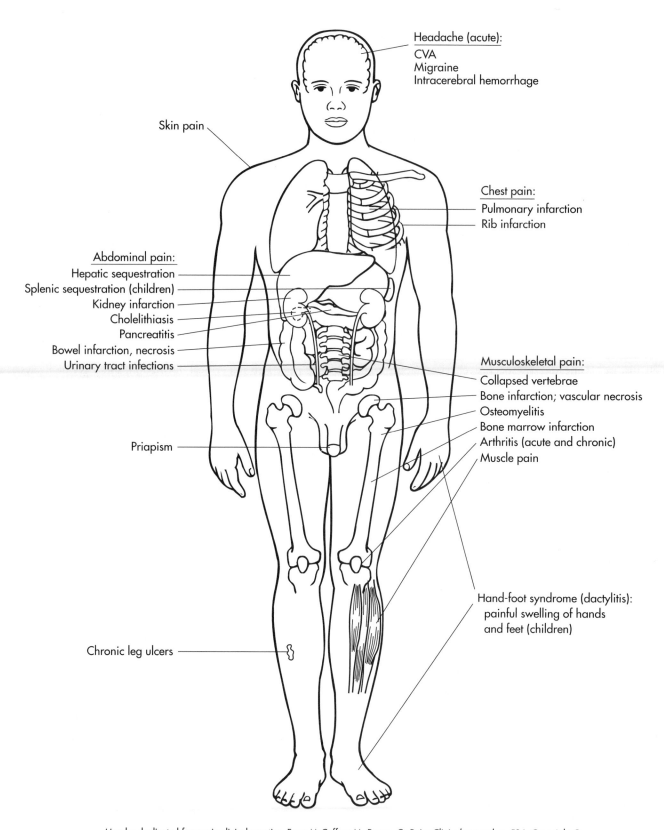

Headache (acute):
CVA
Migraine
Intracerebral hemorrhage

Skin pain

Chest pain:
Pulmonary infarction
Rib infarction

Abdominal pain:
Hepatic sequestration
Splenic sequestration (children)
Kidney infarction
Cholelithiasis
Pancreatitis
Bowel infarction, necrosis
Urinary tract infections

Musculoskeletal pain:
Collapsed vertebrae
Bone infarction; vascular necrosis
Osteomyelitis
Bone marrow infarction
Arthritis (acute and chronic)
Muscle pain

Priapism

Hand-foot syndrome (dactylitis):
painful swelling of hands
and feet (children)

Chronic leg ulcers

May be duplicated for use in clinical practice. From McCaffery M, Pasero C: *Pain: Clinical manual*, p. 586. Copyright © 1999, Mosby, Inc.

F I G U R E 12.18   Examples of pain that may occur in patients with sickle cell disease. A vasoocclusive crisis may disrupt blood flow to virtually any area of the body. Repeated vasoocclusive crises (acute pain) may result in progressive organ failure (chronic pain) from ischemia and infarction.

of being addicted, and grossly undertreated the pain. Therefore clinicians must make a special effort to reverse this adversarial relationship by providing prompt, consistent, and effective pain management in a respectful manner that involves the patient and family.

Home care

Many patients manage crises at home. Patient and family need simple written instructions that include telephone numbers and names to access health care professionals, specific instructions for adequate hydration, a list of analgesics with the number of tablets and milligrams, a stepwise approach to increasing analgesic doses, and criteria for emergency room visits. Heating pads and hot baths are also helpful to many patients; cold usually makes the sickle cell pain worse.

Many patients who have frequent crises are never pain free. Although the painful crisis resolves, the patient may be left with a variety of chronic, painful conditions such as arthritis or leg ulcers. These may require daily oral opioids in addition to nonopioid and adjuvant analgesics.

Emergency department care

The severity of the pain demands immediate attention, preferably within 15 minutes. The unpredictability of the painful crises engenders loss of control and underscores the necessity for consistency in treating the pain.

Treatment is facilitated if the patient has a "passport" document (small booklet or plasticized card) that summarizes the initial comprehensive clinical assessment and contains a written pain treatment plan that has been developed and agreed on by patient, family, and caregivers (Beyer, Platt, Kinney et al., 1994). The emergency department may also develop and have on file a protocol or individualized treatment plan for patients seen regularly (Nichols, 1996).

Opioid management begins with IV boluses of morphine or hydromorphone with the dose based on intensity of pain and what has been effective in the past. At the peak effect, approximately 10 to 15 minutes, another IV dose is administered (50% to 100% of previous dose) if the patient is still in moderate to severe pain and is responsive to verbal stimuli. Some patients require high opioid doses (e.g., twice the dose ordinarily required to relieve postoperative pain) (Shapiro, Cohen, Howe, 1993) and even higher doses (e.g., morphine, 50 mg IV/hour). Subcutaneous continuous infusion is an option if venous access is problematic.

Meperidine is avoided because of its active metabolite normeperidine that may accumulate, especially if renal dysfunction exists, and cause central nervous system excitatory toxicity, including seizures.

After pain is reduced to a mild intensity, a decision is made as to whether the patient is to be admitted or discharged home. Analgesia must be maintained, usually by the IV route if admitted and the oral route if discharged. Oral morphine or hydromorphone may be necessary if pain is moderate to severe. If pain is inadequately treated in the emergency department or if the patient is discharged without adequate analgesia, the patient unfortunately may need to return to the emergency department.

Inpatient care

Consistency of care is facilitated by admitting the patient to the same clinical unit each time and by developing an individualized care plan that builds on previously effective interventions. IV PCA is appropriate for most patients once the pain is brought under control with clinician-administered IV boluses. The PCA continuous infusion mode, if used, should be low, at least initially, and the bolus dose should be high enough to produce significant analgesia after one or two doses (Shapiro, Cohen, Howe, 1993).

After a few days, severe crisis pain may decrease rapidly, but weaning off of IV opioids easily frightens the patient unless it is done slowly, with the patient's cooperation, and in a carefully planned manner that the patient understands. In addition, slow tapering is necessary to avoid precipitating withdrawal syndrome and perhaps another crisis in those patients who have become physically dependent on the opioid (Benjamin, 1989). An effective plan includes obtaining pain ratings from the patient, establishing comfort/function goals, changing the analgesic doses rather than the intervals, decreasing doses by only 20% to 25%, and determining whether oral analgesics are adequate before the IV route is discontinued.

A study of 50 patients who frequented the emergency room demonstrated how more effective and less expensive pain management can be achieved for these patients. Change from IM meperidine to IV morphine or another strong mu agonist, such as hydromorphone (Dilaudid), was successfully accomplished in all but one patient (Brookoff, Polomano, 1992). Patients were switched to controlled-release morphine as soon as pain was controlled. The results were that the number of hospital admissions decreased by 44%, length of hospital stay decreased by 23%, and number of emergency department visits decreased by 67% with no evidence that patients used other hospitals.

SUMMARY

In sickle cell disease–related pain, vasoocclusive crises cause acute pain and may result in progressive organ failure that causes chronic pain. The hallmark of the disease is the vasoocclusive crisis. Treatment considerations for a crisis are as follows:

- Painful crises require immediate attention.
- Guard against undertreatment and unfounded fears of addiction.

- As is true for all types of pain, placebos are never appropriate for the assessment or treatment of pain related to sickle cell disease.
- Meperidine (Demerol) is avoided if at all possible because of its active metabolite. IM meperidine is avoided because it rapidly causes fibrosis.
- IV route is preferred to IM.
- Morphine or hydromorphone (Dilaudid) is an alternative to meperidine.
- As pain decreases, the patient may be switched to oral opioids, including morphine or hydromorphone.

Text reviewed by Patrick J. Coyne; figure reviewed by Rhonda Nichols.

Resources

Sickle Cell Disease Association of America Inc.
200 Corporate Pointe, Suite 495
Culver City, CA 90230-7633
(800) 421-8453

Educational resources, annual meetings, newsletter.

Publications for laypeople and clinicians regarding pain associated with sickle cell disease:

Odesina VF, Spurlock-McLendon J: *Sickle cell disease related pain assessment and management: A guide for patients and parents*, Mt. Desert, Me 1994, New England Regional Genetics Groups.

Shapiro BS, Schechter NL, Ohene-Frempong K: *Sickle cell disease related pain assessment and management: Quick reference guide for clinicians*, Mt. Desert, Me, 1994, New England Regional Genetics Groups.

Shapiro BS, Schechter NL, Ohene-Frempong K, editors: *Sickle cell disease related pain assessment and management: Conference proceedings*, Mt. Desert, Me, 1994, New England Regional Genetics Groups.

To order the above:
New England Regional Genetics Groups
P.O. Box 670
Mt. Desert, ME 04660
(207) 288-2704
Fax: (207) 288-2705

American Pain Society (APS): *Guidelines for the management of acute and chronic pain in sickle cell disease*, Glenview, Ill, 1999, APS.

To order the above:
American Pain Society
4700 W. Lake Ave.
Glenview, IL 60025
(847) 375-4715
Fax: (847) 375-4777

Guideline Panel: *Clinical practice guideline for sickle cell disease: Screening, diagnosis, management, and counseling in newborns and infants*, Rockville, Md, Agency for Health Care Policy and Research (AHCPR), 1993 (No. 93-0562). Also available is a guide for parents (No. 93-0564) and a quick reference guide for clinicians (No. 93-0563).

To order:
AHCPR Publications Clearinghouse
P.O. Box 8547
Silver Spring, MD 20907
(800) 358-9295

References

Armstrong FD, Pegelow CH, Gonzalez JC et al.: Impact of children's sickle cell history on nurse and physician ratings of pain and medication decisions, *J Pediatr Psychol* 17(5):651-664, 1992.

Benjamin LJ: Pain in sickle cell disease. In Foley KM, Payne RM, editors: *Current therapy of pain*, pp 90-104, Philadelphia, 1989, BC Decker.

Beyer JE, Platt A, Kinney T et al.: Assessment of pain in adults and children with sickle cell disease. In Shapiro BS, Schechter NL, Ohene-Frempong K, editors: *Sickle cell disease related pain assessment and management: conference proceedings*, pp 10-17, Mt. Desert, Me, 1994, New England Regional Genetics Groups.

Brookoff D, Polomano R: Treating sickle cell pain like cancer pain, *Ann Intern Med* 116(5):364-368, 1992.

Brozovic M, Davies S, Yardumian A et al.: Pain relief in sickle cell crisis, *Lancet* 2:624-625, 1986.

Cole TB, Sprinkle RH, Smith SJ et al.: Intravenous narcotic therapy for children with severe sickle cell pain crisis, *Am J Dis Child* 140:1255-1259, 1986.

Nichols R: Pain during sickle-cell crises, *Am J Nurs* 96:59-60, 1996.

Payne R: Pain management in sickle cell disease: rationale and techniques, *Ann NY Acad Sci* 565:189-206, 1989.

Platt OS, Thorington BD, Brambilla DJ et al.: Pain in sickle cell disease: rates and risk factors, *N Engl J Med* 325:11-16, 1991.

Shapiro BS: Pain related to sickle cell disease. In Lefkowitz M, Lebovits AH, editors: *A practical approach to pain management*, pp 280-289, Boston, 1996, Little Brown & Co.

Shapiro BS, Cohen DE, Howe CJ: Patient-controlled analgesia for sickle cell related pain, *J Pain Symptom Manage* 8(1):22-28, 1993.

Shapiro BS, Schechter NL, Ohene-Frempong K: *Sickle cell disease related pain assessment and management: quick reference guide for clinicians*, Mt. Desert, Me, 1994, New England Regional Genetics Groups.

Vichinsky EP, Johnson R, Lubin BH: Multidisciplinary approach to pain management in sickle cell disease, *Am J Pediatr Hematol Oncol* 4:328-333, 1982.

TEMPOROMANDIBULAR DYSFUNCTION

Warren P. Vallerand and April Hazard Vallerand

Description

Chronic pain in the orofacial region may have many causes and can be quite difficult to diagnose. Patients may have multiple pain complaints, often with a confusing constellation of signs and symptoms. Headache pain, odontogenic (tooth) pain, or sinus disease as a cause of pain must be ruled out. Peripheral or central neuropathic pain involving the trigeminal or glossopharyngeal nerves can also be severe and debilitating (Vallerand, 1996 a,b). Having ruled out these other causes of chronic facial pain, the resulting diagnosis of exclusion is very commonly temporomandibular dysfunction (TMD).

TMD is a collective term, encompassing a number of medical and dental conditions affecting the temporomandibular joint (TMJ) and/or the muscles of mastication, as well as contiguous tissue components. It is considered a subclassification of musculoskeletal disorders.

Although specific causes such as degenerative arthritis and trauma underlie some TMD, as a group these disorders have no common cause or biologic explanation and comprise a heterogeneous group of painful conditions whose signs and symptoms are overlapping but not necessarily identical. The reported prevalence of TMDs differs from study to study because of lack of standardized definitions of TMDs and their characteristics (De Kanter, Truin, Burgersdijk et al., 1993; Goulet, Lavigne, Lund, 1995). Most studies suggest the prevalence of clinically significant TMD-related facial pain to be ≥5% in the general population, with a peak prevalence in young adults (20 to 40 years of age). A number of clinical case series studies have reflected an overwhelming predominance of TMD in women in the third to fourth decades. Nearly 2% of the general population seek treatment of TMD symptoms. Data from epidemiologic studies often suggest a much higher prevalence of TMD-related signs and symptoms and a corresponding need for treatment (de Bont, Dijkgraff, Stegenga, 1997).

Pain Characteristics

The term "TMD" has been used to describe a constellation of signs and symptoms that includes pain in the face or jaw joint; earache; headache; limited mouth opening; clicking, grinding, or popping sounds in the jaw joint; "locking" of the jaw in a closed or open position; and fatigue, pain, or tenderness of the masticatory muscles. The major sources and sites of pain for patients with TMD are the temporalis muscle, TMJ, and the masseter muscle (Figure 12.19). The severity of the signs or symptoms can be highly variable, ranging from noticeable but clinically insignificant signs to seriously debilitating pain or dysfunction. The intensity of the pain and the resultant impairment of function are also highly variable between individuals. In any given patient the pain and impairment is dynamic, varying over time from minimal to incapacitating. Infrequent pain of moderate to severe intensity is likely to be perceived as a nuisance, whereas persistent chronic pain of even lesser severity can cause significant disruption of lifestyle. Chronic pain with acute exacerbations is common in patients with TMD. TMD pain may be self-limiting and episodic and/ or progressive.

Assessment

Laboratory studies or diagnostic tests are of little value in most cases of TMD. No suitable biomarkers have been validated for identifying TMD patients as a group or for classifying any subsets. Carefully collected symptoms and signs combined with physical examination make up the most sensitive and specific diagnostic "tool" (Clark, Tsukiyama, Baba et al., 1997; Vallerand, Sirois, 1995). In patients with signs or symptoms suggestive of systemic disease in addition to their facial pain reports, it is important to investigate and rule out connective tissue

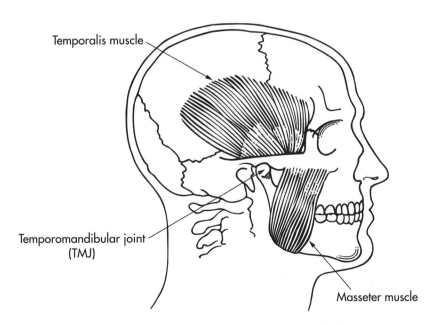

Temporalis muscle

Temporomandibular joint (TMJ)

Masseter muscle

May be duplicated for use in clinical practice. From McCaffery M, Pasero C: *Pain: Clinical manual*, p. 589. Copyright © 1999, Mosby, Inc.

FIGURE 12.19 The temporalis muscle, temporomandibular joint, and the masseter muscle are the major sources and sites of pain for patients with temporomandibular dysfunction.

diseases such as lupus erythematosus, Sjögren's syndrome, and rheumatoid disorders, which may present with non-specific pain in and about the facial musculature and jaw joints. An initial screening for connective tissue disease, consisting of a complete blood count with differential, erythrocyte sedimentation rate, antinuclear antibody, and rheumatoid factor titers is adequate in those cases. More specific serologic tests may be indicated on the basis of the results of the initial screening battery.

Radiographic abnormalities on CT scan or MRI may be seen in TMD associated with degenerative arthritis or internal derangement of the TMJ (Christiansen, Thompson, 1995; Westesson, 1995). Analysis of inflammatory mediators and cartilage degradation products in aspirated synovial fluid from the TMJ has provided some interesting research results but is of little clinical usefulness at this time. Arthroscopy of the TMJ may be used to directly visualize the joint and obtain synovial tissue biopsy specimens in cases where significant intraarticular disease is suspected.

Pain Management

As with any initial assessment of pain, when planning a management strategy for TMD pain, it is important to evaluate the patient's perception of the pain and dysfunction and the impact of these on the patient's quality of life and functional status (Vallerand, 1997). Currently available epidemiologic evidence suggests that TMD is usually benign and self-limiting. In the absence of overt jaw joint pathology, with mild pain and minimal dysfunction, initial management should consist of supportive patient education regarding the benign nature of most TMDs and self-management and elimination of behaviors that may contribute to or exacerbate the pain. Stress reduction, rest, and dietary modification, restricting the intake of hard or chewy foods, is helpful for many patients. Application of moist heat or cool compresses directly over painful muscles or jaw joints is also often beneficial.

Pharmacologic agents

NSAIDs are the first-choice agents for the control of mild to moderate TMD pain. The NSAIDs as a group share similar side effect profiles, and patients vary greatly with their response to and ability to tolerate one agent over another. A series of analgesic trials may be necessary to find the best drug for a patient. Initially, OTC formulations of aspirin, ibuprofen, or naproxen sodium may be adequate for mild pain. Because of the chronic nature of TMD pain, dosing should be continuous and time contingent rather than PRN. Doses should be titrated to effect, up to the analgesic ceiling dose for the agent chosen. Prescription formulation NSAIDs may be required for patients receiving no relief or unmanageable side effects from OTC agents. When choosing an OTC or pre-scription NSAID, factors such as the patient's experience or history with a given drug, cost, and half-life must be considered. In patients with chronic, stable pain, choosing an agent with a longer half-life can help improve compliance by decreasing the number of doses per day. The addition of an H_2 blocker such as famotidine (Pepcid) or a prostaglandin analogue such as misoprostol (Cytotec) may be necessary in patients with a history of gastric intolerance to NSAIDs.

An opioid should be added to the regimen when TMD pain cannot be adequately controlled with a NSAID alone. Opioids may be the first-line choice in moderate to severe pain or in patients in whom the use of NSAIDs is contraindicated. As with the NSAIDs, because of the chronic nature of TMD, use of continuous, time-contingent dosing provides the most effective pain control with the lowest possible doses. Once the patient's 24-hour opioid requirement is known, use of a sustained-release formulation of oxycodone, morphine, or transdermal fentanyl, with rescue doses of an immediate-release agent, is recommended.

Adjuvants such as tricyclic antidepressants, anticonvulsants, and antiarrhythmics such as mexiletine can also be helpful in the management of TMD-related pain when added to a regimen including a nonopioid and an opioid. This is especially true in patients who have undergone one or more surgical procedures involving the TMJ in an attempt to decrease their pain and dysfunction. Stepwise addition of individual agents with gradual upward dose titration is required with careful monitoring for side effects.

Intraoral appliances

Many hypotheses regarding the TMD etiology propose a discoordination of function of the masticatory muscles, with resulting muscle fatigue and spasm as causal factors for the resultant facial pain. Others suggest abnormal stress loading of the TMJ, resulting in excessive pressures being placed on the pain-sensitive structures of the joint. The use of intraoral occlusal orthotic appliances, sometimes referred to as "splints" or "night guards," is often recommended as a means of decreasing masticatory muscle pain and spasm and decreasing loading of the TMJ. Extensive clinical experience and case records suggest that intraoral appliances can be helpful in reducing TMD-related facial pain and TMJ dysfunction. The mechanism of action is not understood, and many studies have suggested placebo effect to play a strong role. Appliances that stabilize the patient's current bite are considered reversible and noninvasive and are recommended. Splints designed with the intention to attempt to "reposition" the lower jaw or the TMJ may produce detrimental changes in the bite or TMJ function and should not be used (National Institutes of Health Technology Assessment Conference Statement, 1996).

Occlusal or orthodontic therapy

Dental malocclusion or "abnormal bite" has long been assumed to be a major causal factor in TMD. This had been used as the empirical framework to suggest extensive occlusal adjustment, dental restorations, or orthodontic treatment as means of treating TMD. There is little evidence that orthodontic treatment or prophylactic occlusal adjustment prevents TMD, and critical review of published data indicates the relationship between TMD and dental occlusion to be a weak causal inference at best. For this reason, and given the invasive, irreversible nature of such treatment, orthodontic treatment, occlusal adjustment, or dental restorative work aimed at correcting occlusion to treat TMD is not recommended.

Physical therapy

Numerous physical therapy modalities such as ultrasound, iontophoresis, vapocoolant spray-stretch, and active and passive range of motion exercises may be used in the management of TMD. Although all these modalities have been documented to be helpful on the basis of clinical reports and case records, these effects appear to be limited to the period during the treatment and shortly thereafter, with questionable sustained benefit. Randomized, prospective studies documenting their efficacy are needed. Physical therapy appears to be most beneficial in the acute setting after injury, surgical intervention, or acute exacerbation. Because of the reversible, noninvasive nature of these modalities, no contraindication to their use exists in the management of TMD, provided that defined endpoints and goals of therapy are identified. Passive and active range of motion exercise instruction, when indicated, should be included in the initial self-management patient education (Feine, Widmer, Lund, 1997).

Surgery

A spectrum of surgical procedures has been applied to those instances of TMD with significant TMJ pathology. Surgical intervention may be considered for a small percentage of patients who have persistent and significant pain and dysfunction and for whom more conservative treatment has failed. Procedures range from arthrocentesis (percutaneous needle irrigation of the joint) to total joint replacement. Although numerous studies have documented significant symptom and function improvement after TMJ surgery, randomized controlled clinical trials to support the efficacy of individual procedures have not been performed. Indications for surgery include one or more of the following: moderate to severe pain localizable to the TMJ, joint dysfunction (clicking, locking, limited opening, or chewing ability) causing significant disability, or radiographic evidence of significant joint pathology (National Institutes of Health Technology Assessment Conference Statement, 1996).

SUMMARY

- "Gold standard" for assessment = thorough history and examination.
- Severity of signs and symptoms and their effect on functional status are highly variable.
- Most TMD pain is benign and nonprogressive.
- Analgesic management with WHO pyramid for pain control (see p. 117).
- Chronic low-dose opioid therapy is appropriate and effective in a number of cases.
- Orthodontic, occlusal, restorative therapy is not recommended.
- Stabilizing (nonrepositioning) oral orthotic appliance therapy may be helpful.
- Physical therapy modalities may be helpful.
- Surgery is appropriate for severe, persistent cases refractory to conservative care.

Resources

American Academy of Head, Neck, and Facial Pain
    520 W. Pipeline Road
    Hurst, TX 76053
    (817) 282-1501

American Academy of Orofacial Pain
    10 Joplin Court
    Lafayette, CA 94549
    (510) 945-9229

TMJ Association
    6418 W. Washington Boulevard
    Milwaukee, WI 53213
    (414) 259-3223
    Fax: (414) 259-8112

References

Christiansen E, Thompson JR: Radiographic evaluation of the TMJ. In Pertes RA, Gross SG, editors: *Clinical management of temporomandibular disorders and orofacial pain*, pp 161-174, Chicago, 1995, Quintessence.

Clark GT, Tsukiyama Y, Baba K et al.: The validity and utility of disease detection and of occlusal therapy for temporomandibular disorders, *Oral Surg* 83:101-106, 1997.

de Bont L, Dijkgraff LC, Stegenga B: Epidemiology and natural progression of articular temporomandibular disorders, *Oral Surg* 83: 72-76, 1997.

De Kanter RJAM, Truin GJ, Burgersdiijk RCW et al.: Prevalence in the Dutch population and a meta-analysis of signs and symptoms of temporomandibular disorders, *J Dent Res* 72:1509-1518, 1993.

Feine JS, Widmer CG, Lund JP: Physical therapy: a critique, *Oral Surg* 83:123-127, 1997.

Goulet JP, Lavigne GJ, Lund JP: Jaw pain prevalence among French-speaking Canadians in Quebec and related symptoms of temporomandibular disorders, *J Dent Res* 74:1738-1744, 1995.

McNamara JA: Orthodontic treatment and temporomandibular disorders, *Oral Surg* 83:107-117, 1997.

National Institutes of Health technology assessment conference statement: management of temporomandibular disorders, April 29-May 1, 1996, *J Am Dent Assoc* 127:1595-1603, 1996.

Vallerand AH: Measurement issues in the comprehensive assessment of cancer pain, *Semin Oncol Nurs* 13(1): 16-24, 1997.

Vallerand WP: Trigeminal neuralgia. In Hupp JR, Williams T, Vallerand WP, editors: *The five minute clinical consult for dental professionals*, pp 546-547, Baltimore, 1996a, Williams & Wilkins.

Vallerand WP: Glossopharyngeal neuralgia. In Hupp JR, Williams T, Vallerand WP, editors: *The five minute clinical consult for dental professionals*, pp 220-221, Baltimore, 1996b, Williams & Wilkins.

Vallerand WP, Sirois DA: Examination procedures for orofacial pain. In Pertes RA, Gross SG, editors: *Clinical management of temporomandibular disorders and orofacial pain*, pp 315-328, Chicago, 1995, Quintessence.

Westesson PL: Magnetic resonance imaging of the temporomandibular joint. In Pertes RA, Gross SG, editors: *Clinical management of temporomandibular disorders and orofacial pain*, pp 175-196, Chicago, 1995, Quintessence.

WOUND PAIN

Lia van Rijswijk

Description

Every day, thousands of people sustain acute surgical or nonsurgical wounds that are expected to heal within a reasonable amount of time. When wound healing problems develop (e.g., the surgical wound becomes infected) or when the wound's primary cause is an underlying condition (e.g., vascular insufficiency), it is classified as a chronic wound. In the United States 1 in 800 people have leg ulcers (McGuckin, Stineman, Goin et al., 1997), approximately 10% of patients in acute care facilities have a pressure ulcer (Barczak, Barnett, Childs et al., 1997), and an estimated 15% of patients with diabetes mellitus will develop a foot ulcer during their lives (Palumbo, Melton, 1985). Unfortunately, research on wound pain, particularly pain experienced by patients with chronic wounds, is scarce.

Pain Characteristics

The assumption that not all wounds are painful is in stark contrast with nursing research findings, which suggest that pain is "the worst thing about having an ulcer" (Hofman, Ryan, Arnold et al., 1997; Lindholm, Bjellerup, Christensch et al., 1993). After interviewing patients with venous ulcers, Krasner (1997a) observed how ironic it is that patients often do not report pain because they expect to have to "grit their teeth" and "carry on," whereas health care professionals assume that wounds are not painful. Undertreatment of pain is common in patients with chronic wounds. Studying patients with pressure ulcers, Dallam, Smyth, Jackson and others (1995) found that 59% of patients reported having wound pain of some type and only 2% were given analgesics for the pain (within 4 hours of the interview). Pain and the presence of a wound also affect patients' quality of life. Patients with chronic wounds have been reported to feel socially isolated, depressed, and anxious (Lindholm, Bjellerup, Christensch et al., 1993; Phillips, Stanton, Provan et al., 1994).

Considering the skin's rich supply of sensory receptors, it is not surprising that *all* skin trauma and breakdown causes pain. (See Figure 12.4 for layers of skin tissues.) Even when the dermis and its sensory receptors

are absent, as may be the case in full-thickness wounds (such as deep pressure ulcers and third-degree burns, see pp. 527-531), the wound edges and the underlying tissues still contain sensory receptors. Also, sensations such as pressure (e.g., from sitting or wound packing materials) and movement (e.g., wound manipulation) will be perceived by the proprioceptive receptors in the underlying fascia, muscles, tendons, and ligaments. Finally, when the wound starts to heal, peripheral nerves will regenerate, sending out immature sprouts of nerve tissue that are hypersensitive to stimuli such as wound care procedures and topical agents used (Rook, 1996).

Neuropathic pain, described as burning, stinging, or pins and needles, has not only been documented in patients with peripheral neuropathy as a result of diabetes mellitus, but also in patients with venous ulcers (Krasner, 1997a). Although not directly related to the wound, it is important to remember that other conditions commonly associated with chronic wounds (e.g., arterial or venous insufficiency) may cause pain and discomfort.

Assessment

Clinicians should assume that all wounds are painful. Chronic wound pain usually encompasses three aspects, and each must be assessed separately (Krasner, 1997b):

- Noncyclic acute wound pain (manipulations such as debridement or drain removal)
- Cyclic acute wound pain (recurring manipulations including movement and dressing changes)
- Chronic wound pain (persistent pain in the absence of manipulations)

Patients should be asked if the pain causes sleep problems. More than 60% of patients with venous ulcers have been reported to have trouble sleeping because of ulcer pain (Hofman, Ryan, Arnold et al., 1997).

As the wound condition changes, continue assessing pain. Results of most chronic wound care studies indicate that pain diminishes when the wound is managed appropriately and is healing (Arnold, Stanley, Fellows et al., 1994; Scurr, Wilson, Coleridge Smith, 1994).

Pain Management

Reducing nociceptive input from the wound has been found to make a significant difference in the levels of pain experienced by patients with acute and chronic wounds. Nociceptive pain is most often caused by chemicals, physical factors, or a combination of both (Table 12.11). Most people know from experience that antiseptics (e.g., hydrogen peroxide, povidone iodine) and styptics cause pain. In general, their use should be avoided unless the wound is anesthetized (e.g., cleansing traumatic wounds).

Chemical irritation can also be caused by the presence of devitalized tissue because damaged tissues release or

● ● ● ● ●

TABLE 12.11 **Nociceptive Wound Pain**

CAUSE	PAIN CATEGORY MOST AFFECTED*	WOUND CARE STRATEGIES TO REDUCE NOCICEPTIVE INPUT
1. Chemical • Irritating topical treatments • Release of nociceptive substances/chemicals from damaged tissue	• Cyclic acute • Chronic	• Use nontoxic, nonirritating wound cleansers (e.g., saline and topical ointments). • Remove devitalized tissue. • Use moisture retentive dressing (e.g., hydrocolloid or film dressing) to protect exposed nerve endings and prevent tissue dessication.
2. Physical • Pressure • Movement • Procedures	• Noncyclic acute • Cyclic acute • Chronic	• Reduce pressure from surfaces. • Pack deep wounds lightly with soft, nonadherent materials (e.g., hydrofiber or alginate when wound is wet or gel dressing when wound is dry). • Reduce edema (e.g., compression bandages). • Use anesthetic (e.g., local infiltration or topical anesthetic/analgesic such as EMLA) before painful procedures (e.g., sharp debridement, drain removal) • Use dressing that supports (adheres to surrounding skin) without adhering to the wound itself (e.g., hydrocolloid or film dressing).

May be duplicated for use in clinical practice. From McCaffery M, Pasero C: *Pain: Clinical manual*, p. 593. Copyright © 1999, Mosby, Inc.
*Based on Krasner, 1997b.

synthesize chemicals that irritate nociceptive nerve terminals (Rook, 1996). This is one of the reasons that wounds in the inflammatory phase of the healing process are more painful than wounds that have started to repair. Measures to reduce chemical irritation include removal of the source (dead tissues) and wound care strategies that prevent drying of the wound bed, which causes cell death and prolongs the inflammatory process. Drying of the wound bed by exposing it to air or using nonmoisture-retentive dressings is also painful because the nerve endings are exposed instead of protected by the dressing and by a mixture of growth factors, infection-fighting cells, and wound fluid (Field, Kerstein, 1994).

Physically, dried tissue ("scab") irritates sensory receptors because it is not as flexible as healthy, well-hydrated tissues. Also, when a deep wound contains necrotic tissue, the dead tissue will actually splint the wound and keep it open.

Other physical factors that cause wound pain include movement, pressure, and procedural pain. Common causes of noncyclic acute or procedural pain include sharp debridement or the removal of dressings that adhere to the wound bed or edges (e.g., wet-to-dry dressings). For example, when patients with abscess cavities were asked to rate pain, removal of gauze-type dressings was significantly more painful (5.1 on a 0 to 10 scale) than removal of dressings that do not adhere to exudating wounds (1 on a 0 to 10 scale) (Dawson, Armstrong, Fulford et al., 1992). Similarly, assessing the pain of patients undergoing surgical debridement of their leg ulcer, researchers found that the median pain rating

when a mixture of lidocaine and prilocaine was applied before the procedure was 1.85 on a 0 to 10 scale compared with 8.4 in the control group (Holm, Andren, Grafford, 1990).

Pressure, which may be associated with chronic and cyclic acute pain, can be caused by putting the wrong type or too much dressing material in a wound (overpacking), pressure from a surface (chair, bed), or edema. Swelling secondary to inflammation (see also chemical causes of nociceptive pain, Table 12.11) and edema secondary to an underlying condition (e.g., venous insufficiency) puts pressure on the wound. In fact, patients with venous ulcer have been found to equate swelling with pain (Krasner, 1997a), and most patients with venous ulcer report a reduction in wound pain when appropriate local wound care and compression therapy are initiated (Arnold, Stanley, Fellows et al., 1994; Scurr, Wilson, Coleridge Smith, 1994). Patients with pressure ulcers will benefit from careful positioning and transfer techniques and the use of pressure-relieving devices.

The effect of movement on wound pain varies greatly and has been found to be related to the type of wound care provided. Sutured wounds may hurt when movement occurs because the sutures will pull or because the approximated edges rub against each other. Examining the relationship between dressing adhesion and surgical wound pain, researchers have found a significant relationship between dressing adhesion and pain. Dressings that adhere well to the surrounding skin but not to the wound cause significantly less pain than dressings that adhere to the wound bed and not, or very little, to the skin (Murharyo, 1996). This explains the tradition of "splinting" surgical wounds and why support bandages (e.g., abdominal binders) can be helpful when pain during movement is severe.

In addition to protecting exposed nerve endings, the "splinting" effect of some dressings may explain the results of clinical studies in patients with nonsutured wounds. For example, skin graft donor sites dressed with moisture-retentive hydrocolloid dressings are less painful than those covered with gauze-type dressings and significantly less painful when patients are ambulating (Madden, Nolan, Finkelstein et al., 1989). Gauze not only allows the wound bed to dry out, but it also "pulls" when moving.

Reducing nociceptive input from the wound should always be part of the patient care plan. However, particularly during the early phases of the healing process and when neuropathic pain is suspected, these measures may have to be supplemented with pharmacologic or other nonpharmacologic interventions (e.g., relaxation strategies, transcutaneous electric nerve stimulation).

Pharmacologic pain management recognizes that wound pain may be nociceptive, neuropathic, or both. Nonopioid and adjuvant medications (e.g., tricyclic antidepressants) and opioid analgesics may be needed to manage the acute and/or chronic wound pain.

Before painful wound care, the patient should be adequately medicated. An oral combination of opioid and nonopioid, such as acetaminophen and oxycodone, may be sufficient. However, when oral medications are used, enough time must be allowed for peak effect to occur. Usually the patient is instructed to take the oral analgesic at least 1 hour before painful wound care.

Controlled studies have shown that the pain associated with sharp debridement of leg ulcers is significantly reduced by application of a topical lidocaine-prilocaine cream before the procedure (Hansson, Holm, Lillieborg et al., 1993; Holm, Andren, Grafford, 1990). The use of other topical preparations such as lidocaine, benzocaine, or prilocaine may also be helpful (Fowler, van Rijswijk, 1995).

SUMMARY

Pain reduction should always be included as one of the goals of wound care. In addition to increasing patient comfort, most measures to reduce nociceptive wound pain have also been shown to benefit the wound healing process. For example, many painful antiseptic agents in commonly used dilutions are toxic to the cells needed for repair (Bergstrom, Bennett, Carlson et al., 1994), whereas the use of moisture-retentive dressings reduces pain and facilitates healing (Field, Kerstein, 1994; Madden, Nolan, Finkelstein et al., 1989). Similarly, eradicating a painful infection allows a wound to heal, and edema reduction, which reduces pain in patients

with venous ulcers, is strongly associated with ulcer healing (Cherry, Hofman, Cameron et al., 1996). When wounds are painful, they are trying to communicate that something is wrong. All we have to do is listen.

Resources

Bergstrom N, Bennett MA, Carlson CE et al.: *Treatment of pressure ulcers*, Clinical Practice Guideline No. 15, Rockville, Md, U.S. Department of Health and Human Services, Public Health Service, Agency for Health Care Policy and Research, AHCPR Publication No. 95-0652, Dec 1994.

Treatment of pressure ulcers—Consumer Version, AHCPR Publication No. 95-0654.

  To order the two above: (free)
  AHCPR
  Publications Clearinghouse
  P.O. Box 8547
  Silver Spring, MD 20907
  Web site: //www.ahcpr.gov/guide/
  (800) 358-9295

Association for the Advancement of Wound Care (AAWC)
320 E. Towsontown Boulevard, Suite 207
Baltimore, MD 21212
(410) 321-5557
E-mail: *AAWCLINE@aol.com; aaschelp@voicenet.com*

  Interdisciplinary organization; membership open to health care professionals and laypersons. Benefits include networking directory and newsletter.

Wound, Ostomy and Continence Nurses Society
1550 S. Coast Highway, Suite 201
Laguna Beach, CA 92651
(888) 224-WOCN

  Membership includes journal, newsletter, and membership directory.

References

Arnold TE, Stanley JC, Fellows EP et al.: Prospective, multicenter study of managing lower extremity venous ulcers, *Ann Vasc Surg* 8:356-362, 1994.

Barczak CA, Barnett RI, Childs EJ et al.: Fourth national pressure ulcer prevalence study, *Adv Wound Care* 10(4):18-26, 1997.

Bergstrom N, Bennett MA, Carlson CE et al.: *Treatment of pressure ulcers*, Clinical Practice Guideline No. 15, Rockville, Md, U.S. Department of Health and Human Services, Public Health Service, Agency for Health Care Policy and Research, AHCPR Publication No. 95-0652, Dec 1994.

Cherry GW, Hofman D, Cameron J et al.: Bandaging in the treatment of venous ulcers: a European view, *Ostomy/Wound Manage* 42(10A): 13S-18S, 1996.

Dallam L, Smyth C, Jackson B et al.: Pressure ulcer pain: assessment and quantification, *J WOCN* 22(5):211-218, 1995.

Dawson C, Armstrong MWJ, Fulford SCV et al.: Use of calcium alginate to pack abscess cavities: a controlled clinical trial, *J R Coll Surg* 37:177-179, 1992.

Field CK, Kerstein MD: Overview of wound healing in a moist environment, *Am J Surg* 167(Suppl 1A):2S-6S, 1994.

Fowler E, van Rijswijk L: Using wound debridement to help achieve the goals of care, *Ostomy/Wound Manage* 41(7A):23S-25S, 1995.

Hansson C, Holm J, Lillieborg S et al.: Repeated treatment with lidocaine/prilocaine cream (EMLA) as a topical anaesthetic for the cleansing of venous ulcers: a controlled study, *Acta Dermatol Venereol (Stockh)* 73:231-233, 1993.

Hofman D, Ryan TJ, Arnold F et al.: Pain in venous leg ulcers, *J Wound Care* 6(5):222-224, 1997.

Holm J, Andren B, Grafford K: Pain control in the surgical debridement of leg ulcers by the use of a topical lidocaine-prilocaine cream, EMLA, *Acta Dermatol Venereol (Stockh)* 70:132-136, 1990.

Krasner D: *Carrying on despite the pain: living with painful venous ulcers—a Heideggerian Hermeneutic Analysis*, Doctoral thesis, School of Nursing, University of Maryland at Baltimore, 1997a.

Krasner D: Chronic wound pain. In Krasner D, Kane D, editors: *Chronic wound care: a clinical source book for healthcare professionals*, ed 2, pp 336-343, Wayne, Penn, 1997b, Health Management Publications.

Lindholm C, Bjellerup M, Christensch O et al.: Quality of life in leg ulcer patients: an assessment according to the Nottingham profile, *Acta Dermatol Venereol (Stockh)* 73:440-443, 1993.

Madden MR, Nolan E, Finkelstein J et al.: Comparison of an occlu-sive and a semi-occlusive dressing and the effect of the wound exudate upon keratinocyte proliferation, *J Trauma* 29:924-931, 1989.

McGuckin M, Stineman MG, Goin JE et al.: *Venous ulcer guideline*, Philadelphia, 1997, University of Pennsylvania.

Murharyo P: Dressings following circumcision: results of a controlled, clinical study, *Singapore Paediatr J* 38(3):125-130, 1996.

Palumbo PJ, Melton LJ III: Peripheral vascular disease in diabetes. In *Diabetes in America: diabetes data compiled in 1984*, NIH Pub. No. 85-1468, Washington, DC, 1985, U.S. Government Printing Office.

Phillips T, Stanton B, Provan A et al.: A study of the impact of leg ulcers on quality of life, *J Am Acad Dermatol* 31:49-53, 1994.

Rook JL: Wound care pain management, *Adv Wound Care* 9(6):24-31, 1996.

Scurr JH, Wilson LA, Coleridge Smith PD: A comparison of calcium alginate and hydrocolloid dressings in the management of chronic venous ulcers, *Wounds* 6(1):1-8, 1994.

section 2
BRIEF DESCRIPTIONS OF SELECTED PAIN PROBLEMS

Karen P. Kettelman

The following serve as a brief introduction to selected pain problems and provide basic resources for learning more. The discussion of each includes a definition of the condition, cause (if known), characteristics of the pain, methods of assessing the problem and associated pain, pain management specific to the condition, resources, and references.

ANKYLOSING SPONDYLITIS
Definition/Cause

Ankylosing (fusing together) spondylitis (inflammation of the spine) (AS) is one of a group of inflammatory diseases affecting joints. AS is uncommon; it is not as easily identified as other types of arthritis and is often missed or incorrectly diagnosed. The cell marker HLA-B27 is present in about 90% of ankylosing spondylitis cases (Halverson, 1997). The causal relationship between HLA-B27 and AS is unclear. It is known that AS is strongly associated with this genetic cell marker. This link helps to explain the susceptibility that runs in families. Men are affected with AS three times as often as women.

Pain Characteristics

AS begins insidiously in adolescence and during the 20s with dull, aching stiffness in the back. Pain increases gradually over time, sometimes restricting motion in the back, rib cage, and neck. Classic symptoms include spondylitis or inflammatory back pain, especially in the low back, and inflammation at sites where ligaments and tendons attach. Some variability may exist in symptoms of the disease and in its severity. The initial inflammation and pain in the spine may cause muscle spasms that can, if left untreated, lead to scarring and stooped posture.

The disease often has a milder course in women, and peripheral joints and the neck may be affected rather than the low back. Women can experience normal pregnancy and childbirth with the treatments available today.

Late in the disease progression abnormalities related to posture may include flexion contractures of the hips. Disability is common as deformities become severe.

Assessment

Diagnosis is made primarily on the basis of physical findings such as the amount of restricted back motion with reduced extension, lateral flexion, and forward flexion, as well as x-ray films showing sacroiliitis. Early in the disease, x-ray films may be completely normal. No specific laboratory tests are conclusive, but an elevated erythrocyte sedimentation rate or mild anemia may be detected.

Pain Management

Treatments for the pain of AS target the maintenance of health and mobility. Physical therapists play an important role in providing instruction in exercises for stretching the back, neck, and chest. Patients are encouraged to sleep flat on their back on a very firm surface to promote a more functional position if fusion of the neck and back occur. Prevention of deformities allows for a normal lifestyle. Good posture and exercise are essential as a part of the regular regimen for health maintenance and control of pain.

NSAIDs are often prescribed for pain relief in the AS patient. Indomethacin (Indocin) has been shown to be the most effective NSAID for AS patients. Patients with intractable pain may respond to methotrexate. Corticosteroids are sometimes prescribed, but use is limited because of severe side effects with long-term use.

Physical agents such as heat, ultrasound, and massage can also be useful in providing relief of pain for the patient with AS.

Opioid pain medication may be indicated for the patient with pain that cannot be controlled with other analgesics. Many patients tolerate long-term opioid therapy and are able to function normally.

With severe AS, surgery is sometimes indicated. Total joint replacements are performed when deterioration is significant. Surgery to correct severe flexion deformities of the spine is sometimes done although it is a risky procedure that can lead to spinal cord injury and paralysis.

Resources

Spondylitis Association of America
P.O. Box 5872
Sherman Oaks, CA 91413
(800) 777-8189

Available from the above:

Straight Talk on Spondylitis—a comprehensive book to help patients understand and manage spondylitis.

Exercise tapes—demonstrating flexibility and strengthening exercises.

References

Halverson PB: The spondyloarthropathies, *Orthop Nurs* 16(4):21-25, 1997.
Swezey RL: *Straight talk on spondylitis,* ed 2, Sherman Oaks, Calif, 1992, Spondylitis Association of America.
Thomas MA, Kahan B: Physical examination of the patient in pain. In Kanner R, editor: *Pain management secrets,* pp 16-17, Philadelphia, 1997, Hanley & Belfus.

ARACHNOIDITIS
Definition/Cause

Arachnoiditis is a painful, inflammatory response, resulting in a thickening of the arachnoid meningeal layer, or covering of the spinal cord, around the nerve root. This inflammatory response may be accompanied by ischemia and deterioration or atrophy of the nerve root. Arachnoiditis can occur after infection or trauma. Sources of infection include syphilis or local tubercular infection. The most common traumatic causes of arachnoiditis are failed back surgery, lumbar puncture, ruptured disk, and spinal anesthesia. Additional sources of irritation may be blood or chemical, as with the use of contrast media for diagnostic radiologic procedures.

Pain Characteristics

Patients with arachnoiditis describe pain in the back and neck and radicular pain in the distribution of the nerve root involved in the inflammatory process. This process can progress to spinal cord dysfunction and in some patients to paraplegia.

Assessment

When examined by MRI the nerve roots appear matted together in a clump in the center of the spinal canal or on the sides of the canal (Kanner, 1997). Diagnosis may also be established with myelography, revealing spotty and irregular collections of contrast material and impaired flow through the subarachnoid space.

Pain Management

No cure exists for this sometimes disabling disease. Treatment options are aimed at returning the patient to functional status through conservative measures. Surgery can be done in an attempt to remove the adhesions but may be minimally effective because the scar tissue will continue to develop and the already irritated spinal cord is exposed to additional trauma. In addition, treatment may include antibiotics if a specific infectious organism can be identified.

Pharmacologic interventions include the use of tricyclic antidepressants and anticonvulsants to treat the neuropathic pain component. Baclofen (Lioresal) is helpful for spasmodic-type pain.

Opioid and nonopioid analgesics may also be used. Treating the pain both centrally and peripherally may be the most effective, with a minimum of side effects.

Resources

Arachnoiditis Information Network
P.O. Box 1166
Baldwin, MO 63022

References

Kanner R: Low back pain. In Kanner R, editor: *Pain management secrets,* pp 76-83, Philadelphia, 1997, Hanley & Belfus.
National Institute of Neurological Disorders and Stroke: NIH, Bethesda, MD 20892 *www.ninds.nih.gov/healinfo/disorder/arachnoi/arachnoi.htm*

CHRONIC FATIGUE SYNDROME/CHRONIC FATIGUE IMMUNE DEFICIENCY SYNDROME
Definition/Cause

The hallmark of chronic fatigue syndrome (CFS)/ chronic fatigue immune deficiency syndrome (CFIDS) is pronounced, severe fatigue that comes on suddenly and is relentless or relapsing. Persons who have no apparent reason for feeling this way have debilitating tiredness or exhaustion that is not cured with a few good nights' sleep. Impairment of memory and concentration often accompanies the symptoms of CFS/CFIDS.

CFS is two to four times more common in women younger than 45 than in any other group. The cause of CFS/CFIDS is unknown, but theories include HHV-6 or other viruses, including herpesvirus, terovirus, and retrovirus. CFIDS has been associated with increased levels of Epstein-Barr virus antibodies, and it is now believed that the increase may be a result of the disease rather than a cause. Development of CFS often follows an acute infection such as a cold, bronchitis, hepatitis, or mononucleosis. It can also occur more gradually and with no triggering event. The estimated number of people suffering from CFS in the United States is approximately 4 to 10 cases per 100,000 adults, although it also occurs in children.

CFIDS carries with it a stigma of not being real. Patients often have to learn to cope with not only their physical condition and pain but also with not being believed by health care providers, insurers, family, friends, employers, and people in general.

Pain Characteristics

Patients often feel as if they have a flu syndrome that will not go away. Symptoms include headache, tender lymph nodes, sore throat, muscle and joint aches in addition to the fatigue, weakness, fever, and allergic manifestations.

Assessment

Research in the area of CFS/CFIDS is attempting to define the disease by use of strict symptom and physical criteria. Until that definition is established, the first rule is to rule out similar diseases such as multiple sclerosis, lupus erythematosus, and fibromyalgia.

Pain Management

Because to date no specific CFS/CFIDS treatments exist, patients are treated symptomatically. NSAIDs help the headache, sore throat, muscle and joint aches, and fever. Cyclobenzaprine (Flexeril) has also been useful for the treatment of muscle spasms. Antidepressants can increase the feeling of fatigue. Benzodiazepines are sometimes used to treat the acute anxiety and sleep problems.

Studies testing antiviral drugs, such as acyclovir, have been inconclusive as to their benefit in the treatment of CFS/CFIDS.

Some people with CFS/CFIDS spontaneously recover, and others wax and wane after their initial episode.

Resources

The National CFIDS Foundations newsletter *The Forum*. Membership and informational materials available from:

National CFIDS Foundation
103 Aletha Road
Needham, MA 02192

On the internet: *www.cdc.gov/ncidod/diseases/cfs/ support.htm;* support groups across the country.

References

Rich KD: Book and media reviews: Clinical management of chronic fatigue syndrome, *J Pharmaceut Care Pain Symptom Manage* 5(2): 105-106, 1997.
Web sites at the National Institutes of Health/National Institute of Allergy and Infectious Diseases @ *www.niaid.nih.gov/factsheets/cfs.htm; www.cdc.gov/ncidod/diseases/cfs/treatmen.htm.*

CROHN'S DISEASE
Definition/Cause

Crohn's disease is a chronic inflammatory bowel disease that is characterized by remissions and relapses. Diarrhea and abdominal pain are the earliest symptoms and may be accompanied by perianal pain-related sores. Joint pain, weight loss, and loss of appetite are also common. No cause is known. Some evidence shows that certain major histocompatibility complex (MHC) genes play a role in the development of Crohn's disease. MHC genes are part of the immune response. Some researchers believe that an environmental stimulus such as a virus or bacterium causes Crohn's disease in patients who are genetically predisposed.

Crohn's disease tends to run in families, and it affects men and women equally. The disease usually develops between the ages of 15 and 40.

Neither emotional stress nor certain foods are believed to be the cause of Crohn's disease. Emotional stress does influence the course of the disease, however.

Pain Characteristics

The pain that accompanies Crohn's disease comes in many forms. Abdominal pain, soreness, and cramping are the most common and troublesome. Abdominal cramping often occurs after a meal. Inflamed joints and arthritis are frequently experienced later in the illness. Although sufferers of Crohn's disease experience acute episodes of pain and chronic pain, they usually are able to function normally much of the time and lead productive lives.

Assessment

Signs and symptoms of Crohn's disease mimic other gastrointestinal conditions and may be difficult to diagnose. Diagnosis is made primarily by a suggestive history and a physical examination. Laboratory values may reflect blood loss and malabsorption.

The abdominal pain and tenderness may be a result of obstruction or inflammation narrowing the lumen of the bowel.

Pain Management

The pain and other symptoms are usually controlled by the appropriate management of the underlying inflammation. The drugs most commonly used today include corticosteroids, aminoglycosides, antibiotics, and immunosuppressive drugs. Opioids are sometimes used to treat the pain, but care should be taken because of the risk of toxic megacolon, a condition of nonobstructive dilatation of the colon that sometimes occurs in patients with inflammatory bowel diseases because of decreased motility.

The patient's dietary intake is important as well. Patients are advised to eat low-residue foods, and many are advised to limit milk products because patients with Crohn's disease tend to have lactose intolerance.

For patients in whom these conservative treatments are not effective, surgery can be done. A segment of the bowel is removed and the ends of the bowel are anastomosed, or sometimes an ileostomy or colostomy is performed. Although this relieves the symptoms of the disease, it may recur in tissue previously believed to be disease free.

Resources

For information and a variety of educational brochures and books contact:

Crohn's and Colitis Foundation of America, Inc.
National Headquarters
386 Park Avenue South, 17th Floor
New York, N.Y. 10016-8804
(800) 932-2423

For brochures only call (800) 343-3637.

References

Anonymous: Inflammatory bowel disease: making sense of a mystery ailment, *Harvard Health Letter*, 22(2):4-6, 1996.
Kimmey MB, Silverstein FE, Bonica JJ: Diseases of the gastrointestinal tract. In Bonica JJ, editor: *The management of pain*, ed 2, pp 1186-1213, Penn, 1990, Lea & Febiger.

HEMOPHILIA

Definition/Cause

Hemophilia, a disorder of blood coagulation, occurs in approximately 1 in 5000 male births (Mosher, 1996). The primary type of hemophilia, hemophilia A, is associated with a deficiency of factor VIII. The degree of the deficiency and the frequency of significant bleeding with normal activity helps to classify the hemophilia as mild, moderate, or severe.

The pain associated with hemophilia is caused by intraarticular bleeding. This intraarticular hemorrhage causes both acute and chronic pain. The pain is often used as an indicator that bleeding has occurred.

HIV/AIDS-related pain is common in hemophilia patients as well. Many of these patients contracted HIV through blood transfusions before regular screening of blood for HIV.

Pain Characteristics

The acute joint pain of hemophilic arthropathy, or disease of the joint, may begin as fullness and stiffness and later may be described as nagging, burning, or bursting. During the acute phase of bleeding into the joint, the pain is incapacitating and severely impairs activity, depending on the degree of pressure and swelling in the capsule of the joint. The chronic pain experienced by patients with this disorder is related to the joint degeneration that occurs later in the disease process. This chronic pain is described as aching, gnawing, or grating, and it becomes more severe with movement. The joints most commonly affected are the knees, ankles, and elbows. Shoulders, hips, and wrist joints are affected next most often.

HIV-related pain is commonly caused by associated neuropathies and is usually described as burning pain.

Assessment

X-ray films show little in the affected joints other than soft tissue swelling. In patients with chronic pain and destruction of the joint, a narrowing of the joint space may be evident. The diagnosis is clear when there is a severe hemophilic factor deficiency. In patients with a lesser deficiency other causes of degenerative arthritis should be considered before diagnosis can be confirmed.

Obtaining an accurate history from the patient is essential. The history should include frequency and severity of bleeding episodes, nature and severity of the pain, posture, balance, and the need for assistive devices and activity limitation.

Pain Management

Pain management in the patient with hemophilia varies greatly depending on the phase of the disease and the type of pain. For patients with acute bleeding, immobility, ice, assistive devices, and appropriate positioning are important. In subacute disease with chronic pain, mild exercises can be done, and biofeedback, hydrotherapy, and mobilization may be indicated.

Pharmacologic management of the pain of hemophilia is somewhat controversial. There is great reluctance to use opioids because of the fear of addiction in patients with chronic painful conditions. However, only rarely does addiction occur as a result of chronic opioid use for pain relief. It is important to clarify for patients and families the difference between addiction, tolerance, and physical dependence. Opioids can be safely used in these patients for relief of painful episodes and, with supervision and careful patient selection, for long-term use in patients with chronic pain.

Drugs of the benzodiazepine class, such as diazepam (Valium) and lorazepam (Ativan), are helpful if muscle spasms are a problem. It is important to remember that these drugs do not otherwise have analgesic properties.

Acetaminophen and NSAIDs are often used for pain relief in these patients. It is important to choose NSAIDs that do not interfere with platelet aggregation, such as choline magnesium salicylate (Trilisate) and salsalate (Disalcid), to prevent increased risk of bleeding in the already compromised patient.

For hemophilia patients with HIV/AIDS, neuropathic pain may be a problem, and the use of adjuvant medications such as tricyclic antidepressants and anticonvulsants may be beneficial.

Resources

The National Hemophilia Foundation
110 Greene St., Suite 303
New York, NY 10012
(800) 42 HANDI

The National Hemophilia Foundation of Nevada
P.O. Box 90158
Henderson, NV 89009
(702) 564-HFNV (4368)

References

Gilbert MS, Wiedel JD: *The treatment of hemophilia: current orthopedic management,* New York, 1996, The National Hemophilia Foundation.
Mosher DF: Disorders of blood coagulation. In Bennett JC, Plum F, editors: *Cecil textbook of medicine,* ed 20, pp 987-1003, Philadelphia, 1996, WB Saunders.

LOW BACK PAIN

Definition/Cause

There are many causes of low back pain (LBP), and this fact contributes to the controversy surrounding its treatment. Patients with LBP are often labeled as malingerers or are not believed. Their reports of pain may be discounted because the exact cause can be difficult to define and analgesics are required for long periods of time, adding to the controversy.

LBP may be of a superficial nature because of trauma or ulceration, or LBP may be caused by deeper processes that interrupt the mechanics of the back itself, processes that might include structural injuries to tendons, muscles, ligaments, fascia, bones, or joints. Another type of LBP is radicular, or arising from an injury to spinal nerve roots. Other causes of radicular pain may be related to ischemia or decreased blood flow to spinal nerves. LBP may also be neurogenic, arising from abnormalities in the central nervous system with damage to the sensory portion of the nerve. LBP may occur as referred pain from an internal organ that shares innervation with structures in the area of the lumbosacral spine.

Whatever the cause of LBP, it is the most frequent cause of activity limitation in people younger than 45. Back pain occurs most often in men. In the postmenopausal period a larger percentage of women suffer from LBP than do women before menopause. The magnitude of the problem of LBP is enormous. It is the second most common reason for visiting a physician, the fifth most common reason for hospitalization, and the third most common reason for surgery (Borenstein, Wiesel, Boden, 1995). There are approximately 400,000 back injuries covered by workers compensation claims in the United States each year.

Pain Characteristics

Symptoms of LBP vary somewhat according to the cause but may not be specific to the cause. Pain associated with the mechanics of the back itself, such as muscle or tendon damage, causes pain with activity and significant superficial soreness and tenderness. It rarely appears to radiate to a more distant location or follow a dermatomal pattern that may correspond with an affected spinal nerve root as in radiculopathy.

Radicular pain is often lancinating, shooting, sharp, and burning-type pain and radiates to another area. Sciatica is a common form of radicular pain that radiates, shooting pain into the buttock and down the back of the leg. In patients who have LBP with CNS damage, light touch may induce excruciating pain.

Assessment

Assessment of LBP must first focus on ruling out causes that might be serious, requiring immediate intervention, as in a leaking aortic aneurysm, cauda equina syndrome, fractures, or malignant tumors. Beyond this, a thorough history of the problem is paramount to an accurate diagnosis and development of an appropriate treatment plan. The history should include the patient's description of the pain, past history, social history, review of systems, family history, and history of the present condition. A thorough physical examination is the next step. When examining the patient with LBP, it is important to believe his or her report of pain and its intensity. It may be difficult to determine the source of the LBP through physical examination, but it will help to determine the patient's level of functioning.

Myelography, computed tomography, and magnetic resonance imaging are often used to establish the nature and extent of disease and the level of spinal involvement.

In young adults, muscle or ligament strain, congenital abnormalities, injury, or spondyloarthropathies might be considered. In older adults, osteoporosis and degenerative conditions, including spinal stenosis and malignant lesions, are common.

Pain Management

The care of superficial LBP may be simple and may require local or topical treatment only. Treatment for mechanical injuries should be conservative and may include NSAIDs, muscle relaxants, and sometimes a brief course of opioid analgesics along with bedrest. Some patients, however, obtain great relief from opioid therapy and are able to function very well on long-term use of opioids. Bedrest beyond a couple of days can lead to deconditioning and may prolong the recovery time. It is believed now that traction does not contribute to recovery any more than resting supine. Physical modalities such as heat and massage can contribute to the comfort of the patient with LBP as can the application of TENS units. Stretching and strengthening exercises can be helpful to prevent future injuries to the low back. Most LBP resolves without intervention within the first 2 weeks and most of the remainder within 6 to 12 weeks.

A controversial treatment for LBP is injection therapy. Local or regional injections of local anesthetics and steroids may provide pain relief but do not absolutely confirm the source of the pain. Injections can be made in soft tissue, trigger points along the muscle, and ligaments supporting the lumbar spine. In patients for whom conservative therapy has failed, steroids may be injected into the epidural space at the level of the pain to decrease the inflammation and relieve the pain. On occasion, a differential spinal block may be indicated to isolate or confirm the origin.

For patients who have pain that persists despite the above measures, evaluation for surgical intervention may be done. Only 1% to 2% of LBP conditions require surgical interventions such as decompression of the nerve root, diskectomy, or fusion with or without the application of hardware for stability. After surgery, patients experience significant postoperative pain that will require aggressive opioid therapy. These patients will also require a brace for stability for a period of months to a year after surgery. Some patients experience persistent pain even after surgical intervention.

The controversy surrounding the treatment of LBP intensified with the publication of the AHCPR guidelines Acute Low Back Problems in Adults: Assessment and Treatment (1994) and Back Pain in the Workplace (Fordyce, 1995). The concerns raised by specialists in pain management include worries about treatment being determined by these guidelines when patients do not have physical signs of definable, measurable pain but do report pain nevertheless. A problem exists when we treat all LBP the same. Patients with acute LBP versus refractory or chronic LBP may require very different approaches to their problem. It should also be noted that there was not a pain specialist on the AHCPR panel responsible for the development of the back pain guidelines and that *Back Pain in the Workplace* (1995) was rejected by the Canadian Pain Society (1996).

Resources

Back Pain Association of America
    P.O. Box 135
    Pasadena, MD 21223

Understanding acute low back problems, patient guide.

Acute low back problems in adults: Assessment and treatment, quick reference for clinicians.

  Above two are available free from the Agency for Health Care Policy and Research:

    Publications Clearinghouse
    P.O. Box 8547
    Silver Spring, MD 20907
    (800) 358-9295

References

Acute low back problems in adults: assessment and treatment, Rockville, Md, Agency for Health Care Policy and Research Clinical Practice Guideline, 1994.

Borenstein DG, Wiesel SW, Boden SD: *Low back pain medical diagnosis and comprehensive management,* ed 2, Philadelphia, 1995, WB Saunders.

Canadian Pain Society: Statement approved by the executive of the Canadian Pain Society on 2 December, 1995, *Pain* 65:114, 1996.

De Jong RH: Backlash: AHCPR practice guideline for acute low back pain, *Pain Digest* 6:1-2, 1996.

Fordyce WE, editor: *Back pain in the workplace,* Seattle, 1995, IASP Press.

Loeser J: Back pain in the workplace II, *Pain* 65:7-8, 1996.

LYME DISEASE

Definition/Cause

Pain is one of many troubling symptoms of Lyme disease. People suffering from Lyme disease also may experience severe fatigue and neurologic manifestations that range from disorientation and loss of the ability to concentrate to cranial nerve palsy, radiculoneuritis, nerve root inflammation, and meningitis. Cerebrovascular accidents (CVAs) and Guillain-Barré syndrome have also been associated with Lyme disease.

Lyme disease is caused by a spirochetal bacterium spread through the bite of a tick. It is a progressive disease and is unpredictable in its pattern of progression, but basically the stages are as follows. In the earliest stage of the disease the patient may have only a localized rash at the site of the bite. This rash is known as the EM rash, or "erythema migrans," and may be the only sign of the disease. Sometimes disseminated early disease develops, and patients may have widespread inflammation with flulike symptoms. This stage can begin even before the localized rash is present. The severity of the symptoms at this stage may be predictive of how severe the disease may become. Disseminated late disease results in organ infiltration and damage to organ systems. Late disease may start about 3 months after the initial bite, but it often takes longer for the symptoms to become apparent. Lyme disease, or the spirochetal bacterium, can be transmitted through the placental barrier, making unborn children at risk for the disease.

Assessment

The stages of Lyme disease may not be distinct, and therefore it is important to concentrate on the symptoms themselves. The list of symptoms of Lyme disease is extensive; many are related to painful conditions. The pain may take the form of headaches, including migraines, muscle aches, joint pain and arthritis, chest pain and rib soreness, breast pain, abdominal pain, sore throat, and testicular or pelvic pain. Patients with neurologic involvement may experience burning or stabbing sensations. Inflammation of the nerve root, or radiculoneuritis, may start as severe pain radiating down the extremities. Radiculoneuritis is the most common neurologic symptom of Lyme disease.

Lyme disease may affect one or more body systems. There may be cardiac manifestations and pulmonary, gastrointestinal, bladder, and kidney involvement as well. Patients experiencing headache and neck pain should be evaluated for the possibility of meningitis.

Psychiatric manifestations of Lyme disease are common and may include depression, mood swings, paranoia, dementia, and psychosis. Patients with late manifestations of Lyme disease are sometimes incapacitated and unable to function in their daily lives.

Pain Management

When treating patients with Lyme disease, the primary objective is to eradicate the organism that causes the disease. Antibiotics have been useful in eliminating the pain and other manifestations. Corticosteroids are sometimes used for patients with congestive heart failure or complete heart block when antibiotic therapy alone is not successful.

Other treatments include symptomatic relief as with analgesics such as NSAIDs and opioids as needed for pain.

Healthy living habits such as eating a healthy diet, avoiding alcohol, and smoking cessation contribute to recovery from this sometimes devastating disease.

Resources

Lyme Disease Foundation, Inc.
　One Financial Plaza
　Hartford, CT 06103
　(800) 525-2000
　24-hour hot line (800) 886-LYME
　Web site: *http://www.lyme.org*

References

Lang D, Territo J: *Coping with Lyme disease: a practical guide to dealing with diagnosis and treatment,* ed 2, New York, 1997, Henry Holt.
Vanderhoof-Forchner K: *Everything you need to know about Lyme disease and other tickborne disorders,* New York, 1997, John Wiley & Sons.

MUCOSITIS
Definition/Cause

Mucositis (also called stomatitis) affects approximately 400,000 patients per year. It affects 40% of those cancer patients who do not have head or neck cancer. The percentage is much higher in head and neck patients and other high-risk groups, such as those undergoing treatment for leukemia and bone marrow transplantation.

Mucositis is most often caused by chemotherapy for the treatment of malignancy. Administering radiation to the head and neck for treatment of cancer is also a common cause of mucositis and other oral complications. Patients undergoing very high-dose chemotherapy and radiation for bone marrow or stem cell transplantation are especially at risk for mucositis.

The rapid turnover of epithelial cells in the mucous membranes makes them vulnerable to the effects of chemotherapy and radiation. The mucositis is caused by inflammation or dryness induced by these treatments and secondary infections. Poor oral hygiene contributes to the development of mucositis and makes it more difficult to manage. The development of mucositis after chemotherapy is somewhat predictable and usually begins 3 to 5 days after the treatment has started. With head and neck radiation, the mucositis begins in about the second week of treatment and plateaus during the fourth week of treatment.

Head and neck cancer patients undergoing radiation therapy commonly have oral yeast infections severe enough to interfere with the continuation of their radiation treatments if not prevented or treated promptly.

Pain Characteristics

Superficial sloughing, decreased thickness of the mucosa, and ulcerations occur in the mouth and on the tongue. The pain of mucositis is often severe, interfering with the patient's oral intake. Swallowing may be impaired, and oral intake may need to be restricted until healing begins. Patients typically describe a burning sensation related to the inflammation.

Assessment

The extent of the tissue damage or injury contributes to the severity of the pain. Mucositis is graded according to level of severity, and several scales exist for this purpose (see example in Iwamoto, 1996). The Oncology Nursing Society clinical practice committee developed the Stomatitis Grading Scale to assess the severity of mucositis after transplantation (Madeya, 1996). The scale takes into account the number of positive *Candida* cultures and the use of morphine, among other variables.

Severe mucositis can lead to airway obstruction when the cheeks, lips, tongue, and throat become edematous.

Pain Management

Many approaches to the treatment of the pain of mucositis exist. A multitude of topical treatments have been used. Viscous xylocaine can be used but is often refused by patients because of its consistency. Dyclone, an extremely effective topical anesthetic, is well tolerated by patients and works especially well in combination with topical diphenhydramine in a very small quantity. Hydroxypropylcellulose film (Zilactin) can be applied to lesions to serve as a protective coating and pain-relieving measure. Topical application of cocaine is effective for pain relief but rarely used because of its potential side effects of agitation and confusion, and an increase in blood pressure and heart rate.

Artificial saliva products help with the dryness that accompanies mucositis. Rinses with a variety of solutions are used, such as a mixture of hydrogen peroxide and povidone iodine, half-strength hydrogen peroxide alone, or chlorhexidine. A rinse including an antifungal agent may be used if an oral yeast infection is identified. These rinses are administered using a "swish-and-spit" technique but are not harmful if swallowed. Therapy for the treatment of mucositis is aimed at maintaining good oral hygiene while controlling pain. Rinses with any alcohol content are avoided because of the drying effect. Success has been described using water only as a rinsing agent.

Treatment of mucositis pain often requires the use of opioid analgesics in addition to the topical treatments mentioned. Aggressive use of opioid analgesics such as opioids with a PCA device may be indicated.

Resources

Oncology Nursing Society
    501 Holiday Dr.
    Pittsburgh, PA 15220-2749
    (412) 921-7373

References

Ganley BJ: Mouth care for the patient undergoing head and neck radiation therapy: a survey of radiation oncology nurses, *Oncol Nurs Forum* 23:1619-1623, 1996.

Goodman M, Ladd L, Purl S: Integumentary and mucus membrane alterations. In Groenwald SL, Goodman M, Frogge MH et al., editors: *Cancer nursing principles and practice*, pp 763-781, Boston, 1993, Jones & Bartlett.

Iwamoto RR: Alterations in oral status. In McCorkle R, Grant M, Frank-Stromborg M et al.: *Cancer nursing*, pp 944-962, Philadelphia, 1996, WB Saunders.

Madeya ML: Oral complications from cancer therapy. 2. Implications for assessment and treatment, *Oncol Nurs Forum* 23(5)808-819, 1996.

MULTIPLE SCLEROSIS
Definition/Cause

Multiple sclerosis (MS) is a disease of unknown cause affecting the central nervous system. The disease involves an inflammatory process that produces a demyelination of nerves, the brain, and the spinal cord. Symptoms often include some degree of weakness or paralysis along with impaired speech or vision. Manifestations vary depending on the location of the lesions on the brain and spinal cord. Women are affected more often than men, and onset usually occurs between the ages of 20 and 50. The course of the disease is unpredictable, and patients often have remissions and exacerbations of their symptoms. Over time new symptoms appear, old symptoms recur, and residual symptoms may increase.

MS at one time was thought to be a painless disease. In reality, most MS sufferers experience clinically significant pain at some time during the course of their illness.

Pain Characteristics

Some MS sufferers have episodes of sudden onset, severe pain, but continuous chronic pain affects 23% to 80% of patients with MS. The sudden onset, severe episodes of pain may present as trigeminal neuralgia or stabbing pain in the face, stabbing or shock-like pains in the head, down the back (called Lhermitte's sign), or in the extremities. The tightness of a girdle-like band around the waist or chest can be felt. Patients often report acute burning in the extremities.

Continuous chronic pain syndromes may include a burning or pricking feeling, like pins and needles, in the extremities. Spasticity is often a significant source of pain for patients, described as painful muscle spasms and a sensation of tightness and aching in the joints and muscles. Back pain and shooting pain down the leg similar to sciatica can also be caused by MS. Headaches occur in about 10% of MS patients.

Assessment

Assessment begins with ruling out any other sources of the pain. For example, low back pain may indicate a coexisting herniated disk. MRI is used widely to diagnose MS and to rule out other conditions that may be the cause of the symptoms, such as tumor with spinal cord compression. Increase in temperature may reduce neurologic functioning in the multiple sclerosis sufferer and increase or worsen symptoms. A return to normal temperature reverses this phenomenon, and the new symptoms disappear.

Pain Management

The sudden onset, severe burning pain of MS responds very well to anticonvulsants such as carbamazepine (Tegretol) and diphenylhydantoin (Dilantin) and is sometimes treated with corticosteroids.

Continuous chronic pain syndromes in MS patients are often treated with antidepressants such as amitriptyline (Elavil) with some success. TENS units have been used to treat chronic MS pain. For patients with spasticity, baclofen (Lioresal) is the drug of choice to improve function and comfort. In patients with intractable spasticity, an implanted pump can deliver a continuous infusion of baclofen into the spinal fluid through a tiny tunneled catheter. Although baclofen is a muscle relaxant, it has been found to work directly on nerve pathways and has a low incidence of side effects.

The back pain of MS has been treated a number of ways, including the use of antispasticity drugs, NSAIDs, physical therapy, and wheelchair supports and cushions.

Some MS patients have undergone a surgical procedure for the implantation of an electric stimulator in the spinal cord. This treatment has been found ineffective and sometimes dangerous and is therefore not recommended. For rare cases of intractable pain and spasticity, nerve roots that carry sensation have been cut (dorsal rhizotomy), as well as tendons (tenotomy). These are irreversible procedures and are only performed when all other therapies have failed.

Patients may benefit most from a multidisciplinary approach to the management of their pain. There may be a role for the use of opioids and a variety of other approaches to the management of pain in the patient with MS.

Resources

The National Multiple Sclerosis Society
    733 Third Avenue
    New York, NY 10017
    (800) Fight-MS ([800] 344-4867)
    E-mail: *info@nmss.org.*

References

The National Multiple Sclerosis Society Web site: *www.nmss.org*
Rudick RA: Multiple sclerosis and related conditions. In Bennett JC, Plum F, editors: *Cecil textbook of medicine*, ed 20, pp 2106-2113, Philadelphia, 1996, WB Saunders.

PHANTOM LIMB PAIN

Definition/Cause

Phantom pain can occur after the removal of a body part and is very common after the removal or loss of a limb or breast. The focus here is pain after the loss of a limb. Up to 100% of amputees have "phantom sensations." These phantom sensations may include a pleasant tingling sensation or the perception of motion of the absent limb, which may affect balance. Phantom limb pain occurs in up to 85% of limb amputees. The incidence of phantom limb pain is significantly higher in patients who had preoperative pain in that limb. Research on the cause of phantom sensations and pain is ongoing. It is believed that the brain can act in the absence of input from an extremity. Another theory proposes that phantom sensa-

tions and pain arise in the periphery, especially in the amputated stump. Some researchers believe that these sensations are like hallucinations and arise from the sufferer's psyche.

Pain Characteristics

The intensity and frequency of phantom pain varies greatly among amputees. Those with phantom limb pain typically suffer burning, cramping, or shocking/shooting qualities of pain. Treatment differs according to the quality of the pain. Amputees are often reluctant to report phantom pain for fear of being thought insane. In a study of 2700 veteran amputees, 69% reported that their physicians directly or indirectly told them that it was "just in their heads."

Pain Management

Phantom pain is exceedingly difficult to treat effectively after it has persisted for longer than 1 year. Many interventions have been tried, mostly without success.

The most promising and successful treatment to date is prevention. Preemptive intervention 1 to 3 days before amputation with an infusion of epidural opioids and/or local anesthetic has been shown to minimize and in many cases eliminate postoperative pain and later phantom pain in amputees.

Biofeedback techniques have been helpful as an adjunct to medications. For example, the use of muscle relaxant medications and muscle tension biofeedback has been effective for cramping pain; vasodilators and the use of temperature biofeedback are useful for burning-type pain. Long-term opioids are effective for some patients, allowing them to function and perform activities of daily living. Other options include sympathetic blocks, which may provide minimal or transitory relief. Surgical neurolysis has been used, but it is high risk and may actually increase pain.

When examining treatment options with the patient, it is important to share realistic expectations for relief. It is misleading to tell patients that their pain is likely to go away.

Resources

National Amputation Foundation (NAF)
    73 Church St.
    Malverne, NY 11565
    (516) 887-3600

The amputee's guide to the amputation and the recovery process available from the Department of Orthopedics, Madigan Army Medical Center, Tacoma, WA 98431-5000. (Reprinted in Sherman RA: *Phantom pain*, New York, 1997, Plenum Press.)

References

Bach S, Noreng MF, Tjellden NU: Phantom limb pain in amputees during the first 12 months following limb amputation, after postoperative lumbar epidural blockade, *Pain* 33:297-301, 1988.

Jensen TS, Rasmussen P: Phantom pain and other phenomena after amputation. In Portenoy RK, Kanner RM, editors: *Pain management: theory and practice,* pp 651-665, Philadelphia, 1996, FA Davis.

Sherman RA: *Phantom pain,* New York, 1997, Plenum Press.

POSTMASTECTOMY PAIN

Definition/Cause

Injury to the intercostobrachial nerve with axillary dissection is the most common cause of the pain after mastectomy. This injury results in neuropathic pain in the distribution of the nerve to the axilla and the medial aspect of the arm. Other nerves in the chest wall may be injured as well. Causes of pain not related to the surgery might include radiation from another area and metastasis of the cancer as to the ribs.

Research shows that patients who have undergone autologous reconstruction have the same incidence of pain as those patients who have not had reconstruction. When implants are used, however, the incidence of pain is increased. Patients who have undergone autologous reconstruction, such as with an abdominal flap, also report abdominal pain as a problem. This may be caused by damage to the nerves that serve the flap.

The incidence of postmastectomy pain is as high as 28%, starting 2 weeks to 6 months after the removal of the breast. Of the 10% to 64% of women reporting phantom sensations after mastectomy, about 80% of those sensations are said to be painful to some degree. If the patient had breast pain before its removal, the incidence of postmastectomy pain is higher.

Pain Characteristics/Assessment

Postmastectomy pain is neuropathic in nature and may be described as burning, stinging, electric, or shooting. This type of pain may be worse at night or with activity. Allodynia, or pain elicited by a normally nonpainful stimulus such as light touch, may be present. Dysesthesia may also occur, which is an unpleasant sensation that occurs with little outside stimulus.

Patients who report pain after insertion of implants describe sharp pain around the area of the implant. This pain may be due to nerve compression from fibrosis around the implant itself.

Pain Management

Treatment for the management of postmastectomy pain may involve a trial of many pharmacologic and nonpharmacologic options.

Topical application of capsaicin cream three to four times per day can be used. This cream burns at first, but this subsides with continued use. TENS units and acupuncture have been used with success in some patients.

Tricyclic antidepressants (TCAs) are often the treatment of choice for neuropathic postmastectomy pain. The choice of TCA depends on the patient's sleep pattern and tolerance. If the patient has difficulty sleeping, a sedating antidepressant such as amitriptyline may be appropriate. If sleep is not a problem, a less sedating TCA like nortriptyline may be a better choice.

For pain that is maintained by the sympathetic nervous system, α_1-blockers, such as prazosin (Minipress) and terazocin (Hytrin), titrated to effect have been effective. α_2-agonists such as clonidine (Catapres) may improve postmastectomy pain by blocking the release of norepinephrine and inhibiting the central pain pathways. Baclofen (Lioresal), an antispasmodic, is also known to be effective for neuropathic pain. Improvement should be seen in 2 weeks if these treatments are effective.

Opioids may be beneficial and should be tried but are often not effective alone for neuropathic pain.

Resources

Managing cancer pain. Patient guide

Available from:

AHCPR Publications Clearinghouse
P.O. Box 8547
Silver Spring, MD 20907
(800) 4-CANCER

References

Irving GA, Wallace MS: Postmastectomy and post-breast-surgery pain. In *Pain management for the practicing physician,* ed 1, pp 209-216, New York, 1997, Churchill Livingstone.

Mauskop A: Painful neuropathies. In Lefkowitz M, Lebovits AH, editors: *A practical approach to pain management,* pp 228-232, New York, 1996, Little, Brown & Co.

POSTPOLIO SYNDROME

Definition/Cause

Some patients who have had poliomyelitis experience further deterioration later in life. Postpolio syndrome (PPS) is manifested by an insidious onset of progressive weakness beginning 30 or more years after the initial attack of acute poliomyelitis. Approximately 20% to 30% of previously paralyzed patients are affected by PPS. The weakness of PPS usually affects the already weak muscles but may involve muscles not previously affected. Some patients experience a neuromuscular problem called postpolio progressive muscular atrophy (PPMA). New progressive weakness is the primary symptom of PPMA, and it may be accompanied by new atrophy. Fatigue is the most prominent symptom experienced by individuals with PPS.

Most polio survivors in the United States are between 45 and 60 years of age and are among the growing aging population that will require extensive health care resources.

Pain Characteristics

The pain involved in PPS is related to the instabilities of the musculoskeletal system. This musculoskeletal pain is often the result of long-term overstress of joints because of residual weakness that leads to joint deterioration. There can be progressive scoliosis, poor posture, deformed joints, and uneven limb size contributing to the stress on the musculoskeletal system and pain in patients with PPS. Pain from tendons that have been stressed because of joint deformities from long-standing muscle weakness is common. Individuals often experience muscle pain from overuse of weak muscles or overcompensation with another muscle, joint, or extremity. Scar tissue that has entrapped nerve tissue can also be a source of pain in the PPS patient. PPS patients are commonly intolerant to cold. All this pain and stress on the muscles, tendons, and joints can lead to immobility, requiring a return to previously used assistive devices.

PPS patients also have an increased risk for fractures in their affected limbs.

Assessment

Patients with PPS may have had pain for such a long time it can be difficult to differentiate the pains that they do have. A careful assessment includes their description of the pain and its qualities, whether muscle spasms are present or if the pain is burning, tingling, sharp, or stabbing. The assessment of laboratory values in patients with PPS may reveal a slight increase in muscle enzyme levels from overuse of muscles or at times a mildly elevated protein level in the CSF; otherwise laboratory studies are usually normal. Electromyelography shows signs of denervation with or without new areas of weakness but is not specific to PPS patients. Muscle biopsies can be done to help distinguish between existing and new muscle weakness.

It is important to rule out the possibility that the weakness, fatigue, and pain experienced by the PPS patient could be caused by a different disease.

Pain Management

The treatment of pain in the PPS patient may include a variety of measures. It is important for the patient with PPS to listen to his or her own body and slow down. Historically, PPS patients have focused on maximum exertion and working through pain. This became a lifelong characteristic of polio survivors. They also are generally well-educated, high-achieving individuals. Lifestyle adjustments allowing for periods of rest interspersed with periods of activity may be necessary. Activities that decrease stress on joints and muscles, such as swimming in a warm pool, assist in controlling pain. Strengthening exercises that are nonfatiguing or those that are of short duration and submaximal in effectiveness over time have been shown to improve strength. Heat and massage are helpful nondrug treatments. PPS patients frequently use assistive and supportive devices. Supportive care and symptomatic relief are primary considerations for treatment along with preventing the overuse of joints and muscles. Patients should be advised to stop or take a break from activity that produces pain or fatigue.

NSAIDs are commonly prescribed for relief of pain in the patient with PPS. Opioids and muscle relaxants are not commonly used because of the increased risk of respiratory depression in these patients. Whenever the use of these drugs is necessary, as with surgery, caution must be exercised and short-acting agents should be used.

Surgical intervention for the relief of pain and deformity is sometimes necessary. Procedures to improve function include muscle transfers, tendon lengthening, and osteotomy. Positioning of the patient during surgical procedures is extremely important, as well as the careful use of opioids and anesthetic agents as previously mentioned.

Resources

Polio network news, an international newsletter for polio survivors, available through:

> The International Polio Network
> 4207 Lindell Boulevard, Suite 110
> St. Louis, MO, 63108
> (314) 534-0475

Reviewed by John Smith, Birmingham, Ala, a post-polio patient.

References

Habel M, Strong P: Providing excellent care for patients with post-polio syndrome part I and part II, *Nurseweek,* pp 10-11, Jan 20, 1997, and Feb 3, 1997.
Jubelt B, Drucker J: Post-polio syndrome: an update, *Semin Neuro* 13(3):283-290, 1993.

POSTTHORACOTOMY PAIN
Definition/Cause

Patients who have undergone major thoracic surgery experience severe pain in the immediate postoperative period requiring aggressive intervention; 26% to 67% have pain that continues for 6 months or longer. Many of those (estimated to be 9% to 66%) require medical intervention. This lasting pain is usually a result of surgical trauma to the intercostal nerve during rib retraction and is often unavoidable. Even though the cause of postthoracotomy pain is usually evident, it can be very difficult to treat.

Other causes of postthoracotomy pain include pain along the scar, including the development of neuromas, and myofascial pain of the chest wall. It is important to rule out tumor recurrence as the cause of the pain.

Pain Characteristics

Pain is excruciating in the immediate postoperative period and, if left untreated or undertreated, may severely compromise the patient's pulmonary status and delay recovery. The most characteristic chronic pain of postthoracotomy patients is intermittent, severe, lancinating pain.

Other forms of chronic pain that postthoracotomy patients experience, such as neuromas along the surgical scar, may be acutely painful to the touch. They may also experience burning sensations or dysesthesias.

Assessment

Assessment requires a focus on the individual characteristics of the patient's pain. The immediate postoperative pain should subside as healing takes place. If pain recurs after a pain-free period, it is important to rule out the possibility of tumor recurrence. If the patient is found to be cancer free, the pain is usually neuropathic in nature.

Pain Management

The acute postoperative pain is most effectively treated with epidural opioids, with or without local anesthetics such as bupivicaine.

The chronic pain syndromes of postthoracotomy patients are more difficult to treat and may require a variety of interventions. Tricyclic antidepressants (TCAs) are often the treatment of choice. If the patient has difficulty sleeping, a sedating antidepressant such as amitriptyline may be appropriate. If sleep is not a problem, a less sedating TCA like nortriptyline may be a better choice.

Sometimes TENS units and acupuncture provide effective relief of postthoracotomy pain. The application of capsaicin cream to the scar can be effective for the treatment of pain in that area. Capsaicin usually burns at first, but this symptom subsides with repeated applications.

For pain that is maintained by the sympathetic nervous system, alpha$_1$-blockers, such as prazosin (Minipress) and terazocin (Hytrin), titrated to effect have been effective. Alpha$_2$-agonists such as clonidine (Catapres) may relieve postthoracotomy pain by blocking the release of norepinephrine and inhibiting the central pain pathways. Baclofen (Lioresal), an antispasmodic, is also known to be effective for neuropathic pain. Improvement should be seen in 2 weeks if these treatments are effective.

Opioids may be beneficial. Many patients do well with long-term use of opioids.

Resources

American Chronic Pain Association
P.O. Box 850
Rocklin, CA 95677
(916) 632-0922

National Chronic Pain Outreach Association
7979 Old Georgetown Road
Suite 100
Bethesda, MD 20814-2429

References

Irving GA, Wallace MS: *Post-thoracotomy pain management for the practicing physician*, pp 217-221, New York, 1997, Churchill Livingstone.

Mauskop A: Painful neuropathies. In Lefkowitz M, Lebovits AH, editors: *A practical approach to pain management*, pp 228-232, New York, 1996, Little, Brown & Co.

SPINAL CORD INJURY
Definition/Cause

Pain is a common and difficult problem for patients with spinal cord injuries (SCIs). The pain experienced by these patients varies in quality and generally falls into one of three categories: mechanical or acute pain related to the physical nature of the injury or some other primary disease process; radicular pain associated with injury to nerve tissue; or the most common and often disabling, dysesthetic pain, also called "central pain," which is most often perceived below the level of the injury. Pain after SCI is more often a problem after an incomplete injury of the spinal cord such as a gunshot wound to the spine or a spine injury that has not been surgically stabilized. Patients with complete or total SCI such as transection may not experience chronic pain as much as those with incomplete injury. Complete SCI has been associated with phantom pain, however.

Pain Characteristics

The pain experienced by the patient with an SCI may be mild to severe and disabling, and often interferes with the performance of activities of daily living.

Most often the pain experienced by spinal cord-injured patients is felt internally or in the lower extremities. Dysesthetic pain syndrome is the most common of the pain syndromes associated with SCI, and it is often described as burning, piercing, radiating, or tightness. Dysesthetic pain syndrome usually presents within 1 year of the injury. The role of the level of injury and completeness of the lesion in the development of dysesthetic pain syndrome is somewhat controversial.

Acute or mechanical pain is usually described as a sharp pain localized to the area of injury. Radicular pain is more difficult to characterize and variable, but it tends to follow a dermatomal path.

Assessment

The assessment of pain in the patient with SCI is difficult because of the coexisting problems and the psychologic impact of the SCI itself. Pain is associated with an element of suffering, as is the SCI itself. Dysesthetic pain syndrome affects a fairly small group of individuals, but it has a profound effect on their quality of life. Assessment of pain in the patient with SCI begins with a history, including factors that influence the pain (What makes it better? What makes it worse?), pain ratings, questions about coping responses and functional status, a medical evaluation, and a psychologic evaluation. Involve the patient in monitoring his or her own behavior related to the pain experience. Integration of the neurologic, functional, and rehabilitation factors that may affect the SCI patient will assist with complete assessment and providing appropriate pain care. Additional research is needed to understand the mechanism of pain below the level of the injury.

Pain Management

A variety of treatments have been used in an attempt to alleviate the pain experienced by the patient with SCI, most of which have shown little promise. Treatments that have been used include TENS units, biofeedback, acupuncture, implanted dorsal column stimulators, and a variety of analgesic medications. Because of the limited success of treatment of SCI-related pain, it is still best to start with the conservative treatments before moving on to more invasive surgical options. Treatment options include (1) general health promotion and relief from exacerbating factors; (2) nonopioid drug treatments (NSAIDs and acetaminophen, tricyclic antidepressants, anticonvulsants); (3) physical treatments (physical and occupational therapy aimed at improving function and preventing deformity); (4) surgical procedures (neuroablative procedures such as dissection of a nerve root: rhizotomy); and (5) opioid therapy. The most effective treatments are promoted by an interdisciplinary team, including physicians with experience in pain management, rehabilitation nursing staff, psychologists, and physical, occupational, and recreational therapists.

Resources

Spinal Cord Injury Hotline, (800) 526-3456, through the Spine and Nerve Center at Massachusetts General Hospital/Harvard.

On the internet:
neurosurgery.mgh.harvard.edu/spine-hp.htm.

References

Balazy TE: Clinical management of chronic pain in spinal cord injury, *Clin J Pain* 8:102-110, 1992.

Davidoff G, Roth E, Guarracini M et al.: Function-limiting dysesthetic pain syndrome among traumatic spinal cord injury patients: a cross-sectional study, *Pain* 29:39-48, 1987.

Mariano AF: Chronic pain and spinal cord injury, *Clin J Pain* 8:87-92, 1992.

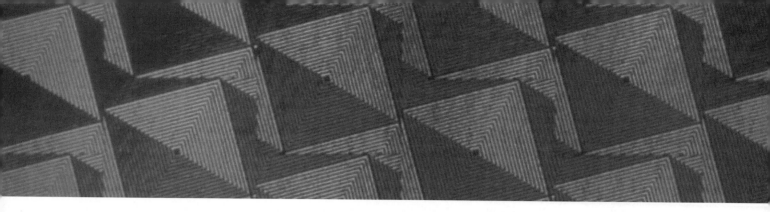

chapter thirteen

PREGNANCY, CHILDBIRTH, POSTPARTUM, AND BREAST FEEDING
Use of Analgesics

Robin Britt and Chris Pasero

CHAPTER OUTLINE

TERMINOLOGY

Abstinence syndrome: A manifestation of physical dependence; occurrence of withdrawal symptoms when the opioid is abruptly stopped or an opioid antagonist is given.

Antenatal: Occurring before or formed before birth.

Dystocia: Prolonged, painful, or otherwise difficult delivery.

Involution: Return of uterus to prepregnancy size and condition.

Multigravida: Woman who has been pregnant two or more times.

Multipara: Woman who has carried two or more pregnancies to viability, whether they have ended in live births or stillbirths.

"Natural childbirth": Term applied generally to the exclusive use of nondrug methods and no analgesics or anesthetics for pain during childbirth.

Nulliparous: Woman who has not yet carried a pregnancy to viability.

Perinatal: Of or pertaining to the time and process of giving birth.

Preterm: Delivery before 37 weeks' gestational age.

Primigravida: Woman who is pregnant for the first time.

Primipara: Woman who has carried a pregnancy to viability, whether a live or still birth.

Teratogenesis: The origin or mode of the production of a malformed fetus.

Trimester: Time period of 3 months; first, conception to 13 weeks from last menstrual period; second, 13 weeks to 26 weeks from last menstrual period; third, 27 weeks after last menstrual period to delivery of the infant.

Research shows that unrelieved pain in the pregnant patient markedly increases the release of a number of hormones, including cortisol, glucagon, and catecholamines (Bonica, McDonald, 1995) (see Chapter 2). These hormones in turn impose stress, which increases metabolism and oxygen consumption. Most important, a prolonged increase in stress hormones, particularly catecholamines, has been shown to cause uterine hypoperfusion and decrease placental blood flow. This can result in uterine irritability and preterm labor, dystocia, and/or fetal asphyxia. In addition, pain can suppress breast milk production and hinder breast feeding and maternal-infant bonding. The goal of perinatal pain management is to find a balance between relief of pain for the mother and the degree of risk to her, the fetus, or the infant (Benedetti, 1995).

This chapter discusses the various types of pain women experience during pregnancy, childbirth, postpartum, and breast feeding. It presents analgesics and techniques that can be used safely and those that should be avoided during these times. Also included is the management of pain unrelated to or exacerbated by pregnancy. Controversies regarding the use of both pharmacologic and nondrug interventions are addressed. Selected terms and definitions are listed under Terminology at the beginning of this chapter to facilitate an understanding of the content. Misconceptions related to the use of analgesics during pregnancy, childbirth, postpartum, and breast feeding are presented in Table 13.1. Box 13.1 lists resources available to both consumers and clinicians for obtaining information on pain and its management during pregnancy, childbirth, postpartum, and breast feeding.

PAIN MANAGEMENT DURING PREGNANCY

Pain management can be complicated in women who are pregnant because nearly all drugs they take eventually reach the fetus/infant. One of the main issues to consider in the use of analgesics during pregnancy is their potential to increase vascular resistance or decrease placental blood flow. Another important consideration is an analgesic's potential to cause transient or permanent harm to the fetus or infant. Although adverse reproductive and developmental events can occur at any time during gestation, the most susceptible time for teratogenesis (fetal deformity) to occur is during the third through the twelfth week after implantation, when the embryo's organs are developing (postimplantation organogenesis) (Ward, Mirkin, 1994).

Studies of analgesic use during pregnancy are limited or lacking because of concerns about producing maternal, fetal, or infant harm during trials. Some drugs are not recommended for use during pregnancy, not because they have been found to produce harm but because they have not been studied adequately.

Under the Federal Food, Drug, and Cosmetic Act, the Food and Drug Administration (FDA) has responsibility for ensuring that prescription drugs and biologic products are accompanied by labeling that contains narrative information on the drug's teratogenic effects, other effects on reproduction and pregnancy, and, when relevant, effects on later growth, development, and functional maturation of the child. The regulation also requires that each product be classified under one of five pregnancy categories (A, B, C, D, or X) on the basis of risk of adverse reproductive and developmental effects or, for certain categories, on the

TABLE 13.1 ● ● ● ● ●

Misconceptions	Use of Analgesics During Pregnancy, Childbirth, Postpartum, and Breast Feeding
MISCONCEPTION	CORRECTION
1. Pregnancy, childbirth, and breast feeding are natural processes that are not painful.	Pregnancy, childbirth, and breast feeding are accompanied by varying degrees of pain, ranging in intensity from mild to excruciating.
2. Taking any medication during pregnancy will produce fetal deformity.	Many medications, including analgesics, have been studied for use during pregnancy without evidence of risk for causing fetal deformity or transient or permanent harm. Some drugs are not recommended for use during pregnancy, not because they have been found to produce harm but because they have not been studied adequately.
3. The use of any analgesics during pregnancy, childbirth, or breast feeding is more harmful than the pain.	A number of analgesics, including acetaminophen and many of the opioids and adjuvant drugs, can be taken safely during pregnancy, childbirth, and breast feeding. Unrelieved pain, on the other hand, has several very harmful effects, including uterine hypoperfusion, preterm labor, suppression of breast milk production, and interference with maternal-infant bonding.
4. It is unsafe to use opioid analgesics on a long-term basis to treat severe pain during pregnancy (e.g., in patients with sickle cell crises, burns, or trauma).	No well-controlled studies suggest a relationship between fetal malformations and exposure to any opioids. The best evidence that long-term opioid use does not result in fetal harm is that no higher incidence of congenital abnormalities has been found in babies born to addicted mothers than in those born to nonaddicted mothers. Appropriate supportive and medical therapies (gradual tapering of opioid) for infants born to mothers receiving long-term opioid treatment results in little short-term consequence to these infants.
5. Nondrug methods (i.e., "natural childbirth") are sufficient for pain relief during labor and delivery.	Although nondrug methods can be effective in helping the woman in labor relax, few well-controlled studies demonstrate that these methods actually reduce pain. Many women experience excruciating pain with the exclusive use of nondrug methods during labor. As with the management of other types of pain, the use of nondrug interventions should complement, not replace, pharmacologic interventions for the management of labor and delivery pain.

May be duplicated for use in clinical practice. From McCaffery M, Pasero C: *Pain: Clinical manual,* p. 610. Copyright © 1999, Mosby, Inc.

basis of such risk weighed against potential benefit. Each drug manufacturer assigns a pregnancy category, which is then examined by the FDA review panel (Box 13.2).

According to a public hearing held late in 1997 (FDA Public Hearing, Sept 12, 1997), the current FDA categories appear to be misleading and may not accurately reflect reproductive and developmental risk. A comprehensive evaluation of the FDA process for assessing reproductive and developmental toxicities and how this information is communicated to clinicians is underway. At the time of this publication, the FDA is seeking public comment and conducting a preliminary review of the pregnancy category designations for marketing drugs. Until clearer guidelines are established, it is recommended that clinicians also consult references and resources like the ones provided in Box 13.3 when selecting analgesics for their patients during pregnancy and breast feeding.

Maternal-Placental-Fetal Drug Transfer

The placenta is an endocrine organ. It transfers nutrients to and waste away from the fetus, and it also functions as an organ of metabolism and respiration for the fetus. For years, the placenta was thought to provide a protective barrier similar to the blood-brain barrier. However, it is now known that the placenta acts as a simple membrane and is not a highly selective barrier for the fetus against substances taken during pregnancy (Spencer, 1993).

The placental cell membrane is composed of lipids (fats) combined with proteins. Drugs cross the placental cell membrane by means of diffusion; the more lipid soluble the drug, the easier and faster it can cross the membrane (Bissonnette, 1995). The electrical charge of a drug molecule also influences how rapidly it can cross the placental membrane. Uncharged (nonionized) drugs usually are lipophilic and rapidly penetrate the placental cell membrane (Benet, Kroetz, Sheiner, 1996; Wong, Sundin,

BOX 13.1

Resources for Materials Containing Information on Pain and Pain Management During Pregnancy, Childbirth, Postpartum, and Breast Feeding

- Childbirth Graphics
  A Division of WRS Group, Inc.
  P.O. Box 21207
  Waco, TX 21207
  Telephone: (800) 299-3366, extension 287
  Fax: (888) 977-7653
  E-mail: sales@wrsgroup.com
  Web site: http://www.wrsgroup.com

  Free catalog with extensive list of resources related to childbirth and childbirth education for consumers and professionals. Includes charts, brochures, slides, and posters related to pain management and prevention during pregnancy, childbirth, postpartum, and breast feeding. Also lists titles of obstetric analgesia/anesthesia references.

- La Leche League International
  9616 Minneapolis Ave.
  P.O. Box 1209
  Franklin Park, IL 60131-8209
  Telephone: (800) LaLeche (525-3243)
         or (708) 455-7730

  Free material on nondrug and alternative pain management techniques during breast feeding, including information on correct technique and management of problems, such as breast engorgement and nipple pain.

- March of Dimes Birth Defects Foundation
  (inquire about materials available)
  1275 Mamaroneck Ave.
  White Plains, NY 10605
  Telephone: (914) 428-7100
  Fax: (914) 997-4410
  Web site: http//www.modimes.org

- March of Dimes Birth Defects Foundation
  (warehouse for ordering materials)
  P.O. Box 1657
  Wilkes-Barre, PA 10605
  Telephone: (800) 367-6630
  Fax: (717) 825-1987

  Numerous free consumer and professional brochures, handouts, and videos related to the use of medications during pregnancy.

May be duplicated for use in clinical practice. From McCaffery M, Pasero C: *Pain: Clinical manual*, p. 611. Copyright © 1999, Mosby, Inc.

Box 13.1 lists resources available for both consumers and professionals.

BOX 13.2 **FDA Pregnancy Risk Classification Categories for Medications Used in Pain Management**

Category A: Well-controlled studies in pregnant women show no fetal risk (e.g., multivitamins).
Category B: No evidence of risk in human studies or animal studies are negative (e.g., ibuprofen, morphine).
Category C: Risk cannot be ruled out because human studies are lacking and animal studies are either lacking or demonstrate fetal risk. However, potential benefits may justify potential risk (e.g., aspirin, lidocaine).
Category D: Positive evidence of risk as demonstrated by investigation or postmarketing data; however, the potential benefits may outweigh the potential risks (e.g., diazepam, phenytoin).
Category X: Contraindicated in pregnancy; animal and human studies (investigational or postmarketing data) show fetal risk that clearly outweighs any benefit to the patient.

May be duplicated for use in clinical practice. As appears in McCaffery M, Pasero C: *Pain: Clinical manual*, p. 611, 1999, Mosby, Inc.

FDA, Food and Drug Administration.

Drugs have been categorized by the FDA according to their potential to cause teratogenic effects. Opioids are classified category D when used for prolonged periods or in large doses near term.

Modified from *Federal Register* 44:37434-37467, 1980; in Rathmell JP, Viscomi CM, Asburn MA: Management of nonobstetric pain during pregnancy and lactation, *Anesth Analg* 85:1074-1087, 1997.

1995). Drugs with high molecular weight are slowly diffused (Ward, Mirkin, 1994). For example, heparin and insulin do not pass readily through the placental membrane because they are large molecular weight drugs (see Chapter 6 for more on the pharmacokinetics of drugs). Almost all opioid analgesics and nonsteroidal antiinflammatory drugs (NSAIDs) pass readily through the placental membrane. Figure 13.1 depicts drug disposition in the maternal-placental-fetal unit.

Analgesic Use During Pregnancy

Traditionally, clinicians instruct pregnant patients with pain to use nondrug pain–relieving measures and caution against the use of analgesics. In fact, after the clinician confirms pregnancy, the first warning given to the patient usually is to take no medications for pain except acetaminophen during the pregnancy. However, a number of analgesics can be taken safely during this time. Following are comments about selected analgesics as they relate to use during pregnancy. For more on specific analgesics, see Chapters 5, 6, and 7.

Acetaminophen and nonsteroidal antiinflammatory drugs

Acetaminophen is considered to be safe for use during pregnancy in therapeutic doses. Although less effective than NSAIDs, acetaminophen has no known teratogenic

References and Resources for Clinicians Selecting Analgesics and Other Drugs for Their Patients During Pregnancy and Lactation

- Briggs GG, Freeman RKD, Yaffe SJ: *A reference guide to fetal and neonatal risk: Drugs in pregnancy and lactation,* ed 4, Baltimore, 1994, Williams & Wilkins.

  This reference guide presents much of the existing research regarding the teratogenic, reproductive, and developmental effects of a variety of drugs in the fetus/neonate/infant when taken during pregnancy and lactation. The drug evaluations weigh the therapeutic effects of the various drugs against their potential to cause harm to the fetus/neonate/infant.

- The *Federal Register*

  The *Federal Register* reports all FDA actions and can be found on line by GPO access at Web site address: *http://www.wais.access.gpo.gov.* The FDA hearing September 12, 1997, which initiated the evaluation of the current pregnancy labeling categories, can be found in its entirety at this Web site.

- The Food and Drug Administration (FDA)

  The FDA provides press releases, copies of lectures, and back issues of the publication *FDA Consumer.* It also has a list of recently approved drugs. The web site URL is *http://www.fda.gov/*

- Friedman JM, Polifka JE: *Teratogenic effects of drugs: A resource guide for clinicians (TERIS),* Baltimore, 1994, The Johns Hopkins University Press.

  This book compiles the research data on numerous drugs. A risk assessment for use during pregnancy, based on a consensus of ratings from the authors and five internationally recognized authorities in clinical teratology, is provided for each drug and agent in the book.

- Scialli AR, Lione A, Boyle Padgett GK: *Reproductive effects of chemical, physical and biologic agents,* p. 891, Baltimore, 1995, The Johns Hopkins University Press.

  This book provides information on the reproductive toxicology of more than 2800 physical and chemical agents. Summaries of agents include their effects on male and female fertility, embryonic and fetal development, and breast feeding infants when taken by women during lactation.

- Shephard TH: *Catalog of teratogenic agents,* ed 8, Baltimore, 1995, The Johns Hopkins University Press.

  This catalog is a comprehensive compilation of animal and human research from countries worldwide on the teratogenicity of more than 2500 chemical and environmental agents.

On-line Computerized Databases

- The Organization of Teratology Information Services (OTIS) is a comprehensive state-by-state listing of Teratology Information Service (TIS) organizations that is available at URL:*http://orpheus.ucsd.edu/otis.* Member programs of OTIS are located throughout the United States and Canada, and a collaborative relationship exists with the European Network of Teratology Information Services (ENTIS). Services are free and vary among programs. Some provide extensive services, including on-line consultation regarding agent exposure during pregnancy. OTIS also compiles "fact sheets" on various agents, which can be obtained on line free of charge. Many TIS groups provide free TERIS summaries.

- REPRORISK is a commercially based system produced by Micromedix, Inc., in Denver, Colorado, and consists of a CD-ROM program that contains electronic versions of *REPROTEXT, the Reproductive Hazard Reference* by Betty Dabney, and *REPROTOX, Reproductive Hazard Information* by Anthony R. Scialli, which is a frequently updated version of *Reproductive effects of chemical, physical and biologic agents* (see earlier entry). Micromedex, Inc. can be reached at (800) 525-9083 or at URL: *http://www.micromedex.com.*

- Teratogen Information Service (TERIS) is designed to assist health care professionals in assessing the teratogenic risk associated with various drugs and other agents during pregnancy. It consists of a series of agent summaries, each based on a thorough review of published clinical and experimental literature. Summaries include a risk assessment derived by consensus of an advisory board comprised of nationally recognized authorities in clinical teratology. Summaries can be accessed by generic, domestic, or foreign proprietary names. TERIS provides the on-line version of the *Catalog of teratogenic agents* (see previous entry). At present, subscribers must pay $1000/year for access to the database.

- The Teratology Society provides links and information to TIS groups and is available at URL: *http://www.teratology.org.*

- The TERIS Program at the University of Washington in Seattle, Washington also has a Web site entitled the Clinical Teratology Web at URL: *http://weber.u.washington.edu/~terisweb/teris/index.html.* This site offers links to computerized databases, teratology information services, lactation information, training programs, organizations, societies, meetings, resources, and books related to teratology.

Box 13.3 provides resources that clinicians may find helpful for evaluating the effects of various drugs and other agents when taken during pregnancy and lactation.

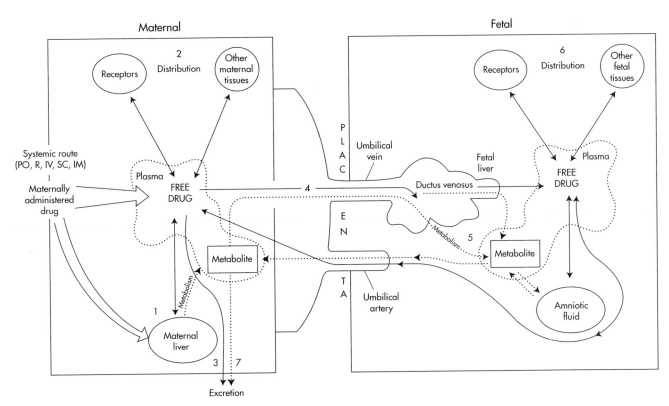

May be duplicated for use in clinical practice. As appears in McCaffery M, Pasero C: *Pain: Clinical manual*, p. 613, 1999, Mosby, Inc.
IM, intramuscular; *IV,* intravenous; *PO,* oral; *R,* rectal; *SC,* subcutaneous.

●●●●● FIGURE 13.1 **Drug disposition in the maternal-placental-fetal unit.** This figure depicts the processes involved in the transfer of drug to the fetus after maternal systemic administration: (1) maternal liver metabolism of drug and metabolite formation; (2) distribution of drug to maternal tissues and drug receptors; (3) maternal elimination of drug; (4) transfer of drug and metabolites across the placental membrane; (5) fetal drug metabolism and metabolite formation; (6) distribution of drug to fetal tissues and drug receptors; (7) fetal elimination of drug.

Redrawn from Mirkin BL: Drug distribution in pregnancy. In Boreus L, editor: *Fetal pharmacology,* New York, 1973, Raven Press.

effects, relatively few side effects, and does not inhibit prostaglandin synthesis or platelet function (Viscomi, Rathmell, 1998) (see Chapter 5).

NSAIDs generally are not recommended for use during pregnancy. Short-term use is probably safe (Viscomi, Rathmell, 1998). However, a literature review revealed a few reports about maternal use of indomethacin being associated with renal failure in the newborn (Merry, Power, 1995). Indomethacin given to treat preterm labor has been linked to premature antenatal closure of the fetal ductus arteriosus (Viscomi, Rathmell, 1998).

The relationship between aspirin (salicylate) and congenital effects is controversial (Briggs, Freeman, Yaffe, 1994). Large trials examining the use of low-dose (80 mg/day) aspirin during pregnancy to prevent preeclampsia point to its safety (Collaborative Low-Dose Aspirin Study in Pregnancy [CLASP], Collaborative Group, 1994). Although no evidence exists that moderate doses of aspirin damage the fetus, even during the first trimester (Viscomi, Rathmell, 1998), long-term use is associated with reduced birth weight (Insel, 1996). Still,

aspirin is the drug of choice in pregnant women with rheumatoid arthritis; with carefully titrated doses, deleterious effects can be managed (Bonica, 1995a). In general, avoiding chronic use or intermittent high doses of aspirin during pregnancy is recommended (Briggs, Freeman, Yaffe, 1994). Close medical monitoring is warranted if NSAIDs of any kind are used on a long-term basis during pregnancy.

During the third trimester of pregnancy, salicylates, such as aspirin, and other NSAIDs should be avoided because they delay onset of labor, increase the possibility of prepartum and postpartum hemorrhage, and, as mentioned, have a relationship to early ductus arteriosus closure. Misoprostol, a synthetic prostaglandin gastroprotective therapy that is often coadministered with NSAIDs to prevent ulcers, should not be used during pregnancy because it may induce spontaneous abortion (Bjorkman, 1996).

Opioid analgesics

Opioid analgesics have a long history of safely relieving perinatal pain. When opioids are necessary to control pain during pregnancy, the mu opioid agonists, such as morphine, hydromorphone (Dilaudid), fentanyl, methadone, oxycodone, and hydrocodone, are recommended. Animal studies with the newly synthesized receptor-selective opioids have demonstrated that the mu opioid agonists are best tolerated during pregnancy and have the least side effects (Clapp, Kett, Olariu et al., 1998). Although commonly used in obstetrics, agonist-antagonist opioids are not recommended as first-line analgesics for any type of pain and offer no advantages over the mu opioid agonist analgesics (AHCPR, 1992; APS, 1992; Viscomi, Rathmell, 1998) (see Chapter 6, p. 188).

A large collaborative perinatal study found no congenital anomalies occurred in babies born of women who took the opioids hydrocodone, meperidine, methadone, morphine, or oxycodone during pregnancy (Heinomen, Slone, Shapiro, 1977). Anomalies were observed in infants born of women who took the opioids codeine and propoxyphene (Darvon); however, with the exception of respiratory malformation associated with codeine use, the incidence of anomalies was not statistically greater than in the general population (Viscomi, Rathmell, 1998).

Lipophilic (attracted to fatty tissue) opioids, such as fentanyl and sufentanil, traverse the lipoprotein placental membrane faster than hydrophilic (attracted to aqueous solution) opioids, such as morphine and hydromorphone. However, this is of little consequence because almost all opioid analgesics eventually pass through the placental membrane.

Meperidine is widely prescribed for the treatment of pain during pregnancy. However, it is not recommended as a first-line opioid for any type of pain, including perinatal pain. Meperidine produces a toxic metabolite, normeperidine, which can produce irritability, tremors, seizures, and even death (see p. 618, p. 623, and Chapter 6, p. 183).

Local anesthetics often are combined with epidural opioids. Although studies are lacking on the potential for local anesthetics to produce teratogenic effects, bupivacaine (Marcaine) has been used extensively in pregnant surgical patients without posing significant risk. Only mepivacaine has been linked to teratogenic effects; however, the number of patient exposures to this local anesthetic limits the drawing of any conclusions (Viscomi, Rathmell, 1998).

Long-Term Use of Opioids During Pregnancy

Some coexisting conditions (e.g., burns) and chronic diseases (sickle cell disease, HIV) may require extended use of opioid analgesics. No studies could be found that confirm long-term use of opioids during pregnancy to be a safe practice, and all opioids are classified FDA category D when used for prolonged periods or in large doses near term. However, no well-controlled studies suggest a relationship between fetal malformations and exposure to

any opioids. The best evidence that long-term opioid use does not result in fetal harm is that no higher incidence of congenital abnormalities occurs in babies born to addicted mothers than in those born to nonaddicted mothers. For example, no increase in congenital defects has been observed in the offspring of methadone-consuming patients (Viscomi, Rathmell, 1998).

Long-term use of nalbuphine (Nubain) and pentazocine (Talwin) is not recommended during pregnancy because they can precipitate abstinence syndrome in both mother and baby (Rathmell, Viscomi, Ashburn, 1997) (see p. 616 and Chapter 14, pp. 631-632, for management of neonatal abstinence syndrome). When opioid analgesics are used on a long-term basis, it is particularly important to avoid the use of opioids with active metabolites, which can accumulate and produce toxicity. For example, both propoxyphene and meperidine have toxic metabolites and should be avoided.

Adjuvant analgesics

Adjuvant analgesics are used to treat pain of a neuropathic origin (pain that is described as sharp, shooting, burning [e.g., as in reflex sympathetic dystrophy, some chronic back pain]). These include local anesthetics, antidepressants, anticonvulsants, corticosteroids, and benzodiazepines. Following are comments about adjuvant analgesics as they relate to pregnancy. See Chapter 7 for more on the use of adjuvant analgesics.

Local Anesthetics

As mentioned, studies are lacking on the potential for local anesthetics to produce teratogenic effects. Mexiletene and lidocaine, used for some chronic pain syndromes, do not appear to present a significant risk to the fetus, but little data are available to assess the safety of these agents during pregnancy (Briggs, Freeman, Yaffe, 1994).

Antidepressants

Antidepressants are used to treat depression and a number of chronic pain conditions. Most of the selective serotonin reuptake inhibitors (SSRIs) (e.g., sertraline, paroxetine) are classified as FDA category C drugs primarily because animal studies have shown an association between taking the SSRIs and an increase in rat pup deaths during the first few days after birth (*Drug Facts and Comparisons,* 1997). The tricyclic antidepressants, amitriptyline and imipramine, are more effective analgesics but generally are not recommended during pregnancy. However, the benefits of their use may outweigh the risks involved in some cases (Viscomi, Rathmell, 1998).

Antidepressants appear to produce no long-term effects. Global intelligence quotient, language development, and behavioral development in preschool children whose mothers received tricyclic antidepressants or fluoxetine during pregnancy were compared with those of children whose mothers had not been exposed to any agents known to affect the fetus adversely. No significant differences were found between the children (Nulman, Rovey, Stewart et al., 1997).

Anticonvulsants

Most of the data on the potential for fetal harm from the use of anticonvulsants have been taken from infants born of women treated for epilepsy with anticonvulsants. The risk of congenital defects in their offspring was approximately 5%, or twice that of the general population. Although anticonvulsants have been described as having teratogenic risk, epilepsy itself may be responsible for the higher incidence of congenital defects seen in these patients. Research is lacking on the safety during pregnancy of the relatively new anticonvulsant gabapentin (Viscomi, Rathmell, 1998).

Corticosteroids

Most corticosteroids cross the placenta. Prednisone and prednisolone are inactivated by the placenta and have not been linked to fetal malformations (Viscomi, Rathmell, 1998).

Benzodiazepines

Benzodiazepines are used as analgesics for muscle spasm only, and their use during pregnancy can seldom be justified. First trimester use of benzodiazepines may increase the risk of congenital deformities. Diazepam (Valium) has been linked to cleft lip/palate and other abnormalities (Viscomi, Rathmell, 1998).

Pain Related to or Affected by Pregnancy

Addressing pain during pregnancy is extremely important because prolonged unrelieved pain increases the risk of preterm labor and may decrease perfusion to the uterus. Round ligament pain, migraine and nonmigraine headaches, low back pain, pyrosis (heartburn), and Braxton Hicks uterine contractions are among the most common causes of pain related to pregnancy (Martin, Martin, Morrison, 1991).

Round ligament pain

The round ligaments are attached on either side of the uterus just below and in front of the fallopian tubes. These ligaments both hypertrophy and stretch during pregnancy as the uterus rises in the abdomen. This stretching and pressure on the ligaments by the uterus can cause pain. Most clinicians recommend nondrug pain relief measures, including position changes, warm baths, and applications of a heating pad to the lower abdomen (Varney, 1987). Acetaminophen or short-term use of low-dose aspirin, ibuprofen, or naproxen during the first and second trimesters may be helpful (Viscomi, Rathmell, 1998).

Headache

Migraine headaches rarely begin with pregnancy, but they can occur during pregnancy (Viscomi, Rathmell, 1998). Seventy percent of women with a history of migraine headache report improvement or remission with pregnancy, suggesting an estradiol effect (Hainline, 1994).

Treatment of both migraine and nonmigraine headache includes acetaminophen as a first-line drug; aspirin, ibuprofen, or naproxen may be used short term in the first and second trimesters. If pain is unrelieved with these nonopioids, short-term use of hydrocodone in combination with acetaminophen may be helpful. For severe unrelieved headache, parenteral opioids may be necessary (Viscomi, Rathmell, 1998).

Sometimes beta-blockers are used to treat both migraine and nonmigraine vascular headaches. The use of beta-blockers has not been shown to cause an increase in teratogenic effects; however, propranolol is associated with decreased fetal weight (Viscomi, Rathmell, 1998).

Sumatriptan is used extensively for treatment of migraine headache in nonpregnant patients. To date, the birth defect rate associated with the use of sumatriptan is similar to that of the general population (Viscomi, Rathmell, 1998).

Ergotamine is used for treatment of migraine headache; however, it is contraindicated during pregnancy because it has significant teratogenic risk. High doses have caused uterine contractions and abortion (Viscomi, Rathmell, 1998).

Back pain

Back pain is common in pregnancy, so common that many inappropriately consider it to be a normal part of pregnancy that requires no treatment. Three types of back pain are reported by pregnant women: high back pain (10% of pregnant women), low back pain (40%), and sacroiliac pain (50%) (Ostgaard, Andersson, Karlsson, 1991).

Back pain tends to increase in intensity as the pregnancy progresses because of the weight of the uterus and a shift in the center of gravity that predisposes the woman to severe lordosis. Back problems before pregnancy, young age, obesity, and multiparity have been reported to increase the risk of back pain developing during pregnancy (Breen, Ransil, Groves et al., 1994; Ostgaard, Andersson, Karlsson, 1991). The higher incidence in multipara women is thought to be due to less-toned abdominal rectus muscles.

Relief measures for back pain include acetaminophen or short-term use of aspirin, ibuprofen, or naproxen during the first and second trimesters; pelvic tilt and muscle toning exercises; use of good body mechanics; massage; and application of heat or cold to the painful back area. Severe back pain may require treatment with short-term oral or parenteral opioids and physical therapy (Viscomi, Rathmell, 1998).

Pyrosis (heartburn)

In the late second and third trimesters, the hormones relaxin and progesterone can slow gastric motility and cause the cardiac sphincter to relax, resulting in pyrosis (heartburn). Avoiding large, fatty meals and maintaining good posture along with low-sodium antacids may help to prevent and relieve pyrosis. Chewing gum for a half hour before meals (four to five sticks a day) has been found to significantly reduce the frequency and severity of heartburn (Jancin, 1996).

Braxton Hicks contractions

Braxton Hicks contractions are intermittent, infrequent, irregular uterine contractions that typically begin in the third trimester (sometimes earlier in multipara women). They are thought to be caused by the growth of the uterus during pregnancy. The pain intensity of Braxton Hicks contractions is similar to that of labor contractions. Braxton Hicks contractions can be distinguished from labor contractions because Braxton Hicks contractions usually dissipate with ambulation, position change, hydration, and/or use of acetaminophen, whereas labor contractions do not. Women experiencing more than six contractions per hour should be evaluated for preterm labor.

Pain Unrelated to Pregnancy

Some pregnant women have coexisting conditions (e.g., burns) and diseases (e.g., sickle cell disease, arthritis, cardiac disease, HIV, and collagen diseases) that can cause pain and require analgesics. Some diseases are exacerbated by pregnancy, such as cholelithiasis and cholecystitis, and require short-term pain relief. Nonobstetric surgery during pregnancy, which occurs in 0.2% to 2.2% of pregnancies (Martin, Martin, Morrison, 1991), mandates the need for postoperative pain management.

Pain in the pregnant patient with sickle cell disease

In patients with sickle cell disease, vasoocclusive crisis occurs when the sickle-shaped erythrocytes occlude the patient's microvasculature. Crisis is accompanied by sudden attacks of varying intensities of pain. Vasoocclusive crisis is the most common complication during pregnancy in women with sickle cell disease (Viscomi, Rathmell, 1998). Because crises often are precipitated by urinary tract infections, patients are encouraged to maintain hydration with an adequate fluid intake during

pregnancy. Prophylactic blood transfusion sometimes is used to reduce the incidence of severe sickling during pregnancy (Viscomi, Rathmell, 1998).

Management of crises is supportive and symptomatic, beginning with aggressive hydration and pain control by use of a variety of methods depending on the severity of pain. These may include acetaminophen and opioids, transcutaneous electric nerve stimulation (TENS), exercise, splinting, and local heat application. (Cold is contraindicated because it can promote blood cell clumping.)

Intravenous (IV) patient-controlled–analgesia (PCA) opioids frequently are used for pain control during vasoocclusive crisis. The first choice opioid is morphine; fentanyl or hydromorphone is used if morphine is not tolerated. Higher doses than typically used to control postoperative pain often are necessary (Viscomi, Rathmell, 1998). Meperidine should not be used because most patients with sickle cell disease also have some degree of renal insufficiency, which increases the risk of meperidine and normeperidine accumulation (APS, 1992) (see Chapter 6, p. 183).

Low-dose epidural local anesthetics increase microvascular blood flow. This may be particularly beneficial in sickle cell patients with pain localized in the trunk or lower extremities who are unable to tolerate opioids (Viscomi, Rathmell, 1998).

After resolution of vasoocclusive crisis, patients receiving opioids are transitioned to controlled-release oral opioids (e.g., MS Contin, OxyContin). The dose of oral opioid is then tapered over the next several days (Viscomi, Rathmell, 1998). See also quick guide to managing pain related to sickle cell disease, pp. 585-588.

Substance Abuse During Pregnancy

Mothers who abuse substances such as alcohol and opioids during pregnancy warrant monitored treatment for their addiction to prevent withdrawal syndrome. Drug withdrawal is not advisable during the perinatal period (Jacoby, McDonald, 1995). Withdrawal syndrome can predispose women to preterm labor and can cause deleterious stress and possibly uterine hypoperfusion, resulting in fetal asphyxia. Most studies suggest that pregnant women on methadone maintenance and their babies have much better outcomes than untreated opioid abusers (Rathmell, Viscomi, Ashburn, 1997). Withdrawal from opioids after pregnancy is the same as it is for other patients. See Chapter 10 for more on pain management in the substance abuser.

Neonatal abstinence syndrome

Expecting addicted newborns to endure withdrawal syndrome without appropriate treatment is unethical, dangerous, and not recommended. To prevent withdrawal symptoms after birth, opioid doses are tapered very slowly over several days (as low as 10% reduction every third day). These infants require close monitoring during this period. Appropriate supportive and medical therapy of this nature results in few short-term consequences to the infant (Viscomi, Rathmell, 1998). See Chapter 14, pp. 631-632, for management of neonatal abstinence syndrome.

PAIN MANAGEMENT DURING CHILDBIRTH

Incidence and Factors Influencing Childbirth Pain and Suffering

In the past the pain experienced during childbirth was depicted as a comparable experience among women, gradually and predictably worsening as labor progresses. Today it is known that there is wide variability in the location, intensity, quality, and predictability of labor pain (Bonica, 1995a,b; Waldenstrom, Bergman, Vasell, 1996).

Described as severe to excruciating and intolerable by a large number of women, labor pain is considered to be among the most agonizing of pain syndromes (Bonica, 1995a,b; James, 1997; Melzack, 1985). In a classic study Robert Melzack (1984) found that only 10% of primiparas and 24% of multiparas rated their labor pain as mild to moderate; 30% of both groups rated it as severe, and 38% of primiparas and 35% of multiparas reported having extremely severe labor pain and 23% of primiparas and 11% of multiparas rated it as horrible or excruciating. It is estimated that only 1% of women do not feel any labor pain (Waldenstrom, Bergman, Vasell, 1996).

Many factors are thought to contribute to the suffering associated with labor pain. The lack of appropriate analgesic use is perhaps the biggest contributing factor to suffering during childbirth. Others include lack of a support person, hunger, fatigue, and low self-confidence (Bonica, 1995a). The lack of childbirth preparation often is cited as a cause for increased suffering during labor (Simkin, 1995); however, a review of studies comparing labor pain intensity in women who had received childbirth preparation with those who did not showed mixed results (Bonica, 1995a,b; Simkin, 1995). The vast differences between patients in terms of physiologic, emotional, and motivational characteristics and analgesic requirements mandate an individual approach to pain management during childbirth.

Patterns of Labor Pain

Labor pain is nociceptive (a result of normal pain transmission; see Chapter 2). It is often referred to according to the dermatomes (skin areas) innervated by the spinal nerves receiving the noxious stimuli (see Chapter 6, p. 214). For example, during the first stage of labor (0 to 10 cm cervical dilatation), pain is mainly visceral (noxious stimuli are received from the uterus and surrounding structures). The pain of the very early part of the first stage (1 to 3 cm cervical dilatation) affects dermatomes at the thoracic level (T10-T12). As labor progresses to the active phase of the first stage (3 to 4 cm cervical dilatation), sensory input from the cervix increases and the affected dermatomes extend from T10 to low lumbar (L1-L2) (Bonica, 1995a).

Although noxious stimulation arising from the cervix diminishes in the second stage of labor (complete dilatation to delivery), the contractions and distention of the uterus continue to cause pain in the same areas as during the first stage of labor. However, the pain becomes more somatic (musculoskeletal) and is felt most sharply in the perineum, thighs, sacrum, and anus (S1-S4) (Bonica, 1995a).

Use of Nondrug Methods During Childbirth

In the past the use of nondrug methods, such as relaxation breathing, distraction, imagery, effleurage, water, heat, and even acupuncture, were promoted as the safest and most acceptable methods for controlling pain during childbirth (Simkin, 1995). Practitioners hoped that by learning these methods in childbirth preparation classes, women could use the methods to eliminate pain during labor.

Unfortunately, childbirth preparation classes do not result in pain-free childbirth or even consistently reliable pain relief. Although nondrug methods can be effective in helping patients in labor relax, few well-controlled studies demonstrate that these methods actually reduce pain (see Chapter 9 for more on nondrug techniques). "Controlled" expression of pain and a reduction in analgesic use do not mean that patients necessarily experience less pain. Many women can describe experiencing excruciating labor pain when nondrug measures were used exclusively (Bonica, 1995a).

The tendency of caregivers, family, and friends to promote "natural childbirth" as the only safe and acceptable method for controlling pain is presumptuous and not based on research. Furthermore, it can lead to feelings of inadequacy and failure in women who are unable to accomplish labor and delivery without analgesics. Encouraging patients to put off taking analgesics or avoid them entirely is outdated, inappropriate, and has the same harmful consequences for patients in labor and their babies as it does for other patients (see Chapter 2 and the introductory material in this chapter).

As with the management of other types of pain, the use of nondrug interventions should complement, not replace, pharmacologic interventions for the management of labor and delivery pain (AHCPR, 1992, 1994). Today, women have many safe choices for the management of pain during childbirth, which may be used with or without nondrug methods. Caregivers, family, and friends should respect the right of each woman to choose the method of pain control that best suits her.

Use of Opioid Analgesics During Childbirth

The mu opioid agonist analgesics, such as fentanyl, morphine, and hydromorphone, are recommended for pain during labor (Viscomi, Rathmell, 1998). Although commonly administered for labor pain, meperidine is not recommended. Meperidine has been found to produce a dysphoric, rather than analgesic, effect on women in labor (Olofsson, Ekblom, Ekman-Ordeberg et al., 1996) (see Chapter 6, p. 183, for more on meperidine).

Studies point to the adverse effects of meperidine and normeperidine accumulation on the fetus/neonate. Maternal plasma levels indicate that both meperidine and normeperidine (half-life 15 to 20 hours) accumulate after multiple dosing of meperidine during labor (Kuhnert, Philipson, Kuhnert et al., 1985). Fetal accumulation of normeperidine occurs also, and the mean half-life of normeperidine in neonatal tissues is up to 85 hours (Kuhnert, Kuhnert, Philipson et al., 1985). This is because plasma protein binding does not approach adult levels (in both the fetus and neonate) until the first year of life. This characteristic allows more drug to remain active and markedly prolongs drug half-life in the fetus and neonate (Rice, 1996). When repeated doses of meperidine are given, uptake into fetal tissues is continuous but without time for clearance before the next injection (Kuhnert, Kuhnert, Philipson et al., 1985). Fetal accumulation of normeperidine has been implicated as the cause of respiratory depression in neonates after multiple dosing of meperidine during labor (Kuhnert, Kuhnert, Tu et al., 1979).

The use of the partial agonist opioid buprenorphine (Buprenex) should be avoided in patients during labor and delivery. Respiratory depression and other side effects associated with buprenorphine are not readily reversed by naloxone; very high doses (10 to 12 mg) of naloxone may be required (APS, 1992).

Nalbuphine (Nubain) has been delivered by IV PCA in the first stage of labor. However, its use is limited to the first stage of labor because it produces significant maternal sedation and PCA alone does not provide sufficient analgesia for the later stages of labor (Wittels, Sevarino, 1992).

Despite widespread use of parenteral agonist-antagonist opioids, such as nalbuphine and butorphanol (Stadol), for pain management during childbirth, they are not recommended as first-line drugs for any type of pain (AHCPR, 1992, 1994; APS, 1992) (see Chapter 6, p. 188). Some clinicians use agonist-antagonist opioid analgesics believing that they cause no respiratory depression or less than the mu agonist opioid analgesics. However, at equianalgesic doses all opioids produce equal respiratory depression. Agonist-antagonist opioids do have a ceiling on the respiratory depression they produce, but they also have a ceiling on their analgesia. When the analgesic ceiling is reached, any increase in dose will not produce an increase in analgesia (APS, 1992). This is why they are especially inappropriate for severe, escalating pain. In addition, maternal administration of nalbuphine can cause a sinusoidal fetal heart rate (FHR) pattern, which can make assessment of fetal well-being difficult (Viscomi, Rathmell, 1998).

Combinations of opioids and antiemetics (e.g., meperidine and promethazine [Phenergan], called Mepergan; fentanyl and droperidol, called Innovar) are not suitable for use during labor. No scientific evidence exists that drugs such as promethazine enhance the analgesic effects of opioids. In addition, droperidol and the phenothiazines, such as promethazine, are sedative, dysphoric, and can produce tachycardia, bradycardia, and increases and decreases in blood pressure (McGee, Alexander, 1979) (see Chapter 6, p. 264).

Use of Local Anesthetics During Childbirth

The long-acting local anesthetic bupivacaine (in concentrations up to 0.5%) is used most often for epidural analgesia and anesthesia during labor and delivery. Ropivacaine (in concentrations up to 0.5%), with characteristics similar to bupivacaine, also is used for obstetric pain. Comparative studies show little difference between ropivacaine and bupivacaine in onset, duration, or maximum sensory block height, but ropivacaine appears to produce a motor blockade that is less intense and shorter in duration. Ropivacaine also is less cardiotoxic than bupivacaine, making it ideal for pain relief in the obstetric patient. Lidocaine 1% to 2% sometimes is used when particularly intense analgesia is required, such as for instrumental delivery (Brownridge, Cohen, Ward, 1998).

As mentioned, all local anesthetic drugs cross the placenta. Fetal dose depends on maternal dose, rate of maternal absorption, and placental perfusion (Brownridge, Cohen, Ward, 1998). The factors that influence maternal toxicity also influence fetal toxicity (see p. 228).

Both lidocaine and mepivacaine have been implicated in reduction of muscle tone in the neonate. Bupivacaine does not seem to have this effect, most likely because it binds to maternal plasma proteins better than lidocaine and mepivacaine. Because bound drugs do not cross the placental membranes readily, lower fetal blood levels are possible (Woods, Difazio, 1995).

Use of Benzodiazepines During Childbirth

Benzodiazepines are analgesic for muscle spasm only, and their use during childbirth is not recommended. If used immediately before delivery, benzodiazepines can cause fetal hypothermia, hyperbilirubinemia, and respiratory depression (Viscomi, Rathmell, 1998).

Parenteral Pain Relief During Childbirth

The parenteral route of administration includes the IV, intramuscular (IM), and subcutaneous (SC) routes. Chapter 6 discusses in detail the pros and cons of the various routes of opioid administration. It bears repeating that, although commonly used, the IM route of administration is not recommended for any type of pain management (AHCPR, 1992; APS, 1992). Unreliable absorption makes it difficult to predict peak times for the opioid administered. This is of particular concern in patients in labor because the time of birth is unpredictable.

Pain and anxiety can inhibit gastrointestinal motility and function and produce a significant delay in gastric emptying; therefore analgesics usually are not administered by the oral route during labor (Bonica, 1995a). Mu agonist opioid analgesics given by the IV route are preferred. The IV route is most efficient when an immediate analgesic effect is required, such as for acute, severe escalating pain. It allows for rapid titration.

The bolus method is used most often to administer IV opioids during labor. Duration of analgesia by bolus administration is dose dependent; the higher the dose, usually the longer the duration. Of all routes of administration, IV produces the highest peak concentration of the drug, and the peak concentration is associated with the highest level of toxicity (e.g., sedation, nausea). To decrease the peak effect and lower the level of toxicity, IV boluses should be administered very slowly (e.g., 10 mg of morphine over 15 minutes every 3 hours) or in smaller doses at closer intervals (e.g., 2 to 5 mg every 60 to 90 minutes). An alternative to clinician-administered IV boluses is IV PCA, which has been used with success during the first half of labor (Wittels, Sevarino, 1992).

The timing of opioid administration is an issue of concern. An excessive dose of opioid given early in labor can decrease uterine contractions and slow labor. However, optimal doses of opioids given after 4 cm dilation have been shown to have little or no depressant effect and may even enhance labor by reducing pain and anxiety. The depressant effect of opioids is less evident in multigravida than primigravida patients and after membranes are ruptured in all patients (Benedetti, 1995).

It is unclear whether there is an optimal time to inject an IV opioid during labor. Theoretically, the amount of drug transferred to the fetus would be minimized if injected during a contraction because blood flow to the placenta decreases during a contraction. Research is needed to determine whether the timing of an IV opioid injection during labor is relevant.

To avoid neonatal opioid-induced respiratory depression from opioid administration just before delivery, an opioid's onset of action and peak times are considered. For example, IV fentanyl should not be administered immediately before delivery because its onset is 1 to 5 minutes and its peak is 3 to 5 minutes (Viscomi, Rathmell, 1998).

Regional Techniques for Pain Relief During Childbirth

Because labor pain is regional (localized to specific areas of the body) in nature, it is ideally suited for treatment with regional analgesia and anesthesia techniques. Examples of regional techniques include epidural and intrathecal analgesia, pudendal block, field blocks, and paracervical block.

Intraspinal analgesia

The reader is asked to refer to Chapter 6, pp. 213-236, where intraspinal analgesia is discussed in detail, including analgesics, side effects, spinal anatomy, catheter placement techniques, and patient assessment.

As discussed in Chapter 6, analgesics can be delivered into the subarachnoid space (intrathecal or spinal analgesia) or the epidural space (epidural analgesia) by single bolus technique or by placing an indwelling catheter and administering intermittent bolus doses or a continuous analgesic infusion. The most common analgesics used for intraspinal analgesia and anesthesia during labor and delivery are local anesthetics alone or in combination with mu agonist opioids. Combining local anesthetics and opioids with low doses of the alpha$_2$-agonist clonidine (see Chapter 6, p. 229) is gaining in popularity for use in obstetrics (Brownridge, Cohen, Ward, 1998). Both intrathecal and epidural analgesia have long histories of effectiveness and safety for both mother and fetus (Bonica, McDonald, 1995).

Intrathecal Analgesia

Various terms have been applied to the delivery of analgesics into the subarachnoid space (e.g., "spinal block" is the same as a subarachnoid block; "saddle block" is a subarachnoid block that provides complete relief only in the sacral area). As with other types of acute pain, when intrathecal analgesia is used to manage labor and delivery pain, it is delivered most often by a single bolus dose (see Chapter 6, p. 220). In settings where access to continuous epidural analgesia is limited or unavailable, single-dose intrathecal analgesia has particular appeal. It is safe, effective, and relatively simple and can be administered rapidly in the active phase of labor; it has a low failure rate, and a low incidence of side effects (McDonald, Mandalfino, 1995; Wildman, Mohl, Cassel et al., 1997).

The most common analgesics delivered by the intrathecal route for labor pain are the mu agonist opioids.

The use of intrathecal local anesthetics generally is reserved to produce anesthesia in obstetric patients. Avoiding the use of local anesthetics prevents the occurrence of respiratory and/or circulatory collapse and motor block from the local anesthetic. However, when intrathecal opioids alone are administered, a pudendal block should be used to help control pain during the second stage of labor.

Although used less often than epidural analgesia, intrathecal analgesia offers a unique benefit. By delivering opioids directly to the receptors in the spinal cord, the dose required for analgesia by the intrathecal route is nearly 10 times less than that of the epidural route (DuPen, DuPen, 1998). Lower maternal doses result in lower fetal doses. A shortcoming of the subarachnoid block is that its analgesia is relatively brief (approximately 100 minutes). Other disadvantages are rapid-onset maternal hypotension (management is discussed later) and postdural puncture headaches (see Chapter 6, p. 232).

Epidural Analgesia and Anesthesia

Lumbar epidural block by continuous infusion of a mu agonist opioid and local anesthetic is a highly effective method for controlling labor and delivery pain. The comparative ease and safety of maintaining an indwelling epidural catheter and infusion has made continuous epidural analgesia the most commonly used intraspinal technique for obstetric pain relief (Bonica, 1995a).

The lumbar level of epidural administration is recommended because the dermatomes affected by noxious stimuli during active labor and throughout delivery are below T10. To avoid the spinal cord, many clinicians prefer to place the catheter below the L3 vertebral interspace. As discussed in Chapter 6, pp. 228-229, problems can arise from lumbar administration of local anesthetics. If high doses of concentrated local anesthetics (0.25% to 0.5%) are used, a dense sensory and motor block of the dermatomes of the lower extremities is produced. This mandates bedrest for the laboring patient. Significant sensory and motor blockade also interferes with the woman's ability to bear down and push during the second stage. This can lead to an extended second stage and often is blamed for an increase in the need for cesarean section delivery (see following discussion on controversies). Finally, high concentrations of epidural local anesthetics produce a sympathetic blockade resulting in vasodilatation. This, in turn, can produce maternal hypotension, endangering both mother and fetus (management is discussed later).

To address these issues, a number of variations in traditional intrathecal opioid and epidural local anesthetic techniques are used. The most common is to combine low doses of opioid (e.g., 2 μg/ml of fentanyl) with weaker concentrations of local anesthetic (e.g., 0.0625% to 0.125% of bupivacaine) for epidural analgesia. By combining the two drugs, lower doses of each are possible without jeopardizing pain relief (see Chapter 6 for more). The lack of adverse fetal effects with combination local anesthetic and opioid epidural infusions during labor is well documented (Bader, Gragnetto, Terui et al., 1995). In addition to lower maternal and fetal doses of both opioid and local anesthetic, a primary benefit to laboring patients is improved analgesia from the opioid with less local anesthetic blockade (Brownridge, Cohen, Ward, 1998; Ferrante, Barber, Segal et al., 1995).

The almost exclusive use of low-dose bupivacaine (Marcaine) and, increasingly, ropivacaine (Naropin) has been helpful in reducing sensory and motor blockade (Brownridge, Cohen, Ward, 1998). Compared with other local anesthetics, these are better able to block nerve fibers that carry noxious stimuli with minimal effect on sensory and motor fibers (Gianino, York, Paice, 1996).

Another variation is the epidural administration of opioids alone or in combination with "ultra low dose" local anesthetics (e.g., 0.04% bupivacaine). The lower local anesthetic dose allows patients to ambulate during labor ("walking epidurals"). One study found 70% of women who received "ultra low dose" epidural analgesia were able to ambulate during labor (Breen, Shapiro, Glass et al., 1993).

Patient-controlled epidural analgesia (PCEA) with or without a basal rate (continuous infusion) is used frequently in obstetric patients. PCEA allows the woman to control the amount of pain relief and motor and sensory block and other side effects experienced (Brownridge, Cohen, Ward, 1998; Vandermeulen, Van Aken, Vertommen, 1995). Better analgesia at lower total local anesthetic doses than with continuous epidural infusion alone is possible in laboring patients (Ferrante, Barber, Segal et al., 1995).

Combined Spinal-Epidural Analgesia

Combined spinal-epidural analgesia (CSEA) for childbirth, cesarean section, and postcesarean section pain relief is used primarily to minimize the shortcomings of both intrathecal and epidural analgesia while taking advantage of their benefits (Cousins, Veering, 1998).

Because CSEA uses the intrathecal route to administer very low doses of local anesthetic for laboring patients, less motor block is produced. The epidural route is used for supplemental boluses. With appropriate assessment, CSEA allows patients to safely and comfortably ambulate during labor (Brownridge, Cohen, Ward, 1998; Gautier, Debry, Fanard et al., 1997). CSEA is discussed in Chapter 6, p. 231.

Other regional anesthetic techniques

When an intraspinal local anesthetic is not used or parenteral opioids alone are used during labor, other appropriate regional anesthetic techniques should be administered during the delivery process to control pain. Examples include the pudendal block, field blocks, and paracervical block.

The pudendal nerve block involves anesthetizing the pudendal nerves bilaterally and indiscriminately infiltrating the perineum. This provides anesthesia of the perineum and lower part of the vagina during the second stage. Also used during the second stage, field blocks are SC local infiltrations that block minor nerves that supply a particular area (e.g., perineum, episiotomy site) (Bonica, McDonald, 1995).

After extensive use during the 1950s and 1960s, the paracervical block is rarely used today. The block involves local infiltration of the pelvic neural plexus and provides analgesia for the first stage of labor. Because of limited duration, repeated blocks are necessary; maintaining a catheter for continuous infusion is technically difficult. The primary disadvantage and probable reason for diminished use of this block is a high incidence of fetal arrhythmia (particularly bradycardia). Fetal deaths have occurred with the paracervical block (Brownridge, Cohen, Ward, 1998).

Controversies Related to Analgesic/Anesthetic Use During Childbirth

Parenteral versus neuraxial opioids

One drawback of administering opioids parenterally is that by this route, opioids bind to both supraspinal (outside of the CNS) and spinal opioid receptors. Supraspinal opioid binding can result in a higher incidence of side effects than when opioids bind primarily in the spinal cord, such as occurs with intraspinal opioids. In other words, parenteral opioids tend to be associated with more side effects than intraspinal opioids; this can limit the dose of opioid that can be given to the patient. For example, a small but very carefully controlled study revealed that after repeated doses of IV opioids during labor, pain relief was inadequate and patients were excessively sedated (Olofsson, Ekblom, Ekman-Ordeberg et al., 1996).

Another shortcoming of the parenteral route is that it cannot target specific dermatomes that are affected by the noxious stimuli producing labor and delivery pain. This is possible only with regional analgesic and anesthetic techniques.

Does epidural analgesia increase the incidence of cesarean section?

Controversy is ongoing over whether the use of epidural analgesia/anesthesia prolongs labor and contributes to a higher incidence of cesarean section deliveries than when it is not used. The research is conflicting on this issue. Some studies show an increase in operative deliveries as a result of epidural analgesia (Ramin, Gambling, Lucas et al., 1995; Thorp, Breedlove, 1996); others show no relationship. For example, when compared with women receiving IV analgesia, even early administration of epidural block to nulliparous (no previous live births) women in spontaneous labor (Chestnut, McGrath, Vincent et al., 1994) and to nulliparous women receiving IV oxytocin (Chestnut, Vincent, McGrath et al., 1994) did not prolong labor or significantly increase the cesarean section rate.

Weaker concentrations of epidural local anesthetics (0.0625% to 0.125% bupivacaine) and the use of restricted ("segmental") block during the first stage of labor may be helpful in increasing the likelihood of spontaneous delivery (Brownridge, Cohen, Ward, 1998). Further research is needed to clarify the relationship between epidural analgesia during labor and the incidence of cesarean section delivery.

Adverse fetal effects

During labor, fetal heart rate (FHR) variability is monitored to assess the dynamic relationship between the fetus' sympathetic and parasympathetic systems. A pattern of variability between the two systems indicates fetal wellness. The loss of FHR variability is a signal of possible fetal hypoxia. Although opioid administration during childbirth can cause loss of FHR variability, opioids often are inappropriately blamed for its occurrence. A number of other factors influence FHR variability, including fetal maturity, maternal and placental health, maternal hydration, and maternal positioning. These should be considered and ruled out or managed before abruptly discontinuing opioids and local anesthetics. In many cases, when loss of FHR variability is thought to be due to the analgesic, reducing the analgesic dose may be a more reasonable approach.

Maternal hypotension as a result of aggressive analgesia during labor can lead to fetal hypoxia and acidosis. However, when maternal hypotension is short lived and treated promptly with IV fluids and an IV pressor drug (e.g., ephedrine), it appears to be of little consequence. Prophylactic IV administration of at least 1 L of crystalloid solution is recommended. Dextrose infusions are avoided because of the possibility of disturbances in maternal, fetal, and neonatal glucose levels (Brownridge, Cohen, Ward, 1998).

PAIN MANAGEMENT DURING THE POSTPARTUM PERIOD

Effective pain management is particularly important during the postpartum period for a number of reasons. Because clotting factors are elevated in the postpartum period, women are at high risk for thrombophlebitis during this time. Therefore postpartum and postcesarean section pain relief should be directed toward maximizing the patient's mobility. In addition to bonding with her baby, the new mother must learn a tremendous amount of new information about how to care for herself and her baby in a very brief period of time. The health care team must make pain management a priority to ensure that pain does not interfere with the new mother's important responsibilities.

Pain From Uterine Contractions

Involutionary uterine contractions continue after delivery and can be quite painful. This is particularly true when frequent fundal massage and the use of oxytocin is necessary to prevent or manage excessive uterine bleeding from lax uterine musculature (common in multigravida and obese women). Uterine contractions also intensify during breast feeding. In most cases, pain is relieved by a combination of acetaminophen and/or ibuprofen, ambulation, and application of a very warm heating pad or bottle to the abdomen. Combination opioids, such as acetaminophen and hydrocodone or oxycodone, may be needed and are especially warranted for women with the combined pain of uterine contractions and an episiotomy (see following discussion for use of acetaminophen and opioids during breast feeding).

Episiotomy Pain

An episiotomy is a vertical perineal cut used to facilitate delivery of the baby. The primigravida patient is the most likely candidate for episiotomy because she has not been subjected to previous perineal stretching. Because episiotomies are painful and carry the risk of becoming infected during the postpartum period, attempts are made to limit their use. Despite this, episiotomies are performed frequently (Reynolds, Yudkin, 1987).

Episiotomies are categorized according to the degree of incision: first degree involves incision of the epidermis, dermis, and fascia only; second degree includes incision of muscle; third degree includes the anal sphincter; and fourth degree extends through the rectal wall. The higher the degree of episiotomy, usually the more severe the pain. It is not unusual to treat third-degree and fourth-degree episiotomy pain with IV opioids.

A preventive approach to treatment of episiotomy pain is recommended (e.g., an ice pack is placed immediately after delivery and reapplied at regular intervals ATC). Perineal cleansing spray after elimination, rather than using toilet paper, is recommended. Local anesthetic sprays provide relief and result in negligible maternal local anesthetic blood concentrations, making them safe for use during breast feeding (Harrison, Brennan, Reed et al., 1987). Acetaminophen alone or in combination with hydrocodone or oxycodone is recommended (see

the following discussion on the use of opioids and local anesthetics during breast feeding).

Patients have been burned with the use of heat treatments for episiotomies (e.g., heat lamps, warm sitz baths), resulting in the diminished use of these treatments over the past few years. However, empirically, these methods do reduce edema and inflammation, and many women find them to be comforting.

Breast and Nipple Pain

Breast and nipple pain can occur whether a woman breast feeds or not. For example, sometimes attempts to suppress milk production in the non–breast-feeding woman are unsuccessful, leading to breast engorgement and pain. No medications are recommended to suppress milk production.

First and second time breast feeding mothers and their babies often experience difficulty adjusting to the breast feeding process. Frequently, infants latch on to the breast incorrectly and/or suck vigorously, causing pain that can lead to decreased breast feeding time. This, in turn, leads to breast engorgement and reduced milk production, which causes the baby to suck harder, and the cycle repeats itself (Hill, Humenick, 1993).

Methods used to relieve nipple and breast pain in breast feeding mothers include more frequent but shorter breast feeding sessions, applying modified lanolin and warm water compresses to the nipples and areola, expressing breast milk manually, and leaving breasts open to air. Women who are not breast feeding are advised to wear a snug bra and not to express milk. Acetaminophen also may help to relieve discomfort for both breast feeding and non–breast-feeding women.

Post–Cesarean Section Pain

Women with the most severe postpartum pain are those who deliver their babies by cesarean section. The type of abdominal and uterine incisions can influence the severity of postoperative pain. The upper portion (fundus) is the most contractile part of the uterus. A low transverse abdominal incision and transverse uterine incision ("low cervical") involve incising a smaller area away from the fundus and are usually associated with less pain than other incisions. The "classical" incision is either a vertical or transverse abdominal incision and a vertical uterine incision. This approach is simple and often used for emergency cesarean sections. Generally, pain is more severe because the classical incision is larger and closer to the fundus (Pernoll, Mandel, 1995). Regardless of the type of incision, the reader is reminded that pain and analgesic requirements are highly individual and all reports of unrelieved pain require attention.

When epidural anesthesia is provided for the cesarean section, the epidural catheter often is used to administer a single bolus dose of preservative-free morphine (e.g.,

5 mg) to provide pain relief for up to 24 hours after delivery. After the bolus dose is administered, the epidural catheter is removed. The epidural catheter also may be left in place to treat postoperative pain with intermittent bolus dosing, continuous epidural analgesic infusion, or PCEA. When general anesthesia is used during the surgery, typically IV PCA morphine, hydromorphone, or fentanyl is recommended. See Chapter 6 for more on IV PCA and epidural analgesia.

ANALGESIC USE DURING BREAST FEEDING

A number of drugs can be taken safely while breast feeding. In 1994 the American Academy of Pediatrics (AAP) Committee on Drugs categorized various drugs according to their safety during breast feeding (Box 13.4).

High lipid solubility, low molecular weight, and the nonionized state all facilitate secretion of medications into breast milk. It is estimated that the neonate receives approximately 1% to 2% of the maternal dose of a drug (Viscomi, Rathmell, 1998). Taking medications right before or after breast feeding may minimize drug transfer through breast milk. These dosing times result in lower plasma concentrations of the drug.

Acetaminophen and NSAIDs

Acetaminophen is safe for use during breast feeding; however, NSAIDs generally are not recommended because of the possible adverse effects (e.g., inhibition of prostaglandin production) on the infant. If a NSAID is required, an appropriate choice is one with a short half-life and inert metabolites that are rapidly excreted, such as

● ● ● ● ●

BOX 13.4	**AAP Classification of Maternal Medication Use During Lactation**

Category 1: Should not be consumed during lactation. Strong evidence that serious effects to the infant can occur with maternal ingestion.
  Examples: Ergotamine
Category 2: Infant effects in humans are unknown; caution is urged.
  Examples: Amitriptyline, desipramine, doxepin, fluoxetine, imipramine, trazodone
Category 3: Compatible with breast feeding.
  Examples: Codeine, fentanyl, methadone, morphine, butorphanol; acetaminophen, ibuprofen, ketorolac, naproxen; caffeine, carbamazepine, phenytoin, valproic acid, propranolol, lidocaine, mexiletine

May be duplicated for use in clinical practice. As appears in McCaffery M, Pasero C: *Pain: Clinical manual,* p. 623, 1999, Mosby, Inc.

Drugs have been categorized by the American Academy of Pediatrics (AAP) according to their potential to cause adverse effects in breast feeding infants. Box 13.4 lists opioid, nonopioid, and adjuvant analgesics according to the AAP categories.

Drug categories from the AAP Committee on Drugs: The transfer of drugs and other chemicals into human milk, *Pediatrics* 93:137-150, 1994. Drug examples from Rathmell JP, Viscomi CM, Ashburn MA: Management of nonobstetric pain during pregnancy and lactation, *Anesth Analg* 85:1074-1087, 1997.

ibuprofen (Brooks, Needs, 1992) (see Box 13.4). Again, drug exposure for the child can be minimized by taking the drug just before or after breast feeding. Aspirin should be used only occasionally and for brief periods while breast feeding because infants eliminate salicylates very slowly. Indomethacin should be avoided entirely during breast feeding (Viscomi, Rathmell, 1998).

Opioid Analgesics

Opioids are secreted in breast milk, ingested by the baby, and absorbed after undergoing hepatic metabolism. Codeine, fentanyl, methadone, and morphine are classified as AAP Category 3 drugs and approved for use during breast feeding (see Box 13.4). To minimize sedation from exposure to opioids in breast feeding infants, mothers who are receiving IV PCA can be encouraged to self-administer a dose just after nursing. Intraspinal analgesia provides post–cesarean section pain relief with lower doses of opioids than when given by parenteral routes of administration (see Chapter 6). When carefully titrated, drug exposure to breast feeding infants whose mothers are receiving analgesics by the intraspinal routes of administration is minimal (Rathmell, Viscomi, Ashburn, 1997).

Meperidine is a particularly poor choice for use during lactation. In a study comparing nursing neonates whose mothers were receiving meperidine to those whose mothers were receiving morphine, significant neurobehavioral depression occurred in neonates in the meperidine group. Nursing infants exposed to morphine were more alert and oriented to animate human cues than those exposed to meperidine (Wittels, Glosten, Faure et al., 1997).

Epidural bupivacaine commonly is combined with opioids for treatment of post–cesarean section pain without posing problems to breast feeding neonates. In fact, one study demonstrated a link between the excellent pain control afforded by continuous epidural bupivacaine and an improvement in the amount of breast feeding and infant weight gain (Hirose, Hara, Hosokawa et al., 1996).

Adjuvant Analgesics

Adjuvant analgesics are used to treat pain of a neuropathic origin (described as sharp, shooting, burning pain [e.g., as in reflex sympathetic dystrophy, some chronic back pain]). These include local anesthetics, antidepressants, anticonvulsants, corticosteroids, and benzodiazepines (for muscle spasm). Following are comments about adjuvant analgesics as they relate to use in breast feeding women. See Chapter 7 for more on use of adjuvant analgesics.

The local anesthetics lidocaine and mexiletine are sometimes used for chronic pain. They both are classified as Category 3 drugs and safe for use during breast feeding (see Box 13.4).

Most of the antidepressants are classified as Category 2 drugs for use during lactation (see Box 13.4). Less than 1% of the dose of amitriptyline, nortriptyline, and desipramine is passed to the nursing infant without any adverse effects. These are recommended as the antidepressants of choice during breast feeding. Maternal doxepin has been associated with respiratory depression in nursing infants (Rathmell, Viscomi, Ashburn, 1997).

Anticonvulsants are safe for use during lactation (see Box 13.4). Research is lacking on the safety of the relatively new anticonvulsant, gabapentin, during lactation (Rathmell, Viscomi, Ashburn, 1997).

Very low doses of steroids (e.g., <1% prednisone) are passed to neonates in breast milk and are unlikely to have an adverse effect (Viscomi, Rathmell, 1998) (see Box 13.4).

Benzodiazepines sometimes are used for muscle spasm. Diazepam (Valium) and its metabolite desmethyldiazepam are found in the breast feeding infant's blood for up to 10 days after one maternal dose. These infants also can be sedated and can be poor feeders (Viscomi, Rathmell, 1998) (see Box 13.4).

Studies are lacking on most of the analgesics used for treatment of migraine headache during breast feeding. Sometimes propranolol, atenolol, and clonidine are used to treat both migraine and nonmigraine vascular headaches. Customary maternal doses of these drugs appear to have minimal neonatal effect. Only 0.24% of the maternal dose of sumatriptan is passed to the nursing infant. Moderate use of caffeine (≤2 cups coffee/day) has not demonstrated any increased risk of fetal malformation or posed a problem in breast feeding infants. Ergotamines are contraindicated during breast feeding because they can cause neonatal convulsions and severe gastrointestinal disturbances (Viscomi, Rathmell, 1998) (see Box 13.4).

References

Agency for Health Care Policy and Research (AHCPR): *Acute pain management: Operations or medical procedures and trauma—clinical practice guideline,* AHCPR Pub No. 92-0032, Rockville, Md, Feb 1992, U.S. Public Health Service, AHCPR.

Agency for Health Care Policy and Research (AHCPR): *Management of cancer pain: Clinical practice guideline,* No. 9, AHCPR Pub No. 94-0592, Rockville, Md, March 1994, U.S. Department of Health and Human Services, Public Health Service.

American Academy of Pediatrics (AAP) Committee on Drugs: The transfer of drugs and other chemicals into human milk, *Pediatrics* 93:137-150, 1994.

American Pain Society (APS): *Principles of analgesic use in the treatment of acute pain and cancer pain,* ed 3, Glenview, Ill, 1992, APS.

Bader AM, Gragnetto R, Terui K et al.: Maternal and neonatal fentanyl and bupivacaine concentrations after epidural infusion during labor, *Anesth Analg* 81:829-832, 1995.

Benedetti C: Opioids, sedatives, hypnotics, ataractics. In Bonica JJ, McDonald JS, editors: *Principles and practice of obstetric analgesia and anesthesia,* ed 2, pp 575-614, Baltimore, 1995, Williams & Wilkins.

Benet LZ, Kroetz DL, Sheiner LB: Pharmacokinetics. In Hardman JG, Limbird LE, editors: *Goodman and Gilman's the pharmacological basis of therapeutics,* ed 9, pp 3-27, New York, 1996, McGraw-Hill.

Bissonnette JM: Placental transfer of anesthetics and related drugs and effects. In Bonica JJ, McDonald JS, editors: *Principles and practice of obstetric analgesia and anesthesia,* ed 2, pp 225-242, Baltimore, 1995, Williams & Wilkins.

Bjorkman DJ: Nonsteroidal anti-inflammatory drug-induced gastrointestinal injury, *Am J Med* 101(Suppl 1A):25S-32S, 1996.

Bonica JJ: The nature of the pain of parturition. In Bonica JJ, McDonald JS, editors: *Principles and practice of obstetric analgesia and anesthesia,* ed 2, pp 243-273, Baltimore, 1995a, Williams & Wilkins.

Bonica JJ: Evolution and current status. In Bonica JJ, McDonald JS, editors: *Principles and practice of obstetric analgesia and anesthesia,* ed 2, pp 5-41, Baltimore, 1995b, Williams & Wilkins.

Bonica JJ, McDonald JS: Epidural analgesia and anesthesia. In Bonica JJ, McDonald JS, editors: *Principles and practice of obstetric analgesia and anesthesia,* ed 2, pp 344-470, Baltimore, 1995, Williams & Wilkins.

Breen TW, Ransil BJ, Groves PA et al.: Factors associated with back pain after cesarean section, *Anesthesiology* 81:29-34, 1994.

Breen TW, Shapiro T, Glass B et al.: Epidural anesthesia for labor in an ambulatory patient, *Anesth Analg* 77:919-924, 1993.

Briggs GG, Freeman RK, Yaffe SJ: *A reference guide to fetal and neonatal risk: Drugs in pregnancy and lactation,* ed 4, pp 1-974, Baltimore, 1994, Williams & Wilkins.

Brooks PM, Needs CJ: NSAIDs in lactating women. In Famaey JP, Paulus HE, editors: *Therapeutic applications of NSAIDs subpopulations and new formulations,* pp 157-162, New York, 1992, Marcel Dekker.

Brownridge P, Cohen SE, Ward ME: Neural blockade for obstetrics and gynecologic surgery. In Cousins MJ, Bridenbaugh PO, editors: *Neural blockade,* pp 557-604, Philadelphia, 1998, Lippincott-Raven.

Chestnut DH, McGrath JM, Vincent RD et al.: Does early administration of epidural analgesia affect obstetric outcome in nulliparous women who are in spontaneous labor? *Anesthesiology* 80(6):1201-1208, 1994.

Chestnut DH, Vincent RD, McGrath JM et al.: Does early administration of epidural analgesia affect obstetric outcome in nulliparous women who are receiving intravenous oxytocin? *Anesthesiology* 80(6):1195-1200, 1994.

Clapp JF, Kett A, Olariu N et al.: Cardiovascular and metabolic responses to two receptor-selective opioid agonists in pregnant sheep, *Am J Obstet Gynecol* 178(2):397-401, 1998.

Collaborative Low-Dose Aspirin Study in Pregnancy (CLASP), Collaborative Group: CLASP: a randomized trial of low-dose aspirin for the prevention and treatment of preeclampsia among 9364 pregnant women, *Lancet* 343:619, 1994.

Cousins MJ, Veering BT: Epidural neural blockade. In Cousins MJ, Bridenbaugh PO, editors: *Neural blockade,* pp 243-321, Philadelphia, 1998, Lippincott-Raven.

Drug Facts and Comparisons, St. Louis, 1997, Wolters Kluwer.

DuPen SL, DuPen AR: Spinal analgesia. In Ashburn MA, Rice LJ, editors: *The management of pain,* pp 171-186, New York, 1998, Churchill Livingstone.

Ferrante FM, Barber MJ, Segal M et al.: 0.0625% bupivacaine with 0.0002% fentanyl via patient-controlled epidural analgesia for pain of labor and delivery, *Clin J Pain* 11:121-126, 1995.

Food and Drug Administration (FDA) Public Hearing, Sept 12, 1997: *Content and format of labeling for human prescription drugs. Part II. Pregnancy labeling categories* (on-line). Available: http://www.fda.gov/cder/meeting/part15tr.htm.

Gautier PE, Debry F, Fanard L et al.: Ambulatory combined spinal-epidural analgesia for labor: influence of epinephrine on bupivacaine-sufentanil combination, *Regional Anesth* 22(2):143-149, 1997.

Gianino JM, York MM, Paice JA: *Intrathecal drug therapy for spasticity and pain,* New York, 1996, Springer.

Hainline B: Neurologic complications of pregnancy: headache, *Neurol Clin* 12:443-460, 1994.

Harrison RF, Brennan M, Reed JV et al.: A review of post-episiotomy pain and its treatment, *Curr Med Res Opin* 10(6):359-363, 1987.

Heinomen OP, Slone S, Shapiro S: *Birth defects and drugs in pregnancy,* Littleton, Mass, 1977, Publishing Science Group.

Hill PD, Humenick SS: Nipple pain during breastfeeding: the first two weeks and beyond, *J Perinat Educ* 2(2):21-35, 1993.

Hirose M, Hara Y, Hosokawa T et al.: The effect of postoperative analgesia with continuous epidural bupivacaine after cesarean section on the amount of breast feeding and infant weight gain, *Anesth Analg* 82:1166-1169, 1996.

Insel PA: Analgesic-antipyretic and antiinflammatory agents and drugs employed in the treatment of gout. In Hardman JG, Limbird LE, editors: *Goodman and Gilman's the pharmacological basis of therapeutics,* ed 9, pp 617-657, New York, 1996, McGraw-Hill.

Jacoby J, McDonald JS: Unusual case management problems in obstetric anesthesia. In Bonica JJ, McDonald JS, editors: *Principles and practice of obstetric analgesia and anesthesia,* ed 2, pp 1162-1195, Baltimore, 1995, Williams & Wilkins.

James CF: Pain management for labor and delivery in the 90's, *J Florida Med Assoc* 84(1):28-36, 1997.

Jancin B: For pregnancy-associated heartburn, *Obstet Gynecol News* 31(14):21, 1996.

Kuhnert BR, Kuhnert PM, Philipson EH et al.: Disposition of meperidine and normeperidine following multiple doses during labor. II. Fetus and neonate, *Am J Obstet Gynecol* 151:410-415, 1985.

Kuhnert BR, Kuhnert PM, Tu AL et al.: Meperidine and normeperidine levels following meperidine administration during labor. II. Fetus and neonate, *Am J Obstet Gynecol* 133:909-913, 1979.

Kuhnert BR, Philipson EH, Kuhnert PM et al.: Disposition of meperidine and normeperidine following multiple doses during labor. I. Mother, *Am J Obstet Gynecol* 151:406-409, 1985.

Martin JN, Martin RW, Morrison JC: Surgical diseases and disorders in pregnancy. In Pernoll ML, editor: *Current obstetric and gynecologic diagnosis and treatment,* pp 480-492, Norwalk, Conn, 1991, Appleton & Lange.

McDonald JS, Mandalfino DA: Subarachnoid block. In Bonica JJ, McDonald JS, editors: *Principles and practice of obstetric analgesia and anesthesia,* ed 2, pp 344-496, Baltimore, 1995, Williams & Wilkins.

McGee JL, Alexander MR: Phenothiazine analgesia: Fact or fantasy? *Am J Hosp Pharm* 36:633-640, May 1979.

Melzack R: The myth of painless childbirth, *Pain* 19:321-337, 1984.

Merry A, Power I: Perioperative NSAIDs: towards greater safety, *Pain Rev* 12:268-291, 1995.

Nulman I, Rovey J, Stewart DE et al.: Neurodevelopment of children exposed in utero to antidepressant drugs, *N Engl J Med* 336:258-262, 1997.

Olofsson C, Ekblom A, Ekman-Ordeberg G et al.: Lack of analgesic of systemically administered morphine or pethidine on labour pain, *Br J Obstet Gynaecol* 103:968-972, 1996.

Ostgaard HC, Andersson GBJ, Karlsson K: Prevalence of back pain in pregnancy, *Spine* 16:549-552, 1991.

Pernoll ML, Mandel JE: Cesarean section. In Bonica JJ, McDonald JS, editors: *Principles and practice of obstetric analgesia and anesthesia,* ed 2, pp 968-1009, Baltimore, 1995, Williams & Wilkins.

Ramin SM, Gambling DR, Lucas MJ et al.: Randomized trial of epidural versus intravenous analgesia during labor, *Obstet Gynecol* 86:783-789, 1995.

Rathmell JP, Viscomi CM, Ashburn MA: Management of nonobstetric pain during pregnancy and lactation, *Anesth Analg* 85:1074-1087, 1997.

Reynolds JL, Yudkin PL: Changes in the management of labour. II. Perineal management, *Can Med Assoc J* 136:1045-1048, 1987.

Rice L: Regional anesthesia and analgesia. In Motoyama EK, Davis PJ, editors: *Smith's anesthesia for infants and children,* ed 6, pp 403-442, St. Louis, 1996, Mosby.

Simkin P: Psychologic and other nonpharmacologic techniques. In Bonica JJ, McDonald JS, editors: *Principles and practice of obstetric analgesia and anesthesia,* ed 2, pp 715-746, Baltimore, 1995, Williams & Wilkins.

Spencer RT: Pharmacodynamics and pharmacokinetics. In Spencer RT, Nichols LW, Lipkin GB et al., editors: *Clinical pharmacology and nursing management,* ed 4, pp 62-90, Philadelphia, 1993, JB Lippincott.

Thorp JA, Breedlove G: Epidural analgesia in labor: an evaluation of risk and benefits, *Birth: issues Perinat Care Educ* 23(2):63-83, 1996.

Vandermeulen EP, Van Aken H, Vertommen JD: Labor pain relief using bupivacaine and sufentanil: patient controlled epidural analgesia versus intermittent injections, *Eur J Obstet Gynecol Reprod Biol* 59 (Suppl):S47-S54, 1995.

Varney H: *Nurse-midwifery,* ed 2, p 846, Boston, 1987, Blackwell Scientific Publications.

Viscomi CM, Rathmell JP: Pain management issues in the pregnant patient. In Ashburn MA, Rice LJ, editors: *The management of pain,* pp 363-381, New York, 1998, Churchill Livingstone.

Waldenstrom U, Bergman V, Vasell G: The complexity of labor pain: experiences of 278 women, *J Psychom Obstet Gynec* 17:215-228, 1996.

Ward RM, Mirkin BL: Perinatal/neonatal pharmacology. In Brody TM, Lamer J, Minneman KP et al., editors: *Human pharmacology: molecular to clinical,* pp 843-853, St. Louis, 1994, Mosby.

Wildman KM, Mohl VK, Cassel JH et al.: Intrathecal analgesia for labor, *J Fam Prac* 44(6):535-540, 1997.

Wittels B, Glosten B, Faure EAM et al.: Postcesarean analgesia with both epidural morphine and intravenous patient-controlled analgesia: neurobehavioral outcomes among nursing neonates, *Anesth Analg* 85:600-606, 1997.

Wittels B, Sevarino FB: PCA in the obstetric patient. In Sinatra RS, Hord AH, Ginsberg B et al., editors: *Acute pain: mechanisms and management,* pp 175-181, St. Louis, 1992, Mosby.

Wong KC, Sundin JR: Pharmacology of inhalational and intravenous anesthetics. In Bonica JJ, McDonald JS, editors: *Principles and practice of obstetric analgesia and anesthesia,* ed 2, pp 615-646, Baltimore, 1995, Williams & Wilkins.

Woods AM, Difazio CA: Pharmacology of local anesthetics and related drugs. In Bonica JJ, McDonald JS, editors: *Principles and practice of obstetric analgesia and anesthesia,* ed 2, pp 297-323, Baltimore, 1995, Williams & Wilkins.

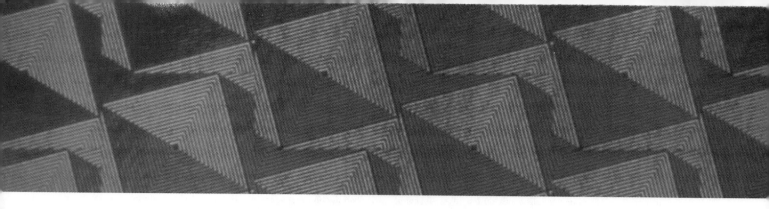

chapter fourteen
PAIN IN INFANTS

Bonnie Stevens

CHAPTER OUTLINE

TERMINOLOGY*

Extremely-low-birth-weight (ELBW) infant: An infant whose birth weight is less than 1000 g regardless of gestational age.

Infant: A baby who is less than 12 months of age.

Low-birth-weight (LBW) infant: An infant whose birth weight is less than 2500 g, regardless of gestational age.

Neonatal period: The period of time between birth and 1 month of age.

Neonate: Newborn infant who is less than 1 month postnatal age.

Perinatal period: The period of time between 20 weeks' gestation to 7 days after birth. A different definition is between 28 weeks' gestation to 28 days after birth.

Preterm neonate: An infant born before completion of 37 weeks' gestation, regardless of birth weight.

Term (full-term) neonate: An infant born between the beginning of the 38th week and the completion of the 42nd week of gestation, regardless of birth weight. After 42 weeks' gestation, the infant is considered postmature.

Very-low-birth-weight (VLBW) infant: An infant whose birth weight is less than 1500 g, regardless of gestational age.

*Terminology for the different age groups in infants is not yet standardized.

TABLE 14.1 ● ● ● ● ●

Misconceptions Pain in Infants

MISCONCEPTION	CORRECTION
1. Infants are incapable of feeling pain.	Infants have the anatomic and functional requirements for pain processing by mid to late gestation (Anand, 1993).
2. Infants are less sensitive to pain than older children and adults.	Term neonates have the same sensitivity to pain as older infants and children. Preterm neonates may have a greater sensitivity to pain than term neonates or older children (Anand, 1995).
3. Infants are incapable of expressing pain.	Although infants cannot verbalize pain, they respond with behavioral cues and physiologic indicators that can be observed by others (Anand, Craig, 1996).
4. Infants must learn about pain from previous painful experiences.	Pain requires no prior experience; it need not be learned from earlier painful experience. Pain is present with the first insult (Anand, Craig, 1996).
5. Pain cannot be accurately assessed in infants.	Behavioral cues (i.e., facial expressions, cry, body movements) and physiologic indicators of pain can be reliably and validly assessed either alone (univariate approach) or in combination (multivariate approach). The most valid univariate approach is facial expression (Craig, 1998). The most valid multivariate approach is through the use of a composite pain measure (Stevens, 1998).
6. Infants are incapable of remembering pain.	Early exposure to noxious stimuli may have an effect on the infant's future responses to painful events (Grunau, Whitfield, Petrie, 1994; Grunau, Whitfield, Petrie et al., 1994; Taddio, Goldbach, Ipp et al., 1995; Taddio, Katz, Ilersich et al., 1997).
7. Analgesics and anesthetics cannot be safely given to infants and neonates because of their immature capacity to metabolize and eliminate drugs and their sensitivity to opioid-induced respiratory depression.	Infants older than 1 month of age metabolize drugs in the same manner as older infants and children. Careful selection of the agent, dosage, administration route and time, and frequent monitoring for desired and undesired effects, and drug titration and weaning can minimize the adverse effects of opioids and nonopioids for pain management in neonates (Stevens, 1997; Yaster, Krane, Kaplan et al., 1997).

May be duplicated for use in clinical practice. From McCaffery M, Pasero C: *Pain: Clinical manual*, p. 627. Copyright © 1999, Mosby, Inc.

Information from Anand KJS: Analgesia and sedation in ventilated neonates, *Neonatal Respir Dis* 5:1-11, 1995; Anand KJS: The applied physiology of pain. In Anand KJS, McGrath PJ, editors: *Pain in neonates*, pp 39-66, Amsterdam, 1993, Elsevier; Anand KJS, Craig KD: New perspectives on the definition of pain, *Pain* 67:3-6, 1996; Craig KD: The facial display of pain in infants and children. In Finley GA, McGrath PJ, editors: *Measurement of pain in infants and children*. In *Pain research and management*, Vol 10, pp 103-121, Seattle, 1998, IASP Press; Grunau RVE, Whitfield M, Petrie J: Pain sensitivity and temperament in extremely-low-birth-weight premature toddlers and preterm and full-term controls, *Pain* 58:341-346, 1994; Grunau RVE, Whitfield M, Petrie J et al.: Early pain experience, child and family factors, as precursors of somatization: A prospective study of extremely premature and full-term children, *Pain* 56:353-359, 1994; Stevens B: Composite measures of pain. In Finley GA, McGrath PJ, editors: Measurement of pain in infants and children, *Progress in pain research and measurement*, Vol 10, pp 161-178, Seattle, 1998, IASP Press; Stevens B: Pain assessment in children: Birth through adolescence. In Weisman S, editor: *Pain management in children: Child and adolescent psychiatric clinics of North America*, pp 725-743, Philadelphia, 1997, W.B. Saunders; Taddio A, Goldbach M, Ipp M et al.: Effect of circumcision on pain responses during vaccination in male infants, *Lancet* 345:291-292, 1995; Taddio A, Katz J, Ilersich AL et al.: Neonatal circumcision and pain response during routine vaccination 4 to 6 months later, *Lancet* 349:599-603, 1997; Yaster M, Krane EJ, Kaplan RF et al.: *Pediatric pain management and sedation handbook*, St. Louis, 1997, Mosby.

See text for further references.

OVERVIEW

Pain in infants poses a major challenge for health professionals and parents. Although infants, especially preterm neonates, are particularly vulnerable to pain and its consequences, pain is less adequately controlled in this group than any other. Many reasons account for the undertreatment of pain in infants, but most relate to a lack of knowledge rather than inadequate human compassion. Fortunately, in the past decade interest in pain in infants has increased dramatically. In addition to rapid growth in the number of research papers published in a wide variety of the most prestigious professional and research journals, pain in infants is now the focus of several research review articles, book chapters, books, and scientific databases. However, despite this increase in knowledge, we are still far from an optimal approach for assessing and relieving pain in infants. The purpose of this chapter is to present the most relevant and recent research and to provide the best practical information for assessing and relieving pain in infants. The specific purposes of this chapter are:

- To define pain as it relates to infants
- To explore the undertreatment of pain in infants and its consequences
- To determine the sources and settings of pain in infants
- To describe pain assessment approaches in infants
- To evaluate pharmacologic and nonpharmacologic pain interventions for infants
- To examine the roles of health professionals and parents in management of pain in infants
- To list resources for health professionals and parents

Chapter terminology for age and weight groups is located at the beginning of this chapter.

Throughout this chapter, the reader will be referred to previous chapters and will also be introduced to new material. The level of material presented assumes that the reader has basic knowledge about the growth and development of infants and about the care of infants during health and illness in the home and in a variety of health care settings.

However, this chapter is neither a complete nor a thorough guide to pain in infants. The limitations of this chapter are as follows:

- Discussion of pain is limited to term and preterm neonates and infants. Older children including toddlers and preschoolers are not included in this chapter.
- Discussion of pain is not related to specific diagnostic categories (e.g., colic), but rather is referred to from a broad source (i.e., pain from procedures, surgery, medical conditions).
- This chapter is an introduction to some of the many possible ways of assessing and managing pain in infants for health professionals and parents. Because of space limitations, many methods of assessment and

relief that are included in this chapter are not discussed in detail.

References at the end of the chapter are offered to guide the reader in pursuit of additional information and more depth in various specialty areas. Furthermore, considerable research is in progress and the reporting of newly completed research may be in press. The reader is encouraged to refer to the current professional and research literature for the most recent advances in the care of infants with pain.

Definition of Pain in Infants

Pain is defined by the International Association for the Study of Pain (IASP) as an unpleasant sensory and emotional experience associated with actual or potential tissue damage or described in terms of such damage. Pain is always subjective (Merskey, Albe-Fessard, Bonica et al., 1979). Two reasons why this definition is not appropriate for infants are: First, infants are incapable of self-report in the usual sense. Therefore the term "nociception" frequently has been used interchangeably with pain for infants. Nociception is defined as the detection of a noxious stimulus and transmission and transduction of that stimulus from the site of tissue damage to the brain (McGrath, 1990). Nociception is thought to occur in a less organized way in the preterm infant than in the child or adult (Fitzgerald, 1993). Nociception incorporates the physiologic and behavioral responses of infants to a painful stimulus but not the cognitive responses that are part of pain perception. Anand and Craig (1996) suggest that pain perception is an inherent quality of life that appears early in infant development to serve as a signaling system for tissue damage. This signaling includes behavioral and physiologic responses that are considered valid indicators of pain. However, pain must be inferred by others, such as health care professionals and parents.

Second, the IASP definition states that pain is an association based on previous actual or potential tissue damage. In neonates and infants, most often no opportunity has existed for gaining previous experience. Anand and Craig (1996) dispute that pain is a learned experience and state that it can be expressed by all individuals in the first experience. This notion is supported by studies that describe the pain responses of neonates during the first few days of life (Grunau, Craig, 1987; McIntosh, van Veen, Brameyer, 1993; Stevens, Johnston, 1994). This rethinking of how pain is defined in infants provides a possible new starting point that enhances valid pain assessment for researchers and clinicians alike (McIntosh, 1997).

Undertreatment of Pain

Undertreatment of pain in infants results from misconceptions and inappropriate knowledge regarding the infant's capabilities for pain, valid pain assessment approaches, and effective and safe implementation of pharmacologic and nonpharmacologic treatment interventions. The existence of pain in infants tends to be doubted to a greater degree than pain in older children and adults. Infants with pain are subjected to the many misconceptions that exist about pain in individuals of all ages but also to the misconceptions specific to their age and stage of growth and development. In an attempt to clarify confusion about pain and its treatment in infants, some of the most common misconceptions are presented in Table 14.1 at the beginning of this chapter. Each misconception is accompanied by correct information.

Misconception

Infants are incapable of feeling pain.

Correction

Health care professionals historically believed that infants were unable to feel pain because of (a) an immature or incompletely myelinated nervous system that would not allow for transmission of noxious stimuli from the site of injury to the central nervous system (CNS), (b) inadequate CNS development, and (c) inadequate development of the peripheral nervous system. An abundance of evidence refutes these beliefs and demonstrates that infants have the anatomic and functional requirements for pain processing by mid to late gestation (Anand, 1993). By 20 weeks' gestational age (GA) sensory receptors have spread to all cutaneous and mucous surfaces. At birth the density of nociceptive nerve endings in the newborn's skin is similar to or greater than in adults. Also, by 20 weeks' GA, the fetal neonatal cortex has a full complement of neurons, suggesting fetuses are capable of pain. Lack of myelination does not support the argument that infants are incapable of feeling pain. Even in adults, nociceptive impulses are carried through unmyelinated fibers. Incomplete myelination affects impulse transmission by slowing the conduction speed of pain impulses. However, this decrease in conduction speed is offset in infants by the shorter distances traveled by impulses to the CNS (Anand, Hickey, 1987). All these data suggest that infants have the capacity for pain at birth, even if that birth is preterm or premature.

Misconception

Infants are not as sensitive to pain as children and adults.

Correction

Infants born at term are equally as sensitive to pain as older children and adults, whereas preterm infants have an increased sensitivity to pain (Anand, 1995; Fitzgerald, 1993). Anand (1995) has summarized the following evidence to support this thinking. First, development of neurotransmitters in the dorsal horn of the spinal cord (that facilitate pain transmission) has been associated with

nociception and increased somatosensory excitability in the premature spinal cord. The presence of these transmitters supports transmission of pain signals to the CNS for pain processing. In contrast, neurotransmitters contained in descending inhibitory fibers from supraspinal centers were only found to be present after birth. The lack of neurotransmitters in the descending tracts implies poorly developed inhibitory mechanisms for pain in preterm neonates, thus making these infants more sensitive to pain (Anand, Carr, 1989). Second, pharmacokinetic studies on anesthetic agents demonstrated that higher plasma concentrations were required to maintain effective surgical anesthesia in preterm neonates than older age groups (Yaster, 1987). Serum morphine concentrations required for producing analgesia in neonates are twice those required in older children and adults (Chay, Duffy, Waler, 1992). Third, prolonged hypersensitivity occurs after an acute painful stimulus in preterm neonates, decreasing the pain threshold and making even nonnoxious stimuli (i.e., handling) be perceived as noxious and producing stress responses (Evans, Vogelpohl, Bourguignon et al., 1997). Finally, the cutaneous flexor reflex (i.e., a clear distinct withdrawal of the leg that can be evoked by a painful stimulus to the heel) has a much lower threshold in preterm infants, suggesting that preterm infants are more sensitive to pain. This threshold was further decreased (i.e., caused by sensitization) after repeated stimulation or local tissue injury and was abolished by topical analgesia (Fitzgerald, Shaw, McIntosh, 1988). In light of this body of evidence, repeated painful stimulation may have substantially greater biologic and clinical importance for very-low-birth-weight (VLBW) infants than for older preterm or term neonates.

Misconception

Infants are incapable of expressing their pain.

Correction

This misconception has been pervasive because of the belief that pain is subjective and must be expressed through self-report. This lack of self-report is thought to contribute to inadequate pain assessment and management in infants. Although infants are incapable of verbalizing their pain, with Anand and Craig's (1996) reconceptualization of the definition of pain, behavioral cues and physiologic indicators can also be considered valid pain indicators. However, these indicators must be inferred by others. Physiologic indicators, including increases in heart rate and decreases in oxygen saturation, frequently have been assessed in infants to provide precise, objective, quantifiable information concerning the child's response to a noxious stimulus (McIntosh, van Veen, Brameyer, 1993; Stevens, Johnston, 1994). However, these indicators alone cannot necessarily be interpreted as pain (Craig, Grunau, 1993) because they are more clearly associated with stress than pain. Conversely, behavioral cues such as facial activity are more consistent indicators of pain, although they vary in intensity, frequency, and nature with age and other contextual factors such as behavioral state. Specific facial actions, including brow bulge, eye squeeze, nasolabial furrow, and open lips, are the most frequently described in response to painful procedures by very preterm infants (i.e., 25 weeks' GA) (Craig, Whitfield, Grunau et al., 1993), preterm infants of greater GA (i.e., 32 to 34 weeks' GA) (Stevens, Johnston, Horton, 1994), and term neonates (Taddio, Stevens, Craig et al., 1997) and older infants (Johnston, Stevens, Craig et al., 1993). These results all serve to refute the misconception that infants are incapable of expressing their pain. In addition, the belief that pain is learned from early experiences in childhood is also refuted by these results because newborn infants with no previous experience demonstrate reactions to painful stimuli during their first days of life that are clearly indicative of pain.

Misconception

Pain in infants cannot be reliably or accurately assessed.

Correction

The skill and accuracy of recognizing pain is challenging for health care professionals and caregivers. To meet this challenge, an overabundance of pain measures for infants has been developed. These measures incorporate both univariate and multivariate approaches (Abu-Saad, Bours, Stevens et al., in press; Franck, Miaskowski, 1997; Stevens, 1997, 1998). Of the univariate approaches, change in facial expression (i.e., individual facial actions) has been the most reliable and consistent indicator of pain across situations and ages (Craig, 1998). Physiologic indicators that are present during acute pain are nonspecific indicators of stress. Although pain is known to be stressful, stress is not necessarily painful. The relationship between behavioral cues and physiologic indicators has not been strong, indicating that pain is complex and multidimensional (Stevens, 1998). To capture the complexity and multidimensionality of pain, a multidimensional approach that uses composite measures combining behavioral cues, physiologic indicators, and taking context into consideration have recently been developed. Of these measures, a few have adequate reliability, validity, and clinical usefulness to be useful in clinical situations. These include the CRIES (Krechel, Bildner, 1995) and the PIPP (Stevens, Johnston, Petryshen et al., 1996).

Misconception

Infants are incapable of remembering pain.

Correction

The issue of whether infants remember pain has long been a topic of heated debate. Memory and learning de-pend on brain plasticity, which is particularly evident during the late prenatal and neonatal periods. Although the structures and functional capacity for memory are thought to be present in the neonate, there is no evidence to support that infants remember pain. However, a growing number of research studies suggest that early exposure to unrelieved pain and the stress related to the event may mediate altered behavioral responses at a later time (Grunau, Whitfield, Petrie, 1994; Grunau, Whitfield, Petrie et al., 1994; Taddio, Goldbach, Ipp et al., 1995; Taddio, Katz, Ilersich et al., 1997).

Penticuff (1987) reported that infants display signs of memory "by exhibiting defensive maneuvers when painful procedures that occurred in the past are about to occur again" (p. 8). Defensive maneuvers displayed by infants included stiffening and withdrawal. Fitzgerald, Millard, and McIntosh (1989) have provided evidence of hypersensitivity to repeated heel lance procedures in premature infants born 27 to 32 weeks' GA.

Barba, Gatto, Valenza and others (1991) hypothesized that a repeated painful experience may cause the newborn to eventually recognize the activities of the event and demonstrate altered behaviors. They analyzed the behavioral and physiologic responses of 20 term newborns to repeated heel lancing. With another 20 term newborns as a control group, they repeated the same steps of the heel lance procedure but without puncturing the skin. As hypothesized, the experimental groups demonstrated responses indicating awareness of the forthcoming painful event, whereas the control group did not.

Indirect evidence for infants' memory of pain is found in two published case histories. Both children were born prematurely and spent extended time in an intensive care unit undergoing repeated painful procedures. Both children subsequently developed an aversion to human contact. The physician parents of one infant described their son's irritability and crying when others attempted to cuddle, caress, rock, or hold him. The child was most comfortable lying alone in his crib for the first 6 months at home. The parents believed that premature infants acquire an aversion to human contact because they associate it with pain (Langland, Langland, 1988).

The second study appears to confirm this belief. The infant had been hospitalized from birth for 6 months for numerous painful medical conditions and was withdrawn, noncommunicative, had no eye contact, and was developmentally at $3\frac{1}{2}$ months of age. Those caring for this child speculated that through the process of stimulus generalization, the infant had equated all human contact with negative stimulation and responded by withdrawing and crying. To help the infant learn to discriminate between pleasant and unpleasant experiences, auditory conditioning was used. The conditioning stimulus (white noise) did not accompany pleasant experiences. Within a few weeks the infant cried before the unpleasant contact but was not agitated during pleasant contacts. Within 5 months, his development improved but remained less than the expected norm (Sexson, Schneider, Chamberlin et al., 1986).

Nurses' anecdotal reports suggest that infants exhibit defensive behaviors when painful procedures are repeated. Nurses often describe infants who stiffen when touched because human touch has repeatedly been associated with pain. Such infants often become hypervigilant, gazing intently at the hands of people who approach them, rather than at the eyes (Penticuff, 1987; Sparshott, 1997). Not only do these reports indicate infants remember painful events, but they also show that continual exposure to pain affects response to human contact.

A study by Wong (1992) specifically investigated the effect of prior pain experiences on the physiologic and behavioral responses of infants to an injection. Infants with high pain history scores had significantly more physical distress or anger expressions than infants with low pain history scores. An implication of this study is the preliminary evidence that past pain influences present pain responses. These studies emphasize the need for good pain management for all painful procedures experienced early in life.

Misconception

Opioid analgesics and anesthetics cannot be safely given to infants and neonates because of their immature capacity to metabolize and eliminate drugs and their sensitivity to opioid-induced respiratory depression.

Correction

If the pharmacokinetics and pharmacodynamics of analgesics are properly understood and if the infant is carefully monitored in a setting where health care professionals are trained in resuscitation, administration of analgesics, including opioids, and anesthetics can be implemented safely for pain in infants, newborns, and preterm infants (Yaster, Krane, Kaplan et al., 1997).

All drugs have potential side effects. But despite the risk of anaphylactic shock from allergy to antibiotics, children continue to receive them when they are indicated. Therefore the potential for side effects from opioids should not preclude their use because the most dangerous side effects, such as respiratory depression, can be easily monitored. Furthermore, should respiratory depression or any other life-threatening side effects from opioids occur, they are almost always easily and quickly reversed by the antidote naloxone (Narcan).

Another concern that influences the use of analgesics in infants and young children is the fear of physical dependence, tolerance, and addiction with prolonged administration. Physical dependence is not synonymous with addiction (Yaster, Krane, Kaplan et al., 1997). *Physical dependence* can occur with prolonged opioid, benzo-

diazepine, steroid, and adrenergic drug administration. Physical dependence or "neuroadaptation" is a normal, natural, physiologic state of adaptation characterized by withdrawal symptoms after abrupt discontinuation of the drug. Any individual who has received opioid analgesics for more than 5 to 10 days should be considered physically dependent on opioids and may require a weaning protocol to prevent opioid withdrawal (Yaster, Krane, Kaplan et al., 1997). *Tolerance* occurs when a need exists to increase the dose of an opioid or benzodiazepine agonist to achieve the same analgesic or sedative effect that was previously achieved with a lower dose. Tolerance may develop after 10 to 21 days of morphine administration (Yaster, Krane, Kaplan et al., 1997).

Addiction implies the psychologic dependence on a particular drug and a cause-effect mode of thinking (e.g., I need the drug because it makes me feel better). Infants are incapable of this higher level cognitive recognition and therefore cannot become addicted. No evidence suggests that use of opioid analgesics early in life increases risk for addiction later in life. Parents need to be made aware of these differences between physical dependence, tolerance, and addiction because they may express concerns about the use and duration of opioids and other pain-relieving drugs. Infants appropriately treated with morphine and other opioids can become tolerant and physically dependent. They cannot, however, become psychologically dependent or addicted.

Withdrawal occurs when opioids (or benzodiazepines) are suddenly discontinued. Symptoms of withdrawal usually begin with 24 hours of drug cessation and reach their peak within 72 hours. The clinical features of withdrawal include the following:

- Neuralgic excitability (irritability, hyperactive deep tendon reflexes, tremors, seizures, increased motor tone, and insomnia)
- Gastrointestinal dysfunction (nausea, vomiting, diarrhea, abdominal cramps)
- Autonomic dysfunction (sweating, fever, chills, tachypnea, nasal congestion, and rhinitis) (Yaster, Krane, Kaplan et al., 1997)

Withdrawal can be anticipated and can be easily prevented by weaning patients from opioids rather than by abrupt cessation. When pain relief is no longer required, weaning by reducing the dosage 20% per day and discontinuing after 5 to 10 days is recommended (Yaster, Berde, Billet, 1996).

To assess the efficacy of opioid weaning, the Children's Hospital Oakland Opioid Weaning Flowsheet (Franck, 1991) can be used (Form 14.1).

Consequences of Pain

Pain is stressful and results in immediate biochemical, physiologic, and behavioral responses. Biochemical responses are the most direct measure of the stress responses

Children's Hospital Oakland Opioid Weaning Flowsheet and Guidelines for Use of the Form
Analgesia/sedation orders (drug/dose/frequency)

Date			
Drug			
Administration time			
Dose ↑ or ↓ or freq change			

Time:

Choose one: Crying/agitated 25%-50% of interval / Crying/agitated >50% of interval	2 / 3		
Choose one: Sleeps ≤25% of interval / Sleeps 26%-75% of interval / Sleeps >75% of interval	3 / 2 / 1		
Choose one: Hyperactive Moro / Markedly hyperactive Moro	2 / 3		
Choose one: Mild tremors, disturbed / Moderate/severe tremors, disturbed	1 / 2		
Increased muscle tone	2		
Temperature 37.2°-38.4°C	1		
Temperature >38.4°C	2		
Respiratory rate >60 (extubated)	2		
Suction >twice/interval (intubated)	2		
Sweating	1		
Frequent yawning (>3-4/interval)	1		
Sneezing (>3-4/interval)	1		
Nasal stuffiness	1		
Emesis	2		
Projectile vomiting	3		
Loose stools	2		
Watery stools	3		
TOTAL SCORE			
ADJUSTED SCORE			
INITIALS OF PERSON SCORING			

Directions: Score every 2-4 hours per guideline
Score greater than 8-12 may indicate withdrawal

Guidelines for use of the flow sheet

Use of form

Use the flowsheet for all infants who have received continuous or around-the-clock opioid medication for 3 days or more, or more than 3 doses per day for more than 5 days. This patient population will most often include postoperative patients, agitated intubated infants, and all post-ECMO patients.

Instructions

1. Write drug, dose, and frequency of analgesics and sedatives ordered
2. Enter date, name of drug (abbreviated MS=morphine sulfate or FENT=fentanyl), and administration time of drugs given in the appropriate boxes; indicate if dose frequency given is an increase or decrease from the ordered dose
3. Scoring must be performed every 4 hours during weaning of opioids, every 2 hours if score is 8 or greater. The score for each item indicates the presence of the sign during the previous 2-4 hours (depending on the scoring interval). Every 4-hour scoring should continue until the patient is off all opioids for 48-72 hours. Place a "0" in the column after the sign if it is not seen during the scoring period.

Central nervous system

Crying behavior: Score 2 points if patient exhibits crying or cry behavior for a duration of ≤50% of the scoring interval. Score 3 points if cumulative crying behavior totals >50% of the scoring interval.
NOTE: Crying behavior is accompanied by the facial expressions associated with crying, but without audible sounds because of endotracheal intubation.

Sleeping: Score 3 points if patient sleeps for ≤25% of the scoring interval. Score 2 points if patient sleeps for 26%-75% of the scoring interval. Score 1 point if patient sleeps for >75% of the scoring interval.

Moro (startle) reflex: Score 2 points if patient has some arm and/or leg extension when touched or when disturbed by loud noises. Score 3 points if patient has marked arm and/or leg extension that is accompanied by crying behavior, hyperalert state, or continued arm and/or leg tremors after being startled.

Tremors—disturbed: Score 1 point if patient has mild tremors when disturbed. Score 2 points if patient has moderate to severe tremors when disturbed. NOTE: Tremors are alternating movements that are rhythmic, of equal rate and amplitude, and can usually be stopped by flexion of the limb.

Increased muscle tone: Score 2 points if patient exhibits fisting or tight flexion of extremities that are difficult to extend.

Metabolic

Temperature: Score 1 point if patient's temperature is 37.2°-38.4°C. Score 2 points if patient's temperature is >38.4°C.

Respiratory rate: Score 1 point if patient's spontaneous respiratory rate is >60/minute. Score 2 points if patient's spontaneous respiratory rate is >60/minute and accompanied by retractions.

Suction: Score 2 points if patient is suctioned more than twice during a 4-hour period.

Sweating: Score 1 point if patient exhibits any type of sweating, including beads of sweat, or if skin is moist to touch.

Yawning: Score 1 point if patient yawns >3-4 times in succession or yawns 1-2 times often during a 4-hour period.

Sneezing: Score 1 point if patient sneezes >3-4 times in succession or sneezes 1-2 times during a 4-hour period.

Nasal stuffiness: Score 1 point for nasal stuffiness.

Gastrointestinal

Emesis of formula/stomach contents: Score 2 points if patient has 1 or more episodes of emesis during a 4-hour period.

Projectile vomiting: Score 3 points if patient has 1 or more episodes of projectile vomiting.

Loose stools: Score 2 points if patient has loose stools characterized by a water ring around some solid stool. The stools will often be frequent. NOTE: Do not score for "breast milk" stools: frequent, small, seedy, yellow stools.

Watery stools: Score 3 points if patient has stools that consist of only liquid. The stools will often be frequent.

Total score: Add up all the scores in the column and place the total score in this box. Clinical signs that appear continuously, such as respiratory rate >60 or regular poor feeding, should be included in the total score.

Adjusted score: The adjusted score is used when a sign is detected that is expected to occur independently of withdrawal, due to a preexisting condition (high respiratory rate in infant with bronchopulmonary dysplasia). The decision to adjust the score should be made after discussion with the healthcare team during rounds, and the rationale should be recorded in a problem-oriented note. Circle the signs to be excluded and deduct the points from the total score to obtain the adjusted score.

Initials of person scoring: The person scoring should write his/her initials in this space.

in infants. These responses result from a complex pattern of catabolic hormone release characterized by increases in cortisol, epinephrine, norepinephrine, growth hormone, and endorphins, as well as a decrease in insulin production (Schmeling, Coran, 1991). Although these responses provide precise data on the infant's response to stress and pain, the availability of information on these responses is limited because of the lack of available assays to perform the tests, minimal data on the normal ranges of these hormones in neonates under stressful conditions, and the feasibility of obtaining data on these indicators in the clinical setting (Franck, Miaskowski, 1997).

Physiologic indicators of pain include (a) increases in heart rate, respiratory rate and blood pressure, and heart rate and intracranial pressure variability; (b) decreases in vagal tone, transcutaneous oxygen saturation levels, transcutaneous carbon dioxide levels and peripheral blood flow, and palmar sweating; and (c) autonomic changes in skin color, nausea, vomiting, gagging, hiccoughing, diaphoresis, and dilated pupils. Most research on pain indicators includes measurement of vital signs (i.e., heart rate, respiratory rate, and blood pressure) because data are readily available and easy to observe in the clinical setting. However, changes in vital signs are difficult to interpret because they are influenced by nonnoxious stimuli, particularly in ill or preterm infants (Cabal, Siassi, Hodgman, 1992; Evans, Vogelpohl, Bourguignon et al., 1997). Also, their usefulness is limited to the immediate poststimulus period because they are the result of activation of the sympathetic nervous system and, as such, are inconsistent and unsustainable by the infant over time. Therefore because of their lack of specificity and inconsistency, vital signs alone cannot determine the presence or absence of pain or the efficacy of interventions. However, in combination with other behavioral and contextual indicators of pain (e.g., as in a composite measure), they may add significant information to the infant's response to acute pain. Other physiologic indicators such as vagal tone index, palmar sweat, and skin blood flow, although more specific physiologic indicators of pain, are not feasible for clinical use and therefore will not be discussed here. (For a more detailed discussion of biochemical and physiologic pain responses of infants, please see Anand, Grunau, Oberlander, 1997; Franck, Miaskowski, 1997).

Behavioral indicators of pain include facial expression, cry, gross motor movement, the flexor reflex threshold, and changes in behavioral state and functions (e.g., sleeping and eating patterns). Changes in behavioral indicators are commonly used as indicators of pain by researchers, clinicians, and parents. Facial expression is more commonly studied in infants than older children and is considered the most consistent (Craig, Grunau, 1993; Stevens, 1997) and convincing (McIntosh, van Veen, Brameyer, 1993) indicator of pain across age

groups. The typical facial expression of pain in infants has the brows and forehead bulging, eyes squeezed tightly closed, cheeks raised to form a nasolabial furrow, and the mouth opened and stretched both horizontally and vertically. Support for the validity of facial activity is provided by its correlation with cry latency and duration in the term neonate (Rushforth, Levene, 1994). Because behavioral indicators of pain have been incorporated into many of the pain assessment measures in infants, they are further discussed in the pain assessment section on pp. 639-651.

Infants of many species cry in response to painful stimuli. Pain is thought to induce stress that causes activation of the neuroendocrine stress response, muscle contraction, and physiologic disorganization that results in an atypical cry (Lester, 1984). Although infants cry when they are angry, fearful, and hungry, the pain cry is distinctive in terms of time (i.e., latency, duration), frequency (i.e. pitch, melody, phonation, jitter, tenseness), and intensity (i.e., loudness) (Fuller, 1991; Johnston, O'Shaughnessy, 1987). The typical pain cry is highly pitched, tense, harsh, nonmelodious, short, sharp, and loud. These attributes can be detected by adult listeners and parents, as well as health professionals in term neonates and older children. However, although cry assumes an important role in alerting adults to infant distress and often provides clues to the severity of distress, facial activity (Figure 14.1) has had a greater impact than cry on adults in judging pain in children (Craig, Grunau, Aquan-Assee, 1988; Hadjistavropoulos, Craig, Grunau

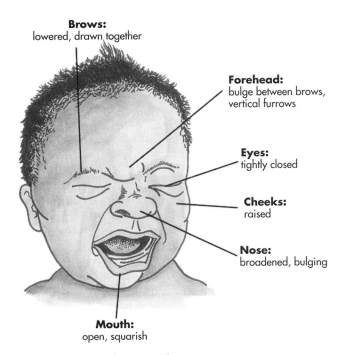

Brows: lowered, drawn together

Forehead: bulge between brows, vertical furrows

Eyes: tightly closed

Cheeks: raised

Nose: broadened, bulging

Mouth: open, squarish

F I G U R E 14.1 Facial expression of pain.
From Wong DL: *Whaley and Wong's nursing care of infants and children*, ed 6, St. Louis, 1999, Mosby.

et al., 1994) and infants (Craig, 1998; Hadjistavropoulos, Craig, Grunau et al., 1997). Preterm infants less than 32 weeks' GA frequently do not cry during painful procedures (Stevens, Johnston, Horton, 1994). Therefore absence of cry cannot be interpreted as absence of pain. Rather, nonresponse may reflect the infant's conservation of energy for more vital functions, such as growth and healing. Also, intubated infants, who may experience the most frequent and intense painful stimuli, are unable to cry because of mechanical or pharmacologic inhibition. However, these infants do express a silent cry in which no sound is made (Figure 14.2) and demonstrate facial action consistent with pain (Sparshott, 1997).

Gross body movements often are used as indicators of pain in older infants and toddlers who display vigorous gross motor movements and attempts to withdraw from a painful stimulus (Franck, 1986; Mills, 1989). In contrast, preterm or sick infants may become limp and flaccid in response to noxious stimuli. Similarly, inhibition of motor responses has been noted in children 3 to 7 years of age after surgery (Beyer, McGrath, Berde, 1990). Taylor (1983) observed that toddler and preschool children were less active as they became more awake after surgery and realized that movement increased pain. Gross body movements are not frequently used as pain indicators because of the difficulties in controlling stimulus intensity or behavioral state and the lack of objective measurement approaches. However, similar to facial expression, changes in body movements have been incorporated into composite or multidimensional indices of pain.

In contrast to gross motor movements, the flexor withdrawal reflex of the neonate is a clear, distinct withdrawal of the leg that can be evoked by a noxious stimulus to the heel (Fitzgerald, Andrews, 1998). In human adults the amplitude of the reflex is linearly correlated with the perception of pain (Willer, 1977). The neonatal flexor reflex threshold (FRT) can be assessed by applying von Frey filaments or hairs (calibrated in size and graded mechanical stimulation) to the sole of the foot and recording the force required to elicit the response (Fitzgerald, Shaw, McIntosh, 1988). The FRT has been shown to be a discrete and reproducible response in the neonate (Andrews, Fitzgerald, 1994) but is evoked by stimuli of much lower intensity than in the adult. Although the flexion withdrawal reflex in the neonate does not have all the same properties as in the adult, it can be used to study sensory processing and pain in the clinical setting. Fitzgerald and Andrews (1998) state that quantitative changes in the flexion withdrawal reflex can be used to study the effects of opioid analgesics, hyperalgesia after surgery or NICU trauma or chronic illness, and the effects of cerebral damage on spinal sensory processing. As such, this response holds a lot of promise for future research. However, it has not been widely used by researchers or clinicians to date.

Pain can also affect behavioral state changes in term infants. Behavioral states are a cluster of discrete behavioral and physiologic elements representing the infant's arousal level. States are usually stable, occur in regular cycles, and influence the infant's ability to respond to stimulation (Prechtl, 1974). Changes in sleep and wakefulness patterns have been noted in infants after circumcision (Anders, Chalemain, 1974; Emde, Harmon, Metcalf et al., 1971; Gunnar, Fisch, Korsvik et al., 1981). Changes in parent-infant interaction and feeding patterns also have been noted in 2-day-old infants after painful stimuli (Marshall, Porter, Rogers et al., 1982). Similarly, infants who underwent circumcision without the benefit of analgesia from dorsal penile nerve block (DPNB) were reported to have less attention, poorer self-soothing ability, and greater motor activity for up to 24 hours after surgery compared with infants who had received DPNB (Dixon, Snyder, Holve et al., 1984). Most clinicians are familiar with the concept and assessment of behavioral state and can make assessments based on how pain affects sleeping and feeding patterns. However, extensive training is required to detect subtle changes in state. Because of its importance in influencing behavioral response, behavioral state must be considered as part of the context in which pain is experienced in the measurement of all neonatal behavioral pain indicators.

Changes in the biochemical, physiologic, and behavioral responses to noxious stimulation may produce acute and long-term consequences of pain. These changes increase the breakdown of fat and carbohydrate stores, prolong hyperglycemia, and increase serum lactate, pyruvate, total ketone bodies, and nonesterified fatty acids (Anand,

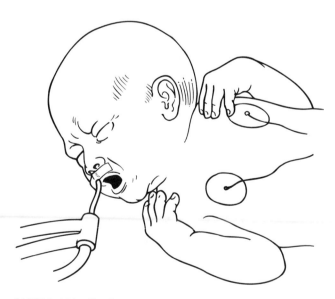

FIGURE 14.2   The silent cry.

Hickey, 1987). Such consequences can contribute to a greater morbidity for neonates in the NICU and a significant decrease in the above-mentioned responses when analgesia and adequate anesthesia are used before the painful procedures. With the standardization of postoperative pain management strategies for infants in the NICU, decreased length of time to extubation, decreased length of stay, improved fluid balance, and reduced side effects of opioids have been noted. Improved pain management documentation, decreased cost, and less nursing time also have been reported (Furdon, Eastman, Benjamin et al., in press).

Pain has significant consequences for preterm infants. For severe pain from surgery, an overwhelming stress response leading to serious complications and even death has been reported (Anand, 1997; Anand, Phil, Hickey, 1992). Less serious complications have also been identified. Taddio and others (1995) reported that male term infants circumcised without analgesia had increased pain from immunization at 2 months compared with uncircumcised infants. A further study indicated that infants treated with placebo-eutetic mixture of local anesthetics (EMLA) had greater pain at 4 and 6 month immunization than circumcised infants treated with EMLA (Taddio, Stevens, Craig et al, 1997). Although no evidence exists that pain is remembered, stress related to the event may mediate altered behavioral responses at a later time.

Peripheral neural structural changes have also been reported after repeated tissue injury (Anand, Plotsky, 1996; Andrews, Fitzgerald, 1994; Fitzgerald, 1993). These changes resulted in heightened sensitivity or tenderness of the affected area (Anand, Plotsky, 1996; Andrews, Fitzgerald, 1994) and the potential for long-term hyperalgesia (Shortland, Woolf, Fitzgerald, 1989; Wolff, 1987). Parents of VLBW infants who had prolonged NICU care have reported decreased infant pain sensitivity at 18 months of age compared with those born at term or those who were preterm but had less complicated care (Grunau, Whitfield, Petrie et al., 1994). The inconsistency of these results may be attributed to the parent's ability to assess pain accurately in this age child. Increased somatization at age $4\frac{1}{2}$ years in children who had repeated NICU procedures as infants also has been reported (Grunau, Whitfield, Petrie et al., 1994).

As discussed in Chapter 2, repeated pain in neonates, especially preterm neonates, can have numerous adverse effects. Exposure to frequent painful procedures associated with neonatal illness can result in hypoxemia, ischemia, and insufficient energy for metabolism, all contributing to higher neonatal morbidity and mortality (Brazy, Goldstein, Oehler et al., 1993). Long-term effects include reduced vigor and strength required to perform neurobehavioral functions later in infancy (Brazy, Goldstein, Oehler et al., 1993; Korner, Stevenson, Kraemer et al., 1993).

Early repetitive pain and environmental stress for children with a history of extremely low birth weight (ELBW) are associated with increased prevalence of neurologic deficits, cognitive defects, learning disorders, poor motor performance, psychosocial problems, inability to adapt and cope in new situations, and impulsive behavior and lack of control in social situations (Anand, Grunau, Oberlander et al., 1997). Increased physiologic responses to neonatal heelsticks have been linked to infant distress behavior at 6 months of age (Gunnar, Porter, Wolf et al., 1995).

In animal studies, repetitive neonatal pain was associated with a decreased pain threshold during later development and a greater preference for alcohol in adulthood (Anand, 1996; Anand, Grunau, Oberlander et al., 1997). Long-term effects were altered development of the pain system and increased vulnerability to stress disorders, addictive behavior, and anxiety states in rats. Repeated, prolonged noxious stimuli can result in a state of hyperexcitability and hypersensitivity at the spinal cord level called "windup" (see Chapter 2), which can lead to chronic neuropathic pain states in which stimuli that are normally innocuous produce pain (allodynia). For example, light stroking of the skin may be felt as extremely painful (Eide, Stubhaug, Stenehjem, 1995; Portenoy, Kanner, 1996). This helps to explain the incidence of chronic pain in premature infants who are exposed to repetitive painful stimuli. Long-term unrelieved chronic pain may have even more biologic and clinical consequences than unrelieved acute pain for these infants (Anand, Grunau, Oberlander et al., 1997).

The harmful effects of undertreated and unrelieved prolonged pain in neonates continues to be studied and much is yet to be learned. However, it is known that prevention of acute pain and effective treatment of acute and chronic pain in neonates can help to reduce the morbidity associated with exposure to repetitive pain (Anand, Carr, 1989; Anand, Phil, Hickey, 1992).

Sources and Settings of Pain

Before and including birth

"Pain is much more than a medical problem—it is part of everyone's life" (Kuttner, 1996, p. 256). As such, pain has the potential to begin within fetal life, continue through birth, and then through all the stages of growth and development throughout life. Fortunately, fetuses, for the most part, enjoy a narcissistic existence within a womb that is warm, cushioned by fluid, dim, and muffled from the outside world. However, for some infants the fetal environment is disturbed when mothers undergo amniocentesis or fetal surgery is performed to correct life-threatening fetal malformations or conditions. This disturbance is rarely accompanied by the benefit of analgesia for the infant, thus rendering the infant susceptible to the consequences of stress and pain that the infant has the capacity for from mid to late gestation.

Although there is a large body of research on the pain of labor suffered by the mother, there is little research on the travail of the infant during this process (Sparshott, 1997). The passage between the harmony that is experienced in the womb and the discordance of a world that demands to be noticed is a trauma at least as shocking for the baby as the mother (Sparshott, 1997). This trauma is created by passage through the birth canal and the contrast between the total dependence of existence in the womb and the quasi-dependence of life outside the womb. If the birth is gentle, the effect of this trauma may be minimized for the newborn infant. However, if the delivery is prolonged or difficult, the infant may be subjected to many hours of painful contractions followed by a delivery that includes surgery for cesarean sectioning, forceps, or vacuum extraction. All of these procedures have the potential to be very painful for the infant. However, due to the rapid course of events, concern for the well-being of the infant and mother and the physical inaccessibility of the infant during the birth process, there is frequently little intervention for the infant until after the birth. At that time, the infant can be comforted by being placed in close contact with the mother to initiate sucking, covered with blankets to maintain warmth, and provided with tactile and vestibular stimulation by gentle stroking and rocking.

Immediately after birth and during the neonatal period

For the healthy term infant, the sources of pain immediately after birth are minimal and are usually limited to one or two heel lances to procure blood for laboratory samples and an injection to administer vitamin K. These procedures are usually performed within the first 24-72 hours of life prior to the infant's discharge home. If the infant is jaundiced and is treated with hyperbilirubinemia therapy (e.g., phototherapy), further heel lances may be necessary to assess bilirubin levels and the infant's hospital stay may be lengthened.

Circumcision

One of the most painful procedures physicians perform is circumcision, yet many physicians continue to perform this procedure without providing any anesthesia or analgesia whatsoever. A number of unsupported explanations are offered for this lack of attentive analgesic care, including myths that babies do not feel pain or remember pain and will not be able to urinate if the penis is anesthetized (see Table 14.1, p. 627).

Several researchers have studied the responses of neonates during circumcision (Maxwell, Yaster, Wetzel et al., 1987; Williamson, 1997; Williamson, Williamson, 1983). In these studies blinded observers had no difficulty distinguishing neonates who did not receive anesthesia from those who did. Neonates not only demonstrated signs of excruciating pain during circumcision but also a number of disturbing and dangerous physiologic stress reactions, including breath holding, apnea, cyanosis, gagging, vomiting, and accelerated glucose consumption (Maxwell, Yaster, Wetzel et al., 1987; Rice, 1996; Williamson, 1997; Williamson, Williamson, 1983).

In a recent study it was noted that both anesthetized and unanesthetized neonates cried during application of restraints and surgical scrubbing before circumcision (Williamson, 1997). Both groups of neonates also demonstrated similar decreases in oxygen saturation and increases in heart rate during this time. All the anesthetized neonates in this study cried during the 30-second interval while lidocaine was injected for the dorsal penile nerve block, but crying subsided immediately afterward and throughout the circumcision procedure. However, all the unanesthetized neonates cried in a high-pitched screeching manner, typical of a pain cry, from the beginning of the glans dissection until the dressing was applied at the end of the circumcision procedure. Unanesthetized neonates exhibited breath holding, apnea, hyperventilation, and a heart rate mean peak of 60 beats/min greater than baseline during dissection of the foreskin from the glans and placement of the Gomco clamp.

Other findings from this study counter objections regarding the safety of anesthesia during circumcision. The anesthetized infants urinated earlier (2.2 to 11.7 hours) than the unanesthetized infants (2.7 to 18.2 hours), and peak serum lidocaine levels in the anesthetized infants were lower than those seen in infants whose mothers receive epidural anesthesia for labor or cesarean section. In neither group was there abnormal bleeding, swelling, inflammation, exudate, or postoperative vital signs. Williamson concludes that "humane care" of babies must include appropriate anesthesia and analgesia during procedures for which older children and adults would receive such treatment and urges informing parents of the availability of penile block for anesthesia during circumcision (Williamson, 1997).

Various anesthetic techniques were compared with placebo (representative of current practice) for circumcision (Lander, Brady-Fryer, Metcalfe et al., 1997). One- to 3-day-old males received ring block, dorsal penile nerve block, topical EMLA, or topical placebo before circumcision. Newborns in the placebo group demonstrated sustained elevation of heart rate and high-pitched crying throughout the entire circumcision procedure; two newborns in the placebo group choked and became apneic after circumcision. The three other groups had significantly less crying and lower heart rates during and after the procedure. The ring block proved to be the most effective of all treatments. Methemoglobin levels were highest in the EMLA group, but no infants required treatment (see p. 657 for more on EMLA and methemoglobinemia).

There are alternatives to lidocaine for penile block for circumcision. Chloroprocaine was found to be as effective as lidocaine for reducing "neonatal stress" during circumcision. Neonatal stress in this study was evaluated by noting changes from baseline cry duration, tissue oxygenation, and heart rate. Ideal anesthesia was found at 3 minutes, and the researchers cited the more rapid onset of chloroprocaine as a major benefit (Spencer, Miller, O'Quin et al., 1992). However, the short duration of chloroprocaine also must be considered. It is rapidly metabolized and has a plasma half-life of 25 seconds, therefore leaving the infants with no (or minimal) postoperative analgesia (Catterall, Mackie, 1996).

A lidocaine-prilocaine 5% cream (EMLA, Astra USA Inc.) has also been used for pain control during neonatal circumcision in two other studies (Benini, Johnston, Faucher et al., 1993; Taddio, Stevens, Craig et al., 1997). Benini and others (1993) applied one half gram of EMLA or petroleum jelly placebo for 45 to 65 minutes before circumcision. For both physiologic (i.e., heart rate, oxygen saturation) and behavioral (i.e., facial expressions, crying) pain indicators, EMLA was associated with a significantly reduced response compared with placebo during the most painful phases of the procedure. The average heart rate for the EMLA group compared with the control group was 25 beats/min less, and the average oxygen saturation was 5% higher. Facial activity was significantly less (i.e., 20%), and less crying (i.e., 15%) was observed in the EMLA compared with the placebo group.

Taddio et al. (1997) also tested the efficacy of EMLA by randomly assigning infants to receive either one third of a 1-g dose of EMLA or EMLA placebo applied to the lower abdomen. Next, the penis was extended upward and folded against the abdomen. Then the rest of the EMLA or EMLA placebo dose was applied to an occlusive dressing, which was placed over the penis and taped to the abdomen. After 60 to 80 minutes, the dressing and cream were removed. Compared with infants who received the placebo EMLA cream, infants who received EMLA had less facial activity, spent less time crying, and had smaller increases in heart rate during the most invasive phases of the circumcision. Blood methemoglobin concentrations were similar in both groups. Although EMLA decreased pain during circumcision in both of these studies, the risk of methemoglobinemia associated with EMLA use is an important consideration for neonates and infants. The efficacy and safety of EMLA for procedural pain have been systematically reviewed (Taddio, Ohlsson, Einarson et al., 1998) and are further discussed on p. 657.

Patient Example

Mrs. S. had her baby yesterday and plans to have him circumcised. She is concerned about the baby's pain during and after the circumcision. Recently, the hospital's pain care committee established a protocol for circumcision pain control. Mrs. S.'s nurse tells Mrs. S. that the physician will numb the baby's penis with lidocaine before the circumcision. She assures Mrs. S. that nondrug comfort measures also will be used during the procedure, such as giving the baby a pacifier to suck on, talking softly or singing to him, and keeping him warm with a carefully placed heat lamp during the procedure. The nurse asks Mrs. S. if she would like to be present during the circumcision. If she decides not to be present, the baby will be taken immediately to her afterward for comforting. A dose of acetaminophen elixir will be given at the end of the procedure so that it can take effect as the local anesthetic wears off. Because Mrs. S. and her baby will be discharged today, the nurse teaches Mrs. S. to give the baby the acetaminophen elixir in scheduled ATC doses for 48 hours after the circumcision. After watching the nurse, Mrs. S. practices measuring and putting dextrose water into a nipple for the baby to suck just as she will when she administers the acetaminophen elixir. The baby tolerated the circumcision very well. Although he objected at first to being restrained for the procedure, his CRIES pain rating was 0 during and after the procedure (see pp. 642-644 for more on the CRIES pain rating scale).

The Preterm and/or Ill Infant

For the preterm infant or term infant who is sick, the sources of pain suffered during hospitalization immediately after birth and during the neonatal period may be considerable. Barker and Rutter (1995) described the nature and number of invasive procedures in 54 infants admitted consecutively to the NICU. In this group of infants more than 3000 procedures were recorded, 74% in infants less than 31 weeks' GA. One infant of 23 weeks' GA experienced 488 procedures. Similarly, Stevens et al. (in press) noted that in a randomized crossover trial, infants in the NICU between 27 to 31 weeks' GA at birth experienced an average of 134 painful procedures (SD 144, range 0 to 821) within the first two weeks of life. Furthermore, approximately 10% of the youngest and/or sickest infants received more than 300 painful procedures. Painful procedures in the NICU can either be tissue damaging or nontissue damaging. Tissue-damaging procedures include heel lances, intravenous and arterial insertions, lumbar punctures, and bladder taps, whereas non-tissue-damaging procedures include insertion of feeding tubes, suctioning, intubations, and tape removal.

Evans and others (1997) have also reported facial grimacing, slight cry expression, increased cry expression, and knee/leg flexion after known painful procedures and after "nonpainful" procedures such as total position change, addition or withdrawal of fluid from an umbilical catheter, and IV administration of medication.

Findings from a recent survey (Porter, Wolf, Gold et al., 1997) completed by 374 clinicians indicated that although health professionals believe that infants feel as much pain as adults and that 9 of 12 specified procedures were thought to be moderately to very painful, neither pharmacologic nor comfort measures were believed to be used frequently, even for the most painful procedures. These results are consistent with two studies that indicated that although infants in the NICU receive adequate pain relief for postoperative pain, we have made little progress in managing procedural pain for these NICU infants who undergo multiple painful procedures and experience significant physiologic stress related to pain (Anand, Selanikio, 1996; Johnston, Collinge, Henderson et al., 1998). Additional findings in this study were that physicians and nurses believed that both pharmacologic and comfort measures should be used more frequently. Compared with physicians, nurses believed comfort measures should be used more frequently. Physicians who had experienced significant personal pain tended to rate infant pain higher compared with physicians who had not experienced significant pain.

Much less is known about the pain associated with specific conditions experienced during the perinatal period (e.g., intracranial hemorrhage, posthemorrhage hydrocephalus). However, no evidence suggests that this pain is of a lower magnitude in the fetus or neonate than the older child or adult with similar tissue injury (Anand, Carr, 1989). Also a lack of information exists on recurrent or chronic pain (i.e., conditions with extensive tissue damage such as epidermolysis bulbosa, necrotizing enterocolitis) in infants. Research on chronic and recurrent pain in infants needs to be undertaken to fill these gaps in knowledge.

During the first year of life

After the infant leaves the hospital, the instances of pain from procedures diminish dramatically. However, because immunizations are the most effective way of preventing common childhood diseases such as diphtheria, whooping cough, tetanus, polio, meningitis, measles, mumps, and rubella, infants have painful injections during visits to the pediatrician or outpatient clinic at approximately 2 months, 4 months, 6 months, 12 months, and 18 months. Immunization injections are most often given in the thigh muscle in infants and toddlers. Clinicians can teach parents how to diminish their child's pain and ease their anxieties during these situations. Strategies for management of pain from immunization injections are described in Table 14.2.

The home is the place where the infant will grow, develop, and gain independence. Although most infants enjoy a pain-free home environment, some infants require continuation of painful procedures after discharge from

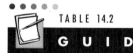

TABLE 14.2

GUIDELINES

DECREASING PAIN FROM IMMUNIZATIONS

Strategy	Rationale
Use a local anesthetic cream (e.g., EMLA) 60-90 min before the injection on the thigh site.	The anesthetic cream creates a numb area so the pain from injection is decreased.
Give the infant the recommended dose of analgesic (e.g., acetaminophen) $\frac{1}{2}$ to 1 h before the injection. This may also be repeated q4h after the injection for up to 24 h.	There is adequate time for the medication to be absorbed into the system, thus minimizing pain at the time of the injection and for the 24 h after the injection if the site is red, swollen, or painful.
Use a cool cloth or ice wrapped in a cloth for 5-10 min after injection.	This will reduce inflammation and swelling.
Have the parent hold the baby during the immunization.	Having someone familiar present will decrease the anxiety associated with the experience and will promote soothing.
Use breast or bottle feeding immediately after the injection (not during).	This is an expedient way of having the infant regain security after the painful event.
Allow extra time for sleep.	Sleep promotes healing and recovery from a stressful situation.

the hospital. Some of these procedures may include injections, tube insertions, suctioning, dressing changes, and stoma care. These procedures may be performed by a visiting home care nurse but most often eventually are taken over by the mother. The impact on mothers of performing painful procedures on their infants at home has not been researched. However, given what is known about the developing maternal-infant relationship in early life (Wynn, 1997), inflicting pain by the person whom the infant normally seeks protection from could be highly problematic. This is an area that requires research at a time when, because of fiscal constraints and cost-cutting measures, more and more infants still requiring painful procedures will be discharged home to the care of their parents.

Home is also the place where minor injuries, such as cuts, bruises, and scrapes, and more serious injuries, including fractures, dislocations, burns, and other injuries, may occur. For infants, minor injuries most often occur as the child becomes mobile and is learning how to crawl or walk. These injuries, although painful, can most likely be managed at home with nonpharmacologic strategies such as cleaning the wound, applying a bandage, distraction, and soothing. More serious injuries such as fractures, dislocations, and burns may cause severe pain for the infant and need to be assessed and treated in the ED of the hospital. Parents need to have a plan for injury and pain management that is familiar and agreeable to parents, baby-sitters, and other caregivers because they often feel guilty when a child is hurt and may not act appropriately. This plan needs to include emergency telephone numbers of parents, doctors, and the hospital; knowledge of normal procedures for managing injuries; and the location of supplies. It is also important to develop an open and trusting relationship between parents and caregivers that includes open discussion of all occurrences and accidents.

The healthy infant who requires minor surgical or diagnostic procedures such as hernia repair, cystoscopy, or bronchoscopy may receive these services or procedures in the ambulatory or outpatient setting. Because of limited time for contact with the child, these admissions need to be planned well in advance. If the short stay experience involves procedures that will be painful, plans for analgesic administration before, during, and after the event need to be determined and discussed with the parents before admission to prepare both themselves and the infant for the event and to help them make plans for afterwards. In particular, parents need to know how to assess whether the infant has pain and how to manage it. Although a measure exists for parents to assess postoperative pain at home in children aged 7 to 12 (The Postoperative Pain Measure for Parents; Chambers, Reid, McGrath et al., 1996), it has not been validated for use with infants and no similar infant pain measure is available for parents. Therefore parents need to be taught how to carefully observe for behavioral and physiologic cues that may indicate pain in their child after discharge from the ambulatory setting. These include (1) changes in sleep, play, eating, and elimination patterns; (2) increased irritability and crying, moaning, groaning, and clinginess; (3) decreased energy and consolability; and (4) pallor, flushing, fever, and/or swelling in the surgical area. Parents need to be clear on how much pain is "normal" after minor surgical procedures that are performed in ambulatory settings and how to manage pain should it occur by use of both pharmacologic and nonpharmacologic interventions.

PAIN ASSESSMENT IN INFANTS

Pain assessment is the first step in pain relief. Valid assessment of pain facilitates diagnosis, defines the impact of procedures on the individual, and determines the efficacy of pain management interventions. However, pain assessment is challenging in infants because of the subjective and complex nature of the phenomenon, cognitive and language limitations that preclude comprehension and self-report, the variability and inconsistency of pain expression, and the dependence on others to infer pain from behavioral and physiologic indicators. The quality of pain measurement is highly dependent on the pain assessment measures and those using them. Therefore the focus of this section will be to:

- Distinguish between assessment and measurement of pain in infants
- Identify assumptions and beliefs that influence pain assessment in infants
- Describe univariate versus multivariate approaches to pain assessment in infants
- Evaluate measures of infant pain in terms of their purpose (acute versus chronic), validity, reliability, clinical use, and feasibility, which are described in depth in Chapter 3, Box 3.6, p. 66.

Assessment Versus Measurement

Assessment and measurement of pain are different processes. Measurement is the quantifiable aspect of assessment and answers the question, How much? The emphasis is on the quantity, extent, and degree of pain judged by a standard unit. Measurement provides data to support the comparison of more or less to a standard of some kind (Johnston, 1998). Physiologic indicators of pain can be measured in an objective, bias-free manner. For infants in pain, health care professionals can determine how much heart rate increases or how much oxygen saturation decreases from monitors. Clinical decisions are often made on the basis of the actual units being measured or changes in the magnitude of values.

Assessment is a broader concept than measurement. Assessment may include measurement but also involves clinical judgments that are made on the basis of observations on the nature, significance, and other relevant properties of pain. Precise numbers usually are not associated with assessment, although quantifiable terms, such as *more* or *less,* can be used. For infants incapable of self-report, assessment including the intensity, location, duration, unpleasantness, and contextual and situational factors that may influence measurement is crucial for clinical decision making.

Assumptions and beliefs

Assessment of pain in children, especially the very young, requires active use of educated assumptions and beliefs. On the basis of certain assumptions, decisions about the presence or absence of pain are made, action is taken, and the outcome is evaluated, recognizing that once again certain assumptions must be made.

Our approach to infant pain assessment is made on the basis of the following assumptions or beliefs:

- All infants, including neonates and preterm infants, have the ability to feel pain.
- Anything that causes pain in adults also causes pain in infants.
- Some things that do not cause pain in adults may cause pain in infants.
- Assessment encompasses responses at the moment and over time. Assessments are made at regular intervals and compared, and a written record is kept.
- Infants respond to pain not only with a variety of physiologic and behavioral indicators but also without exhibiting any observable responses. Lack of response does not necessarily mean lack of pain.
- In infants, pain must be assessed by use of multiple indicators, with special attention being paid to changes in these indicators.
- Opinions about pain are best obtained from parents and caretakers familiar with the infant.
- An ongoing, open dialog between staff and parents about the infant's pain is encouraged in the hope that increasingly accurate assessments and insights will occur.

Infant Pain Measurement Approaches

Acute versus chronic pain

Most research on infant pain assessment has focused on acute or procedural pain. This is largely due to the pressing need to have measures for assessing procedural and postoperative pain and the effectiveness of pain-relieving interventions. Over the past 5 years, more than a dozen pain measures for assessing pain in infants have been developed. However, almost all these measures have been developed for assessing acute pain. Little understanding exists about the measurement of long-term effects of repeated pain or chronic pain or stress. Indicators of chronic and acute pain differ in that behavior associated with chronic pain may be more passive or neutral, and decreases in physiologic change and variability may be minimal. However, an increase in depression, insomnia, change in feeding patterns, and impaired coping responses may occur.

Sparshott (1997) describes the infant who, after weeks or months of illness and a constant bombardment of traumatic procedures, presents as a picture of inertia, diminished alertness, withdrawal, and hostility. These infants have given up trying to defend themselves against repeated episodes of pain, but their resignation may be difficult to recognize. However, attempts by familiar caregivers or a parent will be met with indifference, visual aversion, or the expression of "frozen watchfulness" (p. 50).

Unidimensional versus multidimensional approaches

Unidimensional and multidimensional approaches to measurement are both used for assessing pain in infants. Unidimensional measures may have one indicator (e.g., heart rate), one type of indicator (e.g., facial expression), or a unitary approach to pain assessment (e.g., behavioral). Multidimensional assessment combines a variety of subjective and objective univariate measurement approaches or uses a composite measure. Composite pain measures include a variety of physiologic, behavioral, sensory, affective, and cognitive dimensions and contextual factors within one instrument. Multidimensional assessment is particularly appropriate when self-report is not possible or generally with children who have developmental, cognitive, and verbal limitations or with children less than 5 years old (McGrath, 1995).

In the past decade more than a dozen infant pain measures have been developed. Because the major impetus during this time has been to understand how to assess and manage pain in this age group, most of these measures have been developed for research purposes. No one measure has been shown to be adequate for use in the clinical setting for infants of all ages and in all situations. However, some measures that have established reliability and validity are more promising than others in terms of feasibility and clinical usefulness for particular groups of infants and particular situations. These measures include the CRIES (Krechel, Bildner, 1995) and the PIPP (Stevens, Johnston, Petryshen et al., 1996). They are multidimensional measures shown in Forms 14.2 and 14.3, respectively (see pp. 644-645). Other unidimensional and multidimensional pain measures are also briefly described. Their specific indicators and psychometric properties are summarized in Tables 14.3 (unidimensional) and 14.4 (multidimensional) (see pp. 643 and 650).

Unidimensional Pain Measures

Unidimensional pain measures in infants include physiologic and behavioral indicators. Physiologic indicators include increases in heart rate, respiratory rate, blood pressure, palmar sweating, intracranial pressure, and stress hormones; decreases in transcutaneous oxygen saturation levels, transcutaneous carbon dioxide levels, or vagal tone; and autonomic changes including changes in skin color, nausea, vomiting, gagging, hiccoughing, diaphoresis, and dilated pupils. These indicators support the activation of the sympathetic nervous system but are inconsistent among children. Physiologic indicators alone cannot unequivocally be interpreted as pain because they are more clearly associated with stress.

The most predominant unidimensional approach to pain assessment is behavioral and the most frequently assessed behavioral indicator in infant pain measures is facial activity. Facial activity is more commonly studied in infants than older children and is considered the most consistent indicator of pain in this age group. Prkachin and Craig (1995) have used either the *Facial Action Coding System* (FACS; Ekman, Friesen, 1978) or its adaptation to the study of facial activity in infants, *Baby FACS,* because of the infant's different facial structure (Oster, Rosenstein, 1993). These measures require trained coders to identify the presence or absence, intensity, and temporal features of 45 different discrete facial actions from videotapes and therefore are best suited to research rather than ongoing clinical evaluation (Craig, 1998).

Less demanding measures of facial activity have been developed to assess neonatal pain. *The Neonatal Facial Coding System* (NFCS; Grunau, Craig, 1990) is one of two anatomically based systems for assessing facial expression in infants. This 10-item measure is the basis of the FACS (Ekman, Friesen, 1978) but is adapted for use with neonates. Facial actions that are most consistently associated with pain include a bulging brow, eyes squeezed tightly shut, deepening of the nasolabial furrow, open lips, mouth stretched vertically and horizontally, and a taut or dished tongue, although there can be substantial individual variation in these actions and in the vigor of the infant's response (Craig, 1998) (see Figure 14.1, p. 633).

The Maximally Discriminative Facial Coding System (MAX; Izard, 1979) is a more global judgment measure that consists of templates for patterns of facial activity associated with specific emotional states derived from differential emotions theory. Three parts of the face are scored separately: the forehead and brow, the eyes and nose ridge, and the mouth. These assessments are used to identify, from photographs, 10 different emotions, including anger, fear, surprise, joy, and pain. The pain pattern has the brows lowered and drawn together, bulging and/or vertical furrows between brows, nasal root broadening and bulged, eye fissures tightly closed, and an angular squarish mouth. Similar to the FACS, the NFCS

and the MAX were developed primarily for use in research, require intensive training and time for coding, and have minimal clinical use.

Other behaviors can also form the basis of a pain assessment approach. *The Infant Body Coding System* (IBCS; Craig, McMahan, Morison et al., 1984) is a behavioral measure for assessing gross motor activity in infants. Movements of the hand, foot, arm, leg, head, and torso are scored as either present or absent. The IBCS has been used with the NFCS to determine the effect of gestational age on the newborn infant's response to heel lance. The IBCS was more sensitive with increasing levels of activity in term compared with preterm infants, but less specific to the painful event.

Three univariate measures have incorporated more than one type of behavioral indicator for the assessment of pain. *The Clinical Scoring System* (Attia, Amiel-Tison, Mayer et al., 1987; Barrier, Attia, Mayer et al., 1989) combines a variety of behavioral indicators for evaluating postoperative pain. Higher scores (less pain) were associated with infants who had received fentanyl versus a placebo postoperatively. This scoring system is somewhat confusing because higher scores indicate lower pain, whereas lower scores equal higher pain. This scale has had minimal testing for reliability and validity and has limited feasibility for use in the clinical setting because indicators are scored over the previous hour or hours.

The *Behavioral Pain Score* (Pokela, 1994) consists of four indicators that assess facial expression, body movements, response to handling/consolability, and rigidity of the limbs and body. The scale was developed from the Children's Hospital of Eastern Ontario Pain Scale to determine the effectiveness of pharmacologic therapy (i.e., opioids) in reducing pain and hypoxemia in ventilated preterm and full-term neonates during painful procedures. This scale has not been tested for reliability and validity, and the clinical use of the measure is unknown.

The *Modified Behavioral Pain Scale* (MBPS; Taddio, Nulman, Koren et al., 1995) was adapted from CHEOPS; (McGrath, Johnson, Goodman et al., 1985) for use with infants. Reliability and validity of the measures were assessed in a study of 96 infants undergoing vaccination, in which infants were randomized to receive either an EMLA or placebo treatment. Infants' behavioral responses were videotaped before, during, and after the procedure and were found to be lower in infants who received the EMLA treatment. Pain scores from the MBPS were highly and significantly correlated with a visual analog scale (VAS) rating assessed by health care professionals during the vaccination session.

Two additional pain scales can be described as multimodal-item behavioral pain scales. Within each item, several modes of behavior are included. The *Pain Rating Scale* (PRS; Joyce, Schade, Keck et al., 1994) includes six multimodal categories of behavior that increase in intensity. The no pain category has several behaviors that the authors suggest indicate no pain, including smiling, sleeping, and no change in behavior when moved or touched. Conversely, the worst pain category includes sleeping prolonged periods interrupted by jerking, continuous crying, and rapid shallow respirations. A second measure, the *Riley Infant Pain Scale* (RIPS; Schade, Joyce, Gerkensmeyer et al., 1996), was developed in a similar manner by the same group of investigators for use with children less than 36 months of age and children with cerebral palsy. The RIPS has four categories of multimodal behavior, with 0 = no pain and 3 = worst pain. The "no pain" category indicators include neutral face/smiling, calm, sleeping quietly, no cry, consolable, moves easily. The "worst pain" category includes full cry expression, thrashing/flailing, sleeping prolonged periods interrupted by jerking or no sleep, screaming/high-pitched cry, inconsolable, and screaming when touched or moved.

In summary, behavioral measurement with univariate measures has made significant strides but much remains to be done. No single indicator is reliable, valid, sensitive, specific, practical, or feasible for identifying the existence, intensity, location, and impact of pain in any given population or situation. Although a few of the unidimensional measures have well-established psychometric properties, the lack of reported validity and reliability for most of the unidimensional measures for assessing pain in infants frequently precludes their use in the clinical setting. These limitations are the basis for the development and use of multidimensional approaches or composite measures of pain. A summary of the pain indicators for unidimensional infant pain measures is included in Table 14.3, along with reliability and validity and clinical usefulness.

Multidimensional Pain Measures

The complex and multidimensional nature of pain suggests that it is best assessed by more than a single indicator or by multiple dimensions that provide as much information as possible about individual pain responses. Multidimensional pain assessment can include combining a number of subjective and objective univariate measurements or by use of a composite measure that includes a variety of self-report, physiologic, behavioral, and contextual indicators within one instrument. Several composite measures for assessing pain in infants have been recently developed. Of these, two have been tested more thoroughly for reliability and validity than the others. These include the CRIES (Krechel, Bildner, 1995), which was developed for assessing postoperative pain in infants, and the PIPP (Stevens, Johnston, Petryshen et al., 1996), which was developed for assessing pain in preterm and term neonates. Both of these measures have also undergone either formal or informal initial testing for clinical use. Other multidimensional measures will also be discussed briefly.

The *CRIES* (Krechel, Bildner, 1995) is a neonatal postoperative pain measure (Form 14.2) that consists of five physiologic and behavioral indicators. Each indicator is rated on a 3-point scale (0, 1, 2) that results in a total score ranging from 0 to 10. The title of the measure CRIES is an acronym created to stimulate memory of the indicators on the scale.

- **C**rying
- **R**equires O_2 for saturation >95
- **I**ncreased vital signs (heart rate and blood pressure)
- **E**xpression
- **S**leepless

The psychometric properties of the measure were established with a group of 24 infants (32 to 60 weeks' gestational age) admitted to the neonatal and pediatric intensive care units after surgery. Construct validity was established by comparing CRIES scores at the time analgesia was administered and 1 hour later. The decrease in scores between the two time points was significantly different. Concurrent validity was established by correlating the CRIES scores and subjective nurse ratings. To establish convergent validity, the same two nurses independently rated the infant's pain using the CRIES and the Objective Pain Scale (OPS) (Hannalah, Braodman, Belman et al., 1987). Although nurses generally stated that they had a preference for the CRIES over the OPS, the feasibility and clinical usefulness of the measures have not been formally assessed. However, to date, the CRIES is the most promising measure available for assessment of postoperative pain in infants.

The *Premature Infant Pain Profile* (PIPP; Stevens, Johnston, Petryshen et al., 1996) was specifically developed to assess acute pain in preterm and term neonates (Form 14.3, p. 645). PIPP is a 7-indicator pain measure that includes behavioral, physiologic, and contextual indicators. Initially 15 indicators were selected from the literature and clinical expertise suggesting face validity. The number of indicators was reduced to seven after principal components analysis and a sensitivity/specificity analysis. These seven indicators were reviewed by a group of multidisciplinary experts to establish content validity. Each indicator is evaluated on a 4-point scale (0, 1, 2, 3) for a possible total score of 21 for infants of lesser gestational age and a total score of 18 for infants of greater gestational age at birth. For all age groups, a total score of 6 or less generally indicates minimal or no pain, whereas scores greater than 12 indicate moderate to severe pain.

Several methods were used to establish construct validity. First, the same group of preterm infants (32 to 34 weeks' gestational age) was assessed for pain in divergent situations (handling versus heelstick). Second, two different groups of the same gestational age were assessed in the same two divergent situations (handling versus heelstick). Third, a group of lesser gestational age (28 to 32 weeks' gestation) was assessed in a different situation (heelstick versus sham heelstick), and finally a group of

● ● ● ● ●

TABLE 14.3 **Unidimensional Infant Pain Measures**

MEASURE	INDICATORS	VALIDITY	RELIABILITY
NFCS (Grunau, Craig, 1990)	Facial actions: • Brow bulge • Eye squeeze • Nasolabial furrow • Open lips • Vertical mouth stretch • Horizontal mouth stretch • Lip purse • Taut tongue • Tongue protrusion • Chin quiver	Face Content Construct	Interrater Intrarater
MAX (Izard, 1979)	Templates for patterns of facial activity associated with 10 specific emotional states (e.g., pain, anger)	Face Content Construct	Interrater
Infant Body Coding System (Craig, McMahan, Morison et al., 1984)	Movements of • Hand/foot • Arm/leg • Head/torso	Face Content	Interrater
Clinical Scoring System (Attia, Amiel-Tison, Mayer et al., 1987; Barrier, Attia, Mayer et al., 1989)	Sleep in previous hour Facial expressions Quality of cry Spontaneous motor activity Spontaneous excitability Flexion of fingers/toes Sucking Global evaluation of tone Consolability Sociability	Construct	
Behavioral Pain Score (Pokela, 1994)	Facial expression Movements Response to handling/consolability Rigidity of limbs/body	Construct	
Modified Behavioral Pain Score (Taddio, Nulman, Koren et al., 1995)	Facial expression Crying Movements	Content Construct	Interrater
Pain Rating Scale (Joyce, Schade, Keck et al., 1994)	Six multidimensional behavioral items	Construct	Interrater
Riley Infant Pain Scale (Schade, Joyce, Gerkensmeyer et al, 1996)	Four multidimensional behavioral items	Construct	Interrater

May be duplicated for use in clinical practice. From McCaffery M, Pasero C: *Pain: Clinical manual*, p. 643. Copyright © 1999, Mosby, Inc.
Information from Attia J, Amiel-Tison C, Mayer M-N et al.: Measurement of postoperative pain and narcotic administration in infants using a new clinical scoring system, *Anesthesiology* 67:532A, 1987; Barrier G, Attia J, Mayer M-N et al.: Measurement of post-operative pain and narcotic administration in infants using a new clinical scoring system, *Intens Care Med* 15:S37-S39, 1989; Craig KD, McMahan RJ, Morison JD et al.: Developmental changes in infant pain expression during immunization injections, *Soc Sci Med* 19:1331-1337, 1984; Grunau RVE, Craig KD: Facial activity as a measure of neonatal pain expression. In Tyler DC, Krane EJ, editors: *Advances in pain research and therapy, pediatric pain*, vol 15, pp 147-56, New York, 1990, Raven Press; Izard CE: The maximally discriminative facial movement coding system (MAX), Newark, 1979, University of Delaware Instructional Resources Center; Joyce BA, Schade JG, Keck JF et al.: Reliability and validity of preverbal pain assessment tools, *Iss Comprehens Pediat Nurs* 17:121-135, 1994; Pokela M: Pain relief can reduce hypoxemia in distressed neonates during routine treatment procedures, *Pediatrics* 93:379-383, 1994; Schade JG, Joyce BA, Gerkensmeyer J et al.: Comparison of three preverbal scales for postoperative pain assessment in a diverse pediatric sample, *J Pain Symptom Manage* 12:348-359, 1996; Taddio A, Nulman I, Koren BS et al.: A revised measure of acute pain in infants, *J Pain Symptom Manage* 10:456-463, 1995.

older gestational age (term neonates) was assessed during a control and experimental intervention for circumcision. In all situations and age groups, the PIPP score accurately reflected differences between pain and nonpain situations. In the circumcision situation the PIPP reflected a differ-

ence in interventions to assist in determining the efficacy of the pain management strategy being tested.

To determine the clinical validity, preterm and term neonates received three randomly ordered events: baseline, handling, and painful. The infant's responses were

● ● ● ● ●

FORM 14.2 **CRIES Neonatal Postoperative Pain Measurement Score**

		0	1	2
	Crying	No	High pitched	Inconsolable
	Requires O_2 for sat >95	No	<30%	>30%
	Increased vital signs	HR and BP = or <preop	HR or BP ↑ <20% of preop	HR or BP ↑ >20% of preop
	Expression	None	Grimace	Grimace/grunt
	Sleepless	No	Wakes at frequent intervals	Constantly awake

Neonatal pain assessment tool developed at the University of Missouri-Columbia. Copyright S. Krechel, MD, and J. Bildner, RNC, CNS.

CODING TIPS FOR USING CRIES

Crying	The characteristic cry of pain is *high pitched*. If no cry or cry that is not high pitched, score 0. If cry high pitched but baby is easily consoled, score 1. If cry is high pitched and baby is inconsolable, score 2.
Requires O_2 for sat >95%	Look for *changes* in oxygenation. Babies experiencing pain manifest decreases in oxygenation as measured by TCo_2 or oxygen saturation. If no oxygen is required, score 0. (Consider other causes of changes in oxygenation, If <30% O_2 is required, score 1. such as atelectasis, pneumothorax, over-sedation) If >30% is required, score 2.
Increased vital signs	NOTE: Take blood pressure last as this may wake child, causing difficulty with other assessments. Use baseline preoperative parameters from a nonstressed period. Multiply baseline HR × 0.2 and then add this to baseline HR to determine the HR, which is 20% over baseline. Do likewise for BP. Use mean BP. If HR and BP are both unchanged or less than baseline, score 0. If HR or BP is increased but increase is <20% of baseline, score 1. If either one is increased >20% over baseline, score 2.
Expression	The facial expression most often associated with pain is a grimace. This may be characterized by brow lowering, eyes squeezed shut, deepening of the nasolabial furrow, open lips and mouth. If no grimace is present, score 0. If grimace alone is present, score 1. If grimace and noncry vocalization grunt are present, score 2.
Sleepless	This parameter is scored based on the infant's state during the hour preceding this recorded score. If the child has been continuously asleep, score 0. If he or she has awakened at frequent intervals, score 1. If he or she has been awake constantly, score 2.

May be duplicated for use in clinical practice. As appears in McCaffery M, Pasero C: *Pain: Clinical manual*, p. 644, 1999, Mosby, Inc.
From Krechel SW, Bildner J: CRIES: A new neonatal postoperative pain measurement score. Initial testing of validity and reliability, *Pediatr Anesth* 5:53-61, 1995.

independently rated by four raters (two nurses at the bedside and one nurse and one expert coder in the research laboratory using a videotape). No significant difference was found between the raters, but a significant difference was found between the events, suggesting that the PIPP had construct validity when used by raters in the clinical setting. Interrater and intrarater reliability was high. Use of the PIPP was facilitated by a set of instructions for users and implementation of individual practice sessions before use. Training nurses at the bedside to use the PIPP to assess pain in the infant took approximately 1 minute and another 2 to 3 minutes for practice. This measure has had more validity and reliability testing than any other measure of pain in infants. However, its use has been primarily limited to procedural pain in preterm neonates. Testing of the PIPP for more enduring pain (e.g., postoperative pain, pain from medical conditions) is currently underway, but its usefulness in these situations has not been determined.

The *Neonatal Infant Pain Scale* (NIPS; Lawrence, Alcock, McGrath et al., 1993) is composed of six indicators of pain (five behavioral and one physiologic) that were identified by nurses. The NIPS was adapted from CHEOPS (McGrath, Johnson, Goodman et al., 1985),

FORM 14.3 **Premature Infant Pain Profile (PIPP)**

Infant ID Number: _____

Date/time: _____

Event: _____

PROCESS	INDICATOR	0	1	2	3	SCORE
Chart	Gestational age (at time of observation)	36 weeks and more	32 weeks to 35 weeks, 6 days	28 weeks to 31 weeks, 6 days	Less than 28 weeks	
Observe infant 15 sec Observe baseline: Heart rate _____ Oxygen saturation _____	Behavioral state	Active/awake Eyes open Facial movements Crying (with eyes open or closed)	Quiet/awake Eyes open No facial movements	Active/sleep Eyes closed Facial movements	Quiet/sleep Eyes closed No facial movements	
Observe infant 30 sec	Heart rate Max. _____	0 to 4 beats/minute increase	5 to 14 beats/minute increase	15 to 24 beats/minute increase	25 beats/minute or more increase	
	Oxygen saturation Min. _____	0% to 2.4% decrease	2.5% to 4.9% decrease	5.0% to 7.4% decrease	7.5% or more decrease	
	Brow bulge	None 0%-9% of time	Minimum 10%-39% of time	Moderate 40%-69% of time	Maximum 70% of time or more	
	Eye squeeze	None 0%-9% of time	Minimum 10%-39% of time	Moderate 40%-69% of time	Maximum 70% of time or more	
	Nasolabial furrow	None 0%-9% of time	Minimum 10%-39% of time	Moderate 40%-69% of time	Maximum 70% of time or more	
					TOTAL SCORE	

May be duplicated for use in clinical practice. As appears in McCaffery M, Pasero C: *Pain: Clinical manual,* p. 645, 1999, Mosby, Inc.

Form and scoring method from Stevens B, Johnston CC, Petryshen P et al.: Premature infant pain profile: Development and initial validation, *Clin J Pain* 12:13-22, 1996.

● ● ● ● ●

Scoring Method for the PIPP

1. Familiarize yourself with each indicator and how it is to be scored by looking at the measure.
2. Score gestational age (from the chart) before you begin.
3. Score behavioral state by observing infant for 15 seconds immediately before the event.
4. Record baseline heart rate and oxygen saturation.
5. Observe the infant for 30 seconds immediately after the event. You will have to look back and forth from the monitor to the baby's face. Score physiologic and facial changes seen during that time and record immediately after the observation period.
6. Calculate the final score.

which was developed for assessing postoperative pain in children aged 1 to 7 years. Reliability and validity for the scale were established during painful procedures in both preterm and full-term infants. Although there is adequate establishment of these psychometric properties, the NIPS has not been used in practice. No data are available on the feasibility or clinical usefulness of the measure.

The *Distress Scale for Ventilated Newborn Infants* (DSVNI, Sparshott, 1996) was developed to assess the behavioral and physiologic responses of the ventilated newborn infant to painful procedures (Form 14.4,*A*). This measure is based on five previously developed scoring systems, including the Neonatal Behavioral Assessment Scale (NBAS; Brazelton, Nugent, 1995), the Assessment of Preterm Infant's Behavior (APIB; Als, Lester, Tronick et al., 1984), the NFCS (Grunau, Craig, 1987, 1990), the IBCS (Craig, McMahon, Morison et al., 1984), and the Gustave-Roussy Child Pain Scale developed by Gauvain-Piquard (1987). Physiologic responses are assessed by monitor readings. Behavioral responses are visually observed and include changes in facial expression, body movement, and color (Forms 14.4,*B*, 14.4,*C*, 14.4,*D*). Detailed scoring instructions accompany this measure. This measure looks very promising for this population of infants that require special consideration.

FORM 14.4A Distress Scale for Ventilated Newborn Infants (DSVNI)

DSVNI score sheet

Name: Date: Time: Hospital number:

Gestation: Age: Birth weight:

Main diagnosis:

Type of ventilation: Duration of ventilation:

Analgesia or local   Dose:
   anaesthetic:

Bolus/infusion: Time since last given:

Traumatic procedure: No. of attempts:

                                 Duration of procedure:

Score	Baseline	During procedure	After procedure At 3 min	At 1 h	Time taken to return to baseline
Facial expression					
Body movement					
Color					
Heart rate*					
Blood pressure*					
Oxygen saturation*					
Temperature – skin* – toe*					
Total					

Code for invasive procedures:

CD	Chest drain insertion	LP	Lumbar puncture
INT	Intubation	VP	Venipuncture
ETS	Endotracheal suctioning	AS	Arterial stab
OPS	Oropharangeal suctioning	HL	Heel lance
CPAP	Continuous positive airway pressure		Other

*To avoid more disturbance to the baby, these observations need only be made if monitoring equipment is already in place.

May be duplicated for use in clinical practice. As appears in McCaffery M, Pasero C: *Pain: Clinical manual,* pp. 646-648, 1999, Mosby, Inc.

From Sparshott M: *Pain, distress and the newborn baby,* pp 164-167, Oxford, 1997, Blackwell Science; Sparshott M: The development of a clinical distress scale for ventilated newborn infants: Identification of pain and distress based on validated behavioral scores, *J Neonatal Nurs* 2:5-11, 1996.

FORM 14.4B DSVNI Scoring System

Behavioral score

Facial expression

0   "relaxed"   Smooth muscled; relaxed expression; either in deep sleep or quietly alert

1   "anxious"   Anxious expression; frown; REM behind closed lids; wandering gaze; eyes narrowed; lips parted; pursed lips as if "oo" is being pronounced

2   "anguished"   Anguished expression/crumpled face; brow bulge; eye-squeeze; nasolabial furrow pronounced; square-stretched mouth; cupped tongue; "silent cry"

3   "inert"   (Only during or immediately after traumatic procedure) no response to trauma; no crying; rigidity; gaze avoidance; fixed/staring gaze; apathy; diminished alertness

Body movement

0   "relaxed"   Relaxed trunk and limbs; body in tucked position; hands in cupped position or willing to grasp a finger

1   "restless"   Moro reflex; startles; jerky or uncoordinated movement of limbs; flexion/extension of limbs; attempt to withdraw limb from site of injury

2   "exaggerated"   Abnormal position of limbs; limb/neck extension; splaying of fingers and/or toes; flailing or thrashing of limbs; arching back; side swiping/guarding site of injury

3   "inert"   (Only during or immediately after traumatic procedure) no response to trauma; inertia; limpness/rigidity; immobility

Color

0   Normal skin color (depending on skin type)

1   Redness; congestion

2   Pallor; mottling; grey

Physiologic changes

Physiologic changes are not scored but read directly from the monitors. Changes indicative of stress read from baseline are:

Heart rate   Increase; decrease; bradycardia frequent in fragile infants

Blood pressure   Increase

Oxygenation   Commonly decrease; occasionally increase because of crying and consequent increased intracranial pressure

Temperature differential   Widening gap in core and peripheral temperature; decrease in peripheral temperature

May be duplicated for use in clinical practice. As appears in McCaffery M, Pasero C: *Pain: Clinical manual,* pp. 646-648, 1999, Mosby, Inc.

Behavioral score	0	1	2	3
Facial expression	*"Relaxed"* Smooth muscled; unlined, relaxed expression; deep sleep/quiet alert state	*"Anxious"* Anxious expression; frown; REM; wandering gaze/eyes narrowed; lips parted/pursed	*"Anguished"* Anguished expression/crumpled face; brow bulge; eye-squeeze; nasolabial furrow; square/stretched mouth; cupped tongue; "silent cry"	*"Inert"* (No response to trauma) No crying; gaze avoidance; fixed/staring gaze; rigidity; diminished rigidity
	Deep sleep state / Quiet alert state	Eyes tightly closed; pursed lips / Eyes narrowed/wandering gaze; lips pursed/slightly parted	Silent cry / Cupped tongue	Gaze avoidance / Fixed/staring gaze
Body movement	*"Relaxed"* Relaxed trunk and limbs; tucked position; cupped hands/finger grasp	*"Restless"* More reflex; startles; jerky/uncoordinated movements; limb flexion/extension; limb withdrawal	*"Exaggerated"* Limb/neck extension; finger/toe splay; flailing; thrashing of limbs; arching back; side-swiping; guarding	*"Inert"* (No response to trauma) Inertia; immobility; limpness/rigidity
	Relaxed trunk and limbs / Tucked position	Limb withdrawal	Exaggerated neck extension; flailing; arching back / Exaggerated limb extension; finger/toe splay	Rigidity
Color	Normal skin color according to type	Redness; congestion	Pallor; mottling; grey	Baseline color; pallor, mottling, grey

May be duplicated for use in clinical practice. As appears in McCaffery M, Pasero C: *Pain: Clinical manual*, pp. 646-648, 1999, Mosby, Inc.

0	"Relaxed"—infant comfortable, not distressed.
1-2	Some transitory distress caused; returns immediately to "relaxed."
3-4	Transitory distress, likely to respond to consolation.
5	Infant experiences pain; if no response to consolation, may require analgesia.
6	"Anguished" and "exaggerated"—infant experiencing acute pain; is unlikely to respond to consolation, will probably benefit from analgesia.
6-8	"Inert"—(no response to traumatic procedure) infant is habituated to pain; will not respond to consolation; systematic pain control by analgesia should be considered.

May be duplicated for use in clinical practice. As appears in McCaffery M, Pasero C: *Pain: Clinical manual*, pp. 646-648, 1999, Mosby, Inc.
Form 14.4 A-D modified from the Distress Scale for Ventilated Newborn Infants (DSVNI).

However, no psychometric properties or clinical usefulness have been reported. This testing is underway (personal communication with the author).

The *Pain Assessment Tool* (PAT; Hodgkinson, Bear, Thorn et al., 1994) includes a variety of behavioral and physiologic indicators, as well as the nurse's perception of pain. The scoring system ranges between 0 and 20 with a score of 4 or less equaling no pain and a score of 20 indicating the worst pain. No reports of the validity, reliability, or clinical usefulness of this measure have been made to date.

Composite measures have also been developed to assess the broader concept of behavioral distress in children. With these measures, pain is conceptualized as the major construct that is interwoven with other related phenomena such as anxiety, fear, or depression. These measures were either developed for the pediatric intensive care patients or pediatric oncology patients. In the latter group the measures were used to assess distress associated with repeated painful procedures such as bone marrow aspirations.

The *COMFORT Scale* (Ambuel, Hamlett, Marx et al., 1992) is an example of a more general distress measure. The COMFORT scale is an 8-dimension scale that was developed for pediatric intensive care patients (newborn to 24 months) to measure distress. Distress for this measurement includes all behaviors of negative affect associated with pain, anxiety, and fear. Potential indicators were developed through a literature review and a survey of critical care nurses to ensure content validity. Concurrent validity was established by correlating the total COMFORT scale with the expert clinical judgment of a nurse using a VAS. Interrater reliability was reported as moderate, and internal consistency was reported as high. The scale is reported to be clinically useful. The authors report that administration time is approximately 3 minutes, and training of health professionals takes about 2 hours (Ambuel, Hamlett, Marx et al., 1992).

In summary, currently a growing number of both unidimensional and composite measures for assessing pain in infants exist. These measures have been described in detail and evaluated in several review papers (Abu-Saad, Bours, Stevens et al., in press; Craig, 1998; McGrath, 1998; Stevens, 1997; Stevens, 1998), which should be consulted for a more detailed and critical analysis of the measures. Composite measures discussed previously are summarized in Table 14.4. Even though a number of reliable and valid composite measures are now available to assess pain in infants, the importance of a multidimensional pain assessment in infants/individuals incapable of self-report cannot be underestimated. Box 14.1 provides guidelines for a multidimensional pain assessment for infants.

Factors that affect pain assessment in infants

Several factors have been reported to influence pain response in infants. Gestational age (GA) has been explored in two recent studies as a factor that influences pain responses in premature infants (Craig, Whitfield, Grunau et al., 1993; Johnston, Stevens, 1996). In both of these studies, the responses of preterm infants 26 weeks' GA were similar but significantly less robust than infants of older GA. In general, behavioral pain responses of VLBW infants are of lesser magnitude than infants of more advanced GA, thus depriving caregivers of important behavioral cues that signal pain.

Postnatal age (PNA), or the number of days of life since birth, has been associated with a decrease in behavioral response to painful stimuli when newborn and 4-week-old infants of the same GA (i.e., 32 weeks' GA) were compared during routine heel lance (Johnston, Stevens, 1996). When the responses of 32-week GA infants who were born at 28 weeks' GA were compared in a cross-sectional study with newborn infants born at 32 weeks' GA, they exhibited less behavioral and greater physiologic response to pain than the newborns born and tested at 32 weeks' GA. Similarly, increased PNA was found to be highly correlated with the number of painful procedures, resulting in decreased pain response for some interventions (Stevens, Johnston, Franck et al., in press).

Behavioral state (BS) has been shown to be a modifier of facial expression in several studies (Owens, Todt, 1984; Stevens, Johnston, Horton, 1994). Infants in the sleep states exhibited less facial expression immediately after painful procedures such as heel lance compared with infants in the awake alert states. GA, PNA, and BS are included as indicators in one of the composite measures of pain (i.e., PIPP; Stevens, Johnston, Petryshen et al., 1996) to account for their modifying influence on pain response.

Severity of illness (SOI) involves cry responses of healthy and sick term infants. It was found that more preterm and sick infants exhibited shorter cry duration and higher pitch (Michelsson, 1971; Michelsson, Jarvenpaa, Rinne, 1983). Stevens, Johnston, and Horton (1994) corroborated these findings in newborn premature infants of 32 to 34 weeks' GA. However, the influence of SOI was limited to cry outcomes and did not modify facial activity or physiologic pain indicators, such as heart rate or oxygen saturation, during painful procedures. Johnston and Stevens (1996) also reported that SOI, frequency of therapeutic procedures, and birth weight were not responsible for changes in facial actions.

Studies examining gender differences in pain responses of neonates have yielded inconsistent findings. In early studies by Bell and others (Bell, Costal, 1964; Bell, Waylayer, Waldrop, 1971) female neonates were found to show greater reaction when compared with males in behavioral response to an air jet to the abdomen. Lipsitt and Levy (1959) also found that female neonates demonstrated a greater reaction to electrotactual stimulation. Conversely, Gullickson and Crowell (1964) found no gender differences in responses to

● ● ● ● ●

TABLE 14.4   **Multidimensional Infant Pain Measures**

MEASURE	INDICATORS	VALIDITY	RELIABILITY
CRIES (Krechel, Bildner, 1995)	Crying O_2 saturation >95% Increased vital signs: • Heart rate • Blood pressure Expression Sleeplessness	Face Content Criterion Construct	Interrater
PIPP (Stevens, Johnston, Petryshen et al., 1996)	Gestational age Behavioral state Heart rate Oygen saturation Brow bulge Eye squeeze Nasolabial furrow	Face Content Content	Interrater Intrarater Internal consistency
NIPS (Lawrence, Alcock, McGrath et al, 1993)	Facial expression Cry Breathing patterns Arm movement Leg movement State of arousal	Face Content Criterion Construct	Interrater Internal consistency
DSVNI (Sparshott, 1996)	Physiologic changes: • Heart rate • Blood pressure • Oxygenation • Temperature differential Behavioral responses Body movements Color		
PAT (Hodgkinson, Bear, Thorn et al., 1994)	Posture/tone Sleep patterns Expression Color Cry Respirations Heart rate Saturations Blood pressure Nurses' perceptions of pain		
COMFORT Scale (Ambuel, Hamlett, Marx et al., 1992)	Mean arterial blood pressure Heart rate Muscle tone Facial tension Alertness Calmness/agitation Respiratory behavior Physical movement	Face Content Criterion	Interrater Internal consistency

Information from Ambuel B, Hamlett KW, Marx CM et al.: Assessing distress in pediatric intensive care environments: The Comfort Scale, *J Pediatr Psychol* 17:95-109, 1992; Hodgkinson K, Bear M, Thorn J et al.: Measuring pain in neonates: Evaluating an instrument and developing a common language, *Aust J Adv Nurs* 12:17-22, 1994; Krechel SW, Bildner J: CRIES: A new neonatal postoperative pain measurement score: Initial testing of validity and reliability, *Pediatr Anesth* 5: 53-61, 1995; Lawrence J, Alcock D, McGrath P et al.: The development of a tool to assess neonatal pain, *Neonatal Network* 12:59-66, 1993; Sparshott M: The development of a clinical distress scale for ventilated newborn infants: Identification of pain and distress based on validated behavioural scores, *J Neonatal Nurs* 2: 5-11, 1996; Stevens B, Johnston C, Petryshen P et al.: Premature infant pain profile: Development and initial validation, *Clinical J Pain* 12:13-22, 1996.

electrotactual stimulation. More recently, Owens and Todt (1984) found no gender differences in response to heel lance for PKU in healthy neonates. Grunau and Craig (1987) found gender differences in the speed of behavioral response, with boys showing shorter time to cry and to display facial action after heel lance. Stevens and others (1994) found no effect of gender, frequency of therapeutic interventions, or PNA on pain responses

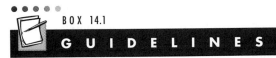

BOX 14.1

GUIDELINES

MULTIDIMENSIONAL PAIN ASSESSMENT FOR INFANTS

• Initiate discussions about pain between parents, caregivers, and health care professionals. Emphasize to the family that health team members cannot always determine when the infant is in pain and it is important for parents to let the caregiver know when they notice changes in their child's behavior. These changes could include alterations in sleeping, feeding, activity level, or parent-infant interactions. Help parents become sensitive to behaviors the infant may use to express pain and explain that severe pain may exist in the absence of any obvious behavioral indicators, especially if the pain is prolonged.

• Obtain frequent reports from parents or other caregivers *about* the infant's pain. Parents can be asked to rate their perception of their infant's pain on a scale of 0 to 10, where 0 equals no pain and 10 equals the worst pain imaginable. This is often referred to as a proxy pain rating. Remind parents that when the infant is critically ill and/or receiving muscle-paralyzing agents (e.g., pancuronium bromide) extra attention must be given to assessing pain because the infant's methods of expressing pain may be severely limited.

• Identify whether pathologic processes or procedures that are known to cause pain in older children and adults are occurring in the infant. All caregivers need to understand that some infants, particularly preterm neonates, may be more sensitive to pain and therefore some things that do not normally cause pain in older children may cause pain in preterm neonates.

• Observe for behavioral indicators of pain in the infant's cry, facial expression, and body movements. These indicators may include a high-pitched, harsh, brief loud cry; moaning; grunting; screaming or breath holding. Facial expression that reflects a grimace (bulging brow, eyes tightly shut, the mouth open and stretched wide) probably indicates pain or discomfort. Body movements including splaying of hands and fingers, clenched fists, rigid posturing, guarding of a body part, agitation, moving the head from side to side, jerking, pulling back, kicking, waving arms, fidgeting, or clinging to the parent may all indicate pain in the infant.

• Note changes in physiologic indicators such as increases in heart rate, breathing, sweating, pallor, cyanosis, or a rise or fall in blood pressure. Remind caregivers that these indicators most likely will only be observable immediately after a painful event. Absence of these indicators does not mean that the child is not in pain.

• Consider a trial of an appropriate dose of analgesic and note the responses as discussed previously. This approach may be very helpful when trying to decide whether the infant has pain or agitation. Agitation may be characterized by restlessness, whimpering, and inconsolability. A trial dose of analgesic may help clarify the difference between pain and agitation (e.g., the whimpering and restlessness may resolve).

May be duplicated for use in clinical practice. From McCaffery M, Pasero C: *Pain: Clinical manual*, p. 651. Copyright © 1999, Mosby, Inc.

---

of 32- to 34-week GA neonates. In summary, although some factors such as gestational age of the infant at birth and behavioral state have been shown to influence pain response in neonates, other factors such as gender and severity of illness are inconsistent in how they modify pain responses. In addition, no studies have examined the influence of factors such as ethnicity or race.

Summary of pain assessment in infants

The number of validated unidimensional and multidimensional or composite measures for assessing pain in infants has grown dramatically over the past decade. However, no one measure stands out as "the best" for all situations. The most promising measures in terms of feasibility and clinical usefulness appear to be the CRIES (Krechel, Bildner, 1995) for assessing postoperative pain in term and preterm neonates and the PIPP (Stevens, Johnston, Petryshen et al., 1996) for assessing procedural pain in term and preterm neonates. The DSVNI (Sparshott, 1996) also may be useful for assessing pain in ventilated infants, although very little psychometric data or evidence of clinical usefulness supports this measure at this time. Most measures and measurement approaches

have been developed to assess acute pain, and none have been sufficiently evaluated to determine their applicability to infants with chronic pain caused by congenital abnormalities, birth defects, or intense and complicated medical treatment (e.g., extracorporeal membrane oxygenation). Further validation of existing measures for acute pain in VLBW infants who are critically ill is needed. Additional measures are required for assessing pain with infants who are in chronic pain or who are developmentally, physically, mechanically, or pharmacologically compromised. An accurate pain assessment measure provides the means to determine the safety and efficacy of interventions that may relieve pain and decrease suffering in children.

MANAGEMENT OF PAIN IN INFANTS

Pain management strategies can be classified as pharmacologic and nonpharmacologic. These strategies, described in detail in previous chapters for use with adults, are also appropriate for relieving pain in infants. Therefore the purpose of this section is to present the following:

• Strategies and interventions that can be implemented either alone or in combination to reduce or

relieve pain from minor procedures (e.g., heel lances, injections) and major procedures (e.g., surgery) in infants
- Considerations for managing special populations of infants (e.g., VLBW infants, critically ill infants, developmentally and physically compromised infants)
- Relevant research on the efficacy and safety of non-pharmacologic interventions and directions for future research

As is true with adults, several methods of pain management may need to be used for adequate pain relief and control of accompanying emotional states in infants. For example, an infant who is to receive an immunization injection may benefit from an oral analgesic or a topical anesthetic, distraction, relaxation, a cold compress, and emotional support from his or her mother or father used simultaneously or alternatively.

Because assessment of the infant with pain is challenging and complex, it may be difficult at times to individualize pain relief measures on the basis of the infant's responses to painful stimuli. For example, adjusting the dose of an analgesic and interval between doses is not as easy to do with an infant who cannot verbally comment on the effectiveness of the intervention. However, as with all pain assessment in infants, pain indicators must be assessed regularly and frequently by health care professionals to provide information for making a best guess as to the intensity, location, and nature of their pain. Despite assessment difficulties, every attempt must be made to tailor pain relief interventions to the individual child and situation.

Some health care professionals have suggested that failure to try to provide pain relief for infants is both abusive and unethical (Rana, 1987; Stang, Gunnar, Snellman et al., 1988). This failure to take appropriate and humane action is often influenced by individual and societal attitudes about children that have decreased the attention paid to children's pain. Unlike the misconceptions previously described, which can be corrected with accurate information, these attitudes are embedded in sociocultural beliefs and cannot be proven or disproven. Common attitudes toward pain management in children include the following:
- Throughout all eras, humane and compassionate child-rearing has existed alongside cold and inhumane practices (McGrath, Unruh, 1987). It is generally clear, however, that during eras and cultures when disease or circumstance have devalued individual life, concerns about quality of life, such as decreasing pain, have received decreased attention in *favor* of concern for survival.
- Strong societal biases against pain expression in children exist. For example, pain is often seen as character building, in that enduring a noxious event and mastering or overcoming it serves to improve

one's emotional strength and the ability to compete (Schechter, Berde, Yaster, 1993). This thinking is consistent with the "no pain, no gain" philosophy and the idea that it is admirable to withstand pain without protesting (e.g., crying) during painful events.
- Pain has religious and cultural connotations such that it may acquire personal levels of meaning that are greater than the meaning attributed to other symptoms. For example, the expression of pain may be unacceptable in some cultures and therefore attention to pain management would go against acceptable cultural or religious practices.
- Personal attitudes of health care professionals may influence their pain management practices toward infants and children. In a recent survey, Porter, Wolf, Gold et al. (1997) noted that physicians' attitudes toward pharmacologic pain management of procedures in infants was highly influenced by their own personal pain experiences.

Together, these societal and individual attitudes about children and pain management have denigrated the importance of providing adequate pain relief (Schechter, Berde, Yaster, 1993).

Pharmacologic Pain Management

Management of pain after surgery and for some medical conditions has improved considerably for infants over the past decade. The use of continuous infusions of opioids, epidural analgesia, and peripheral nerve blockade has enhanced the ability of health care professionals to treat postoperative and medical pain safely and effectively. Local anesthetics and nonopioids have also been instituted in many settings for the treatment of pain from some procedures. However, despite these advances, pharmacologic management of infant pain remains less than optimal.

Pharmacokinetics and pharmacodynamics

The metabolism of the newborn is significantly different than that of the older child or adult. An understanding of newborn pharmacokinetics (movement of drugs in the body over time) and pharmacodynamics (dose-response relationship) provides the basis for safe and effective dosing for anesthesia, analgesia, or both. Pharmacokinetics are affected by the quality of absorption, distribution, and elimination of medications by the infant. Gastrointestinal absorption is determined by gastric acidity and gastric emptying. The gastric pH of the newborn is between 6 and 8 and falls to a pH between 1 and 3 within the first day of life. The gastric environment of the newborn does not maintain an acidic stability until 3 years of age. Drugs that are acid labile are affected by the neutral or alkaline gastric environment of the neonate and therefore reach higher levels of concentration than in children and adults (Koren, Jacobson,

1993). Gastric emptying is also significantly slower in the newborn than in older children and adults. Preterm infants have even slower gastric emptying than term infants. Delayed gastric emptying contributes to delayed and incomplete absorption of some medications. Gastric absorption improves after birth and continues to improve by 3 months of age. At this time, gastric absorption in the infant may be as efficient or more efficient than in the adult (Koren, Jacobson, 1993).

Intramuscular absorption of medications is influenced by the perfusion of the area of injection, the rate of penetration of the drug throughout the capillary endothelium, and the apparent volume into which the drug has been distributed. Neonatal physiology includes vasomotor instability, smaller muscular mass and subcutaneous fat, and a higher proportion of water. The documented research on intramuscular absorption of drugs is somewhat incomplete. Although some medications are absorbed within a similar time period in infants, children, and adults, some medications are absorbed more slowly in infants. Therefore this physiologic difference must be considered as a precaution when administering intramuscular medications to the neonate. The impact of the physiologic differences in infants' skin on the absorption of percutaneous medications is also unknown and should be considered a precaution for administering transdermal preparations (Koren, Jacobson, 1993).

The distribution of medications is determined by protein binding and compartmentalization of body water. Protein binding in the newborn is lower than in older children and adults. This results in higher proportions of medications left free to penetrate different tissue compartments, causing higher distribution volumes. Various analgesics and antiinflammatory drugs are potent displacers of bilirubin from albumin binding and hence may increase the risk of hyperbilirubinemia in the neonate (Koren, Jacobson, 1993). Infants have proportionally more water weight, more extracellular water, less fat, and less muscle tissue than adults. Drugs that are distributed in body water therefore have a larger distribution in infants than in adults. As a result, the same dose of a medication given to an infant and an adult will produce lower peak levels in the infant than in the adult. The mean serum concentration however is more affected by drug clearance rates than by distribution (Koren, Jacobson, 1993).

In infants, brain and viscera account for a greater proportion of body mass, whereas muscle and fat account for smaller amounts of body mass than in adults. Therefore passage of opioids such as morphine into the brain is increased. In neonates, and particularly preterm neonates, this leads to diminished ventilatory responses to hypoxemia and hypercarbia. Studies on newborn rats suggest that they also have a greater propensity toward respiratory depression and higher analgesic requirements than

older rats (Pasternak, Zhang, Tecott, 1980). This may lead to a significantly increased risk of respiratory depression at opioid doses necessary for adequate analgesia.

Drug clearance rates depend on hepatic and renal metabolism. Most analgesics are conjugated in the liver. Neonates, and particularly preterm neonates, have delayed maturation of the enzyme systems involved in drug conjugation, including sulfation, glucuronidation, and oxidation. The cytochrome P_{450} system, which catalyzes these reactions in the liver, is quite immature at birth and does not reach adult levels until the first months of life (Houck, 1998). Therefore hepatic metabolism is much slower in the neonate, causing a slower drug clearance rate. Consequently, therapeutic or toxic levels of opioids, acetaminophen, NSAIDs, and local amide anesthetics are achieved with lower unit doses or longer dose intervals.

Likewise, the glomerular filtration rate (GFR) and tubular secretion processes of the neonatal kidneys are diminished during the first week of life but generally are sufficiently mature to clear medications and metabolites by 2 weeks of age (Houck, 1998). However, newborns have delayed excretion, and, therefore, most analgesic medications used in the neonatal period have significantly longer half-lives. Preterm infants have fewer glomeruli than term infants. As the tubules prolongate and mature and renal perfusion improves, renal filtration improves. GFR depends on GA and postnatal age. The renal functions reach adult values by approximately 6 to 12 months (Koren, Jacobson, 1993).

Because of the differences in preterm and term renal functioning, the preterm infant requires lower doses or longer dose intervals than the term infant to maintain similar therapeutic concentrations. A reasonable starting dose of opioids for the neonate who is not mechanically ventilated is between one quarter and one third the recommended starting dose for children. The neonate should be closely monitored with a cardiorespiratory monitor and pulse oximetry, and the dose titrated for effect. Neonates may develop opioid tolerance rapidly, and therefore very large doses may be required to achieve adequate pain control for infants with continual severe pain (AHCPR, 1992).

Nonopioid analgesics

The pharmacodynamics of acetaminophen, salicylates, and NSAIDs in infants older than 1 month of age are not much different than in older children and adults. The choice of drug depends on the availability of the route (i.e., oral, rectal, or intravenous), potential side effects, duration of use, purpose of use, and cost (Houck, 1998).

Acetaminophen

Acetaminophen is the most popular nonopioid analgesic prescribed for the treatment of mild pain. Acetaminophen is a centrally acting analgesic and antipyretic agent that has been found to be safe and effective in all age groups, including newborns. In fact, the immaturity of hepatic enzyme systems in the neonate may be protective in that production of the toxic metabolites of this drug is diminished. Children gradually excrete more acetaminophen as the glucuronide metabolite until age 12 when the glucuronide/sulfate ratio approaches adult values. This leads to a dramatic increase in liver toxicity after acetaminophen overdose in children older than 12 years of age compared with younger children (Rumack, Peterson, 1978). Doses of 10 to 15 mg/kg every 4 hours given orally are generally sufficient to provide analgesia for 3 to 4 hours (Kelley, Watson, Edge et al., 1992). The appropriate rectal dosage is somewhat controversial because of the longer half-life and highly variable absorption rate, which depends on the child and the placement of the suppository. The analgesic dose of rectally administered acetaminophen is higher than the oral recommended dosage (e.g., 20 to 25 mg/kg every 4 to 6 hours). Although these doses have been recommended for the term neonate, no research suggests efficacy and/or safety in preterm neonates.

Nonsteroidal Antiinflammatory Drugs (NSAIDs)

Acetylsalicylic acid is rarely used to treat pain in young children because of its association with Reye syndrome (Giannini, Brewer, Miller et al., 1990), increased incidence of gastrointestinal side effects, and platelet dysfunction (Houck, 1998). Acetylsalicylic acid also has the ability to displace bilirubin from albumin. Other more common NSAIDs used in children include ibuprofen, naproxen, indomethacin, and choline magnesium trisalicylate. For children who are unable to tolerate oral medications, intravenous ketorolac is available. However, NSAIDs are not recommended for use in neonates because clinical guidelines and safety have not been adequately established (Berde, Anand, Sethna, 1989).

Indomethacin is a NSAID that has been used frequently in neonates for promoting closure of the patent ductus arteriousus. Although elimination is delayed in preterm neonates, volume of distribution and elimination half-life approach that of adults by 1 year of age. Associated side effects that have been noted in preterm infants include oliguria, weight gain, and hyponatremia. These effects have not been noted in children older than 1 year of age. Indomethacin was investigated for use as a continuous infusion after major surgery in older children. Results indicate that excellent adjunctive pain relief and greater patient satisfaction were achieved over opioids alone (Maunuksela, Olkkola, Korpela, 1988). With the advent of intravenous ketorolac, further investigation of the analgesic properties of indomethacin have ceased. Safety and efficacy data are insufficient to recommend the use of indomethacin as an analgesic in infants.

Opioid analgesics

Opioids act as agonists for endogenous opioid receptors in the CNS (For a further discussion of opioids, single bolus technique, and doses see Chapter 8, Box 8.4, p. 379.) The most common opioids prescribed for newborns are morphine and fentanyl. Although the analgesic effects are thought to be similar, morphine may provide greater sedation, less risk of chest wall rigidity, and less rapid tolerance than fentanyl. However, fentanyl causes minimal histamine release and concomitant hemodynamic instability (Franck, 1991). The use of these drugs has been severely limited in the past because of the belief that the newborn is particularly sensitive to opioid-induced respiratory depression (Yaster, Krane, Kaplan et al., 1997). However, with the use of monitoring and dosing based on the most recent pharmacokinetic and pharmacodynamic modeling data, the use of these opioids for neonates has increased.

Morphine

Morphine is the standard mu-receptor agonist to which all other opioids are compared. Morphine pharmacokinetics differ more significantly in preterm and term neonates than in older infants in the following ways:

- The elimination half-life in term neonates less than 4 days of age is seven times greater than in older infants, resulting in plasma morphine levels that are three times higher than in older infants.
- Preterm neonates have slower clearance and longer elimination half-lives of morphine than term infants.

Because of these differences, use of morphine in preterm and term neonates requires adjustment of dosages to

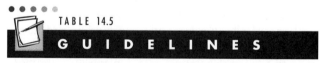

TABLE 14.5

G U I D E L I N E S

MORPHINE AND FENTANYL INFUSION RATES FOR NEWBORN AND OLDER INFANTS

Population	Pain Level	Morphine (μg/kg/h)	Fentanyl (μg/kg/h)
Preterm newborn	Severe	5–10	1
	Moderate	2–5	0.5
	Mild	0–2	0.5
Term newborn	Severe	10–20	1–2
	Moderate	5–10	0.5–1
	Mild	0–5	0–0.5
Older infant	Severe	15–30	1–2
	Moderate	10–20	1
	Mild	0–10	0–1

May be duplicated for use in clinical practice. As appears in McCaffery M, Pasero C: *Pain: Clinical manual*, p. 654, 1999, Mosby, Inc.

From Yaster M, Krane EJ, Kaplan RF et al: *Pediatric pain management and sedation handbook*, p. 199, St. Louis, 1997, Mosby.

account for pharmacokinetic differences. This is especially true in infants with a history of apnea (Leith, Weisman, 1997). Recommended infusion rates of morphine for preterm and term neonates and older infants are summarized in Table 14.5 (Yaster, Krane, Kaplan et al., 1997).

Fentanyl

The increased volume of distribution of fentanyl in term and preterm neonates leads to lower peak plasma levels of fentanyl after bolus dosing, a longer half-life of elimination, and lower drug clearance than in older infants. However, metabolism of fentanyl in the liver appears to be similar in the newborn compared with the older patient. Yaster and others (1997) recommend that continuous fentanyl infusions in the newborn should be reduced by 25% to 50% compared with the older infant. Dose recommendations for continuous infusion of morphine and fentanyl for term, preterm, and older infants are summarized for mild, moderate, and severe pain in Table 14.5 (Yaster, Krane, Kaplan et al., 1997). Sufentanil and alfentanil are synthetic opioids that have little practical clinical use for the management of pain in infants because inadequate pharmacokinetic and pharmacodynamic studies have been completed.

Codeine

Codeine is usually administered by the oral route and is most commonly used for mild to moderate pain. Codeine may be used for postoperative pain in older infants because it is available in an elixir form. Codeine is not usually administered to neonates. Codeine is often given in combi-nation with acetaminophen because it is more effective than either single drug alone. The recommended dose for oral codeine is approximately 1 mg/kg (Leith, Weisman, 1997) but may range from 0.5 to 1.2 mg/kg (Yaster, Krane, Kaplan et al., 1997); higher doses are frequently associated with nausea, pruritus, and constipation.

Adverse Effects

The adverse effects of opioids are partially related to the dosage or infusion time. Therefore the drug must be carefully selected, and infants must be carefully monitored with a cardiorespiratory monitor and observation for both desired effect and adverse effects. Appropriate titration and weaning of the drug can also prevent undesirable adverse effects, including respiratory depression, excessive sedation, nausea, vomiting, pruritus, constipation, brady-cardia, hypotension, muscle rigidity, seizures, urinary retention, tolerance, and physiologic dependence.

Respiratory depression is often of most concern to health care professionals caring for infants receiving opioids. Signs of respiratory depression from opioid administration include the following:

- Unresponsiveness (i.e., hard to arouse without tactile stimulation, responds to pain only, or no response)
- Decrease in respiratory rate (i.e., <12 breaths/min in children less than 2 years of age) (Yaster, Krane, Kaplan et al., 1997)

Respiratory depression should be considered a medical emergency and the actions summarized in Box 14.2 need to be undertaken immediately (Yaster, Krane, Kaplan et al., 1997).

BOX 14.2

G U I D E L I N E S

EMERGENCY TREATMENT OF RESPIRATORY DEPRESSION

Respiratory Depression From Opioids

- Stop the infusion of opioids.
- Call for *help.*
- Establish an airway and assist ventilation as required. Call a *code.*
- Administer naloxone per standing order (0.001 to 0.1 mg/kg) IV or IM (Yaster et al., 1997, p. 49).
- Notify the child's primary medical and nursing care provider immediately.
- Stay with the child; do not leave the child alone for any reason.
- Assess the child's vital signs every 5 minutes until the level of consciousness and respiratory rate return to baseline. Note that small doses of naloxone may only last for 15 minutes. Therefore the child may become renarcoticized

and require additional treatment. For additional information on how to determine when naloxone is necessary and how to administer it, refer to Box 6.29, p. 270.

Respiratory Depression From Agonists or Benzodiazepines

Follow all the same steps as above, except instead of naloxone, administer flumazenil (Romazicon). Pediatric dosing is unknown. Yaster et al. (1997) suggest a starting dose of 0.01 mg/kg. If no (or inadequate) response occurs within 1 to 2 minutes, the dose can be repeated every minute until a maximum total dose of 1 mg is given. Other health care professionals suggest an initial dose of 0.01 mg/kg with increments of 0.005 mg/kg/min until awake or to a maximum of 1 mg (Jones et al., 1991). No clinical guidelines are established for appropriate doses for neonates.

Use of Opioids in Critically Ill Preterm Neonates

IV administration of opioids is the most common analgesic intervention in the NICU. IV opioids are administered to critically ill infants to provide analgesia during mechanical ventilation, invasive monitoring of vital functions, and surgical procedures. Although bradycardia, hypotension, and respiratory depression are anticipated effects, minimal data exist regarding the prevalence and severity of cardiorespiratory side effects associated with opioid use in these infants (Franck, Miaskowski, 1998). For critically ill ventilated neonates within the first 3 days of life, plasma beta-endorphins, cortisol, and blood glucose were measured before and after administration of a single dose of opioid analgesia. After opioid administration, cortisol levels decreased significantly within 2 hours, glucose levels decreased to preadministration levels within 12 hours, and beta-endorphin levels decreased by 24 hours, suggesting that the stress responses of critically ill neonates can be attenuated with opioid analgesia (Pokela, 1994).

Although fears of opioid-induced side effects persist, IV opioids are now used in the NICU for management of stress and for analgesia. However, methods to evaluate opioid effects and the prevalence and severity of cardiorespiratory side effects are needed. Until better methods are available to accurately monitor drug effects and associated toxicities, underuse of opioids in the critically ill neonate will continue to be a significant problem (Franck, Miaskowski, 1998).

Sedatives

Sedatives including benzodiazepines (lorazepam, midazolam) are often used in combination with opioid analgesics for procedural and postoperative pain management. Sedatives should not be used as a replacement for analgesics because they suppress the behavioral responses to pain and because of their lack of analgesic effect. They are commonly used in some NICUs for term and preterm neonates in combination with opioids to manage stress because animal and human studies suggest that opioid/benzodiazepine interaction is additive for sedation but synergistic for hypnotic effects (Kissin, Brown, Bradley, 1990; Tverskoy, Fleyshman, Ezry et al., 1989). However, little research supports the safety and efficacy of combining these drugs in the neonatal population.

Midazolam (Versed) has been approved by the FDA for use in neonates. However, only one research study demonstrated the sedative effects of midazolam in neonates (Jacqz-Aigrain, Daoud, Burtin et al., 1994). Also, adverse hemodynamic effects and abnormal movements have been associated with its use (Harte, Gray, Lee et al., 1997; Magny, Zupan, Dehan et al., 1994). Midazolam (Versed) and lorazepam (Ativan) can be used with older infants for their sedative, anxiolytic, and amnestic effects and are the drugs of choice for children in inten-

sive care units. Recommended pediatric equisedating benzodiazepine doses are summarized in Table 14.6. Similar to opioid-induced respiratory depression, benzodiazepines can also cause respiratory depression and sedation. These effects can be reversed with flumazenil. See Box 14.2 for a summary of emergency actions for treating respiratory depression caused by opioids or benzodiazepines.

Chloral hydrate is a hypnotic drug that is frequently used for sedation or hypnosis in infants. Although the mechanism of action is unknown, chloral hydrate produces mild cerebral depression and quiet, deep sleep. However, the major metabolite, tricholorethanol, accumulates with repeated dosing and may be associated with adverse effects such as CNS depression, cardiorespiratory changes, respiratory depression, development of metabolic acidosis, and the potential to predispose newborns to conjugated and uncongugated hyperbilirubinemia. Therefore, although single doses have been used safely in the neonatal period, there is a need for vigilance long after the procedure has been completed. The half-life of one dose of chloral hydrate is as great as 40 hours in preterm infants, 30 hours in term infants, and 10 hours in toddlers (Mayers, Hindmarsh, Sankaran, 1991; Yaster, Krane, Kaplan et al., 1997). Therefore older infants and toddlers receiving repeated doses need to be very carefully monitored. Repeated doses should be avoided in preterm and term neonates.

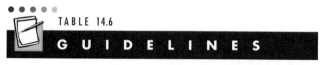

TABLE 14.6

GUIDELINES

EQUISEDATING BENZODIAZEPINE DOSES

Name	Equipotent IV dose (mg/kg)	Equipotent oral dose (mg/kg)	Equipotent rectal dose (mg/kg)
Diazepam*	0.1-0.2	0.2-0.3	0.2-0.3
Lorazepam*,†	0.03-0.05	0.05-0.2	0.1-0.2
Midazolam*	0.05-0.15	0.5-0.75‡	0.3-1.0‡
Oxazepam*	—	0.2-0.5§	—

May be duplicated for use in clinical practice. As appears in McCaffery M, Pasero C: *Pain: Clinical manual,* p. 656, 1999, Mosby, Inc.

*There are clinically important age-related pharmacodynamic effects. Younger patients require higher mg/kg doses than older patients.

†Lorazepam, like all benzodiazepines, is a respiratory depressant and has been associated with the urgent need for airway intervention during treatment of status epilepticus.

‡The enteral dose of midazolam is 3-10 times the intravenous dose. The maximum oral and rectal dose is 20 mg.

§The pediatric (mg/kg) dose of oxazepam has not been clearly established. The adult dose, 15-30 mg, was divided by an average adult weight (50-80 kg).

From Yaster M, Krane EJ, Kaplan RF et al.: *Pediatric pain management and sedation handbook,* p. 350, St. Louis, 1997, Mosby.

Regional anesthesia and analgesia

With outpatient and community care becoming more prevalent, many procedures are now performed outside the traditional hospital setting. This practice has greatly increased the use of regional anesthetic techniques to decrease anesthetic requirements and to manage pain. In infants, these techniques most commonly include the use of local anesthetics or opioids along the neuraxis (e.g., epidural), topical anesthesia, and peripheral nerve blocks.

Local and Topical Anesthesia

Lidocaine and bupivacaine are two local amide anesthetics that are frequently used for postoperative pain management in children. Bupivacaine has a more prolonged duration of action than lidocaine and perhaps, in dilute concentrations, a relative preference for sensory blockage over motor blockade (Houck, 1998). Because of its slow onset and long duration, bupivacaine is not recommended for use by nonanesthetists (Leith, Weisman, 1997). Lidocaine, which has a more rapid onset and shorter duration, has been used for management of procedural pain in infants, but data on its safety and efficacy are limited. Suggested maximal doses of local anesthetics for peripheral or subcutaneous nerve blockage are summarized by Yaster and others (1997) in Table 14.7. Local anesthetics must be used cautiously in neonates. Neonates have low concentrations of albumin and alpha$_1$-acid glycoprotein that can lead to decreased protein binding of local anesthetics and increases in the plasma concentrations of the unbound drug. Amide local anesthetics are also metabolized by the enzyme systems in the liver, which are not fully active for weeks after birth. In sick infants with respiratory diseases and cardiac insufficiency, liver blood flow may also be decreased, which can

● ● ● ● ●
TABLE 14.7

SUGGESTED MAXIMUM DOSES OF LOCAL ANESTHETICS FOR PERIPHERAL OR SUBCUTANEOUS NERVE BLOCKADE			
Drug	Concentration	Without epinephrine (mg/kg)	With epinephrine (mg/kg)
Chloroprocaine	1%–2%	8	10
Procaine	1%–2%	7	8.5
Bupivacaine	0.25%	2	3
Etidocaine	0.5%–1.0%	3	4
Lidocaine	0.5%–1.0%	5	7
Mepivacaine	1%–1.5%	5	6
Prilocaine	4%	5	7

May be duplicated for use in clinical practice. As appears in McCaffery M, Pasero C: *Pain: Clinical manual*, p. 657, 1999, Mosby, Inc.

From Yaster M, Krane EJ, Kaplan RF et al.: *Pediatric pain management and sedation handbook*, p 65, St. Louis, 1997, Mosby.

lead to a significantly prolonged half-life of these agents (Houck, 1998).

Ester local anesthetics (procaine, chloroprocaine, and tetracaine) are also broken down by enzyme systems in the liver. Because the activity of these enzymes is diminished in the first 6 months of life, liver clearance may theoretically be prolonged. However, research has indicated that neonates can clear these drugs effectively (Henderson, Sethna, Berde, 1993).

EMLA has been demonstrated as an effective and safe pain-reducing strategy for procedures in a number of pediatric and neonatal studies. (For a complete review on the efficacy and safety of EMLA for procedural pain in neonates, see Taddio, Ohlsson, Einarson et al., 1998). EMLA 5% cream is a 2.5% lidocaine and 2.5% prilocaine mixture; when the two drugs are combined they melt at a lesser temperature than they do separately. This interaction permits a higher effective concentration on the skin and increases the rate of drug uptake (Bodin, Nyqvist-Mayer, Wadsten et al., 1984).

The manufacturers of EMLA warn against its use in infants less than 1 month of age and in infants less than 12 months of age who are receiving treatment with methemoglobin-inducing agents, such as acetaminophen and sulfonamides (ASTRA, 1997). Methemoglobinemia is a condition in which more than 1% of the blood hemoglobin has been oxidized to the ferric form, which is incapable of binding molecular oxygen for transfer to cells (Wong, 1997). Very young patients and those with glucose-6-phosphate deficiency are more susceptible to methemoglobinemia than others. The signs of methemoglobinemia include cyanosis, dyspnea, dizziness, lethargy, and coma. It is reversible when treated promptly with IV methylene blue 1%, 1 to 2 mg/kg (Yaster, Krane, Kaplan et al., 1997).

Methemoglobinemia associated with EMLA is relatively rare in infants. One reported case was a 3-month-old prematurely born male weighing 5.3 kg who had 5 g of EMLA applied to the back of his hands and cubital region for 5 hours. The infant was receiving sulfonamides concomitantly. In another situation, a 2-month-old infant who had EMLA for removal of a port-wine stain took acetaminophen postoperatively. Both of these infants developed methemoglobinemia and responded satisfactorily to treatment (ASTRA, 1997; Wong, 1995).

These cases have led many practitioners to avoid the use of EMLA for painful procedures in infants less than the age of 12 months. However, researchers have found EMLA to be safe and efficacious for this age group but only for certain procedures. In a systematic review and meta-analyses by Taddio and others (1998), EMLA was found to be effective for reducing pain from circumcision. Limited data also suggest that EMLA was effective in decreasing pain from venipuncture, arterial puncture, and venous catheter placement. However, EMLA was not effective in relieving the pain from heel lance in term or preterm neonates. Data to recommend EMLA for other procedures are insufficient. Single doses, 0.5 to 2.0 g, of 5% EMLA cream administered for 60 to 90 minutes for procedures in term neonates were found to be safe (Taddio, Ohlsson, Einarson et al., 1998).

Summary of Pharmacologic Interventions

Researchers are beginning to have a better understanding of the anatomy and physiology of pain transmission, the hormonal and metabolic response to pain, and the assessment of pain in infants. Because of these advances, they are able to begin to address the safety and efficacy of pharmacologic interventions for acute pain. However, significant gaps still exist in the treatment of chronic pain and the safety and efficacy of many pharmacologic interventions, both alone and in combination with nonpharmacologic strategies.

Nonpharmacologic Pain Management

Health professionals are often reluctant to administer analgesia to infants because of concerns about side effects and toxicity. Although this reluctance is frequently decreased for the management of postsurgical pain and pain from chronic medical conditions, the pain from procedures that are considered "minor" often goes untreated or undertreated. Nonpharmacologic pain management strategies, administered alone or in combination with pharmacologic interventions, are feasible alternatives to analgesic administration for procedural pain to reduce pain, ameliorate stress, and induce comfort. The two most common approaches to nonpharmacologic pain management in infants are the developmentally sensitive behavioral interventions and sucrose.

Developmentally sensitive behavioral interventions

An individualized developmentally sensitive care delivery approach for hospitalized preterm infants, developed by Dr. Heidi Als and colleagues (Als, Lawhon, Brown et al., 1986; Als, Lawhon, Duffy et al., 1994), has gained widespread support. The goal of "developmental care" is to enhance comfort and stability and to reduce the stress and untoward consequences associated with the environment and therapeutic procedures. Box 14.3 provides guidelines for developmental care.

When these interventions are consistently incorporated into a developmental approach to care, the number of days on assisted ventilation was reduced; the incidence of intraventricular hemorrhage, bronchopulmonary dysplasia, and retinopathy of prematurity was decreased; and time to full feedings, accelerated weight gain, and improved parent/infant interaction was shorter. Although the philosophy of developmental care is consistent with

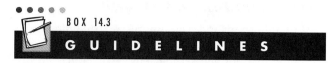

BOX 14.3

GUIDELINES

DEVELOPMENTAL CARE

- Decrease excess light and noise in the NICU.
- Darken the incubators by covering them.
- Decrease the ambient noise in the NICU.
- Speak softly to the infant.
- Use positioning aids, such as boundary supports, nests, and buntings, to promote a balance of flexion and extension postures.
- Handle the infant slowly and smoothly.
- Work around sleep/wake patterns and try not to interrupt sleep if possible.
- Cluster caregiving and therapeutic encounters to reduce stress and provide "time-outs" as needed.
- Promote self-regulatory behaviors, such as holding, grasping, and sucking.
- Involve parents in the care of their infants as much as possible.

May be duplicated for use in clinical practice. From McCaffery M, Pasero C: *Pain: Clinical manual,* p. 658. Copyright © 1999, Mosby, Inc.

the goals of pain relief, only a few of the developmental care interventions have been specifically evaluated to determine their efficacy for the management of pain. These include positioning, containment, and nonnutritive sucking (alone and in combination with sucrose administration).

Positioning

Proper positioning can affect many physiologic and neurobehavioral parameters in the infant (Blackburn, VandenBerg, 1993). When the infant is positioned with a midline orientation, hand-to-mouth activity and proper flexion, self-soothing, and self-regulatory behaviors can be promoted. Side-lying or lateral positioning has been found to support oxygenation while decreasing the incidence of external rotation of the extremities. Side-lying further promotes flexion and midline opportunities. Prone positioning has been reported to increase oxygenation, tidal volume, and the compliance of the lungs compared with infants in a supine position (Crane, Snyder, Knight et al., 1990; Masterson, Zucker, Schulze, 1998; Wagman, Shutack, Moomjian et al., 1979). However, prone positioning was not effective in reducing pain during single heel lances in preterm infants (Stevens, Johnston, Franck et al., in press). Corff and others (Corff, 1993; Corff, Seideman, Venkataraman et al., 1995) have reported that "facilitated tucking" (holding the infant's extremities flexed and contained close to the trunk) during heel lance lowered mean heart rate and resulted in less crying time and more stability in the sleep-wake cycles after the lance.

Containment

Over the ages infants have been swaddled or bundled to decrease stress. Containment through positioning and blanket rolls to provide a "nest" facilitates the VLBW infant's attempts to self-regulate. Containment also increases the infant's feelings of security and self-control and decreases stress. Babies who are contained tend to be calmer and gain weight more rapidly (Cole, Jorgensen, 1997). Swaddling combined with vestibular interventions (rocking, water beds) has been effective in promoting stability in physiologic indicators, growth, and behavioral state in preterm infants (Deireggi, 1990; Korner, Thoman, 1972). Swaddling premature infants (between 27 and 34 weeks' GA) after a routine heelstick procedure was also found to quiet crying infants immediately, decrease heart rate, and facilitate return to a sleep state (Ferran, Kisilevsky, Tranmer et al., 1997). When the same infants were not swaddled, they took a minimum of 10 minutes to return to baseline physiologic and behavioral state levels.

Nonnutritive Sucking

The pacifying effect of nonnutritive sucking has been well studied in infants, but the nature of the mechanism(s) underlying this effect remain unclear. Nonnutritive sucking has been found to be antinociceptive and reduce vocalizations by opioid and nonopioid mechanisms in neonatal rats (Blass, Ciaramitaro, 1994). In human neonates nonnutritive sucking has been associated with increases in oxygenation, respiratory and gastrointestinal function (Burrows, Asonye, Anderson-Shanklin et al., 1978; Paludetto, Robertson, Hack et al., 1984), decreased restlessness (Field, Ignatoll, Stringer et al., 1982; Gill, Behnek, Conlon et al., 1988), more time in awake states (Gill, Behnek, Conlon et al., 1988), decreased heart rate and energy expenditure (Chessex, Reichman, Verellen et al., 1981; Woodson, Hamilton, 1986), and greater feeding success and less feeding stress, as well as a more rapid return to sleep after feeding (Pickler, Higgins, Crummette, 1993).

Nonnutritive sucking has also been used as a pain management strategy. Franck (1987) reported that neonatal nurses ranked a pacifier as their first choice to manage pain. However, the effectiveness of nonnutritive sucking as a pain-relieving intervention has only recently been studied rigorously (Campos, 1989, 1994; Field, Goldson, 1984; Gunnar, Fisch, Malone, 1984; Marchette, Main, Redick et al., 1991; Miller, Anderson, 1994). Pacifiers during circumcision in term infants reduced behavioral distress (Gunnar, Fisch, Malone, 1984; Marchette, Main, Redick et al., 1991), although indicators of physi-

ologic arousal were only reduced in premature infants with less severe postnatal complications. Campos (1989) compared the effectiveness of swaddling and pacifiers and found that pacifiers soothed infants more rapidly than swaddling, but a rebound in distress occurred when the pacifier was removed. Swaddling was less immediately effective but was less subject to rebound on termination of the intervention. Campos (1994) also compared the efficacy of rocking and pacifiers during heel lance in healthy term neonates. Both reduced crying, but pacifiers predominantly produced sleep states, whereas rocking produced alert states. Pacifiers were more effective in reducing physiologic responses. Field and Goldson (1984) reported decreased crying with nonnutritive sucking in both term and preterm infants during heel lancing procedures. Miller and Anderson (1994) studied the effectiveness of nonnutritive sucking in 10 intubated premature and term infants in a randomized crossover study. All infants demonstrated crying (nonvocalized) and sucking. Infants cried less and had lower heart rates when in the nonnutritive sucking condition. Most recently, nonnutritive sucking was effective in reducing pain in preterm infants during single heel lances (Stevens, Johnston, Franck et al., in press).

To provide a positive, supportive nonnutritive sucking experience for the infant, it is important to choose a pacifier that fits the infant's mouth in size and shape. Pacifiers that are too short and/or bulbous can lead to abnormal tongue movement that can impede sucking. Conversely, pacifiers that are too long can cause the infant to gag or choke. Pacifiers with a soft exterior shield facilitate positive perioral stimulation and enhance proper placement when the infant is in the side-lying position. Although the use of pacifiers may be challenged for infants in general because of their perceived interference with feeding, they have been shown to enhance the transition to oral feeding in preterm infants and/or infants with feeding difficulties (Wolf, Glass, 1992). Pacifiers are also a simple and feasible alternative that can be used alone or with sucrose or pharmacologic interventions for the management of procedural pain.

Sucrose

The administration of sucrose alone and in combination with nonnutritive sucking (pacifiers) has been the most frequently studied nonpharmacologic intervention for relief of procedural pain in neonates. Sucrose has been examined in relation to its calming effects in crying newborns (Barr, Quek, Cousineau et al., 1994; Blass, Ciaramitaro, 1994; Blass, Fillion, Rochat et al., 1989) and its pain-relieving effects for single invasive procedures in term and preterm neonates (Abad, Diaz, Domenech et al., 1993, 1996; Allen, White, Walburn, 1996; Blass, Hoffmeyer, 1991; Blass, Shah, 1995; Bucher, Moser, von Siebenthal et al., 1995; Field, Goldson, 1984; Gormally,

Barr, Young et al., 1996; Haouari, Wood, Griffith et al., 1995; Johnston, Stremler, Stevens et al., 1997; Ramenghi, Griffith, Wood et al., 1996; Ramenghi, Wood, Griffith et al., 1996; Rushforth, Levene, 1994; Stevens, Johnston, Franck et al., in press). The pain-relieving effects of sucrose are thought to be the result of both the endogenous opioid and nonopioid systems (Blass, Fitzgerald, Kehoe, 1987), but the underlying mechanisms may differ. The coadministration of sucrose with nonnutritive sucking may be additive or synergistic. Indirect evidence for endogenous opioid mediation has been derived through studies with animal models.

Kehoe and Blass (1986) demonstrated that rat pups had diminished distress vocalizations after an electrical charge to their hindpaw after the administration of sucrose. Pain responses were markedly attenuated after intraoral infusion of sucrose. Such infusions decreased the distress vocalization and increased the pain threshold. Similar reduction in vocalization was reproduced by exogenous morphine administration. These distress vocalizations were reversed with the administration of naltrexone (an opioid antagonist), which suggests an opioid mediation. Similarly, Panksepp and others (1986) demonstrated that the administration of opioids to young chicks decreased their vocalizations after a painful stimulus. The results of Kehoe and Blass (1986) and Panksepp and others (1986) studies suggest that sucrose is (1) antinociceptive, (2) effective with a short latency, and (3) effective after the painful stimulus has ceased.

Two systematic reviews of existing randomized controlled trials support the efficacy of sucrose in decreasing procedural pain in human neonates. In the first review (Stevens, Taddio, Ohlsson et al., 1997) of 13 studies, 4 studies of term and 1 study of preterm infants ($n = 271$) were combined in a meta-analysis and indicated that sucrose was associated with a statistically and clinically significant reduction in the proportion of crying after a painful stimulus. Although effective doses varied from 0.01 to 2 ml, the most commonly used dose was 2 ml of 12% to 24% sucrose (0.24 to 0.48 g), given by syringe, dropper, or with a pacifier approximately 2 minutes before a painful stimulus. In a second systematic review of 15 studies (Stevens, Ohlsson, 1998), two additional studies indicated that much smaller doses of sucrose were also shown to be effective in decreasing behavioral indicators of pain when administered in either single (Johnston, Stremler, Stevens et al., 1997) or triple (Johnston, Stremler, Horton et al., 1997) oral applications to preterm infants between 26 and 34 weeks' GA. The most recent research on procedural pain in preterm infants indicated that pain, as assessed with the PIPP (Stevens, Johnston, Petryshen et al., 1996), was significantly reduced for single heel lance procedures compared with a control intervention.

The systematic reviews and meta-analysis provide support for ongoing research for the safety and efficacy of sucrose. Although no adverse effects of sucrose were reported in any study, it is not clear whether the investigators monitored for adverse effects or for how long (Stevens, Johnston, Franck et al., in press). Only one 20-year-old study (Willis, Chabot, Radde et al., 1977) has concluded that 20% sucrose concentrations could predispose preterm infants to necrotizing enterocolitis (NEC). The authors suggest that the hyperosmolarity of sucrose resulted in local trauma to the upper gut wall, which initiated the pathologic process resulting in NEC. This study administered small concentrations of sucrose (8 to 12 times per day) in small volumes delivered directly into the stomach by means of a No. 5 nasogastric tube. The sucrose was mixed with calcium lactate. Infants were nonrandomly assigned to one of three groups: (1) sucrose/calcium lactate was given with each feeding; (2) sucrose/calcium lactate was given 20 minutes before each feeding; and (3) sucrose/calcium lactate was dispersed in water and given at the end of each feeding. Infants in group 2 were more likely to develop NEC. Limitations in this study include the lack of demographic data on subjects. More importantly, it is not clear whether the route of delivery, frequency of doses, or the hyperosmolarity of calcium lactate was the causative factor in the development of NEC. Volumes of 0.5 to 1.0 ml sucrose/calcium lactate in addition to feedings given through a nasogastric tube every 2 hours may be excessive for preterm infants. Other pathogenetic mechanisms such as prematurity, alteration of bowel flora, and the presence of umbilical lines must also be considered as causative agents for NEC.

In summary, several nonpharmacologic interventions hold promise as feasible pain-relieving strategies for procedural pain or for use in combination with pharmacologic interventions for postoperative or chronic pain in infants. In addition, developmentally sensitive strategies that have not been specifically evaluated for their pain-relieving effects have been shown to decrease stress in neonates. One such promising intervention that is designed to decrease stress and promote stability is kangaroo care (Anderson, 1991; Whitelaw, 1990; Whitelaw, Sleath, 1985).

Kangaroo care is a skin-to-skin intervention that has been used with stable preterm infants to provide contact, warmth, and closeness between the infant and parent. Kangaroo care was introduced in 1979 in Bogota, Colombia by two neonatologists (Ray and Marinez) to decrease the neonatal mortality rate. With its implementation, a significant drop in mortality occurred, as well as reduced morbidity and abandonment, enhanced maternal-infant attachment, prolonged lactation, and increased weight gain (Field, 1995). Kangaroo care has been reported to have several behavioral benefits, including decreased crying, improved state organization, increased frequency and duration of quiet sleep, decreased motor activity, and physiologic benefits, including improved growth and decreased oxygen requirements with no compromise in skin temperature (Acolet, Sleath, Whitelaw, 1989; deLeeuw, Colin, Dunnebier et al., 1991; Ludington, 1990; Ludington-Hoe, Hadeed, Anderson, 1991; Ludington-Hoe, Thompson, Swinth et al., 1994). Since its introduction and reported success, kangaroo care has attracted widespread interest, including the involvement of the World Health Organization and UNICEF. Although it continues to be promoted and implemented, it is only beginning to be researched in relation to pain management (Stremler, Johnston, Garand et al., in press).

ROLES OF HEALTH CARE PROFESSIONALS AND PARENTS IN THE MANAGEMENT OF PAIN IN INFANTS

Roles of Health Care Professionals

Health care professionals, because of frequency of contact, experience, and interest, are in a unique position to prevent, assess, and manage pain in infants. More specifically, health care professionals have a moral and ethical obligation to prevent pain when possible, assess pain in infant patients who cannot verbalize pain themselves, provide relief or reduction of pain, and assist the infant and family in coping when pain cannot be prevented (Franck, 1993). This mandate is especially relevant for critically ill or preterm infants in the NICU. Strategies for health professionals to prevent or minimize pain in critically ill or preterm infants are summarized in Box 14.4.

By preventing or ameliorating pain in sick and preterm infants, health care professionals can assist in healing, growth, and improved quality of life. However, health care professionals must be knowledgeable about the potential risks of pain to make adequate and unbiased management decisions to achieve these goals. Health care professionals also have a responsibility to integrate previously discussed knowledge about pain assessment and pharmacologic and nonpharmacologic methods of pain relief in a manner that improves the daily care of infants with pain. One practical approach is to develop and use protocols, standards, algorithms, and other simple guides for staff. The pain, distress, agitation algorithm (the first part of Figure 14.3) is an example of a method developed by Franck for systematically assessing the need for analgesia and sedation in neonates. The second part of the figure is the step-by-step process for creating the pain, distress, agitation algorithm for an NICU.

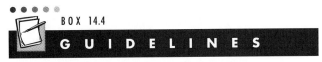

BOX 14.4

GUIDELINES

STRATEGIES TO PREVENT OR MINIMIZE PAIN IN THE CRITICALLY ILL OR PREMATURE INFANT

- Group blood draws to minimize the number of venipunctures per day.
- Use noninvasive monitoring devices when possible.
- Establish central vessel access to minimize vein and artery punctures.
- Have only expert staff attempt IV access on the most unstable patients.
- Use minimal amount of tape and remove it gently.
- Ensure proper premedication before invasive procedures.

May be duplicated for use in clinical practice. As appears in McCaffery M, Pasero C: *Pain: Clinical manual,* p. 661, 1999, Mosby, Inc.

From OGN *nursing practice resource: Prevention, recognition and management of neonatal pain,* pp 3-4, Washington, DC, 1991, NAACOC.

Although great strides have been made in our knowledge through research of the pain substrate for infants, the consequences of pain, the use of assessment measures, and the value of pharmacologic and nonpharmacologic pain management interventions, effective pain management is still less than optimal and consistent. This is largely due to the attitudes and beliefs of health care professionals, persistent fears of addiction, and disproportionate concern for side effects and toxicities. These issues have promoted undertreatment of pain despite emerging scientific evidence and have maintained a wide research practice gap.

Integrating research into practice is an integral component of evidenced-based practice. Once there is a sound basis for particular management strategies, patient care standards can be developed, implemented, and evaluated, and clinical patient outcomes can be determined. Steps to develop patient care standards include reviewing current pain practices, acknowledging that current practices may be less than ideal, developing groups of interested practitioners to review current research literature, and developing written guidelines. These guidelines provide standardized pain management strategies, protocols, or standards.

Two standardized pain management protocols or standards recently have been developed for postoperative pediatric patients. The first, developed by Furdon et al. (in press) is summarized in Box 14.5, p. 664. A chart review of infants in the NICU who had abdominal surgery was conducted to compare patient outcomes before and after use of the standardized pain

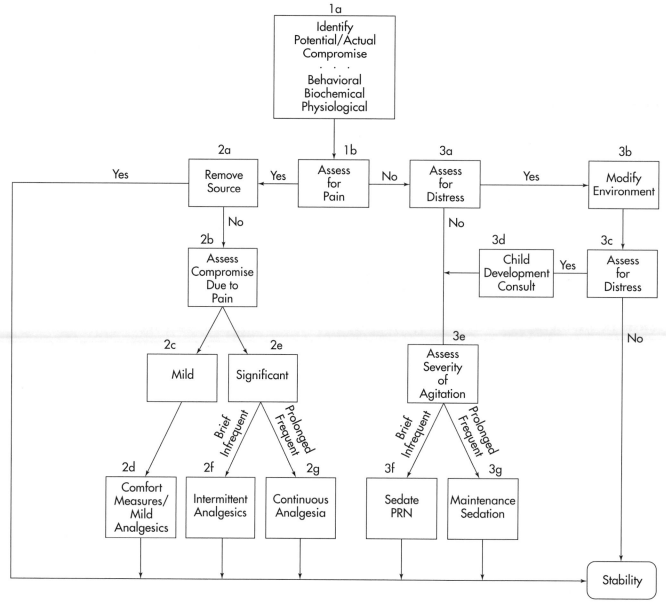

May be duplicated for use in clinical practice. As appears in McCaffery M, Pasero C: *Pain: Clinical manual,* p. 662, 1999, Mosby, Inc.

● ● ● ● ● FIGURE 14.3   Pain, distress, agitation: An algorithm for neonatal intensive care unit interventions.

Modified from Franck LS: Issues regarding the use of analgesia and sedation in critically ill neonates, *AACN* 2:709-719, 1991.

management protocol. Results indicated that with the standardization of pain management strategies for infants in the NICU, there was decreased length of time to extubation, decreased length of stay, better fluid management, and reduced side effects of opioids. Additional benefits included improved pain management documentation, decreased cost of patient care, and decreased nursing time.

A second research-based standard for the assessment, intervention, and evaluation of pain after neonatal and pediatric cardiac surgery has been developed by McRae

and others (1997). In this two-phase project, pain management practices in the pediatric cardiothoracic intensive care unit were retrospectively analyzed in 100 children 0 to 18 years of age and prospectively analyzed in 32 children 3 to 18 years of age. Data from these two analyses, observation by health care professionals of opioid tolerance and withdrawal, and review of guidelines from the AHCPR (1992) led to the development of the standard pain protocol. This comprehensive protocol has been implemented in clinical practice but has not yet been evaluated in relation to patient outcomes.

Interpretation of Algorithm

1a. The first step in the process is to identify the actual or potential compromise to the infant. This may include disruption of behavioral, biochemical, or physiologic states. Examples include excessive gross motor movement and caloric expenditure, poor feeding, inability to sleep, increased catecholamine and stress hormone release, or unstable blood pressure and decreased oxygenation.

1b. The clinician then attempts to identify a source of pain, either external (e.g., invasive procedures, irritating infusion) or internal (e.g., fracture, edema, otitis).

2a. For the patient in whom a source of painful stimuli is identified, ideally the source of pain can be removed. This should result in alleviation of the actual or potential compromise to the patient.

2b. If the source of pain cannot be removed, the degree of compromise to the infant must be assessed.

2c. Mild compromise to the infant, such as occasional fussiness and crying during procedures that does not affect oxygenation, may be managed by providing comfort measures.

2d. Consider providing pacifier, swaddling, holding, etc., or mild analgesics.

2e. Painful stimuli that cause significant compromise to the infant, resulting in the potential for unstable vital signs and oxygenation, require opioid analgesics.

2f. Intermittent administration of morphine or fentanyl may be used before invasive procedures, possibly in conjunction with a local anesthetic.

2g. When pain is frequent and prolonged, ATC administration or a continuous infusion should be considered.

3a. If a source of pain cannot be identified, the environment should be examined for stressors (i.e., bright lights, noise, lack of physical boundaries).

3b. The environment is then modified to remove or diminish the stressors.

3c. The infant can then be reassessed for signs of distress. If the infant's distress is reduced and actual or potential compromise resolved, the environmental modifications should be maintained.

3d. If the infant remains distressed, a consultation with an expert in infant development is suggested to identify any additional stressor in the environment. NOTE: These individuals vary from hospital to hospital and represent a variety of disciplines: nursing, occupational therapy/physical therapy, early childhood education.

3e. If the infant remains distressed, an assessment of the severity and temporal quality of the distress should be made. Are the episodes of the distress brief and infrequent, perhaps precipitated by handling or occurring only during certain times of the day? Or is the distress prolonged and frequent, without any identifiable precipitating factors? Is the infant's oxygenation compromised?

3f. If the distress is brief and infrequent but represents compromise to the infant and is unrelieved by environment modification, intermittent sedation is recommended on an as-needed basis. A sedative such as chloral hydrate may be effective in this instance, as long as the frequency and the total number of doses are monitored closely.

3g. If the distress is prolonged and frequent and represents significant compromise to the infant, unrelieved by environmental modification, continuous sedation may be required. This may be particularly necessary for the chronically ventilated infant who is otherwise stable and does not require painful procedures, but who breathes out of synchrony with the ventilator, causing air hunger and respiratory distress. A benzodiazepine such as lorazepam may be appropriate for such maintenance sedation.

May be duplicated for use in clinical practice. As appears in McCaffery M, Pasero C: *Pain: Clinical manual*, p. 663, 1999, Mosby, Inc.

● ● ● ● ●
F I G U R E 14.3—cont'd

Health care professionals can also decrease infant pain through improved communication and advocacy. "The best technical ability can never replace the actual power of seeing and inquiring and speaking" (Heidegger, 1959). Effective communication includes verbal dialog with members of the multidisciplinary health care team to discuss the current assessment of an infant's pain and the effectiveness of particular pharmacologic and non-pharmacologic strategies. This may be done informally but has also been done in more organized approaches such as "pain rounds" or by "pain teams." Charting the effectiveness of successful and nonsuccessful interventions is also crucial. Because infants most often require an individualized tailored plan of pain management, valuable information and time is lost—"what works" is not communicated effectively from one caregiver to the next.

Health care professionals also need to be advocates for the infant in pain who cannot speak for himself or herself. This involves not only communicating the infant's pain needs to peers but also means representing the infant's best interests on committees, teams, and groups that are responsible for decisions, policies, and procedures that affect infant pain assessment and management (e.g., quality control committees). Teaching parents how to advocate along with the health professional for optimal management of their child's pain also may be effective. For example, when parents are asked for their permission to perform a procedure that may be painful, they need to be taught in a comfortable manner to ask how much pain is

Text continued on p. 668.

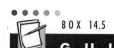

BOX 14.5

G U I D E L I N E S

PAIN MANAGEMENT PROTOCOL FOR NEONATES/INFANTS/TODDLERS

Purpose: To outline the nursing management of the neonate/infant/toddler requiring pain management.

Level: Interdependent (*requires MD order).

Initiated	Discontinued
Date: _____	Date: _____
Time: _____	Time: _____
RN: _____	RN: _____

Supportive Data

CNS elements required for transmission of painful stimuli are present at 24 weeks GA. Organization and maturation then continue after birth. Newborns have the ability to respond to pain and have memory of pain. This protocol is for the management of pain for neonates and preverbal children.

Infant response to the environment is complex. It is a major challenge to interpret the significance of infant behavior. Assessment of pain can be made with information gathered from behavioral and physiologic responses. The absence of overt responses may indicate that the infant is too ill to respond, sedated, or pharmacologically paralyzed. Lack of response does not indicate lack of pain perception.

In conjunction with physiologic parameters, the Neonatal Infant Pain Scale (NIPS) should be used to assess behavioral parameters related to pain in infants. NIPS is an objective tool for use in assessing pain. It cannot be used in isolation. The overall status and environment must be taken into account. Zero on the NIPS may indicate that the infant is too ill to respond.

Pain Relief Strategies

1. *Use* the following as guidelines for management of pain:

Procedure	Interventions
Minor procedures (venipuncture, heelsticks)	Provide the following nonpharmacologic measures if possible: • Swaddling, holding, rocking • Vocalization • Tactile stimulation • Pacifiers
Circumcision	• Apply lidocaine/prilocaine (EMLA) cream if infant >36 wk GA or >2 wk of age if GA <36 wk • Apply 2 h before procedure • Give acetaminophen, 15 mg/kg/dose PO q 4-6h × 24 h (20 mg/kg/dose PR)
PICC insertion	• Apply lidocaine/prilocaine (EMLA) cream if infant >36 wk GA or >2 wk of age if GA <36 wk
Lumbar puncture	• If lumbar puncture nonemergent, apply lidocaine/prilocaine (EMLA) cream if infant >36 wk GA or >2 wk if GA <36 wk • If lumbar puncture emergent, prepare lidocaine/sodium bicarbonate solution (see No. 6)

Chest tubes	• Prepare lidocaine/sodium bicarbonate solution (see No. 6)
	Collaborate with MD for:
	    Morphine sulfate, 0.1 mg/kg/dose IV × 1
	    Acetaminophen, 15 mg/kg/dose PO q 4-6h (20 mg/kg/dose PR)

Postoperatively	Collaborate with MD for ATC pharmacologic measures as outlined below.

EMLA Cream

2. *Verify* that patient does not have the following:
   a. Known allergy to local anesthetics of the "amide" type (e.g., bupivacaine, dibucaine, lidocaine)
   b. Condition associated with methemoglobinemia
3. *Consider* EMLA cream for the following:
   a. Needle insertion (LP, PICC, bone marrow aspiration, Port-a-Cath access, venous access)
   b. Superficial surgical procedures (circumcision, preputial adhesion separation, biopsies, cutdowns)
   c. Laser treatments for removal of warts/nevi

May be duplicated for use in clinical practice. As appears in McCaffery M, Pasero C: *Pain: Clinical manual*, pp. 664-667, 1999, Mosby, Inc.   *Continued.*
Courtesy AMCH (Albany Medical Center Hospital), 1994.

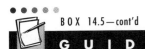

BOX 14.5—cont'd

GUIDELINES

PAIN MANAGEMENT PROTOCOL FOR NEONATES/INFANTS/TODDLERS

EMLA Cream—cont'd

4. *Verify* that MD/NP order includes:
   a. Site and time of application (at least 90 minutes before procedure)
   b. Time procedure is to be performed
5. *Apply* lidocaine/prilocaine (EMLA) cream to intact skin and place under occlusive dressing for at least 90 minutes before procedure. Avoid mucous membranes, open wounds, areas near eyes/ears.

Sodium Bicarbonate/1% Lidocaine Solution

6. *Consider* sodium bicarbonate/1% lidocaine solution for emergent invasive procedures (lumbar punctures, chest tube insertion).
7. *Draw up* 2 mEq sodium bicarbonate and place in 20-ml vial of 1% lidocaine. Label. May store at room temperature for 24 h.
8. *Provide* solution to MDs for their use during sterile procedure.

Assessment

9. *Discuss* pain assessment/management on return from the OR and qd on rounds with medical team.
10. *Review* the following in relation to pain management:
    a. Type of procedure
    b. Analgesics ordered
    c. Type of analgesia/dose appropriate for pain experienced/expected
    d. Timing of administration appropriate for pain experienced/expected
    e. Route of administration
    f. Monitoring of side effects
11. *Assess* for pain/effectiveness of pain relief measures by use of the following Neonatal Infant Pain Scale (NIPS) (Lawrence, Alcock, McGrath et al., 1993):
    a. q 1 while on continuous morphine/fentanyl drip (unable to use with neuromuscular blocking agents)
    b. q 1 after major operative procedure × 24 h, then at each assessment interval × 48 h
    c. At each assessment interval after minor operative procedure × 36 h

	0	1	2
Facial expression	Relaxed muscles Neutral expression	Tight facial muscles Furrowed brow, chin, jaw	—
Cry	Quiet—not crying	Mild moaning, intermittent cry	Loud scream, rising, shrill, continuous Silent cry (intubated) as evidenced by facial movement
Breathing patterns	Relaxed	Changed in breathing: irregular, faster than usual, gagging, breath holding	—
Arms	Relaxed No muscular rigidity Occasional random movements of arms	Flexed/extended Tense, straight arms, rigid and/or rapid extension, flexion	—
Legs	Relaxed No muscular rigidity Occasional random movements of legs	Flexed/extended Tense, straight leg, rigid and/or rapid extension, flexion	—
State of arousal	Sleeping/awake Quiet, peaceful, sleeping or alert and settled	Fussy Alert, restless, and thrashing	—

As appears in McCaffery M, Pasero C: *Pain: Clinical manual*, pp. 664-667, 1999, Mosby, Inc. *Continued.*

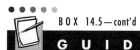

BOX 14.5—cont'd

GUIDELINES

PAIN MANAGEMENT PROTOCOL FOR NEONATES/INFANTS/TODDLERS

Assessment—cont'd

12. *In addition,* assess the following parameters as needed:
    a. Saturations, color (pallor/flushing)
    b. HR, BP
    c. Capillary glucose
    d. Activity level
    e. Environmental effects (light, noise) on physiologic changes

S/P Minor OR Procedures

13. *Collaborate* with MD for acetaminophen, 15 mg/kg/dose PO q4-6 h × 24 h (20mg/kg/dose PR).
14. *Assess* pain relief effectiveness.

S/P Major OR Procedures

15. *Collaborate* with MD for narcotic bolus q2-4 h.
16. *Consider* initiation of drip based on the following:
    a. Type of procedure
    b. Frequency/amount of bolus administration
    c. Assessment of infant
    d. Use of neuromuscular blocking agents
17. *Consider* use of lorazepam in conjunction with continuous infusion and neuromuscular blocking agents.

Morphine Continuous Infusions

*18. *Load* with 0.1 mg/kg × 1 and then start drip at closest port to patient as follows:
    a. *Add* 4 mg morphine sulfate to 39 ml $D_5W/D_{10}W$.
    b. *Begin* at 0.01mg/kg/h-0.02 mg/kg/h. Avoid beginning doses of 0.03-0.04 mg/kg/h in neonates (may induce seizures)
19. *Use* minimum dose to achieve desired effect with minimal side effects.
*20. *Infuse* according to the following guidelines:

	0.01 mg/kg/h	0.02 mg/kg/h
1 kg	0.1 ml/h	0.2 ml/h
1.5 kg	0.15 ml/h	0.3 ml/h
2 kg	0.2 ml/h	0.4 ml/h
2.5 kg	0.25 ml/h	0.5 ml/h
3 kg	0.3 ml/h	0.6 ml/h
3.5 kg	0.35 ml/h	0.7 ml/h
4 kg	0.4 ml/h	0.8 ml/h
5 kg	0.5 ml/h	1 ml/h
6 kg	0.6 ml/h	1.2 ml/h
7 kg	0.7 ml/h	1.4 ml/h
8 kg	0.8 ml/h	1.6 ml/h
9 kg	0.9 ml/h	1.8 ml/h
10 kg	1 ml/h	2 ml/h

21. For infants/toddlers with chronic pain/sickle cell anemia, *collaborate* with MD to titrate up to higher doses.
22. *Assess* vital signs (BP, HR, RR) q1h.
23. *May* piggyback drip into TPN.

BOX 14.5—cont'd

GUIDELINES

PAIN MANAGEMENT PROTOCOL FOR NEONATES/INFANTS/TODDLERS

Fentanyl Continuous Infusion

*24. Load with 1–2 mcg/kg fentanyl and then start drip of 2–4 mcg/kg/h as follows:
  a. Add 100 mcg fentanyl to 48 ml $D_5W/D_{10}W$.
  b. Begin at 2 mcg/kg/h. Infuse according to the following guidelines:

	2 mcg/kg/h	*3 mcg/kg/h*	*4 mcg/kg/h*
1 kg	1 ml/h	1.5 ml/h	2 ml/h
1.5 kg	1.5 ml/h	2.2 ml/h	3 ml/h
2 kg	2 ml/h	3 ml/h	4 ml/h
2.5 kg	2.5 ml/h	3.8 ml/h	5 ml/h
3 kg	3 ml/h	4.5 ml/h	6 ml/h
3.5 kg	3.5 ml/h	5.2 ml/h	7 ml/h
4 kg	4 ml/h	6 ml/h	8 ml/h
5 kg	5 ml/h	7.5 ml/h	10 ml/h
6 kg	6 ml/h	9 ml/h	12 ml/h
7 kg	7 ml/h	10.5 ml/h	14 ml/h
8 kg	8 ml/h	12 ml/h	16 ml/h
9 kg	9 ml/h	13.5 ml/h	18 ml/h
10 kg	10 ml/h	15 ml/h	20 ml/h

25. *Assess* vital signs q1h (BP, HR, RR).
26. *Assess* for pain effectiveness. May develop tolerance and dosage may need to be increased.

Weaning Drips

27. *Collaborate* with MD to wean patient from dose. Wean no more rapidly than by 50% q24h.

Reportable Conditions

28. *Report* the following:
  a. Assessment (physiologic/behavioral) indicates pain (VS [HR, respiratory effort, BP] deviate from baseline/NIPS >4).
  b. Assessment indicates no pain relief with measures prescribed.
  c. Respiratory depression: apnea requiring stimulation or bag/mask ventilation; desaturation <92%.
  d. Suspected ileus (↓ BS, abdominal distention).
  e. Urinary retention.

Parent Instruction

29. *Inform* parents that pain management is an important part of treatment.
30. *Teach* parents infant cues related to pain/pain relief.
31. *Elicit* from parents their beliefs about pain.
32. *Encourage* parents to comfort infant as possible and to vocalize their concerns.

Documentation

33. *Document* implementation of protocol on standard flowsheet (SFS).
34. *Document* assessment of pain score (NIPS)/sedation in activity level column of patient care data record (PCDR).
35. *Document* administration of medication on MAR (Medication Administration Record).
36. *Document* management of pain related to:
  a. Absence/presence of pain according to NIPS/physiologic parameters
  b. Effectiveness of pharmacologic agents
  c. Modifications in pain relief strategies
  d. Presence of complications

anticipated and what interventions will be implemented to prevent or minimize the pain.

In summary, health care professionals have the ability to ensure that the infant has the best pain management possible. This can be achieved through education, examination of personal beliefs and attitudes, improving formal and informal communication, becoming an advocate, developing and using standardized pain management approaches, and offering decision-making algorithms arrived at on the basis of scientific knowledge to narrow the research practice gap.

Roles of Parents

Parents can play a key role in the assessment and management of their infant's pain. Parents usually know their child better than the health care professional, although they may not have seen their child in moderate to severe pain before. Parents are invaluable when taking a pain history and can contribute to what is usual behavior for their infant, how he or she normally expresses pain, and what has an impact on the pain including the following:

- Precipitating events (those events that cause or increase the pain such as injections, parental absence)
- Relieving events (those that lessen or decrease the pain such as medications, a favorite toy, rocking, parental presence)
- Temporal events (times when the pain is relieved or increased)
- Positional events (e.g., being held, lying down, sitting up)
- Associated events (e.g., feeding, hiccoughing)

Parents can also be taught how to assess their infant's pain from behavioral and physiologic cues. Because of their excellent observation skills of their own infants, parents are often able to describe subtle changes in facial expression, body movement, cry, disruptions in feeding and sleeping patterns, and changes in normal interactions with their infants. Although pain assessment by parents may not lead to effective pain management, it will assist health professionals. A postoperative pain measure for parents has been developed for children ages 7 to 12 (Chambers, Reid, McGrath et al., 1996). Although this measure has been reported to help parents identify when their child's pain is clinically significant and requires medication, it has not been validated for use with infants.

Health care professionals also need to explore with parents their feelings about pharmacologic management of pain. A study by Finley et al. (1996) indicated that approximately half of the parents believed that their children could become addicted when opioids were used for pain relief and approximately one third thought that children who have to take pain medicine regularly might learn to use drugs at a later time to solve other problems.

This type of rationale may prevent parents from medicating their child appropriately for pain, although the reasons why parents undermedicate their child for pain are largely unknown.

Parents who participate in the care of their sick infant in the hospital or who are sent home with an infant after surgery need to know specific information about the amount, location, and kind of pain their child may experience and information about each medication the child is taking. More precisely, parents need to know how much pain to expect during or after major or minor procedures, the best pain management and comfort strategies to attempt, the correct methods of administering medications (if caring for the child at home), and the appropriate health care professionals to contact if the pain is not relieved as anticipated.

In summary, pain in infants is a problem that affects infants, their families, and the health care professionals who provide care to them. All these individuals have a role to play in ensuring that pain in infants is either prevented, minimized, or managed in the most optimal manner. If pain is addressed through the available research by caring and knowledgeable health professionals and families, infants will reap the clinical benefits of optimal pain management and an improved quality of life.

RESOURCES FOR HEALTH PROFESSIONALS AND PARENTS

Resources

Acute Pain Management in Infants, Children, and Adolescents: Operative and Medical Procedures
Quick Reference Guide for Clinicians, 1992. DHHS Pub. No. AHCPR 92-0020. To obtain free copies:
    AHCPR, Publications Clearinghouse
    PO Box 8547,
    Silver Spring, MD 20907
    (800) 358-9295
    (From outside the United States, call [410] 381-3150)
    To get copies off Web site: //www.ahcpr.gov/guide/

A Child in Pain: How to Help, What to Do
Book written by Leora Kuttner, 1996, for consumers. Some sections address pain in infants. To order:
    Hartley & Marks Publishers
    PO Box 147
    Roberts, WA 98281
    (800) 277-5887

Dollops
A newsletter for nurses on pain management in pediatrics. To obtain complimentary subscription:
    Dollops
    c/o Leverte Associates Inc.
    50 Washington St.
    Norwalk, CT 06854-9847

How to Raise Professional Awareness of the Need for Adequate Pain Relief for Infants

An article by N.B. Butler in *Birth* 12(1):38-41, 1988. Contains a list of questions parents and concerned professionals might ask of their local health care institutions.

Pain in Infants: Confronting the Challenges

A videotape by Bonnie J. Stevens describing assessment strategies and analgesic intervention for neonates and infants. To order:

Williams & Wilkins Electronic Media
428 E. Preston St.
Baltimore, MD 21202
(800) 527-5597, ext. 4466

Pain in Infants, Children, and Adolescents

A book edited by Neil L. Schechter, Charles B. Berde, and Myron Yaster, 1993 that addresses neurophysiology, pharmacology, psychologic aspects, ethical issues, a variety of interventions, and special pain problems. To order:

Williams & Wilkins
428 E. Preston St.
Baltimore, MD 21202
(800) 527-5597

Pain in Neonates

A book by K.J.S. Anand and P.J. McGrath, 1993 on the anatomy and physiology of pain in infants, pain assessment and management, and moral, ethical, social, legal and research issues. To order:

Elsevier Science Inc.
PO Box 945
New York, NY 10159-0945
(212) 633-3650

Pain, Pain, Go Away: Helping Children With Pain

Book by Patrick J. McGrath, G. Allen Finley, and Judith Ritchie, 1994 teaches parents about pain and helps them request better pain care. To order ($3.00):

Dr. Patrick J. McGrath
Dalhousie University Department of Psychology
Halifax, NS B3H 4J1
Canada

Pediatric Pain Awareness Initiative (PPAI)

A multidisciplinary group of health care professionals whose purpose is to raise the awareness of parents and professionals about managing pain in children. Will provide information to parents about pain management. To obtain information packets: (888) 569-5555

Pediatric Pain Letter

Newsletter that publishes abstracts and commentaries on pain in infants, children, and adolescents. To subscribe ($25.00):

Pediatric Pain Letter
Managing Editor
Dalhousie University
Psychology Department
Halifax, Nova Scotia B3H 3W4
Canada
Fax: (902) 494-6585

Pediatric Pain Network

An electronic mail list for participants to address clinical and research issues on pain in infants and children. To subscribe (free of charge):

E-mail: *Mailserv@ac.dal.ca*
First line must read: subscribe PEDIATRIC-PAIN

References

Abad NM, Diaz E, Domenech M et al.: Attenuation of pain related behavior in neonates given oral sweet solutions, *Abstracts 7th World Congress on Pain,* Paris, France, August, 1993.

Abad NM, Diaz E, Domenech M et al.: Oral sweet solution reduces pain-related behavior in preterm infants, *Acta Paediatr* 85:854-858, 1996.

Abu-Saad HH, Bours G, Stevens B et al.: Assessment of pain in the neonate: a critical review. In press.

Abu-Saad HH, Bours G, Stevens B et al.: Pain assessment in infants: a critical evaluation, *Semin Perinatol.* In press.

Acolet D, Sleath K, Whitelaw A: Oxygenation, heart rate, and temperature in very low birthweight infants during skin-to-skin contact with their mothers, *Acta Paediatr* 78:189-193, 1989.

Acute Pain Management Guideline Panel: *Acute pain management in infants, children, and adolescents: operative and medical procedures. Quick reference guide for clinicians.* AHCPR Pub. No. 92-0020, Rockville, Md, 1992, Agency for Health Care Policy and Research, Public Health Service, U.S. Dept. of Health and Human Services.

Allen K, White D, Walburn J: Sucrose as an analgesic agent for infants during immunization injections, *Arch Pediatr Adolesc Med* 150:270-274, 1996.

Als H, Lawhon G, Brown E et al.: Individualized behavioral and environmental care for the very low-birth-weight preterm infant at risk for bronchopulmonary dysplasia: neonatal intensive care unit and developmental outcome, *Pediatrics* 78:1123-1132, 1986.

Als H, Lawhon G, Duffy FH et al.: Individualized developmental care for the very low-birth-weight-preterm infant, *JAMA* 272:853-858, 1994.

Als H, Lester BM, Tronick E et al.: Manual for the Assessment of Preterm Infants' Behavior (APIB). In Fitzgerald HE, Lester BM, MW Youngman, editors: *Theory and research in behavioral pediatrics,* New York, 1984, Plenum.

Ambuel B, Hamlett KW, Marx CM et al.: Assessing distress in pediatric intensive care environments: The Comfort Scale, *J Pediatr Psychol* 17:95-109, 1992.

Anand KJS: The applied physiology of pain. In Anand KJS, McGrath PJ, editors: *Pain in neonates,* pp 39-66, Amsterdam, 1993, Elsevier.

Anand KJS: Analgesia and sedation in ventilated neonates, *Neonatal Respir Dis* 5:1-11, 1995.

Anand KJS: Long-term effects of pain in neonates and infants. Special Lecture Abstract 110. *Abstracts 8th World Congress on Pain,* Seattle, August, 1996, IASP Press.

Anand KJS: Long-term effects of pain in neonates and infants. In Jenson TS, Turner JA, Wiesenfeld-Hallin Z, editors: *Proceedings of the 8th World Congress on Pain, Progress in pain research and management,* vol 8, pp 881-892, Seattle, 1997, IASP Press.

Anand KJS, Carr DB: The neuroanatomy, neurophysiology, and neurochemistry of pain, stress, and analgesia in newborns and children, *Pediatr Clin North Am* 36:795-822, 1989.

Anand KJS, Craig KD: New perspectives on the definition of pain, *Pain* 67:3-6, 1996.

Anand KJS, Grunau RVE, Oberlander TF: Developmental character and long-term consequences of pain in infants and children. In Weisman SJ, editor: Pain management in children, *Child Adolesc Psychiat Clin North Am* 6:703-724, 1997.

Anand KJS, Hickey PR: Pain and its effects in the human neonate and fetus, *N Engl J Med* 317:1321, 1987.

Anand KJS, Phil D, Hickey PR: Halothane-morphine compared with high-dose sufentanil for anesthesia and postoperative analgesia in neonatal cardiac surgery, *N Engl J Med* 326:1-9, 1992.

Anand KJS, Plotsky PM: Neonatal pain alters weight gain and pain threshold during development in infant rats, *Crit Care Med* 23:A222, 1996.

Anand KJS, Selanikio JD: SOPAIN Study Group: Routine analgesic practices in 109 neonatal intensive care units (NICUs), *Pediat Res* 39:192A, 1996.

Anders TF, Chalemain RJ: The effects of circumcision on sleep-wake cycles in human neonates, *Psychosom Med* 36:174-179, 1974.

Anderson GC: Current knowledge about skin-to-skin (kangaroo) care for preterm infants, *J Perinatol* 11:216-226, 1991.

Andrews K, Fitzgerald M: The cutaneous withdrawal reflex in human neonates: sensitization, receptive fields, and the effects of contra lateral stimulation, *Pain* 56:95-102, 1994.

ASTRA USA, Inc: EMLA cream package insert, *Dollops* 4(1), 1997.

Attia J, Amiel-Tison C, Mayer M-N et al.: Measurement of postoperative pain and narcotic administration in infants using a new clinical scoring system, *Anesthesiology* 67:532A, 1987.

Barba B, Gatto C, Valenza E et al.: Pain memory in full-term newborns, *J Pain Symptom Manage* 6:206, 1991.

Barker D, Rutter N: Exposure to invasive procedures in neonatal intensive care unit admissions, *Arch Dis Child* 72:F47-F48, 1995.

Barr R, Oberlander T, Quek V et al.: *Dose-response analgesic effect of intraoral sucrose in newborns*, Program of the Society for Research in Child Development, Abstract No. 68, 1993.

Barr R, Quek V, Cousineau D et al.: Effects of intraoral sucrose on crying, mouthing and hand-mouth contact in newborn and six-week old infants, *Dev Med Child Neurol* 36:608-618, 1994.

Barrier G, Attia J, Mayer M-N et al.: Measurement of post-operative pain and narcotic administration in infants using a new clinical scoring system, *Intens Care Med* 15: S37-S39, 1989.

Bell RQ, Costal NS: Three tests for sex differences in tactile sensitivity in the newborn, *Biol Neonate* 7:335-347, 1964.

Bell RQ, Waylayer GM, Waldrop MF: Newborn and preschooler: organization of behavior and relation between periods, *Monogr Soc Res Child Dev* 36:1-145, 1971.

Benini F, Johnston CC, Faucher D et al.: Topical anesthesia during circumcision in newborn infants, *JAMA* 270:850-853, 1993.

Berde CB, Anand KJS, Sethna NF: Pediatric pain management. In Gregory GA, editor: *Pediatric anesthesia*, vol 2, ed 2, pp 679-727, New York, 1989, Churchill Livingstone.

Beyer JE, McGrath PJ, Berde CB: Discordance between self-report and behavioural pain measures in children aged 3-7 years after surgery, *J Pain Symptom Manage* 5:350-356, 1990.

Blackburn ST, VandenBerg KA: Assessment and management of neonatal neurobehavioral development. In Kenner C, Bruggemeyere A, Gunderson LP, editors: *Comprehensive neonatal nursing: a physiological perspective*, pp 1094-1133, Philadelphia, 1993, WB Saunders.

Blass EM, Ciaramitaro V: A new look at some old mechanisms in human newborns: taste and tactile determinants of state, affect and action, *Monogr Soc Res Child Dev* 59:1-80, 1994.

Blass EM, Fillion TJ, Rochat P et al.: Sensorimotor and motivational determinants in hand-mouth coordination in 1-3 day old human infants, *Dev Psychol* 25:963-975, 1989.

Blass EM, Fitzgerald E, Kehoe P: Interactions between sucrose, pain and isolation distress, *Pharmacol Biochem Behav* 26:483-489, 1987.

Blass EM, Hoffmeyer LB: Sucrose as an analgesic for newborn infants, *Pediatrics* 87:215-218, 1991.

Blass EM, Shah A: Pain-reducing properties of sucrose in human newborns, *Chem Senses* 20:29-35, 1995.

Bodin A, Nyqvist-Mayer A, Wadsten T et al.: Phases diagram and aqueous solubility of the lidocaine-prilocaine binary system, *J Pharm Sci* 73:481, 1984.

Brazelton TB, Nugent KN: *The neonatal behavioral assessment scale*, ed 3, Holborn, London, 1995, Mac Keith Press.

Brazy JE, Goldstein R, Oehler J et al.: Nursery neurobiologic risk score: levels of risk and relationships with nonmedical factors, *J Behav Pediatr* 14:375-380, 1993.

Bucher HU, Moser T, von Siebenthal K et al.: Sucrose reduces pain reaction to heel lancing in preterm infants: a placebo-controlled, randomized and masked study, *Pediatr Res* 38:332-335, 1995.

Burrows A, Asonye U, Anderson-Shanklin G et al.: The effect of nonnutritive sucking on transcutaneous oxygen tension in noncrying preterm neonates, *Res Nurs Health* 1:69-75, 1978.

Cabal LA, Siassi B, Hodgman JE: Neonatal clinical cardiopulmonary monitoring. In Fanaroff AA, Martin RJ, editors: *Neonatal-perinatal medicine: diseases of the fetus and infant*, pp 437-455, St. Louis, 1992, Mosby.

Campos R: Soothing pain-elicited distress in infants with swaddling and pacifiers, *Child Dev* 60:781-792, 1989.

Campos R: Rocking and pacifiers: two comforting interventions for heelstick pain, *Res Nurs Health* 11:321-331, 1994.

Catterall W, Mackie K: Local anesthetics. In Hardman JG, Limbird LE, editors: *Goodman and Gilman's the pharmacological basis of therapeutics*, ed 9, pp 331-347, New York, 1996, McGraw-Hill.

Chambers CT, Reid GJ, McGrath PJ et al.: Development and preliminary validation of a postoperative pain measure for parents, *Pain* 68:307-313, 1996.

Chay PCW, Duffy BJ, Waler JS: Pharmacokinetic-pharmacodynamic relationships of morphine in neonates, *Clin Pharmacol Ther* 51:334-342, 1992.

Chessex P, Reichman B, Verellen G et al.: Relation between heart rate and energy expenditure in the neonate, *Pediatr Res* 15:1077-1082, 1981.

Cole JC, Jorgensen KM: Medical, developmental, and pharmacologic intervention: the essence of collaboration, *Neonatal Network* 16:56-58, 1997.

Corff KE: An effective comfort measure for minor pain and stress in preterm infants: facilitated tucking, *Neonatal Network* 12:74, 1993.

Corff KE, Seideman R, Venkataraman P et al.: Facilitated tucking: a nonpharmacologic comfort measure for pain in preterm infants, *J Obstet Gynecol Neonatal Nurs* 24:143-147, 1995.

Craig KD: The facial display of pain in infants and children. In Finley GA, McGrath PJ editors: *Measurement of pain in infants and children. In pain research and management*, vol 10, pp 103-121, Seattle, 1998, IASP Press.

Craig KD, Grunau RVE: Neonatal pain perception and behavioural measurement. In Anand KJS, McGrath PJ, editors: *Pain in neonates*, pp 67-105, Amsterdam, 1993, Elsevier.

Craig KD, Grunau RVE, Aquan-Assee J: Judgement of pain in newborns: facial activity and cry as determinants, *Can J Behav Sci* 20:442-451, 1988.

Craig KD, McMahan RJ, Morison JD et al.: Developmental changes in infant pain expression during immunization injections, *Soc Sci Med* 19:1331-1337, 1984.

Craig KD, Whitfield MF, Grunau RVE et al.: Pain in the preterm neonate: behavioral and physiological indices, *Pain* 52:287, 1993.

Crane L, Snyder J, Knight P et al.: Effects of position changes on transcutaneous carbon dioxide tension in neonates with respiratory distress, *J Perinatol* 10:35, 1990.

Deiriggi PM: Effects of waterbed flotation on indicators of energy expenditure in preterm infants, *Nurs Res* 39:140-146, 1990.

deLeeuw R, Colin EM, Dunnebier EA et al.: Physiological effects of kangaroo care in very small preterm infants, *Biol Neonate* 59:149-155, 1991.

Dixon S, Snyder J, Holve R et al.: Behavioral effects of circumcision with and without anesthesia, *Dev Behav Pediatr* 5:246-250, 1984.

Eide PK, Stubhaug A, Stenehjem AE: Central dysthesia pain after traumatic spinal cord injury is dependent on N-methyl-D-aspartate receptor activation, *Neurosurgery* 37:1080, 1995.

Ekman P, Friesen WV: *Facial action coding system: a technique for the measurement of facial movement*, Palo Alto, Calif, 1978, Consulting Psychologists Press.

Emde RN, Harmon RJ, Metcalf D et al.: Stress and neonatal sleep, *Psychosom Med* 33:491-497, 1971.

Evans JC, Vogelpohl DG, Bourguignon CM et al.: Pain behaviors in LBW infants accompany some "nonpainful" caregiving procedures, *Neonatal Network* 15:33-39, 1997.

Fearon I, Kisilevsky B, Hains S et al.: Swaddling after heel lance: Age-specific effects on behavioral recovery in preterm infants, *Develop Behav Pediatr* 18:222-232, 1997.

Field T: *Touch in early development*, Mahwah, NJ, 1995, Lawrence Erlbaum Associates.

Field T, Goldson E: Pacifying effects of nonnutritive sucking on term and preterm neonates during heelsticks, *Pediatrics* 74:1012-1015, 1984.

Field T, Ignatoff E, Stringer J et al.: Nonnutritive sucking during tube feedings: effects on preterm neonates in an intensive care unit, *Pediatrics* 70:381-384, 1982.

Finley GA, McGrath PJ, Forword SP et al.: Parents' management of children's pain following 'minor' surgery, *Pain* 64:83-87, 1996.

Fitzgerald M: Development of pain pathways and mechanisms. In Anand KJS, McGrath PJ, editors: *Pain in neonates,* pp 19-33, Amsterdam, 1993, Elsevier.

Fitzgerald M, Andrews K: Flexion reflex properties in the human infant: a measure of spinal sensory processing in the newborn. In Finley GA, McGrath PJ: *Management of pain in infants and children: progress in pain research and management,* vol 10, pp 47-57, Seattle, 1998, IASP Press.

Fitzgerald M, Millard C, McIntosh N: Cutaneous hypersensitivity following peripheral tissue damage in newborn infants and its reversal with topical anaesthesia, *Pain* 39:31-36, 1989.

Fitzgerald M, Shaw A, McIntosh N: Postnatal development of the cutaneous flexor reflex: comparative study of preterm infants and newborn rat pups, *Dev Med Child Neurol* 30:520-526, 1988.

Franck LS: A new method to quantitatively describe pain behavior in infants, *Nurs Res* 35:28-31, 1986.

Franck LS: A national survey of assessment and treatment of pain and agitation in the neonatal intensive care unit, *J Obstet Gynecol Neonatal Nurs* 16:387-393, 1987.

Franck LS: Identification, management, and prevention of pain in the neonate. In Kenner C, Brueggemeyer A, Gunderson L, editors: *Comprehensive neonatal nursing: a physiologic perspective,* pp 913-925, Philadelphia, 1993, WB Saunders.

Franck LS: Issues regarding the use of analgesia and sedation in critically ill neonates, *AACN* 2:709-719, 1991.

Franck LS, Miaskowski C: Measurement of neonatal responses to painful stimuli: a research review, *J Pain Symptom Manage* 14:343-378, 1997.

Franck LS, Miaskowski C: The use of intravenous opioids to reduce nociceptive stress responses in critically ill, premature neonates: a research critique, *J Pain Symptom Manage* 15:41-69, 1998.

Fuller BF: Acoustic discrimination of three types of infant cries, *Nurs Res* 40:156-160, 1991.

Furdon SA, Eastman M, Benjamin K et al: Outcome measures after standardized pain management strategies in postoperative patients in the NICU, *J Perinatal Neonatal Nurs,* in press.

Gauvain-Pichard A: Comment reconnaitre la douleur d'un enfant, *Revue de l'infirmiere* 15:19-24, 1987.

Giannini EH, Brewer EJ, Miller ML et al.: Ibuprofen suspension in the treatment of juvenile rheumatoid arthritis: Pediatric Rheumatology Collaborative Study Group, *J Pediatr* 117:645, 1990.

Gill N, Behnek M, Conlon M et al.: Effect of non-nutritive sucking on behavioral state in preterm infants before feeding, *Nurs Res* 37:347-350, 1988.

Gormally SM, Barr RG, Young SN et al.: Combined sucrose and carrying reduces newborn pain response more than sucrose or carrying along, *Arch Pediatr Adolesc Med* 150:47, 1996.

Grunau RVE, Craig KD: Pain expression in neonates: facial action and cry, *Pain* 28:395-410, 1987.

Grunau RVE, Craig KD: Facial activity as a measure of neonatal pain expression. In Tyler DC, Krane EJ, editors: *Advances in pain research and therapy, pediatric pain,* vol 15, pp 147-56, New York, 1990, Raven Press.

Grunau RVE, Whitfield M, Petrie J: Pain sensitivity and temperament in extremely low-birth-weight premature toddlers and preterm and full-term controls, *Pain* 58:341-346, 1994.

Grunau RVE, Whitfield M, Petrie J et al.: Early pain experience, child and family factors, as precursors of somatization: a prospective study of extremely premature and fullterm children, *Pain* 56:353-359, 1994.

Gullickson GR, Crowell DH: Neonatal habituation to electrotactual stimulation, *J Exper Child Psychol* 1:388-396, 1964.

Gunnar MR, Fisch RO, Korsvik S et al.: The effects of circumcision on serum cortisol and behavior, *Psychoneuroendocrinology* 6:269-275, 1981.

Gunnar MR, Fisch R, Malone S: The effects of a pacifying stimulus on behavioral and adrenocortical responses to circumcision, *J Am Acad Child Psychiatry* 23:34-38, 1984.

Gunnar MR, Porter FL, Wolf CM et al.: Neonatal stress reactivity: predictions to later emotional temperament, *Child Dev* 66(1):1-13, 1995.

Hadjistavropoulos HD, Craig KD, Grunau RVE et al.: Judging pain in newborns: facial and cry determinants, *J Pediatr Psychol* 19:305-318, 1994.

Hadjistavropoulos HD, Craig KD, Grunau RVE et al.: Judging pain in infants: behavioural, contextual, and developmental determinants, *Pain* 73:319-124, 1997.

Hannallah RS, Broadman LM, Belman AB et al.: Comparison of caudal and ilioinguinal/iliogastric nerve blocks for control of post-orchiopexy pain in pediatric ambulatory surgery, *Anesthesiology* 66:832-834, 1987.

Haouari N, Wood C, Griffiths et al.: The analgesic effect of sucrose in full term infants: a randomised controlled trial, *BMJ* 310:1498-1500, 1995.

Harte GJ, Gray PH, Lee TC et al.: Hemodynamic responses and population pharmacokinetics of midazolam following administration to ventilated, preterm neonates, *J Pediatr Child Health* 33:335-338, 1997.

Heidegger M: The fundamental questions. In *An introduction to metaphysics,* pp 1-51, New Haven, CT, 1959, Yale University Press.

Henderson K, Sethna NF, Berde CB: Continuous caudal anesthesia for inguinal hernia repair in former preterm infants, *J Clin Anesth* 5:129, 1993.

Hodgkinson K, Bear M, Thorn J et al.: Measuring pain in neonates: evaluating an instrument and developing a common language, *Aust J Adv Nurs* 12:17-22, 1994.

Houck CS: The management of acute pain in the child. In Ashburn MA, Rice LJ, editors: *The management of pain,* pp 651-666, New York, 1998, Churchill Livingstone.

Izard CE: *The maximally discriminative facial movement coding system (MAX),* Newark, 1979, University of Delaware Instructional Resources Center.

Jacqz-Aigrain E, Daoud P, Burtin P et al.: Placebo-controlled trial of midazolam sedation in mechanically ventilated newborn babies, *Lancet* 344:646-650, 1994.

Johnston C: Psychometric issues in the measurement of pain. In Finley GA, McGrath PJ, editors: Measurement of pain in infants and children, *Progr Pain Res Measurement,* 10:5-20, Seattle, 1998, IASP Press.

Johnston C, Collinge J, Henderson S et al.: A cross sectional survey of pain and analgesia in Canadian neonatal intensive care units, *Clin J Pain* 13:308-312, 1998.

Johnston C, O'Shaughnessy D: Acoustical attributes of infant pain cries: discriminating features, *Pain (Suppl)* 4:S233, 1987.

Johnston C, Stevens B: Experience in the NICU affects pain responses, *Pediatrics* 98:925-930, 1996.

Johnston C, Stevens B, Craig KD et al.: Developmental changes in pain expression in premature, full-term, two- and four-month-old infants, *Pain* 52:201, 1993.

Johnston C, Stremler RL, Horton LJ et al.: Single vs. triple dose of sucrose for pain in preterm neonates, *Pain Res Manage* 2(1), 60A, 1997.

Johnston C, Stremler RL, Stevens B et al.: Effectiveness of oral sucrose and simulated rocking on pain response in preterm neonates, *Pain* 72:193-199, 1997.

Jones RDM et al.: Antagonism of the hypnotic effect of midazolam in children: a randomized double-blind study of placebo and flumazenil administered after midazolam-induced anaesthesia, *Br J Anaesth* 56:560-566, 1991.

Joyce BA, Schade JG, Keck JF et al.: Reliability and validity of preverbal pain assessment tools, *Issues Comprehens Pediatr Nurs* 17:121-135, 1994.

Kehoe P, Blass EM: Behaviorally functional opioid systems in infant rata. II. Evidence for pharmacological, physiological and psychological mediation of pain and stress, *Behav Neurosci* 10:624-630, 1986.

Kelley MT, Watson PD, Edge JH et al.: Pharmacokinetics and pharmacodynamics of ibuprofen isomers and acetaminophen in febrile children, *Clin Pharmacol Ther* 52:181, 1992.

Kissin I, Brown P, Bradley E: Sedative and hypnotic midazolam-morphine interactions in rats, *Anesth Analg* 71:137-143, 1990.

Koren G, Jacobson S: Developmental considerations in the clinical pharmacology of analgesics. In Schechter NL, Berde CB, Yaster M, editors: *Pain in infants, children, and adolescents,* Baltimore, 1993, Williams & Wilkins.

Korner A, Stevenson D, Kraemer H et al.: Prediction of the development of low birth weight preterm infants by a new neonatal medical index, *Dev Behav Pediatr* 14:105-111, 1993.

Korner A, Thoman EB: The relative efficacy of contact and vestibular-proprioceptive stimulation on soothing neonates, *Child Dev* 2:443-453, 1972.

Krechel SW, Bildner J: CRIES: a new neonatal postoperative pain measurement score: initial testing of validity and reliability, *Pediatr Anesth* 5:53-61, 1995.

Kuttner L: *A child in pain: how to help, what to do,* Roberts, WA, 1996, Hartley & Marks Publishers.

Lander J, Brady-Fryer B, Metcalfe JB et al.: Comparison of ring block, dorsal penile nerve block, and topical anesthesia for neonatal circumcision, *JAMA* 278:2157-2162, 1997.

Langland J, Langland P: Pain in the neonate and fetus (letter to the editor), *N Engl J Med* 318:1398, 1988.

Lawrence J, Alcock D, McGrath P et al.: The development of a tool to assess neonatal pain, *Neonatal Network* 12:59-66, 1993.

Leith PJ, Weisman SJ: Pharmacologic interventions for pain management in children, *Child Adolesc Psychiat Clin North Am* 6:797-815, 1997.

Lester BM: A biosocial model of infant crying. In Lipsitt LP, editor: *Advances in infancy research,* pp 167-212, New York, 1984, Academic.

Lipsitt LP, Levy N: Electrotactual threshold in the neonate, *Child Dev* 30:547-544, 1959.

Ludington-Hoe SM, Hadeed AJ, Anderson GC: Physiologic responses to skin-to-skin holding contact in hospitalized premature infants, *J Perinatol* 11:19-24, 1991.

Ludinton SM: Energy conservation during skin-to-skin contact between premature infants and their mothers, *Heart Lung* 19:445-451, 1990.

Ludington-Hoe SM, Thompson C, Swinth J et al.: Kangaroo care: research results and practice implication guidelines, *Neonatal Network* 13:19-27, 1994.

Magny JF, Zupan V, Dehan et al.: Midazolam and myoclonus in neonates, *Eur J Pediatr* 153:389-392, 1994.

Marchette L, Main R, Redick E et al.: Pain reduction interventions during neonatal circumcision, *Nurs Res* 40:241-244, 1991.

Marshall RE, Porter FL, Rogers AG et al.: Circumcision. II. Effects upon mother-infant interaction, *Early Hum Dev* 7:367-374, 1982.

Masterson J, Zucker C, Schulze K: Prone and supine positioning effects on energy expenditure and behavior of low birth weight infants, *Pediatrics* 5:689, 1988.

Maunuksela E-L, Olkkola KT, Korpela R: Does prophylactic intravenous infusion of indomethacin improve the management of postoperative pain in children? *Can J Anaesth* 35:123, 1988.

Maxwell LG, Yaster M, Wetzel RC et al.: Penile nerve block for newborn circumcision, *Obstet Gynecol* 70:415, 1987.

Mayers DJ, Hindmarsh KW, Sankaran et al.: Chloral hydrate disposition following single-dose administration to critically ill neonates and children, *Dev Pharmacol Ther* 16:71-77, 1991.

McGrath PA: *Pain in children,* New York, 1990, Guilford Press.

McGrath PJ: There is more to pain measurement in children than "ouch," *Can Psychol* 37:63-75, 1995.

McGrath PJ, Johnson G, Goodman JT et al.: CHEOPS: A behavioral scale for rating postoperative pain in children. In Fields HL, Dubner R, Cerveri F, editors: *Advances in pain research and therapy,* p 395-402, vol 9, New York, 1985, Raven Press.

McGrath PJ, Unruh A: *Pain in children and adolescents,* Amsterdam, 1987, Elsevier.

McIntosh N: Pain in the newborn, a possible new starting point, *Eur J Pediatr* 156:173-177, 1997.

McIntosh N, van Veen L, Brameyer H: The pain of heel prick and its measurement in preterm infants, *Pain* 52:71-74, 1993.

McRae ME, Rourke DA, Imperial-Perez FA et al.: Development of a research-based standard for assessment, intervention, and evaluation of pain after neonatal and pediatric cardiac surgery, *Pain Med J Club J* 3:281-285, 1997.

Merskey H, Albe-Fessard DG, Bonica JJ et al.: Pain terms: a list with definitions and notes on usage: recommended by the IASP Subcommittee on Taxonomy, *Pain* 6:249-252, 1979.

Michelsson K: Cry analysis of symptomless low birth weight neonates and of asphyxiated newborn infants, *Acta Pediatr Scand* 19:309-315, 1971.

Michelsson K, Jarvenpaa AL, Rinne A: Sound spectrographic analysis of pain cry in preterm infants, *Early Hum Dev* 8:141-149, 1983.

Miller H, Anderson GC: Nonnutritive sucking: effects on crying and heart rate in intubated infants requiring assisted mechanical ventilation, *Neonatal Intens Care* May/June:46-48, 1994.

Mills N: Pain behaviors in infants and toddlers, *J Pain Symptom Manage* 4:184-190, 1989.

Oster H, Rosenstein D: *Baby FACS: analyzing facial movement in infants,* Paper presented at the Annual Meeting of the Society for Research in Child Development, New Orleans, LA, March 1993.

Owens ME, Todt EH: Pain in infancy: neonatal reaction to a heel lance, *Pain* 20:77-84, 1984.

Paludetto R, Robertson S, Hack M et al.: Transcutaneous oxygen tensions during nonnutritive sucking in preterm infants, *Pediatrics* 74:539-542, 1984.

Panksepp J, Siviy S, Normansell L: Brain opioids and social emotion. In Reite M, Fields T, editors: *The psychobiology of attachment and separation,* pp 3-39, San Diego, 1986, Academic Press.

Pasternak GW, Zhang AZ, Tecott L: Developmental differences between high and low affinity opiate binding sites: their relationship to analgesia and respiratory depression, *Life Sci* 27:1185, 1980.

Penticuff J: Neonatal nursing ethics: toward a consensus, *Neonatal Network* 5:7-16, 1987.

Pickler RH, Higgins KE, Crummette BD: The effect of non-nutritive sucking on bottle-feeding stress in preterm infants, *J Obstet Gynecol Neonatal Nurs* 22:230-243, 1993.

Pokela M: Pain relief can reduce hypoxemia in distressed neonates during routine treatment procedures, *Pediatrics* 93:379-383, 1994.

Portenoy RK, Kanner RM: Definition and assessment of pain. In Portenoy RK, Kanner RM, editors: *Pain management: theory and practice,* pp 3-18, Philadelphia, 1996, FA Davis.

Porter FL, Wolf CM, Gold J et al.: Pain and pain management in newborn infants: a survey of physicians and nurses, *Pediatrics* 100:625-632, 1997.

Prechtl HFR: The behavioral states of the newborn infant (review), *Brain Res* 76:185-212, 1974.

Prkachin KM, Craig KD: Expressing pain: the communication and interpretation of facial pain signals, *J Nonverbal Behav* 19:191-205, 1995.

Ramenghi L, Griffith G, Wood C et al.: Effect of non-sucrose sweet-tasting solution on neonatal heel prick responses, *Arch Dis Child* 74:F129-F131, 1996.

Ramenghi L, Wood C, Griffith G et al.: Reduction of pain response in premature infants using intraoral sucrose, *Arch Dis Child* 74:F126-F128, 1996.

Rana SR: Pain: a subject ignored (letter to the editor), *Pediatrics* 79:309-310, 1987.

Rice LJ: Regional anesthesia and analgesia. In Motoyama EK, Davis PJ, editors: *Smith's anesthesia for infants and children,* pp 403-442, St. Louis, 1996, Mosby.

Rumack BH, Peterson RG: Acetaminophen overdose: incidence, diagnosis, and management in 416 patients, *Pediatrics* (Suppl) 62:898, 1978.

Rushforth JA, Levene MI: Behavioural response to pain in healthy neonates, *Arch Dis Child* 70:F174-F176, 1994.

Schade JG, Joyce BA, Gerkensmeyer J et al.: Comparison of three preverbal scales for postoperative pain assessment in a diverse pediatric sample, *J Pain Symptom Manage* 7:348-359, 1996.

Schechter NL, Berde CB, Yaster M: *Pain in infants, children and adolescents,* Baltimore, 1993, Williams & Wilkins.

Schmelling DJ, Coran AG: Hormonal and metabolic responses to operative stress in the neonate, *J Parenteral Enteral Nutr* 15:215-238, 1991.

Sexon W, Schneider P, Chamberlin J et al.: Auditory conditioning in the critically ill neonate to enhance interpersonal relationships, *J Perinatol* VI:20-23, 1986.

Shortland P, Woolf CJ, Fitzgerald M: Morphology and somatotropic organization of the central terminals of hindlimb hair follicle afferents in the rat lumbar spinal cord, *J Comprehens Neurol* 289:416-433, 1989.

Sparshott M: The development of a clinical distress scale for ventilated newborn infants: identification of pain and distress based on validated behavioural scores, *J Neonatal Nurs* 2:5-11, 1996.

Sparshott M: *Pain, distress and the newborn baby,* Oxford, 1997, Blackwell Science.

Spencer DM, Miller KA, O'Quin M et al.: Dorsal penile nerve block in neonatal circumcision: chloroprocaine versus lidocaine, *Am J Perinatol* 9:214-218, 1992.

Stang HJ, Gunnar MR, Snellman L et al.: Local anesthesia for neonatal circumcision, *JAMA* 259:1507-1511, 1988.

Stevens B: Pain assessment in children: birth through adolescence. In Weisman S, editor: Pain management in children, *Child Adolesc Psychiatr Clin North Am,* pp 725-743, Philadelphia, 1997, WB Saunders.

Stevens B: Composite measures of pain. In Finley GA, McGrath PJ, editors: Measurement of pain in infants and children, *Progress in pain research and measurement*, vol 10, pp 161-178, Seattle, 1998, IASP Press.

Stevens B, Johnston CC: Physiologic response of premature infants to a painful stimulus, *Nurs Res* 43:226-231, 1994.

Stevens B, Johnston CC, Franck LS et al.: The efficacy of developmentally sensitive interventions and sucrose for relieving procedural pain in very low birth weight neonates, *Nurs Res* in press.

Stevens B, Johnston CC, Horton L: Factors that influence the behavioral response of premature infants, *Pain* 59:101-109, 1994.

Stevens B, Johnston CC, Petryshen P et al.: Premature infant pain profile: development and initial validation, *Clin J Pain* 12:13-22, 1996.

Stevens B, Ohlsson A: The efficacy of sucrose to reduce procedural pain in neonates as assessed by physiologic and/or behavioral outcomes. In Sinclair JC, Bracken MB, Soll RS et al.; editors: *Neonatal modules of the Cochrane data base of systematic reviews* (Updated February, 1998). Available in the Cochrane Library. The Cochrane Collaboration; Issue 2, Oxford, 1998, Update Software.

Stevens B, Taddio A, Ohlsson A et al.: The efficacy of sucrose for relieving pain in neonates: a systematic review and meta-analysis, *Acta Paediatr* 86:837-842, 1997.

Stremler R, Johnston C, Garand, L et al.: *Kangaroo care as a means of decreasing pain from routine heelstick in preterm neonates: a pilot study,* in press.

Taddio A, Goldbach M, Ipp M et al.: Effect of circumcision on pain responses during vaccination in male infants, *Lancet* 345:291-292, 1995.

Taddio A, Katz J, Ilersich AL et al.: Neonatal circumcision and pain response during routine vaccination 4 to 6 months later, *Lancet* 349:599-603, 1997.

Taddio A, Nulman I, Koren BS et al.: A revised measure of acute pain in infants, *J Pain Symptom Manage* 10:456-463, 1995.

Taddio A, Ohlsson A, Einarson T et al.: A systematic review of lidocaine-prilocaine cream (EMLA) in the treatment of acute pain in neonates, *Pediatrics* 101:e1-14, 1998.

Taddio A, Stevens B, Craig K et al.: Efficacy and safety of lidocaine-prilocaine cream for pain during circumcision, *N Engl J Med* 336:1197-1201, 1997.

Taylor P: Post-operative pain in toddler and pre-school age children, *Matern Child Nurs J* 12:35-50, 1983.

Tverskoy M, Fleyshman G, Ezry J et al.: Midazolam-morphine sedative interaction in patients, *Anesth Analg* 68:282-285, 1989.

Wagman MJ, Shutack JG, Moomjian AS et al.: Improved oxygenation and lung compliance with prone positioning of neonates, *J Pediatr* 94:787-791, 1979.

Whitelaw A: Kangaroo baby care: just a nice experience or an important advance for preterm infants? *Pediatrics* 85:604-605, 1990.

Whitelaw A, Sleath K: Myth of the marsupial mother: home care of very low birthweight babies in Bogota, Columbia, *Lancet* May:25:1206-1208, 1985.

Willer JC: Comparative study of perceived pain and nociceptive flexion reflex in man, *Pain* 3:69-80, 1977.

Williamson ML: Circumcision anesthesia: a study of nursing implications for dorsal penile nerve block, *Pediatr Nurs* 23:59-63, 1997.

Williamson PS, Williamson ML: Physiologic stress reduction by a local anesthetic during newborn circumcision, *Pediatrics* 71:36-40, 1983.

Willis DM, Chabot J, Radde IC et al.: Unsuspected hyperosmolarity of oral solutions contributing to necrotizing enterocolitis in very low birth weight infants, *Pediatrics* 60:535-538, 1977.

Wolf LS, Glass RP: *Feeding and swallowing disorders in infancy.* Tucson, 1992, Therapy Skill Builders.

Wolff PH: *The development of behavioral states and the expression of emotions in early infancy,* Chicago, 1987, The University of Chicago Press.

Wong D: EMLA's safety for small infants (response to letter to the editor), *Am J Nurs* 95:18-19, 1995.

Wong D: *Physiological responses, facial expressions, and cry of infant during immunization in relation to their pain history,* University Microfilms, Ann Arbor, MI, 1992.

Wong D: *Wong and Whaley's essentials of pediatric nursing,* ed 5, St. Louis, 1997, Mosby.

Woodson R, Hamilton C: Heart rate estimates of motor activity in preterm infants, *Infant Behav Dev* 9:283-290, 1986.

Wynn F: The embodied chiasmic relationship of mother and infant, *Hum Studies* 19:253-270, 1997.

Yaster M: The dose response of fentanyl in neonatal anesthesia, *Anesthesiology* 66:433-435, 1987.

Yaster M, Berde C, Billet C: The management of opioid and benzodiazepine dependence in infants, children, and adolescents, *Pediatrics* 98:135-140, 1996.

Yaster M, Krane EJ, Kaplan RF et al.: *Pediatric pain management and sedation handbook,* St. Louis, 1997, Mosby.

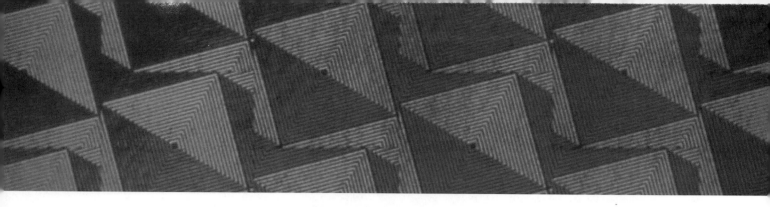

chapter fifteen
PAIN IN THE ELDERLY

Chris Pasero, Barbara A. Reed, and Margo McCaffery

CHAPTER OUTLINE

TERMINOLOGY

Alzheimer's disease: Most common cause of dementia in older adults; caused by a degenerative process with large loss of cells from cerebral cortex and other brain areas; prominent early symptom is memory loss.

Cognitive impairment: Disordered thinking, deficits in memory, attention, visual/spatial skills, and language.

Confusion: Acute confusion is a transient syndrome characterized by abnormalities in attention and cognition, fluctuating levels of consciousness, disordered psychomotor behavior, sleep-wake disturbances, and disturbance of the autonomic nervous system.

Debilitated: Weak, feeble, exhausted, worn out, deprived of strength, impaired, decrepit, diminished, crippled.

Delirium: Disturbed intellectual function, disorientation to time and place but usually not to person, altered attention span, worsened memory, labile mood, meaningless chatter, poor judgment, altered level of consciousness.

Dementia: Progressive, degenerative disease characterized by brain atrophy; loss of intellect; decline of memory, recall, and retention; disorientation; deterioration of motor ability; loss of verbal communication skills; incontinence; and physical deterioration leading to death.

Elderly: Culturally determined classification of people made on the basis of age in years.

Frail: Not robust, delicate, weak, easily broken, at risk.

Neuropathic pain: Pain initiated or caused by a primary lesion or dysfunction in the peripheral or central nervous system.

Nursing home: Institution providing long-term custodial care, primarily for elderly patients; usually isolated from other elements of the health care system; also referred to as long-term care facility.

TABLE 15.1 ● ● ● ● ●

Misconceptions **Pain Management in the Elderly**

MISCONCEPTION	CORRECTION
1. Pain is a natural outcome of growing old.	It is true that the elderly are at greater risk (as much as twofold) than younger adults for many painful conditions; however, pain is not an inevitable result of aging. The illogical nature of this misconception is best illustrated by the comment of a 101-year-old male participant in a study on aging. When he stated that his left leg hurt, the physician suggested that it was to be expected at age 101. The man then asked the physician to explain why his right leg, which was also 101 years old, did not hurt a bit.
2. Pain perception, or sensitivity, decreases with age.	This assumption is unsafe. Although there is evidence that emotional suffering specifically related to pain may be less in older than in younger patients, no scientific basis exists for the assertion that a decrease in perception of pain occurs with age or that age dulls sensitivity to pain. Assessment and intervention for pain in the elderly should begin with the assumption that all neurophysiologic processes involved in nociception are unaltered by age.
3. If the elderly patient does not report pain, he or she does not have pain.	Elderly patients commonly underreport pain. Reasons include expecting to have pain with increasing age; not wanting to alarm loved ones; being fearful of losing their independence; not wanting to distract, anger, or bother caregivers; and believing caregivers know they have pain and are doing all that can be done to relieve it. The absence of a report of pain does not mean the absence of pain.
4. If an elderly patient appears to be occupied, asleep, or otherwise distracted from pain, he or she does not have pain.	Older patients often believe it is unacceptable to show pain and have learned to use a variety of ways to cope with it instead (e.g., many patients use distraction successfully for short periods of time). Sleeping may be a coping strategy or indicate exhaustion, not pain relief. Assumptions about the presence or absence of pain cannot be made solely on the basis of a patient's behavior.

May be duplicated for use in clinical practice. From McCaffery M, Pasero C: *Pain: Clinical manual,* pp. 675-676. Copyright © 1999, Mosby, Inc. *Continued.*

TABLE 15.1—cont'd ● ● ● ● ●

Misconceptions | Pain Management in the Elderly

MISCONCEPTION	CORRECTION
5. The potential side effects of opioids make them too dangerous to use to relieve pain in the elderly.	Opioids may be used safely in the elderly. Although the opioid-naïve elderly may be more sensitive to opioids, this does not justify withholding the use of them in the management of pain in this population. The key to use of opioids in the elderly is to "start low and go slow." Potentially dangerous opioid-induced side effects can be prevented with slow titration; regular, frequent monitoring and assessment of the patient's response; and adjustment of dose and interval between doses when side effects are detected. If necessary, clinically significant respiratory depression can be reversed by an opioid antagonist drug.
6. Alzheimer's patients and others with cognitive impairment do not feel pain, and their reports of pain are most likely invalid.	No evidence exists that the cognitively impaired elderly experience less pain or that their reports of pain are less valid than individuals with intact cognitive function. It is probable that patients with dementia, progressive deficits of cognition, apraxias, and agnosia, particularly those in long-term care facilities, suffer significant unrelieved pain and discomfort. Assessment of pain in these patients is challenging but possible. The best approach is to accept the patient's report of pain and treat the pain as it would be treated in an individual with intact cognitive function.
7. Elderly patients report more pain as they age.	Even though elderly patients experience a higher incidence of painful conditions, such as arthritis, osteoporosis, peripheral vascular disease, and cancer, than younger patients, studies have shown that they underreport pain. Many elderly patients grew up valuing the ability to "grin and bear it," and, unfortunately, have been heavily influenced by the "Just Say No" to drugs campaign.

May be duplicated for use in clinical practice. From McCaffery M, Pasero C: *Pain: Clinical manual,* pp. 675-676. Copyright © 1999, Mosby, Inc.

Information from Butler RN, Gastel B: Care of the aged: Perspectives on pain and discomfort. In Ng LK, Bonica J, editors: *Pain, discomfort and humanitarian care,* pp 297-311, New York, 1980, Elsevier; Harkins SW, Price DD: Assessment of pain in the elderly. In Turk DC, Melzack R, editors: *The handbook of pain assessment,* pp 315-331, New York, 1992, Guilford Press; Harkins SW, Price DD: Are there special needs for pain assessment in the elderly? *APS Bull* 3:1-5, January/February 1993; Harkins SW, Price DD, Bush FM et al.: Geriatric pain. In Wall PD, Melzack R, editors: *Textbook of pain,* pp 769-784, London, 1994, Churchill Livingstone.

For many years the elderly have been the fastest growing segment of the population. In 1900, life expectancy in the United States was 49 years. In less than 100 years, life expectancy has increased 65% to 76 years. In 1996 there were 37,000 people older than 100 years of age in the United States. This number is expected to increase to 1,200,000 by 2050 (Gaines, 1994) (Figure 15.1). The projected number of people older than 65 years by the year 2020 has been adjusted from earlier projections of 33 million to 52 million (Harkins, Price, 1993).

Pain is common in the elderly population. It is estimated that the prevalence of pain is twice as high in individuals older than 60 compared with those less than age 60 (Crook, Rideout, Browne, 1984). Among elderly people living in the community, 25% to 50% have pain (Gloth, 1996). Among the institutionalized elderly, 71% to 83% report at least one pain problem (Gagliese, Melzack, 1997).

With the rapid growth in the number of elderly and the prevalence of pain in this population, one would expect to see a strong emphasis placed on assessing and treating pain in this age group. Instead, the elderly are among the most undertreated for pain (AHCPR, 1992).

The reasons for the undertreatment of pain in the elderly include those associated with the undertreatment of pain in other age groups and have been discussed in earlier chapters of this book. In addition, for the elderly, caregivers appear to have heightened fears of possible drug interactions and adverse effects (Gagliese, Melzack, 1997; Novy, Jagmin, 1997). Undertreatment of pain may also result from the belief that the perception of pain diminishes with age or that it is not possible to safely provide complete pain relief to the elderly. These and other misconceptions associated with the undertreatment of pain in the elderly are discussed in Table 15.1. Although much is still to be learned about pain management in the elderly, current knowledge and technology can be applied to develop and implement pain treatment plans that are both safe and effective for elderly patients.

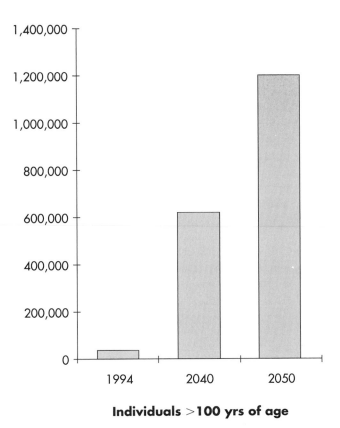

May be duplicated for use in clinical practice. As appears in McCaffery M, Pasero C: *Pain: Clinical manual,* p. 677, 1999, Mosby, Inc.

● ● ● ● ●
F I G U R E 15.1 Illustrates the rapid growth in the number of individuals older than 100 in the United States.

Modified from Gaines JE: Here comes everybody, *Adv Pract Nurse,* p 42, Spring/Summer 1994.

This chapter addresses special considerations in the assessment and relief of pain in the elderly, including the involvement and teaching of family and caregivers in a variety of clinical settings. Common types of pain in the elderly are presented. The special characteristics of the elderly and how these influence the approach that health care providers take to assess and to manage pain in this population are discussed. This chapter includes the use of analgesics with a focus on the physiologic differences between the elderly and younger adults, an overview of nondrug interventions that are particularly effective in the elderly, and the assessment and management of pain in complex elderly patients.

AGE CLASSIFICATIONS FOR THE ELDERLY

To ensure a comprehensive approach to improving pain in all the elderly, it is necessary to identify groups of individuals within age classifications who are at extremely high risk for undertreatment or overtreatment of pain. Elderly patients are often classified according to three groups: the younger old (age 65 to 75), the older old (age 75 to 85), and the oldest old (age >85), also called the

"elite-old" (Eliopoulos, 1997). It is estimated that 78% of the younger old and 64% of the older old report a recurrent pain problem (Gagliese, Melzack, 1997).

Individuals older than 85 years now represent approximately 40% of the elderly, and their numbers are steadily growing. In a large study of the oldest-old during hospitalization, 46% reported pain and 19% reported moderately severe pain at least half of the time or extremely severe pain at various times during their hospitalization. Those at greatest risk for pain were those admitted for orthopedic reasons (e.g., fractures). Nearly 13% were dissatisfied with their pain control during hospitalization and 54% had pain at 1 year after hospitalization (Desbiens, Mueller-Rizner, Connors et al., 1997).

A limitation of age classifications is that they provide no information about a person's physical condition, and age alone does not determine how healthy or frail an elderly person may be. Many individuals remain healthy and active after age 75, whereas others younger than 75 are frail and debilitated. Elderly patients, regardless of age classification, who are at extremely high risk for undertreated pain include those who are frail and debilitated, are cognitively impaired, abuse alcohol or drugs, or are reluctant to report their pain.

COMMON TYPES OF PAIN IN THE ELDERLY

Like younger people, the elderly experience acute pain, cancer pain, and chronic nonmalignant pain. The causes of these types of pain may differ somewhat in the elderly.

Acute Pain

Little systematic research exists on the different forms of acute pain in the elderly. It is known that the acute pain associated with cutaneous structures; fractures; and muscle, joint, and tendon strain does not change with age in otherwise healthy, elderly people. Acute pain is most likely to occur as a symptom of a disease or injury (e.g., fracture from a fall) (Harkins, Price, Bush et al., 1994; Sternbach, 1981). Regardless of its cause, age-induced physiologic changes and coexisting diseases (e.g., chronic obstructive pulmonary disease, coronary artery disease) place the elderly at particularly high risk for the adverse effects of unrelieved acute pain (e.g., atelectasis, pneumonia, thromboembolism) (Egbert, 1996).

Older adults are more likely than younger adults to have what is referred to as atypical acute pain (Harkins, Price, Bush et al., 1994). For example, silent acute myocardial infarction (MI) occurs more often in the old than in the young. Whereas acute pain may be the primary presenting symptom in a young person with MI or appendicitis, it may be completely absent in the older person. It is unknown whether the reason for atypical acute pain in the elderly is due to physiologic or anatomic changes or from unrecognized disease processes. However, experts warn that atypical pain is not to be taken as evidence that age dulls sensitivity to pain because it can occur in persons of any age (Harkins, Price, Bush et al., 1994).

As common recipients of surgical procedures, the elderly are also exposed to acute postoperative pain. The types of surgery commonly performed in the elderly are listed in Table 15.2. Some of the surgical procedures performed on the elderly are life-saving, such as aortic aneurysm resection and coronary artery bypass graft, whereas others, such as cataract extraction, are performed to improve quality of life. Increasingly, surgery in the elderly is undertaken in the hope of reducing chronic pain and improving quality of life (e.g., joint replacement).

Many instances occur in which surgery can relieve pain in the elderly. For example, many elderly individuals have spinal stenosis, a particularly disabling condition that can cause leg pain, numbness, and weakness. Pain is increased with ambulation, posing a high risk of falling. However, surgical intervention has been shown to improve both existing pain and quality of life for elderly people with spinal stenosis (Keller, Atlas, Singer et al., 1996). In a large prospective study, patients (mean age, 66 years) with spinal stenosis treated surgically were compared with those treated with nonsurgical methods, such as back exercises, physical therapy, and spinal manipulation. Evaluation at 1 year after treatment showed greater improvement in the predominant symptom, low back or leg pain, in patients with severe spinal stenosis who were treated surgically compared with those who were treated nonsurgically. Quality of life was reported to be at least moderately improved in 81% of the surgically treated patients compared with 49% of the nonsurgically treated patients (Atlas, Deyo, Keller et al., 1996).

Cancer Pain

The typical patient with cancer is described as being approximately 60 years old, having multiple medical problems, taking several different medications, and being cared for by a family member who also is older than 60 (Ferrell, 1995). The most common cancers in the elderly are breast and prostate (Stein, 1996). The probability for developing invasive cancers in all sites (Table 15.3) increases with age, and nearly half of patients with cancer experience moderate to severe pain at the time of their cancer diagnosis and at the intermediate stages of the disease (AHCPR, 1994). Consequently, cancer pain is common in the elderly.

● ● ● ● ●

TABLE 15.2 Common Types of Surgery in the Elderly

Site	Surgical procedure
Eye	Cataract extraction, corneal transplant, iridectomy
Orthopedic	Diskectomy, laminectomy, spinal fusion, joint replacement, hip pinning after fracture, limb amputation
Thoracic	Lobectomy, lung volume reduction
Cardiac	Coronary artery bypass graft
Vascular	Abdominal aortic aneurysm repair, femoral-popliteal bypass graft, embolectomy, varicose vein resection
Gastrointestinal	Cholecystectomy
Urologic	Transurethral prostatectomy, bladder suspension
Multiple sites: Cancer treatment	Head and neck resection, mastectomy, gastrectomy, colon resection, hysterectomy, lung lobectomy, prostatectomy

May be duplicated for use in clinical practice. As appears in McCaffery M, Pasero C: *Pain: Clinical manual*, p. 678, 1999, Mosby, Inc.

From Short LM, Burnett ML, Egbert AM et al.: Medicating the postoperative elderly: How do nurses make their decisions? *J Gerontol Nurs* 16: 12-17, 1990.

● ● ● ● ●

TABLE 15.3 Probability of Invasive Cancers Developing at Certain Ages

Site	Gender	Birth to 39	40–59	60–79
All sites	Male	1 in 58	1 in 13	1 in 3
	Female	1 in 52	1 in 11	1 in 4
Breast	Female	1 in 217	1 in 26	1 in 15
Colon and rectum	Male	1 in 1667	1 in 108	1 in 23
	Female	1 in 2000	1 in 137	1 in 30
Prostate	Male	<1 in 10,000	1 in 103	1 in 8
Lung	Male	1 in 2500	1 in 65	1 in 15
	Female	1 in 3333	1 in 93	1 in 28

May be duplicated for use in clinical practice. As appears in McCaffery M, Pasero C: *Pain: Clinical manual*, p. 678, 1999, Mosby, Inc.

Table 15.3 shows that the probability of invasive cancers developing increases with age.

Modified from Stein WM: Cancer pain in the elderly. In Ferrell BR, Ferrell BA, editors: *Pain in the elderly*, pp. 69-80, Seattle, 1996, IASP Press.

In addition to pain related to the disease itself, elderly patients with cancer may be subjected to surgical pain because procedures for curative and/or palliative purposes often are necessary. Some of the more common types of cancer treated surgically in elderly patients are cancers of the breast, prostate, lung, colon, and rectum (Stein, 1996) (see Table 15.2).

Chronic Nonmalignant Pain

Elderly people often suffer persistent chronic nonmalignant pain (CNP), typically of the joints, legs, and back (Herr, Mobily, Wallace et al., 1991). Pain is usually the result of a degenerative condition, such as osteoarthritis, which is thought to afflict more than 80% of individuals older than 65 (Davis, 1988). Other painful and disabling conditions to which the elderly are prone include diabetic neuropathy, osteoporosis with vertebral body collapse, temporal arteritis, polymyalgia rheumatica, post stroke, peripheral vascular disease, and postherpetic neuralgia (Ferrell, 1991). The incidence of postherpetic neuralgia after herpes zoster (shingles) has been reported to be as high as 75% in the elderly compared with 10% to 15% in younger people (Baumel, Eisner, 1991; Rowbotham, 1994) (see Chapter 12 for more on some of these conditions). Table 15.4 lists the common nonmalignant pain conditions in the elderly.

● ● ● ● ●

TABLE 15.4 **Common Nonmalignant Pain Conditions in the Elderly**

SITE	PAIN CONDITION
Head, neck	Trigeminal neuralgia, occipital neuralgia, cluster headache, temporal arteritis, cervical osteoarthritis
Joints	Osteoarthritis of shoulder, hip, knee, or hand; rheumatoid arthritis
Spine	Lumbar disk disease, lumbar stenosis, lumbar osteoarthritis, osteoporosis, vertebral body collapse
Extremities	Peripheral neuropathy, peripheral vascular disease, reflex sympathetic dystrophy, phantom limb pain
Heart	Angina
Trunk	Postsurgical intercostal neuralgia, diabetic neuropathy, postherpetic neuralgia, postmastectomy pain, postthoracotomy pain
Gastrointestinal	Hiatal hernia, acute cholecystitis, irritable bowel syndrome, chronic constipation

May be duplicated for use in clinical practice. As appears in McCaffery M, Pasero C: *Pain: Clinical manual,* p. 679, 1999, Mosby, Inc.

Table 15.4 lists some of the chronic nonmalignant pain conditions common in the elderly population.

Modified from Hewitt DJ, Foley KM: Pain and pain management. In Cassel CK, Cohen HJ, Larson EB et al., editors: *Geriatric medicine,* ed 3, New York, 1997, Springer-Verlag.

Poorly controlled acute pain can predispose patients to debilitating chronic pain syndromes (Bach, Noreng, Tjellden, 1988; Dworkin, 1997; Tasmuth, Estlanderb, Kalso, 1996). Many of these syndromes are the result of surgical procedures that are performed most often in the elderly, such as limb amputation (phantom limb pain), mastectomy (postmastectomy pain syndrome), and thoracotomy (postthoracotomy pain syndrome).

SETTINGS IN WHICH THE ELDERLY RECEIVE CARE

The elderly receive health care in a variety of settings, including the acute care hospital, multidisciplinary pain care programs, hospice, long-term care facilities, and the home.

Acute Care Hospital

Approximately half of all hospital beds are filled by patients older than 65 years, and one fourth of all inpatient hospital days are used by patients older than 75 (Eliopoulos, 1997). The most common reason for the elderly person's admission to the hospital is for an emergency or elective surgical procedure. With advancements in surgical technology and techniques aimed at improving function and quality of life for the elderly, many hospitals have experienced an increase in surgical procedures performed in this age group (Eliopoulos, 1997).

Even with improvements in surgical techniques and methods for controlling pain, the elderly do not receive adequate pain management during hospitalization. It is quite common for elderly patients to be given less postoperative opioid than younger patients (Faherty, Grier, 1984). Studies show that only 24% to 27% of prescribed analgesics were administered to elderly postoperative patients (Faherty, Grier, 1984; Short, Burnett, Egbert et al., 1990).

These findings are particularly bothersome in light of the research linking aggressive pain control with improved outcomes, decreased length of stay, and reduced cost of care in the elderly population (Carli, Phil, Halliday, 1997; Kehlet, 1998; Liu, Carpenter, Mackey et al., 1995; Pati, Perme, Trail, 1994; Tuman, McCarthy, March et al., 1991). Institutions and health care providers are challenged to commit to a concentrated interdisciplinary effort to improve their approach to managing pain in elderly hospitalized patients. Although much is still to be learned about pain management in the elderly, current knowledge and technology can be applied to develop and implement pain treatment plans that are both safe and effective for elderly patients.

Clinical pathways

One approach to improving pain treatment plans for the elderly is the use of clinical pathways (also called critical pathways or care maps). Clinical pathways standardize as much as possible the day-to-day care of hospitalized patients with the same medical or surgical diagnosis. They are developed by multidisciplinary teams in an effort to reduce variations in practice, thereby reducing error and improving quality. Other expected outcomes include prudent use of resources, decreased cost of care, and shorter length of hospital stay (Williamson, 1997) (see Chapter 16).

Diagnoses associated with high patient morbidity, mortality, and cost of care generally are targeted for clinical pathway development. Because the elderly often enter the hospital with this type of diagnosis, they often receive care guided by clinical pathways. For example, the clinical pathway for care of the elderly patient after hip fracture is one of the most commonly used in hospitals.

Fractures are a major source of morbidity and mortality in the elderly (Harkins, Price, Bush et al., 1994). Fractured hips account for more than 225,000 acute care admissions annually involving Medicare recipients older than 65 at an annual cost of $7.3 billion. These figures are estimated to double by the year 2040. Morbidity and mortality associated with hip fracture is particularly high, with 48% of the elderly dying or being institutionalized within 6 months of the injury (Anders, Ornellas, 1997).

A review of the literature found that when managed by interdisciplinary clinical pathway guidelines, patients with fractured hips had significantly fewer postoperative complications, better physical and psychiatric outcomes, and more were returned to a home setting and in a shorter period of time than those cared for without a clinical pathway (Anders, Ornellas, 1997).

A major predictor of patient morbidity and mortality associated with elderly hip fracture was postoperative ambulation, and a high level of preoperative ambulation was found to be a positive predictor of postoperative ambulation (Anders, Ornellas, 1997). This underscores the importance of good pain management and other types of care that keep the elderly active.

Postoperative rehabilitation

The elderly are at particularly high risk postoperatively for organ dysfunction from restricted nutritional intake and for loss of muscle function and fatigue from immobilization (Kehlet, 1998). Providing good pain relief is insufficient in attenuating these effects. However, an integrated approach that combines aggressive preoperative teaching, effective pain control methods, enforced mobilization, and early nutrition may provide a means for reducing this risk. The reader is referred to Chapter 16 for more on postoperative rehabilitation.

Multidisciplinary Pain Care Programs

Over the past 30 years multidisciplinary pain care programs for the management of complex chronic pain have increased in the United States (MacDonell, 1998). Given that pain problems increase with advancing age, one would expect that older patients constitute a significant proportion of the client population using these multidisciplinary facilities. However, this does not seem to be the case. It is estimated that less than 10% of the patients seen in multidisciplinary pain care clinics are older than 65 (Harkins, Price, 1992).

The low percentage of older patients being treated at multidisciplinary pain care centers is probably due to a number of factors (Gagliese, Melzack, 1997). Most pain care programs require referral from patients' primary physicians. However, not all primary physicians know how to accurately diagnose some of the chronic pain syndromes that could benefit from the treatment offered by a multidisciplinary pain care program. As pointed out, many clinicians believe pain is a natural part of aging and are unaware of advances in pain treatment (Harkins, Price, 1993). Because many elderly patients share the belief that pain is inevitable, they fail to report symptoms to their primary care physicians and rarely expect referral to other professionals for help in managing pain.

Although most pain treatment centers do not provide primary care for patients, such care may be necessary if older adults with chronic nonmalignant pain are to receive effective pain management. Many of the elderly have coexisting illnesses and multiple needs. The use of a coordinated interdisciplinary management approach may be ideal in this population. In addition to treating pain, the team can manage the other common problems affecting the elderly, such as cognitive impairment, decreased personal care and mobility, incontinence, depression, and social isolation (Gagliese, Melzack, 1997). Many multidisciplinary pain programs have case managers who coordinate access to clinical, psychologic, and social resources in the community and hospital setting. This approach may reduce the need for institutionalizing some elderly people (Gibson, Farrell, Katz et al., 1996) (see also Chapter 11).

Pain care has been successfully incorporated into services offered by comprehensive geriatric rehabilitation facilities (Gibson, Farrell, Katz et al., 1996; Helme, Katz, Gibson et al., 1996). Professionals available for elderly patients include geriatricians, neurologists, clinical psychologists, physical therapists, occupational therapists, and nurses. Pain therapies are provided on both an outpatient and inpatient basis, depending on patient need. A team conference is the forum for developing an individualized treatment plan for the patient, which may include a wide variety of therapies. The patient becomes an active member of the health care team and is encouraged to develop goals for improvement. The focus of treatment in most cases is on rehabilitation and functional independence rather than cure.

Although published outcome studies on the multidisciplinary approach to managing pain in the elderly are few, their results are promising. Elderly patients appear to benefit from this approach, showing improvements in pain control, increases in activity and function, and reduction in depression and anxiety (Farrell, Gibson, 1993; Gibson, Farrell, Katz et al., 1996; Helme, Katz, Gibson et al., 1996; Kotler-Cope, Gerber, 1993). An additional noteworthy benefit of using the multidisciplinary approach is increased family involvement (Sandin, 1993).

Hospice

Hospice programs offer individuals who are terminally ill an alternative to the high-technology, interventional care found in an acute care or skilled nursing setting. Most patients who need hospice care are elderly and have cancer. More than 70% of hospice patients are Medicare-eligible, although this percentage is changing because of the growing number of younger individuals with AIDS in need of hospice care (Richardson, 1990).

It is estimated that one third of all hospices are Medicare-certified. By the end of 1987 there were 417 Medicare-certified hospices, with 91,475 admissions. This reflects an increase of 89,000 hospice admissions over a 5-year period and is thought to be due primarily to increased federal and private insurance reimbursement (Richardson, 1990). Clearly, the rationale for allocating Medicare funds for hospice care is that it is less costly than funding care in other settings. The guidelines for admission reinforce this with provisions that at least 80% of the days in a hospice program be spent outside of the inpatient setting (Richardson, 1990). (A list of Medicare-certified hospices can be obtained from the local Social Security Administration office.)

In the United States, general guidelines for admission to and reimbursement for hospice care are that the patient has a life expectancy of 6 months or less, the patient and family know of the terminal illness, the patient has a primary care person, and the patient and family waive Medicare benefits for curative or duplicate services. Because no effective treatment exists to halt or reverse the progression of Alzheimer's disease, a patient in the advanced stage of the disease may be considered terminally ill and thereby eligible for hospice care (Volicer, Volicer, Hurley, 1993).

Unfortunately, the concept of dying in the home surrounded by family and other supportive individuals is not a reality for many elderly people. Today, family members often live far distances away, elderly spouses may have died or may also be ill, and children of the very old sometimes are elderly themselves (Watt, 1996). For those who are candidates for hospice and without family, care can be provided by a public agency or private organization that is primarily engaged in furnishing services to terminally ill individuals and their families.

Long-Term Care Facilities

Long-term care facilities (LTCFs) (referred to traditionally as "nursing homes") are housing facilities for the elderly and/or the chronically ill or disabled. In 1995 more than 1.5 million frail elderly persons were living in approximately 20,000 LTCFs in the United States (Ferrell, Ferrell, Rivera, 1995). It is thought that approximately one in four adults will spend some time in a LTCF during the last years of their lives (Eliopoulos, 1997).

Until recently, the LTCF has been somewhat isolated from the other health care settings in the United States. However, the current trend toward shorter hospital stays and admission to LTCFs of elderly patients with a higher acuity of care has resulted in the evolution of comprehensive geriatric centers. Many of these centers are capable of providing a continuum of health care programs ranging from skilled nursing to a relatively high level of independent living (Burton, 1994).

Pain in elders who require care in LTCFs is common. Although as many as 80% have painful conditions (Ferrell, 1995, Gloth, 1996), only 40% to 50% are given analgesics (Gloth, 1996). Pain causes impaired mobility, decreased socialization, depression, and sleep disturbances in elderly LTCF residents as well as an increased use of health care resources. In addition, gait disturbances, falls, slowed rehabilitation, multiple medications, cognitive dysfunction, and malnutrition are among the conditions that are potentially worsened by the presence of pain, and they complicate pain assessment and management (Ferrell, 1991).

Research shows that many of the elderly people living in LTCFs have become resigned to their pain, are reluctant to express it, and are ambivalent about the benefit of any intervention to control it (Yates, Dewar, Fentiman, 1995). These findings underscore the urgent need to improve pain assessment and management in the LTCF setting. As in the hospital setting, the key to improvement lies in breaking down the numerous barriers to effective pain management that exist in institutional settings. These barriers and how to conquer them are addressed in Chapter 16.

In addition to improving the pain management knowledge and practice of clinicians and caregivers in the LTCF setting, elderly LTCF residents and their families must be informed of the resident's right to attentive pain care, including the appropriate use of analgesics. Patients and families must know that signs of inadequate or inappropriate pain management must be reported immediately to the LTCF supervisor and the patient's physician.

Taking a step-by-step approach to selecting a LTCF and discussing pain assessment and management practices with the LTCF administrator are recommended (Box 15.1). State health departments can answer inquiries about specific LTCFs, and survey results of individual facilities are available to the public through the local health department. Local Medicaid or Medicare offices, the American Association of Retired Persons, and the National Citizens' Coalition for Nursing Home Reform

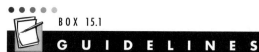

BOX 15.1

GUIDELINES

SELECTION OF A LONG-TERM CARE FACILITY (LTCF)

1. Compile a list.
   a. Request a list of local nursing homes from the social services department of your local hospital or the discharge planner.
   b. Eliminate places that are not conveniently located or that you know do not meet your loved one's health care needs.
2. Call the LTCFs on this list to see whether there is an opening or if your loved one must be placed on a waiting list.
3. Schedule telephone conferences with the administrators of the LTCFs on your list and ask the following questions:
   a. Available services.
      i. Level of care: residential, intermediate, skilled.
      ii. Is temporary convalescent care or permanent placement offered?
      iii. What ancillary services are available? (e.g., OT, PT, podiatry, speech therapy, pain treatment, ambulance service)
      iv. Is there an activities director? What activities are planned?
      v. Is the facility linked to a hospital?
      vi. Is medical care provided by the resident's physician or a house physician?
      vii. How often is the physician required to visit?
      viii. Can LTCF care for patients with IVs, ventilators, Alzheimer's disease?
      ix. What is the LTCF's policy on advance directives?
      x. Are necessary medications administered? (e.g., blood pressure, insulin, heart medication, pain medication)
   b. Cost.
      i. What is the daily rate and what does it include?
      ii. Is a deposit required?
      iii. Is it necessary to sign the family home over to the facility?
      iv. What is the refund policy?
      v. Does the LTCF accept Medicare or Medicaid if insurance runs out, or will the patient be transferred to another facility?
      vi. What costs must be paid out-of-pocket (e.g., toiletries, laundry, medications, incontinence pads, dietary supplements, special equipment)
      vii. Who pays for ancillary services?
4. Eliminate LTCFs that do not meet your loved one's needs.
5. Schedule on-site meetings with administrators and tours of the LTCFs remaining on your list.
6. Tour the facility with your loved one if possible.
   a. If it is not possible to take your loved one, take pictures of the facility, including an unoccupied resident's room, the dining room, lounge, and physical therapy room. Show these pictures and any brochures of the LTCF to your loved one to provide an idea of what the facility is like.
   b. Get copies of admission agreements.
   c. Ask about, and whenever possible, see or get a copy in writing:
      i. Philosophy of care
      ii. Patient rights (Is there a residents' council to voice concerns?)
      iii. Care planning (Are there conferences with the family?)
      iv. Quality of life (Is resident independence and individuality encouraged?)
      v. Pain management policy (Is pain assessed systematically? Are pain medications given to those who need them?)
   d. Determine who provides care.
      i. Who is the medical director? Credentials? On-site?
      ii. Is a gerontologic nurse practitioner employed? On site?
      iii. How many RNs are on staff? Each shift?
      iv. Student nurses? Residents? Volunteers?
      v. Is the staff regularly trained in fire and disaster safety? CPR certified?
   e. Evaluate visiting hours and telephone contact.
      i. How do visiting hours compare with state requirements?
      ii. Are leaves for home visits possible?
      iii. Are there telephones in the residents' rooms? Additional cost?
      iv. Are there rooms available for private visits?
   f. Evaluate the food service.
      i. Is there a registered dietitian?
      ii. Are special diets available?
      iii. Can residents select food and snacks they like?
      iv. Do residents eat in dining room?
      v. Are residents allowed to eat in their room?
      vi. Can family and friends eat with residents?
   g. Other questions:
      i. Are residents able to have personal possessions (photos, furniture)?
      ii. How much money can residents keep? How is it kept safe?
      iii. How do residents get access to their money?
      iv. How often are residents checked? Is contact made at least daily with residents who live independently in residential quarters?
   h. Evaluate the environment and atmosphere of the LTCF during the tour.
      i. The residents: Do they speak freely? Are they happy? Do they appear to trust the staff? Do they wear hospital gowns or personal clothing? Are they shaved and groomed? Are they encouraged

Continued.

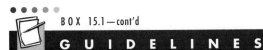

BOX 15.1—cont'd

GUIDELINES

SELECTION OF A LONG-TERM CARE FACILITY (LTCF)

to move around? Are any residents restrained in chairs or lined up in the lounge? Are they involved in activities? Outside if weather is nice?

ii. The staff: Are they friendly? Do they speak freely and interact with residents or are they sitting at the nursing station most of the time? Do they answer call bells promptly? Do they seem to treat residents with dignity? Do they respect privacy by knocking on doors before entering?

iii. Cleanliness: Is the air free of heavy smells such as urine and deodorants? Are window sills and floor corners clean?

iv. Safety: Are halls free of clutter? Do halls and rooms have good lighting? Are exits clearly marked? Are exits secured so residents cannot wander away? Can they be opened quickly and easily in case of fire? Are fire extinguishers and alarms clearly marked and easily accessible? Are

there handrails in the halls, grab bars in the bathrooms, and bedrails on the beds?

v. Look for clearly displayed and up-to-date information:
   a. Licensure
   b. Ombudsman phone number
   c. Health department inspection report

7. Make your choice.
   a. Include your loved one in the decision-making process.
   b. Ask yourself if this is a place you could live? If your answer is "no," keep looking.

8. After your loved one takes residence in the LTCF, stop by unannounced to see what life is really like.
   a. Visit during evening or weekend hours when an administrator is not on duty.
   b. Note all aspects of care you evaluated in No. 6 above.

9. Act on your concerns. Talk with the supervising nurse, contact the LTCF administrator or physician if warranted.

May be duplicated for use in clinical practice. As appears in McCaffery M, Pasero C: *Pain: Clinical manual*, pp. 682-683, 1999, Mosby, Inc.

Box 15.1 provides a step-by-step guide to aid families selecting a long-term care facility.

Modified from Selecting a nursing home: A step-by-step guide, *RN* pp 39-40, March 1997.

---

also can be of assistance in determining the availability of LTCFs in a particular area. These resources and others are listed in Box 15.2. (See also resources listed in Chapter 11 for chronic nonmalignant pain and Chapter 12 for selected pain problems.)

Home Care

It is reported that as many as 50% of community-dwelling elderly people suffer pain (Gloth, 1996). Higher survival rates have resulted in a higher percentage of elderly people living with disabilities. A 1993 survey found that a remarkable 90% of disabled elderly were cared for by their families in the home setting (Gaines, 1994).

In addition to disabled elderly, more patients with cancer are cared for at home and more elderly patients are having surgery and coming home from acute care settings with a long period of recovery ahead of them. All these patients may be dependent for indefinite periods on elderly spouses or children who must also manage their own families and careers (Ferrell, Grant, Chan et al., 1995).

In 1982, approximately 2.2 million people in the United States were acting as primary caregivers to disabled elderly persons in their homes (Stone, Cafferata, Sangl, 1987). Caregivers were usually women (72%), and their mean age was 57 years. Interestingly, 25% of these were 65 to 74 years old and 10% were older than 75,

meaning that approximately one third of the caregivers were elderly themselves.

Added to the caregiver's burden is the fact that pain accompanies many of the conditions prevalent in the elderly population. This has resulted in caregivers assuming the added responsibility of managing the elderly person's pain, a role for which most family caregivers are inadequately prepared (Ferrell, Dean, 1994).

The family caregiver as pain manager

Researchers have consistently found pain to be a major concern and source of distress for family caregivers (Ferrell, Cohen, Rhiner et al., 1991; Ferrell, Rhiner, Cohen et al., 1991; Ferrell, Taylor, Grant et al., 1993). Many caregivers consider pain to be an indicator of the patient's status and equate worsening pain with advancing disease and impending death. Some caregivers view death as a welcome relief from pain, and others avoid thinking about death by denying both the pain and the progressing illness (Ferrell, Rhiner, Cohen et al., 1991).

Caregivers tend to perceive pain and associated distress as worse than the patients perceive their pain and distress. Fears of addiction, tolerance, uncontrolled pain, and analgesic side effects are sources of constant worry for caregivers and present a conflict in terms of providing pain relief (Ferrell, Rhiner, Cohen et al., 1991). Despite

Resources for Patients, Caregivers, and Clinicians

Organizations and Support Groups

- Alzheimer's Disease and Related Disorders Association, Inc.
  919 N. Michigan Ave. Suite 1000
  Chicago, IL 60611-1676
  (800) 272-3900
  Educational materials, support services, local chapters

- American Association of Homes for the Aging
  901 E. Street, N.W., Suite 500
  Washington, DC 20036
  (202) 783-2242

- American Association of Retired Persons (AARP)
  Criminal Justice Services Program Department
  601 E St., N.W.
  Washington, DC 20049
  (202) 434-2222
  Free pamphlet: Domestic Mistreatment of the Elderly, Towards Prevention, Some Dos and Don'ts

- American Geriatrics Society (AGS)
  Panel on Chronic Pain in Older Persons: The management of chronic pain in older persons. Clinical practice guidelines. *J Am Geriatr Soc* 46:635-651, 1998.

- American Nurses Association, Inc.
  Council on Gerontological Nursing
  2420 Pershing Road
  Kansas City, MO 64108

- Arthritis Foundation National Office
  1314 Spring Street, N.W.
  Atlanta, GA 30309
  (404) 872-7100 or (800) 283-7800

- Legal Services for the Elderly
  130 West 42nd Street, 17th floor
  New York, NY 10036
  (212) 391-0120

- National Arthritis, Musculoskeletal and Skin Disease Information Clearinghouse (NAMSIC)
  9000 Rockville Pike, Box AMS
  Bethesda, MD 20892
  (301) 495-4484

- National Center on Elder Abuse
  American Public Welfare Association
  810 First Street, N.E., Suite 500
  Washington, DC 20002-4267
  (202) 682-2470
  Information, provider training

- National Citizens Coalition for Nursing Home Reform
  1424 16th Street, N.W.
  Washington, DC 20036
  (202) 332-2275

- National Coalition for Cancer Survivorship
  1010 Wayne Avenue, 5th floor
  Silver Spring, MD 20910
  (301) 650-8868

Information on Support Groups

- National Council on the Aging, Inc.
  409 Third Street, S.W., Suite 202
  Washington, DC 20024

- National Family Caregivers Association
  9621 E. Bexhill Drive
  Kensington, MD 20895-3104
  (800) 896-3650
  Quarterly newsletter, educational pamphlets, caregivers' network

- National Hospice Organization
  1901 North Moore Street, Suite 901
  Arlington, VA 22209
  (800) 658-8898 for a directory of hospices

- National Institute on Adult Day Care
  600 Maryland Ave., S.W.
  Washington, DC 20024
  (202) 479-1200

- National Organization for Victim Assistance
  (800) TRY-NOVA or (202) 232-6682
  Referrals, resources in every state

- National Osteoporosis Foundation
  2100 M Street, N.W., Suite 602
  Washington, DC 20037
  (503) 223-2226 or (503) 297-1545

- *Pathways: Exercise Video for People with Limited Mobility* (48 minutes).
  This video is a nonaerobic, yoga-based exercise routine, including breathing techniques and a 10-minute guided relaxation, designed specifically for seniors, people with MS, mild arthritis, and other limitations. To order:
  Mobility Limited
  475 Arbutus Ave.
  Morro Bay, CA 93442
  (800) 366-6038

Free Medications for Indigent Elderly Patients

- Janssen Pharmaceutica No. 2 (Duragesic)
  Patient Assistance Program
  (800) 554-2987

- SmithKline Beecham: Program No. 1 (all SmithKline prescription products)
  Contact: SB Access to Care Program
  SmithKline Beecham Pharmaceuticals
  (800) 546-0420 (patient requests)
  (215) 751-5722 (physician requests)

- Upjohn Company (Ansaid, Motrin)
  Contact: Patient Consumer Information
  Upjohn Company
  (616) 323-6004

Continued.

● ● ● ● ●
B O X 15.2—cont'd

Written Resources and Teaching Materials

- *The Cancer Pain Education Program: A Comprehensive Approach to Pain Management in the Home*
  Marketing Department
  City of Hope National Medical Center
  1500 East Duarte Road
  Duarte, CA 91010-0269
- List of publications and services of the Arthritis Foundation
  Arthritis Foundation
  P.O. Box 19000
  Atlanta, GA 30326
  (800) 283-7800

- *Pain Facilities Directory*
  American Pain Society
  4700 W. Lake Ave.
  Glenview, IL 60125-1485
  (847) 375-4715
  Fax: (847) 375-4777
- *Pocket Guide to Geriatric Assessment*
  Sepulveda VA Medical Center, GRECC (11E)
  16111 Plummer Street
  Sepulveda, CA 91343
  (818) 895-9311
  (Make check for $1.50 payable to: UC Regents)

May be duplicated for use in clinical practice. From McCaffery M, Pasero C: *Pain: Clinical manual*, pp. 684-685. Copyright © 1999, Mosby, Inc.

---

wanting to help and comfort the family member, they often are afraid of causing harm (Ferrell, Dean, 1994).

Box 15.3 provides an overview of how family caregivers see their role in managing pain in the home setting and how the clinician can help. The comments listed indicate that caregivers play a very important role in the pharmacologic and nonpharmacologic management of pain in the home setting. It is clear that both patients and caregivers carry a significant burden and have many concerns and unanswered questions about the principles of pain management. The need for consistent responses and practice on the part of caregivers with regard to issues such as physical dependence, tolerance, and addiction is evident (see Table 6.18, pp. 275-276, on talking with patients and families about addiction).

Research shows that patients and caregivers benefit from structured pain management education (Ferrell, Grant, Chan et al., 1995; Ferrell, Rhiner, Ferrell, 1993). One educational program exposed caregivers and elderly patients to the basic principles of pain assessment and pharmacologic and nondrug pain relief and addressed fears of addiction and respiratory depression (Ferrell, Rhiner, Ferrell, 1993). Follow-up evaluations during home visits at 1 and 4 weeks showed an increase in knowledge and improvement in attitudes regarding pain management. Most important, changes in practice were evident with adequate doses of analgesics being given ATC. Beyond changing practice, pain management education of this sort has translated into improved quality of life with more patient reports of feeling useful, having more strength, improved appetite, less worry, and greater sense of control (Ferrell, Ferrell, Ahn et al., 1994; Ferrell, Grant, Chan et al., 1995).

The emotional and physical demands of caring for a loved one with pain at home can be overwhelming and are likely to increase in the future. Advances in pain technology now require that families manage complex medication

● ● ● ● ●
B O X 15.3 **The Family Caregiver Burden**

CAREGIVER ROLE IN MANAGING PAIN

1. Deciding what medications to give and when to give them
2. Awakening at night to assess pain and administer pain medications
3. Reminding and encouraging reluctant patients to take pain medication
4. Keeping complex records of multiple medications
5. Guarding or limiting medications because of fear of addiction
6. Taking total responsibility for pain medication

CAREGIVER CONCERNS AND QUESTIONS ABOUT PAIN

1. Will pain get worse in the future?
2. Why does the patient have to have pain and suffer?
3. Why is pain so difficult to control?
4. Does worsening pain indicate death?
5. What if the pain cannot be controlled?
6. What if tolerance develops?
7. What if the side effects of the medications cause more discomfort?

WHAT PHYSICIANS AND NURSES CAN DO TO HELP

1. Remain hopeful and do not give up.
2. Explain symptoms and treatments.
3. Be honest about diagnosis and prognosis.
4. Listen to the patient and family.
5. Address ongoing patient and caregiver concerns about addiction (one explanation is not enough) and act consistently. Caregivers express frustration with clinicians who hesitate to give medications because of their own fears of addiction.
6. Answer questions about giving medications.

May be duplicated for use in clinical practice. As appears in McCaffery M, Pasero C: *Pain: Clinical manual*, p. 685, 1999, Mosby, Inc.

Box 15.3 illustrates the family caregiver's burden. It also shows that caregivers have many unanswered concerns about pain and its management.

From Ferrell BR, Cohen MZ, Rhiner M et al.: Pain as a metaphor for illness, part II. Family caregivers' management of pain, *Oncol Nurs Forum* 18(8):1315-1321, 1991.

regimens, parenteral infusion devices, and even intraspinal analgesia at home (Ferrell, Taylor, Grant et al., 1993).

SUPPORT GROUPS AND RESOURCES

Many individuals find the experience and empathy of people who suffer from the same condition helpful and may benefit from group support. Support groups can be a source of social identity, emotional support, and access to information (AHCPR, 1994). Box 15.2, p. 684, lists some of the support groups available to the elderly and to caregivers. It is important to remember that, although some elderly people find comfort in belonging to a peer support group, others may not feel comfortable discussing their feelings with others or listening to others discuss their problems. The elderly person's right to refuse this option must be respected.

PAIN ASSESSMENT IN THE ELDERLY

The principles of pain assessment and the pain assessment tools discussed in Chapter 3 can be used in the same manner in cognitively intact elderly patients as in cognitively intact younger patients. However, pain assessment in the elderly may be more complex than in younger patients. Poor memory, depression, and sensory impairment may make getting pain information from the patient difficult (Ferrell, 1995). Elderly patients with cancer pain may not report pain because they fear that worsening pain means progression of disease. Elderly people in the home setting may not want to worry their loved ones or risk jeopardizing their independence by admitting that they have pain (Ward, Goldberg, Miller-McCauley et al., 1993).

The reader is referred to Chapter 3, p. 89, for discussion of the reasons patients are reluctant to report pain and the Barriers Questionnaire (BQ) on p. 93. The Pain Control Record (p. 87) is designed for the home care of patients with pain related to progressive disease, typically patients who are terminally ill. To avoid burdening the patient and family, the record is kept only until an effective pain management plan is developed.

Pain Assessment in Cognitively Impaired Elders

Because self-report is the most reliable indicator of pain, every effort should be made to obtain pain ratings. Sometimes clinicians prematurely conclude that a cognitively impaired patient cannot report pain or use a pain-rating scale. In a study of 758 cognitively impaired nursing home residents, investigators concluded that, although these patients "may slightly underreport experienced pain, their self-reports are generally no less valid than those of cognitively intact individuals" (Parmelee, Smith, Katz, 1993).

Furthermore, even patients with substantial cognitive impairment may be able to use a pain-rating scale. A study of 217 patients in skilled nursing homes with a mean age of 85, who were dependent in most activities of daily living and had substantial cognitive impairment (Mean Folstein Mini-Mental State examination score = 12.1), revealed that many reported pain and were able to use a pain-rating scale (Ferrell, Ferrell, Rivera, 1995). Of these patients, 62% reported pain, mostly musculoskeletal and neuropathic, and 83% of those reporting pain could complete at least one of five pain-rating scales that were explained to them. The pain-rating scale completed by the most patients (65%) was the McGill's Present Pain Intensity scale, a 0 to 5 scale with word anchors. Before patients were considered unable to respond to a specific scale, they were given at least 30 seconds to reply, and the scale was repeated at least three times.

These findings suggest that teaching cognitively impaired patients to use a pain-rating scale is best accomplished by allowing sufficient time for the patient to process the information and then respond. It also appears that a 0 to 5 scale may be preferable to a 0 to 10 scale for these patients. Although developed for use with infants, the Neonatal Infant Pain Rating Scale (NIPS) (Givens Bell, 1995; Lawrence, Alcock, McGrath et al., 1993) has been used successfully with the nonverbal elderly in a home for the aged (Toth-Fisher, 1996).

The importance of asking about pain more than once and in more than one way was reinforced by findings in another study (Sengstaken, King, 1993). Eighty percent of patients answered affirmatively to the single question, "Has the pain relief been adequate since surgery?" But with further questioning, 45% admitted to pain sufficient to cause them to cry out.

When it is not possible to obtain the patient's self-report of pain, other information may be helpful. The presence of a stimulus that causes pain, such as an incision, is sufficient to justify the assumption that the patient has pain. Behavioral indicators of pain may also be present but are not likely to be vigorous. Rather than flailing or screaming, the frail elderly patient in pain may only exhibit a slight frown or maintain a rigid body posture. Families may be helpful in pointing out behavioral clues that may indicate pain.

Behavioral indicators

The practicality of using behavioral indicators in patients who are unable to provide a self-report is illustrated in a pilot study using a list of 25 observable pain behaviors to assess pain in nonverbal elderly patients (Simons, Malabar, 1995). In all instances the nurses were able to identify one of the behaviors to support their belief that the patient was in pain. (The behavioral list is included in the published article.) Furthermore, when analgesics were administered, the behaviors either changed or the analgesic was modified, resulting in behavior change. In most instances, attempts at pain relief changed the pain behaviors to nonpain behaviors.

A scale to assess pain in patients with advanced Alzheimer's disease has been developed. The tool consists of nine items: noisy breathing, absence of a look of contentment, looking sad, looking frightened, frowning, absence of relaxed body posture, looking tense, and fidgeting. These behaviors are observed for frequency, intensity, and duration over a 5-minute period. The researchers note that a 5-minute observation period is adequate to identify discomfort and rule out transitory and meaningless gestures or postures (Hurley, Volicer, Hanrahan et al., 1992).

In patients with dementia (impairment of intellectual function), however, caution is necessary when using behavioral and physiologic indicators of pain. Increased dementia is associated with blunting of physiologic responses to pain, and facial expressions may be difficult to interpret (Porter, Malhotra, Wolf et al., 1996).

Chapter 3 provides a number of tools that are helpful for coordinating the information that may be used to assess pain in patients who are unable to provide a self-report (see Pain Screen, p. 96).

ANALGESIC USE IN THE ELDERLY

The reader is referred to Chapter 6 for a broad discussion of drug pharmacokinetics and pharmacodynamics and to Chapters 4 through 7 for information on the three analgesic groups. The following is an overview of the alterations in pharmacokinetics and pharmacodynamics induced by aging and how these influence analgesic selection and use in the elderly patient.

Physiologic Changes Influencing Analgesic Therapy

Compared with race, site of pain, and intensity of pain, age is the most important variable to influence analgesic response (Kaiko, Wallenstein, Rogers et al., 1982). Even in healthy people, organ function begins to decline in the late 20s or early 30s. The rate of decline seems to be relatively steady until approximately 85 years of age. Anecdotal data suggest that decline in function accelerates after age 85 (Joyner, 1991). This normal aging process changes how the body metabolizes and eliminates drugs. As a result, the elderly are more sensitive to both the therapeutic and toxic effects of analgesics. Table 15.5 summarizes how the various analgesics are influenced by age-induced changes. Following is a brief explanation of the effects of aging on drug absorption, distribution, metabolism, and elimination.

● ● ● ● ● ●

TABLE 15.5 Influence of Age-Induced Changes on Analgesics

AGE-RELATED CHANGE	DRUG	IMPLICATION
ABSORPTION		
↓ gastric pH, ↓ motility	NSAIDs	↑ GI irritation, ↑ GI bleeding, ↑ GI ulceration
DISTRIBUTION		
↓ lean body mass, ↑ body fat, ↓ muscle tissue mass, ↓ soft tissue mass, ↓ total body water	NSAIDs, opioids, benzodiazepines	For lipid-soluble drugs: ↑ distribution area, ↑ risk of accumulation, slightly delayed onset of action For water-soluble drugs: ↓ distribution area, higher peak and slower decrease in plasma concentrations = ↑ toxicity, slightly faster onset, and longer duration of action
↓ production of albumin	NSAIDs, opioids, benzodiazepines	↑ therapeutic effect, ↑ toxicity
METABOLISM		
↓ hepatic function	NSAIDs, opioids, benzodiazepines	Cumulation of drugs and metabolites, ↑ toxicity, need for ↑ interval between doses
ELIMINATION		
↓ hepatic blood flow, ↓ renal mass, ↓ renal blood flow, ↓ glomerular filtration rate, ↓ tubular reabsorption	NSAIDs, opioids, benzodiazepines	↓ clearance, ↓ elimination, ↑ half-life, cumulation of drugs and metabolites, ↑ therapeutic effect, ↑ toxicity
Prostaglandin-mediated blood flow	NSAIDs	Renal failure resulting from reduced prostaglandins

May be duplicated for use in clinical practice. From McCaffery M, Pasero C: *Pain: Clinical manual*, p. 687. Copyright © 1999, Mosby, Inc.

Table 15.5 lists the many age-induced pharmacokinetic alterations of analgesics. ↓, decreased; ↑, increased; *NSAIDs*, nonsteroidal antiinflammatory drugs.

Information from Gloth FM: Concerns with chronic analgesic therapy in elderly patients, *Am J Med* 101 (Suppl 1A):19S-24S, 1996; Hughey JR: Pain medications and the elderly, *Top Emerg Med* 11:3, 1989; Lee ML: Drugs and the elderly: Do you know the risks? *Am J Nurs* 96:25-32, 1996; Popp B, Portenoy RK: Management of chronic pain in the elderly: Pharmacology of opioids and other analgesic drugs. In Ferrell BR, Ferrell BA, editors: *Pain in the elderly*, pp 21-34, Seattle, 1996, IASP Press; Tollison JW, Longe, RL: Special considerations in pharmacologic pain management. Part II: The elderly, *Pain management*, pp. 29-34, May/June 1991.

Absorption

In the absence of disease, the absorption of most analgesics is basically unimpaired in the elderly despite decreased gastric surface area and blood flow, increased acidity (decreased gastric pH), and diminished GI motility (Bressler, Katz, 1993; Lee, 1996; Popp, Portenoy, 1996; Reidenberg, 1982; Tollison, Longe, 1991). Decreased motility of the GI tract may cause problems in absorption of NSAIDs and increased GI bleeding and ulceration (Oppeneer, Vervoren, 1983; Tollison, Longe, 1991); however, in most cases, the changes in GI function as a result of aging are not significant enough to warrant avoiding a medication (Lee, 1996) (see Table 15.5).

Some elderly individuals have conditions, such as malabsorption and diarrhea, that can cause a significant reduction in drug absorption. Some pharmaceutical preparations, such as antacids, that the elderly are prone to take can also reduce the absorption of drugs. To minimize this effect, it is recommended that patients be told to take other drugs at least 2 hours before taking an antacid if possible (Lee, 1996).

Distribution

A number of factors affecting the distribution of drugs are altered by increasing age. Body composition changes with age reflect a decrease in the ratio of lean body mass to body weight with an increase in the proportion of body fat from 15% to approximately 30% by the age of 70 (Tollison, Longe, 1991). However, the ratio of lean body mass to total body weight may increase again in the oldest-old, who experience a reduction in the proportion of body fat (Popp, Portenoy, 1996). Muscle and soft tissue mass decrease by 25% to 30%, and body water volume declines about 18% (Tollison, Longe, 1991).

As a result of these changes, lipid-soluble drugs, such as methadone (Dolophine) and fentanyl, have a larger distribution and may have a delayed onset of action and accumulate with repeated dosing. Conversely, water-soluble drugs, such as morphine and hydromorphone (Dilaudid), have a lower volume of distribution and a higher peak and slower decrease in plasma concentrations (Popp, Portenoy, 1996). The onset of action after a single dose of a hydrophilic opioid may be slightly faster and duration of action slightly longer in the elderly. Higher peak concentrations make the elderly more susceptible to toxicity (side effects) than younger adults (Gloth, 1996; Popp, Portenoy, 1996) (see Table 15.5).

Protein Binding

Many drugs bind to plasma protein, leaving a portion of the drug circulating unbound or free for pharmacologic activity. Albumin is the major circulating protein to which drugs bind, and the production of albumin generally declines with age. This change alone is probably not clinically significant. However, in the presence of chronic disease (e.g., diabetes, liver disease, cancer), poor nutrition, immobility, or surgery, or with the coadministration of some drugs that also reduce albumin and albumin drug binding, a greater drug effect and risk of toxicity from higher concentrations of unbound drug can occur (Popp, Portenoy, 1996). For example, elderly patients taking phenytoin (Dilantin) who develop a condition that produces hypoalbuminemia can experience toxicity (e.g., confusion, sleepiness, ataxia) from their usual dose (Lee, 1996).

Metabolism

Elderly patients are at risk for accumulating many of the drugs used to control pain. With advancing age, functional liver tissue diminishes and hepatic blood flow decreases. Consequently, the capacity of the liver to break down and convert drugs and their metabolites declines (Lee, 1996). This may be exacerbated by other age-induced changes and medical conditions (e.g., cancer, heart failure, malnutrition, cirrhosis). Many of the drugs commonly prescribed for the elderly, such as verapamil (Calan, Isoptin), diltiazem (Cardizem), and allopurinol (Zyloprim), further slow drug metabolism (Lee, 1996). The practical application of these findings may be to allow for a longer period of metabolism by anticipating the need for a longer interval between doses and observing for signs of toxicity from accumulation in patients with these risk factors (see Table 15.5).

Elimination

Elimination of drugs and their metabolites is impeded by the age-related reduction in renal mass and blood flow and the accompanying declines in glomerular filtration and tubular reabsorption rates. This may result in prolonged analgesic effects, both therapeutic and toxic ((Popp, Portenoy, 1996; Tollison, Longe, 1991). Dehydration and heart failure may further reduce renal function (Lonergan, 1988; Pagliaro, Pagliaro, 1986).

The measurement of creatinine clearance reflects the capacity of the kidneys to filter and excrete substances. After age 40, creatinine clearance drops by 10% for every 10 years of life. Typically, a 70-year-old man has a creatinine clearance of approximately 70 ml/min. When creatinine clearance falls to less than 30 ml/min, the excretion of drugs that are eliminated mainly by the kidney decreases and the risk of accumulation of the drug and its metabolites increases (Lee, 1996). Because a significant reduction in glomerular flow rate must occur before serum creatinine increases, elderly patients with normal serum creatinine levels should be assumed to have substantially lower renal drug clearance than younger patients with the same laboratory values (Popp, Portenoy, 1996) (see Box 6.1, p. 170, for formula for calculating creatinine clearance).

The elderly are at higher risk for drug accumulation and toxicity with long-term analgesic administration, especially if the analgesic has a long half-life. A drug's half-life (the time it takes for the amount of drug in the body to be reduced by 50%) changes with the body's ability to eliminate the drug. Therefore, when developing a regimen for long-term opioid analgesic administration, both half-life and clearance (the ratio between rate of drug elimination and drug concentration in plasma or blood) are important considerations (Popp, Portenoy, 1996). Because half-life and clearance are interrelated, both are influenced by age. With advanced age, drug clearance can be expected to decrease and drug half-life to increase (Benet, Kroetz, Sheiner, 1996; Foley, 1995). If a drug is eliminated at a slower rate than it is absorbed, accumulation occurs (see Table 15.5).

Selected Analgesics

With some adjustments, the same analgesics and principles for using them to treat pain in younger individuals are used to treat pain in older individuals. With the elderly, the saying is "analgesics are 'stronger and longer' so 'start low and go slow.'" Analgesics with short half-lives and the fewest side effects are generally the best choices for elderly patients.

Nonopioid analgesics

Nonopioid analgesics include NSAIDs and acetaminophen (Tylenol). They are widely used to treat a variety of types of pain suffered by the elderly ranging from "aches" to postoperative pain.

Acetaminophen is the most commonly prescribed analgesic for elderly individuals in nursing homes (Ferrell, 1995). It is well tolerated by most elderly patients and does not affect platelets or cause GI side effects. The rate of hepatic metabolism of acetaminophen may be decreased in the elderly (Pagliaro, Pagliaro, 1986). Long-term use of acetaminophen must be closely monitored because it has been shown to cause a cumulative dose-dependent increase in the risk of end-stage renal disease (Ferrell, 1995) and liver damage (Tollison, Longe, 1991). Even at therapeutic doses, patients with chronic alcoholism or impaired liver function can have severe liver damage develop from acetaminophen (APS, 1992).

All NSAIDs must be used with caution in the elderly. Administering NSAIDs can be more unsafe than administering opioids to elders because of the increased risk of GI problems, renal insufficiency, and platelet dysfunction. No difference exists between the elderly and younger patients in terms of absorption, distribution, and metabolism of NSAIDs unless hepatic impairment is involved. However, a higher prevalence of renal insufficiency is seen in the elderly, which may result in drug accumulation because NSAIDs are eliminated by the kidneys and excreted in the urine. Avoiding piroxicam (Feldene) because of its extremely long half-life (50 hours) is recommended (Egbert, 1996). Box 15.4 lists several of the

BOX 15.4 **Possible Adverse Effects From Long-Term NSAID Use in the Elderly**

GASTROINTESTINAL EFFECTS
- Dyspepsia, nausea, vomiting, diarrhea, constipation
- Esophagitis, esophageal ulcer
- Gastric and duodenal mucosal erosions, ulcers, bleeding, perforation
- Small and large bowel ulcers, diaphragm-like strictures (uncommon)

RENAL EFFECTS
- Hemodynamic renal failure (ranging from increased creatinine clearance to acute renal failure)
- Interference with salt or water excretion (e.g., hypertension, heart failure, pedal edema)
- Hypercalcemia
- Interstitial nephritis (uncommon)

HEMATOLOGIC EFFECTS
- Increased bleeding time (decreased platelet aggregation)
- Bone marrow depression (rare)

CENTRAL NERVOUS SYSTEM EFFECTS
- Sedation, confusion, headache
- Depression, psychosis (especially with indomethacin, but rare)
- Tinnitus (especially with salicylates)
- Coma (salicylate intoxication)

HEPATIC EFFECTS
- Increased transaminase levels (common)
- Clinical hepatitis (uncommon)
- Hepatic failure (rare)

PULMONARY EFFECTS
- Worsening chronic obstructive pulmonary disease
- Asthma

OTHER EFFECTS
- Rash
- Confusion (rare)
- Photosensitivity

May be duplicated for use in clinical practice. As appears in McCaffery M, Pasero C: *Pain: Clinical manual*, p. 689, 1999, Mosby, Inc.
From Conaway DC: Using NSAIDs safely in the elderly, *Hosp Med*, May 1995.

adverse effects that can occur with long-term use of NSAIDs in the elderly.

Elderly individuals who take NSAIDs daily are four times as likely to have peptic ulcer disease (Griffin, Piper, Daugherty et al., 1991) and five times as likely to die from GI bleeding as those who do not take NSAIDs (Griffin, Ray, Schaffner, 1988). Risk for peptic ulcer disease increases with increases in NSAID dose.

The NSAID most likely to produce GI irritation is aspirin, followed closely by piroxicam, indomethacin (Indocin), sulindac (Clinoril), meclofenamate (Meclomen), tolmetin (Tolectin), and naproxen (Naprosyn, Anaprox). Patients with a history of GI disturbances, concomitant corticosteroid therapy, tobacco use, alcohol abuse, and those taking high doses of NSAIDs are at greater risk than others for developing adverse GI effects from NSAIDs (Kennedy, Small, 1997). It is important for clinicians to realize that GI irritation can result from NSAIDs, regardless of the route of administration, because they reduce prostaglandin formation in the stomach.

For both short-term and long-term NSAID therapy, lower NSAID doses and coadministration of misoprostol (Cytotec) are the only methods thus far that have been shown to reduce the occurrence of gastric and duodenal ulcers (Bjorkman, 1996; Higa, 1997; Raskin, White, Jackson et al., 1995). Ranitidine (Zantac) provides partial protection against gastric ulcers (Ehsanullah, Page, Wood, 1988); doses greater than 300 mg/day and use for more than 12 weeks should be avoided (Beers, Ouslander, Rollingher et al., 1991).

The highest risk for GI irritation occurs within the first 90 days of NSAID treatment. Monitoring hemoglobin and hematocrit and testing for occult blood in the stool during this time is recommended. It is important to tell patients to always take NSAIDs with food and plenty of water and to report black, tarry stools and any increased need for antacids. Complete blood count, liver function tests, and a renal function profile every 6 to 12 months are recommended for ongoing monitoring of long-term NSAID treatment in the elderly (Kennedy, Small, 1997). Table 15.6 lists alternative approaches that can be used when an elderly patient is unable to tolerate NSAIDs.

NSAIDs that are highly protein bound and likely to be associated with greater pharmacologic effect and toxicity include aspirin, diflunisal (Dolobid), ibuprofen (Motrin), naproxen, indomethacin, meclofenamate, and piroxicam (Flower, Moncada, Vane, 1985; Lee, 1996). Signs of toxicity from highly protein-bound NSAIDs include headache, severe confusion, pruritus, sodium and water retention, blood dyscrasias, and renal dysfunction (Sager, Bennett, 1992).

A major drawback of NSAIDs is their ceiling on analgesia (dose increases will not yield further increases in analgesia) (Ferrell, 1995). A dose of acetaminophen (4000 mg/day) resulted in analgesia equal to ibuprofen whether ibuprofen was administered as an analgesic at 1200 mg/day or as an antiinflammatory agent at 2400 mg/day (Bradley, Brandt, Katz et al., 1991). The practical application of this is that acetaminophen with its low side effect profile may be a better analgesic for patients without inflammation and who are at high risk for the adverse effects of NSAIDs.

Postoperative Use of NSAIDs

When NSAIDs are used to treat postoperative pain in the elderly, the course of treatment will be short, perhaps 2 to 4 days. The risks associated with short-term NSAID prescription may be outweighed by benefits of reduced

● ● ● ● ●	
TABLE 15.6	**Alternative Approaches to NSAID Therapy**
CONDITION	**ALTERNATIVES**
Osteoarthritis	Acetaminophen, 650 mg qid Local deep heat (20-minute applications) Walking supports, weight loss Nonweight-bearing/isometric exercises Orthopedic surgery
Back pain	Acetaminophen, 650 mg qid Adequate rest, improve posture Rectus abdominus strengthening Exercise (e.g., rowing machine) TENS therapy, ultrasonography (deep heat) Trigger point injections
Bursitis/ tendinitis	Acetaminophen, 650 mg qid Rest, cold packs, splints Local corticosteroid injections Range-of-motion exercises Work-site alterations
Fibromyalgia	Acetaminophen, 650 mg qid Tricyclic antidepressants Education Fluori-Methane spray and stretching Sleep restoration Muscle reconditioning Trigger point injections
Rheumatoid arthritis	Acetaminophen, 650 mg qid Low-dose prednisone Local injections Disease modifying drugs (e.g., gold)
Gout	Acetaminophen, 650 mg qid Short course of prednisone Colchicine Prophylactic normalization of serum uric acid

May be duplicated for use in clinical practice. As appears in McCaffery M, Pasero C: *Pain: Clinical manual,* p. 690, 1999, Mosby, Inc.

Table 15.6 presents approaches that may be helpful for managing painful conditions in elderly patients who are unable to take NSAIDs.

qid, four times daily; *mg,* milligram; *TENS,* transcutaneous electrical nerve stimulation.

Modified from Sager DS, Bennett RM: Individualizing the risk-benefit ratio of NSAIDs in older patients, *Geriatrics* 47(8):24-31, 1992.

opioid-induced side effects and improved patient outcome from better pain control (Dahl, Kehlet 1991; Egbert, 1996; Kehlet, Dahl, 1992). Rather than deny the elderly the benefits of NSAIDs for short-term pain management, it may be wiser to guard against the risk of adverse effects from NSAIDs.

IV ketorolac (Toradol) may be used safely in elderly patients provided caregivers screen very carefully for contraindications and prescribe appropriately. Although renal failure is rare (Aiken, Burns, McArdle et al., 1992), frail elderly patients with dehydration, preexisting renal dysfunction, cirrhosis, or heart failure are at increased risk and should not receive ketorolac (Egbert, 1996).

Ketorolac should be used for no more than 5 days. For patients older than 65, the recommended adult dose must be decreased by 50%, and the total daily dose of IV ke-torolac should not exceed 60 mg (Strom, Berlin, Kinman et al., 1996). Some practitioners provide satisfactory pain control with ketorolac at a lower total 24-hour dose by administering 7.5 to 15 mg every 8 hours instead of every 6 hours. Many also discontinue it in the elderly patient af-ter the first 24 to 48 postoperative hours, depending on the type of surgery and the patient's pain intensity.

Opioid analgesics

Opioids are effective for many of the types of pain the elderly have and, unlike NSAIDs, they have no analgesic ceiling. Yet many health care providers are reluctant to administer opioids to elderly patients. Many erroneously believe that elders cannot tolerate opioids, especially when they are given intravenously or epidurally. This has led to a double standard of pain care. For example, it is not uncommon to find practitioners who willingly ad-minister IV PCA and epidural opioid infusions to their younger patients for severe postoperative pain but deny them to their elderly patients.

It is true that elderly patients may be more sensitive to the analgesic effects of opioid drugs because they may experience a higher peak effect and a longer duration of pain relief. However, by initially reducing the recom-mended adult opioid dose by 25% to 50%, carefully titrating doses, and closely monitoring patient response, opioids can be safely administered to elderly patients in any setting (AHCPR, 1992).

There is no justification for withholding opioids for fear of producing life-threatening opioid-induced respi-ratory depression in elderly patients receiving long-term opioid therapy. After approximately 72 hours of opioid administration, significant tolerance to the respiratory depressant effects develops. In fact, tolerance to most of the opioid side effects, except constipation, develops over time (AHCPR, 1994).

Many elderly patients have concerns that pose barri-ers to the use of opioids. They often fear experiencing side effects, such as constipation, confusion, sedation, and respiratory depression. Also, they worry about addiction, perhaps in part because many have lived through the prohibition era. It is not uncommon to find elders who refuse pain medication and suffer pain needlessly because they believe they are protecting themselves from possible addiction. The fears that elders have of drug overdose, IV lines, and mechanical technology can interfere with the use of effective postoperative pain control with methods like PCA. Many elderly are hesitant to learn to use un-familiar equipment, such as PCA pumps (see PCA dis-cussion following).

Selecting the Right Opioid Analgesic

For most elderly people, morphine is the opioid anal-gesic of choice (Ferrell, 1995). However, when establish-ing an analgesic regimen, it is important to know that plasma clearance of morphine decreases with age (Kaiko, Wallenstein, Rogers et al., 1982). As a result, morphine may remain in the body longer and at higher concentra-tions, suggesting that its effects could be greater and last longer in the elderly compared with younger patients. In clinical situations these findings alert us to the fact that individual patient responses need to be assessed for ad-justments that may include lower doses of opioid given less frequently.

In addition, morphine produces two metabolites, morphine-6-glucuronide (M6G) and morphine-3-glucuronide (M3G), which are excreted by the kidneys. M6G is a potent analgesic; M3G is not analgesic (Sjogren, 1997). The use of morphine in patients with impaired re-nal or hepatic function can result in prolonged effects and toxicity because of the accumulation of M6G and M3G (Bressler, Katz, 1993; Forman, 1996; Sjogren, 1997). Dur-ing long-term use of morphine, patients with poor renal function may initially respond favorably to morphine but could experience increasing side effects, including respi-ratory depression, over the next several days as M6G and M3G accumulate (Sjogren, 1997).

Hydromorphone is an acceptable alternative to mor-phine for the elderly (Dellasega, Keiser, 1997). It has a short half-life, and no evidence exists that hydromor-phone's metabolites are clinically relevant. Its analgesia and side effects are similar to morphine (Popp, Portenoy, 1996).

The oral bioavailability of morphine and hydromor-phone is unaffected by age. Thus the equianalgesic doses and conversion ratios discussed in Chapter 6 remain the same for the elderly as for younger patients (Forman, 1996).

Fentanyl has no known active metabolites (Foley, 1995), and studies show that, by the IV route, the pharmacokinetics of fentanyl are unchanged by age (Cartwright, Prys-Roberts, Gill et al., 1983; Houde, 1979). However, fentanyl is a lipophilic opioid, and, with continuous administration, may accumulate over time in the elderly. After repetitive dosing or continuous in-fusion of fentanyl, a steady state is approached. Al-though fentanyl is reported to have a terminal half-life of approximately 3 to 4 hours, at steady state, slow removal of fentanyl from storage sites can result in a longer ter-minal half-life (up to 15 hours) (Mather, Denson, 1992; Willens, Myslinski, 1993). This can lead to accumula-tion and late, prolonged duration of sedation and respi-ratory depression (Marshall, Longnecker, 1996; Mather, Denson, 1992; Willens, Myslinski, 1993). Elderly patients, in particular, may be subject to this effect (Willens, Myslinski, 1993).

Reports of less constipation (Donner, Zenz, Tryba et al, 1996; Korte, de Stoutz, Morant, 1996) and sedation (Ahmedzai, Brooks, 1997) and greater patient conve-nience and preference (Donner, Zenz, Tryba et al., 1996; Hammack, Mailliard, Loprinzi, 1996; Korte, de Stoutz,

Morant, 1996) compared with other extended-release opioid preparations makes transdermal fentanyl an appealing option for the elderly. For elderly patients who are unable or unwilling to take oral analgesics, transdermal fentanyl may provide an alternative. However, at least one study showed a marked increase in the transdermal delivery rate of fentanyl in normal elderly patients compared with younger patients (Holdsworth, Forman, Nystrom, 1994). The increased rate of drug delivery was accompanied by respiratory depression, nausea, and pruritus.

A common misconception is that patients who have minimal body fat, such as some elderly and those who are cachetic, will not be able to absorb fentanyl by the transdermal route. However, no studies demonstrate that the pharmacokinetics of transdermal fentanyl change depending on the amount of a patient's body fat (see Chapter 6, pp. 206-209, for more information about transdermal fentanyl).

Controlled-release oxycodone has been found to produce excellent pain relief with minimal side effects in elderly individuals. One study of healthy young and elderly patients showed small, nonsignificant age-related differences in the pharmacokinetics of controlled-release oxycodone (Grandy, Fitzmartin, Kaiko et al., 1995). The researchers of this study suggested that no special dosage adjustment of controlled-release oxycodone is needed for the healthy elderly patient.

A study of elderly patients with chronic osteoarthritis showed a 20-mg dose of controlled-release oxycodone every 12 hours significantly reduced pain without impairment of ability to conduct common daily activities over the 2-week study period (Roth, Burch, Fleischmann et al., 1995). Therapy at this dose improved quality of life with significant weekly reductions in the negative impact of pain and improved enjoyment of life, mood, and sleep pattern (Patt, 1996). In a long-term trial, patients with osteoarthritis received a daily dose of 40 mg of oral oxycodone (Purdue Pharmaceutica LP, 1996). Adverse effects, such as sleepiness, pruritus, and dizziness, declined over time. Acceptability of treatment was high in these patients. As with all controlled-release medications, supplemental doses are indicated (see Chapter 6, pp. 198-199).

Opioids with a long half-life, such as methadone and levorphanol, must be used with caution in the elderly. Their safe use requires careful monitoring during the period before steady state is reached (Popp, Portenoy, 1996). These opioids have a propensity to accumulate and cause toxicity, especially in the elderly with impaired hepatic or renal function.

Tramadol

Tramadol (Ultram) is a relatively new analgesic in the United States marketed for moderate to moderately severe pain. Tramadol is unique in that it has both opioid and nonopioid analgesic mechanisms. It is not a NSAID. Although its mode of action is not completely understood, tramadol and its main metabolite, o-demethyl tramadol (M1), exert an analgesic effect through two mechanisms: they bind to the mu opioid receptors as agonists (opioid effect) and weakly inhibit the reuptake of serotonin and norepinephrine (nonopioid effect), similar to the effect of tricyclic antidepressants (Barnung, Treschow, Borgbjerg, 1997; Dayer, Collart, Desmeules, 1994; Stubhaug, Grimstad, Breivik, 1995) (see Chapter 6, pp. 190-191).

According to one study of elderly patients with chronic pain, 50 mg of tramadol was equal to acetaminophen, 300 mg, and codeine, 30 mg (Rauck, Ruoff, McMillen, 1994). However, researchers comparing oral tramadol (50 and 100 mg), acetaminophen (1000 mg) plus codeine (60 mg), and placebo in patients (group mean ages 59 to 61) after orthopedic surgery found acetaminophen plus codeine to be significantly superior to placebo and both strengths of tramadol (Stubhaug, Grimstad, Breivik, 1995). Side effects, especially vomiting, were more common in the tramadol groups and appeared to be unrelated to the dose of tramadol.

Other reports confirm the high incidence of significant nausea and vomiting associated with the use of tramadol (Grond, Meuser, Zech et al., 1995; Katz, 1995). For this reason, it is recommended that tramadol therapy be initiated at a dose of 25 to 50 mg daily for the first 2 or 3 days (Katz, 1995).

Other side effects of tramadol include dizziness, constipation, headache, nausea, vomiting, sedation, and orthostatic hypotension. Anaphylaxis has been reported after the first dose in patients with a history of allergy to codeine, and spontaneous seizures and convulsions have been reported with the first dose of tramadol at the recommended dose range and higher (Emory University Hospital Drug Information Center, 1996).

The risk of respiratory depression with tramadol appears to be low. However, caution is recommended when multiple doses are administered to patients with hepatic or renal impairment. In these patients, the elimination half-life of tramadol is increased twofold; therefore the interval of administration should be increased if administered in multiple doses (Lee, McTavish, Sorkin, 1993). Dose reduction is recommended in patients with creatinine clearances of <30 ml/min and in patients with cirrhosis of the liver. The half-life of tramadol may be prolonged in patients older than 65. The daily dose of tramadol should not exceed 300 mg in patients older than 75 because serum concentrations may be elevated in this age group (Katz, 1995).

Opioids to Avoid in the Elderly

Meperidine (Demerol) remains one of the most commonly used opioid analgesics in the elderly despite recommendations against its use in this population (AHCPR, 1992). Besides the fibrosis that rapidly occurs when it is administered IM, it has an active metabolite that may accumulate regardless of the route of administration. Normeperidine, the active metabolite, is eliminated by the kidneys; therefore meperidine is contraindicated in patients with compromised renal function. This excludes many elderly patients because renal function decreases with aging. It should not be given by continuous infusion (Hunt, 1989) and is also contraindicated for long-term administration, specifically over 48 hours (AHCPR, 1992; APS, 1992) (see Chapter 6, pp. 183-185, for more on normeperidine toxicity).

Propoxyphene (Darvon) is another commonly prescribed but poor choice opioid analgesic for the elderly (Beers, Ouslander, Rollingher et al., 1991; Willcox, Himmelstein, Woolhandler, 1994). Like meperidine, propoxyphene has a toxic metabolite (norpropoxyphene) that relies on renal clearance (Forman, 1996). Propoxyphene's analgesia is no more effective than aspirin or acetaminophen, and it can produce renal injury (Beaver, 1988) (see p. 187).

Pentazocine (Talwin) causes delirium and agitation in the elderly (Ferrell, 1991) and should be avoided. Other opioids are much safer and more effective. Oral pentazocine's analgesia is no more effective than aspirin or acetaminophen (see p. 189).

Route of Administration

Regardless of the type of pain being treated, analgesics should be administered by the least invasive and safest route capable of producing satisfactory analgesia, and generally only one route of administration at a time should be used. The oral route is the preferred route of administration for opioids and should always be considered before other routes because it is relatively safe, convenient, and inexpensive (AHCPR, 1992, 1994; Coyle, Cherny, Portenoy, 1995). For patients unable or unwilling to take medications by the oral route, noninvasive alternatives are available, such as the rectal and transdermal routes. In some cases, the IV or subcutaneous route may be necessary for long-term opioid administration.

The IV route is indicated for most postoperative patients because of its quick onset and ease of titration. Avoiding IM injections is especially important for elderly patients because they have muscle wasting and less fatty tissue than younger patients (AHCPR, 1992). IV opioids given by bolus injections or PCA can provide excellent pain control for moderate to severe postoperative pain. For major thoracic, abdominal, and joint surgeries, which are associated with severe postoperative pain, intraspinal opioids are indicated (see Chapter 6, pp. 194-239, for discussion of routes of administration).

Patient-Controlled Analgesia

IV PCA has been shown to be safe in elderly patients (Bedder, Soifer, Mulhall, 1991; Duggleby, Lander, 1992; Egbert, Parks, Short et al., 1990), but practitioners often hesitate to prescribe it for fear of producing confusion in these patients. In cases when IV or epidural PCA is war-

ranted, elderly patients should not be denied access to this modality simply because they are elderly. Instead, they should be carefully screened for their cognitive and physical ability to manage their pain by PCA (see Box 6.3 on considerations and patient selection guidelines for the use of IV PCA, p. 176). As mentioned earlier, elderly patients may be intimidated by the PCA pump, so it is important to spend extra time preoperatively teaching them how to use it and reinforcing its correct use postoperatively (Pasero, McCaffery, 1996).

The addition of a continuous background basal rate to IV PCA boluses helps maintain a stable analgesic blood level but should be used cautiously with opioid-naive elderly patients. The decision to add a basal rate to PCA for an elderly patient should be made on the basis of patient response rather than a preconceived notion that the elderly cannot tolerate basal rates. Hourly monitoring of sedation and respiratory status by the nurse is warranted, and the basal rate must be promptly decreased if increased sedation is detected (see Chapter 6, p. 251, for more on use of basal rate in opioid-naive patients).

If a patient is not physically or cognitively able to activate PCA, family-controlled analgesia or ATC nurse-activated dosing may be instituted. With family-controlled analgesia, *one* family member or significant other is designated to be the patient's primary pain manager and has the responsibility of pressing the PCA button. With nurse-activated dosing, the patient's primary nurse has that responsibility (see Box 6.4, p. 177, on alternative uses of PCA technology). Some institutions have even adapted their PCA equipment for patients who are cognitively able to use PCA but are physically unable to press the button, such as patients with rheumatoid arthritis (Pasero, 1994; Pasero, McCaffery, 1993).

Intraspinal Analgesia

The reader is referred to Chapter 6, pp. 213-236, for a discussion of spinal anatomy and the pharmacology and management of intraspinal analgesia and its side effects and complications. The concepts regarding intraspinal analgesia presented in Chapter 6 apply to patients in all age groups.

Although intraspinal analgesia is safe and effective in elderly patients, the indications for its use must be determined by weighing its benefits against associated risks, such as infection and hematoma. Many practitioners find that the benefits of intraspinal analgesia outweigh the risks for major thoracic, abdominal, and joint surgeries, which, when treated with traditional pain management techniques, are associated with much higher rates of morbidity. Many elderly patients have coexisting chronic pulmonary dysfunction, which adds significantly to the morbidity and mortality associated with these procedures. However, aggressive intraoperative and postoperative pain control, including the use of epidural analgesia, has improved surgical outcomes for these high-risk patients (de Leon-Casasola, Lema, 1992; Liu, Carpenter, Neal, 1995) (see Box 6.14, p. 215, for patient selection considerations for intraspinal analgesia and Chapter 2 for more on harmful effects of unrelieved pain).

A significant reduction in postoperative morbidity parameters and cost of care was found in high-risk elderly (average age 71) surgical patients experiencing intrathoracic, intraabdominal, or major vascular surgery who received epidural anesthesia and analgesia (Yeager, Glass, Neff et al., 1987). The average American Society of Anesthesiologists (ASA) classification of patients in this study was III. (ASA classification is a means for anesthesiologists to rate a patient's preoperative condition from a classification I [healthy] to V [moribund]. Classification III describes a patient with severe systemic disease; definite functional limitation) (Ross, Tinker, 1990).

The effect of epidural anesthesia and analgesia on postoperative outcome in elderly (average age 68) patients with atherosclerotic vascular disease undergoing major vascular surgery was studied (Tuman, McCarthy, March et al., 1991). The rates of cardiovascular, infectious, and several other types of postoperative complications, as well as the duration of ICU stay, were significantly reduced in the patients who received epidural anesthesia and analgesia compared with those who received PRN parenteral opioids.

The perioperative courses of more than 200 patients who underwent coronary artery bypass surgery over a 9-month period were studied retrospectively (Turfrey, Ray, Sutcliffe et al., 1997). The average age of patients in this study was 60 years old. Patients received general anesthesia with either continuous IV opioids until they were able to manage IV PCA postoperatively or general anesthesia with thoracic epidural anesthesia and postoperative epidural analgesia. New arrhythmias occurred in 32% of the patients receiving IV PCA compared with 18% receiving epidural analgesia. A significant decrease in time to tracheal extubation in patients receiving epidural analgesia and a trend toward reduced incidence of respiratory complications also was found.

A fourfold reduction of the risk of postoperative myocardial ischemia and tachycardia was found in elderly patients with cardiac risk factors who received epidural anesthesia and analgesia after elective major intraabdominal, vascular, or orthopedic total joint surgery (Beattie, Buckley, Forrest, 1993). Another study looked at older (average age, 70) patients with both cardiac and pulmonary risk factors who had received abdominal aneurysmectomy (Major, Greer, Russell, 1996). Those who received postoperative epidural analgesia had a significant decrease in both cardiac and pulmonary complications compared with those who received IV PCA or IV PRN morphine postoperatively.

Another surgical procedure common in the elderly is the total knee replacement. Again, epidural analgesia was shown to significantly improve rehabilitation parameters, such as range of motion, ease of mobility, and independence compared with IV PCA (Mahoney, Noble, Davidson et al., 1990; Pati, Perme, Trail, 1994).

Limb amputation and phantom limb and stump pain are threats to the elderly (see Chapter 2, pp. 30-31). However, a number of studies have demonstrated the effectiveness of neural blockade techniques in reducing or eliminating phantom limb and stump pain in elderly patients (Bach, Noreng, Tjellden, 1988; Jahangiri, Jayatunga, Bradley et al., 1994; Shug, Burrell, Payne et al., 1995). The results of these studies stress the importance of considering the use of preemptive techniques before surgery, painful procedures, and whenever pain management is expected to be difficult, such is so often the case with the elderly (Portenoy, 1992).

Combination of local anesthetic and opioid epidurally. As discussed in Chapter 6, p. 227, it is possible to reduce the amount of opioid administered epidurally by adding low doses of local anesthetic to the opioid infusion. Long-acting local anesthetics, such as bupivacaine (Marcaine) and ropivacaine (Naropin), are used most often. Ropivacaine may be the best choice for the elderly because it is reported to produce less motor blockade and CNS and cardiac toxicity than equipotent doses of bupivacaine (Covino, Wildsmith, 1998; Scott, Emanuelsson, Mooney et al., 1997). Whenever epidural local anesthetics are administered, nurse monitoring for motor and sensory deficits, adverse hemodynamic effects, and urinary retention is necessary. Precautions such as the use of side rails and assisted ambulation should be enforced.

Because of altered drug clearance in the elderly, systemic accumulation of local anesthetics must be monitored. Significant blood levels of local anesthetics can result in orthostatic hypotension, which can cause clumsiness and cognitive impairment (AHCPR, 1992) (see Table 6.11, pp. 230-231, for tips on monitoring for unwanted effects of epidural local anesthetics).

Starting Opioid Doses and Titration

Individualization of the dose is the key principle of pain management (Popp, Portenoy, 1996). Because elderly patients may experience a higher peak effect and a longer duration of pain relief from an opioid, it is wise to start with a 25% to 50% reduction in the opioid dose recommended for younger adults and titrate upward slowly as needed (AHCPR, 1992). Caregivers often are reluctant to increase doses in elderly patients (McCaffery, Ferrell, 1991). However, this can be done safely when dose increases are made on the basis of patient response in terms of comfort and side effects rather than a preconceived notion of what milligram amount the patient "should" require (see Chapter 6, pp. 240-253).

As discussed, the elderly often are reluctant to ask for pain medication, so opioids should be administered ATC if pain is present most of the day. Continuous administration also avoids the toxicity associated with the high peak effect (toxicity) typical of PRN bolus doses (Popp, Portenoy, 1996). Dosing PRN is appropriate only when pain is intermittent. In these cases, pain must be assessed and analgesics offered regularly.

Treatment of Opioid-Induced Side Effects

The potential for side effects is greater in the elderly because of altered distribution and excretion of drugs (AHCPR, 1992). In addition, the medications commonly prescribed to treat side effects can cause side effects themselves. However, the increased risk of side effects in the elderly should not be allowed to interfere with providing them with the best possible pain relief.

Several of the medications that are traditionally prescribed for the treatment of other opioid-induced side effects are not tolerated well by the elderly. For example, the elderly are particularly sensitive to the anticholinergic side effects of phenothiazines, such as promethazine (Phenergan), which often is used for nausea, and antihistamines and diphenhydramine (Benadryl), which is often used for pruritus (AHCPR, 1992). Because nausea and vomiting are actually less likely in the elderly than in younger patients (Quin, Brown, Wallace, 1994), routine use of antiemetics is not recommended.

The most effective strategy to use in managing any opioid-induced side effect is to decrease the dose of the opioid causing the side effect. If the patient has satisfactory pain relief, the opioid dose can be decreased by 25% to 50%, depending on the severity of the side effect. Administration of a medication to relieve the immediate symptoms of the side effect may be indicated while the dose is decreased. But, by decreasing the opioid dose, the side effects are being eliminated rather than treated repeatedly with medications (Pasero, McCaffery, 1994) (see Chapter 6, pp. 261-271).

For patients who have side effects *and* are in pain, a NSAID, such as ibuprofen or ketorolac, should be considered when decreasing the opioid dose. Acetaminophen can be given if the patient cannot tolerate a NSAID. A cold pack or TENS may also be useful. These measures will produce additive analgesia without opioid side effects and may allow a decrease in the opioid dose (Pasero, McCaffery, 1994).

The incidence of constipation unrelated to opioid use in patients older than 65 is twice that of the general population (Levy, 1991). Unfortunately, constipation is the one opioid-induced side effect to which patients do not develop tolerance, and it is a particularly distressing side effect to the elderly. A laxative and stool softener should be initiated prophylactically as soon as opioid therapy is started in most patients and continued until regular bowel elimination is established after opioid therapy is stopped. Many older people are accustomed to their own methods of treating constipation and may be reluctant to

try new suggestions for handling this side effect. Use of the patient's customary treatment, if feasible, may increase compliance (see Table 6.17, p. 262, for bowel management suggestions).

Respiratory depression is probably more feared than any other side effect when opioids are administered to elderly patients for pain control. Tolerance to the respiratory depressant effects of opioids develops over time, and no clinical evidence exists that tolerance to the respiratory depressant effects develops slower in the elderly than in younger individuals (Popp, Portenoy, 1996). Therefore fear of respiratory depression in opioid-tolerant elderly people should not pose a barrier to appropriate use of opioids.

Appropriate monitoring of sedation levels can help prevent clinically significant respiratory depression. Because more opioid is required to produce respiratory depression than is required to produce sedation, patients with clinically significant opioid-induced respiratory depression usually are also sedated (APS, 1992). When increased sedation is detected, clinically significant opioid-induced respiratory depression can be averted by simply reducing opioid doses and increasing the frequency of monitoring respiratory status (Pasero, McCaffery, 1994).

Nursing observation is the best method of monitoring sedation level and respiratory status in patients of all age groups. Mechanical monitoring, such as pulse oximetry, usually is warranted only if patients have preexisting conditions that require it (de Leon-Casasola, Parker, Lema et al., 1994; Pasero, McCaffery, 1994; Scherer, Schmutzler, Geibler et al., 1993; Sullivan, Muir, Ginsberg, 1994). Close monitoring is warranted in elderly patients who require rapid dose escalation because of severe persistent pain. Elderly patients with coexisting pulmonary conditions must be observed particularly closely during dose stabilization, and doses should be increased very gradually in these patients to ensure safety (Popp, Portenoy, 1996). (See Chapter 6, pp. 267-270, for more on opioid-induced sedation and respiratory depression and its prevention and treatment.)

Adjuvant analgesics

The term *adjuvant analgesic* describes any drug that has a primary indication other than pain but is analgesic in some painful conditions. Adjuvant analgesics may be added to a treatment plan that includes nonopioid and opioid analgesics or as primary therapy in certain painful disorders. The following is a discussion of adjuvant analgesics with regard to their indications and use in the elderly. The reader is referred to Chapter 7 for a thorough discussion of adjuvant analgesics and for complete references for the information discussed in this chapter.

Painful Conditions Responsive to Adjuvant Analgesics

Temporal arteritis is a systemic disease that afflicts the elderly and causes inflammation of the cranial arteries.

Evaluation for this condition is warranted in anyone older than 50 reporting a sudden onset headache that persists and worsens with time. The headache is described as aching, throbbing, or burning, and often jaw pain is present. Patients also may report scalp tenderness over inflamed arteries, fever, weight loss, sweating, and polymyalgia rheumatica (see following). The treatment of temporal arteritis is considered a medical emergency because permanent blindness from retinal and optic nerve ischemia and stroke can occur. Treatment includes the use of corticosteroids (Bressler, Katz, 1993).

Polymyalgia rheumatica is almost exclusively a disease of patients older than 55 and frequently occurs in conjunction with temporal arteritis, but its cause is unknown. It is characterized by pain in the muscles of the shoulders and hip girdle regions without signs of inflammatory disease in these areas. Pain can be severe and accompanied by stiffness and usually temporary weakness in proximal muscle groups. A markedly increased sedimentation rate is common in patients with polymyalgia. Treatment includes low-dose corticosteroids, sometimes for months to years (Bressler, Katz, 1993).

Pain after stroke is a poorly recognized symptom occurring immediately after a stroke or many months later in some elderly patients. It is a major cause of long-lasting disability (Leijon, Boivie, Johansson, 1989). Pain after stroke may be both nociceptive and neuropathic in nature. The most common poststroke nociceptive pain is shoulder pain caused by musculoskeletal changes as a result of paresis. The most common neuropathic pain is central pain caused by the brain lesion.

Both nociceptive and neuropathic poststroke pain cause major treatment challenges in the elderly patient. Analgesics seem to provide little relief, so it is important to address physical and psychologic rehabilitation from the beginning of treatment. Some success has been reported with the use of amitriptyline (Elavil) for central poststroke pain (Leijon, Boivie, 1989; Portenoy, 1996). The oral local anesthetic mexiletine has been reported anecdotally to provide sustained pain relief for some patients (Edmondson, Simpson, Stubler et al., 1993).

Atherosclerotic peripheral vascular disease (PVD) is the most common vascular disease of old age. At least 10% of adults older than 70 have symptomatic PVD. The pain associated with PVD usually is severe and cramping, occurring initially with exercise, but eventually may occur at rest if the arterial insufficiency becomes severe. The pain may be so excruciating that it is unrelieved even by opioids. Occasionally, amputation of the affected limb is the only option in cases unresponsive to medical treatment (Cantwell-Gab, 1996) (see Chapter 2, pp. 30-31, and Chapter 4 on preemptive analgesia).

Painful polyneuropathy is associated with many metabolic diseases that are common to the elderly, such as diabetes, nutritional deficiencies, and uremia. The pathogenesis of the polyneuropathy often is unknown or unclear. Patients uniformly describe burning or other uncomfortable sensations in the feet and distal legs, spontaneous or provoked paroxysmal lancinating pains, deep aching in the feet and legs, and muscle cramping; the hands are involved when the lesion is advanced (Portenoy, 1996). Pain from polyneuropathy usually is responsive to tricyclic antidepressants and anticonvulsants.

The pain of herpes zoster usually resolves spontaneously with time (Kost, Straus, 1996). However, approximately 10% to 15% of those who have acute herpes zoster develop postherpetic neuralgia (PHN), which is characterized by persistent severe pain and is more common in older than younger individuals. Advanced age is the strongest predictor of PHN developing (Rowbotham, 1994). The pain is described as burning dysesthesia (altered, painful sensitivity to touch), deep aching, itching, stabbing, and paroxysmal (Portenoy, 1996). Treatment may include antidepressants, anticonvulsants, and local anesthetics (see quick guide on PHN, Chapter 12, p. 561).

Selecting the Right Adjuvant Analgesic

The selection of a specific adjuvant analgesic is usually determined by the characteristics of the pain the person reports, such as continuous burning neuropathic pain versus sharp and shooting pain. In many situations multiple drug options exist. The initial choice is made on the basis of a comprehensive assessment of the patient and one's best clinical judgment. Adjuvant analgesics with short half-lives and minimal side effects are the best choices for the elderly. However, responses vary considerably from one patient to another, and it may be necessary to try more than one adjuvant analgesic before finding one that is both effective and well tolerated.

Low initial doses and gradual dose escalation may avoid early side effects or allow tolerance or adjustment to the side effects of adjuvant analgesics. In the elderly with coexisting diseases or major organ failure, this precaution is especially appropriate when adjuvant analgesics are initiated. Sedation, confusion, and constipation may be compounded by the sedative and anticholinergic effects of many of the adjuvant medications.

Because low doses and slow titration are recommended to optimize the balance between pain relief and adverse effects, patients must be forewarned that onset of analgesia is likely to be delayed. Otherwise, they may become discouraged and stop taking the drug.

Antidepressants

Traditionally, first-line treatment for continuous burning neuropathic pain is tricyclic antidepressants. When tricyclic antidepressants are indicated, an initial dose of 10 mg is given instead of the recommended 25 mg for younger adults. Doses are increased by 10 mg every 4 to 7 days to minimize side effects. Although amitriptyline

(Elavil) is the most effective of the tricyclic antidepressants, it is associated with a high incidence of side effects. Nortriptyline or desipramine may be better choices for the elderly.

The elderly are particularly sensitive to the anticholinergic side effects of the tricyclic antidepressants. These include dry mouth, confusion, dizziness, blurred vision, tachycardia, constipation, and urinary retention. These side effects are not only uncomfortable for the older person but also potentially dangerous. They may also cause a patient to stop taking the medication.

Side effects may be reduced with bethanechol (Urecholine), 10 mg three times daily (Rosen, Pollock, Altieri et al., 1993). Sucking on hard candy, chewing gum, rinsing the mouth frequently, increasing fluid intake if not contraindicated, and staying inside on hot, humid days may help to reduce mouth dryness. Ensuring dentures fit appropriately will help to prevent them from rubbing on dry gums and mouth sores from developing. Good oral hygiene is important to prevent long-term dental problems in patients taking antidepressants. Prevention rather than treatment of constipation is recommended and can be accomplished with a laxative and stool softener and increasing dietary bulk and fluids (see also Table 6.17, pp. 262-264, on treatment of opioid-induced side effects). Many elderly patients are sexually active, so it is important to discuss the possibility of sexual dysfunction that sometimes occurs with antidepressants (see Chapter 7, p. 309). Changes in vision and sensorium and difficulty voiding should be addressed promptly. Safety precautions to prevent falls may be necessary until side effects pass. Persistent side effects may require a change to another antidepressant.

Orthostatic hypotension is one of the most common and serious cardiovascular adverse effects of the tricyclic antidepressants (Peabody, Whiteford, Hollister, 1986; Rosen, Pollock, Altieri et al., 1993). Nortriptyline (Pamelor) is the least likely of the tricyclic antidepressants to cause orthostatic hypotension and should be considered for use with elderly patients who are considered at risk for falling (Roose, Glassman, Giardina et al., 1986). The elderly patient must be cautioned to get up out of bed in stages, to "dangle" before standing, and to always have something to hold on to such as a cane or a piece of furniture when first standing up.

Elderly patients who are predisposed to orthostatic hypotension may be better candidates for a selective serotonin reuptake inhibitor (SSRI) antidepressant. Although less effective as analgesics than the tricyclic antidepressants, the SSRIs are less likely to cause sedation and mental clouding (Spiegel, Kalb, Pasternak, 1983) and may even give some patients more energy.

Anticonvulsants

Traditionally, first-line treatment for lancinating, shooting neuropathic pain is anticonvulsants. Gabapentin (Neurontin), an anticonvulsant, is a good choice for a multipurpose analgesic for neuropathic pain in the elderly because it has minimal side effects (Dichter, Brodie, 1996; McLean, 1995; Morris, 1995) and drug interactions. It has been found to control aching, burning continuous neuropathic pain as well as sharp, shooting neuropathic pain. As a result, gabapentin is effective for a variety of neuropathic pain syndromes, including postherpetic neuralgia (Rosner, Rubin, Kestenbaum, 1996; Segal, Rordorf, 1996) and reflex sympathetic dystrophy (Mellick, Mellick, 1995).

The most common side effects associated with gabapentin are dizziness followed by drowsiness or sedation. These usually decrease with continued use. Occasionally patients report changes in mood, such as dysphoria, or cognitive impairment, which may be subtle. Movement disorders have been reported but appear to cease when the drug is discontinued (Buetefisch, Gutierrez, Gutmann, 1996; Reeves, So, Sharbrough et al., 1996) (see pp. 321-324).

Corticosteroids

Corticosteroids are considered multipurpose adjuvant analgesics. Accumulated experience in the treatment of reflex sympathetic dystrophy (RSD) and diverse types of cancer pain, including bone pain, neuropathic pain from infiltration or compression of neural structures, headache caused by increased intracranial pressure, and arthralgia, establishes the analgesic potential of corticosteroid drugs in a variety of chronic pain syndromes.

Corticosteroid drugs have additional indications in the palliative care setting. Numerous studies have suggested that these drugs may improve appetite, nausea, malaise, and overall quality of life.

Well-recognized adverse effects are associated with short-term and long-term administration of corticosteroids and with the withdrawal of these drugs after chronic use (Haynes, 1990; Weissman, Dufer, Vogel et al., 1987). The risk of serious toxicity increases with the dose of the drug, the duration of therapy, and predisposing factors associated with the medical condition of the patient.

Although short-term corticosteroid therapy is usually well tolerated, the potential toxicities include adverse neuropsychologic effects, hyperglycemia, fluid retention (which can lead to hypertension or volume overload in predisposed patients), and GI disturbances ranging from dyspepsia to bowel perforation. The neuropsychologic toxicity associated with corticosteroid therapy ranges from delirium to relatively isolated changes in mood, cognitive functioning, or perception.

The adverse effects associated with chronic administration of a corticosteroid that are of greatest concern in the elderly are hypertension, severe osteoporosis, myopathy, increased risk of infection, hyperglycemia, gastrointestinal toxicity, and late neuropsychologic effects. The risk of peptic ulcer is increased by coadministration of a corticosteroid and a NSAID (Piper, Ray, Daugherty et al., 1991). This potentiation of GI toxicity relatively contraindicates the combined use of a corticosteroid and a NSAID in the elderly. Steroid use also increases the risk of GI perforation, even during short-term therapy (Fadul, Lemann, Thaler et al., 1988; ReMine, McIlrath, 1980). An increased risk of perforation during treatment has been associated with constipation (see pp. 311-313).

Local Anesthetics

Systemic local anesthetics (oral or parenteral) are appropriate as second-line analgesics for some types of continuous neuropathic pain in the elderly. For example, they may be effective in patients with continuous dysesthesias, such as burning pain, who do not respond adequately to antidepressants or anticonvulsants or who cannot tolerate them. (See Chapter 7, pp. 317-320, for a thorough discussion of and references for studies regarding the use of local anesthetics for painful conditions.)

Mexiletine may be the oral local anesthetic least likely to produce serious toxicity and so the best choice for use in the elderly person. If mexiletine does not provide relief to a patient with severe neuropathic pain that has already proved refractory to opioids and other adjuvants, trials with tocainide or flecainide are justified. In controlled trials, tocainide was effective for trigeminal neuralgia (Lindstrom, Lindblom, 1987) and mexiletine lessened the pain of diabetic neuropathy (Dejgard, Petersen, Kastrup, 1988). Mexiletine has also been reported anecdotally to provide sustained pain relief for some patients with poststroke pain (Edmondson, Simpson, Stubler et al., 1993).

Surveys suggest that a brief IV infusion of lidocaine or procaine can be effective in a variety of chronic pains and that analgesia may continue for a prolonged period after the infusion. Types of pain that have responded favorably to IV infusions of local anesthetics include neuropathic pains, arthritis, musculoskeletal pains, poststroke pain, pain of postherpetic neuralgia, and painful diabetic neuropathy.

The major dose-dependent toxicities associated with the local anesthetics affect the CNS and the cardiovascular system, the existence of which mandates caution in dose selection and titration, especially in the elderly. The CNS effects generally occur at a lower concentration than cardiac changes. Dizziness, perioral numbness (numbness surrounding the mouth), other paresthesias (abnormal sensations), and tremors usually occur first. At higher plasma concentrations, progressive encephalopathy develops and seizures may occur (Covino, 1993). Toxic concentrations of local anesthetic drugs can also produce cardiac conduction disturbances and myocardial depression (Covino, 1993).

All local anesthetic drugs must be used cautiously in patients with preexisting heart disease. It is prudent to avoid this therapy in those patients with cardiac rhythm disturbances, those who are receiving antiarrhythmic drugs, and those who have cardiac insufficiency. Patients who have significant heart disease should undergo cardiologic evaluation before local anesthetic therapy is administered.

Troublesome side effects occur commonly during therapy with mexiletine or tocainide (Kreeger, Hammill, 1987). A survey of patients administered tocainide for arrhythmia noted nausea, dizziness, light-headedness, tremors, palpitations, vomiting, and paresthesias (Horn, Hadidian, Johnson et al., 1980). Serious but rare reactions include interstitial pneumonitis, severe encephalopathy, blood dyscrasia, hepatitis, and dermatologic reactions (Horn, Hadidian, Johnson et al., 1980; Kreeger, Hammill, 1987; Stein, Demarco, Gamsu et al., 1988; Vincent, Vincent, 1985).

Mexiletine often produces nausea and vomiting (diminished by ingesting the drug with food), tremors, dizziness, unsteadiness and paresthesias, which may induce discontinuation of dosing in up to 40% of patients (Campbell, 1987; Kreeger, Hammill, 1987). Serious side effects, including liver damage and blood dyscrasias, are very rare, however.

Benzodiazepines

Benzodiazepines, sometimes used to treat anxiety or agitation, are not tolerated well by elderly people. One study showed that benzodiazepines tripled the risk of delirium and that long-acting agents appear riskier than short-acting ones (Marcantonio, Juarez, Goldman et al., 1994). An investigation of elderly Canadian residents revealed that benzodiazepines with long half-lives like chlordiazepoxide (Librium), clorazepate (Tranxene), diazepam (Valium), and flurazepam (Dalmane) were associated with a 70% greater risk of hip fracture than benzodiazepines with shorter half-lives like alprazolam (Xanax), lorazepam (Ativan), and oxazepam (Serax) (Ray, Griffin, Downey, 1989).

Motor vehicle accidents involving elderly drivers are of increasing concern as people live longer and drive longer. A study from Quebec showed that although no increased risk of motor vehicle accidents for elderly people was associated with the initiation and continued use of benzodiazepines with short half-lives, increased risk was associated with taking benzodiazepines with long half-lives (Hemmelgam, Suissa, Huang et al., 1997).

Issues Related to Analgesic Use in the Elderly

Polypharmacy

Elderly people often take multiple medications, a phenomenon referred to as "polypharmacy." Polypharmacy increases the potential for additive side effects, unpredictable adverse effects, and drug interactions, to which the elderly are already sensitive. A survey of analgesic use in the elderly found that 72% of the medications elderly persons obtained were without prescription, 14% of women and 11% of men were taking at least two analgesics, and 6% of women and 11% of men were taking both prescription and nonprescription medications (Chrischilles, Lemke, Wallace et al., 1990).

This survey underscores the importance of taking a thorough medication history from elderly patients, which includes specific questions about all OTC and prescription medications before beginning analgesic treatment. Patients should be cautioned against adding any OTC and prescribed medications without first discussing them with their physician. If admitted for surgical procedures, patients should be told that they should not resume taking any of their medications postoperatively without the approval of their primary physician (Pasero, McCaffery, 1996). A system for regular communication between all the individuals involved in the care of the elderly patient regarding issues such as medication use will increase the safety and effectiveness of the pain treatment plan.

Inappropriate medication use

Studies show that physicians prescribe inappropriate medications for as many as 25% of community-dwelling elderly people (Beers, Ouslander, Rollingher et al., 1991; Willcox, Himmelstein, Woolhandler, 1994). One group of researchers estimated that, over the course of 1 year, almost one quarter of older Americans were unnecessarily exposed to potentially hazardous prescribing practices (Willcox, Himmelstein, Woolhandler, 1994). Many of the drugs listed in Table 15.7 should be avoided altogether in

● ● ● ● ●
TABLE 15.7

INAPPROPRIATE MEDICATIONS FOR THE ELDERLY	
Drug	**Comments**
Opioids	
Meperidine (Demerol)	Avoid use; metabolite produces CNS toxicity; other opioids are safer and more effective.
Propoxyphene (Darvon, Darvocet)	Avoid use; metabolite causes CNS and cardiac toxicity; can cause renal injury; analgesia equal to aspirin or acetaminophen; other opioids are safer and more effective.
Pentazocine (Talwin)	Avoid use; causes delirium and agitation in elderly, potential for renal injury; oral analgesia equal to aspirin or acetaminophen; other opioids are safer and more effective.
NSAIDs	
Indomethacin (Indocin)	↑ CNS toxicity; may be indicated for acute gout, Reiter's syndrome, and ankylosing spondylitis only.
Phenylbutazone	Avoid use; risk of bone marrow toxicity.
Antidepressants	
Amitriptyline (Elavil)	Avoid use; use less anticholinergic antidepressant if needed.
Combination Antidepressants-Antipsychotics	
Amitriptyline-perphenazine (Triavil)	Avoid all use; if these types of drugs are needed, avoid amitriptyline and prescribe individual components at proper geriatric doses.
Sedatives and Hypnotics	
Diazepam (Valium), flurazepam (Dalmane), meprobamate (Miltown, Equanil), chlordiazepoxide (Limbitrol), pentobarbital (Nembutal), secobarbital (Seconal)	Avoid all use; ↑ CNS depressant effects (e.g., sedation), especially in conjunction with analgesics; ↑ risk of falls.
Histamine Blockers	
Cimetidine (Tagamet)	Avoid doses > 900 mg/d or use beyond 12 wk; ↑ action of benzodiazepines.
Ranitidine (Zantac)	Avoid doses > 300 mg/d or use beyond 12 wk.
Dementia Treatment	
Cyclandelate, isoxsuprine	Avoid all use; no demonstrated efficacy for either drug.

May be duplicated for use in clinical practice. From McCaffery M, Pasero C: *Pain: Clinical manual*, p. 699. Copyright © 1999, Mosby, Inc.

Table 15.7 lists several medications that are frequently prescribed but inappropriate and not recommended for use in the elderly.

Information from Beaver WT: Impact of non-narcotic oral analgesics on pain management, *Am J Med* 84:3-15, 1988; Beers MH, Ouslander JG, Rollingher I et al.: Explicit criteria for determining inappropriate medication use in nursing home residents, *Arch Intern Med* 151:1825-1832, 1991; Willcox SM, Himmelstein DU, Woolhandler S: Inappropriate drug prescribing for the community-dwelling elderly, *JAMA* 272:292-296, 1994.

the elderly, yet are among the most commonly ordered for this population (diazepam, propoxyphene). These drugs are not only prescribed inappropriately, but also they are often prescribed in combination, which greatly increases the risk of additive side effects, adverse effects, and drug interactions.

Medications such as methocarbamol (Robaxin), chlorzoxazone (Parafon Forte) and carisoprodol (Soma) often are prescribed for elderly patients as "muscle relaxants"; however, no evidence exists that they relax tense skeletal muscles and they are extremely sedative. Although diazepam and cyclobenzaprine (Flexeril) may have some antispasmodic properties, their anticholinergic and sedative effects make them inappropriate for use with the elderly. One of the most commonly prescribed analgesics, propoxyphene, provides no more analgesia than aspirin or acetaminophen, produces a toxic metabolite, and can cause renal injury (Beaver, 1988).

NONDRUG PAIN RELIEF

Although analgesics are the mainstay of pain management, a more systematic use of nondrug pain relief methods may be beneficial to the elderly patient. Most nondrug interventions tend to be initiated by the patient and are based on home remedies and past experiences. Being in settings other than the home can deprive the patient of access to these methods.

Elderly patients often have experience and preferences in the type of nondrug methods that work well for them. For example, they may be accustomed to using music or television to distract themselves from their chronic pain conditions and may find that these same methods are helpful in relieving acute pain as well.

Research on use of nondrug pain relief methods by cancer patients (>60 years old) cared for at home sheds some light on the potential preferences of elders undergoing surgery (Rhiner, Ferrell, Ferrell et al., 1993). Heat and massage/vibration were rated by the patients as the most effective methods. The authors noted that anxious patients seemed to prefer physical nondrug methods over cognitive (see Chapter 9).

Transcutaneous Electrical Nerve Stimulation

TENS certainly is not a first-line treatment choice for pain in the elderly. However, it may be worthy of consideration as a method of reducing the opioid dose required for satisfactory pain relief or as a method of stimulating peristalsis.

In the 1980s postoperative use of TENS was widespread in the United States. Today it is rarely used, in part because of a lack of well-controlled research studies to support its use. Nevertheless, TENS may be a helpful adjunct to other efforts to relieve postoperative pain in an elderly patient who is at high risk for respiratory depression from opioids and also at risk for poor recovery if pain relief is inadequate.

TENS use for relief of postoperative pain is relatively simple. Electrodes are usually placed parallel to the incision, about 1 inch or more from it. The settings on the TENS unit are adjusted to a level that is felt by the patient but that is also comfortable (Lampe, Mannheimer, 1984).

One of the most important potential benefits of TENS postoperatively is stimulation of peristalsis and prevention of ileus. A few research studies along with clinical experience indicate that TENS may be a very simple, low-risk way of stimulating peristalsis (Hymes, 1984; Hymes, Yonehiro, Raab et al., 1974; Richardson, Cerullo, 1979). The elderly patient is prone to decreased peristalsis, and this is further complicated by several aspects of the surgical experience, such as the use of opioids, decreased activity, and reduced fluid intake.

The best sites for electrode placement for stimulation of peristalsis are probably over the ascending and descending colon. Stimulation is set at a comfortable level. Bowel sounds may be heard within 30 minutes of beginning stimulation, but longer periods of stimulation treatment are necessary in the prevention and treatment of ileus (Hymes, 1984).

TENS therapy has also been used successfully in a variety of chronic pain conditions in older patients. Pain associated with diabetic neuropathies, bursitis, and fractured ribs may respond to TENS therapy (Ferrell, 1991).

CARING FOR COMPLEX ELDERLY PATIENTS

Within the elderly population, some groups of individuals are at extremely high risk for undertreatment or overtreatment of pain. These include elders who are frail, debilitated, cognitively impaired, or misusing alcohol.

Elders Who Are Frail and Debilitated

Elderly patients of any age who are frail and debilitated and have chronic medical problems face a greater risk of complications. Their poor health places them at particularly high risk for the harmful effects of unrelieved pain (see Chapter 2), yet they present special challenges in providing safe and effective pain control without producing adverse side effects. They are at risk for undertreated pain because caregivers are reluctant to administer analgesics to them for many reasons, including fear of producing confusion, excessive sedation, and respiratory depression. At the same time, they are also at risk for overtreated pain because they experience a higher peak effect and a longer duration of pain relief (AHCPR, 1992).

It is possible to provide safe and effective pain control for this subset of elderly patients if pain management plans are developed and implemented with extra attention and caution (Egbert, 1996). In postoperative frail elderly patients it is wise to assume the presence of pain and administer a NSAID and an opioid on an ATC schedule. The use of preemptive analgesic techniques, starting with low initial analgesic doses, titrating doses gradually, and assessing pain and patient response to treatment frequently and systematically (e.g., every hour for at least the first 24 to 48 hours of treatment) helps to ensure the frail elderly are given the best possible pain relief.

Elders Who Are Cognitively Impaired or Confused

It is estimated that between 10% and 60% of elderly medical-surgical patients will experience acute confusion during hospitalization (Parikh, Chung, 1995; Welch-McCaffrey, Dodge, 1988). The confusion is characterized by an abrupt onset of disturbances in attention, memory, and perception. In surgical patients the reduction in mental functioning typically occurs on the second postoperative day, usually with full recovery of cognitive function within 1 week. Transient reduction in cognitive function during hospitalization is associated with increased morbidity, delayed functional recovery, and prolonged hospital stay (Liu, Carpenter, Neal, 1995).

The administration of opioids often is implicated as the cause of cognitive impairment. When confusion is detected, especially in the elderly, opioids are likely to be abruptly discontinued. However, little evidence supports the assertion that opioids directly cause cognitive impairment (Parikh, Chung, 1995). In fact, pain (Duggleby, Lander, 1994; Lorenz, Beck, Bromm, 1997) and many other factors, including hypoxemia and sleep disturbance, have been directly linked to cognitive impairment (Parikh, Chung, 1995).

Patients of all ages who are treated with opioids and some of the adjuvant analgesics (e.g., amitriptyline) may experience some degree of cognitive impairment for a short period of time after therapy is started or a dose is increased (Bruera, Macmillan, Hanson et al., 1989). Long-term opioid use is not believed to have a sustained effect on normal cognitive functioning. However, changes in reaction time have been detected in cancer patients receiving long-term systemic or spinal opioid therapy (Banning, Sjogren, 1990; Sjogren, Banning, 1989).

The effects of controlled-release morphine on pain, mood, and basic components of cognitive function at the beginning of long-term opioid treatment in patients with chronic nonmalignant pain were studied (Lorenz, Beck, Bromm, 1997). Findings concluded that even with sedation, the dosage of opioid required for subjective pain relief did not induce any signs of cognitive decline. Researchers suggested that pain relief may temper the sedative side effects of morphine and even lead to improved cognitive performance.

Duggleby and Lander (1994) studied the influences of postoperative pain and analgesics on mental status and the relationships among age, mental status, and pain in patients aged 50 to 80 years. Mental status declined after surgery for more than one third of the patients in this study. Pain was poorly managed in these patients. The researchers found that pain, not analgesic intake, predicted mental decline. Another interesting finding is that no correlation was found between age and pain, indicating that age is not a factor in pain perception. This study suggests that one reason for acute confusion in older patients after surgery is unrelieved pain and that improving pain management practices is one way to reduce confusion in these patients after surgery.

Sleeplessness after surgery may contribute to altered mental status (Duggleby, Lander, 1994; Rosenberg, Rosenberg-Adamsen, Kehlet, 1995). A number of factors contribute to sleeplessness, but patients most often cite incisional pain as the cause (Simpson, Lee, Cameron, 1996). Other causes include inability to get comfortable in the hospital bed and inability to perform usual routine activities before sleep. Several researchers have suggested changes be made in the patient's environment and nursing care routines that disturb sleep patterns (Rosenberg, Rosenberg-Adamsen, Kehlet, 1995; Simpson, Lee, Cameron, 1996). Such changes may include providing better pain control with scheduled doses of analgesics, reducing environmental lighting and noise, encouraging patients to perform their usual routines before sleep, and coordinating nursing care activities to accommodate patients' sleep time as much as possible.

Postoperative hypoxemia and the development of mental confusion were studied in patients undergoing minor and major surgery (Rosenberg, Kehlet, 1993). Those having minor surgery (average age 55) did not develop postoperative hypoxemia and mental deterioration, but patients undergoing major surgery (average age 65) experienced severe constant and episodic hypoxemia followed by decreased mental function. Increased use of neural block techniques with local anesthetics, reduced use of opioids to improve oxygenation, early ambulation, and avoiding the supine position have been recommended to reduce the incidence of cognitive impairment after surgery. Routine postoperative oxygenation may be beneficial for the first 2 to 4 days in high-risk surgical patients (Kehlet, 1997).

Theoretically, the use of epidural anesthesia, rather than general anesthesia, would benefit cognitive functioning because it would reduce the direct toxic effect of general anesthetics on the cerebral cortex (Kehlet, 1998). It also is possible to produce superior postoperative analgesia with less opioid by the epidural route compared with other routes of administration. Unfortunately, it is quite common for practitioners to deny epidural analgesia to cognitively impaired or confused patients, but for some types of surgery the epidural route may actually be preferable to others. Liu, Carpenter, and Neal (1995), point out that, ". . . previous studies have demonstrated less sedation in patients receiving epidural analgesia (local anesthetic or opioid) than those receiving parenteral opioid . . . these data suggest potential for reduction in postoperative cognitive dysfunction from use of epidural analgesia" (p. 1492).

Support for avoiding the IM route of administration in the elderly was found in a study comparing elderly men receiving IV PCA morphine with those receiving IM morphine postoperatively (Egbert, Parks, Short et al., 1990). Fewer complications, including mental confusion, occurred in patients who received IV PCA.

PCA fentanyl was found to produce less depression in cognitive function than PCA morphine in postoperative elderly patients (Herrick, Ganapathy, Komar et al., 1996). Urinary retention was less with fentanyl, but no differences were found in other side effects, such as pruritus, nausea and vomiting, excessive sedation, and respiratory depression in this study. Further investigation is needed regarding the differences in cognitive effects of the various opioids in the postoperative period.

Other factors implicated in the development of confusional states in the elderly include alcohol and sedative-hypnotic drug withdrawal, endocrine and metabolic problems, preoperative depression, type of anesthesia during surgery, use of drugs with anticholinergic effects, heightened sensitivity to drug interactions, and sepsis. Clearly, many possible explanations can be given for cognitive impairment in the elderly that must be evaluated before blame can be placed on analgesics.

Expected mental status changes related to aging

Frequently the elderly are labeled as confused or senile when caregivers fail to consider the expected changes of aging such as mild recent memory loss, slowed thinking, and impaired sight and hearing (Welch-McCaffrey, Dodge, 1988). Ensuring that older patients have their eyeglasses and functioning hearing aids and allowing them adequate time to respond to questions will help reduce the likelihood of mislabeling patients.

The Mini-Mental State examination is a simplified test of cognitive function that clinicians can administer to help distinguish patients with cognitive disturbance from those without cognitive disturbance (Folstein, Folstein, McHugh, 1975). It may be especially useful for serial testing when the patient's mental condition fluctuates (Parikh, Chung, 1995). This test has proven validity and reliability, and use of a standardized form (Form 15.1) has been found to be quick, easy to use, and acceptable to both patients and clinicians. The Mini-Mental State examination is not intended to replace thorough evaluation in forming a diagnosis.

Dementia

Dementia, unlike acute confusion, is an insidious, progressive cognitive loss caused by changes in the brain (Breitbart, Passik, 1993; Welch-McCaffrey, Dodge, 1988). Most prominent symptoms are difficulties in short-term and long-term memory, impaired judgment and abstract thinking, and disturbed higher cortical functions such as voluntary movements (apraxia) and ability to communicate (aphasia) (Breitbart, Passik, 1993). Dementia usually is irreversible. Elderly patients with dementia appear to be particularly predisposed to the opioid side effects of somnolence and cognitive impairment (Popp, Portenoy, 1996) and so must be closely monitored during opioid therapy. Some of the characteristics of chronic dementia are similar to those of acute confusion. Table 15.8 provides information that may help clinicians distinguish between acute confusion and dementia.

Implications of caring for the confused elder

Acute confusion usually is reversible once the underlying problem is resolved. Interventions include ensuring adequate fluid and nutritional intake, attending to elimination needs, providing pain relief, promoting activity and self-care, and offering psychologic support.

Family members are especially helpful in orienting confused patients to their surroundings and should be encouraged to communicate calmly and frequently with the confused patient, provide orienting devices such as clocks and calendars, ensure that the patient's eyeglasses and hearing aid are in place, provide an organized approach and environment, and talk with the patient in concrete terms and in the here and now. Many hospitals provide family members with in-room accommodations so that they can stay with the elderly patient as much as possible. Some hospitals have found it cost-effective, in terms of preventing injury, to assign staff members to stay during their off-time with elders who have no family or friends. If the patient is bedridden, passive or active range-of-motion exercises should be done every shift (Hall, Wakefield, 1996; Welch-McCaffrey, Dodge, 1988).

Haloperidol (Haldol) may help to control symptoms of agitation, paranoia, fear, or delirium should they occur (Breitbart, Passik, 1993; Breitbart, Marotta, Platt et al., 1996; Welch-McCaffrey, Dodge, 1988). Treatment with haloperidol should be viewed as a short-term measure to relieve symptom distress only (Welch-McCaffrey, Dodge, 1988). Unless the patient is at risk for self-harm and no one can stay at the bedside to prevent injury, restraints should be avoided because their use is likely to increase agitation (Hall, Wakefield, 1996).

Patient _____   Examiner _____   Date _____

MINI-MENTAL STATE

Maximum
Score   Score

ORIENTATION

5   ( ) What is the (year) (season) (date) (day) (month)?
5'   ( ) Where are we: (state) (county) (town) (hospital) (floor)?

REGISTRATION

3   ( ) Name 3 objects: 1 second to say each. Then ask the patient all 3 after you have said them. Give 1 point for each
            correct answer. Then repeat them until he learns all 3. Count trials and record.

                                                                          Trials _____

ATTENTION AND CALCULATION

5   ( ) Serial 7's. 1 point for each correct. Stop after 5 answers. Alternatively spell "world" backwards.

RECALL

3   ( ) Ask for the 3 objects repeated above. Give 1 point for each correct.

LANGUAGE

9   ( ) Name a pencil and watch. (2 points)
            Repeat the following: "No ifs, ands, or buts." (1 point)
            Follow a 3-stage command:
                 "Take a paper in your right hand, fold it in half, and put it on the floor." (3 points)
            Read and obey the following: CLOSE YOUR EYES (1 point)
            Write a sentence. (1 point)
            Copy design. (1 point)
_____   Total score
            ASSESS level of consciousness along a continuum _____
                                                              Alert   Drowsy   Stupor   Coma

INSTRUCTIONS FOR ADMINISTRATION OF MINI-MENTAL STATE EXAMINATION

ORIENTATION

(1) Ask for the date. Then ask specifically for parts omitted. (e.g., "Can you also tell me what season it is?") One point for each correct.
(2) Ask in turn, "Can you tell me the name of this hospital?" (town, county, etc.). One point for each correct.

REGISTRATION

Ask the patient if you may test his memory. Then say the names of 3 unrelated objects, clearly and slowly, about one second for each. After you have said all 3, ask him to repeat them. This first repetition determines his score (0–3) but keep saying them until he can repeat all 3, up to 6 trials. If he does not eventually learn all 3, recall cannot be meaningfully tested.

ATTENTION AND CALCULATION

Ask the patient to begin with 100 and count backwards by 7. Stop after 5 subtractions (93, 86, 79, 72, 65). Score the total number of correct answers.

If the patient cannot or will not perform this task, ask him to spell the word "world" backwards. The score is the number of letters in correct order (e.g., dlrow = 5, dlorw = 3).

RECALL

Ask the patient if he can recall the 3 words you previously asked him to remember. Score 0–3.

LANGUAGE

Naming: Show the patient a wrist watch and ask him what it is. Repeat for pencil. Score 0–2.

Repetition: Ask the patient to repeat the sentence after you. Allow only one trial. Score 0 or 1.

3-Stage Command: Give the patient a piece of plain blank paper and repeat the command. Score 1 point for each part correctly executed.

Reading: On a blank piece of paper print the sentence "Close your eyes" in letters large enough for the patient to see clearly. Ask him to read it and do what it says. Score 1 point only if he actually closes his eyes.

Writing: Give the patient a blank piece of paper and ask him to write a sentence for you. Do not dictate a sentence, it is to be written spontaneously. It must contain a subject and verb and be sensible. Correct grammar and punctuation are not necessary.

Copying: On a clean piece of paper, draw intersecting pentagons, each side about 1 in., and ask him to copy it exactly as it is. All 10 angles must be present and 2 must intersect to score 1 point. Tremor and rotation are ignored.

Estimate the patient's level of sensorium along a continuum, from alert on the left to coma on the right.

From Folstein MF, Folstein SE, McHugh PR: "Mini-mental state": A practical method for grading the cognitive state of patients for the clinician, *J Psychiat Res* 12:189-198, 1975. The copyright in the Mini-Mental State Examination is wholly owned by the Mini-Mental LLC, a Massachusetts limited liability company. For information to obtain permission to use or reproduce the Mini-Mental State Examination, please contact John Gonsalves Jr., Administrator of the Mini-Mental LLC, at 31 St. James Avenue, Suite 1, Boston, MA 02116—(617) 587-4215.

● ● ● ● ○

TABLE 15.8   **Distinguishing Between Acute Confusion and Dementia**

	CONFUSION	DEMENTIA
Symptoms	Cognitive and social inaccessibility; transient and sometimes profound alterations in attention, perception, memory, inhibitions, time sense, sleep/wake cycle, safety comprehension, orientation, cooperation, and ability to communicate; variable psychomotor activity; fear, paranoia, hallucinations possible; symptoms more marked at night than day.	Loss of intellectual function and memory, deficits in time sense, language, reasoning, and ability to carry out daily activities; inability to tolerate fatigue, change, and multiple stimuli; difficulty planning and executing motor function; disinterested, disinhibited; hallucinations not prominent; flat affect; motor deficits late in course.
Onset	Sudden, hours to days.	Usually insidious over months to years, except in rare types or dementia caused by transient ischemic attacks.
Treatment implications	Treat underlying condition; maintain fluid and nutritional intake; monitor renal and bowel function, cardiac status, medications, oxygenation; attend to basic needs (e.g., safety, comfort, self-care); orient frequently to person, place, time; minimize environmental stressors and change.	Attend to basic needs (e.g., safety, comfort, self-care); maximize function, provide activity-based agendas; ensure adequate rest to decrease fatigue; establish routines and avoid change, minimize environmental stressors; monitor for concomitant disorders.
Pain control	Assume presence of pain if circumstances warrant (e.g., surgical incision, chronic painful condition); ATC analgesic dosing, frequent, systematic assessment.	Assume presence of pain if circumstances warrant (e.g., surgical incision, chronic painful condition); ATC analgesic dosing, frequent, systematic assessment; predisposed to opioid side effects of somnolence and cognitive impairment, so must be closely monitored during opioid therapy.
Drug therapy	Short-term haloperidol (Haldol) for agitation, hallucinations, delirium.	Usually none.
Prognosis	Good; usually reversible, but poor if left untreated; tends to recur with acute illness.	Poor; usually irreversible.

May be duplicated for use in clinical practice. From McCaffery M, Pasero C: *Pain: Clinical manual,* p. 704. Copyright © 1999, Mosby, Inc.

Some of the distinguishing characteristics of acute confusion and chronic dementia are similar. Table 15.8 provides information that may help clinicians distinguish between the two conditions.

ATC, around-the-clock.

Information from Hall GR, Wakefield B: Acute confusion in the elderly, *Nursing* 96(7):33-37, July 1996; Welch-McCaffrey D, Dodge J: Acute confusional states in elderly cancer patients, *Semin Oncol Nurs* 4(3):208-216, 1988.

Pain Control

As discussed, cognitively impaired or confused elders are at high risk for undertreated pain. Caregivers often withhold analgesics from patients with mental dysfunction for fear of increasing the impairment or confusion. If a previously oriented patient becomes disoriented while taking analgesics, especially opioids, caregivers usually react by abruptly discontinuing the analgesic. However, a standardized approach to managing cognitively impaired or confused elders may provide a solution to the complexities involved in providing pain relief for these patients. This approach includes using only mu agonist opioid drugs with short half-lives and avoiding meperidine. Nonessential centrally acting drugs should be discontinued when opioid therapy is initiated (Popp, Portenoy, 1996).

If not otherwise contraindicated, cognitively impaired or confused elderly patients with pain can be given acetaminophen or a NSAID and an opioid, if indicated, on an ATC basis and be monitored closely for side effects and safety hazards. If confusion occurs during treatment, a standardized protocol can include decreasing the dose rather than abruptly discontinuing the opioid. Increased monitoring for safety hazards and measures described previously can be instituted, and the patient oriented to person, place, and time during hourly assessments (Pasero, McCaffery, 1993). If confusion continues despite dose decreases, the patient should be switched to another opioid.

If confusion occurs during PCA therapy, reducing the opioid dose and switching patients to family-controlled analgesia or ATC nurse-activated dosing is recommended (see p. 177). PCA can be safely resumed when the patient is oriented and able to self-administer pain medication again (Pasero, McCaffery, 1993).

Elders With Memory Difficulties

Recall of recent events may be unreliable in the elderly so it is best to ask them about their pain in the here and now. Because elders do well with a schedule, pain is assessed frequently and on a routine basis. It is important to orient them to place and time with every assessment and keep them informed of their progress toward recovery.

Patients with memory difficulties may be unable to remember how to use PCA equipment safely and effectively. It is advisable to administer family-controlled analgesia, ATC IV bolusing, or nurse-activated dosing for these patients (Egbert, 1996; Pasero, McCaffery, 1993) (see Box 6.3, p. 176 for alternative uses of PCA technology).

Elders Who Misuse Alcohol

Alcoholism is a serious issue for almost 3 million elderly Americans (Gupta, 1993). Widowers older than 75 have the highest rate of alcoholism in the country (Glass, Prigerson, Kasl et al., 1995). One survey found that 15% of men and 12% of women older than the age of 60 regularly drank >14 drinks per week and >7 drinks per week, respectively (Adams, Barry, Fleming, 1996). Even if the prevalence remains the same, the number of elderly with drinking problems will increase because the general population is aging. An in-depth discussion of alcoholism and withdrawal syndrome is beyond the scope of this chapter. However, following are important points to consider in caring for the elderly person with pain who misuses alcohol (see also Chapter 10).

Of elderly patients seeking medical help, 10% to 15% are thought to have an alcohol-related problem (Gupta, 1993). Elderly patients who misuse alcohol are at higher risk for medical problems and death from illness and injury than those who do not misuse alcohol. For example, the risk of hypertension and certain cancers, such as mouth, tongue, esophagus, and breast cancer, is increased in individuals who drink in excess of two drinks per day (Adams, Barry, Fleming, 1996; Gupta, 1993). Preoperative alcohol misuse is a risk factor for postoperative morbidity (Tonnesen, Petersen, Hojgaard et al., 1992), but it is commonly overlooked by health care providers who interview elderly patients (Gupta, 1993). Failure to diagnose and treat alcohol misuse during hospitalization can result in symptoms of withdrawal syndrome as early as 12 hours after the last drink is taken. IV glucose administration to an alcoholic patient with thiamine deficiency can precipitate a possibly fatal delirious state of alcohol withdrawal psychosis (Parikh, Chung, 1995).

The best way to determine whether a patient is misusing alcohol is to ask about alcohol consumption during the initial interview. The patient may be reluctant to report alcohol misuse or may be unaware that a problem exists. Therefore it is wise to take a nonjudgmental approach, assume that the patient may consume alcohol, and phrase questions in a nonthreatening manner that is likely to elicit accurate information. Questions about caffeine and nicotine use might be followed with questions about alcohol. Rather than asking if the patient drinks alcohol, a better approach is to say, "How much alcohol do you drink?" Also, to gain accurate information on the amount of alcohol the patient consumes, speak in large amounts, such as "Do you drink two six packs of beer over the course of a day?" (Antai-Otong, 1995).

The presence of unexplained conditions, such as incontinence, malnutrition, malaise, insomnia, cognitive impairment, and social isolation, as well as unexplained injuries from cigarette burns and repeated falls, may provide some indications of alcohol misuse (Antai-Otong, 1995; Geroldi, Rozzini, Frisoni et al., 1994). History of epileptic seizures, pancreatitis, gastric bleeding, or liver disease may suggest chronic alcohol intake (Gorman, 1997). Laboratory findings, such as elevated serum amylase and transaminase and less than normal magnesium, phosphate, and potassium levels, also may be helpful in determining an alcohol problem. The CAGE questionnaire is a commonly used assessment tool that can be easily incorporated into initial interviews (Box 15.5). Within

● ● ● ● ●
BOX 15.5

DETECTING ALCOHOLISM: CAGE QUESTIONNAIRE

During the initial history-taking interview, ask elderly patients the following questions:

Cut down
Have you felt you should cut down or stop drinking?

Annoyed
Has anyone annoyed you or gotten on your nerves by telling you to cut down or stop drinking?

Guilt
Have you felt guilty or bad about how much you drink?

Eye opener
Do you wake up in the morning wanting to have an alcoholic drink (eye opener)?

May be duplicated for use in clinical practice. As appears in McCaffery M, Pasero C: *Pain: Clinical manual,* p. 705, 1999, Mosby, Inc.

The CAGE questionnaire is a simple assessment tool that can be used to detect recent alcoholism during the initial patient interview.

From Adams WL, Barry KL, Fleming MF: Screening for problem drinking in older primary care patients, *JAMA* 276(24):1964-1967, 1996; Gorman M: Treating acute alcohol withdrawal, *Am J Nurs* 97(1):22-23, 1997; Mayfield D, McLeod G, Hall P: The CAGE questionnaire, *Am J Psychiatry* 131:1121-1123, 1974.

several hours of the last drink, the patient may be diaphoretic or have tremors that worsen with movement and request medication to "calm the nerves" (Antai-Otong, 1995).

Once the possibility of alcohol misuse has been identified, plans should be made to prevent withdrawal. Benzodiazepines are frequently used. As discussed, short-acting ones, such as lorazepam (Ativan) or chlordiazepoxide (Librium), are preferred in the elderly (Antai-Otong, 1995; Gorman, 1997). These are also the drugs of choice for withdrawal symptoms. Haloperidol (Haldol) is recommended for hallucinations and chlordiazepoxide for delirium tremens. Sometimes patients are simply allowed to drink controlled amounts of alcohol during their hospitalization to prevent withdrawal.

ELDER ABUSE

It is estimated that up to 2,000,000 older adults are abused every year (Lynch, 1997). Researchers expect this number will rise as the elderly population increases. Family members (usually adult children) are the most frequent abusers of older people living in the community. Typically, violence erupts when families are pressured by social, economic, and personal stress. People who are sicker, more impaired, or more isolated are at the greatest risk of mistreatment. This description certainly fits some of the elderly with significant or intractable pain problems.

Neglect is the most common type of mistreatment. Neglectful behaviors may range from failure to meet nutritional and hygienic needs to withholding a hearing aid or eyeglasses, leaving an elder unattended, or failing to provide necessary medical visits. Physical abuse ranges from slapping, bruising, restraining, or sexually molesting to any other action that inflicts pain or injury. Psychologic or emotional abuse includes demeaning behavior with the use of threats, insults, name-calling, or treating the older person like a child (Minaker, Frishman, 1995).

Elders who are admitted to the hospital with confusion, a fracture, extensive bruising, or decubitus ulcers warrant assessment for possible abuse (Minaker, Frishman, 1995), keeping in mind that the elderly have fragile skin and that bruises alone do not necessarily indicate abuse. The elderly also are more at risk for injury from falls because of chronic conditions, such as arthritis and weakness from aging muscles. In any case a thorough physical examination is indicated. A private interview with the patient may reveal important information; however, abused elders may be so dependent on the caregiver that they are afraid to disclose problems. A fragile abused elderly person can be as helpless as an abused child.

There are no simple methods for identifying elder abuse, but inconsistencies in the reports of the cause of an injury and obvious signs of strain between patient and caregiver sometimes are warning signs. Providing the elderly person and the caregiver with information on how to access available community resources, such as adult day-care programs, home health aides, recreation programs, caregiver training, and transportation assistance, may be helpful (Minaker, Frishman, 1995) (see Box 15.2, p. 684, for resources).

All states have agencies that can intervene when an older person is being abused. These agencies can be found in the state government section of the telephone book and usually are listed as Adult Protective Services or Elder Protective Services. The Older Americans Act requires every state to have an ombudsman program to investigate complaints against LTCFs. Nursing homes are required by law to inform clients how to reach an ombudsman (Minaker, Frishman, 1995). The state government section under the Office on Aging in the telephone book usually lists the number for the local ombudsman program.

References

Adams WL, Barry KL, Fleming MF: Screening for problem drinking in older primary care patients, JAMA 276(24):1964-1967, 1996.

Agency for Health Care Policy and Research (AHCPR): Acute pain management: operative or medical procedures and trauma, AHCPR Publication No. 92-0032, Rockville, Md, 1992, U.S. Department of Health and Human Services.

Agency for Health Care Policy and Research (AHCPR); Management of cancer pain, AHCPR Publication No. 94-0592, Rockville, Md, 1994, U.S. Department of Health and Human Services.

Ahmedzai S, Brooks D: Transdermal fentanyl versus sustained-release oral morphine in cancer pain: preference, efficacy, and quality of life, J Pain Symptom Manage 13(5):254-261, 1997.

Aiken HA, Burns, JW, McArdle CS et al.: Effects of ketorolac trometamol on renal function, Br J Anaesth 68:481-485, 1992.

American Pain Society (APS): Principles of analgesic use in the treatment of acute pain and cancer pain, ed 3, Glenview, Ill, 1992, APS.

American Pain Society (APS): Perioperative analgesia: approaching the 21st century, study guide, p 22, Glenview, Ill, 1997, APS.

Anders RL, Ornellas EM: Acute management of patients with hip fracture, Orthop Nurs 16(2):31-46, 1997.

Antai-Otong D: Helping the alcoholic patient recover, Am J Nurs 95(8):23-30, 1995.

Atlas SJ, Deyo RA, Keller RB et al.: The Maine lumbar spine study. Part III. 1-Year outcomes of surgical and nonsurgical management of lumbar spinal stenosis, Spine 21:1787-1794, 1996.

Bach S, Noreng MF, Tjellden NU: Phantom limb pain in amputees during the first 12 months following limb amputation, after preoperative lumbar epidural blockade, Pain 33:297-301, 1988.

Banning A, Sjogren P: Cerebral effects of long-term oral opioids in cancer patients measured by continuous reaction time, Clin J Pain 6:91-95, 1990.

Barnung SK, Treschow M, Borgbjerg FM: Respiratory depression following oral tramadol in a patient with impaired renal function, Pain 71:111-112, 1997.

Baumel B, Eisner LS: Diagnosis and treatment of headache pain in the elderly, Med Clin North Am 75:661-675, 1991.

Beattie WS, Buckley DN, Forrest JB: Epidural morphine reduces the risk of postoperative ischaemia in patients with cardiac risk factors, Can J Anaesth 40(6):532-541, 1993.

Beaver WT: Impact of non-narcotic oral analgesics on pain management, Am J Med 84:3-15, 1988.

Bedder MD, Soifer BE, Mulhall JJ: A comparison of patient-controlled analgesia and bolus PRN intravenous morphine in the intensive care environment, Clin J Pain 7:205-208, 1991.

Beers MH, Ouslander JG, Rollingher I et al.: Explicit criteria for determining inappropriate medication use in nursing home residents, *Arch Intern Med* 151:1825-1832, 1991.

Benet LZ, Kroetz DL, Sheiner LB: Pharmacokinetics. In Hardman JG, Limbird LE, editors: *Goodman and Gilman's the pharmacological basis of therapeutics*, ed 9, pp 3-27, New York, 1996, McGraw-Hill.

Bjorkman DJ: Nonsteroidal anti-inflammatory drug-induced gastrointestinal injury, *Am J Med* 101(Suppl 1A):25S-32S, 1996.

Bradley JD, Brandt KD, Katz BP et al.: Comparison of an antiinflammatory dose of ibuprofen, an analgesic dose of ibuprofen, and acetaminophen in the treatment of patients with osteoarthritis of the knee, *N Engl J Med* 325:87-91, 1991.

Breitbart W, Marotta R, Platt MM et al.: A double-blind trial of haloperidol, chlorpromazine, and lorazepam in the treatment of delirium in hospitalized AIDS patients, *Am J Psychiatry* 153(2):231-237, 1996.

Breitbart W, Passik SD: Psychiatric aspects of palliative care. In Doyle D, Hanks GWC, MacDonald N, editors: *Oxford textbook of palliative medicine*, pp 609-626, New York, 1993, Oxford University Press.

Bressler R, Katz M: *Geriatric pharmacology,* New York, 1993, McGraw-Hill.

Bruera E, Macmillan K, Hanson J et al.: The cognitive effects of the administration of narcotic analgesics in patients with cancer pain, *Pain* 39:13-16, 1989.

Buetefisch CM, Gutierrez MA, Gutmann L: Choreoathetotic movements: a possible side effect of gabapentin, *Neurology* 46:851-852, 1996.

Burton JR: The evolution of nursing homes into comprehensive geriatrics centers: a perspective, *J Am Geriatr Soc* 42:794-798, July 1994.

Campbell RWF: Mexiletine, *N Engl J Med* 316:29-34, 1987.

Cantwell-Gab K: Identifying chronic peripheral arterial disease, *Am J Nurs* 96(7):40-47, 1996.

Carli F, Halliday D: Continuous epidural blockade arrests the postoperative decrease in muscle protein fractional synthetic rate in surgical patients, *Anesthesiology* 86:1033-1040, 1997.

Cartwright P, Prys-Roberts C, Gill K et al.: Ventilatory depression related to plasma fentanyl concentrations during and after anesthesia in humans, *Anesth Analg* 62:966-974, 1983.

Chrischilles EA, Lemke JH, Wallace RB et al.: Prevalence and characteristics of multiple analgesic use in an elderly study group, *J Am Geriatr Soc* 38:979-984, 1990.

Conaway DC: Using NSAIDs safely in the elderly, *Hosp Med* May: 23-34, 1995.

Covino BG: Local anesthetics. In Ferrante FM, Vade Boncouer TR, editors: *Postoperative pain management*, pp. 211-253, New York, 1993, Churchill Livingstone.

Covino BG, Wildsmith JAW: Clinical pharmacology of local anesthetic agents. In Cousins MJ, Bridenbaugh PO, editors: *Neural blockade in clinical anesthesia and management of pain*, pp 97-128, Philadelphia, 1998, Lippincott-Raven.

Coyle N, Cherny N, Portenoy RK: Pharmacologic management of cancer pain. In McGuire D, Yarbro CH, Ferrell BR, editors: *Cancer pain management*, pp. 89-130, ed 2, Boston, 1995, Jones and Bartlett Publishers.

Crook R, Rideout E, Browne G: The prevalence of pain complaints in a general population, *Pain* 18:299-314, 1984.

Dahl JB, Kehlet H: Non-steroidal anti-inflammatory drugs: rationale for use in severe postoperative pain, *Br J Anaesth* 66:703-712, 1991.

Davis MA: Epidemiology of osteoarthritis, *Clin Geriatr Med* 4:241-255, 1988.

Dayer P, Collart L, Desmeules J: The pharmacology of tramadol, *Drugs* 47(Suppl 1):3-7, 1994.

Dejgard A, Petersen P, Kastrup J: Mexiletine for treatment of chronic painful diabetic neuropathy, *Lancet* 1:9-11, 1988.

de Leon-Casasola OA, Lema MJ: Spinal opioid analgesia: influence on clinical outcome. In Sinatra RS, Hord AH, Ginsberg B et al., editors: *Acute pain: mechanisms and management*, pp 293-303, St. Louis, 1992, Mosby-Year Book.

de Leon-Casasola OA, Parker B, Lema MJ et al.: Postoperative epidural bupivacaine-morphine therapy, *Anesthesiology* 81:368-375, 1994.

Dellasega C, Keiser C: Pharmacologic approaches to chronic pain in the older adult, *Nurse Pract* 22:20-35, May 1997.

Desbiens NA, Mueller-Rizner N, Connors AF et al.: Pain in the oldest-old during hospitalization and up to one year later, *J Am Geriatr Soc* 45:1167-1172, 1997.

Dichter MA, Brodie, MJ: New antiepileptic drugs, *N Engl J Med* 334:1583-1590, 1996.

Donner B, Zenz M, Tryba M et al.: Direct conversion from oral morphine to transdermal fentanyl: a multicenter study in patients with cancer pain, *Pain* 64:527-534, 1996.

Duggleby W, Lander J: Patient-controlled analgesia for older adults, *Clin Nurs Res* 1:107-113, 1992.

Duggleby W, Lander J: Cognitive status and postoperative pain: older adults, *J Pain Symptom Manage* 9:19-27, 1994.

Dworkin RH: Which individuals with acute pain are most likely to develop a chronic pain syndrome? *Pain Forum* 6:127-136, 1997.

Edmondson EA, Simpson RK, Stubler DK et al.: Systemic lidocaine therapy for poststroke pain, *South Med J* 86:1093-1096, 1993.

Egbert AM: Postoperative pain management in the frail elderly, *Clin Geriatr Med* 12(3):583-599, 1996.

Egbert AM, Parks LH, Short LM et al.: Randomized trial postoperative patient-controlled analgesia vs. intramuscular narcotics in frail elderly men, *Arch Intern Med* 150:1897-1903, 1990.

Ehsanullah RSB, Page G, Wood RS: Prevention of gastroduodenal damage induced by non-steroidal anti-inflammatory drugs: controlled trial of ranitidine, *BMJ* 297:1017-1021, 1988.

Eliopoulos C: *Gerontological Nursing,* Philadelphia, 1997, Lippincott-Raven.

Emory University Hospital Drug Information Center: Adverse drug reactions: tramadol hydrochloride (Ultram), *Pharmacother Update* 16:5, March/April 1996.

Fadul CE, Lemann W, Thaler HT et al.: Perforation of the gastrointestinal tract in patients receiving steroids for neurologic disease, *Neurology* 38:348-352, 1988.

Faherty BS, Grier MR: Analgesic medication for elderly people postsurgery, *Nurs Res* 33:369-372, November/December 1984.

Farrell MJ, Gibson SJ: Outcomes for geriatric pain clinic patients. In *Proceedings of the 14th Annual Scientific Meeting of the Australian Pain Society*, p 48, Sydney, Australia, 1993, American Pain Society.

Ferrell BA: Pain management in elderly people, *J Am Geriatr Soc* 39:64-73, 1991.

Ferrell BA: Pain evaluation and management in the nursing home, *Ann Intern Med* 123:681-687, November 1995.

Ferrell BR, Cohen MZ, Rhiner M et al.: Pain as a metaphor for illness, part II. Family caregivers' management of pain, *Oncol Nurs Forum* 18:1315-1321, 1991.

Ferrell BR, Dean GE: Ethical issues in pain management at home, *J Palliative Care* 103:67-72, 1994.

Ferrell BR, Ferrell BA, Ahn C et al.: Pain management for elderly patients at home, *Cancer* 74(Suppl):2139-2146, October 1, 1994.

Ferrell BA, Ferrell BR, Rivera L: Pain in cognitively impaired nursing home patients, *J Pain Symptom Manage* 10(8):591-598, 1995.

Ferrell BR, Grant M, Chan J et al.: The impact of cancer pain education on family caregivers of elderly patients, *Oncol Nurs Forum* 22:1211-1218, 1995.

Ferrell BR, Rhiner M, Cohen M et al.: Pain as a metaphor for illness, part I. Impact of cancer pain on family caregivers, *Oncol Nurs Forum* 18:1303-1309, 1991.

Ferrell BR, Rhiner M, Ferrell BA: Development and implementation of a pain education program, *Cancer* 72:3426-3432, 1993.

Ferrell BR, Taylor EJ, Grant M et al.: Pain management at home: struggle, comfort, and mission, *Cancer Nurs* 16:169-178, 1993.

Flower RJ, Moncada S, Vane JR: Drug therapy of inflammation. In Gilman AG, Rall TW, Nies AS et al., editors: *Goodman and Gilman's the pharmacological basis of therapeutics*, ed 7, pp 674-715, New York, 1985, Macmillan.

Foley KM: Misconceptions and controversies regarding the use of opioids in cancer pain, *Anti-Cancer Drugs* 6(Suppl 3):4-13, 1995.

Folstein MF, Folstein SE, McHugh PR: "Mini-mental state": a practical method for grading the cognitive state of patients for the clinician, *J Psychiat Res* 12:189-198, 1975.

Forman WB: Opioid analgesics in the elderly, *Clin Geriatr Med* 12(3):489-500, 1996.

Gagliese L, Melzack R: Chronic pain in elderly people, *Pain* 70:3-14, 1997.

Gaines JE: Here comes everybody, *Adv Pract Nurse*, Spring/Summer: 42-45, 1994.

Geroldi C, Rozzini R, Frisoni G et al.: Assessment of alcohol consumption and alcoholism in the elderly, *Alcohol* 11:513-516, 1994.

Gibson S, Farrell M, Katz B et al.: Multidisciplinary management of chronic nonmalignant pain in older adults. In Ferrell BR, Ferrell BA, editors: *Pain in the elderly*, pp 91-99, Seattle, 1996, IASP Press.

Givens Bell S: Assessing neonatal pain, *Am J Nurs* 95(12):15-16, 1995.

Glass TA, Prigerson H, Kasl SV et al.: The effects of negative life events on alcohol consumption among older men and women, *J Gerontol B Psychol Sci Soc Sci* 50B:S205-S216, 1995.

Gloth FM: Concerns with chronic analgesic therapy in elderly patients, *Am J Med* 101(Suppl 1A):19S-24S, 1996.

Gorman M: Treating acute alcohol withdrawal, *Am J Nurs* 97(1):22-23, 1997.

Grandy R, Fitzmartin RD, Kaiko R et al.: *Pharmacokinetics and pharmacodynamics of controlled release oxycodone (Oxycontin) in healthy elderly and young adult volunteers*, poster presentation, Los Angeles, American Pain Society 14th Annual Scientific Meeting, November 1995.

Griffin MR, Piper JM, Daugherty JR et al.: Nonsteroidal anti-inflammatory drug use and increased risk for peptic ulcer disease in elderly persons, *Ann Intern Med* 114:257-263, 1991.

Griffin MR, Ray WA, Schaffner W: Non-steroidal antiinflammatory drug use and death from peptic ulcer in elderly persons, *Ann Intern Med* 109:359-363, 1988.

Grond S, Meuser T, Zech D et al.: Analgesic efficacy and safety of tramadol enantiomers in comparison with racemate: a randomized, double-blind study with gynaecological patients using intravenous patient-controlled analgesia, *Pain* 62:313-320, 1995.

Gupta KL: Alcoholism in the elderly, *Postgrad Med* 93:203-206, 1993.

Hall GR, Wakefield B: Acute confusion in the elderly, *Nursing* 96(7):33-37, 1996.

Hammack JE, Mailliard JA, Loprinzi CL: Transdermal fentanyl in the management of cancer pain in ambulatory patients: an open label pilot study, *J Pain Symptom Manage* 12(4):234-240, 1996.

Harkins SW, Price DD: Assessment of pain in the elderly. In Turk DC, Melzack R, editors: *The handbook of pain assessment*, pp 315-331, New York, 1992, Guilford Press.

Harkins SW, Price DD: Are there special needs for pain assessment in the elderly? *APS Bull* 3:1-5, January/February 1993.

Harkins SW, Price DD, Bush FM et al.: Geriatric pain. In Wall PD, Melzack R, editors: *Textbook of pain*, pp 769-784, London, 1994, Churchill Livingstone.

Haynes RC: Adrenocorticotrophic hormone: adrenocortical steroids and their synthetic analogs: inhibitors of the synthesis and actions of adrenocortical hormones. In Gilman AG, Rall TW, Nies AS et al. editors: *Goodman and Gilman's pharmacological basis of therapeutics*, ed 8, pp 1431-1462, New York, 1990, Pergamon Press.

Helme RD, Katz B, Gibson S et al.: Multidisciplinary pain clinics for older people: do they have a role? *Clin Geriatr Med* 12(3):563-582, 1996.

Hemmelgam MN, Suissa S, Huang A et al.: Benzodiazepine use and the risk of motor vehicle crash in the elderly, *JAMA* 276:27-31, 1997.

Herr KA, Mobily PR, Wallace RB et al.: Leg pain in the rural Iowa 65+ population: prevalence, related factors, and association with functional status, *Clin J Pain* 7:114-121, 1991.

Herrick IA, Ganapathy S, Komar W et al.: Postoperative cognitive impairment in the elderly, *Anaesthesia* 51:356-360, 1996.

Higa JH: Interventions in nursing home residents receiving NSAIDs: preventing GI damage and complications, *Consultant Pharmacist* 12:304-306, 1997.

Holdsworth M, Forman WB, Nystrom K: Transdermal fentanyl disposition in elderly subjects, *Gerontology* 40:32-37, 1994.

Horn HR, Hadidian Z, Johnson JL et al.: Safety evaluation of tocainide in an American emergency use program, *Am Heart J* 100:1037-1040, 1980.

Houde RW: Analgesic effectiveness of agonist-antagonist, *Br J Clin Pharmacol* 7:297S-308S, 1979.

Hunt RF, Abbott Laboratories, Hospital Products Division: Letter communication to Malcolm Cohen, MD, Mt. Sinai Medical Center, Miami Beach, Fla, July 11, 1989.

Hurley AC, Volicer BJ, Hanrahan PA et al.: Assessment of discomfort in advanced Alzheimer patients, *Res Nurs Health* 15:369-377, 1992.

Hymes A: The therapeutic value of postoperative TENS. In Mannheimer JS, Lampe GN, editors: *Clinical transcutaneous electrical nerve stimulation*, pp 497-510, Philadelphia, 1984, FA Davis.

Hymes AC, Yonehiro EG, Raab DE et al.: Electrical stimulation for the treatment and prevention of ileus and atelectasis, *Surg Forum* 25:222-224, 1974.

Jahangiri M, Jayatunga AP, Bradley JWP et al.: Prevention of phantom pain after major lower limb amputation by epidural infusion of diamorphine, clonidine, and bupivacaine, *Ann R Coll Surg Engl* 76:324-326, 1994.

Joyner MJ: Aging: physiology and anesthetic implications. In Faust RJ, editor: *Anesthesiology review*, pp 160-161, New York, 1991, Churchill Livingstone.

Kaiko RF, Wallenstein SL, Rogers AG et al.: Narcotics in the elderly: symposium on clinical pharmacology of symptom control, *Med Clin North Am* 66(5):1079-1089, 1982.

Katz WA: The role of tramadol in the management of musculoskeletal pain, *Today's Therapeutic Trends* 13(3):177-186, 1995.

Kehlet H: Multimodal approach to control postoperative pathophysiology and rehabilitation, *Br J Anaesth* 78:606-617, 1997.

Kehlet H: Modification of responses to surgery by neural blockade. In Cousins MJ, Bridenbaugh PO, editors: *Neural blockade*, pp 129-175, Philadelphia, 1998, Lippincott-Raven.

Kehlet H, Dahl JB: Are perioperative nonsteroidal anti-inflammatory drugs ulcerogenic in the short term? *Drugs* 44(Suppl 5):38-41, 1992.

Keller RB, Atlas SJ, Singer DE et al.: The Maine lumbar spine study. Part I. Background and concepts, *Spine* 21:1769-1776, 1996.

Kennedy DT, Small RE: Analgesics and elderly patients: the use of nonsteroidal antiinflammatory drugs, *APS Bull* 7(6):4-5, November/December 1997.

Korte W, de Stoutz N, Morant R: Day-to-day titration to initiate transdermal fentanyl in patients with cancer pain: short- and long-term experiences in a prospective study of 39 patients, *J Pain Symptom Manage* 11(3):139-146, 1996.

Kost RG, Straus SE: Postherpetic neuralgia: pathogenesis, treatment, and prevention, *N Engl J Med* 335(1):32-42, 1996.

Kotler-Cope S, Gerber KE: Is age related to response to treatment for chronic pain? In *Abstracts: 7th World Congress on Pain, International Association for the Study of Pain (IASP)*, p 100, Seattle, 1993, IASP Press.

Kreeger W, Hammill SC: New antiarrhythmic drugs: tocainide, mexiletine, flecainide, encainide and amiodarone, *Mayo Clin Proc* 62:1033-1050, 1987.

Lampe GN, Mannheimer JS: Postoperative TENS analgesia: protocol, methods, results, and benefit. In Mannheimer JS, Lampe GN, editors: *Clinical transcutaneous electrical nerve stimulation*, pp 511-528, Philadelphia, 1984, FA Davis.

Lawrence J, Alcock D, McGrath P et al.: The development of a tool to assess neonatal pain, *Neonatal Network* 12:59-66, September, 1993.

Lee CR, McTavish D, Sorkin EM: Tramadol, *Drugs* 46:313-340, 1993.

Lee M: Drugs and the elderly: do you know the risks? *Am J Nurs* 96(7):25-32, 1996.

Leijon G, Boivie J: Central post-stroke pain: a controlled trial of amitriptyline and carbamazepine, *Pain* 36:27-36, 1989.

Leijon G, Boivie J, Johansson I: Central post-stroke pain: neurological symptoms and pain characteristics, *Pain* 36:13-25, 1989.

Levy MH: Constipation and diarrhea in cancer patients, *Cancer Bull* 43:412-422, 1991.

Lindstrom P, Lindblom U: The analgesic effect of tocainide in trigeminal neuralgia, *Pain* 28:45-50, 1987.

Liu SS, Carpenter RL, Mackey DC: Effects of perioperative technique on rate of recovery after colon surgery, *Anesthesiology* 83:757-765, 1995.

Liu SS, Carpenter RL, Neal JM: Epidural anesthesia and analgesia, *Anesthesiology* 82:1474-1506, 1995.

Lonergan ET: Aging and the elderly kidney: adjusting treatment to physiological change, *Geriatrics* 43:27-33, 1988.

Lorenz J, Beck H, Bromm B: Cognitive performance, mood and experimental pain before and during morphine-induced analgesia in patients with chronic non-malignant pain, *Pain* 73:369-375, 1997.

Lynch SH: Elder abuse: what to look for, how to intervene, *Am J Nurs* 97(1):27-32, 1997.

MacDonell C: Accreditation of pain management programs. In Ashburn MA, Rice LJ, editors: *The management of pain*, pp 227-234, New York, 1998, Churchill Livingstone.

Mahoney OM, Noble PC, Davidson J et al.: The effect of continuous epidural analgesia on postoperative pain, rehabilitation, and duration of hospitalization in total knee arthroplasty, *Clin Orthop* 260:30-37, November 1990.

Major CP, Greer MS, Russell WL: Postoperative pulmonary complications and morbidity after abdominal aneurysmectomy: a comparison of postoperative epidural versus parenteral opioid analgesia, *Am Surg* 62:45-51, January 1996.

Marcantonio ER, Juarez G, Goldman L et al.: The relationship of postoperative delirium with psychoactive medications, *JAMA* 272:1518-1522, 1994.

Marshall BE, Longnecker DE: General anesthetics. In Hardman RG, Limbird LE, editors: *Goodman and Gilman's the pharmacological basis of therapeutics,* ed 9, pp 307-330, New York, 1996, McGraw-Hill.

Mather LE, Denson DD: Pharmacokinetics of systemic opioids for the management of pain. In Sinatra R, Hord AH, Ginsberg B et al., editors: *Acute pain: mechanisms and management,* pp 78-92, St. Louis, 1992, Mosby.

McCaffery M, Ferrell BR: Patient age: does it affect your pain control decisions? *Nursing* 91:44-48, 1991.

McLean MJ: Gabapentin, *Epilepsia* 36(Suppl 2):S73-S86, 1995.

Mellick GA, Mellick LB: Gabapentin in the management of reflex sympathetic dystrophy, *J Pain Symptom Manage* 10:265-266, 1995 (letter).

Minaker KL, Frishman R: Elder abuse: love gone wrong, *Harvard Health Letter,* pp 9-12, October 1995.

Morris GL: Efficacy and tolerability of gabapentin in clinical practice, *Clin Ther* 17:891-900, 1995.

Novy CM, Jagmin MG: Pain management in the elderly orthopaedic patient, *Orthop Nurs* 16:51-57, January/February 1997.

Oppeneer RN, Vervoren TM, editors: *Gerontological pharmacology: a resource for health practitioners,* St. Louis, 1983, Mosby.

Pagliaro LA, Pagliaro AM: Age-dependent drug selection and response. In Pagliaro LA, Pagliaro AM, editors: *Pharmacological aspects of nursing,* pp 130-139, St. Louis, 1986, Mosby.

Parikh SS, Chung F: Postoperative delirium in the elderly, *Anesth Analg* 80:1223-1232, 1995.

Parmelee PA, Smith B, Katz, IR: Pain complaints and cognitive status among elderly institution residents, *J Am Geriatr Soc* 41:517-522, 1993.

Pasero C: *Acute pain management policy and procedure guideline manual,* pp 152, Rolling Hills Estates, Calif, 1994, Academy Medical Systems.

Pasero C, McCaffery M: Unconventional PCA: making it work for your patient, *Am J Nurs* 93(9):38-41, 1993.

Pasero C, McCaffery M: Preventing and managing opioid-induced respiratory depression, *Am J Nurs* 94(4):25-31, 1994.

Pasero C, McCaffery M: Postoperative pain management in the elderly. In Ferrell BR, Ferrell BA, editors: *Pain management in the elderly,* pp 45-68, Seattle, 1996, IASP Press.

Pati AB, Perme DC, Trail M: Rehabilitation parameters in total knee replacement patients undergoing epidural vs. conventional analgesia, *J Orthop Sports Phys Ther* 19:88-92, 1994.

Patt RB: Using controlled-release oxycodone for the management of chronic cancer and noncancer pain, *APS Bull* 6(4):1-6, 1996.

Peabody CA, Whiteford HA, Hollister LE: Antidepressants and the elderly, *J Am Geriatr Soc* 34:869-874, 1986.

Piper JM, Ray WA, Daugherty JR et al.: Corticosteroid use and peptic ulcer disease: role of nonsteroidal-antiinflammatory drugs, *Ann Intern Med* 114:735-740, 1991.

Popp B, Portenoy RK: Management of chronic pain in the elderly: pharmacology of opioids and other analgesic drugs. In Ferrell BR, Ferrell BA, editors: *Pain in the elderly,* pp 24-34, Seattle, 1996, IASP Press.

Portenoy RK: Clinical application of opioid analgesics. In Sinatra RS, Hord AH, Ginsberg B et al., editors: *Acute pain mechanisms and management,* pp 93-101, St. Louis, 1992, Mosby.

Portenoy RK: Neuropathic pain. In Portenoy RK, Kanner RM, editors: *Pain management: theory and practice,* pp 83-125, Philadelphia, 1996, FA Davis.

Porter FL, Malhotra KM, Wolf CM et al.: Dementia and response to pain in the elderly, *Pain* 68:413-421, 1996.

Purdue Pharmaceutica LP: *Oxycontin product insert,* Norwalk, Conn, 1996, Purdue Pharmaceutical LP.

Quin AC, Brown JH, Wallace PG: Studies in postoperative sequelae: nausea and vomiting still a problem, *Anaesthesia* 49:62-65, 1994.

Raskin JB, White RH, Jackson JE et al.: Misoprostol dosage in the prevention of nonsteroidal anti-inflammatory drug-induced gastric and duodenal ulcers: a comparison of three regimens, *Ann Intern Med* 123:344-350, 1995.

Rauck RL, Ruoff GE, McMillen JI: Comparison of tramadol and acetaminophen with codeine for long-term pain management in elderly patients, *Curr Ther Res* 55(12):1417-1431, 1994.

Ray W, Griffin M, Downey W: Benzodiazepines of long and short elimination half-life and the risk of hip fracture, *JAMA* 262:3303, 1989.

Reeves AL, So EL, Sharbrough FW et al.: Movement disorders associated with the use of gabapentin, *Epilepsia* 37:988-990, 1996.

Reidenberg MM: Drugs in the elderly, *Med Clin North Am* 66:1073-1089, 1982.

ReMine SG, McIlrath D: Bowel perforation in steroid-treated patients, *Ann Surg* 192:581-586, 1980.

Rhiner M, Ferrell BR, Ferrell BA et al.: A structured non-drug intervention program for cancer pain, *Cancer Pract* 1:137-143, 1993.

Richardson H: Long-term care. In Kovner AR, editor: *Health care delivery in the United States,* ed 4, pp 175-208, New York, 1990, Springer.

Richardson RR, Cerullo LJ: Transabdominal neurostimulation in the treatment of neurogenic ileus, *Appl Neurophysiol* 42:375-382, 1979.

Roose SP, Glassman AH, Giardina EG et al.: Nortriptyline in depressed patients with left ventricular impairment, *JAMA* 256:3253-3257, 1986.

Rosen J, Pollock BG, Altieri L et al.: Treatment of nortriptyline's side effects in elderly patients: a double-blind study of bethanechol, *Am J Psychiat* 150:1249-1251, 1993.

Rosenberg J, Kehlet H: Postoperative mental confusion: association with postoperative hypoxemia, *Surgery* 114:76-81, 1993.

Rosenberg J, Rosenberg-Adamsen S, Kehlet H: Post-operative sleep disturbance: causes, factors, and effects on outcome, *Eur J Anaesth* 12(Suppl 10):28-30, 1995.

Rosner H, Rubin L, Kestenbaum A: Gabapentin adjunctive therapy in neuropathic pain states, *Clin J Pain* 12:56-58, 1996.

Ross AF, Tinker JH: Anesthesia risk. In Miller RD, editor: *Anesthesia,* ed 3, pp 723-724, New York, 1990, Churchill Livingstone.

Roth S, Burch F, Fleischmann R et al.: *The effect of controlled-release oxycodone on pain intensity and activities in patients with pain secondary to osteoarthritis,* poster presentation, Los Angeles, American Pain Society 14th Annual Scientific Meeting, November 1995.

Rowbotham MC: Postherpetic neuralgia, *Semin Neurol* 14(3):247-254, 1994.

Sager DS, Bennett RM: Individualizing the risk-benefit ratio of NSAIDs in older patients, *Geriatrics* 47(8):24-31, 1992.

Sandin KJ: Specialized pain treatment for geriatric patients, *Clin J Pain* 9:60, 1993.

Scherer C, Schmutzler M, Geibler R et al.: Complications related to thoracic epidural analgesia: a prospective study in 1071 surgical patients, *Acta Anaesthesiol Scand* 37:370-374, 1993.

Scott DA, Emanuelsson B-M, Mooney PH et al.: Pharmacokinetics and efficacy of long-term epidural ropivacaine infusion for postoperative analgesia, *Anesth Analg* 85:1322-1330, 1997.

Segal AZ, Rordorf G: Gabapentin as a novel treatment for postherpetic neuralgia, *Am Acad Neurol* 1173-1174, 1996.

Sengstaken EA, King SA: The problems of pain and its detection among geriatric nursing home residents, *J Am Geriatr Soc* 41:541-544, 1993.

Short LM, Burnett ML, Egbert AM et al.: Medicating the postoperative elderly: how do nurses make their decisions? *J Gerontol Nurs* 16:12-17, 1990.

Shug SA, Burrell R, Payne J et al.: Preemptive epidural anaesthesia may prevent phantom limb pain, *Reg Anesth* 20:256, 1995.

Simons W, Malabar R: Assessing pain in elderly patients who cannot respond verbally, *J Adv Nurs* 22:663-669, 1995.

Simpson T, Lee ER, Cameron C: Patients' perceptions of environmental factors that disturb sleep after cardiac surgery, *Am J Crit Care* 5(3):173-181, 1996.

Sjogren P: Clinical implications of morphine metabolites. In Portenoy RK, Bruera, E, editors: *Topics in palliative care,* vol 1, pp 163-175, New York, 1997, Oxford University Press.

Sjogren P, Banning A: Pain, sedation and reaction time during long-term treatment of cancer patients with oral and epidural opioids, *Pain* 39:5-12, 1989.

Spiegel K, Kalb R, Pasternak GW: Analgesic activity of tricyclic antidepressants, *Ann Neurol* 13:462-465, 1983.

Stein MG, Demarco T, Gamsu G et al.: Computed tomography: pathologic correlates in lung disease due to tocainide, *Am Rev Respir Dis* 137:458-460, 1988.

Stein W: Cancer pain in the elderly. In Ferrell BR, Ferrell, BA, editors: *Pain in the elderly*, pp 69-80, Seattle, 1996, IASP Press.

Sternbach RA: Chronic pain as a disease entity, *Triangle* 20:27, 1981.

Stone R, Cafferata GL, Sangl J: Caregivers of frail elderly: a national profile, *Gerontologist* 27:616, 1987.

Strom BL, Berlin JA, Kinman JA et al.: Parenteral ketorolac and risk of gastrointestinal and operative-site bleeding: a postmarketing surveillance study, *JAMA* 275:376-382, 1996.

Stubhaug A, Grimstad J, Breivik H: Lack of analgesic effect of 50 and 100 mg oral tramadol after orthopaedic surgery: a randomized, double-blind, placebo and standard active drug comparison, *Pain* 62:111-118, 1995.

Sullivan F, Muir M, Ginsberg B: A survey on the clinical use of epidural catheters for acute pain management, *J Pain Symptom Manage* 9(5):303-307, 1994.

Tasmuth T, Estlanderb A, Kalso E: Effect of present pain and mood on the memory of past postoperative pain in women treated surgically for breast cancer, *Pain* 68(2,3):343-347, 1996.

Tollison JW, Longe RL: Special considerations in pharmacologic pain management: part II. The elderly, *Pain Manage*, 29-34, May/June 1991.

Tonnesen H, Petersen KR, Hojgaard L et al.: Postoperative morbidity among symptom-free alcohol misusers, *Lancet* 340:334-337, 1992.

Toth-Fisher C: Pediatric tool adapts to elderly patients, *Am J Nurs* 96:18, May 1996 (letter).

Tuman KJ, McCarthy RJ, March RJ et al.: Effects of epidural anesthesia and analgesia on coagulation and outcome after major vascular surgery, *Anesth Analg* 73:696-704, 1991.

Turfrey DJ, Ray DAA, Sutcliffe NP et al.: Thoracic epidural anaesthesia for coronary artery bypass graft surgery, *Anaesthesia* 52:1090-1095, 1997.

Vincent FM, Vincent T: Tocainide encephalopathy, *Neurology* 35:1804-1805, 1985.

Volicer L, Volicer BJ, Hurley AC: Is hospice care appropriate for Alzheimer patients? *CARING Magazine,* pp 50-55, November 1993.

Ward SE, Goldberg N, Miller-McCauley V et al.: Patient-related barriers to management of cancer pain, *Pain* 52:319-324, 1993.

Watt K: Hospice and the elderly: a changing perspective, *Am J Hospice Palliative Care*, pp 47-48, November/December 1996.

Weissman DE, Dufer D, Vogel V et al.: Corticosteroid toxicity in neuro-oncology patients, *J Neurooncol* 5:125-128, 1987.

Welch-McCaffrey D, Dodge J: Acute confusional states in elderly cancer patients, *Semin Oncol Nurs* 4(3):208-216, August 1988.

Willcox SM, Himmelstein DU, Woolhandler S: Inappropriate drug prescribing for the community-dwelling elderly, *JAMA* 272:292-296, 1994.

Willens JS, Myslinski NR: Pharmacodynamics, pharmacokinetics, and clinical uses of fentanyl, sufentanil, and alfentanil, *Heart Lung* 22(3):239-251, 1993.

Williamson V: Clinical pathways for a patient with a total joint replacement, *Orthop Nurs* 16(Suppl 2):41-45, March/April 1997.

Yates P, Dewar A, Fentiman B: Pain: the views of elderly people living in long-term residential care settings, *J Adv Nurs* 21:667-674, 1995.

Yeager MP, Glass DD, Neff RK et al.: Epidural anesthesia and analgesia in high-risk surgical patients, *Anesthesiology* 66:729-736, 1987.

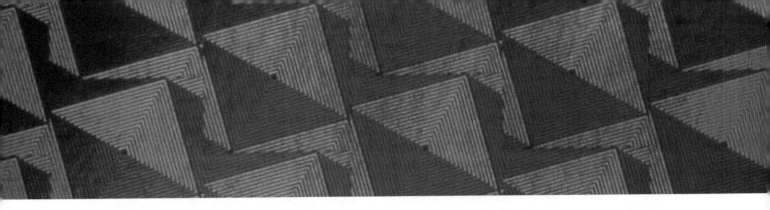

chapter sixteen

BUILDING INSTITUTIONAL COMMITMENT TO IMPROVING PAIN MANAGEMENT

Chris Pasero, Debra B. Gordon, Margo McCaffery, and Betty R. Ferrell

CHAPTER OUTLINE

TERMINOLOGY

Criterion: A standard, rule, or test by which something can be judged or measured. An expected level of achievement or specifications against which performance or quality can be compared (e.g., "Pain ratings *greater than the patient's established comfort goal* will trigger an analgesic dose increase, additional analgesic, or other pain relief intervention").

Data: Information that can be collected and measured or analyzed to define and evaluate a process.

Indicator: A quantitative measure (e.g., ratio, percentage, rate, incidence) used to determine over time performance of functions, processes, and outcomes (e.g., "> 95% of patients will be very satisfied with their pain management during hospitalization").

Institutionalizing pain management: To incorporate basic principles of pain assessment and treatment into patterns of daily practice within institutions.

Opinion leaders: Individuals of any discipline in an organization whose views and beliefs are valued and often followed by others.

Privileging system: A set of rules that allows only specified individuals (usually with special training) to care for patients with a particular condition or receiving a particular treatment such as epidural analgesia.

Processes: A group of sequenced tasks necessary to achieve a particular outcome (e.g., assessing pain, administering and titrating analgesics, and reassessing to achieve pain relief).

Quality assurance: A process of collecting and analyzing data to determine performance; focuses on inspection rather than improvement process.

Quality improvement: A philosophy and process for identifying and eliminating problems to improve the quality of work.

Standard: A level of professional practice to which clinicians are held accountable ("standard of good practice") (e.g., "All patients will be asked about the presence of pain *at least every 8 hours*"). Accreditation bodies define standards as performance expectations, structures, or processes that must be in place to enhance the quality of care.

TABLE 16.1 ● ● ● ● ●

Misconceptions   Improving Institutional Pain Management

MISCONCEPTION	CORRECTION
1. Lack of education is the cause of the undertreatment of pain in institutions.	The undertreatment of pain in institutions is a multifaceted problem. Ingrained and ritualized institutional systems and practices are persistent barriers to effective pain management. Education alone cannot change practice and break down these barriers. An interdisciplinary approach that blends continuous quality improvement with other strategies is most likely to succeed in changing systems and practices that interfere with effective pain management.
2. Poor pain management is a result of physicians underprescribing.	The problem of undertreatment of pain cannot be blamed on one discipline or person. Poor pain management is a multidisciplinary problem. Although it is true that physicians often underprescribe analgesics, nurses often administer inadequate doses.
3. Administrators and upper level managers are responsible for solving the problem of undertreated pain in institutions.	Improving pain management begins at the bedside. Although administrative support for change is essential, practice changes are under the control of clinicians. Nurses, physicians, and pharmacists have a professional and ethical obligation to monitor and improve their practice.

May be duplicated for use in clinical practice. From McCaffery M, Pasero C: *Pain: Clinical manual*, p. 712. Copyright © 1999, Mosby, Inc. See text for references.

Despite the affirmation that pain can be assessed, communicated, and controlled with relatively simple means, pain continues to be an overlooked and neglected institutional problem nationwide (AHCPR, 1992, 1994). The term, "institutional" is defined broadly in this chapter to describe a group of health care providers within an organization working toward a common purpose, that is, to provide health care. Institutional settings include hospitals, home health agencies, hospices, freestanding clinics, physicians' offices, and long-term care facilities.

As pointed out in previous chapters, outdated clinical practices persist, such as failure to accept the patient's report of pain, prescribing PRN IM analgesics, and ignoring the need to titrate and individualize analgesic doses. Over time, these practices have become ingrained and ritualized in the day-to-day activities within health care organizations. In addition, the roles and responsibilities of the numerous disciplines involved in the care of a patient often are unclear when it comes to pain (Max, 1990). Ultimately, no one is held accountable for pain relief.

Compare the assessment and management of pain with the assessment and management of other clinical problems, such as abnormal blood glucose levels. The clinical environment supports both screening and responding to abnormal glucose levels through routine assessment and documentation; most institutions provide patients with monitoring equipment and supplies to ensure regular blood glucose testing and with a nurse to teach them about diabetes and help them control their disease. Authority and accountability for diagnosing and treating diabetes are a part of the inherent rules and ingrained practices in most clinical settings. Considering the multiple adverse effects of unrelieved pain (see Chapter 2), assessment and management of pain deserve at least the same emphasis as the assessment and management of abnormal blood glucose levels.

This chapter presents the use of an interdisciplinary pain care committee as the best method for introducing changes and improving pain management in institutions. A blend of the Agency for Health Care Policy and Research (AHCPR) clinical practice guidelines and the American Pain Society (APS) quality improvement recommendations provides the framework for establishing and guiding the work of the committee. Practical information on getting started and supporting the ongoing work of the pain care committee is offered. A variety of strategies that are used to complement the work of the pain care committee, such as clinical pathways, pain resource nurse programs, and pain services, are discussed. Examples of an institutional needs assessment form, data collection and analysis tools, and educational support materials are provided. Selected terms and definitions are listed at the beginning of this chapter to facilitate an understanding of the content. Table 16.1 corrects some of the misconceptions that have hindered the process of improving pain management in institutions.

INSTITUTIONAL BARRIERS TO EFFECTIVE PAIN MANAGEMENT

Entrenched personal and institutional practices are particularly resistant to change and present, perhaps, the most difficult of all the barriers to overcome. They also are among the most important to conquer. It is clear that no single method, individual, or discipline can conquer these barriers alone (Greco, Eisenberg, 1993). An interdisciplinary approach that uses a variety of methods is recommended to improve pain management within health care organizations (AHCPR, 1992, 1994; APS, 1995).

This interdisciplinary approach has come to be known as "institutionalizing pain management." It involves identifying and breaking down system barriers and using a variety of methods to incorporate the basic principles of pain assessment and treatment into patterns of daily practice. For example, a common barrier in many institutions is the lack of a shared language for communicating about pain. This barrier is overcome by selecting a pain rating scale (see Chapter 3, pp. 62-67), providing clinicians and patients with information about the use of the scale and the negative consequences of pain, and developing a clear, concise system for routine pain assessment and documentation. This approach helps to reinforce the idea that pain can be assessed and documented easily and that pain relief can prevent the occurrence of complications.

Interventions to improve pain management must be sensitive to clinicians' attitudes about pain and their fears regarding the consequences of aggressive pain treatment. For example, strategies that enable clinicians to provide more aggressive pain treatment in a safe, structured manner help to reduce their fears of adverse effects and regulatory scrutiny. Clinicians are likely to view such an approach as helpful rather than threatening.

Finally, every institution has a cultural and political climate. Defining and changing outdated, obstructional "ways of doing things" takes time and requires an individualized approach and support from upper level management. Not all systems within an institution require change; some are designed in a way that can be used or modified slightly to support improvements in pain management. This means that some departments and disciplines may merely have to expand their current responsibilities, whereas others will assume entirely new responsibilities.

CONTINUOUS QUALITY IMPROVEMENT

In addition to using a comprehensive interdisciplinary approach, plans for change must be carefully designed and continuously evaluated and improved to ensure that they are effective and sustained. The rationale for continuous analysis of performance can be found in the principles of total quality management (TQM).

TQM was introduced to the health care industry in the early 1990s when health care organizations began to experience declining profit margins, decreased hospital use, increased competition, and consolidation (Casalou, 1991). TQM blends statistical concepts with a relentless drive for quality and a respect for front-line workers as the product experts (Schiff, Goldfield, 1994). Box 16.1 presents the 14 points of the TQM philosophy, modified to apply to improving pain management.

Central to the concept of TQM is continuous quality improvement (CQI), which is both a philosophy and a process of problem identification and elimination designed to constantly better the work of the organization (Ernst, 1991; Schiff, Goldfield, 1994). The goal of CQI in health care is to reduce wide variations in practices and outcomes of care among patients who receive routine treatment for the same problem (Blumenthal, 1996).

CQI requires the support of an entire organization to succeed. Although administrative support is critical, the

● ● ● ● ●

| BOX 16.1 | **The Fourteen Points of Total Quality Management (TQM) Applied to Improving Pain Management** |

1. *Create constancy of purpose for improvement of care and service.*

   Concentrate on a long-term plan based on a patient-focused mission (e.g., providing patients with attentive analgesic care). Consistently model the vision of the organization (e.g., each person is a unique individual with certain rights). Enable staff to continuously improve costs, services, and patient satisfaction through well-designed pain management plans. Invest in a plan for continuing education and a system of rewards to encourage innovation in staff. Treat continuous improvement of pain management as an ongoing obligation to the patient.

2. *Adopt the new philosophy.*

   Quality pain management must become a driving passion of the organization, so that undertreatment of pain in any care setting is immediately recognized as incompatible with the institution's mission and unacceptable to all of its staff and physicians.

3. *Avoid dependence on inspection only.*

   Traditionally, errors and problems are discovered after the fact through a process of quality assurance (inspection). This inspection process must be replaced with an improvement process that prevents errors and problems. Stop endless data collection on unrelieved pain and establish a pain care committee to analyze and synthesize the data; develop plans to correct current pain problems and prevent the occurrence of new problems.

4. *Avoid the practice of awarding business on price alone.*

   Quality outcomes are possible only when quality materials, supplies, and processes are used. Consider long-term cost and appropriateness of products rather than just their purchase price. Cultivate long-term relationships with vendors, rather than simple short-term purchasing relationships. This requires that the supplier must consistently meet the needs of the organization and commit to continually improving its product (e.g., equipment and supply manufacturers become partners in providing attentive analgesic care by requesting input on how their product can be improved to help clinicians provide better pain care). For example, manufacturers of PCA pumps often rely on suggestions from clinicians who use the pumps to improve the technology. Many suppliers offer a variety of free consultative services and sponsor educational programs for institutions that are interested in improving pain management. This point has implications for the organization's internal "suppliers" (staff and physicians) as well. Cultivating loyalty and trust provides a secure practice environment and long-term relationships with less staff and physician turnover.

5. *Constantly improve every process for planning, implementation, and service.*

   Improving pain management is not a one-time effort. Teamwork is essential. Approve the establishment of an interdisciplinary pain care committee. Empower front-line staff to contribute to the improvement process (e.g., encourage them to serve as members of the pain care committee), to constantly look for ways to reduce waste and improve quality, and to become accountable for pain management (e.g., become a PRN).

6. *Institute teaching and reteaching.*

   On-the-job training alone encourages worker-to-worker propagation of practice. Many practices are faulty and outdated (e.g., promoting the idea that a high risk of addiction when opioids are taken for pain relief). Teach and reteach (continuing education) front-line staff members the important aspects of pain management, give adequate support for providing effective pain relief, and measure the effectiveness of the training. Assign new staff members to trained preceptors who will perpetuate quality performance. Remember to encourage, not drive staff. Adjust the preceptor's workload so that quality training is possible.

7. *Ensure qualified leadership for system improvement.*

   The job of management is to lead. Leading is moving staff toward a vision, managing is helping them do a better job better (e.g., ensure pain care committee members attend meetings, adjust the workload of the PRN to allow time for assisting others with pain problems).

8. *Drive out fear.*

   Many experts consider this the most important of the 14 points because when staff fear failure, embarrassment, or retaliation, they are unwilling to make suggestions and recommendations for change. This results in a lower level of quality. Consider and value all staff suggestions. Appreciate that front-line staff members are "in the trenches" and have invaluable knowledge of how to improve pain management (e.g., extend the concept of the PRN program to all levels of nursing staff).

9. *Break down barriers between departments.*

   The goals of the various departments must complement one another or quality is jeopardized. Foster teamwork by dismantling systems that stop staff from working together to accomplish a project. Help staff understand the needs of other departments and work together toward the organization's vision. Promote processes that support the vision (e.g., initiate postoperative IV PCA in the PACU to avoid the dangerous scenario of patients receiving IM opioid injections on the clinical unit while waiting for IV PCA to be initiated).

10. *Avoid trite slogans, exhortations, and targets.*

    Avoid using derogatory and ambiguous slogans, such as "Just Do It!" These types of slogans provide no direction and may offend and repel some staff and physicians. If slogans and motivational phrases are used, explain them (e.g., "Our slogan is 'Preventing Pain is Easier than Treating Pain.' This means that we remind patients to request analgesia or press their PCA buttons before their pain becomes severe."). Let staff and physicians know exactly what is being done to make it easier for them to provide better pain management (e.g., post in all clinical areas a list of the names and numbers of supervisors and PRNs available to help with pain problems).

11. *Eliminate numeric quotas.*

    Quotas place a cap on productivity and conflict with the continuous nature of quality improvement. Pain issues and problems are ongoing and unending. Encourage staff to look for more than one problem to solve and more than one way to improve pain management. Allow pain improvement workgroups to evolve to a permanent standing interdisciplinary pain care committee.

12. *Remove barriers to pride of workmanship.*

    Delegate authority and responsibility to staff members to foster autonomy while promoting the philosophy of an interdisciplinary, interdepartmental approach to pain management.

● ● ● ● ●

BOX 16.1	**The Fourteen Points of Total Quality Management (TQM) Applied to Improving Pain Management—cont'd**

Avoid focusing on individual or department performance (e.g., pain management is everyone's responsibility); support teaching nurses to titrate analgesics, individualize doses, and manage side effects.

13. *Institute a vigorous program of staff education and continuing education and self-improvement.*

Encourage staff members' ongoing personal development even in areas not related to their jobs. Continually provide updated pain management information to staff and consider the need for updated pain management technology to im-

prove performance (e.g., evaluate and reevaluate the way pain is being assessed and managed and update approaches on the basis of advances in pain knowledge and technology).

14. *Take action to accomplish the transformation.*

Put everyone, including top management, to work on sustaining the organization's new mindset (e.g., discuss the institution's philosophy of providing attentive analgesic care with all new employees during their orientation and update long-time employees during their annual cardiopulmonary resuscitation and fire prevention recertification classes).

May be duplicated for use in clinical practice. From McCaffery M, Pasero C: *Pain: Clinical manual,* pp. 714-715. Copyright © 1999, Mosby, Inc.

Box 16.1 lists the 14 points of the total quality management (TQM) philosophy. The points have been modified to provide a "road map" for management to follow when improving pain management within the organization.

IM, intramuscular; *IV,* intravenous; *PACU,* postanesthesia care unit; *PCA,* patient-controlled analgesia; *PRN,* pain resource nurse; *TQM,* total quality management.

Information from Casalou RF: Total quality management in health care, *Hospital Health Services Admin* 36(1):134-146, 1991; Lopresti J, Whetstone WR: Total quality management: Doing things right, *Nurs Manage* 24(1):34-36, 1993; Pasero C: *Acute pain management service policy and procedure manual,* Rolling Hills Estates, Calif, 1994, Academy Medical Systems; Pasero C, Preble LM: Role of the clinical nurse coordinator. In Sinatra R, Hord AH, Ginsberg B et al., editors: *Acute pain: Mechanisms and management,* pp. 552-559, St. Louis, 1992, Mosby.

creativity and active participation of staff at all levels within the organization makes CQI work. The basic tenets of CQI emphasize: (1) understanding the needs of the customer and linking this knowledge to the day-to-day activities of the organization; (2) molding the culture of the organization to foster pride, critical thinking, and improvements in quality; and (3) using scientific methods of data collection and analysis to understand and control the processes of work (Blumenthal, 1993).

Applying Continuous Quality Improvement to Pain Management

The principles of CQI can be applied easily to pain management. CQI customers include patients with pain and their families, clinicians, administrators, and third-party payers. Each of these groups has unique needs and responsibilities that must be met to achieve safe and effective pain control. CQI offers an approach to tie this chain of customers together in a systematic way. The chain of events for pain management can be mapped out and examined in a scientific way, so that strategies to improve practices can be applied successfully in the clinical setting.

Applying CQI to pain management begins with the understanding that problems with pain management are "process problems" rather than "people problems." A process is defined as a group of sequenced tasks (e.g., pain assessment and administering analgesics) necessary to achieve one particular outcome (e.g., pain relief). Analyzing and correcting problems with the processes (e.g., no place to document pain assessment, recommended analgesics are unavailable) prevents one discipline, clinician, or department from being singled out and blamed for the result (e.g., undertreatment of pain) (see Table 16.1).

BUILDING INSTITUTIONAL COMMITMENT TO IMPROVING PAIN MANAGEMENT

In 1991 the American Pain Society (APS) released recommendations to develop a system to ensure that the occurrence of pain is recognized, and that when pain persists, there is a prompt response within the system to modify treatment (Max, 1991). After applying these recommendations in a number of clinical settings, they were reformatted and released as quality improvement (QI) recommendations for the treatment of acute pain and cancer pain (APS, 1995). The APS QI guidelines complement the AHCPR clinical practice guidelines on acute and cancer pain management and provide an ideal framework for building an institutional commitment to improving pain management. Box 16.2 provides an overview of the APS QI guidelines for pain management.

Establishing a Pain Care Committee

The APS QI guidelines recommend that every health care organization establish an interdisciplinary committee to systematically study and improve the processes involved in pain management. Experience reveals that this is the most efficient and effective method for building institutional commitment to improving pain management.

In many institutions the foundation is laid for a formal committee dedicated to improving pain management when educators, managers, or a group of concerned clinicians recommend the formation of a task force or workgroup to investigate specific pain problems that have been brought to their attention. However, in most institutions the pain management task force or workgroup should evolve into a standing committee.

There are a number of reasons for the workgroup to pursue standing committee status. The most obvious

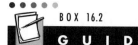

BOX 16.2

GUIDELINES

AMERICAN PAIN SOCIETY (APS) QUALITY IMPROVEMENT GUIDELINES

1. *Recognize and treat pain promptly.*
   Use a variety of mechanisms to ensure that a report of unrelieved pain raises a "red flag" that attracts the clinician's attention.
2. *Make information about analgesics readily available.*
   Teach clinicians about the appropriate use of analgesics and make information about analgesics conveniently accessible where orders and prescriptions are written.
3. *Promise patients attentive analgesic care.*
   Tell patients that reporting unrelieved pain is essential and reassure them that staff will respond promptly. Systematically assess pain using self-reporting pain-rating scales.
4. *Define explicit policies for the use of advanced analgesic technologies.* Implement policies and safeguards for the administration of analgesics and local anesthetics and the use of technology to administer pain treatment
5. *Examine the process and outcomes of pain management with the goal of continuous improvement.*
   Establish an interdisciplinary committee that systematically monitors, evaluates, and improves the processes involved in pain assessment and management.

May be duplicated for use in clinical practice. As appears in McCaffery M, Pasero C: *Pain: Clinical manual,* p. 716, 1999, Mosby, Inc.

Box 16.2 provides an overview of the APS QI guidelines for the treatment of pain. (See also Box 16.6.)

Information from American Pain Society (APS): Quality improvement guidelines for the treatment of acute pain and cancer pain, *JAMA* 274(23):1874-1880, 1995.

reason is that pain issues and problems are ongoing and unending, much the same as the issues and problems other standing committees in institutions face (e.g., pharmacy and therapeutics, ethics). The most important reason is that with standing committee status comes the recognized authority and power to make decisions regarding the committee's focus, that is, pain and its management (Pasero, 1997).

In most institutions standing committee status requires administrative approval. To obtain approval, hospital administrators must be convinced that the impact of the suffering and costs associated with unrelieved pain significantly affect the institution (Pasero, 1997). A formal presentation of several key research studies on the harmful effects of unrelieved pain (see Chapter 2), the data collected from the institution's medical record audits, and the results of physician, staff, and patient surveys is usually met with success.

Composition of the pain care committee

Nurses often lead the effort to form the workgroup and begin the process for improving pain management, but the input and participation of the rest of the health care team is critical to success (Scholtes, Joiner, Streibel,

1996). Without it, the committee risks missing important problems and realistic solutions. It also faces the possibility of physician and staff resistance and noncompliance when solutions to problems are introduced. Therefore multidisciplinary membership is essential (AHCPR, 1992; APS, 1995).

At a minimum, a pain care committee should include representatives from nursing, medicine, and pharmacy. Ideally, the group includes representatives from all disciplines and settings in which patients receive care, including social services, pastoral care, psychology, and physical, respiratory, and occupational therapy. However, committees with too many members have difficulty staying focused and accomplishing work. Instead, a core group of approximately 10 members is recommended.

Most of the committee members should be bedside nurses from the clinical units. The importance of this aspect of committee membership cannot be overemphasized. Clinical nurses have firsthand knowledge of the problems associated with pain and the barriers to managing it. Typically, a 10-member committee is composed of five clinical nurses, one nurse educator, two physicians, one pharmacist, and one manager. Some hospitals include a patient as a member of the core committee. The use of rotating terms, especially for the staff nurses, helps to ensure input from all clinical areas (Pasero, 1997).

Ideally, an anesthesiologist or a certified registered nurse anesthetist (CRNA) should serve on the pain care committee because of his or her specialized knowledge of pain processes and symptom control. This person also plays important roles in providing preemptive analgesia (see Chapter 4, p. 120), intraoperative and postoperative pain management, and nerve blocks for chronic pain syndromes. A pharmacist serves to provide expertise in the pharmacologic management of pain and analgesic side effects. Pharmacists also bring insight into the regulatory and access issues related to the analgesics used to treat pain (Pasero, 1997).

To help keep the size of the committee reasonable, "consultants" (e.g., social workers, physical therapists, religious counselors, patients, and other specialists not represented by the core committee) are asked to participate when the group addresses issues that require a consultant's expertise. Consultants are asked to attend as many meetings as needed to develop a plan of action related to the particular issue (Pasero, 1997). For example, when the committee addresses the purchase of new PCA pumps, representatives from the purchasing and biomedical engineering departments might be asked to attend the meetings and provide guidance in the selection process.

Opinion Leaders

When selecting core committee members, it is wise to look for individuals who are known and respected by others within the organization. These individuals can be from any discipline, and they are commonly referred to as "opinion leaders" (Elliott, Murray, Oken et al., 1997; Rose, Cohen, Yee, 1997). A number of factors, including rank, education, and personality, determine who is recognized as an opinion leader in an organization. The value of having opinion leaders as members of the committee is that their views, beliefs, and practices are likely to be emulated by their colleagues.

However, asking opinion leaders to serve on the pain care committee can have drawbacks. Because of their status, opinion leaders tend to serve on multiple committees and have several other obligations. Typically, physician opinion leaders also are managing thriving practices. As a result, their time is limited and they may miss meetings. This also occurs when upper level managers are asked to serve on committees. Absenteeism and preoccupation with other problems during meetings can adversely affect group morale and become more of a hindrance than a help.

Leading the pain care committee

The responsibilities assigned to members of committees vary among institutions. Formal rules for standing committees often require designating one member of the committee to be the chairperson. Sometimes the hospital administrator appoints this position, and often the rules require that the chairperson be a physician.

In other institutions an informal leadership process is used, and a member of the committee assumes the responsibility for being the "team leader." The team leader's responsibilities include arranging meetings, calling meetings to order, reviewing and moving through the agenda, keeping the team focused, and carrying out administrative details, such as proofing committee reports and meeting minutes. Sometimes the team leader functions in a strictly administrative role as an assistant to the chairperson and is not a member of the committee (Scholtes, Joiner, Streibel, 1996).

In any case the best person to guide the committee, regardless of discipline or title, is one who respects the opinions of others and is identified as a leader among members of the group. For best results, the leader should have a good understanding of pain and its management.

Another important role is that of "coach" (also called facilitator or quality advisor). The coach is not necessarily a member of the team, which makes it possible for him or her to remain neutral. Whether or not he or she is a committee member, the coach should have a good understanding of the problems the committee is addressing (Scholtes, Joiner, Streibel, 1996).

The primary responsibility of the coach is to observe the team's progress and help the members function effectively. The coach ensures that ground rules are followed, teaches the group to use scientific tools, and provides technical expertise. Sometimes the coach assumes additional responsibilities, such as posting ideas on flip charts to keep the team focused on the discussion at hand. In institutions where the use of a coach is not pos-

sible, at least one member of the committee should become expert in the use of scientific tools for data analysis. Box 16.3 provides resources for guidelines and tools that pain care committees may find helpful.

The mission statement and ground rules

The first time the committee meets, time is spent getting to know each other and establishing a mission

---

● ● ● ● ●
BOX 16.3

Resources for Pain Care Committees and Workgroups

- Abbott Northwestern Hospital Resource Manual: *Building clinical improvement for patients: Pain management,* 1996.
  Lori Cassibo, Internal Zip 11404
  Abbott Northwestern Hospital
  800 E. 28th St.
  Minneapolis, MN 55407
  (612) 863-4706
  Fax: (612) 863-2056
  E-mail: lcassibo@allina.com
  Manual available for $45.00; includes shipping and handling.

- Mayday Pain Resource Center
  City of Hope National Medical Center
  Nursing Research and Education
  1500 E. Duarte Rd.
  Duarte, CA 91010
  (626) 359-8111; ext. 3829
  Fax: (626) 301-8941
  Web site: *http://mayday.coh.org*
  Wide variety of materials available for a small fee to cover postage and duplication.

- Scholtes PR, Joiner BL, Streibel BJ: *The team handbook,* ed 2, 1996.
  Oriel Incorporated
  3800 Regent St; P.O. Box 5445
  Madison, WI 53705-0445
  (800) 669-8326 or (608) 238-8134
  Fax: (608) 238-2908
  Manual available for $39.00 plus shipping and handling.

- Wisconsin Resource Manual: *Building an institutional commitment to pain management,* 1996
  Wisconsin Cancer Pain Initiative
  Room 4720 Medical Sciences Center
  1300 University Avenue
  Madison, WI 53706
  (608) 262-0978
  Fax: (608) 265-4014
  E-mail: *kmsteven@facstaff.wisc.edu*
  Manual available for $30 plus $5 shipping; clinical tools available on diskette for $5 plus $1.50 postage.

May be duplicated for use in clinical practice. From McCaffery M, Pasero C: *Pain: Clinical manual,* p. 717. Copyright © 1999, Mosby, Inc.

statement and ground rules. The mission statement helps to define the scope of the process the team will be addressing, the boundaries of the project, the basis of authority, and where the project fits into the institution's overall vision. The mission statement is used to keep the committee members focused on the purpose of their work. It often incorporates the committee's philosophy into a simple patient-centered statement (Box 16.4).

The ground rules are "norms," or what will and will not be tolerated by the team members. These are established by discussing what behaviors members find acceptable and unacceptable. Box 16.5 provides examples and comments about ground rules.

The team leader can save time by planning ahead for the first meeting, sending out reminders to attend, and creating an agenda. Examples of mission statements and a list of common ground rules for members to review and discuss help move the meeting forward. The team coach should explain the purpose of a mission statement and ground rules and guide the group to develop and agree on their content. These are posted prominently at every meeting for reference and review. The mission statement and ground rules must be reaffirmed whenever the core committee composition changes.

Problems with the pain care committee

One of the goals for any committee is to progress from being simply a multidisciplinary committee to an interdisciplinary (multiple disciplines working together toward a goal). This is accomplished over time as committee members begin to feel comfortable with each other and function as a team. However, when projects of the magnitude of improving institutional pain management are undertaken, problems can arise. These may range from minor conflicts between team members to repetitive implementation failures, such as nursing staff and physicians repeatedly ignoring recommendations for change. Table 16.2 lists common group problems, their warning signs, and recommended solutions. The resources listed in Box 16.3 may also be helpful in improving team dynamics and group process.

• • • • •

| BOX 16.5 | **Examples of Ground Rules for Pain Care Committees and Comments for Implementation** |

- Attendance: e.g., "A team member will be asked to resign if the team member and/or alternate misses more than _____ consecutive meetings." One of the most common reasons for committee failure is poor attendance. Team members must place a high priority on attending meetings. Agreeing on a specific number of meetings that can be missed before a replacement is considered helps ensure the process moves forward.
- Promptness: e.g., "Meetings will start and end on time." Make no exceptions and do not take time to update late comers. This will encourage members to make punctuality a priority.
- Meeting place and time: e.g., "Meetings will be the first Thursday of every month at 10 AM in conference room A." As much as is possible, meet regularly and set dates, times, and meeting place in advance.
- Participation: e.g., "Everyone's viewpoint is valuable." Be sure decisions are group decisions and not the decisions of the most verbal members.
- Basic conversational courtesies: e.g., "Team members will listen attentively and will not interrupt." Courtesies help to promote enlightenment and respect for others.
- Assignments: e.g., "Work assignments will be equal." Much work needs to be done outside meetings. Assign work evenly to *all* members and always set and stick to due dates.
- Interruptions: e.g., "The 100 Mile Rule will be in effect for all meetings." The 100 Mile Rule means that there will be no outside interruptions unless it is so important that the disruption would occur even if the meeting was 100 miles away. Decide when interruptions (pagers, telephone calls) will be tolerated.
- Rotations of routine chores: Decide who will be responsible for arranging meeting space, taking minutes, and other housekeeping chores, and how duties will be rotated among members. Although the team leader is responsible for records, many decide to rotate this responsibility. Keeping accurate records and making sure everyone has access to them is important.
- Other norms: What other guidelines are important to the committee?

Ground rules guide what will and will not be tolerated by the team members during meetings. They should be posted prominently at every meeting and reviewed periodically.

Modified from Scholtes PR, Joiner BL, Streibel BJ: *The team handbook*, ed 2, Madison, Wis, 1996, Joiner Associates Inc. (See Box 16.3 for ordering information.)

• • • • •

| BOX 16.4 | **Examples of Mission Statements for Pain Care Committees** |

- An opportunity exists to decrease patients' numeric pain ratings, improve their outcomes, and increase their satisfaction with their pain management during hospitalization.
- Patients of all ages and settings at _____ Medical Center have the right to do the following: (1) express their pain and have that expression accepted and respected as the most reliable indicator of pain, (2) have their pain assessed systematically and thoroughly, (3) have their pain managed according to the most currently accepted, (4) receive a prompt response to unrelieved pain, and (5) be informed and involved in all decisions regarding all aspects of their pain care.

Box 16.4 provides examples of two types of mission statements. The first statement is task oriented and typical of what is used for a one-time quality improvement project; the second reflects a pain care committee's philosophy and that of the institution. Such statements keep team members focused on the purpose of their work.

Information from Pasero C: *Acute pain management service policy and procedure manual*, Rolling Hills Estates, Calif, 1994, Academy Medical Systems.

● ● ● ● ●

TABLE 16.2   **Common Group Problems and Suggested Solutions**

PROBLEM	WARNING SIGNS	SOLUTION
Floundering	False starts, directionless meetings, postponing decisions	Review the mission statement and improvement plan; use a progress checklist to look for clues as to what has stalled the group.
Overbearing participants	Self-appointment as "authority" on a specific issue or area of expertise and discouraging others from discussing it; using technical jargon or referring to existing regulations to intimidate others	Include in ground rules that all members are considered equal and have valuable input for all topics; post and review ground rules at start of meetings; enforce the principle that data drive the improvement process; reinforce that no areas of discussion are "sacred"; talk to the overbearing member outside of meetings and ask for his or her cooperation.
Dominating participants	Talking too much, using long anecdotes, dominating the discussion	Include in ground rules the concept of "balanced participation"; post and review ground rules at the start of meetings; at a pause in dominating member's conversation, ask another member for input on the subject; set a maximum time for a single member to get a point across to the group.
Reluctant participants	Members who rarely speak	Structure participation, divide project tasks into individual assignments; directly ask for input, "Jane, what is your experience?"; conclude meetings by asking each member for input ("round robin").
Unquestioned acceptance of opinions as facts	Personal beliefs and assumptions are presented as facts	Include in ground rules the principle of always using the scientific method; question and clarify, "Is that what you think? "Do you have data?" "How do you know that is true?"; ask member to bring documentation on important issues.
Rush to accomplishment	Impatience about accomplishing a step of project; wanting to solve a problem before it has been analyzed	Review ground rule about using the scientific method; remind members that quality and change take patience; use constructive feedback to confront the rusher.
Attribution	Motives are ascribed to members with different opinions or behaviors, "He just doesn't understand this . . ."	Check it out, ask direct questions: "Do you understand the . . ?"; use the scientific approach, "That may explain why we think he behaves that way, but how do we know?"
Discounts and "plops"	Values or perspectives of others are discounted or not acknowledged (plops)	Include in ground rules the idea that everyone's opinion will be valued and that members will actively listen to each other; post and review ground rules at start of meetings; support the discounted person and acknowledge input; discuss the problem with the discounter outside of the meeting.
Wanderlust: Digression and tangents	Wide-ranging, unfocused conversations that stray from the agenda	Use a written agenda with time estimates for each item; review agenda at start of meeting; redirect the conversation back on track, "We've gotten off track, let's get back to. . . ."
Feuding members	Members feel like spectators at a disagreement between two other members; disagreements are more about winning an argument than the issue at hand	Include in ground rules how differences will be resolved without disrupting the group; deal with feuding members outside of meeting; feuds sometimes predate the group and cannot be resolved, which may require asking one or both members to resign.

May be duplicated for use in clinical practice. As appears in McCaffery M, Pasero C: *Pain: Clinical manual,* p. 719, 1999, Mosby, Inc.

Modified from Scholtes PR, Joiner BL, Streibel BJ: *The team handbook,* ed 2, Madison, Wis, 1996, Joiner Associates Inc. (See Box 16.3 for ordering information.)

The most common reason for repetitive implementation failures is that the committee lacks authority. As discussed, upper level management must authorize the pain care committee to make decisions about how pain will be assessed and treated in the institution. Asking administrators to reinforce the committee's authority periodically may be necessary, especially when the committee is issuing its first few recommendations for change (Pasero, 1997).

Occasionally it is necessary for an ineffective committee to start from the beginning with basic developmental steps. This can be as simple as establishing new ground rules and as difficult as replacing members who do not meet performance standards established by the committee. The most common performance problem is poor attendance. It is essential that representation be adequate from the three major disciplines involved in pain assessment and treatment (i.e., nursing, medicine, and pharmacy). Poor attendance risks ineffectual decision making and adversely affects committee morale. If not handled by swiftly replacing the perpetually absent member, it can cause irreversible damage to the committee's effectiveness and credibility. The ground rules, to which all members of the committee agree, should provide clear guidance for handling this problem (see Box 16.5) (Pasero, 1997).

The composition of the committee may be contributing to its ineffectiveness. If membership is over or under represented by a particular discipline or department, one-sided or impractical plans can result. This is especially true when staff nurses are under represented and when committees lack physician members.

The way in which the committee makes decisions can cause implementation failures. Hasty decision making and plans for change on the basis of hunches and opinions cannot be defended. Staff and physicians are more likely to comply with recommendations for change that are made on the basis of careful problem identification, scientific collection and analysis of institutional data, and consultation with key disciplines and departments. Asking for input from the staff who will be affected by a proposed change is critical to the success of an improvement plan (Pasero, 1997).

Another possible reason for difficulty may be that the committee is trying to accomplish too much too fast. If there are many pain management problems in the institution, the tendency is to try to work on several of them at the same time. A better approach is to tackle just one problem at a time and to work on basic ones before complex ones. For example, a pain assessment standard should be established before a treatment protocol for a complex pain syndrome is developed. Whenever the committee identifies a new problem, goals and objectives should be outlined to define the task at hand. The use of scientific tools, such as flowcharts and fishbone

diagrams (Figures 16.1 and 16.2), to analyze problems and clearly stated assignments and time lines, will help to ensure that important steps in the process are not omitted (Pasero, 1997).

Establishing the Need for Change in Pain Management Practices

The abundance of available research showing inadequate institutional pain management (see Chapter 1) would seem to be justification enough for the need to change pain management practices in all institutions. However, it is recommended that every institution collect and establish its own database to demonstrate the need for change within that institution.

Besides justification of the need for change in practices, institutional data are used to defend the committee's recommendations that outdated pain management practices be abandoned because they are ineffective and harmful. Data also provide insight into the barriers to effective pain management that are unique to the institution. This insight will help to prioritize needs and to focus interventions directly on overcoming those barriers. For example, clinician and patient surveys may reveal that both groups fear and misunderstand addiction more than any other issue related to pain management. This information can be used to develop an educational plan to dispel specific fears and misconceptions. Finally, the initial data establish a baseline for measuring improvements in pain assessment and management after changes are introduced.

Data collection

Performing an institutional needs assessment on the basis of the APS QI guidelines (Form 16.1, pp. 724-726) will help to identify pain management strengths and weaknesses in the institution. This information also can be used to prioritize the activities of the workgroup as it gets started and to ensure important needs are not overlooked.

In addition to the needs assessment, nurses, physicians, pharmacists, and patients should be surveyed for the database. The survey results will provide documentation of the clinicians' basic knowledge, attitudes, practices, and the patients' outcomes and satisfaction with the pain care they received as customers of the institution before any improvements were made.

Observation, case reviews, drug use reviews, and audits of randomly selected medical records (patient charts) can provide the data on pain management practices. Form 16.2, p. 727, provides a simple version of a medical record audit tool that can be used to collect baseline data. A medical record audit helps to identify specific practices that can be targeted for change later, such as inappropriate use of meperidine and the IM route of administration. Different or more indicators

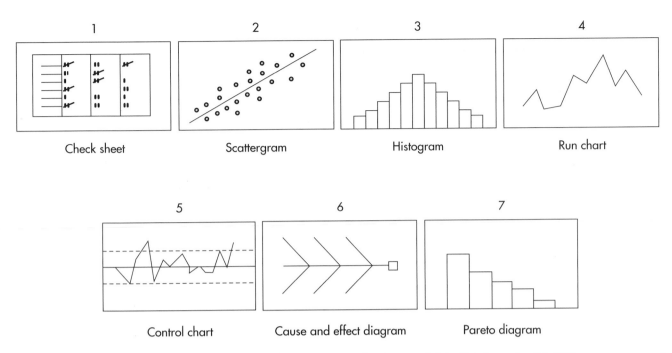

May be duplicated for use in clinical practice. As appears in McCaffery M, Pasero C: *Pain: Clinical manual,* p. 721, 1999, Mosby, Inc.

● ● ● ● ● ●
F I G U R E 16.1 **Quality Improvement Data Analysis Tools.** The use of quality improvement tools to analyze data can prevent faulty and hasty decision making by workgroups and committees. Figure 16.1 shows seven quality improvement data analysis tools: (1) check sheets are simple data collection tools on which tally marks are made; (2) scattergrams are used to show the correlation, but not necessarily the cause and effect relationship, between two variables; (3) histograms are bar graphs that show the distribution of a variance and provide a quick look at the way the data are distributed; (4) run charts plot data over periods of time to show trends, cycles, and other patterns in a process; (5) control charts help to distinguish between normal and abnormal variation, showing how close a process comes to meeting desired objectives. The solid line in the control chart in Figure 16.1 is the average variation, the dotted horizontal lines are the upper and lower limits, the spikes represent abnormal variation; (6) cause and effect diagrams, also known as fishbone or Ishikawa diagrams, help identify potential causes of a problem (see example). They force committee members to consider every possible cause of a problem; (7) Pareto diagrams are a way to display problems or causes by the magnitude of their effect.

Information from Eshelman D, Cooksey C: The quality toolbox, *Quality,* pp 19-20, 27-28, April, 1992; Scholtes PR, Joiner BL, Streibel BJ: *The team handbook,* ed 2, Madison, Wis, 1996, Joiner Associates Inc. (See Box 16.3 for ordering information.)

can be added later to the tool during the QI process. Examples of other medical record audit tools can be obtained from the Mayday Pain Resource Center (see Box 16.3, p. 717).

A number of tools have been developed to assess physician and staff knowledge and attitudes. The same surveys should be used for physicians, pharmacists, and nurses, and it is important that all three disciplines be surveyed. Form 16.3, p. 728, provides an example of a brief knowledge and attitudes survey. The use of this survey plus the "Andrew-Robert" survey described in Chapter 3, p. 40, usually is sufficient for the initial assessment of clinicians' knowledge and attitudes. Other knowledge and attitude surveys can be obtained from the Mayday Pain Resource Center (see Box 16.3, p. 717). Some surveys are quite lengthy and time-consuming to complete, which creates the risk of a poor return rate.

Patients also must be surveyed. As with medical record audits and knowledge and attitude surveys, the more

lengthy and complex the questionnaire, the less likely it is that the survey will be completed and returned. Simplicity and brevity are encouraged in most cases. Form 16.4, p. 729, provides a modified version of the APS patient questionnaire (APS, 1995). Some of the questionnaire items have been adapted from previously validated tools and tested in a number of settings (Bookbinder, Kiss, Coyle et al., 1996; Miaskowski, Nichols, Brody et al., 1994, Ward, Gordon 1994, 1996). The questionnaire can be modified to suit the needs of a particular clinical setting and patient population. It can be completed by the patient or administered to the patient by an unbiased interviewer.

As discussed in Chapter 1, patients often report being satisfied with their pain management despite experiencing poor pain control and levels of pain that interfere with function and quality of life (Miaskowski, Nichols, Brody et al., 1994; Bookbinder, Coyle, Thaler et al., 1996; Ward, Gordon, 1996). It may be that satisfaction

Text continued on p. 730.

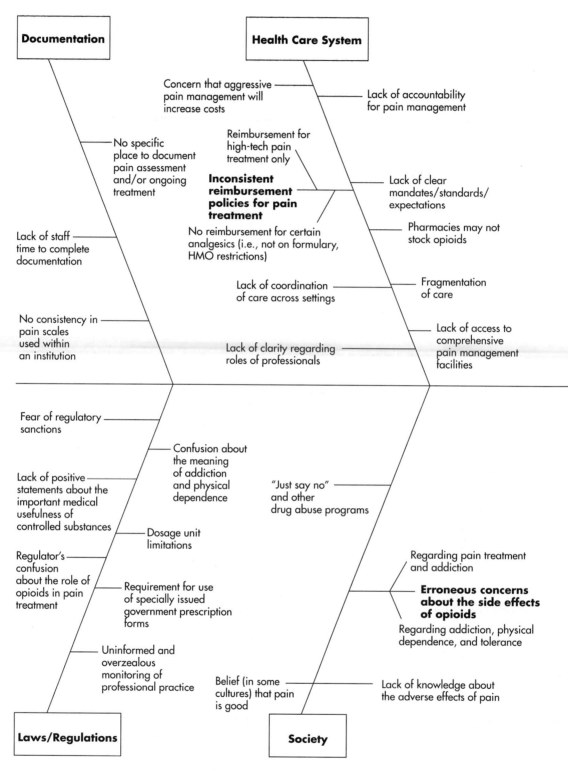

Documentation

Health Care System

Concern that aggressive pain management will increase costs

Lack of accountability for pain management

No specific place to document pain assessment and/or ongoing treatment

Reimbursement for high-tech pain treatment only

Inconsistent reimbursement policies for pain treatment

Lack of clear mandates/standards/expectations

Lack of staff time to complete documentation

No reimbursement for certain analgesics (i.e., not on formulary, HMO restrictions)

Pharmacies may not stock opioids

No consistency in pain scales used within an institution

Lack of coordination of care across settings

Fragmentation of care

Lack of clarity regarding roles of professionals

Lack of access to comprehensive pain management facilities

Fear of regulatory sanctions

Confusion about the meaning of addiction and physical dependence

"Just say no" and other drug abuse programs

Lack of positive statements about the important medical usefulness of controlled substances

Regarding pain treatment and addiction

Erroneous concerns about the side effects of opioids

Dosage unit limitations

Regulator's confusion about the role of opioids in pain treatment

Requirement for use of specially issued government prescription forms

Regarding addiction, physical dependence, and tolerance

Uninformed and overzealous monitoring of professional practice

Belief (in some cultures) that pain is good

Lack of knowledge about the adverse effects of pain

Laws/Regulations

Society

May be duplicated for use in clinical practice. As appears in McCaffery M, Pasero C: *Pain: Clinical manual*, pp. 722-723, 1999, Mosby, Inc.

● ● ● ● ●
FIGURE 16.2   **Example of Cause and Effect Diagram.** The use of a cause and effect diagram prevents hasty decision making by forcing committee members to consider every possible cause of a problem. It is a particularly helpful tool to use when evaluating complex problems that may have many causes or hidden causes.

Reprinted with permission from Patricia Berry, June L. Dahl, Jennifer L. Stiemke: Institutionalizing Pain Management Project, University of Wisconsin Madison Medical School, Madison, Wis, 1998.

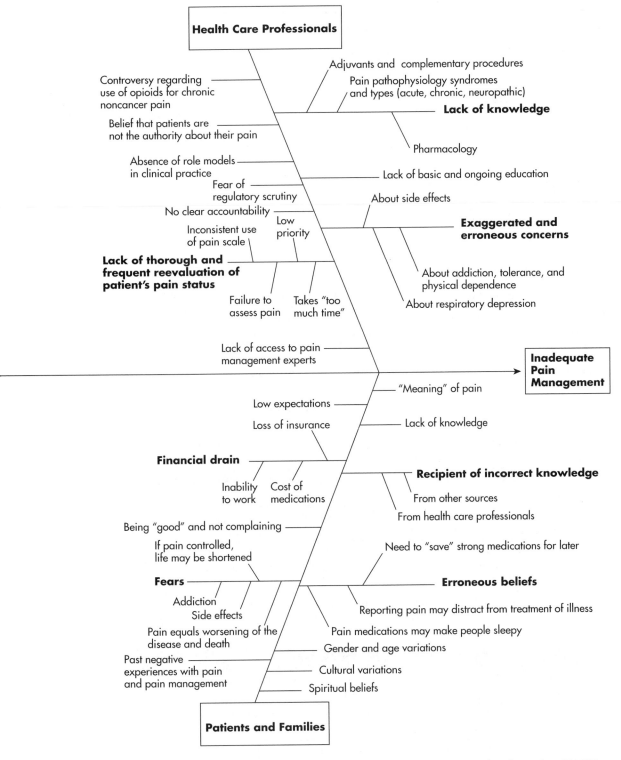

May be duplicated for use in clinical practice. As appears in McCaffery M, Pasero C: *Pain: Clinical manual,* pp. 722-723, 1999, Mosby, Inc.

● ● ● ● ●

F I G U R E 16.2—cont'd **Example of Cause and Effect Diagram.** The use of a cause and effect diagram prevents hasty decision making by forcing committee members to consider every possible cause of a problem. It is a particularly helpful tool to use when evaluating complex problems that may have many causes or hidden causes.

Reprinted with permission from Patricia Berry, June L. Dahl, Jennifer L. Stiemke: Institutionalizing Pain Management Project, University of Wisconsin Madison Medical School, Madison, Wis, 1998.

FORM 16.1 **Institutional Needs Assessment Tool**			
Building an Institutional Commitment to Pain Management	Yes	No	Don't Know
An interdisciplinary workgroup examines and reexamines issues and practices of pain management			
• Is there a process to gain administrative support to develop a pain management improvement workgroup and carry out a work plan?			
• Are there other workgroups or committees already in existence that might be able to support the change efforts?			
• Can you identify and recruit individuals from nursing, medicine, pharmacy, and other disciplines who are interested in improving pain management?			
• Can you identify individual(s) to coordinate and lead the interdisciplinary workgroup?			
• Is there institutional experience or are there training opportunities in continuous quality improvement?			
• Other:			
A standard for pain assessment and documentation ensures that pain is recognized and treated promptly			
• Do current nursing documentation forms screen for pain and provide for the ongoing recording of assessment, interventions, and trends of pain relief?			
• Do current physician documentation forms screen for and address problems with pain?			
• If your system uses clinical pathways, do they incorporate pain assessment, interventions, and outcomes?			
• Is there a written standard of practice that articulates the method and frequency for documenting pain assessments?			
• Does your method for pain documentation place pain in a highly visible and prominent position that encourages regular review by all disciplines?			
• Are there standards/guidelines that define the maximum acceptable pain intensity (comfort goal) that will trigger a change in the pain management plan or consultation?			
• Does your system ensure the communication of the pain management plan as patients transition across settings, e.g., from home to hospital, from clinical unit to clinical unit?			
• Do staff members have access to a variety of pain assessment tools for populations that are at particular risk for undertreatment of pain? (e.g., children, cognitively impaired, patients unable to communicate verbally . . .)			
• Are there written protocols? or do physicians' orders include alternatives when pain is unrelieved by the initial prescription, e.g., titration with supplemental doses, increasing the dose?			
• Other:			
Explicit policies and procedures guide the use of specialized techniques for analgesic administration			
• Are there policies to govern the use of all available specialized techniques such as IV PCA, continuous intravenous, subcutaneous, and intraspinal infusions?			
• Do these policies differentiate roles and responsibilities and describe a mechanism for monitoring competency for all staff involved?			
• Do these policies define appropriate indications and contraindications and the acceptable level of patient monitoring?			
• Are the necessary medications available on the formulary for specialized analgesic techniques?			
a. Preservative-free morphine and fentanyl for intraspinal analgesia			
b. Concentrated doses of morphine or hydromorphone for continuous subcutaneous administration			

May be duplicated for use in clinical practice. From McCaffery M, Pasero C: *Pain: Clinical manual*, pp. 724-726, 1999, Mosby, Inc.   *Continued.*

● ● ● ● ●

FORM 16.1 **Institutional Needs Assessment Tool—cont'd**			
Building an Institutional Commitment to Pain Management	Yes	No	Don't Know
c. Fentanyl or sufentanil for parenteral administration			
d. Long-acting oral opioid preparations and transdermal fentanyl			
e. Other:			
• Other:			
Accountability for pain management is clearly defined			
• Is evaluation of pain management performance integrated into annual staff evaluations?			
• Are there accountability clauses for pain management in existing policies that address procedures known to cause pain? (e.g., venipuncture, nasogastric intubation, invasive procedures . . .)			
• Is there a clear line of consultation for difficult pain problems?			
• Is there a competency-based system for orientation and evaluation of staff performance related to the management of pain?			
• Do policies and procedures that address pain assessment, documentation, and treatment and analgesic technology clearly define the role and responsibilities of all health care providers involved?			
• Is there a privileging system for managing specialized techniques for drug administration? (e.g. IV PCA, spinal analgesia)			
• Other:			
Information about analgesics and nonpharmacologic interventions is readily available to clinicians			
• Are equianalgesic charts available in all clinical areas where orders and prescriptions are written?			
• Do staff have easy access to clinical practice guidelines for pain assessment and management such as the AHCPR clinical practice guidelines and institution-specific guidelines?			
• Are there tools to help clinicians select and dose analgesics such as algorithms, protocols, formulary guidelines, or preprinted orders?			
• Are there quick reference materials available to address pain assessment and treatment, such as pocket reference cards or computer help screens?			
• Are there expert preceptors/role models in pain management (e.g., pain resource nurses, clinical pharmacists) that are readily available to staff?			
• Is there an easily accessible mechanism that informs staff who they can consult with for pain issues?			
• Can staff readily provide nondrug interventions?			
a. Are equipment and supplies available to patients? (e.g., relaxation or music tapes, warm and cold packs, patient education materials)			
b. Are there mechanisms to prompt referral to physical therapy, social work, and pastoral care?			
• Other:			
Patients and families are informed about the importance of pain relief			
• Are all patients informed verbally and in an electronic or printed format that effective pain relief is an important part of their treatment, that it is essential that they report unrelieved pain, and that staff will respond quickly to patients' requests for pain treatment?			

May be duplicated for use in clinical practice. From McCaffery M, Pasero C: *Pain: Clinical manual,* pp. 724-726, 1999, Mosby, Inc.   *Continued.*

FORM 16.1 **Institutional Needs Assessment Tool—cont'd**

Building an Institutional Commitment to Pain Management

	Yes	No	Don't Know
• Is pain management addressed in your Patient's Bill of Rights or the organization's mission statement?			
• Is information about pain integrated in existing classes or educational materials for patients?			
• Does each unit maintain a supply of institutional-specific brochures on pain management, or the AHCPR consumer guidelines for acute and cancer pain, or any other patient pain education materials?			
• Are there opportunities for patients and families to learn about pain management at community forums or support group meetings?			
Staff members have ongoing educational opportunities in pain management			
• Has your institution surveyed its nurses, pharmacists, and physicians to assess prevalent knowledge and attitudes about pain management?			
• Are there ongoing opportunities for case presentations or teaching rounds on patients with pain problems?			
• Does your staff education department offer a variety of resources on pain management (e.g., self-directed learning programs, videos, printed materials?)			
• Is information about pain management incorporated in employee orientation programs?			
• Is there a budget committed to staff and patient education about pain management?			
• Other:			
An ongoing process evaluates the outcomes and works to improve the quality of pain management			
• Are pain assessment and management outcomes monitored and reported through a QA/QI process?			
• Does outcome monitoring involve periodic surveys of patients, including questions about pain intensity, expectations and goals, impact of pain, and satisfaction with the staff?			
• Is staff compliance with documentation standards evaluated?			
• Are there ongoing, frequent opportunities to provide staff members with feedback about improvements in pain and/or areas for future focus?			
• Can you use drug utilization reviews to monitor prescribing practices?			
• Are there avenues to analyze cost issues related to unrelieved pain such as extended length of stay, reimbursement for pain treatment, rates of rehospitalization, or unplanned outpatient visits for pain?			
• Other			

May be duplicated for use in clinical practice. As appears in McCaffery M, Pasero C: *Pain: Clinical manual*, pp. 724-726, 1999, Mosby, Inc.

Form 16.1 provides an example of an institutional pain management needs assessment, which helps to determine institutional strengths and weaknesses and provides direction for pain management improvement efforts.

Reprinted with permission from Gordon D, Stevenson K: *Wisconsin Cancer Pain Initiative,* 1997. Modified from *Pain Audit Tool,* Ferrell B, City of Hope, Duarte, CA, and *Institutional Audit Tool—Pain Management,* Ruzicka D, Tripler Army Hospital, Honolulu, HI.

● ● ● ● ●

FORM 16.2 Medical Record Pain Management Audit

Instructions: Review critical pathway, flow sheets, medication record sheets, histories, and clinical notes for a 24-hour period to obtain the following information:

1. Date of audit: _____

2. Audit start time: _____

3. Medical record number: _____

4. Admission date: _____

5. Discharge date: _____

6. Ethnicity: (1) Caucasian _____ (2) Hispanic _____ (3) African-American _____ (4) Asian _____

   (5) American Indian _____ (6) Other _____

7. Diagnosis (if postoperative, include surgical procedure):

8. Gender: (1) Male _____ (2) Female _____

9. Age: _____

10. Clinical unit: _____

11. Is there evidence of the use of a numeric pain rating scale by an MD?

    (1) Yes _____ (2) Pain documented without scale _____ (3) Pain not documented _____

12. Is there evidence of the use of a numeric pain rating scale by an RN?

    (1) Yes _____ (2) Pain documented without scale _____ (3) Pain not documented _____

13. What was the highest pain rating recorded? _____

14. What was the lowest pain rating recorded? _____

15. What was the pain rating recorded most often? _____

16. What was the patient's comfort goal? _____ Not recorded _____

17. How many times was an analgesic administered? _____

    a. How many times was a pain rating recorded at the time an analgesic was administered? _____

    b. How many times was a pain rating recorded within 1 hour after an analgesic was administered? _____

Analgesic orders	Opioid	NSAID	Combination
Scheduled ATC	18. _____	19. _____	20. _____
PRN	21. _____	22. _____	23. _____

Route of administration (Check all that apply)
24. PO/SL (oral/sublingual) ___ 25. T (transdermal, topical) ___ 26. R (rectal) ___ 27. IM (intramuscular) ___
28. IV (intravenous) ___ 29. SC (subcutaneous) ___ 30. Epidural ___ 31. Intrathecal ___
32. PCA ___ 33. PCEA ___ 34. Intermittent bolus(es) ___ 35. Continuous infusion ___

36. Time audit ended: _____ Signature of auditor: _____

May be duplicated for use in clinical practice. As appears in McCaffery M, Pasero C: *Pain: Clinical manual*, p. 727, 1999, Mosby, Inc.

Form 16.2 is an example of a form used to collect data from the patient's medical record. Examples of other aspects of pain management that some institutions add to the audit tool are the occurrence and treatment of side effects and use of nondrug interventions.

Modified from *Quality improvement medical record audit tool*, Madison, Wis, 1998, University of Wisconsin Hospital and Clinics.

FORM 16.3 Pain Knowledge and Attitude Survey

We are interested in your individual answers. Please complete this survey on your own.

I. Circle *true* (T) or *false* (F) to each of the following statements:

    T F   1. Observable changes in vital signs must be relied on to verify a patient's statement that he or she has severe pain.

    T F   2. Pain intensity should be rated by the clinician, not the patient.

    T F   3. Patients can sleep in spite of moderate or severe pain.

    T F   4. Meperidine (Demerol) IM is the drug of choice for prolonged pain.

    T F   5. Analgesics are more effective when administered PRN rather than around-the-clock.

    T F   6. If the patient can be distracted from the pain, he or she does *not* have as high an intensity of pain as he or she reports.

    T F   7. The patient with pain should be encouraged to endure as much pain as possible before resorting to a pain relief measure.

    T F   8. Opioids (narcotics) act on the central nervous system to decrease the perception of pain, whereas nonopioid analgesics, such as aspirin, act on the peripheral nervous system to decrease the transmission of pain impulses.

    T F   9. Tylenol No. 3 (codeine 30 mg + acetaminophen 300 mg) is equal to approximately one sixth of a dose of meperidine (Demerol), 75 mg IM.

    T F 10. If a patient's pain is relieved by administration of a placebo, the pain is not real.

    T F 11. Beyond a certain dose, increases in the dose of an opioid (narcotic) analgesic, such as morphine, will not increase pain relief.

    T F 12. Research shows that promethazine (Phenergan) is a reliable potentiator of opioid analgesics.

II. Please use the following definitions (American Pain Society, 1992) to answer the questions below:

Opioid (narcotic) *addiction* or psychologic dependence is a pattern of compulsive drug use characterized by continual craving for an opioid and the need to use the opioid for effects other than pain relief. Physical dependence and tolerance are not addiction.

Tolerance to opioid analgesia means that a larger dose of opioid analgesic is required to maintain the original effect.

Physical dependence on opioids is revealed in patients taking opioids long term when the abrupt discontinuation of an opioid or the administration of an opioid antagonist produces an abstinence syndrome (withdrawal).

Circle one number closest to what you consider the correct answer to the following:

When opioids (narcotics) are used for pain relief in the following situations, what percent of patients are likely to develop opioid (narcotic) addiction?

13. All patients—overall	< 1%	5%	25%	50%	75%	100%
14. Patients who receive opioids for 1 to 3 days.	< 1%	5%	25%	50%	75%	100%
15. Patients who receive opioids for 3 to 6 months.	< 1%	5%	25%	50%	75%	100%

Answer key for knowledge and attitude survey:

1. F   2. F   3. T   4. F   5. F
6. F   7. F   8. T   9. T   10. F
11. F 12. F 13. <1% 14. <1% 15. <1%

• • • • •

FORM 16.4 Pain Management Patient Questionnaire

---

1. Have you experienced any pain in the past 24 hours?

    _____ (1) Yes   _____ (2) No

    If you answered "no" to question No. 1, please stop now. If you answered "yes," complete the rest of the questionnaire.

2. On this scale, how much pain are you having right now?

    0 1 2 3 4 5 6 7 8 9 10

    No   *Worst pain*
    pain   *possible*

3. On this scale, please indicate the worst pain you have had in the past 24 hours.

    0 1 2 3 4 5 6 7 8 9 10

    No   *Worst pain*
    pain   *possible*

4. On this scale, please indicate the average (usual) level of pain you have had in the past 24 hours.

    0 1 2 3 4 5 6 7 8 9 10

    No   *Worst pain*
    pain   *possible*

5. Circle the number below that describes how, during the past 24 hours, pain has interfered with your:

    A. General activity

    0 1 2 3 4 5 6 7 8 9 10

    Does not   *Completely*
    interfere   *interferes*

    B. Mood

    0 1 2 3 4 5 6 7 8 9 10

    Does not   *Completely*
    interfere   *interferes*

    C. Walking ability

    0 1 2 3 4 5 6 7 8 9 10

    Does not   *Completely*
    interfere   *interferes*

    D. Sleep

    0 1 2 3 4 5 6 7 8 9 10

    Does not   *Completely*
    interfere   *interferes*

6. Early in your care, did a physician or nurse make it clear to you that the treatment of pain is very important and that you should be sure to tell them when you have pain?

    _____ (1) Yes   _____ (2) No

    a) If yes, what was your comfort goal? _____

    I do not know _____

7. Select the phrase that indicates how satisfied or dissatisfied you are with the way your nurses responded to your reports of pain.

    _____ (1) Very dissatisfied
    _____ (2) Dissatisfied
    _____ (3) Slightly dissatisfied
    _____ (4) Slightly satisfied
    _____ (5) Satisfied
    _____ (6) Very satisfied

8. Select the phrase that indicates how satisfied or dissatisfied you are with the way your physicians responded to your reports of pain.

    _____ (1) Very dissatisfied
    _____ (2) Dissatisfied
    _____ (3) Slightly dissatisfied
    _____ (4) Slightly satisfied
    _____ (5) Satisfied
    _____ (6) Very satisfied

9. If you were **not** satisfied with your pain treatment in any way, please explain why.

10. When you asked for pain medication, what was the longest time you had to wait to get it?

    _____ (1) <10 minutes
    _____ (2) 10-20 minutes
    _____ (3) 20-30 minutes
    _____ (4) 30-60 minutes
    _____ (5) >60 minutes
    _____ (6) Asked for medication but never received it
    _____ (7) Never asked for pain medication

May be duplicated for use in clinical practice. From McCaffery M, Pasero C: *Pain: Clinical manual,* p. 729. Copyright © 1999, Mosby, Inc.

*The following can be added to question No. 5 depending on the setting and type of patient:

E. (For postoperative patients) Other activities that are needed to recover from surgery, such as turning, coughing, deep breathing, physical therapy

    0 1 2 3 4 5 6 7 8 9 10

    Does not interfere   *Completely interferes*

F. (For outpatients with chronic pain) Normal work, including housework

    0 1 2 3 4 5 6 7 8 9 10

    Does not interfere   *Completely interferes*

G. (For patients with chronic pain) Enjoyment of life

    0 1 2 3 4 5 6 7 8 9 10

    Does not interfere   *Completely interferes*

Form 16.4 provides an example of a patient questionnaire. It can be modified to suit the needs of the particular clinical setting and patient population.

Information from American Pain Society (APS): Quality improvement guidelines for the treatment of acute pain and cancer pain, *JAMA* 274(23):1874-1880, 1995.

ratings reflect a reaction to their overall care rather than to the quality of their pain management. No single indicator, including subjective pain assessments, can measure the true quality of pain management. Evaluating other indicators such as patient outcomes and actual reduction in pain, in addition to patient satisfaction, is recommended (Miaskowski, 1996).

Pain care committees can easily become bogged down in endless data collection and analysis. It is recommended that goals, such as a reasonable number of data and a realistic time frame for data collection, be targeted at the outset (e.g., 30 chart audits in 1 month's time). Efficient and expedient data collection and analysis ensure that the QI process moves forward. As discussed, the use of quality improvement tools (see Figures 16.1, p. 721, and 16.2, pp. 722-723) to analyze data and pinpoint problem areas is highly recommended to ensure that all important information, steps, and possible solutions are considered.

Committee Responsibilities

As discussed, the APS QI recommendations (see Box 16.2, p. 716) provide a format for the ongoing work of the pain care committee. The institutional needs assessment (see Form 16.1, pp. 724-726) helps to prioritize activities and to identify those that require immediate attention, such as establishment of standards for pain assessment, treatment, and documentation. Other needs may be less urgent, and many of them are met on a continuous basis, such as developing plans to monitor pain management improvements and provide ongoing pain management educational opportunities for patients and staff.

Most of the activities of the pain care committee require collaboration with several different departments and disciplines to accomplish the many interventions involved in institutionalizing pain management. Committee members must remember to ask for input from the staff who will be affected by a proposed change. As discussed, this approach is more likely to result in staff support and ownership of the improvement plan. It is not always necessary to develop an entirely new way of doing something, and staff members are often particularly skillful and clever at finding ways to modify existing systems to support the improvement effort. Following is an overview of the general committee responsibilities. Box 16.6 provides several suggestions for accomplishing them.

Define and implement standards for pain assessment, treatment, and documentation

The first APS recommendation is for institutional systems to support prompt recognition, treatment, and documentation of pain. To do this, the pain care committee must establish standards for pain assessment, treatment, and documentation (Box 16.7, p. 734). Establishing standards ensures that everyone involved in the care of patients with pain shares exactly the same understanding of what constitutes pain assessment, treatment, and documentation. Standards help to assign accountability and guarantee that what is being measured is done so uniformly over time. Without standards, it is impossible for clinicians to know where to start or when the goal of pain relief has been achieved. Standards provide a "measuring stick" that can be used to demonstrate improvements.

The problem of unrelieved pain has traditionally been invisible to even the most attentive caregiver (Max, 1990). An underlying responsibility of the pain care committee is to make pain more visible in the institution. To do this, some institutions have made pain the "fifth vital sign" and document it on the graphic vital signs record with the other four vital signs (Form 16.5, p. 735).

Make information about analgesics and nondrug interventions readily available

One of the goals of institutionalizing pain management is to confront the many misconceptions surrounding pain and replace them with research-based information. Documents like the AHCPR clinical practice guidelines on acute and cancer pain management and the APS principles of analgesic use (APS, 1992) should be readily available on the clinical units. Pain care committees often find creative and fun ways to disseminate pain management information. Box 16.6 presents several ideas for promoting research-based pain management practice.

Define accountability for pain management

Obviously, patients are likely to receive better pain relief if the health care system holds health care professionals responsible for assessing and relieving pain. Perhaps the most important function of the pain care committee is to establish accountability for pain management. Without it, improvement plans will ultimately fail. Therefore pain care committees must concentrate a great deal of their time and use a variety of approaches to define accountability for pain management. Box 16.6 lists several of these approaches.

The Role of Accreditation in Defining Accountability

Many experts think that widespread accountability for pain management will be elusive until the various agencies responsible for accrediting health care organizations issue clearer standards for pain assessment, treatment, and documentation (Berry, 1997). Accrediting agencies that have potential for increasing institutional accountability for pain management include the Joint Commission on Accreditation of Healthcare Organizations (JCAHO), the National Committee on Quality Assurance (NCQA), and the Commission on Accreditation of Rehabilitation Facilities (CARF).

Text continued on p. 733.

● ● ● ● ●

BOX 16.6	**Pain Care Committee Responsibilities**

DEFINE AND IMPLEMENT STANDARDS FOR PAIN ASSESSMENT AND DOCUMENTATION

1. Clearly state who will assess and document pain and how and when it will be assessed and documented:
   a. Who will assess and document (e.g., nurses, physicians)
   b. Characteristics of pain that will be measured (e.g., intensity, location, quality, onset, duration, aggravating and alleviating factors)
   c. How characteristics will be measured (e.g., self-report, physical examination)
   d. When characteristics will be measured (e.g., during initial examination, at least once every 8 hours, and within 1 hour of analgesic administration or other pain-relieving intervention)
   e. The patient's comfort goal
2. Individualize standards for special patient populations and departments as needed (e.g., pain assessment and documentation at least every 2 hours for first 24 hours after surgery).
3. Select a pain rating scale that can be used to assess pain in most patients with pain; select alternative pain rating scales for special patient populations served by the institution, such as preemies, neonates, infants, young children, non-English speaking patients, cognitively impaired patients, and non-verbal patients (see Chapter 3).
4. Develop a patient teaching plan and written information on the use of the selected pain rating scales, including the scales for special populations served by the institution (see No. 3 above). Determine the best locations to implement the patient teaching plan (where most patients are seen before or on admission, e.g., preadmission testing). Collaborate with the staff in these locations to integrate teaching the use of the pain rating scale and distributing written information to *all* patients and their families into their current teaching plan.
5. Revise medical record to include documentation of teaching patients about pain; use a pain management teaching checklist (see Form 6.2, p. 273) for complex pain management therapies.
6. Revise existing medical record flow sheets to include documentation of pain assessment; designate pain as the "fifth vital sign," e.g., revise vital signs graphic record to include documentation of pain ratings (see Form 16.5, p. 735).
7. Develop or revise flowsheet for analgesic infusion therapies (see Chapter 3, pp. 78-86).
8. Collaborate with management information systems to develop and revise computer programs to include prompts for appropriate pain assessment and documentation.
9. Ensure clinical units include monitoring for compliance with the pain assessment and documentation standards in CQI process.

DEFINE AND IMPLEMENT STANDARDS FOR PAIN TREATMENT

1. Integrate the use of a comfort goal into treatment (see Chapter 3, pp. 67-75):
   a. Clearly state that pain rated above the comfort goal will trigger an analgesic dose increase, additional analgesic, or other pain-relieving intervention.
2. Collaborate with management information systems to develop and revise computer programs to prompt appropriate prescribing and other treatment approaches, including nondrug interventions.

3. Ensure that clinical units include monitoring for compliance with the pain treatment standards in CQI process.
4. Amend policies and procedures to delineate roles and responsibilities for pain assessment, treatment, and documentation for every member of the health care team, including patients.
5. Members of the pain care committee should participate in the development of all clinical pathways to ensure pain is addressed appropriately.
6. Collaborate with the pharmacy and suppliers to ensure that the hospital formulary offers clinicians an appropriate selection of recommended analgesics at a reasonable cost.
7. Develop standardized preprinted physician's orders for analgesic therapies (e.g., IV PCA). Supply appropriate clinical units with copies.
8. Develop protocols to standardize the management of painful conditions such as sickle cell, pancreatitis, HIV-related pain, migraine headache.
9. Amend existing protocols for painful procedures, such as chest tube removal, venipuncture, nasogastric intubation, and circumcision, to include information about assessing and managing pain before, during, and after procedures.
10. Collaborate with appropriate departments (e.g., anesthesia, pain service) to develop policies, procedures, and preprinted orders that direct the safe use of advanced pain management therapies, such as epidural analgesia.
11. Amend conscious sedation protocol to include analgesia for any procedure thought to be painful (see pp. 384-386).

MAKE INFORMATION ABOUT ANALGESICS AND NONDRUG INTERVENTIONS READILY AVAILABLE

1. Supply clinical units with copies of Agency for Health Care Policy and Research clinical practice guidelines and the American Pain Society principles for analgesic use.
2. Provide clinicians with "cheat sheets" and pocket size quick reference guides (Box 16.8, p. 736) explaining key pain assessment and management principles for use at the bedside.
3. Post equianalgesic charts in a convenient location on all clinical units where analgesics are administered.
4. Incorporate the analgesics available in the institution's formulary into a reference guide of recommendations for the appropriate use of analgesics to treat various levels of pain (Table 16.3, p. 737). Post this guide in all areas where prescriptions are written.
5. Use the "form letter" approach to curb or halt unsafe pain management practices (e.g., the first three times a physician prescribes meperidine inappropriately, send a form letter explaining normeperidine toxicity). After the third prescription, ask a pharmacist to talk with the physician to ensure the information on normeperidine toxicity is given.
6. Work with suppliers and central processing department to provide appropriate nondrug equipment and supplies in clinical units.
7. Enlist volunteers to raise funds to purchase radios, cassette and CD players with headphones, and a variety of musical and relaxation selections for patient use; request volunteer assistance in distributing and assisting patients in the use of this equipment.
8. Investigate the possibility of expanding volunteer programs that focus on special populations of patients to other patients (e.g., expand the concept of "preemie cuddling" to

| BOX 16.6 | **Pain Care Committee Responsibilities—cont'd** |

spending time talking and visiting with elderly or isolated patients).

9. Include a pain management "update" in every issue of the hospital newsletter; ask physician members of committee to publish pain management information at regular intervals in the medical staff newsletter.

10. Collaborate with the hospital librarian or education department to develop a "pain management library" (see Box 1.2, p. 7, Box 1.3, p. 8, and Box 16.9, p. 738):
    a. Develop a system for staff to have access to journals with pain content to which the institution subscribes; ask about journals that are kept on clinical units (e.g., anesthesia, oncology).
    b. Subscribe to at least one journal and one book that offer general pain management content.
    c. Preview and consider purchasing audio and video tapes and CD-ROMs on pain management for both patients and staff.
    d. Consider producing customized resources for patients and staff.

11. Include pain management content on in-hospital television channel.

12. Display colorful posters presenting key pain management principles; focus on principles that will refute persistent misconceptions; post the principles in nurses stations and physician and staff lounges and bathroom stalls ("potty training").

13. Frame and post an enlarged pain rating scale in a conspicuous location (e.g., below television set) in every patient room or attach the scale to a long chain affixed to the wall next to the patient beds for easy reference.

14. Supply all appropriate areas, including the hospital's lobbies and waiting rooms, home health agencies, hospices, and physicians' offices, with institution-specific pain management-patient information brochures (see Box 6.38 on IV PCA and Box 6.39 on PCEA, pp. 291-292), the AHCPR consumer guides on acute pain and cancer pain management, and a list of resources such as support groups (see Chapters 5-7 for more on patient education materials).

DEFINE ACCOUNTABILITY FOR PAIN MANAGEMENT

1. Amend, if necessary, the institution's vision or mission statement so that it is compatible with promising patients attentive analgesic care; if an amendment is necessary, ask an upper level manager to attend a pain care committee meeting to address this issue.

2. Amend, if necessary, the Patient's Bill of Rights to include the relief of pain.

3. Promise patients attentive analgesic care. Ensure patients are taught about the harmful effects of unrelieved pain, their role, and the staff's role in achieving the best possible pain relief (see pp. 67-75).

4. Present the institution's pain management philosophy to all new employees during orientation and provide pain management updates to all employees at annual fire prevention and disaster recertification classes.

5. Recommend the appointment of a full-time equivalent registered nurse position to coordinate all the efforts to institutionalize pain management.

6. Provide regular reports to the administration, medicine, nursing, and pharmacy about committee activities and recommendations.

7. Share CQI findings, good and bad, with staff, physicians, upper-level managers, and administrators.

8. Regularly meet with nursing managers at all levels to discuss pain care committee activities and request their input and support of projects.

9. Incorporate accountability for pain assessment, treatment, and documentation into nurses' annual performance evaluations; institute peer review.

10. Collaborate with other committees on pain management issues of mutual concern (e.g., pharmacy and therapeutics, clinical practice, ethics).

11. Develop protocols to address ethical issues related to pain management (e.g., placebo administration); develop a process for employees and patients to report unethical pain management practices; communicate this process to everyone affected by the protocol, including physicians.

12. Establish a mechanism for communicating the pain management plan when patients transition across settings (e.g., from home to hospital, from clinical unit to clinical unit).

13. Establish lines of authority for pain treatment decisions in all settings (e.g., who to contact when the pain management plan fails to relieve pain after discharge).

14. Recommend the development of educational programs for appropriate disciplines aimed at ensuring the highest level of pain management competency.

15. Expand the bedside nurse's role in managing pain; include alternative treatment when initial analgesic prescription fails to relieve pain (e.g., supplemental bolus doses, increase dose); include what to do when this alternative fails.

16. Collaborate with pain service to expand bedside nurse's role in the management of advanced pain management therapies (e.g., administering epidural bolus doses, increasing and decreasing doses, removing epidural catheters).

17. Establish a PRN program and a nurse-based PCA program.

18. Collaborate with the pharmacy to establish a system to enable staff members to request consultation with a clinical pharmacist on difficult pain problems.

19. Establish protocol for requesting consultation or referral to pain team or pain service and support services such as pastoral care, social services, and physical therapy.

20. Prepare for accreditation inspections by outlining how pain assessment, treatment, and documentation standards are implemented.

CONTINUOUSLY MONITOR AND IMPROVE THE QUALITY OF PAIN MANAGEMENT

1. Ensure that clinical units include monitoring for compliance with pain assessment, treatment, and documentation standards in CQI process.

2. Ensure ongoing monitoring of patient satisfaction and outcomes.

3. Ensure ongoing monitoring of advanced pain management therapies (e.g., complications, side effects).

4. Address the cost of providing safe and effective pain management; work with appropriate departments to keep costs reasonable.

5. Regularly review findings (e.g., patient questionnaire findings, clinical pathway outcome data, drug use, adverse effect reports, and clinical unit CQI summary reports) to determine level of compliance with assessment, treatment, and documentation standards.

6. Collect and analyze additional data as needed to evaluate problem areas noted from regular review.

● ● ● ● ●

BOX 16.6 **Pain Care Committee Responsibilities—cont'd**

7. Investigate hunches committee members have about problem areas, including audit analgesic prescribing and administration practices, such as use of meperidine, simultaneous use of multiple opioids, inappropriate routes; commit to long-term monitoring of changes in patient outcomes, such as reduced complications and reduced length of hospital stay.
8. Develop improvement plans and recommendations on the basis of CQI findings.
9. Collaborate with the suppliers, manufacturers, and pharmaceutical representatives to improve pain management products and services.

PROVIDE CONTINUING EDUCATION OPPORTUNITIES FOR STAFF AND PHYSICIANS

1. Assist with the development of a system that will help ensure initial and ongoing competency of all appropriate disciplines in the performance of both basic and advanced skills required to manage pain, including the use of preceptors as needed to teach skills such as titration of analgesics, epidural analgesic administration, and epidural catheter removal.
2. Assist with the development of safe pilot programs to introduce new pain management protocols and therapies.
3. Encourage clinical units to devote a small part of monthly staff meetings to pain management teaching (e.g., a case presentation, explanation of a key principle, CQI findings). Offer to present content.
4. Assist with the planning and presentation of an annual pain management seminar or seek sponsorship for recognized

pain management experts to present during regularly scheduled department meetings once or twice yearly.
5. Provide opportunities for staff to participate in pain management rounds.
6. Enlist the support of suppliers, manufacturers, and pharmaceutical representatives to educate staff and physicians about pain management (e.g., speaker sponsorship, regular participation in annual recertification programs, presentation of new products at department meetings).

PROVIDE CONTINUING EDUCATION OPPORTUNITIES FOR PATIENTS AND OTHER CUSTOMERS

1. Collaborate with marketing department to disseminate pain management information to the public (e.g., development of institution-specific written materials, patient newsletter, media liaison).
2. Use the media to disseminate pain management information to the public (e.g., press releases, feature stories, "health minute" spots).
3. Assist with the planning and presentation of an annual luncheon for third-party payers (e.g., HMO, workers compensation, insurance company representatives) featuring an expert pain management speaker.
4. Develop and participate in pain management programs offered to the public.
5. Extend invitations for attending annual pain management seminar and expert speaker meetings to the physicians' office staff, patients, public, and media.

May be duplicated for use in clinical practice. From McCaffery M, Pasero C: *Pain: Clinical manual*, pp. 731-733. Copyright © 1999, Mosby, Inc.

Box 16.6 lists the general responsibilities of the pain care committee and the various approaches that can be taken to accomplish them.

JCAHO is extremely powerful in terms of influencing institutional accountability for practice. It is a private accrediting body that surveys more than 15,000 health care organizations in the United States, including 5000 hospitals (JCAHO, 1997). Achievement of JCAHO accreditation indicates the health care organization is in compliance with JCAHO standards, which focus on several processes, including patients' rights, assessment and care of patients, patient and family education, continuum of care, and improving organization performance. Although participation in a JCAHO survey is voluntary, there are strong financial incentives for organizations to pursue and achieve accreditation (e.g., Medicare funding). Thus literally every department and discipline in an institution is motivated to comply with the established JCAHO standards.

In the 1992 standards manual issued by JCAHO, effective pain management was stated as one of the rights of a dying patient. In 1994, JCAHO broadened this statement to cover all patients. In 1997 under a grant from the Robert Wood Johnson Foundation, JCAHO began working collaboratively with institutions to improve standards for pain assessment and treatment with plans to conduct national quality improvement programs to help health care facilities meet these standards (Berry, 1997;

JCAHO grasps the initiative on pain: New standards within two years, 1997).

During a JCAHO survey, the survey team looks for evidence of implementation and compliance with JCAHO standards and with institutionally established standards that support optimal quality care. A presentation outlining the pain care committee's improvement plans (see Box 16.6) is a means of demonstrating to surveyors how the standards for pain assessment, treatment, and documentation are implemented. The CQI process is used to demonstrate compliance with the standards.

Continuously monitor and improve the quality of pain management

Sustained improvements in pain management depend on the pain care committee's devotion to the CQI process. Although the pain care committee is not responsible for ongoing data collection and analysis, it is responsible for collaborating with the institution's quality improvement coordinator to amend existing systems for monitoring and evaluating staff performance to include compliance with standards and competency in pain assessment and management. The committee should review

● ● ● ● ●

BOX 16.7	**Example of Standards for Pain Assessment, Treatment, and Documentation**

1. Patients will be promised attentive analgesic care by being informed verbally and in writing at the time of their initial interview that effective pain relief is an important part of their treatment, that their report of unrelieved pain is essential, and that staff will respond quickly to their reports of pain.
⇒ Providing patients with verbal and written information about the institution's promise of attentive analgesic care will be documented in the patient's medical record.

2. Patients will be taught to use a (age-appropriate, condition-appropriate, language-appropriate) pain rating scale to report pain intensity.
⇒ Teaching patients about the use of the pain rating scale, including the type of scale, will be documented in the patient's medical record.

3. When patients are taught to use the pain rating scale, they will be asked to set a comfort (pain relief) goal. The comfort goal is articulated in terms of function and quality-of-life parameters. In setting the comfort goal, patients will be told that pain rated above the goal (e.g., > 3 on scale of 0 to 10) interferes with important activities the patient must be able to perform (e.g., deep breathing, ambulating, visiting with family) and will trigger an analgesic dose increase, additional analgesic, or other pain relief intervention.
⇒ The comfort goal and related patient teaching will be documented in the patient's medical record.

4. At the time of initial evaluation and *at least* once every 8 hours, *all* patients will be asked about the presence and intensity of pain. The initial pain assessment will include pain quality, location, onset, duration, aggravating and alleviating factors, effects of pain on function and quality of life, and response to past interventions.
⇒ Initial and subsequent pain assessments will be documented in the patient's medical record.

5. A pain rating greater than the patient's comfort goal will trigger an analgesic dose increase, additional analgesic, or other pain relief intervention.
⇒ The patient's medical record will show evidence of the use of a pain relief intervention.

6. Pain intensity will be assessed within 1 hour after a pain relief intervention.
⇒ The patient's pain rating within 1 hour after a pain relief intervention will be documented in the patient's medical record.

7. Pain ratings that are persistently above the comfort goal will trigger an interdisciplinary review of the pain management plan and a modification in treatment.
⇒ The patient's medical record will show evidence of an interdisciplinary review of the pain management plan and a modification in treatment.

May be duplicated for use in clinical practice. From McCaffery M, Pasero C: *Pain: Clinical manual*, p. 734. Copyright © 1999, Mosby, Inc.

Information from American Pain Society (APS): Quality improvement guidelines for the treatment of acute pain and cancer pain, *JAMA* 274(23):1874-1880, 1995.

regularly the CQI summaries submitted by the various clinical units monitoring the pain standards and the patients' medical record audits and questionnaire summaries. When problems are identified, the committee must investigate further and recommend corrective actions. The improvement process is ongoing and unending.

Provide ongoing educational opportunities for staff and physicians

The pain care committee is responsible for ensuring that staff and physicians are exposed to ongoing educational opportunities (see Box 16.6). Education is one of the most commonly used methods to effect change. However, although education has been shown to change an individual's knowledge base, changing an individual's behavior and practice are extraordinarily complex endeavors. They are influenced by many factors, including the clinician's training, personality traits, habits, experiences, motivations, social norms, expectations of others (Levin, Berry, Leiter, 1998), reimbursement, and society's concern about and interest in the particular issue (Epstein, 1991). Changes in pain management practice, in particular, are hampered by society's "just say no to drugs" philosophy and the current financial climate of managed care, which emphasizes decreased cost and use of health care services.

It is important for the pain care committee to develop educational opportunities with the understanding that when education alone is used, it often fails to change practice behaviors (Elliott, Murray, Oken et al., 1997; Ferrell, McCaffery, Rhiner, 1992; Levin, Berry, Leiter, 1998; Roenn, Cleeland, Gonin, et al., 1993; Weissman, 1996). The lack of widespread improvement in pain management despite mass dissemination of practice guidelines and consensus statements, such as the AHCPR clinical practice guidelines, demonstrates that increased clinician knowledge and improved attitudes are insufficient to accomplish practice changes (Ellrodt, Conner, Riedinger, 1995, Foley, 1995, Levin, Berry, Leiter, 1998; Lomas, 1991).

In one of the first studies to reveal the inadequacy of inpatient pain management, Marks and Sacher (1973) stated that the undertreatment of pain is much more complex than simple lack of knowledge. This was confirmed recently in a study that showed, even when clinician practice is changed through a combination of approaches, institutional barriers can be insurmountable (Rose, Cohen, Yee, 1997). Anesthesiologists in two hospitals in the same community were studied. Those in the experimental hospital were exposed to multiple educational approaches, including seminars, written literature, feedback, and an opinion leader over an 18-month period; those in the control hospital were given no interventions. Despite sustained significant

FORM 16.5 **Graphic Vital Signs Record**

VITAL SIGNS CHART

TEMPERATURE

Month-Day-Year			
Post Adm/Post-Op (BLACK)			

Hours of day: 4 8 12 4 8 12 4 8 12 4 8 12 4 8 12 4 8 12 4 8 12 4 8 12 4 8 12 4 8 12 4 8 12 4 8 12 4 8 12 4 8 12 4 8 12 4 8 12

Pulse (red) — **Temp C°**

160
150 — 41
140
130 — 40
120
110 — 39
100
90 — 38
80
70 — 37
60
50 — 36
40 — 35

X · TYMPANIC
O · ORAL
● · RECTAL

Respiration
10

Pain Intensity
5
0

Relief acceptable (Y/N)

Weight

N D E N D E N D E N D E N D E N D E N D E N D E N D E

Blood pressure

INTAKE
- Oral
- Tube feeding
- Supplements
- Intravenous
- Blood products
- TPN/PPN/Lipids
- 8-Hour total
- 24-Hour total

OUTPUT
- Urine
- Emesis/NG
- Stool
- 8-Hour total
- 24-Hour total

May be duplicated for use in clinical practice. As appears in McCaffery M, Pasero C: *Pain: Clinical manual*, p. 735, 1999, Mosby, Inc.
Graphing pain intensity ratings on the same form as other vital signs makes pain visible and provides an instant view of trends in the patient's pain.
Courtesy Memorial Sloan-Kettering Cancer Center, 1275 York Avenue, New York, NY 10021.

• • • • •

BOX 16.8   Example of Content for Pain Management "Cheat Sheet" or Pocket Size Quick Reference Guide

PRINCIPLES OF PAIN ASSESSMENT

1. Talk with patients about the benefits of good pain control.
2. Promise patients attentive analgesic care.
   a. Effective pain relief is an important part of their treatment.
   b. Their report of unrelieved pain is essential.
   c. Staff will respond quickly to their reports of pain.
   d. Good pain control leads to faster healing and fewer complications.
3. Teach patients to use the pain rating scale.
4. Help patients set a "comfort goal" (numeric pain rating, e.g., <4 on scale of 0 to 10). Tell them pain rated above the comfort goal must be reported and should trigger an analgesic dose increase, additional analgesic, or other pain-relieving intervention because the pain will interfere with their ability to perform activities such as deep breathing, coughing, and ambulating.
5. Ask patients about the presence of pain at regular intervals.
6. Accept and act on a patient's report of pain. Self-report is the single most reliable indicator of a patient's pain. The absence of behavioral (e.g., restlessness, agitation) and physiologic (e.g., ↑ HR, ↑ BP) signs does not mean that pain is absent.
7. Assess the pain, including intensity (pain rating), location, quality (e.g., aching, burning), onset, duration, what makes the pain better or worse, how pain affects function.
8. If possible, determine the cause of pain (e.g., tissue damage, nerve damage, tumor extension, obstruction).
9. Treat pain while completing evaluation and diagnosis.
10. Discuss goals and limitations of the pain treatment plan.
11. Discuss side effects and complications of analgesics and route of administration.
12. Reassess frequently and modify the pain treatment plan until pain is relieved.

PHARMACOLOGIC MANAGEMENT OF PAIN

1. Base initial choice of analgesic on the severity and type of pain:
   a. Mild pain (pain rating 1 to 3 on scale of 0 to 10): NSAID or acetaminophen or combination oral opioid-nonopioid.
   b. Moderate pain (pain rating 4 to 6 on scale of 0 to 10): NSAID or acetaminophen ± single entity mu-agonist opioid or combination oral opioid-nonopioid.
   c. Severe pain (pain rating 7 to 10 on scale of 0 to 10): Single entity mu agonist opioid + NSAID or acetaminophen.
   d. Mild, moderate, or severe neuropathic pain: May require adjuvant analgesics, such as an antidepressant or anticonvulsant.
   e. Avoid use of multiple opioids or multiple nonopioid analgesics when possible (e.g., when morphine is the mainstay analgesic, use morphine for supplemental [rescue] doses).
2. Increase dose to therapeutic ceiling for nonopioids. There is no analgesic ceiling on opioids. Increase the opioid dose until pain is relieved or side effects become intolerable and unmanageable.
3. Administer analgesics orally whenever possible. Avoid IM injections. Consider the IV route for severe, escalating pain.
4. For ongoing pain, administer analgesics ATC rather than PRN.
5. Anticipate and treat side effects, especially nausea, vomiting, constipation, sedation, and respiratory depression.
6. Consider decreasing the dose of the analgesic to treat a side effect; consider adding a nonopioid to maintain adequate pain relief.
7. Avoid dosing with meperidine (no more than 48 h or at doses greater than 600 mg/24 h). Accumulation of the toxic metabolite normeperidine can lead to CNS excitability and seizures. Meperidine is contraindicated in patients with impaired renal function and those receiving MAO inhibitors. It is a particularly poor choice in the elderly.
8. Addiction occurs very rarely in patients who receive opioids for pain control. Hallmarks of addiction include (1) compulsive use for reasons other than pain relief, (2) loss of control, and (3) use despite harm.
9. Do not use placebos to assess or treat pain.
10. Assess pain, pain relief, and side effects frequently and adjust the dose accordingly.
11. Change to another analgesic if side effects are unmanageable.

NOTE: The pain rating scale can be printed on the backside of the reference guide.

improvement in practice patterns of physicians in the experimental hospital (e.g., increased doses of morphine and increased prescriptions for use of PCA), both the study and control hospitals showed similar declines in postoperative pain ratings and only modest improvements in patient outcomes. Institutional barriers, such as unreliable stock of analgesics and protocols prohibiting the use of PCA outside of designated clinical units, were cited among the reasons for limited success in the experimental hospital; whereas the lack of institutional barriers in the control hospital may

have contributed to the decline in pain scores seen in that hospital.

Several institutions have blended the CQI process with education to improve behaviors and practices of both patients and caregivers (Bookbinder, Coyle, Thaler et al., 1996; Caswell, Williams, Vallejo et al., 1996; Dietrick-Gallagher, Polomano, Carrick, 1994; Ward, Gordon, 1996). For example, clinicians and patients are encouraged to talk with each other about pain and strategies for managing it before it occurs. Patients are asked to report all unrelieved pain, and clinicians are taught to assess it systematically and

● ● ● ● ●

TABLE 16.3 **Format for Formulary Analgesic Reference Guide**

MILD PAIN (PAIN RATING 1-3 ON 0-10 SCALE)	MODERATE PAIN (PAIN RATING 4-6 ON 0-10 SCALE)	SEVERE PAIN (PAIN RATING 7-10 ON 0-10 SCALE)
Select one of the analgesics below.	*Select a NSAID or acetaminophen ± opioid below.*	*Select opioid + NSAID or acetaminophen below.*
ACETAMINOPHEN Trade names: Rχ: Maximum recommended: Cautionary notes:	**ACETAMINOPHEN** Trade names: Rχ: Maximum recommended: Cautionary notes:	**ACETAMINOPHEN** Trade names: Rχ: Maximum recommended: Cautionary notes:
NSAIDS Trade names: Rχ: Maximum recommended: Cautionary notes:	**NSAIDS** Trade names: Rχ: Maximum recommended: Cautionary notes:	**NSAIDS** Trade names: Rχ: Maximum recommended: Cautionary notes:
COMBINATION ORAL OPIOID/NONOPIOID Trade names: Rχ: Maximum recommended: Cautionary notes:	**COMBINATION ORAL OPIOID/NONOPIOID** Trade names: Rχ: Maximum recommended: Cautionary notes:	**SINGLE-ENTITY OPIOIDS** Trade names: Rχ: Maximum recommended: Cautionary notes:
	SINGLE ENTITY OPIOIDS Trade names: Rχ: Maximum recommended: Cautionary notes:	

May be duplicated for use in clinical practice. As appears in McCaffery M, Pasero C: *Pain: Clinical manual,* p. 737, 1999, Mosby, Inc.

The analgesics available in the institution's formulary can be incorporated into a reference guide of recommendations for the appropriate use of analgesics to treat various levels of pain and posted in all areas wherever prescriptions are written.

Modified from St. John Hospital and Medical Center, Department of Pain Management: *Formulary pain medication reference guide,* Detroit, Mich, 1996, author.

make research-based treatment decisions. The QI process is used to monitor outcomes. This blended approach has resulted in modest improvements in pain management.

Provide ongoing educational opportunities for patients and families

Patients' and families' misconceptions and lack of knowledge about pain management are significant barriers to adequate pain relief (Ward, Goldberg, Miller-McCauley et al., 1993; Ward, Gatwood, 1994; Ward, Emery Berry, Misiewicz, 1996). Few patients realize they have the right to aggressive pain treatment, they fail to report their pain unless routinely asked about it (Ward, Gatwood, 1994), and most appear to have low expectations in terms of the health care team's ability to relieve pain. This is supported with research previously discussed that shows patients report satisfaction with their pain management despite poor pain relief (Miaskowski, Nichols, Brody et al., 1994; Ward, Gordon, 1996; Bookbinder, Kiss, Coyle et al., 1996).

To overcome these barriers, patients and families need information about the harmful effects of unrelieved pain and that pain can be relieved with relatively simple and safe methods. They must be taught how and when to communicate their pain. The health care team should seek patient and family input when developing pain management plans to help ensure plans are practical. Plans should include teaching patients and families how to manage both drug and nondrug methods of pain relief, including specific information to help overcome fears of drug addiction, tolerance, and side effects (Ferrell, Rhiner, Ferrell, 1996; Ferrell, Rivera, 1997). Finally, all patients and families should understand the lines of authority and accountability for pain relief and who to contact when pain is unrelieved with the prescribed pain management plan.

BOX 16.9 **Example of an Institutional Pain Management Library**

JOURNALS

Journal of Pain and Symptom Management
Elsevier Science Publishing Co., Inc.
Journals Fulfillment Dept.
P.O. Box 882, Madison Square Station
New York, NY 10160-0200
(212) 633-3730 or (888) 437-4636

Clinical Journal of Pain
Lippincott-Raven Publishers
P.O. Box 1600
Hagerstown, MD 21741-9910
(215) 413-4074

American Journal of Nursing monthly column, "Pain Control"
Subscription Dept.
P.O. Box 50480
Boulder, CO 80322-0480
(303) 604-1464 or (800) 627-0484

Nursing, "Controlling Pain" monthly column
P.O. Box 55338
Boulder, CO 90328-5338
(800) 879-0498

Roxane Pain Institute Reference Materials
Roxane Laboratories, Inc.
P.O. 16532
Columbus, OH 43216-6532
(614) 276-4000 or (800) 327-4865

BOOKS

Ashburn MA, Rice LJ, editors: *The management of pain,* New York, 1998, Churchill Livingstone.
Doyle D, Hanks GWC, MacDonald N, editors: *Oxford textbook of palliative medicine,* ed 2, New York, 1998, Oxford University Press.
Wall P, Melzack R, editors: *Textbook of pain,* New York, 1994, Churchill Livingstone.

VIDEO TAPES

McCaffery on pain: Nursing assessment and pharmacologic intervention in adults
McCaffery on pain: Contemporary issues in pain management
The physiology and pharmacologic management of pain
Pain in infants and children
All of the above video tapes can be obtained for free preview from Williams & Wilkins by calling (800) 527-5597.

May be duplicated for use in clinical practice. From McCaffery M, Pasero C: *Pain: Clinical manual,* p. 738. Copyright © 1999, Mosby, Inc.

An institutional "Pain Management Library" makes resources on general pain management readily available for staff and physicians.

Box 16.6 presents ideas for providing ongoing educational opportunities for patients and families and the public in general. The reader also is referred to previous chapters for specific patient teaching information (Chapter 3 for pain assessment, Chapters 5, 6, and 7 for use of various analgesics; Box 6.18, pp. 275-276, for discussing addiction, physical dependence, and tolerance with patients and their families; and Chapter 9 for the use of nondrug methods).

OTHER STRATEGIES FOR BUILDING INSTITUTIONAL COMMITMENT TO IMPROVING PAIN MANAGEMENT

External pressures, primarily from third-party payers, to improve the quality of health care, decrease costs, and standardize processes have resulted in the use of a number of strategies for changing practice patterns in health care. These include administrative rules, clinical pathways, pain services, and the use of role models and pain resource nurses (Elliott, Murray, Oken et al., 1997; Ellrodt, Conner, Riedinger et al., 1995; Greco, Eisenberg, 1993; Nathanson, 1994; Soumerai, Avorn, 1990; Weissman, Dahl, Beasley, 1993). These strategies can be used to complement the interdisciplinary pain care committee's efforts to institutionalize pain management.

Administrative Rules

When the AHCPR guidelines were released, educators in many institutions brought the problem of unrelieved pain to the attention of upper level management, resulting in a flurry of "administrative rules." Examples of administrative rules include utilization review, standardized protocols and physicians' orders, policies and procedures, and financial incentives and penalties.

The full impact of administrative interventions is difficult to determine. If not used appropriately, they can have an undesirable effect and create barriers to pain management, rather than eliminate them. For example, a policy or utilization review process that creates extra steps may be perceived as burdensome, leading clinicians to completely avoid addressing pain in their patients.

Another drawback to the use of administrative rules is that they may require additional staff and money to implement, both of which are hard to acquire. In addition, some clinicians perceive administrative rules as an intrusion in their practice and discount the recommendation for change entirely. Rather than motivating clinicians, some administrative rules, particularly financial penalties, can anger and repel clinicians. Financial incentives sometimes provide only a "quick fix" for a problem.

When administrative rules are used, simple approaches are recommended, such as altering physician order forms to cue a preferred analgesic and limiting the availability of undesirable analgesic formulations. These approaches have been used successfully to modify other practice behaviors, such as diagnostic testing and the prescribing of antibiotics (Coleman, Rodondi, Kaubisch et al., 1991; Humphries, Counsell, Pediani et al., 1997).

Clinical Pathways

Clinical pathways (also called critical pathways and care maps) are standardized day-to-day plans that guide the care of patients with specific medical or surgical conditions. These pathways are developed by a multidisciplinary team in an effort to decrease variation in practice, thereby reducing error and improving quality. Other expected outcomes include prudent use of resources, decreased cost of care, and shorter length of hospital stay (Gordon, 1996).

When developed correctly, clinical pathways can improve pain assessment and management with a daily treatment plan. However, their effectiveness as a tool for change depends on several factors. If a pain expert or someone who understands accepted pain management guidelines and standards is not included on the pathway development team, inappropriate interventions such as IM analgesics may be incorporated. Even worse, if the team developing a given pathway fails to recognize the impact of unrelieved pain, pain management may be left out completely. A shortcoming of clinical pathways is that they tend to be developed for the high-cost, high-morbidity conditions only, which excludes many patients with pain from care on the basis of these pathways.

Pain Services

The administration of advanced pain management techniques under the supervision of a team of certified and experienced clinicians is recommended (AHCPR, 1992). In 1995 it was estimated that more than half of the hospitals in the United States had acute pain services or had plans to establish one (Warfield, Kahn, 1995). Since the 1980s, growth in the number of chronic pain treatment facilities in the United States has been unprecedented and ranges from clinics that offer only invasive treatments such as nerve blocks to multidisciplinary rehabilitation programs (Kulich, Lande, 1997).

The development of specialized pain management consultation services has improved access to and quality of pain care for many patients (Schug, Torrie, 1993; Stacey, Rudy, Nellhaus, 1997). Often these services are organized as teams of clinicians within a medical department, such as anesthesiology or neurology. Many are developed in conjunction with the nursing department, which assigns one or more nurses to work with the team while remaining under the auspices of nursing (Pasero, Preble, 1992). Chronic pain services usually combine the expertise of multiple disciplines and departments, such as medicine, nursing, psychology, social services, physical rehabilitation, and occupational and respiratory therapy. The team assumes responsibility for training personnel, implementing specialized methods of pain control, and addressing the multiple problems patients with pain face.

Contributions and limitations of pain services

Research has revealed several benefits of providing therapies under the supervision of specialists. One study of more than 3000 postoperative patients showed that a wide range of invasive techniques can be offered and provided safely by an anesthesiology-based pain service

(Schug, Torrie, 1993). Another study compared PCA managed by primary surgeons to PCA managed by a dedicated pain service (Stacey, Rudy, Nellhaus, 1997). Although patients' pain scores were similar in both groups, pain service patients experienced fewer side effects, were more likely to receive a loading dose, and had more individualized therapy than patients managed by surgeons.

Patients with chronic pain also benefit from the specialist team approach. A multicenter evaluation of advanced cancer patients with pain cared for in a variety of settings by multidisciplinary palliative care teams showed a significant reduction in levels of pain and no patients experienced "overwhelming" pain (Higginson, Hearn, 1997). A cost/benefit analysis of a multidisciplinary chronic pain program produced a reduction in posttreatment outpatient visits, a decrease in inpatient length of hospital stay by 3 days, and a decrease in health care dollars over a 5-year period of nearly a half a million dollars for pain treatment for the 30 patients in the study (Kee, Middaugh, Pawlick et al., 1997).

Despite these successes, a dedicated pain management team may not be practical or economical in every institution, such as small or specialized institutions where a small percentage of patients would benefit. By themselves, pain services do not solve the problem of undertreated pain. A small group of experts cannot provide pain management for every patient within the organization. In addition, many pain services tend to provide only invasive pain treatments (e.g., blocks, epidural analgesia), which most patients do not require. Some pain programs focus only on specific types of pain, such as postoperative or chronic pain, and few pain services treat pain in children, infants, and neonates (Broome, Richtsmeier, Maikler et al., 1996). This selectivity has left several groups of patients without access to the same individualized pain management that pain service patients receive. Pain services also tend to provide only treatments that are reimbursed. For example, when third-party payment waned for postoperative IV PCA in the early 1990s, many pain teams abandoned its management.

Although pain teams have brought attention to the need for aggressive pain management in certain populations of patients, pain services also have introduced new barriers to effective pain management. The availability of pain services negates the primary physician's obligation to manage pain. By assuming all the responsibility for managing patients' severe or difficult to manage pain, pain services cause primary physicians to take a secondary role in this important aspect of their patients' care. Sometimes, continuity of care is lost as well. When the pain service completes its course of treatment, which is typically before pain is resolved, patients are referred back to their primary physicians, frequently without follow-up to ensure the patients' ongoing pain care needs are met.

Particularly bothersome is the "hands-off" philosophy many pain services have adopted, deliberately limiting the role of bedside nurses in managing the therapies the pain service offers. For example, in many institutions, bedside nurses are expected to monitor the vital signs of patients receiving epidural analgesia but are prohibited from titrating epidural doses, a function approved by most state boards of nursing. Pain services that impose these types of restrictions lose valuable staff input and risk patient safety. Bedside nurses are in the unique position of being able to provide individualized pain management ATC, an impossible task for the pain service to accomplish alone. Even pain services that offer ATC in-hospital availability cannot be at every bedside at the same time. Rather than restricting the bedside nurses' role, the best pain services expand and support it. Pain services that realize their own limitations and incorporate aspects of the pain resource nurse approach (see following) have met with a high degree of success (Hubbard, 1992, 1994; Pasero, Preble, 1992)

The postoperative rehabilitation program

The harmful effects of inadequate postoperative pain control have been discussed in previous chapters (see Chapters 2 and 6); yet relatively few studies have been able to demonstrate that pain relief alone is sufficient to consistently reduce postoperative complications. The persistent use of outdated, conservative surgical and nursing care practices is thought to contribute to the disappointing research findings (Kehlet, 1997, 1998). However, an exciting and potentially powerful alternative to traditional practice, called postoperative rehabilitation, may provide the key to achieving reliable reductions in postoperative morbidity (Kehlet, 1997, 1998).

The postoperative rehabilitation approach combines effective pain control techniques with aggressive preoperative teaching and early postoperative nutrition and mobilization. It focuses on reducing intraoperative stress, heat and blood loss, postoperative pain, immunosuppression, GI dysfunction, hypoxemia, sleep disturbances, immobilization, catabolism, and muscle wasting. Key recommendations include reducing the use of IVs, drains, and nasogastric tubes and increasing the use of minimally invasive surgical techniques and local anesthetic neural blockade (Kehlet, 1997, 1998).

Preliminary data on this approach suggest considerable improvement in postoperative recovery and reduction in hospital stay (Bardram, Funch-Jensen, Jensen et al., 1995; Moniche, Bulow, Hesselfeldt et al., 1995). The elderly appear to be among those who benefit the most from the postoperative rehabilitation approach.

The establishment of a formal postoperative rehabilitation program (also called managed outcome service or acute recovery services) requires institutional commitment to a goal broader than improving pain management because it mandates a complete change in the way postoperative care is delivered. Development of the program relies on the same processes used to develop clinical pathways and acute pain services, such as collaboration between multiple disciplines and departments and standardization of care. In addition, institutions must support a shift from "bed-oriented" to "activity-oriented" clinical units, which may require architectural design changes in some facilities (Kehlet, 1997). The postoperative rehabilitation program represents an invaluable opportunity for expanding the purpose and role of the acute pain service.

Role Model Programs

The health professional who teaches by example serves as a role model, which is one of the most important tools available to change inappropriate attitudes, validate the importance of providing pain relief, and reinforce the facts about pain and its management (Weissman, Dahl, Beasley, 1993). In 1992 the Wisconsin Cancer Pain Initiative offered the first nationwide formalized role model educational program to physicians and their nonphysician "clinical partners" (Weissman, Dahl, Beasley, 1993). Other versions of the original role model program have put a greater emphasis on institutional rather than individual practitioner change, with a focus on the nurse (Weissman, Griffie, Gordon et al., 1997) or physician/nurse team (Ferrell, Dean, Grant et al., 1995) as leaders of the change effort. Unfortunately, individuals who participated in these programs faced several common institutional barriers when they attempted to implement changes in their institutions, including high staff turnover and lack of time, resources, and appropriate treatments and analgesics (Ferrell, Dean, Grant et al., 1995; Weissman, Griffie, Gordon et al., 1997).

Preceptorships

Preceptorships (also called observerships, fellowships, and internships) provide participants with an opportunity to observe pain management role models in action. During a preceptorship, participants spend days to weeks as apprentices learning pain management and how to institutionalize pain management from an expert group of clinicians. Programs vary in content, but they usually include formal lectures, patient rounds and interaction, observation of procedures, contact with departments and disciplines involved in the delivery of pain management services, group discussions, and problem solving. Some observerships assign mentors to provide private tutorials during the observership and ongoing clinical or research supervision and consultation to participants after they return to their institutions (Breitbart, Rosenfeld, Passik, 1998) (Box 16.10 lists the names of institutions that offer preceptorship programs).

● ● ● ● ●
BOX 16.10

Preceptorships and Pain Resource Nurse (PRN) Programs

Preceptorships, Observerships, Fellowships

Mercy Hospital Medical Center
 Pain Management Services
 400 University Ave.
 Des Moines, IA 50314-1101
 (515) 247-3172 or (515) 247-3239
Comprehensive program focusing on acute, chronic non-malignant, and cancer pain; targeted for nurses, but pharmacists and physicians also may attend.

"Network Project"
Memorial Sloan-Kettering Cancer Center
 Department of Pain and Palliative Care
 1275 York Ave.
 New York, NY 10021
Send written request to attend to address above.
Two-week observership in cancer pain management, psychosocial oncology, and cancer rehabilitation for health care professionals from any discipline. Participants are selected on the basis of their potential to educate and train others within their own institution and community.

Nurse Fellowship in Pain and Palliative Care
Memorial Sloan-Kettering Cancer Center
 Department of Pain and Palliative Care
 1275 York Ave.
 New York, NY 10021
Send written request to attend to address above.
One-year internship in cancer pain management and palliative care for master's prepared nurses.

Palliative Care Nurse Preceptorship Program
Medical College of Wisconsin
 9200 W. Wisconsin Ave.
 Milwaukee, WI 53226
 (414) 257-6117
A three-day clinical and didactic program that focuses on pain and symptom management at end of life.

Beth Israel Hospital
 330 Brookline Ave.
 Boston, MA 02215
 (617) 667-8000; contact person: Kathy Horvath
Preceptorship is arranged on individual request; acute, chronic nonmalignant, and/or cancer pain content tailored to meet participant's needs; nurses, pharmacists, and physicians may attend.

Fox Chase Cancer Center
 7701 Burholme Ave.
 Philadelphia, PA 19111
 (215) 728-3009; contact person: Karen Davis
Preceptorship is arranged on individual request; cancer pain content tailored to meet participant's needs; time is spent with the entire health care team in both the inpatient and outpatient settings; nurses, pharmacists, and physicians may attend.

PRN Programs

City of Hope National Medical Center
 1500 East Duarte Rd.
 Duarte, CA 91010-3012
 (626) 301-8346; contact person: Dr. Betty Ferrell, Nursing Research and Education
Teaches attending nurses how to develop a PRN program in their own institutions.
⇒ City of Hope also offers a pain education program for selected clinical nurse specialists and quality assurance/improvement coordinators.

Mayo St. Luke's Hospital
Anesthesia Department and Training
and Education Department
 4201 Belfort Rd.
 Jacksonville, FL 32224
 (904) 296-3712 or (904) 953-8807
Prepares attending nurses to be PRNs in their own institutions.

May be duplicated for use in clinical practice. From McCaffery M, Pasero C: *Pain: Clinical manual,* p. 741. Copyright © 1999, Mosby, Inc.

Box 16.10 provides the names of institutions that offer preceptorship and/or PRN programs for nurses and other disciplines.

Contributions and limitations of the role model approach

Significant improvements in immediate and long-term knowledge have been demonstrated from using a role model approach, but its impact on actual practice patterns has not been studied (Breitbart, Rosenfeld, Passik, 1998, Ferrell, Dean, Grant et al., 1995; Janjan, Martin, Payne et al., 1996; Weissman, 1996). However, role model programs have shed light on institutional change, confirming that it occurs slowly and requires administrative support, multiple education strategies, and physi-cian input (Ferrell, Dean, Grant et al., 1995; Weissman, Griffie, Gordon et al., 1997). Past programs have shown that acute care hospitals are ideal settings for role model programs and positive change is most likely when the role model is a highly motivated, energetic, and charismatic "champion" (Weissman, Griffie, Gordon et al., 1997).

Although a valuable experience, attending a role model program or preceptorship requires clinicians to take time off from work and can be costly in terms of tuition. Even when tuition is free, the cost of other expenses, such as travel, hotel, and meals, must be considered. Sometimes the institution offering the program limits the number who can attend or has specific requirements to attend. In addition, as mentioned, the difficulties individuals who attend these programs face in transforming their experiences and new knowledge into widespread practice changes in their own institutions often are insurmountable.

Pain Resource Nurse Programs

One of the most innovative strategies to institutionalize pain management is the development of a pain resource nurse (PRN) program. Many are modeled after the original program offered by the City of Hope National Medical Center in Duarte, California, in 1992 (Ferrell, Grant, Ritchey et al., 1993) The purpose of a PRN program is to train a group of decentralized staff nurses to function as pain management experts for other staff members. Additional responsibilities of the PRN include serving as a role model, providing pain management education and consultation, and acting as an agent for change (see Box 16.10 for the names of institutions that provide opportunities to learn how to establish a PRN program).

Some pain services have applied the PRN concept by establishing a partnership with the bedside nurses in an effort to better address all types of pain within the institution (Pasero, 1994; Pasero, Preble, 1992). These programs are comprehensive, providing didactic education and ongoing preceptor experiences and clinical support for all levels of nursing staff (e.g., registered nurses, licensed vocational [practical] nurses, and nursing assistants) within the institution. Comprehensive PRN programs recognize that all members of the bedside nursing staff are crucial to providing safe and effective pain care.

Contributions and limitations of PRN programs

PRN programs are perhaps among the most successful of strategies used to change practice. In a recent survey of existing PRN programs, respondents reported positive impacts within their organization in terms of greater visibility and recognition of the importance of pain management; improvements in knowledge and attitudes of staff; increased patient teaching, pain assessments, and analgesic management; and wider use of nondrug interventions (Ferrell, Virani, 1998).

Although the availability of a PRN on every clinical unit 24 hours a day seems to be an ideal approach to improving pain management, sustained effectiveness depends on institutional commitment to the program. Nurses today face unprecedented staff shortages, pay and work hour reductions, and layoffs (Shindul-Rothschild, 1996). In many institutions PRNs are expected to care for as many patients as their coworkers, which severely limits the amount of time they can spend educating and assisting others with pain management problems. Many

PRNs feel stretched to address their own patients' pain problems during their shift, much less the pain problems of their coworkers' patients.

PRN programs are more likely to succeed in institutions that designate a full-time nursing position to coordinate and oversee the program (Pasero, Preble, 1992). The coordinating nurse is typically responsible for developing and spearheading all the other programs aimed at improving pain management in the institution, such as leading the pain care committee. A primary responsibility of the nurse who assumes this role is to procure incentives to motivate the PRNs, such as education contact hours, adjustments in workload, pay bonuses, extra time off, and formal recognition of the PRN's accomplishments and contributions.

Nurse-Based PCA Programs

Providing IV or SC PCA therapy for hospitalized patients with moderate to severe pain is becoming commonplace. However, most institutions lack an organized approach for teaching patients before initiating PCA therapy, ensuring therapy is initiated promptly, and maximizing its benefits on the clinical units. Some hospitals have solved these problems by centralizing and standardizing the process for providing PCA therapy (Pasero, 1994). Although an interdisciplinary approach is used to manage the patients under this system, it usually is referred to as the nurse-based PCA program.

The concept of the nurse-based PCA program is similar to the PRN program in that it expands the role of the bedside nurse as the patient's primary pain manager. The PCA program staffs one registered nurse in the hospital 24 hours a day who serves as a resource to the bedside nurses in managing patients receiving IV PCA. Other responsibilities of the PCA nurses include teaching patients before therapy is initiated and ensuring smooth initiation of therapy in the PACU for postoperative patients and on the clinical units for nonsurgical patients. The PCA nurses are also responsible for implementing the CQI plan for the program. Like the PRN, the PCA nurse serves as a role model, providing pain management education and consultation to the rest of the health care team.

Most often, the PACU nurse manager provides clinical nursing direction for the PCA program, guided by a protocol set forth by the pain care committee. The protocol standardizes the analgesics and medications used to manage side effects and guides the PCA nurses and bedside nurses in titrating IV PCA, adding adjuvant analgesics, and managing side effects (Pasero, 1994). When developing the protocol, the pain care committee seeks input from the surgeons and physicians who prescribe PCA. Although administrative decisions about the delivery of IV PCA are made by the pain care committee, the primary physicians provide medical direction for their own individual patients if the nurses have difficulty controlling pain or managing side effects based on the protocol. Occasionally, the anesthesiology department provides medical direction for the nurse–based PCA program. In some hospitals anesthesiologists refer their patients who are receiving epidural analgesia to a nurse–based PCA program for nursing management.

References

Agency for Health Care Policy and Research (AHCPR): *Acute pain management operative or medical procedures and trauma*, AHCPR Publication No. 92-0032, Rockville, Md, 1992, U.S. Department of Health and Human Services.

Agency for Health Care Policy and Research (AHCPR): *Management of cancer pain*. AHCPR Publication No. 94-0592, Rockville, Md, 1994, U.S. Department of Health and Human Services.

American Pain Society (APS): *Principles of analgesic use in the treatment of acute pain and cancer pain*, ed 3, Glenview, Il, 1992, APS.

American Pain Society (APS): Quality improvement guidelines for the treatment of acute pain and cancer pain, *JAMA* 274(23):1874-1880, 1995.

Bardram L, Funch-Jensen P, Jensen P et al.: Recovery after laparoscopic colonic surgery with epidural analgesia, and early oral nutrition and mobilisation, *Lancet* 345:763-764, 1995.

Berry P: JCAHO pain management standards, *Cancer Pain Update Issue* 45:2, 14, Fall 1997.

Blumenthal D: Total quality management and physicians' clinical decisions, *JAMA* 269(21):2775-2778, 1993.

Blumenthal D: The origins of the quality of care debate, *N Engl J Med* 335(15):1146-1148, 1996.

Bookbinder M, Coyle N, Thaler H et al.: Implementing national standards for cancer pain management. program model and evaluation, *J Pain Symptom Manage* 12(6):334-347, 1996.

Bookbinder, M, Kiss M, Coyle N et al.: Improving pain management practices. In McGuire DB, Yarbo CH, Ferrell BR, editors: *Cancer pain management*, ed 2, Boston, 1995, Jones and Bartlett Publishers.

Breitbart W, Rosenfeld B, Passik SD: The network project: a multidisciplinary cancer education and training program in pain management, rehabilitation, and psychosocial issues, *J Pain Symptom Manage* 15:18-26, 1998.

Broome ME, Richtsmeier A, Maikler V et al.: Pediatric pain services a national survey of health professionals, *J Pain Symptom Manage* 11:312-320, 1996.

Casalou RF: Total quality management in health care, *Hospital Health Services Admin* 36(1):134-146, 1991.

Caswell DR, Williams JP, Vallejo M et al.: Improving pain management in critical care, *J Quality Improv* 22(10):702-712, 1996.

Coleman RW, Rodondi LC, Kaubisch S et al.: Cost-effectiveness of prospective and continuous parenteral antibiotic control: experience at the Palo Alto Veterans Affairs Medical Center from 1987 to 1989, *Am J Med* 90:439-444, 1991.

Dietrick-Gallagher M, Polomano R, Carrick L: Pain as a quality management initiative, *J Nurs Care Qual* 9:30-42, 1994.

Elliott TE, Murray DM, Oken MM et al.: Improving cancer pain management in communities: main results from a randomized controlled trial, *J Pain Symptom Manage* 13(4):191-203, 1997.

Ellrodt AG, Conner L, Riedinger M et al.: Measuring and improving physician compliance with clinical practice guidelines: a controlled interventional trial, *Ann Intern Med* 122(4):277-282, 1995.

Epstein AM: Changing physician behavior: increasing challenges for the 1990s, *Arch Intern Med* 151:2147-2149, 1991.

Ernst DF: Total quality management in the hospital setting, *J Nurs Care Qual* 8:1-8, 1991.

Ferrell BR, Dean GE, Grant M et al.: An institutional commitment to pain management, *J Clin Oncol* 13(9):2158-2165, 1995.

Ferrell BR, Grant M, Ritchey KJ et al.: The pain resource nurse training program: a unique approach to pain management, *J Pain Symptom Manage* 8:549-556, 1993.

Ferrell BR, McCaffery M, Rhiner M: Pain and addiction: an urgent need for change in nursing education, *J Pain Symptom Manage* 7(2):117-124, 1992.

Ferrell BR, Rhiner M, Ferrell BA: Development and implementation of a pain education program, *Cancer* 72:3426-3432, 1996.

Ferrell BR, Rivera LM: Cancer pain education for patients, *Semin Oncol Nurs* 13(1):42-48, 1997.

Ferrell BR, Virani R: Institutional commitment to improved pain management: sustaining the effort, *J Pharm Care Pain Symptom Control* (6)2:43-55, 1998.

Foley K: Pain relief into practice: rhetoric without reform, *J Clin Oncol* 13(9):2149-2151, 1995.

Gordon DB: Critical pathways: a road to institutionalizing pain management, *J Pain Symptom Manage* 11(4):252-259, 1996.

Greco PH, Eisenberg JM. Changing physicians' practices, *N Engl J Med* 329(17):1271-1274, 1993.

Higginson IJ, Hearn J: A multicenter evaluation of cancer pain control by palliative care teams, *J Pain Symptom Manage* 14(1) 29-35, 1997.

Hubbard L: Community-based pain service. In Sinatra R, Hord AH, Ginsberg B et al., editors: *Acute pain: mechanisms and management,* pp 539-559, St Louis, 1992, Mosby.

Hubbard L: An acute pain management service in a large hospital, *Am J Pain Manage* 4:167-171, 1994.

Humphries CA, Counsell DJ, Pediani RC et al.: Audit of opioid prescribing: the effect of hospital guidelines, *Anaesthesia* 52:745-749, 1997.

Janjan NR, Martin CG, Payne R et al.: Durability of education in cancer pain management principles with the role model program, *Cancer* 77:996-1001, 1996.

JCAHO grasps the initiative on pain: new standards within two years, *Med Ethics Advisor* October: 113-116, 119, 1997.

Kee WG, Middaugh S, Pawlick K et al.: Cost benefit analysis of a multidisciplinary chronic pain program, *Am J Pain Manage* 7(2):59-62, 1997.

Kehlet H: Multimodal approach to control postoperative pathophysiology and rehabilitation, *Br J Anaesth* 78:606-617, 1997.

Kehlet H: Modification of responses to surgery by neural blockade. In Cousins MJ, Bridenbaugh PO, editors: *Neural blockade,* pp 129-175, Philadelphia, 1998, Lippincott-Raven.

Kulich R, Lande SD: Managed care. the past and future of pain treatment, *APS Bull* 7(4):1, 4-5, 1997.

Levin ML, Berry JI, Leiter J: Management of pain in terminally ill patients: physician reports of knowledge, attitudes, and behavior, *J Pain Symptom Manage* 15(1):27-40, 1998.

Lomas J: Words without actions? The production, dissemination, and impact of consensus recommendations, *Ann Rev Public Health* 12: 41-65, 1991.

Marks RM, Sachar EJ: Undertreatment of medical inpatients with narcotic analgesics, *Ann Int Med* 78(2):173-181, 1973.

Max MB: Improving outcomes of analgesic treatment: is education enough? *Ann Intern Med* 113:885-889, 1990.

Max MB: American Pain Society quality assurance standards for relief of acute pain and cancer pain. In Bond MR, Charlton JE, Woolf CJ, editors: *Proceedings of the VIth World Congress on Pain,* Amsterdam 1991, Elsevier.

Miaskowski C: Commentary, *J Pain Symptom Manage* 12(6):331-333, 1996.

Miaskowski C, Nichols R, Brody R et al.: Assessment of patient satisfaction utilizing the American Pain Society's quality assurance standards on acute and cancer related pain, *J Pain Symptom Manage* 9(1): 5-11, 1994.

Moniche S, Bulow S, Hesselfeldt P et al.: Convalescence and hospital stay after colonic surgery with balanced analgesia, early oral feeding, and enforced mobilisation, *Eur J Surg* 161:283-288, 1995.

Nathanson P: Influencing physician practice patterns, *Top Health Care Finance* 20(4):16-25, 1994.

Pasero C: *Acute pain management service policy and procedure manual,* Rolling Hills Estates, Calif, 1994, Academy Medical Systems.

Pasero C: Making your pain care committee effective, *Am J Nurs* 97(3):17-19, 1997.

Pasero C, Preble LM: Role of the clinical nurse coordinator. In Sinatra R, Hord AH, Ginsberg B et al., editors: *Acute pain: mechanisms and management,* pp 552-559, St. Louis, 1992, Mosby.

Roenn JH, Cleeland CS, Gonin R: Physician attitudes and practice in cancer pain management: a survey from the Eastern Cooperative Oncology Group, *Ann Int Med* 119:121-126, 1993.

Rose DK, Cohen MM, Yee DA: Changing the practice of pain management, *Anesth Analg* 84:764-772, 1997.

Schiff GD, Goldfield NI: Deming meets Braverman: toward a progressive analysis of the continuous quality improvement paradigm, *Int J Health Serv* 24:655-673, 1994.

Scholtes PR, Joiner BL, Streibel BJ: *The team handbook,* ed 2, Madison, Wis, 1996, Joiner Associates.

Schug SA, Torrie JJ: Safety assessment of postoperative pain management by an acute pain service, *Pain* 55:387-391, 1993.

Shindul-Rothschild J: Patient care. How good is it where you work? *Am J Nurs* 96(3):22-24, 1996.

Soumerai SB, Avorn J: Principles of educational outreach (academic detailing) to improve clinical decision making, *JAMA* 263(4):549-556, 1990.

Stacey BR, Rudy TE, Nellhaus D: Management of patient-controlled analgesia: a comparison of primary surgeons and a dedicated pain service, *Anesth Analg* 85:130-134, 1997.

Ward S, Emery Berry P, Misiewicz H: Caregiver and patient concerns about analgesics: a comparison of dyads in a hospice setting, *Res Nurs Health* 19(3):205-211, 1996.

Ward S, Gatwood J: Concerns about reporting pain and using analgesics: a comparison of persons with and without cancer, *Cancer Nurs* 17(3):200-206, 1994.

Ward S, Goldberg N, Miller-McCauley V et al.: Patient-related barriers to management of cancer pain, *Pain* 52:319-324, 1993.

Ward S, Gordon DB: Application of the American Pain Society's quality assurance standards, *Pain* 56:299-306, 1994.

Ward S, Gordon DB: Patient satisfaction and pain severity as outcomes in pain management: a longitudinal view of one setting's experience, *J Pain Symptom Manage* 11(4):242-251, 1996.

Warfield CA, Kahn CH: Acute pain management: programs in U.S. hospitals and experiences and attitudes of U.S. adults, *Anesthesiology* 83:1090-1094, 1995.

Weissman DE: Cancer pain education for physicians in practice establishing a new paradigm, *J Pain Symptom Manage* 12(6):364-371, 1996.

Weissman DE, Dahl JL, Beasley JW: The cancer pain role model program of the Wisconsin Cancer Pain Initiative, *J Pain Symptom Manage* 8:29-35, 1993.

Weissman DE, Griffie J, Gordon DB et al.: A role model program to promote institutional changes for pain management of acute and cancer pain, *J Pain Symptom Manage* 14(5):274-279, 1997.

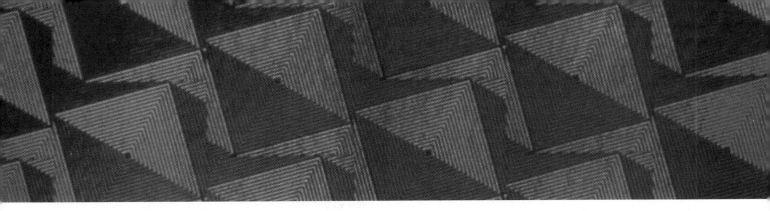

appendix A
PAIN RESOURCES ON THE INTERNET

Jan L. Frandsen

INTRODUCTION

The internet was created in 1969 to provide government scientists with a tool to send and receive information between collaborating sites, although it gradually expanded from being a government entity only. What we now know as the World Wide Web was created by European physicists who needed to send information to each other. They developed the hypertext markup language (HTML), which can be used to send and receive documents, sound, and live pictures—provided one has the software to perform these tasks. As a result of the High-Performance Computing Act of 1991, internet access was made available to the public through telecommunications companies, information services, and other public access systems.

The information that was initially available to the public on the internet was relatively limited, but today the internet has more than 38 million sites on the World Wide Web alone. Over 1000 sites are added to the World Wide Web daily. Furthermore, mailing lists, gopher sites, and other areas are accessible to the general public. One may liken internet access to a gigantic, continuously expanding library. In addition, features such as chat rooms, newsgroups, and mailing lists bring together people from across the world to share and discuss experiences, information, and knowledge. The volume of information—including medical information—is growing rapidly. Consequently the internet attracts both health care professionals and patients.

INFORMATION ABOUT THE INTERNET

As the internet has become more popular, the amount of information found there has grown proportionally. Most well-stocked bookstores or computer stores carry a variety of books written for all levels of usage on the subject of the internet. Numerous magazines about the internet are also available, and most computer magazines have columns, sections, or features devoted to the internet and related topics. Of course, information about the internet is available on the internet itself.

ACCESS TO THE INTERNET

Several ways are available to access the internet. An increasing number of organizations have internal electronic mail (e-mail) with a so-called "gateway" for sending and receiving e-mail via the internet. Most higher educational facilities have internet access, and more public libraries are providing computers for their patrons to access the World Wide Web. Finally, one can subscribe to commercial on-line services or direct internet service providers (ISPs), which can be accessed from a personal computer.

For those who want to access the internet from home, many of the commercial on-line services and ISPs currently offer a flat fee or free access for those who subscribe to their service. These services and their features are reviewed regularly in computer or home/office magazines. A resource guide that is written specifically for nurses on the subject of accessing the internet and has references to usenet groups, mailing lists, and sites on the Web is also available (Nicoll, Oulette, 1997)

SELECTED FEATURES OF THE INTERNET

The features that are most useful for both patients and health care providers are primarily, but not limited to, e-mail, mailing lists, newsgroups, and the World Wide Web.

Electronic Mail

Electronic mail is an effective way of communicating and exchanging information and serves as an alternative to the use of the phone and fax. Because e-mail can be composed, sent, and read at a time convenient for both sender and receiver, it is very convenient and cost effective. Furthermore, e-mail can be saved in an electronic form. For example, communications pertaining to the writing of this part of the book were done with e-mail, and the transcripts of these messages are now saved on a floppy disk, in a process similar to the way documents are filed in a filing cabinet.

If necessary one can also transmit an e-mail with one or more documents attached to the message. This can be highly advantageous when two or more people are collaborating on a project, such as the writing of a scientific paper. The attached document can be formatted in many ways. Word-processing documents, software, slide presentation files, and photos can be transmitted this way. However, one should ensure that the receiver has the correct software to open or translate the attached document.

Mailing Lists

A mailing list contains the names and e-mail addresses of a group of individuals with similar interests for the purpose of sharing information over the internet. The concept of a mailing list can be described as follows:
1. A subscriber posts a question, comment, or some other information.
2. The posting is then distributed to all subscribers.

The members can then act as a group by responding to the posting as though it was a regular e-mail message. The lists of available topics are almost unlimited. The resource list at the end of this appendix includes a few selected mailing lists related to pain management and a Web site where the reader can search for mailing lists geared toward a specific topic.

When subscribing to a mailing list, one must often follow a subscription policy. The subscription process varies a little from one mailing list to another, but when a mailing list is mentioned, details on the subscription procedure are generally included. Nicoll and Oulette (1997) provide some general rules on how to subscribe to mailing lists. Subscriptions to mailing lists are free of surcharges; however, some health care mailing lists require that the subscriber be a health care provider.

Mailing lists transmit information to their subscribers as individual messages or in digest form. The digest form is distributed as one e-mail document containing all the messages sent to the mailing list over a given time period, such as 24 hours. The digest form might be preferable to the individual messages because some mailing lists may send 100 or more messages per day, which can be inconvenient and more time consuming to read.

Newsgroups

Thousands of newsgroups exist on the internet, and as the internet grows, so does the number of these groups. One can compare newsgroups with any public (electronic) bulletin board. Newsgroups are located on a part of the internet known as the Usenet. Unlike mailing lists, one does not subscribe to a newsgroup. Instead access is made through software provided by an ISP or through the use of commercial software.

Newsgroups provide a unique opportunity for individuals to meet and communicate with each other. However, most newsgroups are not moderated, so the quality of information found there may not be as high as that of mailing lists.

Usenet groups related to medical topics are very active and provide a network and means of support for individuals with a particular illness, such as cancer. On some commercial information services, one can access forums that function similarly to the newsgroups. However, participation is limited to members of that particular service only.

As a health care provider, one must be careful when responding to messages related to medical or nursing advice in newsgroups because it could be considered practicing nursing or medicine across state lines. Should someone decide to take legal action based on advice given via the internet, some insurance carriers might not provide coverage in the event of malpractice. Although a disclaimer at the end of a message does not free one from liability, it could be helpful.

File Transfer Protocol

File transfer protocol (FTP) is a method of transferring electronic files to a personal computer from a remote computer. A wide variety of services are available through FTP, and one can obtain everything from the text of Supreme Court opinions to computer freeware and shareware.

Gopher

The gopher is an alternative type of web browser that enables the internet user to browse for resources. The gopher is really an electronic version of the library card catalog. However, once the gopher service locates the needed information, it can retrieve the file on the host computer.

The World Wide Web

Many people think that the World Wide Web (also known as the Web) and the internet are the same entity. However, the Web is only one part of the entire internet. Information on this part of the internet is written in hypertext markup language (HTML) and uses a hypertext transfer protocol (http), a special protocol that allows the user not only to read text, but also to view pictures and movies and hear sound. This information can be transmitted using either regular or cellular telephone lines or fiberoptic lines. In addition, http and HTML enable the user to connect to other areas in the same document, other documents on the same computer, other Web sites, or other file transfer protocol (FTP) servers. For example, if the Web site of the American Pain Society *(http://www.ampainsoc.org)* is accessed (Figure A.1), the user can select a link and move directly to the International Association for the Study of Pain's Web site, and from this site branch out to other sites.

American Pain Society

About APS

Membership

Annual Meeting

Publications

APS Bulletin

Pain Facilities

Advocacy

Resources

Awards and Recognition

Calendar of Events

Site Guide

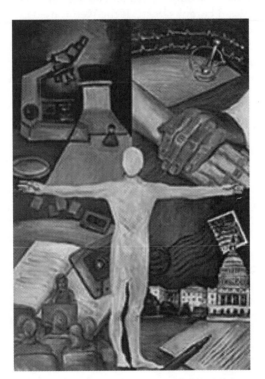

The **AMERICAN PAIN SOCIETY (APS)** is a multidisciplinary educational and scientific organization dedicated to serving people in pain. The society was founded in 1978 as a national chapter of the International Association for the Study of Pain (IASP), and now includes more than 3,200 physicians, nurses, psychologists, dentists, scientists, pharmacologists, therapists and social workers who research and treat pain and advocate for patients with pain.

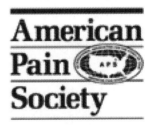

AMERICAN PAIN SOCIETY
4700 W. Lake Avenue • Glenview, IL 60025
Tel 847/375-4715 • Fax 847/375-4777
E-mail info@ampainsoc.org

About APS | Membership | Annual Meeting | Publications
APS Bulletin | Pain Facilities | Advocacy | Resources
Awards and Recognition | Calendar of Events | Site Guide | Home

Copyright © 1996-1998 American Pain Society.
http://www.ampainsoc.org
If you have any technical problems or suggestions regarding these webpages, please contact the WebMaster at webmaster@ampainsoc.org.

FIGURE A.1   The American Pain Society home page. Using links (i.e., the buttons on the left and underlined text), one can access other areas of the APS Web site or Web sites outside the APS server, such as the International Association for the Study of Pain.

The type of software that enables the user to access sites on the internet is called a Web browser. These browsers provide a graphical interface between the personal computer and the internet so that the personal computer can "read" files on the Web.

The places one accesses information on the Web are called Web sites, which consist of one or more Web pages. The first page of a Web site, frequently referred to as the home page, often contains an index from which one can access other pages on the Web site via hyperlinks (see Figure A.1). Web addresses, also known as uniform resource locators (URLs), are used to simplify returning to a site. Because these addresses can be long and complicated, most Web browsers allow users to "bookmark" pages of interest.

A very helpful and comprehensive pain management site for novice pain clinicians is that of C. Richard Chapman at the University of Washington *(http://weber.u. washington.edu:80/~crc/)*. Dr. Chapman has a variety of links to sites with information pertaining to pain management that are of interest to both patients and professionals.

LOOKING FOR INFORMATION ON THE INTERNET

Given the vast amount of information available, looking for information on the internet can be a daunting task, comparable to searching the card catalog at the library. However, because the net is an electronic database, one can search very large amounts of data in a very short time. For example, the keyword "pain" yields an impressive 453,170 sites. When the search is narrowed down to "acute pain," the number of sites decreases to 221,780.

Clearly the search should be narrowed to very specific terms, and more than one search may be necessary. Using the help function of the search engine to maximize its efficiency is strongly recommended. In the selected list of Web sites, some of the search engines' Web sites are listed.

Once the desired Web site has been located, one may wish to return to the site in the future without repeating the search. This can be done with the bookmark, or "favorite places," function on the Web browser. If more than one user is using the same browser, each person should have a different subset of bookmarks. A variety of internet resources are listed at the end of this appendix.

QUALITY OF INFORMATION ON THE INTERNET

In an editorial in the *Journal of the American Medical Association,* Silberg, Lundberg, and Mussachio (1997) wrote, "Health care professionals and patients alike should view with equal parts delight and concern the exponential growth of the internet. . . . The problem is not too little information but too much, vast chunks of it incomplete and not only in the medical arena." (p. 1244) The authors go so far as to call it "the world's largest vanity press," offering the warning *"Caveat lector et viewor*—let the reader and viewer beware."

If the Web is used as an information resource, the user must beware its pitfalls. Much good information can be found on the Web, but the information should be scrutinized at least as carefully as one would do with other sources, such as journals and books. As health care providers, we need to let our patients know that information from the Web may not be supported with sound scientific data, and some of the information may be false or deceptive (McClain, 1997).

The Web is currently a free-for-all, where anyone can post any information about any subject without the protection of the well-established standards applied to books and peer-reviewed journals. The industry is taking a strong stand in developing ways to police this medium without legislation. Several initiatives involving government, industry, and professional organizations are being undertaken to improve the quality of medical information available on the Web.

Mailing lists, Web sites, and e-mail addresses pertaining to pain management clinicians are listed in Table A.1. The listing of a commercial Web site should not be considered an endorsement of the company or its products. The list was checked at the time of submission and found to be accurate, but addresses are subject to change by the provider of the service without prior notice.

References

McClain JD: Hundreds of dubious health claims found on the internet, *Nursing Weekly* November 17, 1997.

Nicoll LH, Oulette TH: *Nurses' guide to the internet,* Philadelphia, 1997, JB Lippincott.

Silberg WM, Lundberg GD, Mussachio RA: Assessing, controlling and assuming the quality of medical information on the internet: *caveat lector et viewor*—let the reader beware, *JAMA* 277(15):1244, 1997.

TABLE A.1   **Selected List of Web Sites and E-mail Addresses With Specific Application to the Pain Management Clinician**

SOURCES FOR PAIN-RELATED INFORMATION

Abbott Laboratories	*http://www.abbott.com*
Agency for Health Care Policy and Research	*http://www.ahcpr.gov*
Am J Nurs/Lippincott Nursing Center	*http://www.nursingcenter.com*
American Academy of Hospice and Palliative Care	*http://www.aahpm.org*
American Academy of Pain Management	*http://www.aapainmanage.org/index.html*
American Association of NeuroScience Nurses	*http://www.aann.org*
American Cancer Society	*http://www.cancer.org*
American Chronic Pain Organization, Inc.	*http://www.coolware/health/medical_reporter/pain.html*
American College of Physician Homecare Guide for Cancer Pain	*http://www.acponline.org/public/homecare*
American Council for Headache	*http://www.achenet.org/index.html*
American Foundation for Pain Research (Interstitial Cystitis)	*http://www.social.com/health/nhic/data/hr2300/hr2313.html*
American Nurses Association	*http://www.nursingworld.org*
American Pain Society	*http://www.ampainsoc.org*
American Society for Action on Pain	*http://www.calyx.net/967Eschaffer/asap/asapain.html*
Arthritis Foundation	*http://www.arthritis.org*
Astra	*http://www.Astra.com*
Baxter Healthcare	*http://www.Baxter.com*
C. Richard Chapman's Home Page	*http://weber.u.washington.edu:80/~crc/*
C. Richard Chapman's Patient Resource Page	*http://weber.u.washington.edu:80/~ crc/CRCPage/patients.html*
Cancer Care	*http://www.cancercare.corr*
Centers for Disease Control	*http://www.cdc.gov*
Chronic Fatigue Immune Deficiency Syndrome Association of America	*http://www.sunflower.org/~cfsdays/fmsfiles.html*
Dee's Pain Management Site	*http://web-shack.com/dee*
Food and Drug Administration	*http://www.FDA.gov*
Gerontological Society of America	*http://www.geron.org*
Healthgate Access to Medline Search	*http://www.healthgate.com*
Helpfull Essential Links to Palliative Care (HELP)	*http://www.dundee.co.uk./MedEd/help/welcome.html*
Hospice Foundation of America	*http://www.hospicefoundation.org*
Hospice Hands (Cyberspace Hospice Resource)	*http://hospice-cares.com*
International Association for the Study of Pain	*http://www.halcyon.com/iasp*
Internet Alcohol Recovery Center	*http://www.med.upenn.edu/~recovery*
Mailing List for Amputees	Send e-mail to: *listserv@sjuvm.stjohns.edu* (in the message write Subscribe AMPUTEE <your first name> <your last name>)
Mailing List for Breast Cancer	Send e-mail to: *listserv@morgan.urcs.mun.ca* (in the message write Subscribe BREAST-CANCER <your first name> <your last name>)
Mailing List for Chronic Fatigue Syndrome	Send e-mail to: *listserv@list.nih.gov* (in the message write Subscribe CFS-MED <your first name> <your last name>)
Mailing List for Ovarian Cancer	Send e-mail to: *listserv@sjuvm.stjohns.edu* (in the message write Subscribe OVARIAN <your first name> <your last name>)

Continued.

TABLE A.1   **Selected List of Web Sites and E-mail Addresses With Specific Application to the Pain Management Clinician—cont'd**

SOURCES FOR PAIN-RELATED INFORMATION—cont'd

Mailing List for Rare Disorders	Send e-mail to: *listserv@sjuvm.stjohns.edu* (in the message write Subscribe RARE-DIS <your first name> <your last name>)
Mayday Pain Resource Center at the City of Hope	Send e-mail to: *mayday_pain@smtplink.coh.org*
Medscape	*http://www.medscape.com*
Morbidity and Mortality Weekly Report (MMWR)	*http://www.cdc.gov/mmwr.mmwr.html*
National Clearinghouse for Alcohol and Drug Information	*http://www.health.org*
National Council on Alcoholism and Drug Dependence	*http://www.ncadd.org*
National Headache Foundation	*http://www.headaches.org*
National Hospice Organization	*http://www.nho.org*
National Institute for Nursing Research	*http://www.nih.gov/ninr*
National Library of Medicine	*http://www.nlm.gov*
National Organization of Rare Diseases (NORDO)	*http://www.pcnet.com/~orphan*
National Rehabilitation Information Center	*http://www.naric.com/naric*
National Vulvodynia Foundation	*http://www.ivf.com/nvabackg.html*
Neurosciences on the Net	*http://lm.com/~nab/*
Newsletter for Chronic Fatigue Syndrome	Send e-mail to: *listserv@list.nih.gov* (in the message write Subscribe CFS-NEWS <your first name> <your last name>)
OncoLink	*http://cancer.med.upenn.edu/*
Oncology Nursing Society	*http://www.ons.org*
Oncopain (mailing list for health care professionals)	Send e-mail to: *oncopain@med.ucalgary.ca* (in message write Subscribe ONCOPAIN <your first name> <your last name> <credential> <title> <department> < institution>)
Project Death	*http://www.soros.org/death*
Purdue-Frederick	*http://www.partnersagainstpain.com*
Reflex Sympathetic Dystrophy Association	*http://www.cyboard.com/rsds*
Roxane Laboratories	*http://www.Roxane.com*
Search engine for more than 60000 mailing lists	*http://www.liszt.com*
Search engine for newsgroups and mailing lists	*http://www.reference.com*
Sigma Theta Tau	*http://stti-iupui.edu*
Simms-Deltec	*http://www.Deltec.com*
University of Iowa Cancer Pain Education	*http://coninfo.nursing.uiowa.edu./www/nursing/apn.cncrpain.toc.html*
USA Fibromylagia Association	*http://www.w2.com/fibro1.html*
World Wide Web search engine	*http://www.altavista.digital.com*
World Wide Web search engine	*http://www.lycos.com*
World Wide Web search engine	*http://www.yahoo.com*
World Wide Web search engine	*http://www.infoseek.com*
Worldwide Congress on Pain	*http://www.pain.com*

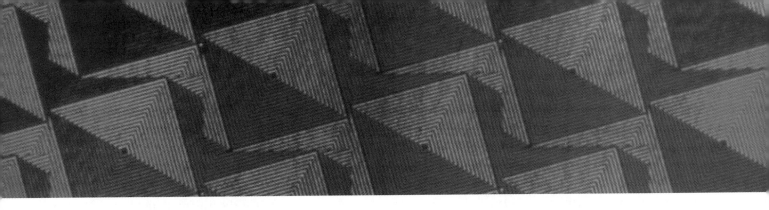

appendix B

WRITTEN AGREEMENTS RELATIVE TO PRESCRIBING OPIOID ANALGESICS

Margo McCaffery

FOCUS AND PURPOSE

Comprehensive care of patients with pain and substance abuse problems is discussed in Chapter 10. Care of patients with chronic nonmalignant pain is discussed in Chapter 11. This appendix addresses agreements and contracts between the following persons:

1. The prescriber of opioid analgesics and the person with chronic nonmalignant pain (CNP). (See Box 11.9, p. 498, for proposed guidelines for the management of opioid therapy for CNP.)
2. The prescriber of opioid analgesics and an actively addicted individual with pain. (See Box 10.9, p. 462, for general guidelines for the management of pain in the patient recovering from addiction.)

Some agreements and contracts include all controlled substances, but the ones discussed here focus only on opioid analgesics.

The issue of agreements between clinicians and persons with pain began to draw attention when aggressive treatment of cancer pain was expanded to include persons infected with human immunodeficiency virus (HIV), some of whom were active or recovering addicts. Interest in agreements also increased as the use of opioid maintenance for CNP became a more acceptable practice. Unfortunately the differences between patients with CNP and patients with pain who are also addicted became confused. Here each issue is discussed separately. Many patients receiving opioids for CNP are clearly not addicted. Moreover, addicted patients may experience a variety of types of acute and chronic pain.

The intent of this section is not to unravel the legal aspects of these agreements, but to explore their usefulness and raise questions about their content and ethical aspects. For example, do written agreements provide any protection or benefits for either the prescriber or the patient? What is the justification for using agreements with some patients who are receiving opioids and not with others? Do agreements have the potential for harming the relationship between the clinician and patient?

Patients have certain rights, such as those stipulated by the Joint Commission on Accreditation of Healthcare Organizations (JCAHO, 1988). These include the right to considerate and respectful care, the right to effective pain management, and the right to make decisions about their medical care. The Bill of Rights for patients in pain (see Chapter 1, Box 1.5, p. 13) states, "I have the right to be treated with respect at all times. When I need medication for pain, I should not be treated like a drug abuser." An important consideration in evaluating written agreements and contracts is whether they violate these or other patient's rights.

TERMINOLOGY

The terms *contract* and *agreement* both suggest an arrangement between two or more parties as to a specific course of action, such as something that is to be done or not done. An agreement can be anything from a mutual understanding to a binding obligation. Contracts are most often used in law and business for agreements that are legally enforceable. Thus contracts usually have legal and punitive connotations, suggesting a level of mistrust, whereas agreements imply that the parties have reached amicable arrangements that are freely accepted by all parties and are open to change (*Webster's College Dictionary*, 1992). Therefore the term *agreement* is used in this discussion, and use of the term *contract* is discouraged.

PATIENT INFORMATION FOR MANAGEMENT OF CHRONIC PAIN IN OUTPATIENT SETTINGS

Most patients with chronic pain, whether malignant or nonmalignant, are cared for on an outpatient basis. All patients should receive certain types of information about their care, including how to access care within the clinical setting. Patients need to know what to expect from their caregivers and what is expected of them. This information may be provided verbally, in writing, or preferably in both forms. Written treatment plans should be developed and shared with all patients. (See Box 3.7, p. 74 for information on how to use a pain rating scale to set goals; see Figure 4.3A, p. 126 for information to be given to the patient about taking medication at home; see Box 11.3, p. 488 for overall goals in the treatment of CNP; see Box 11.12, p. 507 for an example of planning for painful episodes).

Box B.1 provides an example of information that all patients need to know when they are being treated with opioid analgesics in outpatient settings such as an office or clinic. For example, the patient should know whether a new written prescription is required for each refill, whether the prescription can be refilled by telephoning the physician (who in turn telephones the pharmacy), or whether patients can simply telephone the pharmacy themselves. Patients should also receive information about their specific opioid analgesics and any other analgesics or related medications, including the benefits and potential side effects. Examples of pain medication information forms are included in Chapters 5, 6, and 7.

When information is given to the patient verbally or in writing and is documented appropriately in the patient's record, it constitutes informed consent, and the signatures of the patient and clinician are not necessary. However, some states have regulations or acts of law, such as the Intractable Pain Treatment Act, that require or recommend a signed consent form. Regardless of whether the consent is signed, the patient's medical record should reflect that informed consent was given.

● ● ● ● ●

BOX B.1	**Clinic Guidelines: Pain Management**

1. Your physician is Dr. _____. Your doctor is available for pain clinic appointments during the hours of 8:00 AM to 1:00 PM on:

   Monday   Tuesday   Wednesday   Thursday   Friday

   Telephone: _____

2. For emergencies that occur at other times, please call _____.

3. Write down the time and date of your next clinic appointment and double check this with the clerical staff before leaving the clinic.

4. To cancel or reschedule your appointment, please let us know at least 3 days in advance.

5. Please use only one pharmacy for refills of your pain medication. The pharmacy you have chosen is: _____.

   If you wish to change pharmacies, tell your doctor. (Using the same pharmacy helps ensure that it will keep your medication in stock for refills and that it will know that you have a legitimate need for pain medication.)

6. Requests for medication refills will be taken between 8:00 AM and 1:00 PM on Monday, Wednesday, and Thursday. Calling during these hours ensures the most prompt response to your request.

   • Please call in your refill at least 3 days before your last dose of medication. Do not wait until the day your medications run out.

   • Some prescriptions cannot be refilled by phone or mail. A new prescription must be written and picked up at this clinic.

7. Please keep your medications in a secure place. Do not sell, trade, or give away your medication. If your medication is damaged, stolen, or lost, please discuss the problem with your doctor at once.

8. At each clinic visit you and your doctor should decide on the medication, dose, and schedule to be followed to relieve your pain. If you need to change this plan, contact your physician at once.

9. Do not stop taking your pain medication. Contact your doctor first.

10. Please do not seek pain medication from any other doctor. Let us know if at any time another doctor prescribes pain medication for you.

Box B.1. Example of patient information form regarding prescription of opioid analgesics in an outpatient setting. Obviously, specific information will differ from one setting to another. This type of patient information form is recommended for all patients with chronic pain, both malignant and nonmalignant, who are treated with opioids on an outpatient basis.

Modified from University of Texas, MD Anderson Cancer Center, Houston, Texas, 1995.

AGREEMENTS WITH PATIENTS WITH CNP

The prevalence of written agreements with patients receiving opioid analgesics for CNP is unknown, but appears to be widespread. For example, in one issue of a newsletter published by the American Society of Pain Management Nurses, two separate authors state that in their pain care facilities all patients receiving opioid analgesics for CNP are required to sign agreements (Brooke, 1998; Kowal, 1998). The use of similar written agreements with parents of children who have chronic pain, such as pain associated with sickle-cell disease, has also been reported.

Unfortunately very few publications are addressing the contents of such agreements or the criteria for their use. No research was found that examined the benefits or harm resulting from the use of such agreements. Burchman and Pagel (1995) have published the most extensive report to date on the use of contracts with patients with CNP. Over a 3-year period they used a written agreement in the management of 64 patients with CNP. Although these patients were characterized as having a positive response to opioid therapy, they were not compared with a similar group of patients who were managed without the agreement. Therefore identifying harmful or beneficial effects of the agreement is impossible.

The agreement used by Burchman and Pagel (1995) is published in their article. However, a copy is not included in this text because the agreement is being revised (Burchman, 1998). Furthermore, several pain specialists have raised questions about its content. Because this agreement is very similar to other agreements informally obtained from a variety of pain facilities by the author, concerns about some of its content are discussed here.

Some of the conditions in the agreement for patients with CNP are intimidating, convey mistrust, and are inflexible with regard to amount and frequency of opioid analgesic patients are allowed to take (Rose, 1996). The agreement may specify no early prescription refills, no replacement of lost prescriptions or drugs, the threat of discharge from the program for failure to abide by the conditions, and a requirement of random blood or urine tests for alcohol and other drugs.

In contrast, patients with cancer pain are not required to sign such agreements when they receive opioid analgesics for chronic pain. In fact, patients with cancer pain are given considerable latitude in their dosage, including rescue doses prescribed as often as every hour if pain is not relieved by the ongoing analgesic regimen. Compared with CNP, cancer pain is probably more unstable, and certainly the possibility exists that the disease process will escalate quickly, and pain along with it. However, exacerbations of CNP are common and may require adjustment of analgesia.

Does the use of agreements with patients with CNP represent a double standard of care? If two patients—one being terminally ill and the other having CNP—are receiving identical opioid analgesics for pain, why should the one who is not terminally ill be required to sign an agreement? Are patients with CNP less trustworthy than terminally ill patients with pain? Certainly, opioid therapy may last much longer in patients who have CNP. However, does the length of opioid use cause any particular problems that are not encountered with patients who are terminally ill? If so, the use of a written agreement would make sense only after a certain amount of time has elapsed.

The staff's willingness to accept the patient's report of pain and provide analgesic medication sufficient to maintain comfort is crucial to the success of any agreement. Inflexibility in this regard can easily result in inadequate pain control. When patients are asked to sign agreements that provide inadequate pain relief, they are understandably unlikely to abide by the rules. When they violate the agreement, the staff has a tendency to blame the patients rather than realize that the pain management plan was ineffective.

Some behaviors considered to be "red flags" for addiction that patients are asked to avoid are actually indicators of undertreated pain. For example, multiple requests for early refills, repeated episodes of prescription loss, obtaining opioids from multiple providers, and even prescription forgery may be indications that the patient's pain is being undertreated (Pankratz, Hickam, Toth, 1989; Portenoy, 1994; Weissman, Haddox, 1989).

Failure to comply with the terms of the agreement sometimes results in the patient's discharge from the clinic. More appropriate alternatives might be to modify the agreement so that the patient could more easily comply or to continue treatment in the clinic without opioid analgesics.

Requiring patients with chronic cancer pain to submit to random drug testing is not recommended, and it clearly violates one of the points in the patient's Bill of Rights presented in Chapter 1: "When I need medication for pain, I should not be treated like a drug abuser." Random drug testing, coupled with the threat of discharge from the treatment center, is also intimidating and degrading to patients.

Rather than reassuring patients that addiction is a rare consequence of taking opioids for pain relief, as is done in patient teaching materials for patients with cancer pain, patients with CNP are often given erroneous information. For example, they may be told that addiction is a risk rather than a rare occurrence.

Addiction appears to influence the use of contracts with patients with CNP. Yet no evidence exists that the incidence of addictive disease is any greater in patients with CNP than in the general population. Current estimates are that between 3% and 19% of patients with CNP are addicted to alcohol or drugs (Fishbain, Rosomoff, Rosomoff, 1992). This parallels the lifetime prevalence rates (6.1% to 16.7%) of addictive disease in the general population (Regier, Farmer, Rae et al., 1990).

Furthermore, no evidence exists that history of addiction can be used to predict which patients will exhibit problematic drug taking behavior, such as frequent calls for early refills. In a study of 76 patients taking opioid analgesics for CNP, past opioid or alcohol abuse failed to identify which patients would become problematic opioid users (Chabal, Erjavec, Jacobson et al., 1997). Such data should help dispel the myth that patients with a history of substance abuse are predisposed to difficulties when using opioid analgesics (Doleys, 1998). Nevertheless, unlike terminally ill patients with pain, patients with CNP must have no history of or current problems with substance abuse and must have never been involved in illegal activities related to controlled substances to be eligible to receive opioid analgesics from some pain facilities.

In addition, patients who have past or current substance abuse problems do not appear to be more likely to exaggerate their pain than those who do not. Research comparing pain reports and analgesic therapy in acquired immunodeficiency syndrome (AIDS) patients with and without a history of substance abuse showed no significant differences between the two groups' reports of pain and pain intensity (Breitbart, Rosenfeld, Passik et al., 1997). Even among patients who acknowledged continued drug use, no difference was observed in their reports of pain intensity and pain relief compared with those patients who denied recent drug use or were participating in a methadone maintenance program.

The physician's perceptions of regulatory scrutiny is a well-known deterrent to the appropriate prescription of opioids for pain, especially chronic pain. Although some physicians feel that the use of written agreements may offer some protection from inappropriate investigation, no evidence exists to support this belief (Burchman, 1998). Ongoing evaluation and documentation is the best protection. (See Box 10.4, p. 455 for information on documentation of addiction and pain responses.)

The controversial nature of opioid maintenance therapy for patients with CNP seems to be the underlying reason for requiring these patients to sign agreements. Clinicians should remember that the use of opioids for treatment of CNP is in question, not the patients themselves.

AGREEMENTS WITH ACTIVE ADDICTS WITH PAIN

Whether actively addicted patients with pain are cared for in an outpatient or inpatient setting, for acute or chronic pain, the question of contracts or agreements often arises. As is done with all patients, treatment plans should be developed, including specific goals of treatment and potential interventions to accomplish those goals.

Box B.2 presents an example of a written agreement for opioids given by IV PCA to an actively addicted, hospitalized patient. As noted, this action is not necessarily recommended. One reason for caution when using such an agreement is the possibility that it could be considered a double standard of care. Why should patients with addictive disease be treated differently than patients with similar pain problems? One solution would be to use the same format, omitting goal No. 3, not as an agreement, but as written information to be given to all patients whose pain is being treated with IV PCA.

| BOX B.2 | **Patient-Controlled Analgesia (PCA) for Acute Pain** |

GOALS OF TREATMENT

1. To achieve my pain rating and activity goals: _____.
   Example: 2/10 to turn, cough, and deep breathe.

2. To relieve my pain without causing sedation.

3. To keep me from experiencing withdrawal symptoms.

4. Other: _____.

PATIENT AND STAFF RESPONSIBILITIES

1. I will use the pain rating scale to report pain to the staff.

2. The staff will accept and respect my reports of pain as the best indicator of how much pain I have.

3. The staff will be responsible for providing as much analgesia as necessary to relieve my pain, unless it would endanger my health.

4. I will not tamper in any way with the PCA pump.

5. I will not take any unordered medication.

6. I will not allow visitors to bring illicit drugs or alcohol into the hospital setting.

7. The staff will gradually taper the infusion before it is stopped. They will consider my pain ratings and my progress toward recovery to determine when and by how much to reduce doses and to provide other means of pain relief, if necessary.

We mutually agree to the above:

_____   _____   _____
Signature of patient   Signature of clinician   Date

Box B.2.   Example of possible written agreement for use of opioid via IV PCA to treat acute pain in the addicted patient. Although popular, use of such agreements is not necessarily recommended. See text for discussion of this issue.

Adapted from suggestions made by Peggy Compton and Chris Pasero.

Another consideration is that no research has demonstrated that the use of a written agreement in the treatment of acute pain in addicted patients will result in any improvement in patients adhering to the treatment plan. In fact, research has suggested that addicted individuals may be capable of conduct similar to nonaddicted persons being treated with opioids. A small study by Paige and others (1994) found no differences in PCA analgesic use between opioid- or cocaine-abusing patients and normal controls, indicating that addicted patients can use PCA responsibly.

Box B.3 presents an example of a written agreement for an addicted patient with pain being treated with oral opioids on an outpatient basis. The objections related to a double standard of care discussed previously also pertain to this agreement. Many agreements for this patient population contain additional stipulations, such as having the patient submit to blood or urine drug screening and agreeing to refrain from the use of alcohol and other drugs. Such stipulations seem to serve no purpose. Unless an active addict is interested in recovery from substance abuse, the use of alcohol and other drugs most likely will continue and drug tests will be positive.

References

Breitbart W, Rosenfeld B, Passik S et al.: A comparison of pain report and adequacy of analgesic therapy in ambulatory AIDS patients with and without a history of substance abuse, *Pain* 72:235-243, 1997.

Brooke C: Management of the hard to evaluate pain patient, *ASPMN Pathways* 7(1):14, 1998.

Burchman SL: Personal communication, 1998.

Burchman SL, Pagel PS: Implementation of a formal treatment agreement for outpatient management of chronic nonmalignant pain with opioid analgesics, *J Pain Symptom Manage* 10:556-563, 1995.

Chabal C, Erjavec MK, Jacobson L et al.: Prescription opiate abuse in chronic pain patients: clinical criteria, incidence, and predictors, *Clin J Pain* 13:150-155, 1997.

Doleys DM: Commentary, *Pain Med J Club J* 4:18-19, 1998.

Fishbain DA, Rosomoff HL, Rosomoff RS: Drug abuse, dependence, and addiction in chronic pain patients, *Clin J Pain* 8:77-85, 1992.

Joint Commission on Accreditation of Healthcare Organizations: *Hospital Accreditation Standards,* Oakbrook Terrace, Ill, 1998, The Commission.

Kowal N: Evaluate patient outcomes, *ASPMN Pathways* 7(1):7, 1998.

Paige DA, Preble LM, Watrous GA et al.: PCA use in cocaine using patients: a pilot study, *Am J Pain Manage* 4:101-105, 1994.

Pankratz L, Hickam D, Toth S: The identification and management of drug-seeking behavior in a medical center, *Drug and Alcohol Dependence* 24:115-118, 1989.

Portenoy RK: Opioid therapy for chronic nonmalignant pain: current status. In Fields HL, Liebeskind JC: *Progress in pain research and management,* Vol 1, pp. 247-287, Seattle, 1994, IASP Press.

Regier DA, Farmer ME, Rae DS et al.: Comorbidity of mental disorders with alcohol and other drug abuse: results of the epidemiologic catchment area study, *JAMA* 264:2511-2518, 1990.

Rose HL: Re: formal treatment agreements for opioids in nonmalignant pain, *J Pain Symptom Manage* 12:206-207, 1996.

Webster's College Dictionary, New York, 1992, Random House.

Weissman DE, Haddox JD: Opioid pseudoaddiction: an iatrogenic syndrome, *Pain* 36:363-366, 1989.

BOX B.3 Outpatient Opioid Analgesia

GOALS OF TREATMENT

1. To achieve my pain rating and activity goals: _____. Example: 3/10 to return to work.

2. To relieve my pain without causing sedation.

3. To keep me from experiencing withdrawal symptoms.

4. Other: _____.

PATIENT AND STAFF RESPONSIBILITIES

1. I will use the pain rating scale to report pain to the staff.

2. The staff will accept and respect my reports of pain as the best indicator of how much pain I have.

3. The staff will be responsible for providing as much analgesia as necessary to relieve my pain, unless it would endanger my health.

4. I will receive my analgesics from a single provider only, Dr. _____.

   I will not seek medication from a dentist or the emergency room without this doctor's knowledge.

5. I will not sell, trade, or give my pain medication to others.

6. I will not engage in illegal activities to obtain pain medication.

7. I will be responsible for keeping my medication out of the reach of children, pets, and others, and for not misplacing or losing it.

8. I understand that taking my medication when using alcohol or other drugs could be extremely dangerous to my health.

9. I understand that my doctor has supplied me with _____ "rescue doses" per day of medication to take if my pain increases. I will inform my doctor as soon as possible if I need to take more rescue doses than this, and I will come in for reevaluation as instructed.

10. If I have difficulty meeting the above responsibilities, or if other problems occur, I understand that I may need to attend clinic more frequently to pick up prescriptions that cover a shorter time period.

We mutually agree to the above:

_____   _____   _____
Signature of patient   Signature of clinician   Date

Box B.3. Example of possible written agreement for use of oral opioids for outpatient treatment of pain in the addicted patient. Although popular, use of such agreements is not necessarily recommended. See text for a discussion of this issue.

Adapted from suggestions made by Peggy Compton and Chris Pasero.

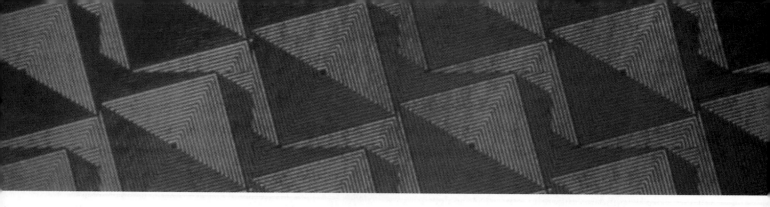

appendix C TERMINOLOGY

The following terms were selected from the terminology sections found at the beginning of some chapters:

- **Abstinence syndrome.** A manifestation of physical dependence; occurrence of withdrawal symptoms when the opioid is abruptly stopped or an opioid antagonist is given.
- **Addiction.** Psychological dependence; a pattern of compulsive drug use characterized by a continual craving for an opioid and the need to use the opioid for effects other than pain relief.
- **Adjuvant analgesic.** A drug that has a primary purpose other than pain relief (e.g., an antidepressant or anticonvulsant) but can also serve as an analgesic for some painful conditions.
- **Agonist.** See mu agonist.
- **Agonist-antagonist.** A type of opioid (e.g., nalbuphine, butorphanol) that binds to the kappa opioid receptor site, where it acts as an agonist (i.e., capable of producing analgesia), and simultaneously binds to the mu opioid receptor site, where it acts as an antagonist (i.e., reversing agonist effects).
- **Allodynia.** A nonpainful stimulus is felt as painful in spite of normal-appearing tissues; common in many neuropathic pain conditions.
- **Analgesic ceiling.** A dose beyond which further increases in dose do not provide additional analgesia.
- **Antagonist.** A drug that competes with agonists for opioid receptor binding sites; can displace agonists, thereby inhibiting their action. Examples include naloxone, naltrexone, and nalmefene.
- **Balanced analgesia.** Also referred to as continuous, multimodal analgesia; often includes drugs from each of the three analgesic groups (i.e., NSAIDs, opioids, and local anesthetics); may be given by several different routes of administration.

- **Bioavailability.** The extent to which a dose of a drug reaches its site of action.
- **Blood-brain barrier.** A barrier that exists between circulating blood and the brain, preventing damaging substances from reaching brain tissue and cerebral spinal fluid.
- **Breakthrough pain.** Pain that increases above the level of pain addressed by the ongoing analgesics; includes incident pain and end-of-dose failure.
- **Central pain.** Pain initiated or caused by a primary lesion or dysfunction in the central nervous system.
- **Crescendo pain.** A period of rapid pain escalation often associated with increasing distress and functional impairment.
- **Deafferentation pain.** Pain following injury to a nerve root or peripheral nerve; inferred to have a predominating central mechanism; a nonspecific term.
- **Dermatome.** An area of skin that is primarily innervated by a single spinal cord segment.
- **Dysesthesia.** An unpleasant abnormal sensation, including allodynia; commonly described as "pins and needles" (e.g., limb "falling asleep"), burning, electrical, tingling; hypersensitive to stimuli; may include area of sensory loss. (Paresthesia, by comparison, is abnormal but not painful.)
- **Efficacy.** The maximum effect that can be produced by a given dose of a drug.
- **Endogenous opioids.** Families of peptides (i.e., enkephalins, endorphins, dynorphins) secreted naturally by the body; capable of producing effects similar to exogenous opioids (e.g., inhibiting pain transmission).
- **Half-life.** The time it takes for the plasma concentration (i.e., the amount of drug in the body) to decrease by 50%. Five half-lives are required for a drug to be effectively eliminated from the body.
- **Hydrophilic.** Readily absorbed in aqueous solution.

- **Hyperalgesia.** An increased response to a stimulus that is normally painful (i.e., increased pain).
- **Lancinating.** Stabbing, knifelike pain.
- **Lipophilic.** Readily absorbed in fatty tissues.
- **Metabolites.** The products of biochemical reactions that occur during drug metabolism.
- **Modulation.** The activation of descending pathways that exert inhibitory effects on the cells responsible for pain transmission.
- **Mu agonist.** A type of opioid; includes morphine and other opioids that relieve pain by binding to the mu receptor sites in the nervous system; used interchangeably with the terms full agonist, pure agonist, and morphine-like drug.
- **Narcotic.** See *Opioid*. An obsolete term used to refer to what are now called opioids. Current usage of the term is primarily in a legal context to refer to a wide variety of substances of potential abuse.
- **Neuralgia.** Pain in the distribution of a nerve (e.g., sciatica, trigeminal neuralgia); often felt as an electrical, shock-like pain.
- **Neuropathic pain.** Pain initiated or caused by a primary lesion or dysfunction in the nervous system.
- **NMDA (*N*-methyl-D-aspartate).** Term used in conjunction with drugs that are NMDA receptor blockers (e.g., ketamine, dextromethorphan).
- **Nociceptive pain.** Pain resulting from the ongoing activation of primary afferent neurons by noxious stimuli. (The nervous system is intact.)
- **Nociceptor.** A receptor that is preferentially sensitive to noxious stimuli or to stimuli that would be noxious if prolonged.
- **Nonopioid.** Preferred to the term "nonnarcotic"; refers to acetaminophen and nonsteroidal antiinflammatory drugs (NSAIDs).
- **Noxious stimulus.** A stimulus that is damaging or potentially damaging to normal tissue.
- **NSAID.** An acronym for nonsteroidal antiinflammatory drug (pronounced "in said"); also referred to as "aspirin-like" drugs.
- **Opioid.** Preferred to the term "narcotic"; refers to natural, semisynthetic, and synthetic drugs that relieve pain by binding to opioid receptors in the nervous system. The term "opioid" is preferred to the term "opiate" because it includes all agonists and antagonists with morphinelike activity, as well as naturally occurring and synthetic opioid peptides.
- **Pain perception.** The process of recognizing, defining, and responding to pain.
- **Parenteral route.** The intramuscular, subcutaneous, and intravenous routes of administration.
- **Paresthesia.** Includes sensations of numbness, prickling, tingling, and heightened sensitivity.
- **Paroxysmal.** Sudden periodic attack or recurrence.
- **Peripheral neuropathic pain.** Pain initiated or caused by a primary lesion or dysfunction in the peripheral nervous system.

- **Physical dependence.** Physical reliance on an opioid evidenced by withdrawal symptoms if the opioid is abruptly stopped or an antagonist is administered.
- **Placebo.** Any medication or procedure, including surgery, that produces an effect in a patient because of its implicit or explicit intent, and not because of its specific physical or chemical properties.
- **Potency.** The dose required to produce a specified effect.
- **Preemptive analgesia.** Preinjury pain treatments (e.g., preoperative epidural analgesia and preincision local anesthetic infiltration) used to prevent the establishment of peripheral and central sensitization of pain.
- **Primary afferent neuron.** See definition of *Nociceptor*.
- **Psychogenic pain.** Pain presumed to exist when no nociceptive or neuropathic mechanism can be identified; term that has a stigmatizing connotation.
- **Refractory.** Resistant to ordinary treatment.
- **Repolarization.** The inside of the cell becoming negative relative to the outside.
- **Somatic pain.** Pain of the musculoskeletal system.
- **Somatization.** The expression of emotion or psychosocial discomfort in the physical language of body symptoms.
- **Substance abuse.** The DSM-IV term for a less severe form of, and often a predecessor to, addiction or substance dependence; distinguished by a shorter duration of impairment and the absence of neurophysiological symptoms.
- **Supraspinal.** Above the level of the spinal cord.
- **Supratentorial pain.** This term is not a recognized diagnosis and has no accepted definition. It is almost always used as a derogatory term to suggest that no physical cause exists for the pain or that the patient is lying about the pain.
- **Synapse.** Point of junction between two neurons.
- **Systemic drug treatment, systemic administration.** Administration of a drug by a route that allows it to be absorbed into the general circulation (e.g., oral, parenteral [intravenous, intramuscular, subcutaneous], rectal, vaginal, topical application, transdermal). By contrast, the intraspinal routes of administration (e.g., epidural, intrathecal) deposit the drug directly into the central nervous system, minimizing the amount of drug that reaches the general circulation.
- **Tabetic pain.** Sharp, lightning-type pain; also called lancinating pain.
- **Titration.** Adjusting the amount (e.g., adjusting the dose of an opioid).
- **Tolerance.** A process characterized by decreasing effects of a drug at the initial dose, or the need for a higher dose of a drug to maintain an effect.
- **Transduction.** Conversion of one form of energy to another.
- **Transmission.** Movement of pain impulses from the site of transduction to the brain.
- **Visceral pain.** Pain of the body's internal organs.

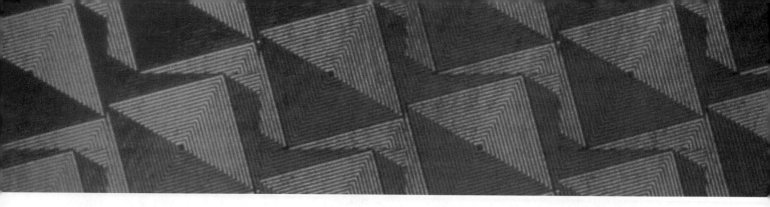

index

t after a page number indicates a table, box, or form; *f* after a page number indicates an illustration.

Generic and Trade Names: Analgesics and Other Medications Used in Conjunction With Analgesics

Nonopioids

acetaminophen (APAP, paracetamol, Tylenol)
choline magnesium trisalicylate (Trilisate)
choline salicylate (Arthropan)
diclofenac (Cataflam [immediate release for acute pain], Voltaren Delayed Release, Voltaren-XR [extended release for chronic therapy])
diflunisal (Dolobid)
etodolac (Lodine)
fenoprofen calcium (Nalfon)
flurbiprofen (Ansaid)
ibuprofen (Motrin, Advil)
indomethacin (Indocin)
ketoprofen (Orudis)
ketorolac (Toradol)
meclofenamate sodium (Meclomen)
mefenamic acid (Ponstel)
nabumetone (Relafen)
naproxen (Naprosyn)
naproxen sodium (Aleve)
oxaprozin (Daypro)
piroxicam (Feldene)
salsalate (Disalcid)
sulindac (Clinoril)
tolmetin (Tolectin)

Opioids

buprenorphine (Buprenex)
butorphanol (Stadol)
codeine (in Tylenol No.3)
dezocine (Dalgan)
dihydrocodeine (DHCplus)
fentanyl (Duragesic, transdermal; Sublimaze, injection)
hydrocodone (in Lortab, Vicodin)
hydromorphone (Dilaudid)
levorphanol (Levo-Dromoran)
meperidine (Demerol)
methadone (Dolophine)
morphine (MS Contin, Oramorph SR, Roxanol, MSIR)
nalbuphine (Nubain)
oxycodone (OxyContin; in Percocet)
oxymorphone (Numorphan)
pentazocine (Talwin)
propoxyphene hydrochloride (Darvon)
propoxyphene napsylate (Darvon-N)
partly mu agonist)

desipramine (Norpramin)
dexamethasone (Decadron)
dextroamphetamine (Dexedrine)
divalproex sodium (Depakote)
doxepin (Sinequan)
fluoxetine (Prozac)
gabapentin (Neurontin)
methotrimeprazine (Levoprome)
methylphenidate (Ritalin)
mexiletine (Mexitil)
nortriptyline (Aventyl, Pamelor)
paroxetine (Paxil)
pemoline (Cylert)
phenytoin (Dilantin)
propranolol (Inderal)
ropivacaine (Naropin)
sertraline (Zoloft)
sumatriptan (Imitrex)
trazodone (Desyrel)
valproic acid (Depakene)
venlafaxine (Effexor)
verapamil hydrochloride (Calan, Isoptin, Verelan)

Other Medications Sometimes Used in Conjunction With Analgesics

This list includes medications used for a variety of problems that may occur in patients with pain, such as anxiety or insomnia; side effects that may accompany analgesic use, such as nausea, agitation, confusion, constipation, and myoclonus; and the need for GI protection during NSAID therapy.

alprazolam (Xanax)
buspirone (Buspar)
carisoprodol (Soma, Rela)
chlorpromazine (Thorazine)
chlorzoxazone (Paraflex)
cimetidine (Tagamet)
cyclobenzaprine (Flexeril)
diazepam (Valium)
diphenhydramine (Benadryl)
dronabinol (Marinol)
droperidol (Inapsine)
haloperidol (Haldol)
hydroxyzine (Vistaril, Atarax)
lorazepam (Ativan)
methocarbamol (Robaxin)
metoclopramide (Reglan)
midazolam (Versed)
misoprostol (Cytotec)
naloxone (Narcan)
ondansetron (Zofran)
prochlorperazine (Compazine)
promethazine (Phenergan)
propofol (Diprivan)
rantidine (Zantac)
temazepam (Restoril)
thiethylperazine (Torecan)
triazolam (Halcion)